2014

the calorie carb and fat bible 2014

Juliette Kellow BSc RD, Lyndel Costain BSc RD & Laurence Beeken

The UK's Most Comprehensive Calorie Counter

The Calorie, Carb & Fat Bible 2014

© Weight Loss Resources 2014
Lyndel Costain's contributions © Lyndel Costain 2007

Published by:
Weight Loss Resources Ltd
2C Flag Business Exchange
Vicarage Farm Road
Peterborough
PE1 5TX.

Tel: 01733 345592
www.weightlossresources.co.uk

Companies and other organisations wishing to make bulk purchases of the Calorie, Carb and Fat Bible should contact their local bookstore or Weight Loss Resources direct.

ISBN 978-1-904512-12-7

Authors: Lyndel Costain BSc RD
         Juliette Kellow BSc RD
         Laurence Beeken, Weight Loss Resources

Database Editor: Laurence Beeken

Design and Layout: Joanne Readshaw

Printed and bound by:
Bookprintinguk.com, Peterborough, PE2 9BF

Contents

Losing weight – the easy way

Juliette Kellow BSc RD

CHINESE TAKEAWAYS, curries, chocolate, chips and a glass of wine! Imagine being told the best diet to help you lose weight includes all these foods and more. It sounds too good to be true, doesn't it? But the truth is, these are exactly the types of foods you can still enjoy if you opt to lose weight by counting calories.

But you'd be forgiven for not knowing you can still eat all your favourite foods *and* lose weight. In recent years, endless trendy diets that cut carbs, boost protein intake or skip entire groups of foods, have helped to make dieting a complicated business. Added to this, an increasing number of celebrities and so-called nutrition experts have helped mislead us into thinking that dieting is all about restriction and denial. Is it any wonder then that most of us have been left feeling downright confused and miserable about what we should and shouldn't be eating to shift those pounds?

Dieting doesn't have to be complicated or an unhappy experience. In fact, there's really only one word you need to remember if you want to shift those pounds healthily and still eat all your favourite foods. And that's CALORIE!

It's calories that count

When it comes to losing weight, there's no getting away from the fact that it's calories that count. Ask any qualified nutrition expert or dietitian for advice on how to fight the flab and you'll receive the same reply: quite simply you need to create a calorie deficit or shortfall. In other words, you need to take in fewer calories than you use up so that your body has to draw on its fat stores to provide it with the energy it needs to function properly. The result: you start losing fat and the pounds start to drop off!

Fortunately, it couldn't be easier to create this calorie deficit. Regardless of your age, weight, sex, genetic make up, lifestyle or eating habits, losing weight is as simple as reducing your daily calorie intake slightly by modifying your diet and using up a few more calories by being slightly more active each day.

Better still, it's a complete myth that you need to change your eating and exercise habits dramatically. You'll notice I've said you need to reduce your calorie intake 'slightly' and be 'slightly' more active. It really is just LITTLE differences between the amount of calories we take in and the amount we use up that make BIG differences to our waistline over time. For example, you only need to consume one can of cola more than you need each day to gain a stone in a year. It's no wonder then that people say excess weight tends to 'creep up on them'.

10 simple food swaps you can make every day (and won't even notice!)

Make these simple swaps every day and in just 4 weeks you'll lose 7lb!

SWAP THIS...	FOR THIS...	SAVE...
300ml full-fat milk (195 calories)	300ml skimmed milk (100 calories)	95 calories
1tsp butter (35 calories)	1tsp low-fat spread (20 calories)	15 calories
1tbsp vegetable oil (100 calories)	10 sprays of a spray oil (10 calories)	90 calories
1tsp sugar (16 calories)	Artificial sweetener (2 calories)	14 calories
1tbsp mayonnaise (105 calories)	1tbsp fat-free dressing (10 calories)	95 calories
Regular sandwich (600 calories)	Low-fat sandwich (350 calories)	250 calories
Can of cola (135 calories)	Can of diet cola (1 calorie)	134 calories
Large (50g) packet of crisps (250 calories)	Small (25g) packet of crisps (125 calories)	125 calories
1 chocolate digestive (85 calories)	1 small chocolate chip cookie (55 calories)	30 calories
1 slice thick-cut wholemeal bread (95 calories)	1 slice medium-cut wholemeal bread (75 calories)	20 calories
	TOTAL CALORIE SAVING:	868 calories

The good news is the reverse is also true. You only need to swap that daily can of cola for the diet version or a glass of sparking water and you'll lose a stone in a year – it really is as easy as that!

Of course, most people don't want to wait a year to shift a stone. But there's more good news. To lose 1lb of fat each week you need to create a calorie deficit of just 500 calories a day. That might sound like a lot, but you can achieve this by simply swapping a croissant for a wholemeal fruit scone, a regular sandwich for a low-fat variety, a glass of dry white wine for a gin and slimline tonic and using low-fat spread on two slices of toast instead of butter. It is also important to become more active and increase your level of exercise. Losing 1lb a week, amounts to a stone in 14 weeks, or just under 4 stone in a year!

Taking control of calories

By now you've seen it really is calories that count when it comes to shifting those pounds. So it should be no surprise that a calorie-controlled diet is the only guaranteed way to help you shift those pounds – and that's a scientific fact! But better still, a calorie-controlled diet is one of the few that allows you to include anything, whether it's pizza, wine or chocolate. A healthy diet means including a wide range of foods *(see 'Healthy Eating Made Easy' page 32).*

And that's where this book can really help. Gone are the days when it was virtually impossible to obtain information about the calorie contents of foods. This book provides calorie information for more than 22,000 different branded and unbranded foods so that counting calories has never been easier.

The benefits of counting calories

- *It's guaranteed to help you lose weight providing you stick to your daily calorie allowance*

- *You can include favourite foods*

- *No foods are banned*

- *It's a great way to lose weight slowly and steadily*

- *Nutrition experts agree that it's a proven way to lose weight*

Calorie counting made easy

Forget weird and wacky science, complicated diet rules and endless lists of foods to fill up on or avoid every day! Counting calories to lose weight couldn't be easier. Quite simply, you set yourself a daily calorie allowance to help you lose between ½-2lb (¼-1kg) a week and then add up the calories of everything you eat and drink each day, making sure you don't go over your limit.

To prevent hunger from kicking in, it's best to spread your daily calorie allowance evenly throughout the day, allowing a certain amount of calories for breakfast, lunch, dinner and one or two snacks. For example, if you are allowed 1,500 calories a day, you could have 300 calories for breakfast, 400 calories for lunch, 500 calories for dinner and two snacks or treats of 150 calories each. You'll find more detailed information on p26-31 (Your step-by-step guide to using this book and shifting those pounds).

QUESTION
What affects the calorie content of a food?

ANSWER:
Fat, protein, carbohydrate and alcohol all provide the body with calories, but in varying amounts:

- *1g fat provides 9 calories*

- *1g alcohol provides 7 calories*

- *1g protein provides 4 calories*

- *1g carbohydrate provides 3.75 calories*

The calorie content of a food depends on the amount of fat, protein and carbohydrate it contains. Because fat provides more than twice as many calories as an equal quantity of protein or carbohydrate, in general, foods that are high in fat tend to contain more calories. This explains why 100g of chips (189 calories) contains more than twice as many calories as 100g of boiled potato (72 calories).

DIET MYTH:
Food eaten late at night stops you losing weight

DIET FACT:
It's not eating in the evening that stops you losing weight. It's consuming too many calories throughout the day that will be your dieting downfall! Providing you stick to your daily calorie allowance you'll lose weight, regardless of when you consume those calories. Nevertheless, it's a good idea to spread your calorie allowance throughout the day to prevent hunger from kicking in, which leaves you reaching for high-calorie snack foods.

Eat for good health

While calories might be the buzz word when it comes to shifting those pounds, it's nevertheless important to make sure your diet is healthy, balanced and contains all the nutrients you need for good health. Yes, you can still lose weight by eating nothing but, for example, chocolate, crisps and biscuits providing you stick to your calorie allowance. But you'll never find a nutrition expert or dietitian recommending this. And there are plenty of good reasons why.

To start with, an unbalanced diet is likely to be lacking in essential nutrients such as protein, vitamins, minerals and fibre, in the long term putting you at risk of nutritional deficiencies. Secondly, research proves that filling up on foods that are high in fat and/or salt and sugar can lead to many different health problems. But most importantly, when it comes to losing weight, it's almost impossible to stick to a daily calorie allowance if you're only eating high-calorie foods.

Filling up on lower-calorie foods also means you'll be able to eat far more with the result that you're not constantly left feeling unsatisfied. For example, six chocolates from a selection box contain around 300 calories, a lot of fat and sugar, few nutrients – and are eaten in just six mouthfuls! For 300 calories, you could have a grilled skinless chicken breast (packed with protein and zinc), a large salad with fat-free dressing (a great source of fibre, vitamins and minerals), a slice of wholemeal bread with low-fat spread (rich in fibre and B vitamins) and a satsuma (an excellent source of vitamin C). That's a lot more food that will take you a lot more time to eat! Not convinced? Then put six chocolates on one plate, and the chicken, salad, bread and fruit on another!

Bottom line: while slightly reducing your calorie intake is the key to losing weight, you'll be healthier and far more likely to keep those pounds off if you do it by eating a healthy diet *(see 'Healthy Eating Made Easy' page 32)*.

Eight steps to a healthy diet

1 *Base your meals on starchy foods.*

2 *Eat lots of fruit and vegetables.*

3 *Eat more fish.*

4 *Cut down on saturated fat and sugar.*

5 *Try to eat less salt - no more than 6g a day.*

6 *Get active and try to be a healthy weight.*

7 *Drink plenty of water.*

8 *Don't skip breakfast.*

SOURCE: www.nhs.uk/Livewell/Goodfood/Pages/eatwell-plate.aspx

Fat facts

Generally speaking, opting for foods that are low in fat can help slash your calorie intake considerably, for example, swapping full-fat milk for skimmed, switching from butter to a low-fat spread, not frying food in oil and chopping the fat off meat and poultry. But don't be fooled into believing that all foods described as 'low-fat' or 'fat-free' are automatically low in calories or calorie-free. In fact, some low-fat products may actually be higher in calories than standard products, thanks to them containing extra sugars and thickeners to boost the flavour and texture. The solution: always check the calorie content of low-fat foods, especially for things like cakes, biscuits, crisps, ice creams and ready meals. You might be surprised to find there's little difference in the calorie content when compared to the standard product.

Uncovering fat claims on food labels

Many products may lure you into believing they're a great choice if you're trying to cut fat, but you need to read between the lines on the labels if you want to be sure you're making the best choice. Here's the lowdown on what to look for:

LOW FAT	by law the food must contain less than 3g of fat per 100g for solids. These foods are generally a good choice if you're trying to lose weight.
REDUCED FAT	by law the food must contain 25 percent less fat than a similar standard product. This doesn't mean the product is low-fat (or low-calorie) though! For example, reduced-fat cheese may still contain 14g fat per 100g.
FAT FREE	the food must contain no more than 0.5g of fat per 100g or 100ml. Foods labelled as Virtually Fat Free must contain less than 0.3g fat per 100g. These foods are generally a good choice if you're trying to lose weight.
LESS THAN 8% FAT	this means the product contains less than 8g fat per 100g. It's only foods labelled 'less than 3% fat' that are a true low-fat choice.
X% FAT FREE	claims expressed as X% Fat Free shall be prohibited.
LIGHT OR LITE	claims stating a product is 'light' or 'lite' follows the same conditions as those set for the term 'reduced'.

10 easy ways to slash fat (and calories)

1 Eat fewer fried foods – grill, boil, bake, poach, steam, roast without added fat or microwave instead.

2 Don't add butter, lard, margarine or oil to food during preparation or cooking.

3 Use spreads sparingly. Butter and margarine contain the same amount of calories and fat – only low fat spreads contain less.

4 Choose boiled or jacket potatoes instead of chips or roast potatoes.

5 Cut off all visible fat from meat and remove the skin from chicken before cooking.

6 Don't eat too many fatty meat products such as sausages, burgers, pies and pastry products.

7 Use semi-skimmed or skimmed milk instead of full-fat milk.

8 Try low-fat or reduced-fat varieties of cheese such as reduced-fat Cheddar, low-fat soft cheese or cottage cheese.

9 Eat fewer high-fat foods such as crisps, chocolates, cakes, pastries and biscuits.

10 Don't add cream to puddings, sauces or coffee.

Getting Ready for Weight Loss Success

Lyndel Costain BSc RD

THIS BOOK not only provides tools to help you understand more about what you eat and how active you are, but guidance on how to use this information to develop a weight loss plan to suit your needs. Getting in the right frame of mind will also be a key part of your weight control journey, especially if you've lost weight before, only to watch the pounds pile back on.

The fact is that most people who want to lose weight know what to do. But often there is something that keeps stopping them from keeping up healthier habits. The same may be true for you. So what's going on? For many it's a lack of readiness. When the next diet comes along with its tempting promises it's so easy to just jump on board. But if you have struggled with your weight for a while, will that diet actually help you to recognise and change the thoughts and actions that have stopped you shifting the pounds for good?

Check out your attitude to weight loss programmes

Before starting any new weight loss programme, including the Weight Loss Resources approach, ask yourself:

Am I starting out thinking that I like myself as a person right now?	(YES or NO)
OR I feel I can only like myself once I lose weight?	(YES or NO)
Do I want to stop overeating, but at the same time find myself justifying it – in other words I want to be able to eat what I want, but with no consequences?	(YES or NO)
Do I believe that I need to take long-term responsibility for my weight?	(YES or NO)
OR Am I relying on 'it' (the diet) to do it for me?	(YES or NO)

Keep these questions, and your replies, in mind as you read through this chapter.

Next Steps

You may have already assessed the healthiness of your weight using the BMI guide on page 37. If not, why not do it now, remembering that the tools are a guide only. The important thing is to consider a weight at which you are healthy and comfortable – and which is realistic for the life you lead *(see opposite - What is a healthy weight?)*.

The next step is to have a long hard think about why you want to lose weight. Consider all the possible benefits, not just those related to how you look. Psychologists have found that if we focus only on appearance we are less likely to succeed in the long-term. This is because it so often reflects low self-esteem or self-worth – which can sabotage success – as it saps confidence and keeps us stuck in destructive thought patterns. Identifying key motivations other than simply how you look - such as health and other aspects of physical and emotional well being - is like saying that you're an OK person right now, and worth making changes for. Making healthy lifestyle choices also has the knock on effect of boosting self-esteem further.

Write down your reasons for wanting to lose weight in your Personal Plan *(see page 42)* – so you can refer back to them. This can be especially helpful when the going gets tough. It may help to think of it in terms of what your weight is stopping you from doing now. Here's some examples: to feel more confident; so I can play more comfortably with my kids; my healthier diet will give me more energy; to improve my fertility.

What is a Healthy Weight?

With all the 'thin is beautiful' messages in the media it can be easy to get a distorted view about whether your weight is healthy or not. However, as the BMI charts suggest, there is no single 'ideal' weight for anybody. Research also shows that modest amounts of weight loss can be very beneficial to health and are easier to keep off. Therefore, health professionals now encourage us to aim for a weight loss of 5-10%. The ideal rate of weight loss is no more than 1-2 pounds (0.5-1kg) per week – so averaging a pound a week is great, and realistic progress.

The health benefits of modest weight loss include:

- *Reduced risk of developing heart disease, stroke and certain cancers*
- *Reduced risk of developing diabetes and helping to manage diabetes*
- *Improvements in blood pressure*
- *Improvements in mobility, back pain and joint pain*
- *Improvements with fertility problems and polycystic ovarian syndrome*
- *Less breathlessness and sleep/snoring problems*
- *Increased self esteem and control over eating*
- *Feeling fitter and have more energy*

Are You Really Ready to Lose Weight?

When you think of losing weight, it's easy just to think of what weight you'd like to get to. But weight loss only happens as a result of making changes to your usual eating and activity patterns – which allow you to consume fewer calories than you burn *(see 'It's calories that count' page 5)*.

So here comes the next big question. Are you really ready to do it? Have you thought about the implications of your decision? If you have lost weight in the past, and put it all back on - have you thought about why that was? And how confident do you feel about being successful this time?

To help you answer these questions, try these short exercises.

Where would you place yourself on the following scales?

Importance

How important is it to you, to make the changes that will allow you to lose weight?

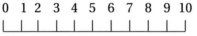

Not at all important   Extremely important

If you ranked yourself over half way along the scale then move on to the next question. If you were half way or less along the scale, you may not be mentally ready to make the required changes to lose weight. To further explore this, go to 'The Pros and Cons of Weight Loss' (page 17).

Confidence

How confident are you in your ability to make the changes that will allow you to lose weight?

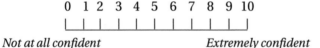

Not at all confident   Extremely confident

Now ask yourself (regarding your confidence ratings):

1. Why did I place myself here?

2. What is stopping me moving further up the scale (if anything)?

3. What things, information, support would help me move further up the scale? (if not near 10)

If you aren't sure about answers to question 3, then keep reading for some pointers.

The Pros and Cons of Weight Loss

Making lifestyle changes to lose weight is simpler if there are lots of clear benefits or pros, for example, clothes fit again, more energy, helps back pain - but there will also be associated downsides or cons. For example, some may feel it interferes with their social life, or don't have the time to plan meals or check food labels. Or overeating can help, if only temporarily, as a way of coping with unwanted feelings. Being overweight allows some people to feel strong and assertive, or to control their partner's jealousy. So in these cases there are downsides to losing weight, even if the person says they are desperate to do it.

If you are aware of the possible downsides, as well as the pros, you will be better prepared to deal with potential conflicts. Understanding what could be (or were with past weight loss efforts) barriers to success gives you the chance to address them. This boosts confidence in your ability to succeed this time, which in turn maintains your motivation.

Have a go at weighing up the pros and cons using the charts below and on page 18. Some examples are included. If you decide that the pros outweigh the cons, then great. You can also use the cons as potential barriers to plan strategies for *(see page 42)*. If you find it's the other way around, this may not be the best time to actively lose weight. Try the exercise again in a month or so.

Making Lifestyle Changes to Lose Weight Now

CONS *e.g. Must limit eating out, take aways*	PROS *e.g. Feel more energetic, slimmer*

Not Making Changes Now – how would I feel in 6 months time?

PROS *e.g. Haven't had to worry about failing;* *Still able to eat take aways a lot*	CONS *e.g. Probably gained more weight;* *Back pain may be worse*

To change your weight, first change your mind

To lose weight you may already have a list of things to change, such as eating more fruit and veg, calculating your daily calorie intake, going for a walk each morning or buying low fat options. Others could also give you tips to try. But knowing what to do isn't the same as feeling motivated or able to do it. To be effective, you have to believe the changes are relevant, do-able and worth it.

What you think, affects how you feel, and in turn the actions you take.

Self-efficacy

In fact, research is telling us that one of the most important factors that influences weight loss success are your feelings of 'self-efficacy'. Self-efficacy is a term used in psychology to describe a person's belief that any action they take will have an effect on the outcome. It reflects our inner expectation that what we do will lead to the results we want. Not surprisingly, high levels of self-efficacy can enhance motivation, and allow us to deal better with uncertainty and conflict, and recovery from setbacks. But low levels, can reduce our motivation. We fear that whatever we do will not bring about our desired goal. This can lead self-defeating thoughts or 'self-talk', which make it hard to deal with set-backs, meaning we are more likely to give up. Here's some examples.

Examples: Low self-efficacy

'No matter how carefully I diet, I don't lose weight ...'

'I have eaten that chocolate and as usual blown my diet, so I may as well give up now.'

'I had a rich dessert – I have no willpower to say no. I can't stand not being able to eat what I want.'

If you have a strong sense of self-efficacy, your mindset and 'self-talk' will be more like:

Examples: High self-efficacy

'I know from previous weight loss programmes, that if I stay focussed on what I am doing I do lose weight. I have always expected to lose too much too quickly which frustrates me. I know that I will lose weight if I keep making the right changes, and this time it is important to me.'

'The chocolate bar won't ruin my diet, but if I think it has and keep on eating, then my negative self-talk will. So I will get back on track.'

'I don't like having to eat differently from others, but losing weight is very important to me, so I **can** stand it. After all, the world won't stop if I say no to dessert, and I will feel great afterwards. If I think about it, I am not hungry so would just feel bloated and guilty if I ate it.'

Willpower is a Skill

Many people feel that they just need plenty of willpower or a good telling off to lose weight. But willpower isn't something you have or you don't have. Willpower is a skill. Like the dessert example on page 19, it's a sign that you've made a conscious choice to do something, because you believe the benefits outweigh any downsides. In reality everything we do is preceded by a thought. This includes everything we eat. It just may not seem like it because our actions often feel automatic *(see 'Look out for trigger eating' page 21).*

When it comes to weight loss, developing a range of skills – including choosing a lower calorie diet, coping with negative self-talk and managing things that don't go to plan - will boost your sense of self-efficacy to make the changes you want. This is especially important because we live in such a weight-promoting environment.

Our weight-promoting environment

We are constantly surrounded by tempting food, stresses that can trigger comfort eating and labour-saving devices that make it easy not to be physically active. In other words, the environment we live in makes it easy to gain weight, unless we stop and think about the food choices we make and how much exercise we do. In fact, to stay a healthy weight/maintain our weight, just about all of us need to make conscious lifestyle choices everyday. This isn't 'dieting' but just part of taking care of ourselves in the environment we live in.

It is also true that some people find it more of a challenge than others to manage their weight, thanks to genetic differences in factors such as appetite control, spontaneous activity level and emotional responses to food – rather than metabolic rate, as is often believed. The good news is that with a healthy diet and active lifestyle a healthier weight can still be achieved. But do talk to your doctor if you feel you need additional support.

Coping with Common Slimming Saboteurs

Lyndel Costain BSc RD

Look out for 'trigger' eating

Much of the overeating we do or cravings we have are actually down to unconscious, habitual, responses to a variety of triggers. These triggers can be external, such as the sight or smell of food, or internal and emotion-led, such as a response to stress, anger, boredom or emptiness. Your food diary (see page 43) helps you to recognise 'trigger' or 'non-hungry' eating which gives you the chance to think twice before you eat (see below).

Get some support

A big part of your success will be having someone to support you. It could be a friend, partner, health professional, health club or website. Let them know how they can help you most.

Make lapses your ally

Don't let a lapse throw you off course. You can't be, nor need to be perfect all the time. Doing well 80-90% of the time is great progress. Lapses are a normal part of change. Rather than feel you have failed and give up, look at what you can learn from a difficult day or week and use it to find helpful solutions for the future.

Understand why you eat

When I ask people what prompts them to eat, hunger usually comes down near the bottom of their list of reasons. Some people struggle to remember or appreciate what true hunger feels like. We are lucky that we have plenty of food to eat in our society. But its constant presence makes it harder to control what we eat, especially if it brings us comfort or joy.

If you ever find yourself in the fridge even though you've recently eaten, then you know hunger isn't the reason but some other trigger. The urge to eat can be so automatic that you feel you lack willpower or are out of control. But it is in fact a learned or conditioned response. A bit like Pavlov's dogs. He rang a bell every time he fed them, and from then on, whenever they heard the bell ring they were 'conditioned' to salivate in anticipation of food.

Because this 'non-hungry' eating is learned, you can reprogramme your response to the situations or feelings that trigger it. The first step is to identify when these urges strike. When you find yourself eating when you aren't hungry ask yourself 'why do I want to eat, what am I feeling?' If you aren't sure think back to what was happening before you ate. Then ask yourself if there is another way you can feel better without food. Or you could chat to your urge to eat in a friendly way, telling it that you don't want to give into it, you have a planned meal coming soon, and it's merely a learned response. Whatever strategy you choose, the more often you break into your urges to eat, the weaker their hold becomes.

Practise positive self-talk

Self-talk may be positive and constructive (like your guardian angel) or negative and irrational (like having a destructive devil on your shoulder).

If you've had on-off battles with your weight over the years, it's highly likely that the 'devil' is there more often. 'All or nothing' self-talk for example, 'I ate a "bad food" so have broken my diet', can make you feel like a failure which, can then trigger you into the action of overeating and/or totally giving up *(see 'Diet-binge cycle' page 23)*. One of the most powerful things about it is that the last thoughts we have are what stays in our mind. So if we think 'I still look fat' or 'I will never be slim', these feelings stay with us.

To change your self-talk for the better, the trick is to first recognise it's happening (keeping a diary really helps, *see Keep a Food Diary, page 29*). Then turn it around into a positive version of the same events *(see Self-efficacy, page 18)* where the resulting action was to feel good and stay on track. Reshaping negative self-talk helps you to boost your self-esteem and feelings of self-efficacy, and with it change your self-definition - from someone who can't 'lose weight' or 'do this or that', to someone 'who can'. And when you believe you can…

The Diet – Binge Cycle

If this cycle looks familiar, use positive self-talk, and a more flexible dietary approach, to help you break free.

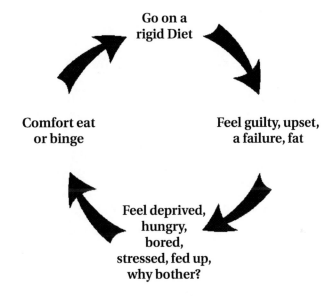

Go on a
rigid Diet

Feel guilty, upset,
a failure, fat

Feel deprived,
hungry,
bored,
stressed, fed up,
why bother?

Comfort eat
or binge

Really choose what you want to eat

This skill is like your personal brake. It also helps you to manage 'trigger/non-hungry' eating and weaken its hold. It legalises food and stops you feeling deprived. It helps you to regularly remind yourself why you are making changes to your eating habits, which keeps motivation high. But it doesn't just happen. Like all skills it requires practise. Sometimes it will work well for you, other times it won't – but overall it will help. Basically, ask yourself if you really want to eat that food in front of you. This becomes the prompt for you to make a conscious choice, weighing up the pros and cons or consequences of making that choice, and feeling free to have it, reject it or just eat some. Remembering all the while that you can eat this food another time if you want to.

Action Planning

Successful people don't just wait for things to happen. They believe in themselves, plan ahead, take action and then refine their plan until it gets, and keeps on getting the results they want. Successful slimmers use a very similar approach. They don't rely on quick-fixes or magic formulas, but glean information from reliable sources to develop a plan or approach that suits their needs, tastes and lifestyle. Thinking of weight management as a lifelong project, which has a weight loss phase and a weight maintenance phase, is also a route to success.

When the Going Gets Tough - Staying on Track

If things start to go off track, don't panic. Learning new habits takes time. And life is never straightforward so there will be times when it all seems too much, or negative 'self- talk' creeps in to try and drag you back into old ways. So if the going gets tough:

- Value what you've achieved so far, rather than only focus on what you plan to do.

- Look back at your reasons to lose weight and refer to the list often.

- Don't expect to change too much, too quickly. Take things a step at a time.

- Accept difficulties as part of the learning and skill building process.

- Enjoy a non-food reward for achieving your goals (including maintaining your weight).

- Use recipes and meal ideas to keep things interesting.

- Talk to your supporters and get plenty of encouragement. This is really vital!

Strategies of Successful Slimmers

Thanks to research conducted by large studies such as the US National Weight Control Registry and the German Lean Habits Study, we now know more about what works best for people who have lost weight and successfully kept it off. So be inspired!

The key elements of success are to:

- Believe that you can control your weight and the changes involved are really worth it.
- Stay realistic and value what you have achieved rather than dwell on a weight you 'dream' of being.
- Be more active – plan ways to fit activity into your daily life – aim for 1 hour of walking daily.
- Plan ahead for regular meals and snacks, starting with breakfast.
- Choose a balanced, low-fat diet with plenty of fruit and vegetables *(see Healthy Eating Made Easy, page 32).*
- Watch portion size and limit fast food.
- Sit down to eat and take time over meals, paying attention to what you are eating.
- Have a flexible approach – plan in and enjoy some favourite foods without guilt.
- Recognise and address 'all or nothing' thinking and other negative 'self-talk'.
- Keep making conscious choices.
- Learn to confront problems rather than eat, drink, sleep or wish they would go away.
- Enlist ongoing help and support from family, friends, professionals or websites.
- Regularly (at least once a week but not more than once daily) check your weight.
- Take action before your weight increases by more than 4-5lb (2kg).
- Accept that your weight management skills need to be kept up long-term.
- Take heart from successful slimmers, who say that it gets easier over time.

Your step-by-step guide to using this book and shifting those pounds

Juliette Kellow BSc RD and Rebecca Walton

1. Find your healthy weight

Use the weight charts, body mass index table and information on pages 36-43 to determine the right weight for you. Then set yourself a weight to aim for. Research shows it really helps if you make losing 10% of your weight your first overall target. It also brings important health benefits too *(see 'What is a Healthy Weight?' page 15)*. You can break this down into smaller manageable steps, for example, 3kg/6.5lbs at a time. If 10% is too much, then go for a 5% loss – this has important health benefits too. In fact, just keeping your weight stable is a great achievement these days, because of our weight-promoting environment *(see page 20)*.

Waist Management

In addition to BMI, another important way to assess your weight is by measuring your waist just above belly button level. It is especially useful for men as they tend to carry more excess weight around their bellies, but women should test it out too. Having excess weight around your middle (known as being 'apple-shaped') increases your risk of heart disease and type 2 diabetes. A simple way to stay aware of your waist is according to how well, or otherwise, skirts and trousers fit. Talk to your doctor about any weight and health concerns.

WAIST MEASUREMENT

	Increased Health Risk	High Risk to Health
Women	32-35in (81-88cm)	more than 35in (88cm)
Men	37-40in (94-102cm)	more than 40in (102cm)

2. Set a realistic time scale

With today's hectic lifestyles, everything tends to happen at breakneck speed, so it's no wonder that when it comes to losing weight, most of us want to shift those pounds in an instant. But it's probably taken years to accumulate that extra weight, with the result that it's unrealistic to expect to lose the excess in just a few weeks! Instead, prepare yourself to lose weight slowly and steadily. It's far healthier to lose weight like this. But better still, research shows you'll be far more likely to maintain your new, lower weight.

If you only have a small amount of weight to lose, aim for a weight loss of around 1lb (½kg) a week. But if you have more than 2 stone (28kg) to lose, you may prefer to aim for 2lb (1kg) each week. Remember though, it's better to keep going at 1lb (½kg) a week than to give up because trying to lose 2lb (1kg) a week is making you miserable! The following words may help you to keep your goal in perspective:

'Never give up on a goal because of the time it will take to achieve it – the time will pass anyway.'

Weight Fluctuations

Weight typically fluctuates on a day to day basis. You know that shock/ horror feeling when you weigh yourself in the morning then later in the day, or after a meal out, and it looks like youve gained pounds in hours! But this is due to fluid not fat changes. Real changes in body fat can only happen more gradually (remember, to gain 1lb you need to eat 3500 calories more than you usually do). Don't be confused either by seemingly very rapid weight loss in the first week or so.

When calorie intake is initially cut back, the body's carbohydrate stores in the liver and muscles (known as glycogen) are used up. Glycogen is stored with three times its weight in water, meaning that rapid losses of 4.5- 6.6lb (2 -3 kg) are possible. These stores can be just as rapidly refilled if normal eating is resumed. True weight loss happens more gradually and this book helps you to lose weight at the steady and healthy rate of no more than 1-2 lbs per week.

3. Calculate your calorie allowance

Use the calorie tables on pages 39-40 to find out how many calories you need each day to maintain your current weight. Then use the table below to discover the amount of calories you need to subtract from this amount every day to lose weight at your chosen rate. For example, a 35 year-old woman who is moderately active and weighs 12 stone (76kg) needs 2,188 calories a day to keep her weight steady. If she wants to lose ½lb (¼kg) a week, she needs 250 calories less each day, giving her a daily calorie allowance of 1,938 calories. If she wants to lose 1lb (½kg) a week, she needs 500 calories less each day, giving her a daily calorie allowance of 1,688 calories, and so on.

TO LOSE...	Cut your daily calorie intake by	In three months you could lose...	In six months you could lose...	In one year you could lose...
½lb a week	250	6.5lb	13lb	1st 12lb
1lb a week	500	13lb	1st 12lb	3st 10lb
1½lb a week	750	1st 5.5lb	2st 11lb	5st 8lb
2lb a week	1,000	1st 12lb	3st 10lb	7st 6lb

TO LOSE...	Cut your daily calorie intake by	In three months you could lose...	In six months you could lose...	In one year you could lose...
¼kg a week	250	3.25kg	6.5kg	13kg
½kg a week	500	6.5kg	13kg	26kg
¾kg a week	750	9.75kg	19.5kg	39kg
1kg a week	1,000	13kg	26kg	52kg

4. Keep a food diary

Writing down what you eat and drink and any thoughts linked to that eating helps you become more aware of your eating habits. Recognising what is going on helps you feel in control and is a powerful way to start planning change. Keeping a food diary before you start to change your eating habits will also help you identify opportunities for cutting calories by substituting one food for another, cutting portion sizes of high-calorie foods or eating certain foods less often. Simply write down every single item you eat or drink during the day and use this book to calculate the calories of each item. Then after a few days of eating normally, introduce some changes to your diet to achieve your daily calorie allowance. Remember to spread your daily calorie allowance fairly evenly throughout the day to prevent hunger. You'll find a template for a daily food and exercise diary on page 43. Try to use it as carefully as you can as research shows that people who do, do best.

 Top Tip

If you only fill in your main food diary once a day, keep a pen and notepad with you to write down all those little extras you eat or drink during the day – that chocolate you ate in the office, the sliver of cheese you had while cooking dinner and the few chips you pinched from your husband's plate, for example! It's easy to forget the little things if they're not written down, but they can make the difference between success and failure.

QUESTION: Why are heavier people allowed more calories than those who have smaller amounts of weight to lose?

ANSWER: This confuses a lot of people but is easily explained. Someone who is 3 stone overweight, for example, is carrying the equivalent of 42 small packets of butter with them everywhere they go – up and down the stairs, to the local shops, into the kitchen. Obviously, it takes a lot more energy simply to move around when you're carrying that extra weight. As a consequence, the heavier you are, the more calories you need just to keep your weight steady. In turn, this means you'll lose weight on a higher calorie allowance. However, as you lose weight, you'll need to lower your calorie allowance slightly as you have less weight to carry around.

5. Control your portions

As well as making some smart food swaps to cut calories, it's likely you'll also need to reduce your serving sizes for some foods to help shift those pounds. Even 'healthy' foods such as brown rice, wholemeal bread, chicken, fish and low-fat dairy products contain calories so you may need to limit the amount you eat. When you first start out, weigh portions of foods like rice, pasta, cereal, cheese, butter, oil, meat, fish, and chicken rather than completing your food diary with a 'guesstimated' weight! That way you can calculate the calorie content accurately. Don't forget that drinks contain calories too, alcohol, milk, juices and sugary drinks all count.

6. Measure your success

Research has found that regular weight checks do help. Weighing yourself helps you assess how your eating and exercise habits affect your body weight. The important thing is to use the information in a positive way – to assess your progress - rather than as a stick to beat yourself up with. Remember that weight can fluctuate by a kilogram in a day, for example, due to fluid changes, premenstrually, after a big meal out, so weigh yourself at the same time of day and look at the trend over a week or two.

People who successfully lose weight and keep it off, also tend to continue weighing themselves at least once a week, and often daily (but not in an obsessive way), because they say it helps them stay 'on track'. Probably because they use it as an early warning system. People who weigh themselves regularly (or regularly try on a tight fitting item of clothing) will notice quickly if they have gained a couple of kilograms and can take action to stop gaining more. Checking your weight less often can mean that you might discover one day that you gained 6kg. That can be pretty discouraging, and it might trigger you to just give up.

Top Tip

Don't just focus on what the bathroom scales say either – keep a record of your vital statistics, too. Many people find it doubly encouraging to see the inches dropping off, as well as the pounds!

7. Stay motivated

Each time you lose half a stone, or reach your own small goal – celebrate! Treat yourself to a little luxury – something new to wear, a little pampering or some other (non-food) treat. It also helps replace the comfort you once got from food and allows you to take care of yourself in other ways. Trying on an item of clothing that used to be tight can also help to keep you feeling motivated. Make sure you keep in touch with your supporters, and if the going gets tough take another look at the *'Coping with Common Slimming Saboteurs' section on page 21*. Once you've reviewed how well you've done, use this book to set yourself a new daily calorie allowance based on your new weight to help you lose the next half stone *(see point 3 - page 28 - Calculate your calorie allowance)*.

8. Keep it off

What you do to stay slim is just as important as what you did to get slim. Quite simply, if you return to your old ways, you are likely to return to your old weight. The great thing about calorie counting is that you will learn so much about what you eat, and make so many important changes to your eating and drinking habits, that you'll probably find it difficult to go back to your old ways – and won't want to anyway. It's still a good idea to weigh yourself at least once a week to keep a check on your weight. The key is to deal with any extra pounds immediately, rather than waiting until you have a stone to lose *(see page 30)*. Simply go back to counting calories for as long as it takes to shift those pounds and enjoy the new slim you. Page 25 has more information about how successful slimmers keep it off.

QUESTION: **Do I need to stick to exactly the same number of calories each day or is it OK to have a lower calorie intake during the week and slightly more at the weekend?**

ANSWER: The key to losing weight is to take in fewer calories than you need for as long as it takes to reach your target, aiming for a loss of no more than 2lb (1kg) a week. In general, most nutrition experts recommend a daily calorie allowance. However, it's just as valid to use other periods of time such as weeks. If you prefer, simply multiply your daily allowance by seven to work out a weekly calorie allowance and then allocate more calories to some days than others. For example, a daily allowance of 1,500 calories is equivalent to 10,500 calories a week. This means you could have 1,300 calories a day during the week and 2,000 calories a day on Saturday and Sunday.

Healthy Eating Made Easy

Juliette Kellow BSc RD

GONE ARE THE DAYS when a healthy diet meant surviving on bird seed, rabbit food and carrot juice! The new approach to eating healthily means we're positively encouraged to eat a wide range of foods, including some of our favourites – it's just a question of making sure we don't eat high fat, high sugar or highly processed foods too often.

Eating a healthy diet, together with taking regular exercise and not smoking, has huge benefits to our health, both in the short and long term. As well as helping us to lose or maintain our weight, a healthy diet can boost energy levels, keep our immune system strong and give us healthy skin, nails and hair. Meanwhile, eating well throughout life also means we're far less likely to suffer from health problems such as constipation, anaemia and tooth decay or set ourselves up for serious conditions in later life such as obesity, heart disease, stroke, diabetes, cancer or osteoporosis.

Fortunately, it couldn't be easier to eat a balanced diet. To start with, no single food provides all the calories and nutrients we need to stay healthy, so it's important to eat a variety of foods. Meanwhile, most nutrition experts also agree that mealtimes should be a pleasure rather than a penance. This means it's fine to eat small amounts of our favourite treats from time to time.

To help people eat healthily, the Food Standards Agency recommends eating plenty of different foods from four main groups of foods and limiting the amount we eat from a smaller fifth group. Ultimately, we should eat more fruit, vegetables, starchy, fibre-rich foods and fresh products, and fewer fatty, sugary, salty and processed foods.

The following guidelines are all based on the healthy eating guidelines recommended by the Food Standards Agency.

Bread, other cereals and potatoes

Eat these foods at each meal. They also make good snacks.

Foods in this group include bread, breakfast cereals, potatoes, rice, pasta, noodles, yams, oats and grains. Go for high-fibre varieties where available, such as wholegrain cereals, wholemeal bread and brown rice. These foods should fill roughly a third of your plate at mealtimes.

TYPICAL SERVING SIZES

* *2 slices bread in a sandwich or with a meal*

* *a tennis ball sized serving of pasta, potato, rice, noodles or couscous*

* *a bowl of porridge*

* *around 40g of breakfast cereal*

Fruit and vegetables

Eat at least five portions every day.

Foods in this group include all fruits and vegetables, including fresh, frozen, canned and dried products, and unsweetened fruit juice. Choose canned fruit in juice rather than syrup and go for veg canned in water without added salt or sugar.

TYPICAL PORTION SIZES

* *a piece of fruit eg: apple, banana, pear*

* *2 small fruits eg: satsumas, plums, apricots*

* *a bowl of fruit salad, canned or stewed fruit*

* *a small glass of unsweetened fruit juice*

* *a cereal bowl of salad*

* *3tbsp vegetables*

Milk and dairy foods

Eat two or three servings a day.

Foods in this group include milk, cheese, yoghurt and fromage frais. Choose low-fat varieties where available such as skimmed milk, reduced-fat cheese and fat-free yoghurt.

TYPICAL SERVING SIZES

* *200ml milk*

* *a small pot of yoghurt or fromage frais*

* *a small matchbox-sized piece of cheese*

Meat, fish and alternatives

Eat two servings a day

Foods in this group include meat, poultry, fish, eggs, beans, nuts and seeds. Choose low-fat varieties where available such as extra-lean minced beef and skinless chicken and don't add extra fat or salt.

TYPICAL SERVING SIZES

* *a piece of meat, chicken or fish the size of a deck of cards*

* *1-2 eggs*

* *3 heaped tablespoons of beans*

* *a small handful of nuts or seeds*

Healthy Eating on a plate

A simple way to serve up both balance and healthy proportions is to fill one half of your plate with salad or vegetables and divide the other half between protein-rich meat, chicken, fish, eggs or beans, and healthy carbs (potatoes, rice, pasta, pulses, bread or noodles).

Fatty and sugary foods

Eat only small amounts of these foods

Foods in this group include oils, spreading fats, cream, mayonnaise, oily salad dressings, cakes, biscuits, puddings, crisps, savoury snacks, sugar, preserves, confectionery and sugary soft drinks.

TYPICAL SERVING SIZES:

- *a small packet of sweets or a small bar of chocolate*
- *a small slice of cake*
- *a couple of small biscuits*
- *1 level tbsp mayo, salad dressing or olive oil*
- *a small packet of crisps*

Useful Tools

Body Mass Index

The Body Mass Index (BMI) is the internationally accepted way of assessing how healthy our weight is. It is calculated using an individual's height and weight. Use the Body Mass Index Chart to look up your BMI, and use the table below to see what range you fall into.

BMI Under 18.5	*Underweight*
BMI 18.5-25	*Healthy*
BMI 25-30	*Overweight*
BMI 30-40	*Obese*
BMI Over 40	*Severely Obese*

This is what different BMI ranges mean.

- **Underweight:** you probably need to gain weight for your health's sake. Talk to your doctor if you have any concerns, or if you feel frightened about gaining weight.

- **Healthy weight:** you are a healthy weight, so aim to stay in this range (note that most people in this range tend to have a BMI between 20-25).

- **Overweight:** aim to lose some weight for your health's sake, or at least prevent further weight gain.

- **Obese:** your health is at risk and losing weight will benefit your health.

- **Severely obese:** your health is definitely at risk. You should visit your doctor for a health check. Losing weight will improve your health.

Please note that BMI is not as accurate for athletes or very muscular people (muscle weighs more than fat), as it can push them into a higher BMI category despite having a healthy level of body fat. It is also not accurate for women who are pregnant or breastfeeding, or people who are frail.

Body Mass Index Table

HEIGHT IN FEET / INCHES

	4'6	4'8	4'10	5'0	5'2	5'4	5'6	5'8	5'10	6'0	6'2	6'4	6'6	6'8	6'10
6st 7	22.0	20.5	19.1	17.8	16.7	15.7	14.7	13.9	13.1	12.4	11.7	11.1	10.6	10.0	9.5
7st 0	23.7	22.1	20.6	19.2	18.0	16.9	15.9	15.0	14.1	13.3	12.6	12.0	11.4	10.8	10.3
7st 7	25.4	23.6	22.0	20.6	19.3	18.1	17.0	16.0	15.1	14.3	13.5	12.8	12.2	11.6	11.0
8st 0	27.1	25.2	23.5	22.0	20.6	19.3	18.1	17.1	16.1	15.2	14.4	13.7	13.0	12.3	11.8
8st 7	28.8	26.8	25.0	23.3	21.8	20.5	19.3	18.2	17.1	16.2	15.3	14.5	13.8	13.1	12.5
9st 0	30.5	28.4	26.4	24.7	23.1	21.7	20.4	19.2	18.1	17.2	16.2	15.4	14.6	13.9	13.2
9st 7	32.2	29.9	27.9	26.1	24.4	22.9	21.5	20.3	19.2	18.1	17.1	16.2	15.4	14.7	14.0
10st 0	33.9	31.5	29.4	27.4	25.7	24.1	22.7	21.4	20.2	19.1	18.0	17.1	16.2	15.4	14.7
10st 7	35.6	33.1	30.8	28.8	27.0	25.3	23.8	22.4	21.2	20.0	18.9	18.0	17.0	16.2	15.4
11st 0	37.3	34.7	32.3	30.2	28.3	26.5	24.9	23.5	22.2	21.0	19.8	18.8	17.9	17.0	16.2
11st 7	39.0	36.2	33.8	31.6	29.6	27.7	26.1	24.6	23.2	21.9	20.7	19.7	18.7	17.8	16.9
12st 0	40.7	37.8	35.2	32.9	30.8	28.9	27.2	25.6	24.2	22.9	21.6	20.5	19.5	18.5	17.6
12st 7	42.3	39.4	36.7	34.3	32.1	30.1	28.3	26.7	25.2	23.8	22.5	21.4	20.3	19.3	18.4
13st 0	44.0	41.0	38.2	35.7	33.4	31.4	29.5	27.8	26.2	24.8	23.5	22.2	21.1	20.1	19.1
13st 7	45.7	42.5	39.6	37.0	34.7	32.6	30.6	28.8	27.2	25.7	24.4	23.1	21.9	20.8	19.8
14st 0	47.4	44.1	41.1	38.4	36.0	33.8	31.7	29.9	28.2	26.7	25.3	23.9	22.7	21.6	20.6
14st 7	49.1	45.7	42.6	39.8	37.3	35.0	32.9	31.0	29.2	27.6	26.2	24.8	23.5	22.4	21.3
15st 0	50.8	47.3	44.0	41.2	38.5	36.2	34.0	32.0	30.2	28.6	27.1	25.7	24.4	23.2	22.0
15st 7	52.5	48.8	45.5	42.5	39.8	37.4	35.2	33.1	31.2	29.5	28.0	26.5	25.2	23.9	22.8
16st 0	54.2	50.4	47.0	43.9	41.1	38.6	36.3	34.2	32.3	30.5	28.9	27.4	26.0	24.7	23.5
16st 7	55.9	52.0	48.5	45.3	42.4	39.8	37.4	35.2	33.3	31.4	29.8	28.2	26.8	25.5	24.2
17st 0	57.6	53.6	49.9	46.6	43.7	41.0	38.6	36.3	34.3	32.4	30.7	29.1	27.6	26.2	25.0
17st 7	59.3	55.1	51.4	48.0	45.0	42.2	39.7	37.4	35.3	33.3	31.6	29.9	28.4	27.0	25.7
18st 0	61.0	56.7	52.9	49.4	46.3	43.4	40.8	38.5	36.3	34.3	32.5	30.8	29.2	27.8	26.4
18st 7	62.7	58.3	54.3	50.8	47.5	44.6	42.0	39.5	37.3	35.3	33.4	31.6	30.0	28.6	27.2
19st 0	64.4	59.9	55.8	52.1	48.8	45.8	43.1	40.6	38.3	36.2	34.3	32.5	30.8	29.3	27.9
19st 7	66.1	61.4	57.3	53.5	50.1	47.0	44.2	41.7	39.3	37.2	35.2	33.3	31.7	30.1	28.6
20st 0	67.8	63.0	58.7	54.9	51.4	48.2	45.4	42.7	40.3	38.1	36.1	34.2	32.5	30.9	29.4
20st 7	69.4	64.6	60.2	56.3	52.7	49.4	46.5	43.8	41.3	39.1	37.0	35.1	33.3	31.6	30.1
21st 0	71.1	66.2	61.7	57.6	54.0	50.6	47.6	44.9	42.3	40.0	37.9	35.9	34.1	32.4	30.9
21st 7	72.8	67.7	63.1	59.0	55.3	51.9	48.8	45.9	43.3	41.0	38.8	36.8	34.9	33.2	31.6
22st 0	74.5	69.3	64.6	60.4	56.5	53.1	49.9	47.0	44.4	41.9	39.7	37.6	35.7	34.0	32.3
22st 7	76.2	70.9	66.1	61.7	57.8	54.3	51.0	48.1	45.4	42.9	40.6	38.5	36.5	34.7	33.1
23st 0	77.9	72.5	67.5	63.1	59.1	55.5	52.2	49.1	46.4	43.8	41.5	39.3	37.3	35.5	33.8
23st 7	79.6	74.0	69.0	64.5	60.4	56.7	53.3	50.2	47.4	44.8	42.4	40.2	38.2	36.3	34.5
24st 0	81.3	75.6	70.5	65.9	61.7	57.9	54.4	51.3	48.4	45.7	43.3	41.0	39.0	37.0	35.3
24st 7	83.0	77.2	71.9	67.2	63.0	59.1	55.6	52.3	49.4	46.7	44.2	41.9	39.8	37.8	36.0
25st 0	84.7	78.8	73.4	68.6	64.2	60.3	56.7	53.4	50.4	47.6	45.1	42.8	40.6	38.6	36.7
25st 7	86.4	80.3	74.9	70.0	65.5	61.5	57.8	54.5	51.4	48.6	46.0	43.6	41.4	39.4	37.5
26st 0	88.1	81.9	76.3	71.3	66.8	62.7	59.0	55.5	52.4	49.5	46.9	44.5	42.2	40.1	38.2
26st 7	89.8	83.5	77.8	72.7	68.1	63.9	60.1	56.6	53.4	50.5	47.8	45.3	43.0	40.9	38.9
27st 0	91.5	85.1	79.3	74.1	69.4	65.1	61.2	57.7	54.4	51.5	48.7	46.2	43.8	41.7	39.7
27st 7	93.2	86.6	80.8	75.5	70.7	66.3	62.4	58.7	55.4	52.4	49.6	47.0	44.7	42.4	40.4
28st 0	94.9	88.2	82.2	76.8	72.0	67.5	63.5	59.8	56.4	53.4	50.5	47.9	45.5	43.2	41.1
28st 7	96.5	89.8	83.7	78.2	73.2	68.7	64.6	60.9	57.5	54.3	51.4	48.7	46.3	44.0	41.9
29st 0	98.2	91.4	85.2	79.6	74.5	69.9	65.8	62.0	58.5	55.3	52.3	49.6	47.1	44.8	42.6
29st 7	99.9	92.9	86.6	80.9	75.8	71.1	66.9	63.0	59.5	56.2	53.2	50.5	47.9	45.5	43.3

WEIGHT IN STONES / LBS

Weight Chart

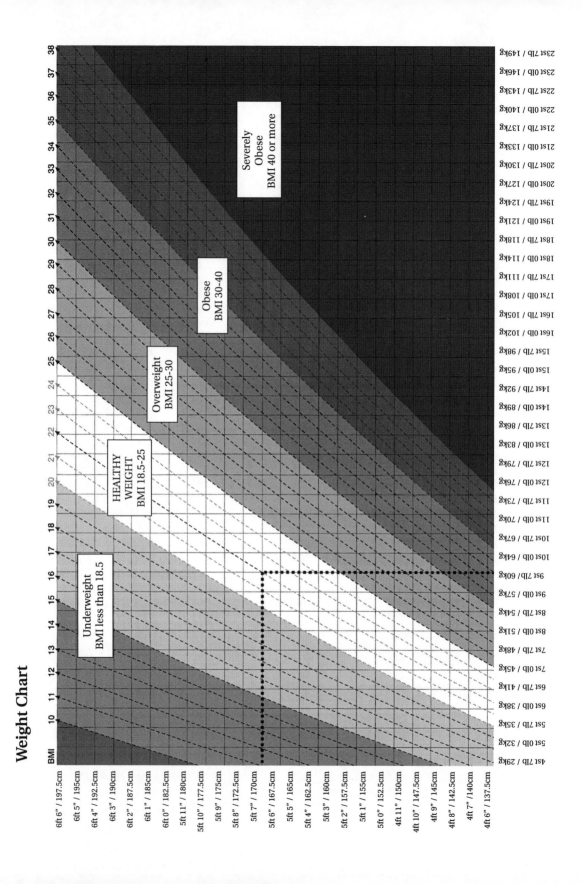

Calories Required to Maintain Weight
Adult Females

ACTIVITY LEVEL / AGE

WEIGHT IN STONES / LBS	VERY SEDENTARY			MODERATELY SEDENTARY			MODERATELY ACTIVE			VERY ACTIVE		
	<30	30-60	60+	<30	30-60	60+	<30	30-60	60+	<30	30-60	60+
7st 7	1425	1473	1304	1544	1596	1412	1781	1841	1630	2138	2210	1956
8st 0	1481	1504	1338	1605	1629	1450	1852	1880	1673	2222	2256	2008
8st 7	1537	1535	1373	1666	1663	1487	1922	1919	1716	2306	2302	2059
9st 0	1594	1566	1407	1726	1696	1524	1992	1957	1759	2391	2349	2111
9st 7	1650	1596	1442	1787	1729	1562	2062	1996	1802	2475	2395	2163
10st 0	1706	1627	1476	1848	1763	1599	2133	2034	1845	2559	2441	2214
10st 7	1762	1658	1511	1909	1796	1637	2203	2073	1888	2644	2487	2266
11st 0	1819	1689	1545	1970	1830	1674	2273	2111	1931	2728	2534	2318
11st 7	1875	1720	1580	2031	1863	1711	2344	2150	1975	2813	2580	2370
12st 0	1931	1751	1614	2092	1897	1749	2414	2188	2018	2897	2626	2421
12st 7	1987	1781	1648	2153	1930	1786	2484	2227	2061	2981	2672	2473
13st 0	2044	1812	1683	2214	1963	1823	2555	2266	2104	3066	2719	2525
13st 7	2100	1843	1717	2275	1997	1861	2625	2304	2147	3150	2765	2576
14st 0	2156	1874	1752	2336	2030	1898	2695	2343	2190	3234	2811	2628
14st 7	2212	1905	1786	2397	2064	1935	2766	2381	2233	3319	2858	2680
15st 0	2269	1936	1821	2458	2097	1973	2836	2420	2276	3403	2904	2732
15st 7	2325	1967	1855	2519	2130	2010	2906	2458	2319	3488	2950	2783
16st 0	2381	1997	1890	2580	2164	2047	2976	2497	2362	3572	2996	2835
16st 7	2437	2028	1924	2640	2197	2085	3047	2535	2405	3656	3043	2887
17st 0	2494	2059	1959	2701	2231	2122	3117	2574	2449	3741	3089	2938
17st 7	2550	2090	1993	2762	2264	2159	3187	2613	2492	3825	3135	2990
18st 0	2606	2121	2028	2823	2298	2197	3258	2651	2535	3909	3181	3042
18st 7	2662	2152	2062	2884	2331	2234	3328	2690	2578	3994	3228	3093
19st 0	2719	2182	2097	2945	2364	2271	3398	2728	2621	4078	3274	3145
19st 7	2775	2213	2131	3006	2398	2309	3469	2767	2664	4162	3320	3197
20st 0	2831	2244	2166	3067	2431	2346	3539	2805	2707	4247	3366	3249
20st 7	2887	2275	2200	3128	2465	2383	3609	2844	2750	4331	3413	3300
21st 0	2944	2306	2235	3189	2498	2421	3680	2882	2793	4416	3459	3352
21st 7	3000	2337	2269	3250	2531	2458	3750	2921	2836	4500	3505	3404
22st 0	3056	2368	2303	3311	2565	2495	3820	2960	2879	4584	3552	3455
22st 7	3112	2398	2338	3372	2598	2533	3890	2998	2923	4669	3598	3507
23st 0	3169	2429	2372	3433	2632	2570	3961	3037	2966	4753	3644	3559
23st 7	3225	2460	2407	3494	2665	2608	4031	3075	3009	4837	3690	3611
24st 0	3281	2491	2441	3554	2699	2645	4101	3114	3052	4922	3737	3662
24st 7	3337	2522	2476	3615	2732	2682	4172	3152	3095	5006	3783	3714
25st 0	3394	2553	2510	3676	2765	2720	4242	3191	3138	5091	3829	3766
25st 7	3450	2583	2545	3737	2799	2757	4312	3229	3181	5175	3875	3817
26st 0	3506	2614	2579	3798	2832	2794	4383	3268	3224	5259	3922	3869
26st 7	3562	2645	2614	3859	2866	2832	4453	3307	3267	5344	3968	3921
27st 0	3618	2676	2648	3920	2899	2869	4523	3345	3310	5428	4014	3973
27st 7	3675	2707	2683	3981	2932	2906	4594	3384	3353	5512	4060	4024
28st 0	3731	2738	2717	4042	2966	2944	4664	3422	3397	5597	4107	4076
28st 7	3787	2768	2752	4103	2999	2981	4734	3461	3440	5681	4153	4128

Calories Required to Maintain Weight
Adult Males

ACTIVITY LEVEL / AGE

WEIGHT IN STONES / LBS	VERY SEDENTARY			MODERATELY SEDENTARY			MODERATELY ACTIVE			VERY ACTIVE		
	<30	30-60	60+	<30	30-60	60+	<30	30-60	60+	<30	30-60	60+
9st 0	1856	1827	1502	2010	1979	1627	2320	2284	1878	2784	2741	2254
9st 7	1913	1871	1547	2072	2026	1676	2391	2338	1933	2870	2806	2320
10st 0	1970	1914	1591	2134	2074	1724	2463	2393	1989	2955	2871	2387
10st 7	2027	1958	1636	2196	2121	1772	2534	2447	2045	3041	2937	2454
11st 0	2084	2001	1680	2258	2168	1820	2605	2502	2100	3127	3002	2520
11st 7	2141	2045	1724	2320	2215	1868	2677	2556	2156	3212	3067	2587
12st 0	2199	2088	1769	2382	2262	1916	2748	2611	2211	3298	3133	2654
12st 7	2256	2132	1813	2444	2310	1965	2820	2665	2267	3384	3198	2720
13st 0	2313	2175	1858	2506	2357	2013	2891	2719	2322	3470	3263	2787
13st 7	2370	2219	1902	2568	2404	2061	2963	2774	2378	3555	3329	2854
14st 0	2427	2262	1947	2630	2451	2109	3034	2828	2434	3641	3394	2920
14st 7	2484	2306	1991	2691	2498	2157	3106	2883	2489	3727	3459	2987
15st 0	2542	2350	2036	2753	2545	2205	3177	2937	2545	3813	3525	3054
15st 7	2599	2393	2080	2815	2593	2253	3248	2992	2600	3898	3590	3120
16st 0	2656	2437	2125	2877	2640	2302	3320	3046	2656	3984	3655	3187
16st 7	2713	2480	2169	2939	2687	2350	3391	3100	2711	4070	3721	3254
17st 0	2770	2524	2213	3001	2734	2398	3463	3155	2767	4155	3786	3320
17st 7	2827	2567	2258	3063	2781	2446	3534	3209	2823	4241	3851	3387
18st 0	2884	2611	2302	3125	2828	2494	3606	3264	2878	4327	3917	3454
18st 7	2942	2654	2347	3187	2876	2542	3677	3318	2934	4413	3982	3520
19st 0	2999	2698	2391	3249	2923	2591	3749	3373	2989	4498	4047	3587
19st 7	3056	2741	2436	3311	2970	2639	3820	3427	3045	4584	4112	3654
20st 0	3113	2785	2480	3373	3017	2687	3891	3481	3100	4670	4178	3721
20st 7	3170	2829	2525	3434	3064	2735	3963	3536	3156	4756	4243	3787
21st 0	3227	2872	2569	3496	3112	2783	4034	3590	3211	4841	4308	3854
21st 7	3285	2916	2614	3558	3159	2831	4106	3645	3267	4927	4374	3921
22st 0	3342	2959	2658	3620	3206	2880	4177	3699	3323	5013	4439	3987
22st 7	3399	3003	2702	3682	3253	2928	4249	3754	3378	5098	4504	4054
23st 0	3456	3046	2747	3744	3300	2976	4320	3808	3434	5184	4570	4121
23st 7	3513	3090	2791	3806	3347	3024	4392	3862	3489	5270	4635	4187
24st 0	3570	3133	2836	3868	3395	3072	4463	3917	3545	5356	4700	4254
24st 7	3627	3177	2880	3930	3442	3120	4534	3971	3600	5441	4766	4321
25st 0	3685	3220	2925	3992	3489	3168	4606	4026	3656	5527	4831	4387
25st 7	3742	3264	2969	4054	3536	3217	4677	4080	3712	5613	4896	4454
26st 0	3799	3308	3014	4116	3583	3265	4749	4135	3767	5699	4962	4521
26st 7	3856	3351	3058	4177	3630	3313	4820	4189	3823	5784	5027	4587
27st 0	3913	3395	3103	4239	3678	3361	4892	4243	3878	5870	5092	4654
27st 7	3970	3438	3147	4301	3725	3409	4963	4298	3934	5956	5158	4721
28st 0	4028	3482	3191	4363	3772	3457	5035	4352	3989	6042	5223	4787
28st 7	4085	3525	3236	4425	3819	3506	5106	4407	4045	6127	5288	4854
29st 0	4142	3569	3280	4487	3866	3554	5177	4461	4101	6213	5354	4921
29st 7	4199	3612	3325	4549	3913	3602	5249	4516	4156	6299	5419	4987
30st 0	4256	3656	3369	4611	3961	3650	5320	4570	4212	6384	5484	5054

Calories Burned in Exercise

This table shows the approximate number of extra* calories that would be burned in a five minute period of exercise activity.

ACTIVITY	CALORIES BURNED IN 5 MINUTES	ACTIVITY	CALORIES BURNED IN 5 MINUTES
Aerobics, Low Impact	25	Situps, Continuous	17
Badminton, Recreational	17	Skiing, Moderate	30
Cross Trainer	30	Skipping, Moderate	30
Cycling, Recreational, 5mph	17	Squash Playing	39
Dancing, Modern, Moderate	13	Tennis Playing, Recreational	26
Fencing	24	Toning Exercises	17
Gardening, Weeding	19	Trampolining	17
Hill Walking, Up and Down, Recreational	22	Volleyball, Recreational	10
Jogging	30	Walking, Uphill, 15% Gradient, Moderate	43
Kick Boxing	30	Walking Up and Down Stairs, Moderate	34
Netball Playing	23	Walking, 4mph	24
Rebounding	18	Weight Training, Moderate	12
Roller Skating	30	Yoga	13
Rowing Machine, Moderate	30		
Running, 7.5mph	48		

*Extra calories are those in addition to your normal daily calorie needs.

My Personal Plan

Date: _____

Weight: _____

Height: _____

Body Mass Index: _____

Waist Measurement: _____

Body Fat % (if known) _____

10% Weight Loss Goal:

Current weight	16stone (224lb)	100kg
- 10% weight	1stone 8½lb (22½lb)	10kg
= 10% loss goal	14stone 5½lb (201½lb)	90kg

My smaller weight targets on the way to achieving my 10% goal will be:

_____ _____ _____

Reasons why I want to lose weight:

_____

Changes I will make to help me lose weight:
Diet:

_____

_____

Activity:

_____

_____

Potential saboteurs or barriers will be:

_____

_____

Ways I will overcome these:

_____

_____

My supporters will be:

_____

I will monitor my progress by:

_____

_____

I will reward my progress with:
In the short term:

_____

_____

In the long term:

_____

_____

Food and Exercise Diary

Date:

/   /

Daily Calorie Allowance: Ⓐ

Food/Drink Consumed	Serving Size	Calories

You are aiming for your Calorie Balance (Box D) to be as close to zero as possible - ie. you consume the number of calories you need.

Your Daily Calorie Allowance (Box A) should be set to lose ½-2lb (¼-1kg) a week, or maintain weight, depending on your goals.

Total calories consumed Ⓑ

Exercise/Activity	No. mins	Calories

Daily Calorie Allowance (A) *plus* Extra Calories used in Exercise (C) *minus* Total Calories Consumed (B) *equals* Calorie Balance (D)

Calories used in exercise Ⓒ $A + C - B = D$

Calorie balance Ⓓ

You can also write down any comments or thoughts related to your eating if you want to.

Food Information

Nutritional Information

CALORIE AND FAT values are given per serving, plus calorie and nutrition values per 100g of product. This makes it easy to compare the proportions of fat, protein, carbohydrate and fibre in each food.

The values given are for uncooked, unprepared foods unless otherwise stated. Values are also for only the edible portion of the food unless otherwise stated. ie - weighed with bone.

Finding Foods

The Calorie, Carb & Fat Bible has an Eating Out section which is arranged alphabetically by brand. In the General Foods and Drinks A-Z most foods are grouped together by type, and then put in to alphabetical order. This makes it easy to compare different brands, and will help you to find lower calorie and/or fat alternatives where they are available.

This format also makes it easier to locate foods. Foods are categorised by their main characteristics so, for example, if it is bread, ciabatta or white sliced, you'll find it under "Bread".

Basic ingredients are highlighted to make them easier to find at a glance. You'll find all unbranded foods in bold - making the index easier to use, whether it's just an apple or all the components of a home cooked stew.

There are, however, some foods which are not so easy to categorise, especially combination foods like ready meals. The following pointers will help you to find your way around the book until you get to know it a little better.

FILLED ROLLS AND SANDWICHES - Bagels, baguettes, etc which are filled are listed as "Bagels (filled)" etc. Sandwiches are under "Sandwiches".

CURRIES - Popular types of curry, like Balti or Jalfrezi, are listed under their individual types. Unspecified or lesser known types are listed under their main ingredient.

BURGERS - All burgers, including chicken-type sandwiches from fast-food outlets, are listed under "Burgers". CHIPS & FRIES - Are listed separately, depending on the name of the particular brand. All other types of potato are listed under "Potatoes".

SWEETS & CHOCOLATES - Well-known brands, eg. Aero, Mars Bar, are listed under their brand names. Others are listed under "Chocolate" (for bars) and "Chocolates" (for individual sweets).

READY MEALS - Popular types of dishes are listed under their type, eg. "Chow Mein", "Casserole", "Hot Pot", etc. Others are listed by their main ingredient, eg. "Chicken With", "Chicken In", etc.

EATING OUT & FAST FOODS - By popular demand this edition has the major eating out and fast food brands listed separately, at the back of the book. They are alphabetised first by brand, then follow using the same format as the rest of the book.

Serving Sizes

Many ready-meal type foods are given with calories for the full pack size, so that an individual serving can be worked out by estimating the proportion of the pack that has been consumed. For example, if you have eaten a quarter of a packaged pasta dish, divide the calorie value given for the whole pack by 4 to determine the number of calories you have consumed. Where serving sizes are not appropriate, or unknown, values are given per 1oz/28g. Serving sizes vary greatly from person to person and, if you are trying to lose weight, it's very important to be accurate – especially with foods that are very high in calories such as those that contain a fair amount of fat, sugar, cream, cheese, alcohol etc.

Food Data

Nutrition information for basic average foods has been compiled by the Weight Loss Resources food data team using many sources of information to calculate the most accurate values possible. Some nutrition information for non-branded food records is from The Composition of Foods 6th Edition (2002). Reproduced under licence from The Controller of Her Majesty's Stationary Office. Where basic data is present for ordinary foodstuffs such as 'raw carrots'; branded records are not included.

Nutrition information for branded goods is from details supplied by retailers and manufacturers, and researched by Weight Loss Resources staff. The Calorie Carb & Fat Bible contains data for over 1400 UK brands, including major supermarkets and fast food outlets.

The publishers gratefully acknowledge all the manufacturers and retailers who have provided information on their products. All product names, trademarks or registered trademarks belong to their respective owners and are used only for the purpose of identifying products.

Calorie & nutrition data for all food and drink items are typical values.

Caution
The information in The Calorie, Carb and Fat Bible is intended as an aid to weight loss and weight maintenance, and is not medical advice. If you suffer from, or think you may suffer from a medical condition you should consult your doctor before starting a weight loss and/or exercise regime. If you start exercising after a period of relative inactivity, you should start slowly and consult your doctor if you experience pain, distress or other symptoms.

Weights, Measures & Abbreviations

ABBREVIATIONS

kcal	*kilocalories / calories*
prot	*protein*
carb	*carbohydrate*
sm	*small*
med	*medium*
av	*average*
reg	*regular*
lge	*large*
tsp	*teaspoon*
tbsp	*tablespoon*
dtsp	*dessertspoon*
gf	*gluten free*

BRAND ABBREVIATIONS USED

ASDA

Good for You	*GFY*
Chosen by You	*CBY*

MARKS & SPENCER *M & S*

Count on Us	*COU*

MORRISONS

Better For You	*BFY*

SAINSBURY'S

Be Good to Yourself	*BGTY*
Way to Five	*WTF*
Taste the Difference	*TTD*

TESCO

Light Choices	*LC*

WAITROSE

Perfectly Balanced	*PB*

	Measure INFO/WEIGHT	per Measure KCAL	FAT	Nutrition Values per 100g / 100ml KCAL	PROT	CARB	FAT	FIBRE
ABALONE								
Cooked, Fried, Weighed without Shells	1 Serving/85g	161	5.8	189	19.6	11.0	6.8	0.0
Raw, Weighed without Shells	1 Serving/85g	89	0.6	105	17.1	6.0	0.8	0.0
ABSINTHE								
Average	*1 Pub Shot/35ml*	*127*	*0.0*	*363*	*0.0*	*38.8*	*0.0*	*0.0*
ACKEE								
Canned, Drained, Average	*1oz/28g*	*43*	*4.3*	*151*	*2.9*	*0.8*	*15.2*	*0.0*
ADVOCAAT								
Average	*1 Pub Shot/35ml*	*91*	*2.2*	*260*	*4.7*	*28.4*	*6.3*	*0.0*
AERO								
Creamy White Centre, Nestle*	1 Bar/46g	244	13.8	530	7.6	57.4	30.0	0.0
Honeycomb, Nestle*	1 Serving/40g	199	10.0	497	5.9	62.2	25.0	0.0
Milk, Eat Later, Bar, Nestle*	1 Bar/29g	156	8.9	539	6.6	57.7	30.9	2.2
Milk, Giant, Bar, Nestle*	1 Bar/125g	674	38.6	539	6.6	57.7	30.9	2.2
Milk, Medium, Bar, Nestle*	1 Bar/43g	232	13.3	539	6.6	57.7	30.9	2.2
Milk, Snacksize, Bar, Nestle*	1 Bar/21g	110	6.5	537	6.6	55.9	31.9	2.2
Milk, Standard, Bar, Nestle*	1 Bar/31g	165	9.6	531	6.3	56.9	30.9	0.8
Minis, Nestle*	1 Bar/11g	57	3.2	518	6.8	58.1	28.7	0.8
Mint, Bubbles, Aero, Nestle*	1 Bubble/3g	16	0.9	538	5.4	60.5	30.1	1.4
Mint, Nestle*	1 Bar/46g	245	13.7	533	4.9	61.2	29.8	0.4
Mint, Snack Size, Nestle*	1 Bar/21g	112	6.7	548	7.7	55.3	32.8	0.9
Mint, Standard, Aero, Nestle*	1 Bar/43g	233	13.2	542	5.2	60.5	30.8	0.9
Orange, Bubbles, Aero, Nestle*	1 Bubble/3g	16	0.9	538	5.4	60.5	30.0	1.4
Orange, Nestle*	6 Squares/22g	119	6.8	542	5.1	60.7	30.7	0.9
Orange Chocolate, Limited Edition, Aero, Nestle*	1 Bar/41g	221	12.3	539	5.1	61.4	29.9	0.9
ALFALFA SPROUTS								
Raw, Average	1 Serving/33g	8	0.3	24	3.0	3.0	0.9	3.0
ALLSPICE								
Ground, Schwartz*	1 Tsp/3g	11	0.1	358	6.1	74.3	4.0	0.0
ALMONDS								
Blanched, Average	*1 Serving/100g*	*617*	*54.3*	*617*	*25.1*	*6.9*	*54.3*	*8.1*
Candied, Sugared	1 Serving/100g	458	16.3	458	8.4	69.2	16.3	2.2
Flaked, Average	*1oz/28g*	*172*	*15.2*	*613*	*24.9*	*6.5*	*54.3*	*7.6*
Flaked, Toasted, Average	*1oz/28g*	*176*	*15.8*	*629*	*24.6*	*5.8*	*56.4*	*7.5*
Ground, Average	*1 Serving/10g*	*62*	*5.6*	*625*	*24.0*	*6.6*	*55.8*	*7.4*
Marcona, Average	*1 Serving/100g*	*608*	*53.7*	*608*	*22.1*	*13.0*	*53.7*	*9.7*
Toasted, Average	*1oz/28g*	*178*	*15.8*	*634*	*25.0*	*6.6*	*56.4*	*6.6*
Whole, Average	*1 Serving/20g*	*122*	*11.0*	*612*	*23.4*	*21.2*	*54.8*	*8.4*
Yoghurt Coated, Holland & Barrett*	1 Pack/100g	536	37.0	536	10.9	45.3	37.0	2.8
ALOO TIKKI								
Average	1 Serving/25g	48	2.0	191	4.5	25.2	8.0	3.5
AMARANTH								
Grain, Cooked	1 Serving/100g	102	2.0	102	4.0	19.0	2.0	2.0
ANCHOVIES								
Drained, Finest, Tesco*	1 Fillets/3g	7	0.4	220	21.3	0.8	14.6	0.5
Fillets, Flat, John West*	1 Can/50g	113	7.0	226	25.0	0.1	14.0	0.0
Fillets, Tesco*	1 Serving/15g	34	2.1	226	25.0	0.0	14.0	0.0
in Oil, Canned, Drained	1 Anchovy/4g	8	0.5	195	23.4	0.0	11.3	0.0
Marinated, Sainsbury's*	¼ Pot/44g	78	4.0	177	22.0	2.0	9.0	0.1
Salted, Finest, Tesco*	1 Serving/10g	9	0.2	93	18.2	0.0	2.2	0.0
ANGEL DELIGHT								
Banana Flavour, Kraft*	1 Sachet/59g	280	12.3	474	2.3	69.3	20.9	0.3
Butterscotch Flavour, No Added Sugar, Kraft*	1 Sachet/47g	226	11.3	480	4.5	61.0	24.0	0.0
Chocolate Flavour, Kraft*	1 Sachet/67g	305	12.1	455	3.7	69.5	18.0	0.4

	Measure INFO/WEIGHT	per Measure KCAL	FAT	Nutrition Values per 100g / 100ml KCAL	PROT	CARB	FAT	FIBRE
ANGEL DELIGHT								
Raspberry Flavour, No Added Sugar, Kraft*	1 Sachet/59g	292	15.3	495	4.8	59.5	26.0	0.0
Strawberry Flavour, Kraft*	1 Sachet/59g	286	12.4	485	2.5	71.0	21.0	0.0
Strawberry Flavour, No Added Sugar, Kraft*	1 Sachet/47g	230	12.5	490	4.8	59.0	26.5	0.0
Vanilla Ice Cream Flavour, Kraft*	1 Sachet/59g	289	12.7	490	2.5	71.5	21.5	0.0
Vanilla Ice Cream Flavour, No Added Sugar, Kraft*	1 Sachet/59g	295	15.9	500	4.8	59.5	27.0	0.0
ANGEL HAIR								
Pasta, Dry	1 Serving/50g	181	1.1	362	12.4	73.6	2.2	4.4
ANTIPASTO								
Artichoke, Sainsbury's*	1 Serving/50g	68	6.2	135	2.0	3.6	12.5	2.3
Coppa, from Selection Platter, TTD, Sainsbury's*	1 Serving/100g	255	17.1	255	25.2	0.1	17.1	0.0
Felino, from Selection Platter, TTD, Sainsbury's*	1 Serving/100g	349	24.9	349	31.1	0.1	24.9	0.0
Mixed, Misto Cotto, Arrosto Erbe, Waitrose*	1 Slice/9g	11	0.4	129	22.2	0.0	4.4	0.0
Mixed Mushroom, Sainsbury's*	¼ Jar/72g	70	6.5	97	2.7	1.4	9.0	3.7
Mixed Pepper, Sainsbury's*	½ Jar/140g	48	1.8	34	1.3	4.2	1.3	3.5
Parma, Salami Milano, Bresaola, Finest, Tesco*	¼ Pack/30g	104	7.9	345	26.4	0.5	26.3	0.0
Parma Ham, from Selection Platter, TTD, Sainsbury's*	1 Serving/100g	236	12.9	236	29.9	0.1	12.9	0.0
Roasted Pepper, Drained, Tesco*	1 Jar/170g	128	9.4	75	0.9	5.5	5.5	4.1
Seafood, Drained, Sainsbury's*	½ Jar/84g	150	9.7	178	14.3	4.1	11.6	1.4
Sun Dried Tomato, Sainsbury's*	¼ Jar/70g	275	25.0	393	4.5	13.4	35.7	6.2
APPLES								
& Grapes, Ready to Eat, Garden Gang, Asda*	1 Bag/80g	46	0.1	58	0.4	12.4	0.1	2.4
Bites, Average	1 Pack/118g	58	0.1	49	0.3	11.6	0.1	2.2
Braeburn, Average	*1 Apple/123g*	*58*	*0.1*	*47*	*0.4*	*11.4*	*0.1*	*2.0*
Cape, Tesco*	1 Apple/100g	50	0.1	50	0.4	11.8	0.1	1.8
Cooking, Baked with Sugar, Flesh Only, Average	*1 Serving/140g*	*104*	*0.1*	*74*	*0.5*	*19.2*	*0.1*	*1.7*
Cooking, Raw, Peeled, Average	*1oz/28g*	*10*	*0.0*	*35*	*0.3*	*8.9*	*0.1*	*1.6*
Cooking, Stewed with Sugar, Average	*1 Serving/140g*	*104*	*0.1*	*74*	*0.3*	*19.1*	*0.1*	*1.2*
Cooking, Stewed without Sugar, Average	*1 Serving/140g*	*46*	*0.1*	*33*	*0.3*	*8.1*	*0.1*	*1.5*
Cox, English, Average	*1 Apple/108g*	*52*	*0.1*	*48*	*0.4*	*11.3*	*0.1*	*2.0*
Crunchy, Snack, Shapers, Boots*	1 Pack/80g	57	0.1	57	0.3	12.0	0.1	2.7
Discovery, Average	*1 Apple/182g*	*82*	*0.9*	*45*	*0.4*	*10.6*	*0.5*	*1.0*
Dried, Average	*1 Pack/250g*	*537*	*0.7*	*215*	*0.8*	*52.8*	*0.3*	*5.9*
Dried, Slices, Love Life, Waitrose*	1 Serving/30g	70	0.1	235	0.9	57.2	0.3	8.7
Dried, Sweetened, Chunks, Snack Pack, Whitworths*	1 Pack/25g	84	0.3	335	0.4	80.3	1.1	1.1
Empire, Average	*1 Apple/120g*	*58*	*0.1*	*48*	*0.4*	*11.8*	*0.1*	*2.0*
Fuji	1 Apple/132g	64	0.1	48	0.4	11.8	0.1	1.8
Gala, Average	*1 Apple/152g*	*73*	*0.2*	*48*	*0.4*	*11.6*	*0.1*	*1.6*
Golden Delicious, Average	*1 Med/102g*	*48*	*0.2*	*48*	*0.4*	*11.2*	*0.2*	*1.8*
Granny Smith, Average	*1 Sm/125g*	*62*	*0.1*	*50*	*0.4*	*11.9*	*0.1*	*2.0*
Grapes & Cheese, Asda*	1 Pack/150g	195	10.6	130	5.3	10.3	7.1	1.7
Green, Raw, Average	*1 Med/182g*	*86*	*0.2*	*48*	*0.4*	*11.3*	*0.1*	*1.8*
Kanzi, Tesco*	1 Apple/134g	71	0.1	53	0.4	11.8	0.1	1.8
Mackintosh, Red, Average	*1 Apple/165g*	*81*	*0.5*	*49*	*0.2*	*12.8*	*0.3*	*1.8*
Pink Lady, Average	*1 Apple/125g*	*62*	*0.1*	*50*	*0.4*	*11.7*	*0.1*	*2.1*
Red, Windsor, Asda*	1 Apple/100g	53	0.1	53	0.4	11.8	0.1	1.8
Sliced, Average	*1oz/28g*	*14*	*0.0*	*49*	*0.4*	*11.6*	*0.1*	*1.8*
Snack Pack, Goodness for Kids, Tesco*	1 Pack/80g	44	0.1	55	0.3	12.3	0.1	1.8
APPLETISER*								
Juice Drink, Sparkling, Appletiser, Coca-Cola*	1 Glass/200ml	94	0.0	47	0.0	11.0	0.0	0.4
APRICOTS								
Bite Size, Dried, Stoned, Ready to Eat, Whitworths*	1 Pack/36g	76	0.1	210	1.6	46.7	0.3	6.6
Canned, in Syrup, Average	*1oz/28g*	*18*	*0.0*	*63*	*0.4*	*16.1*	*0.1*	*0.9*
Dried, Average	*1 Apricot/10g*	*17*	*0.1*	*171*	*3.6*	*37.4*	*0.5*	*6.3*

	Measure INFO/WEIGHT	per Measure		Nutrition Values per 100g / 100ml				
		KCAL	FAT	KCAL	PROT	CARB	FAT	FIBRE
APRICOTS								
Dried, Soft, Average	*1 Serving/50g*	*104*	*0.2*	*208*	*2.4*	*48.5*	*0.4*	*5.2*
Halves, in Fruit Juice, Average	*1 Can/221g*	*87*	*0.1*	*40*	*0.5*	*9.2*	*0.1*	*1.0*
Raw, Flesh Only, Average	*1 Apricot/37g*	*19*	*0.2*	*52*	*1.5*	*12.0*	*0.4*	*2.2*
Raw, Weighed with Stone, Average	*1 Apricot/40g*	*19*	*0.2*	*48*	*1.4*	*11.1*	*0.4*	*2.0*
Ready to Eat, Dried, Organic, Love Life, Waitrose*	1 Serving/40g	97	0.2	243	3.4	55.3	0.5	7.3
Ready to Eat, Everyday Value, Tesco*	1 Serving/30g	55	0.2	180	4.0	36.5	0.6	6.3
Soft, Dried, Love Life, Waitrose*	1 Serving/30g	53	0.2	178	1.8	36.0	0.6	6.3
Yoghurt Coated, Graze*	1 Pack/40g	176	9.0	441	3.4	58.6	22.4	0.0
ARCHERS*								
& Lemonade, Premixed, Canned, Archers*	100ml	86	0.0	86	0.0	13.2	0.0	0.0
Aqua, Peach, Archers*	1 Bottle/275ml	206	0.0	75	0.3	5.1	0.0	0.0
Peach (Calculated Estimate), Archers*	1 Shot/35ml	91	0.0	260	0.0	0.0	0.0	0.0
Vea, Wildberry, Schnapps, Archers*	1 Bottle/275ml	124	0.0	45	0.0	5.8	0.0	0.0
ARTICHOKE								
Chargrilled, in Olive Oil, Cooks Ingredients, Waitrose*	1 Serving/40g	52	4.9	129	1.7	2.7	12.3	2.7
Chargrilled, Italian, Drained, Sainsbury's*	1/3 Tub/43g	40	2.7	92	3.1	2.8	6.1	6.5
Fresh, Raw, Average	*1oz/28g*	*13*	*0.0*	*47*	*3.3*	*10.5*	*0.2*	*5.4*
Hearts, Canned, Drained, Average	*½ Can/117g*	*35*	*0.1*	*30*	*1.9*	*5.4*	*0.0*	*2.2*
Hearts, Marinated & Grilled, Tesco*	½ Pack/100g	340	36.0	340	1.6	1.6	36.0	3.6
Hearts, Marinated & Grilled, Waitrose*	1 Serving/50g	57	5.0	114	3.0	3.0	10.0	3.0
Hearts, Sliced with Extra Virgin Olive Oil, Waitrose*	1 Serving/40g	24	1.6	59	1.3	4.4	4.0	7.0
in Oil, Tesco*	1 Piece/15g	18	1.6	120	2.0	2.2	11.0	7.5
Marinated, Roasted, M&S*	1 Pack/200g	300	26.6	150	1.9	5.0	13.3	2.3
ASPARAGUS								
& Green Vegetables (Steamer Pouch), Waitrose*	½ Pack/125g	28	0.6	22	2.1	2.3	0.5	2.1
Boiled, in Salted Water, Average	*5 Spears/125g*	*32*	*1.0*	*26*	*3.4*	*1.4*	*0.8*	*1.4*
British with Butter, Tesco*	1 Serving/50g	26	2.0	52	2.6	1.6	4.0	2.0
Canned, Average	*1 Can/250g*	*48*	*0.5*	*19*	*2.3*	*2.0*	*0.2*	*1.6*
Tips, Sainsbury's*	1 Pack/125g	36	0.8	29	2.9	2.0	0.6	2.1
Trimmed, Raw, Average	*1 Serving/80g*	*20*	*0.4*	*24*	*2.9*	*1.9*	*0.6*	*1.7*
ASPIRE								
Cranberry Flavoured Soft Drink, Aspire*	1 Can/250ml	12	0.0	5	0.0	1.1	0.0	0.0
AUBERGINE								
Baby, Tesco*	1 Aubergine/50g	8	0.2	15	0.9	2.2	0.4	2.3
Baked Topped, M&S*	1 Serving/150g	165	11.6	110	2.4	7.4	7.7	0.9
Fried, Average	*1oz/28g*	*85*	*8.9*	*302*	*1.2*	*2.8*	*31.9*	*2.3*
in Hot Sauce, Yarden*	1 Serving/35g	96	9.0	273	1.5	8.8	25.8	0.0
Marinated & Grilled, Waitrose*	½ Pack/100g	106	10.0	106	1.0	3.0	10.0	2.0
Parmigiana, M&S*	1 Pack/350g	332	18.6	95	4.6	7.6	5.3	1.1
Raw, Fresh, Average	*1 Sm/250g*	*38*	*1.0*	*15*	*0.9*	*2.2*	*0.4*	*2.0*

INFO/WEIGHT	Measure	per Measure		Nutrition Values per 100g / 100ml				
		KCAL	FAT	KCAL	PROT	CARB	FAT	FIBRE
BACARDI*								
& Diet Cola, Bacardi*	1 Bottle/275ml	85	0.0	31	0.0	1.0	0.0	0.0
37.5% Volume, Bacardi*	**1 Pub Shot/35ml**	**72**	**0.0**	**207**	**0.0**	**0.0**	**0.0**	**0.0**
40% Volume, Bacardi*	**1 Pub Shot/35ml**	**78**	**0.0**	**222**	**0.0**	**0.0**	**0.0**	**0.0**
Breezer, Cranberry, Bacardi*	1 Bottle/275ml	154	0.0	56	0.0	7.1	0.0	0.0
Breezer, Orange, Bacardi*	1 Bottle/275ml	179	0.0	65	0.0	8.2	0.0	0.0
Breezer, Watermelon, Bacardi*	1 Bottle/275ml	100	0.0	36	0.0	3.2	0.0	0.0
BACON								
Back, Dry Cured, Average	**1 Rasher/31g**	**77**	**4.7**	**250**	**28.1**	**0.3**	**15.1**	**0.3**
Back, Dry Fried or Grilled, Average	**1 Rasher/25g**	**72**	**5.4**	**287**	**23.2**	**0.0**	**21.6**	**0.0**
Back, Lean, Average	**1 Rasher/33g**	**57**	**4.0**	**174**	**16.3**	**0.1**	**12.0**	**0.5**
Back, Smoked, Average	**1 Rasher/25g**	**66**	**5.0**	**265**	**20.9**	**0.0**	**19.9**	**0.0**
Back, Smoked, Lean, Average	**1 Rasher/25g**	**41**	**1.2**	**163**	**28.2**	**1.1**	**5.0**	**0.2**
Back, Smoked, Rindless, Average	**1 Rasher/25g**	**60**	**4.3**	**241**	**21.0**	**0.1**	**17.4**	**0.0**
Back, Tendersweet, Average	**1 Rasher/25g**	**63**	**3.6**	**250**	**29.8**	**0.4**	**14.4**	**0.0**
Back, Unsmoked, Average	**1 Rasher/32g**	**78**	**5.5**	**243**	**21.3**	**0.4**	**17.3**	**0.0**
Back, Unsmoked, Rindless, Average	**1 Rasher/23g**	**56**	**3.9**	**241**	**22.5**	**0.0**	**16.9**	**0.0**
Back, Wiltshire, Unsmoked, TTD, Sainsbury's*	1 Rasher/18g	54	3.2	296	34.0	1.0	17.4	0.6
Chops, Average	**1oz/28g**	**62**	**4.2**	**222**	**22.3**	**0.0**	**14.8**	**0.0**
Chops, Coated in American Style BBQ Glaze, Tesco*	1 Serving/200g	480	36.2	240	16.1	2.1	18.1	0.0
Chops, in Cheese Sauce, Tesco*	1 Serving/185g	405	26.5	219	12.6	10.0	14.3	1.1
Collar Joint, Lean & Fat, Boiled	**1oz/28g**	**91**	**7.6**	**325**	**20.4**	**0.0**	**27.0**	**0.0**
Collar Joint, Lean & Fat, Raw	**1oz/28g**	**89**	**8.1**	**319**	**14.6**	**0.0**	**28.9**	**0.0**
Collar Joint, Lean Only, Boiled	**1oz/28g**	**53**	**2.7**	**191**	**26.0**	**0.0**	**9.7**	**0.0**
Cooking, Diced Pieces, Cooked, Basics, Sainsbury's*	1 Pack/200g	332	14.4	166	24.2	0.8	7.2	0.0
Cooking, Pieces, Smart Price, Asda*	1 Serving/100g	215	22.0	215	23.0	0.0	22.0	0.0
Fat Only, Cooked, Average	**1oz/28g**	**194**	**20.4**	**692**	**9.3**	**0.0**	**72.8**	**0.0**
Fat Only, Raw, Average	**1oz/28g**	**209**	**22.7**	**747**	**4.8**	**0.0**	**80.9**	**0.0**
Gammon Rasher, Lean Only, Grilled	**1oz/28g**	**48**	**1.5**	**172**	**31.4**	**0.0**	**5.2**	**0.0**
Lardons, Smoked, Sainsbury's*	1 Serving/200g	476	30.8	238	21.4	0.1	15.4	0.1
Lean, Average	**1 Rasher/33g**	**47**	**2.2**	**142**	**19.6**	**0.9**	**6.7**	**0.2**
Lean Only, Fried, Average	**1 Rasher/25g**	**83**	**5.6**	**332**	**32.8**	**0.0**	**22.3**	**0.0**
Lean Only, Grilled, Average	**1 Rasher/25g**	**73**	**4.7**	**292**	**30.5**	**0.0**	**18.9**	**0.0**
Loin Steaks, Grilled, Average	**1 Serving/120g**	**229**	**11.6**	**191**	**25.9**	**0.0**	**9.7**	**0.0**
Medallions, Average	**1 Rasher/18g**	**27**	**0.6**	**151**	**29.4**	**0.9**	**3.3**	**0.1**
Medallions, Unsmoked, Essential, Waitrose*	1 Slice/25g	35	1.6	139	19.4	0.5	6.5	0.5
Middle, Fried	**1 Rasher/40g**	**140**	**11.4**	**350**	**23.4**	**0.0**	**28.5**	**0.0**
Middle, Grilled	**1 Rasher/40g**	**123**	**9.2**	**307**	**24.8**	**0.0**	**23.1**	**0.0**
Middle, Raw	**1 Rasher/43g**	**104**	**8.6**	**241**	**15.2**	**0.0**	**20.0**	**0.0**
Rashers, Lean Only, Trimmed, Average	1 Rasher/20g	24	0.8	119	20.6	0.0	4.0	0.0
Rindless, Average	**1 Rasher/20g**	**30**	**1.7**	**150**	**18.5**	**0.0**	**8.5**	**0.0**
Smoked, Average	**1 Rasher/28g**	**46**	**2.1**	**166**	**24.8**	**0.2**	**7.4**	**0.0**
Smoked, Crispy, Cooked, Average	**1 Serving/10g**	**46**	**2.7**	**460**	**53.0**	**2.1**	**26.9**	**0.0**
Smoked, Crispy, Pre Cooked, Rashers, Sainsbury's*	½ Pack/27g	148	10.1	547	52.8	0.1	37.3	0.1
Smoked, Rindless, Average	**1 Rasher/20g**	**21**	**0.6**	**106**	**19.8**	**0.0**	**3.0**	**0.0**
Steaks with 3 Cheese Sauce & Mustard Crust, Asda*	½ Pack/175g	390	25.6	223	20.6	2.3	14.6	2.9
Streaky, Average	**1oz/28g**	**76**	**5.9**	**270**	**20.0**	**0.0**	**21.0**	**0.0**
Streaky, Cooked, Average	**1 Rasher/20g**	**68**	**5.6**	**342**	**22.4**	**0.3**	**27.8**	**0.0**
Streaky, Dry Cure, Cooked, TTD, Sainsbury's*	1 Rasher/9g	34	2.5	367	28.4	1.0	27.6	0.6
Streaky, Sweet & Smoky, Grilled, Finest, Tesco*	2 Rashers/28g	105	7.8	375	30.0	1.4	27.9	0.0
Streaky, Unsmoked, Dry Cured, TTD, Sainsbury's*	1 Rasher/20g	61	4.0	305	30.6	0.3	20.1	0.8
Sweetcure, Dry Cured, TTD, Sainsbury's*	1 Rasher/24g	63	3.3	265	33.2	1.5	14.0	0.9
Vegetarian, Rashers	**1 Rasher/16g**	**33**	**1.7**	**206**	**19.5**	**8.6**	**10.4**	**2.8**

	Measure INFO/WEIGHT	per Measure KCAL	FAT	Nutrition Values per 100g / 100ml KCAL	PROT	CARB	FAT	FIBRE
BACON BITS								
Average	**1oz/28g**	**75**	**5.9**	**268**	**18.6**	**0.7**	**21.2**	**0.1**
BACON VEGETARIAN								
Rashers, Cheatin', The Redwood Co*	1 Rasher/16g	32	1.2	196	25.9	7.3	7.3	0.5
Rashers, Tesco*	1 Rasher/20g	41	2.2	203	22.5	3.3	11.1	3.9
Realeat*	1 Rasher/19g	49	1.1	260	27.0	25.0	5.8	1.6
Streaky Style Rashers, Tesco*	1 Rasher/8g	17	0.8	215	23.7	5.0	10.6	2.2
Strips, Morningstar Farms*	1 Strip/8g	30	2.3	375	12.5	12.5	28.1	6.2
BAGEL								
Bacon, & Soft Cheese, Boots*	1 Serving/148g	481	25.2	325	12.0	31.0	17.0	2.2
Cream Cheese, M&S*	1 Bagel/23g	79	4.9	352	7.8	31.0	21.8	1.8
Smoked Salmon, & Cream Cheese, Handmade, Tesco*	1 Bagel/162g	380	12.6	235	13.1	27.7	7.8	1.5
Smoked Salmon, & Cream Cheese, M&S*	1 Bagel/185g	480	18.8	260	12.3	29.5	10.2	1.9
BAGUETTE								
All Day Breakfast, Darwins Deli*	1 Serving/184g	498	21.5	271	13.4	31.9	11.7	0.0
Beef & Horseradish, Freshly Prepared, M&S*	1 Baguette/274g	795	31.0	290	12.1	37.2	11.3	2.0
Brie, Tomato & Rocket, Freshly Prepared, M&S*	1 Baguette/219g	570	21.7	260	10.3	33.2	9.9	1.9
Cheese, & Pickle, Fullfillers*	1 Baguette/280g	767	31.1	274	11.9	35.5	11.1	0.0
Cheese, & Tomato, Tesco*	1 Baguette/108g	243	8.3	225	9.7	29.3	7.7	1.8
Cheese, Mixed, & Spring Onion, Asda*	1 Pack/190g	629	34.8	331	9.5	32.1	18.3	1.3
Cheese & Ham, Average	1 Baguette/203g	593	20.8	292	14.0	35.9	10.3	1.4
Chicken, & Mayonnaise, Asda*	1 Pack/190g	407	16.5	214	9.7	30.5	8.7	1.3
Chicken, & Salad, Asda*	1 Serving/158g	326	9.5	206	9.0	29.0	6.0	2.1
Chicken, & Salad, Boots*	1 Baguette/132g	202	2.4	153	11.0	23.0	1.8	2.0
Chicken, & Stuffing, Hot, Sainsbury's*	1 Baguette/227g	543	16.3	239	13.7	29.6	7.2	0.0
Chicken, Honey & Mustard, BGTY, Sainsbury's*	1 Pack/187g	340	3.7	182	11.0	30.0	2.0	0.0
Chicken, Oakham, Fresh, M&S*	1 Baguette/225g	450	10.8	200	12.4	26.7	4.8	1.5
Chicken, Tikka, Asda*	1 Pack/190g	439	17.9	231	10.4	32.8	9.4	1.3
Egg, Bacon & Tomato, Freshly Prepared, M&S*	1 Baguette/182g	455	17.3	250	12.9	28.0	9.5	1.7
Egg Mayonnaise, & Cress, Cafe, Sainsbury's*	1 Pack/100g	480	20.4	480	13.8	60.2	20.4	0.0
Ham, & Turkey, Asda*	1 Baguette/360g	774	18.4	215	11.6	30.7	5.1	1.3
Ham & Cheese, Freshly Prepared, M&S*	1 Baguette/231g	555	11.3	240	13.4	35.9	4.9	2.4
Ham & Salad with Mustard Mayonnaise, Sainsbury's*	1 Baguette/100g	412	15.9	412	17.6	49.6	15.9	0.1
Mozzarella, Tomato, & Pesto, Darwins Deli*	1 Serving/210g	531	20.4	253	11.7	29.7	9.7	0.0
Prawn, French, Shell*	1 Baguette/63g	171	7.2	272	9.7	32.4	11.5	0.0
Prawn Mayonnaise, Asda*	1 Pack/190g	399	9.3	210	9.1	32.5	4.9	1.3
Smoked Salmon & Egg, Freshly Prepared	1 Baguette/178g	455	17.3	255	13.7	28.4	9.7	1.6
Steak, & Onion, Snack 'n' Go, Sainsbury's*	1 Baguette/177g	398	8.8	225	14.3	30.6	5.0	2.2
Tuna, Crunch, Shapers, Boots*	1 Pack/138g	315	4.8	228	14.0	35.0	3.5	3.1
Tuna, Melt, Sainsbury's*	1 Serving/204g	373	8.0	183	11.3	25.8	3.9	0.0
BAILEYS*								
Glide, Baileys*	1 Serving/200ml	212	2.4	106	0.0	18.0	1.2	0.0
Irish Cream, Original, Baileys*	**1 Serving/50ml**	**164**	**6.5**	**327**	**3.0**	**25.0**	**13.0**	**0.0**
BAKE								
Aubergine & Mozzarella, Finest, Tesco*	1 Pack/400g	288	13.6	72	3.6	6.7	3.4	2.6
Aubergine & Mozzarella Cheese, BGTY, Sainsbury's*	1 Pack/360g	194	7.2	54	3.0	6.0	2.0	1.3
Bean & Pasta, Asda*	1 Pack/450g	598	22.5	133	5.0	17.0	5.0	1.7
Broccoli & Cheese, M&S*	1 Pack/400g	380	22.8	95	4.8	5.6	5.7	1.1
Cauliflower & Broccoli Bake, Tesco*	½ Pack/250g	178	10.2	71	2.8	5.8	4.1	1.0
Chicken Arrabiatta, M&S*	1 Pack/450g	540	13.5	120	7.6	16.0	3.0	2.0
Chicken Pasta, Chilled, LC, Tesco*	1 Pack/400g	425	7.2	106	8.2	13.5	1.8	1.4
Cod & Prawn, COU, M&S*	1 Pack/400g	320	8.0	80	6.5	8.8	2.0	1.0
Fish, Haddock, Average	1 Serving/400g	312	9.2	78	6.4	8.0	2.3	0.9
Fish, Haddock, Smoked, Light & Easy, Youngs*	1 Pack/310g	242	7.1	78	6.4	8.0	2.3	0.9

	Measure INFO/WEIGHT	per Measure		Nutrition Values per 100g / 100ml				
		KCAL	FAT	KCAL	PROT	CARB	FAT	FIBRE
BAKE								
Haddock, Smoked, Light & Easy, Youngs*	1 Pack/300g	234	6.9	78	6.4	8.0	2.3	0.9
Lentil, Spiced, Vegetarian, TTD, Sainsbury's*	1 Bake/132g	245	8.4	186	4.8	27.3	6.4	4.2
Mediterranean Vegetable, CBY, Asda*	1 Bake/120g	279	13.2	232	8.4	22.8	11.0	4.2
Mushroom, Cauldron Foods*	1 Serving/100g	164	12.0	164	6.0	15.0	12.0	6.0
Mushroom, Leek & Spinach, Cumberland, Sainsbury's*	1 Pack/450g	518	24.3	115	3.6	12.9	5.4	1.2
Penne Bolognese, Sainsbury's*	1 Pack/397g	603	27.8	152	7.6	14.8	7.0	2.0
Potato, Cheese, & Bacon, Homepride*	1 Serving/210g	277	26.2	132	1.6	3.2	12.5	0.0
Potato, Cheese, & Onion, Tesco*	1 Pack/400g	376	19.6	94	2.4	10.0	4.9	1.0
Potato, Leek & Gruyere, M&S*	½ Pack/200g	240	15.4	120	2.2	10.3	7.7	1.4
Potato & Vegetable, Co-Op*	1 Bake/340g	425	27.2	125	4.0	11.0	8.0	1.0
Potato with Cheese & Leek, Aunt Bessie's*	½ Pack/275g	300	13.8	109	3.4	12.7	5.0	2.7
Potatoes, Cherry Tomatoes & Mozzarella, M&S*	½ Pack/165g	140	5.6	85	2.2	11.5	3.4	2.6
Roast Onion & Potato, COU, M&S*	1 Pack/450g	338	5.8	75	1.9	13.6	1.3	1.5
Roast Potato, Cheese & Onion, Asda*	½ Pack/200g	288	16.0	144	4.2	14.0	8.0	1.1
Salmon & Prawn, M&S*	1 Bake/329g	460	31.2	140	7.4	6.6	9.5	0.7
Vegetable, M&S*	½ Lg Pack/255g	178	6.9	70	1.9	8.9	2.7	1.6
Vegetable & Lentil, Somerfield*	1 Pack/350g	318	6.3	91	4.9	13.8	1.8	2.5
BAKE MIX								
Potato, Ham & Leek, Colman's*	1 Pack/44g	181	10.6	412	9.9	40.4	24.0	2.1
Tuna & Pasta, Colman's*	1 Pack/45g	149	2.4	331	10.4	60.5	5.3	4.4
BAKING POWDER								
Average	*1 Tsp/2g*	*3*	*0.0*	*163*	*5.2*	*37.8*	*0.0*	*0.0*
BAKLAVA								
Average	2 Pieces/50g	239	14.2	478	8.0	47.4	28.4	2.8
BALTI								
Chick Pea & Spinach, Cauldron Foods*	1 Pack/400g	356	8.0	89	2.3	15.5	2.0	1.0
Chicken, & Naan Bread, Somerfield*	1 Pack/335g	489	16.8	146	10.0	16.0	5.0	0.0
Chicken, & Rice, M&S*	1 Pack/400g	380	6.0	95	6.9	14.1	1.5	1.2
Chicken, Asda*	1 Pack/450g	324	9.9	72	8.0	5.0	2.2	0.0
Chicken, Indian Takeaway, Iceland*	1 Pack/402g	362	19.3	90	7.8	4.0	4.8	0.7
Chicken, M&S*	½ Pack/175g	245	15.2	140	13.0	2.0	8.7	1.7
Chicken, Morrisons*	1 Pack/350g	441	26.6	126	12.1	2.3	7.6	1.5
Chicken, Sainsbury's*	½ Pack/200g	222	11.2	111	11.6	3.6	5.6	1.3
Chicken, Take Away, Tesco*	½ Pack/200g	170	7.6	85	8.1	4.6	3.8	1.9
Chicken, Takeaway, Sainsbury's*	1 Pack/400g	404	18.0	101	10.4	4.8	4.5	1.4
Chicken, Tesco*	1 Pack/460g	662	25.8	144	6.1	17.4	5.6	1.6
Chicken & Mushroom, Tesco*	1 Serving/350g	326	10.5	93	12.3	4.2	3.0	0.7
Chicken Ceylon, Finest, Tesco*	1 Pack/400g	588	38.0	147	14.4	0.9	9.5	5.0
Chicken Tikka, Finest, Tesco*	½ Pack/200g	280	17.2	140	15.8	1.1	8.6	3.2
Chicken with Garlic & Coriander Naan, Frozen, Patak's*	1 Pack/375g	431	18.8	115	6.3	11.1	5.0	1.1
Chicken with Naan Bread, PB, Waitrose*	1 Pack/375g	450	13.5	120	12.1	9.7	3.6	2.8
Chicken with Naan Bread, Sharwood's*	1 Pack/375g	529	23.2	141	7.3	14.1	6.2	2.2
Chicken with Pilau Rice, Asda*	1 Pack/504g	625	24.7	124	5.0	15.0	4.9	1.2
Chicken with Pilau Rice, Weight Watchers*	1 Pack/329g	306	4.3	93	6.9	13.4	1.3	1.2
Chicken with Pilau Rice & Naan Bread, Tesco*	1 Meal/550g	660	19.8	120	6.1	15.5	3.6	1.4
Chicken with Rice, Curry Break, Patak's*	1 Pack/220g	198	6.2	90	4.7	11.6	2.8	0.0
Chicken with Rice, Patak's*	1 Pack/370g	440	13.0	119	6.1	16.7	3.5	1.7
Lamb, Bhuna, Tesco*	1 Pack/400g	360	14.8	90	9.2	4.8	3.7	1.1
Prawn, Budgens*	1 Pack/350g	374	24.8	107	5.6	5.2	7.1	1.3
Vegetable, Asda*	½ Can/200g	206	12.0	103	2.2	10.0	6.0	2.5
Vegetable, Average	1 Serving/200g	182	8.3	91	1.9	11.3	4.1	1.7
Vegetable, Indian Meal for 2, Finest, Tesco*	½ Pack/150g	144	10.8	96	1.6	6.1	7.2	2.9
Vegetable & Rice, Tesco*	1 Pack/450g	378	7.2	84	2.0	15.6	1.6	1.3

	Measure INFO/WEIGHT	per Measure		Nutrition Values per 100g / 100ml				
		KCAL	FAT	KCAL	PROT	CARB	FAT	FIBRE
BAMBOO SHOOTS								
Canned, Average	*1 Can/120g*	*11*	*0.2*	*9*	*1.1*	*0.9*	*0.1*	*0.9*
Canned in Water, Drained, Kingfisher*	1 Can/120g	14	0.2	12	1.5	0.7	0.2	1.4
BANANA								
Raw, Flesh Only, Average	*1 Med/100g*	*95*	*0.3*	*95*	*1.2*	*20.9*	*0.3*	*4.2*
Raw, Weighed with Skin, Average	*1 Med/152g*	*144*	*0.5*	*95*	*1.2*	*20.9*	*0.3*	*4.2*
BANANA CHIPS								
Average	*1oz/28g*	*143*	*8.8*	*511*	*1.0*	*59.9*	*31.4*	*1.7*
BANGERS & MASH								
Asda*	1 Pack/400g	636	28.0	159	9.0	15.0	7.0	1.6
Morrisons*	1 Pack/300g	306	14.7	102	3.0	12.3	4.9	0.8
BARS								
All Bran, Apple, Kellogg's*	1 Bar/40g	158	7.6	395	8.0	48.0	19.0	5.0
All Bran, Honey & Oat, Kellogg's*	1 Bar/27g	99	2.2	366	6.0	67.0	8.0	12.0
All Fruit, Frusli, Strawberry, Jordans*	1 Bar/30g	94	0.1	313	2.3	81.3	0.3	5.0
Almond & Apricot, Weight Watchers*	1 Bar/34g	151	6.6	443	8.6	55.9	19.4	5.2
Almond & Cranberry, Day Break, Atkins*	1 Bar/37g	137	5.9	371	37.0	23.0	16.0	15.0
Am, Cereal, Berry, McVitie's*	1 Bar/30g	146	6.2	486	6.5	68.8	20.5	0.5
Am, Cereal, Fruit & Nut, McVitie's*	1 Bar/35g	167	7.5	477	6.6	64.9	21.4	3.4
Am, Cereal, Raisin & Nut, McVitie's*	1 Bar/35g	148	5.8	422	6.4	62.1	16.4	2.4
Am, Granola, Almond, Raisin & Cranberry, McVitie's*	1 Bar/35g	133	4.0	380	7.1	62.9	11.4	4.0
Am, Muesli Fingers, McVitie's*	1 Bar/35g	154	6.9	440	6.0	59.8	19.6	3.1
Apple, Fruit Bake, Go Ahead, McVitie's*	1 Bar/35g	124	2.5	354	2.7	73.8	7.2	1.2
Apple, Granola, McVitie's*	1 Bar/35g	128	3.4	366	6.6	63.1	9.7	4.3
Apple & Blackberry, Fruit Bakes, Go Ahead, McVitie's*	1 Bar/35g	131	3.0	374	3.5	71.8	8.5	3.9
Apple & Cinnamon, Breakfast Snack, Tesco*	1 Bar/38g	137	4.7	365	4.3	58.8	12.5	2.0
Apple & Raisin, Dorset Cereals*	1 Bar/30g	109	1.1	363	4.0	78.3	3.7	5.3
Apple Pie, Nak'd*	1 Bar/68g	221	5.9	325	6.8	57.2	8.7	7.4
Apricot & Almond, Eat Natural*	1 Bar/50g	202	8.1	403	11.2	53.3	16.1	0.0
Apricot & Almond, Truly Juicy, Raw Health*	1 Bar/45g	182	10.4	405	17.0	49.0	23.0	9.0
Apricot & Almond, Yoghurt Coated, Eat Natural*	1 Bar/50g	228	12.4	456	5.7	52.8	24.7	5.7
Apricot & Orange, Diet Chef Ltd*	1 Bar/25g	97	1.8	388	4.3	75.2	7.0	2.4
Apricot & Sultana Porridge Oat, Stoats*	1 Pack/85g	370	20.8	435	8.2	70.5	24.5	5.6
Banana, Mango & Brazil, Cereal, Dove's Farm*	1 Bar/40g	196	4.6	490	6.5	63.3	11.5	5.3
Banoffee, Weight Watchers*	1 Bar/18g	68	0.9	379	6.3	77.0	5.1	3.0
Berry, Nut Free, Get Buzzing*	1 Bar/62g	173	8.7	279	3.2	50.0	14.0	2.9
Berry Delight, GF, Nak'd*	1 Bar/35g	135	5.2	385	9.0	52.0	15.0	6.0
Biscuit, Chocolate, Penguin, McVitie's*	1 Bar/20g	106	5.6	515	5.1	61.4	27.1	2.4
Biscuit, Chocolate Mint, Penguin, McVitie's*	1 Bar/25g	133	6.9	531	5.4	65.0	27.7	1.5
Biscuit, Chocolate Orange, Penguin, McVitie's*	1 Bar/25g	133	6.9	531	5.4	65.0	27.7	1.5
Biscuit, Medley, Raisin & Chocolate Hob Nob, McVitie's*	1 Bar/31g	131	4.1	422	5.5	69.4	13.3	3.6
Biscuit & Raisin, Reduced Fat, Tesco*	1 Bar/22g	90	2.8	410	4.9	69.5	12.5	1.8
Black Forest, Weight Watchers*	1 Bar/23g	94	2.0	408	3.9	78.4	8.8	1.4
Blue Riband, 99 Calories, Nestle*	1 Bar/19g	99	4.9	513	4.8	66.4	25.3	0.0
Blue Riband, Nestle*	1 Bar/21g	104	5.2	495	4.5	64.5	24.5	1.0
Blueberry, Fruit & Grain, Asda*	1 Bar/37g	124	2.6	335	4.1	64.0	7.0	3.9
Blueberry, Nupo*	1 Bar/29g	99	2.9	343	10.8	41.5	10.0	25.4
Blueberry, Weight Watchers*	1 Bar/25g	91	1.8	365	4.5	74.9	7.4	2.2
Blueberry & Yoghurt Nougat, Shapers, Boots*	1 Bar/23g	89	3.7	385	1.7	58.0	16.0	0.7
Boohbah, Milk & White Chocolate, M&S*	1 Bar/75g	405	24.2	540	7.9	54.7	32.3	1.2
Breakfast, Blueberry, Free From, Sainsbury's*	1 Bar/35g	163	7.8	467	3.8	62.6	22.4	0.2
Breakfast, Cherry, Oats & More, Nestle*	1 Bar/30g	109	2.0	363	6.0	70.2	6.5	3.6
Breakfast, Chocolate Chip Crisp, Morning Start, Atkins*	1 Bar/37g	137	7.0	370	31.8	22.5	18.8	15.0
Breakfast, Muesli, Country Garden Cakes*	1 Bar/25g	94	2.3	376	5.6	67.6	9.2	3.6

	Measure INFO/WEIGHT	per Measure		Nutrition Values per 100g / 100ml				
		KCAL	FAT	KCAL	PROT	CARB	FAT	FIBRE
BARS								
Breakfast with Cranberries, Asda*	1 Bar/28g	105	1.4	376	6.0	77.0	4.9	3.0
Breakfast with Cranberries, Vitality, Asda*	1 Bar/20g	103	1.3	509	8.4	103.7	6.4	4.0
Caramel, Chocolate Nut Roll, Advantage, Atkins*	1 Bar/44g	170	12.0	386	18.2	43.2	27.3	18.2
Caramel, Double, Chocolate, Crunch, Atkins*	1 Bar/44g	160	9.0	364	22.7	50.0	20.4	25.0
Caramel, Nut Chew, Endulge, Atkins*	1 Bar/34g	130	2.7	382	5.0	17.0	8.0	6.0
Caramel Chocolate Peanut Nougat, Advantage, Atkins*	1 Bar/44g	180	11.0	409	22.7	40.9	25.0	25.0
Caramel Crisp Bite, Tesco*	1 Bar/15g	72	3.5	483	4.3	64.4	23.1	1.3
Caramel Crunch, Go Ahead, McVitie's*	1 Bar/24g	106	3.3	440	4.7	76.6	13.8	0.8
Caramel Mighty, Asda*	1 Bar/40g	186	8.0	464	5.0	66.0	20.0	1.5
Caramel Nougat, Soft, Shapers, Boots*	1 Bar/25g	86	2.5	343	2.9	60.4	10.0	0.6
Cashew Cookie, GF, Nak'd*	1 Bar/35g	144	8.0	410	10.0	46.0	23.0	5.0
Cereal, 3 Berries & Cherries, Dorset Cereals*	1 Bar/35g	127	1.7	363	5.7	73.9	4.9	5.2
Cereal, 3 Fruit, Nuts & Seeds, Dorset Cereals*	1 Bar/35g	136	3.6	389	7.4	66.6	10.3	6.2
Cereal, Apple & Blackberry with Yoghurt, Alpen*	1 Bar/29g	117	3.1	404	5.4	71.8	10.6	5.0
Cereal, Apple & Cinnamon, Fruit 'n' Grain, Asda*	1 Bar/37g	131	2.6	353	4.5	68.0	7.0	2.9
Cereal, Apple & Cinnamon, M&S*	1 Bar/24g	84	1.2	350	3.9	68.4	5.2	6.6
Cereal, Apple & Raisin, Harvest, Quaker Oats*	1 Bar/22g	87	2.5	396	5.0	70.0	11.5	4.0
Cereal, Apple & Sultana, Light, Alpen*	1 Bar/20g	63	0.7	330	4.1	59.4	3.6	21.7
Cereal, Apricot & Yoghurt, COU, M&S*	1 Bar/21g	75	0.5	360	5.3	79.6	2.4	3.8
Cereal, Balance with Fruit, Sainsbury's*	1 Bar/25g	100	2.2	401	5.8	75.2	8.6	1.9
Cereal, Banana, Value, Tesco*	1 Bar/21g	80	1.6	387	6.0	73.9	7.5	3.7
Cereal, Banoffee, Vitality, Asda*	1 Bar/22g	73	0.6	331	6.5	69.6	2.9	13.5
Cereal, Benefit with Fruit, Aldi*	1 Bar/27g	108	2.3	401	5.8	75.2	8.6	1.9
Cereal, Chewy & Crisp with Choc Chips, Tesco*	1 Bar/27g	125	6.3	463	9.2	54.0	23.4	3.8
Cereal, Chewy Apple, Fruitus, Lyme Regis Foods*	1 Bar/35g	132	3.8	378	5.4	64.8	10.8	5.4
Cereal, Chewy Pomegranate, Vitality, Asda*	1 Bar/22g	76	0.6	346	4.1	69.3	2.8	13.4
Cereal, Choc Chip, Brunch, Cadbury*	1 Bar/35g	156	6.2	445	6.0	64.0	17.6	4.1
Cereal, Choc Chip & Nut, Chewy & Crisp, Sainsbury's*	1 Bar/27g	129	7.0	476	8.8	51.8	26.0	4.4
Cereal, Chocolate, Double Milk, Special K, Kellogg's*	1 Bar/20g	80	2.0	400	10.0	65.0	10.0	10.0
Cereal, Chocolate, Geobar, Traidcraft*	1 Bar/32g	130	2.7	407	4.3	78.5	8.4	0.0
Cereal, Chocolate & Fudge, Light, Alpen*	1 Bar/18g	62	1.2	344	4.9	55.4	6.5	22.0
Cereal, Chocolate & Orange, Light, Alpen*	1 Bar/21g	71	1.2	339	4.8	56.0	5.5	23.1
Cereal, Chocolate & Orange, Officially Low Fat, Fox's*	1 Bar/19g	54	0.4	286	5.0	61.6	2.3	17.5
Cereal, Chocolate & Orange, Tesco*	1 Bar/22g	78	1.3	355	4.5	70.2	6.0	10.3
Cereal, Chocolate & Raisin, Seeds of Change*	1 Bar/29g	107	2.3	370	5.0	69.6	7.9	3.7
Cereal, Chocolate Chip, Special K, Kellogg's*	1 Bar/21g	84	1.5	401	9.0	76.0	7.0	1.5
Cereal, Citrus Fruits, Light, Alpen*	1 Bar/21g	59	0.9	283	5.6	55.9	4.1	22.4
Cereal, Coconut, Original Crunchy, Jordans*	1 Bar/30g	141	6.8	470	6.5	60.0	22.7	6.2
Cereal, Cranberry, Raisin & Nut, Shapers, Boots*	1 Bar/35g	140	4.4	400	7.1	65.7	12.6	3.7
Cereal, Cranberry & Blackcurrant, LC, Tesco*	1 Bar/25g	75	0.7	295	4.4	62.7	2.9	21.9
Cereal, Cranberry & Orange, Brunch, Cadbury*	1 Bar/35g	154	5.6	440	5.9	67.7	15.9	0.0
Cereal, Crunchy Granola, Apple Crunch, Nature Valley*	1 Bar/21g	92	3.2	440	7.3	69.0	15.0	5.7
Cereal, Crunchy Granola, Ginger Nut, Nature Valley*	1 Bar/42g	189	7.1	451	7.9	64.2	16.9	2.3
Cereal, Dark Chocolate, Le Noir, Orco*	1 Bar/21g	95	3.3	451	7.3	69.9	15.8	0.0
Cereal, Double Milk Chocolate, Special K, Kellogg's*	1 Bar/20g	79	1.8	396	9.0	66.0	9.0	10.0
Cereal, Fruit, Average	1 Bar/34g	130	3.9	382	5.9	64.7	11.5	6.5
Cereal, Fruit & Fibre, Asda*	1 Bar/29g	111	2.8	390	6.0	69.0	10.0	4.1
Cereal, Fruit & Fibre, You Count, Love Life, Waitrose*	1 Bar/25g	88	0.2	351	6.0	76.5	0.9	6.3
Cereal, Fruit & Nut, Alpen*	1 Bar/28g	109	2.3	390	5.8	73.0	8.3	2.9
Cereal, Fruit & Nut, Chewy Trail Mix, Nature Valley*	1 Bar/30g	114	3.2	379	7.7	63.2	10.6	7.3
Cereal, Fruit & Nut Break, Jordans*	1 Bar/37g	138	3.8	374	7.0	63.2	10.4	8.1
Cereal, Fruit & Nut with Milk Chocolate, Alpen*	1 Bar/29g	123	3.8	425	6.4	70.5	13.0	2.2
Cereal, Frusli, Absolutely Apricot, Jordans*	1 Bar/33g	120	3.3	365	5.0	63.8	10.0	6.3

BARS

	Measure INFO/WEIGHT	per Measure KCAL	FAT	Nutrition Values per 100g / 100ml KCAL	PROT	CARB	FAT	FIBRE
Cereal, Frusli, Blueberry, Jordans*	1 Bar/30g	113	2.1	375	5.2	70.2	7.1	4.9
Cereal, Frusli, Cranberry & Apple, Jordans*	1 Bar/30g	113	2.1	376	5.1	75.6	7.1	5.0
Cereal, Frusli, Raisin & Hazelnut, Jordans*	1 Bar/30g	117	3.7	390	5.8	64.3	12.2	4.5
Cereal, Frusli, Red Berries, Jordans*	1 Bar/30g	112	2.2	374	4.8	75.1	7.2	5.4
Cereal, Frusli, Wild Berries, Jordans*	1 Bar/30g	118	2.9	392	5.7	70.0	9.8	5.0
Cereal, Granola, Alpen*	1 Bar/29g	119	3.1	410	5.9	72.4	10.7	0.0
Cereal, Hazelnut, Brunch, Cadbury*	1 Bar/35g	160	7.4	460	7.0	60.5	21.4	2.2
Cereal, Maple, LC, Tesco*	1 Bar/23g	75	0.6	330	4.6	70.6	2.8	12.8
Cereal, Milk Chocolate, Weetos, Weetabix*	1 Bar/20g	88	2.9	440	5.9	70.9	14.7	1.6
Cereal, Milk Chocolate & Apricot, Value, Tesco*	1 Bar/22g	90	2.8	425	6.2	69.5	13.1	3.5
Cereal, Mint Chocolate, Kellogg's*	1 Bar/22g	88	2.2	401	4.5	74.0	10.0	3.5
Cereal, Mixed Berry, Go Ahead, McVitie's*	1 Bar/35g	134	2.2	383	4.6	77.1	6.3	3.1
Cereal, Muesli Break, Breakfast in a Bar, Jordans*	1 Bar/46g	178	5.0	387	5.9	66.6	10.8	4.3
Cereal, Multigrain, Peach & Apricot, BGTY, Sainsbury's*	1 Bar/28g	77	0.6	274	6.4	57.0	2.3	24.2
Cereal, Multigrain Balance, Maple, BGTY, Sainsbury's*	1 Bar/27g	75	0.8	276	6.4	56.2	2.8	25.5
Cereal, Nut & Seed, Organic, Green & Black's*	1 Bar/50g	258	16.3	516	8.4	47.2	32.6	10.0
Cereal, Nutty, Free From, Sainsbury's*	1 Bar/25g	114	5.0	454	6.8	61.8	20.0	2.3
Cereal, Oat & Raisin, Basics, Sainsbury's*	1 Bar/25g	98	2.2	391	5.1	72.8	8.8	3.8
Cereal, Oat & Raisin, Soft Oaties, Nutri-Grain, Kellogg's*	1 Bar/40g	173	6.4	432	6.0	66.0	16.0	3.5
Cereal, Oats & Berries, Crunchy & More, Nature Valley*	2 Bars/42g	190	7.1	453	7.4	64.6	16.9	6.1
Cereal, Oaty, Milk Chocolate, Weetabix*	1 Bar/23g	80	1.5	342	6.9	51.7	6.5	24.3
Cereal, Oaty, Strawberry, Weetabix*	1 Bar/23g	69	1.4	299	6.2	54.7	6.1	24.5
Cereal, Oaty, Toffee Dazzler, Weetabix*	1 Bar/23g	80	1.5	348	6.2	54.9	6.7	21.5
Cereal, Oaty, White Chocolate Flavour, Weetabix*	1 Bar/23g	78	1.4	341	6.4	52.4	6.3	24.3
Cereal, Peanut Butter & Oat, Organic, Meridian Foods*	1 Bar/50g	204	9.2	407	12.6	50.9	18.4	5.0
Cereal, Raisin, Raisin, Cadbury*	1 Bar/35g	150	5.4	430	5.6	66.4	15.5	1.8
Cereal, Raisin & Chocolate Chip, Fairtrade, Co-Op*	1 Bar/49g	185	4.6	378	5.3	69.2	9.4	3.7
Cereal, Raisin & Coconut, Value, Tesco*	1 Bar/21g	84	2.4	400	5.5	67.2	11.6	5.0
Cereal, Roast Hazelnut, Organic, Jordans*	1 Bar/33g	150	7.2	455	8.0	56.7	21.8	7.8
Cereal, Strawberry, Fitness, Nestle*	1 Bar/24g	89	1.6	378	4.9	73.8	7.0	4.1
Cereal, Strawberry, Fruit 'n' Grain, Asda*	1 Bar/37g	126	2.6	340	4.2	65.0	7.0	4.5
Cereal, Strawberry, Value, Tesco*	1 Bar/21g	80	1.1	382	5.5	77.8	5.4	3.3
Cereal, Strawberry with Yoghurt, Alpen*	1 Bar/29g	119	3.1	409	5.7	72.6	10.6	0.0
Cereal, Summer Fruits, Light, Alpen*	1 Bar/21g	70	0.9	334	4.4	58.7	4.1	22.4
Cereal, Super High Fibre, Dorset Cereals*	1 Bar/35g	149	5.6	425	9.6	60.8	16.0	7.1
Cereal, Toffee, Basics, Sainsbury's*	1 Bar/23g	92	1.9	398	4.8	75.8	8.4	2.5
Cereal, Toffee Apple, Chewy, Eat Smart, Morrisons*	1 Bar/25g	88	0.7	354	4.0	78.3	2.8	2.9
Cereal, Very Berry, Weight Watchers*	1 Bar/27g	92	2.7	340	6.6	42.6	9.9	26.8
Cereal, White Chocolate & Strawberry, Value, Tesco*	1 Bar/21g	85	1.7	405	6.2	76.2	8.1	2.4
Cherries, & Almonds, & a Yoghurt Coating, Eat Natural*	1 Bar/45g	200	9.5	444	6.6	58.8	21.1	3.6
Cherry Crunch, Protein Flapjack, Trek*	1 Bar/56g	242	11.1	432	18.3	46.0	19.9	3.1
Chocolate, Caramel, & Biscuit, Asda*	1 Bar/30g	150	8.3	508	8.0	56.0	28.0	2.5
Chocolate, Caramel, Wacko, Belmont, Aldi*	1 Bar/21g	100	4.7	478	4.9	63.8	22.6	1.4
Chocolate, Crisp, Weight Watchers*	1 Bar/25g	92	2.6	369	5.4	75.1	10.2	0.8
Chocolate, Crispy, Free From, Tesco*	1 Bar/30g	132	4.6	440	4.1	71.2	15.4	0.5
Chocolate, Dark, & Almond, Nupo*	1 Bar/29g	99	2.8	343	11.2	41.0	9.8	27.0
Chocolate, Dark, Chewy Delight, Special K, Kellogg's*	1 Bar/24g	97	3.4	404	4.5	57.0	14.0	17.0
Chocolate, Decadence, Atkins*	1 Bar/60g	227	12.2	378	27.1	30.7	20.4	11.6
Chocolate, Double, Dark, Zone Perfect*	1 Bar/45g	190	5.5	422	24.5	44.9	12.2	2.0
Chocolate, Milk, Belgian, Sugar Free, Sweet' N Low*	1 Bar/42g	202	14.3	480	7.1	52.7	34.1	1.8
Chocolate, Milk, Chewy Delight, Special K, Kellogg's*	1 Bar/24g	95	3.1	397	5.0	57.0	13.0	17.0
Chocolate, Milk, Crispy, Endulge, Atkins*	1 Bar/30g	141	9.6	469	13.0	48.0	32.0	2.0
Chocolate, Polar, Sainsbury's*	1 Bar/25g	133	7.2	533	5.5	63.0	28.6	1.2

BARS

	Measure INFO/WEIGHT	per Measure KCAL	FAT	Nutrition Values per 100g / 100ml KCAL	PROT	CARB	FAT	FIBRE
Chocolate, Soya, Dairy Free, Free From, Sainsbury's*	1 Bar/50g	274	17.5	548	10.8	47.5	35.0	4.3
Chocolate, Toffee Pecan, M&S*	1 Bar/36g	179	9.8	498	4.9	58.3	27.3	0.7
Chocolate, Wild & Whippy, Tesco*	1 Bar/18g	78	2.8	447	3.7	72.0	16.0	0.8
Chocolate & Crispy Rice, Organic, Dove's Farm*	1 Bar/35g	147	5.3	421	4.4	66.9	15.1	3.0
Chocolate & Orange, Crispy, Free From, Sainsbury's*	1 Bar/30g	132	4.9	440	4.8	68.2	16.2	1.2
Chocolate & Orange, Diet, Exante Diet*	1 Bar/59g	219	5.6	372	30.3	28.7	9.5	8.4
Chocolate & Peanut Butter, Atkins*	1 Bar/60g	240	12.0	400	31.7	36.7	20.0	16.7
Chocolate Almond Fudge	1 Bar/68g	230	4.5	338	14.7	55.9	6.6	7.4
Chocolate Brownie	1 Bar/68g	240	4.0	353	14.7	60.3	5.9	8.8
Chocolate Caramel, Slim Fast*	1 Bar/26g	95	2.5	365	3.5	61.5	9.6	1.5
Chocolate Caramel, Weight Watchers*	1 Bar/20g	80	2.5	400	5.0	70.0	12.5	0.0
Chocolate Caramel Whip, Weight Watchers*	1 Bar/25g	88	2.7	353	2.7	72.4	10.8	1.0
Chocolate Chip, Snack, Diet Chef Ltd*	1 Bar/27g	99	2.7	367	5.8	63.6	9.9	4.5
Chocolate Chip Granola, Advantage, Atkins*	1 Bar/48g	200	8.0	417	35.4	37.5	16.7	12.5
Chocolate Chip Muesli, Diet Chef Ltd*	1 Bar/50g	191	6.0	382	5.8	59.8	11.9	6.1
Chocolate Creme, Endulge, Atkins*	1 Bar/14g	70	4.8	504	12.5	38.6	34.3	2.5
Chocolate Crisp, Weight Watchers*	1 Bar/25g	94	2.6	378	4.8	66.8	10.2	1.6
Chocolate Crunch, Slim Fast*	1 Bar/60g	210	5.0	350	23.3	51.7	8.3	6.7
Chocolate Flavour, Protein, Diet Chef Ltd*	1 Bar/60g	225	7.1	375	29.3	37.5	11.9	4.2
Chocolate Mint, Cambridge Weight Plan*	1 Bar/50g	174	5.8	348	24.8	30.2	11.6	14.4
Chocolate Muesli, Snack, Slim Fast*	1 Bar/26g	99	3.5	379	4.7	64.5	13.3	6.5
Chocolate Peanut, Slim Fast*	1 Bar/56g	210	7.2	380	24.0	50.0	13.0	5.0
Chocolate Raisin & Cereal, Morrisons*	1 Bar/30g	126	4.4	420	5.4	66.3	14.8	3.8
Club, Fruit, Jacob's*	1 Biscuit/25g	124	6.2	496	5.6	62.2	25.0	2.3
Club, Milk Chocolate, Jacob's*	1 Biscuit/24g	123	6.3	511	5.8	62.6	26.4	2.0
Club, Mint, Jacob's*	1 Biscuit/24g	124	6.5	517	5.6	62.5	27.2	1.7
Club, Orange, Jacob's*	1 Biscuit/23g	117	6.1	509	5.7	61.8	26.5	2.3
Coco Pops, & Milk, Kellogg's*	1 Bar/20g	85	2.6	423	7.0	70.0	13.0	1.0
Cocoa Brownie, Trek, The Natural Health Company*	1 Bar/68g	223	4.1	328	17.0	53.0	6.0	8.0
Cocoa Delight, GF, Nak'd*	1 Bar/35g	135	5.3	386	9.4	49.8	15.1	7.0
Cocoa Loco, Wildly Different, Nak'd*	1 Bar/30g	100	3.0	332	8.0	65.0	10.0	7.0
Cocoa Mint, GF, Raw, Wholefood, Nak'd*	1 Bar/35g	135	5.2	386	9.0	49.0	15.0	7.0
Cocoa Orange, GF, Nak'd*	1 Bar/35g	145	7.0	415	11.0	45.0	20.0	6.0
Cookie, Oreo, Nabisco*	1 Bar/35g	180	10.2	514	2.0	66.0	29.0	0.0
Cranberry, Crunch, Cambridge Weight Plan*	1 Bar/50g	152	5.3	305	23.7	28.7	10.6	17.9
Cranberry, Nupo*	1 Bar/29g	99	2.6	340	11.7	44.4	9.0	21.9
Crazy Caramel, Tesco*	1 Bar/40g	192	9.2	480	3.9	64.0	23.0	1.0
Creme Brulee, Wonka*	2 Pieces/20g	111	6.5	555	5.7	59.1	32.6	1.1
Crunchy Caramel, Tesco*	1 Bar/21g	98	5.2	467	4.6	56.0	25.0	1.4
Crunchy Nut, Chocolate Peanut Crisp, Kellogg's*	1 Bar/35g	169	8.8	483	12.0	53.0	25.0	3.5
Crunchy Nut, Kellogg's*	1 Bar/30g	119	1.5	397	6.0	82.0	5.0	2.5
Dark Chocolate, Cranberry, Organic, Biona*	1 Bar/40g	162	5.9	405	6.2	53.5	14.7	0.0
Dark Chocolate, Crispy Wafer, Tasty Little Numbers*	1 Bar/20g	100	5.1	499	6.4	60.4	25.6	7.0
Date & Walnut, Eat Natural*	1 Bar/50g	220	10.0	441	8.0	57.1	20.1	3.3
Digestive, Milk Chocolate, McVitie's*	1 Bar/23g	118	5.8	511	6.6	64.6	25.1	1.9
Digestive, Milk Chocolate, Tesco*	1 Bar/19g	96	4.9	506	6.8	61.6	25.8	2.4
Digestive, Milk Chocolate, Value, Tesco*	1 Bar/19g	96	4.9	505	6.6	61.8	25.8	3.0
Double Chocolate, Breakfast Snack, Tesco*	1 Bar/37g	144	6.4	385	5.3	52.7	17.0	3.3
Double Chocolate, Light, Alpen*	1 Bar/19g	65	1.2	344	5.0	56.2	6.2	21.8
Double Chocolate Treat, Shapers, Boots*	1 Bar/23g	94	2.5	408	3.3	75.0	11.0	0.7
Echo, Fox's*	1 Bar/25g	126	6.6	513	7.1	60.7	26.7	2.3
Energy, Cocoa Brownie, Natural Balance Foods*	1 Bar/68g	216	4.1	318	17.0	51.0	6.0	0.0
Energy, Cool Mint, Chocolate, Clif*	1 Bar/68g	256	5.0	377	14.7	63.2	7.3	7.4

BARS

INFO/WEIGHT	Measure	per Measure		Nutrition Values per 100g / 100ml				
		KCAL	FAT	KCAL	PROT	CARB	FAT	FIBRE
Energy, Ride, Power Bar*	1 Bar/55g	213	9.1	387	18.6	40.9	16.6	7.4
Energy, Strawberry & Cranberry, Power Bar*	1 Bar/40g	153	3.0	384	7.9	68.7	7.5	4.8
Fair Break, Traidcraft*	1 Bar/22g	116	6.2	528	6.0	63.0	28.0	0.0
Fig & Mango, The Food Doctor*	1 Bar/35g	103	0.9	293	8.6	58.6	2.7	10.3
Flapjack, Apple & Sultana, Organic, Dove's Farm*	1 Bar/40g	178	7.8	446	4.7	61.1	19.6	3.5
Flapjack, Buttery, Traditional, Organic, Dove's Farm*	1 Bar/40g	173	7.5	432	6.1	59.4	18.8	5.7
Food Bar, Apple & Walnut, The Food Doctor*	1 Bar/35g	117	4.0	333	10.8	46.8	11.4	15.3
Forest Fruit, Yoghurt, Breaks, Go Ahead, McVitie's*	2 Slices/36g	144	3.6	402	5.4	72.6	10.0	2.2
Forest Fruit & Raisin, LC, Tesco*	1 Bar/27g	95	0.7	350	4.5	76.8	2.7	3.6
Frosties, & Milk, Kellogg's*	1 Bar/25g	102	2.8	408	7.0	71.0	11.0	1.0
Frosties, Chocolate, Kellogg's*	1 Bar/25g	103	3.0	412	6.0	72.0	12.0	1.6
Frosties, Snack Bar, Kellogg's*	1 Bar/25g	104	2.8	414	7.0	72.0	11.0	1.0
Fruit, Apple, Hellema*	1 Bar/33g	127	2.5	384	4.5	74.0	7.5	2.0
Fruit, Apple, Trimlyne*	1 Bar/27g	92	0.7	342	4.5	69.6	2.7	3.8
Fruit, Fig, Castus*	1 Bar/27g	80	1.3	300	3.0	60.0	5.0	0.0
Fruit, Nut & Seeds Cereal, Eat Well, M&S*	1 Bar/24g	88	2.6	365	6.1	60.8	10.9	6.9
Fruit, Strawberry, Fruitina*	1 Bar/15g	43	0.2	289	1.9	61.9	1.1	12.2
Fruit & Grain, Apple, Aldi*	1 Bar/37g	129	3.0	349	4.2	65.0	8.0	4.5
Fruit & Nut, Eat Natural*	1 Bar/50g	223	11.2	446	11.6	49.8	22.3	5.3
Fruit & Nut, Organic, Eat Natural*	1 Bar/50g	244	15.3	488	10.2	42.9	30.6	0.0
Fruit Muesli, Morning, Oat So Simple, Quaker Oats*	1 Bar/35g	139	3.2	398	7.7	68.1	9.1	6.6
Fruit with Apricot, Castus*	1 Bar/25g	75	1.1	300	2.0	63.0	4.5	9.0
Fruity Cereal, Go, Soreen*	1 Bar/40g	143	1.8	358	6.8	72.6	4.5	0.0
Ginger & Oat, Chocolate Covered, Snack, Waitrose*	1 Bar/27g	120	5.0	444	4.2	65.0	18.6	2.1
Ginger Bread, Nak'd*	1 Bar/35g	158	10.8	450	10.0	35.0	31.0	9.0
Golden Syrup, Morning, Oat So Simple, Quaker Oats*	1 Bar/35g	142	3.5	407	8.2	67.6	10.0	6.8
Granola, Crunchy, Oats & Chocolate, Nature Valley*	2 Bars/42g	195	8.3	464	8.3	59.8	19.8	7.1
Granola, Crunchy, Roasted Almond, Nature Valley*	1 Bar/42g	193	7.6	459	8.1	65.6	18.2	3.7
Granola, Maple Syrup, Twin Pack, Tesco*	2 Bars/42g	204	9.4	485	6.0	64.7	22.3	4.1
Granola, Oats & Hazelnuts, Nature Valley*	2 Bars/42g	195	8.4	465	8.4	58.9	20.1	7.5
Granola, You Can, Dairy Free, Kate's Cakes Ltd*	1 Serving/100g	422	22.0	422	7.2	49.0	22.0	7.1
Groove, Sassy Strawberry, Alpen*	1 Bar/32g	124	1.7	386	5.6	78.8	5.4	1.9
Harvest Cheweee, Apple & Raisin, Quaker Oats*	1 Bar/22g	89	2.6	405	5.5	68.0	12.0	3.0
Harvest Cheweee, Choc Chip, Quaker Oats*	1 Bar/22g	95	3.5	430	5.5	68.0	16.0	3.5
Harvest Cheweee, Toffee, Quaker Oats*	1 Bar/22g	94	3.3	427	5.0	68.0	15.0	3.0
Harvest Cheweee, White Chocolate Chip, Quaker Oats*	1 Bar/22g	94	3.4	425	6.0	67.0	15.5	3.5
Honey Nut, Special K, Special K, Kellogg's*	1 Bar/22g	90	2.0	409	9.1	72.7	9.1	13.6
Honeycomb, Club, Jacob's*	1 Bar/23g	116	6.0	512	5.7	61.9	26.3	2.3
Luxury, Absolute Nut, Jordans*	1 Bar/45g	251	18.6	557	12.7	33.3	41.4	7.0
Macadamia & Fruit, Eat Natural*	1 Bar/50g	242	15.4	485	7.3	44.6	30.8	0.0
Macaroon, Lees*	1 Bar/70g	276	4.7	395	1.2	82.5	6.7	0.0
Marshmallow, Chewy, Rice Krispies Squares, Kellogg's*	1 Bar/28g	119	3.4	424	3.0	76.0	12.0	0.9
Medley, Hazelnuts & Milk Chocolate, McVitie's*	1 Bar/30g	136	5.8	452	6.7	62.0	19.2	4.5
Medley, Hobnobs, Raisins & Milk Chocolate, McVitie's*	1 Bar/30g	127	4.1	422	5.7	71.7	13.7	5.3
Milk Chocolate, Crispy Wafer, Tasty Little Numbers*	1 Bar/20g	100	5.0	499	6.1	61.4	25.1	3.0
Milk Chocolate Whirls, Asda*	1 Bar/26g	116	4.2	447	3.7	72.0	16.0	0.8
Mixed Berry, Trek, Natural Balance Foods*	1 Bar/68g	204	1.5	300	15.6	56.5	2.2	6.0
Mixed Nut Feast, Eat Natural*	1 Bar/50g	278	20.5	556	18.8	28.0	41.0	0.0
Muesli, Apricot & Almond, Carmen's*	1 Bar/45g	190	8.2	423	10.4	50.6	18.2	7.4
Muesli, Cherry & Milk, Sirius*	1 Bar/25g	104	2.8	417	7.2	71.3	11.4	3.9
Multigrain, Fruit & Nut, Jordans*	1 Bar/40g	164	6.5	410	7.0	59.1	16.2	5.7
Natural Energy, Cacao Crunch, Power Bar*	1 Bar/40g	156	3.8	391	8.3	65.5	9.4	5.7
Nine Bar, Mixed Seed with Hemp, Original, Wholebake*	1 Bar/40g	222	16.2	555	18.3	29.2	40.5	5.2

BARS

INFO/WEIGHT	per Measure KCAL	per Measure FAT	Nutrition Values per 100g / 100ml KCAL	PROT	CARB	FAT	FIBRE
Nine Bar, Nutty, Wholebake*	1 Bar/50g	279	20.4	558	15.3	32.3	40.8	4.9
Nougat, Cool Mint, & Dark Chocolate, Shapers, Boots*	1 Bar/23g	83	3.2	362	2.6	70.0	14.0	1.1
Nougat, Summer Strawberry, Shapers, Boots*	1 Bar/23g	83	3.0	361	2.7	73.0	13.0	0.6
Nut, Dark Chocolate & Apricot, Natural, Nice & Natural*	1 Bar/35g	163	10.2	465	15.2	35.2	29.1	5.4
Nutri-Grain, Apple, Kellogg's*	1 Bar/37g	131	3.3	355	4.0	67.0	9.0	4.0
Nutri-Grain, Apple, Soft & Fruity, Kellogg's*	1 Bar/37g	133	3.0	359	4.0	70.3	8.1	4.0
Nutri-Grain, Blackberry & Apple, Kellogg's*	1 Bar/37g	131	3.3	355	4.0	67.0	9.0	4.0
Nutri-Grain, Blackberry & Apple, Soft & Fruity, Kellogg's*	1 Bar/37g	133	3.0	359	4.0	70.3	8.1	4.0
Nutri-Grain, Blueberry, Kellogg's*	1 Bar/37g	133	3.0	359	3.5	69.0	8.0	3.5
Nutri-Grain, Blueberry, Soft & Fruity, Kellogg's*	1 Bar/37g	133	3.0	359	4.0	70.3	8.1	4.0
Nutri-Grain, Cherry, Kellogg's*	1 Bar/37g	129	3.0	348	4.0	67.0	8.0	4.0
Nutri-Grain, Chocolate, Kellogg's*	1 Bar/37g	136	3.7	367	4.5	66.0	10.0	4.0
Nutri-Grain, Chocolate Chip, Chewy, Kellogg's*	1 Bar/25g	103	3.0	413	4.5	73.0	12.0	2.5
Nutri-Grain, Elevenses, Choc Chip Bakes, Kellogg's*	1 Bar/45g	179	5.8	397	4.0	66.0	13.0	2.0
Nutri-Grain, Elevenses, Ginger Bakes, Kellogg's*	1 Bar/45g	168	4.0	373	5.0	68.0	9.0	3.0
Nutri-Grain, Elevenses, Raisin Bakes, Kellogg's*	1 Bar/45g	168	4.0	374	4.5	68.0	9.0	2.5
Nutri-Grain, Honey Oat & Raisin, Chewy, Kellogg's*	1 Bar/25g	98	2.0	393	3.5	78.0	8.0	2.5
Nutri-Grain, Oat Bakes, Totally Oaty, Kellogg's*	1 Bar/50g	206	7.5	411	5.0	64.0	15.0	3.0
Nutri-Grain, Strawberry, Kellogg's*	1 Bar/37g	133	3.0	359	3.5	69.0	8.0	3.5
Nutri-Grain, Strawberry, Soft & Fruity, Kellogg's*	1 Bar/37g	133	3.0	359	4.0	70.3	8.1	4.0
Nutty Crunch Surprise, Wonka*	1 Bar/37g	202	11.9	543	4.9	58.7	32.1	0.9
Nutty Nougat Caramel, Tesco*	1 Bar/40g	200	11.1	490	8.7	52.7	27.2	3.8
Oat, Mixed Berry, Quaker Oats*	1 Bar/38g	137	3.3	360	6.8	64.5	8.8	8.0
Oat, Original with Golden Syrup, Quaker Oats*	1 Bar/38g	139	3.6	366	7.1	64.5	9.5	7.9
Oat, Quaker Oats*	1 Bar/38g	137	3.4	360	6.8	64.5	8.8	8.0
Oaty, Strawberry Crusher, Weetabix*	1 Bar/23g	79	1.4	345	6.1	55.2	6.1	22.2
Orange Crunch, Go Ahead, McVitie's*	1 Bar/23g	99	2.9	430	4.1	78.0	12.8	0.8
Original, Crunchy, Honey & Almond, Jordans*	1 Bar/30g	139	6.8	463	8.3	56.7	22.7	6.7
Original, Nut Free, Get Buzzing*	1 Bar/62g	248	12.0	400	6.8	51.6	19.4	3.7
Original Muesli, Diet Chef Ltd*	1 Bar/50g	199	6.9	398	6.1	59.0	13.8	6.4
Peach & Apricot, Special K, Kellogg's*	1 Bar/21g	80	1.3	383	8.0	75.0	6.0	2.5
Peanut, Mr Toms*	1 Bar/40g	210	13.0	525	20.0	42.5	32.5	2.5
Peanut & Oat, Trek, Nak'd*	1 Bar/68g	239	7.5	352	16.0	49.0	11.0	7.0
Peanut Butter, Chewy, Granola, Slim Fast*	1 Bar/56g	123	3.4	220	8.0	35.0	6.0	0.0
Peanut Fudge Granola, Advantage, Atkins*	1 Bar/48g	210	10.0	438	33.3	35.4	20.8	18.8
Pecan Pie, GF, Nak'd*	1 Bar/35g	156	10.8	447	8.0	36.0	31.0	9.0
Penguin Bigstix, McVitie's*	1 Biscuit/13g	64	3.2	508	6.4	62.8	25.7	2.6
Protein, Chocolate Chewy Crisp, Pro-Bar Xs*	1 Bar/70g	239	4.6	341	44.0	6.0	6.5	12.0
Protein, Flapjack, Oat Crunch, Natural Balance Foods*	1 Bar/56g	249	12.9	444	18.0	43.0	23.0	3.0
Protein, Low Carb, Pro-Lite 25, Peak Body*	1 Bar/50g	177	3.4	354	50.0	7.8	6.8	0.0
Protein, Peanut Blast, Natural Energy, Ball, Bounce*	1 Ball/49g	210	8.0	429	28.6	38.8	16.3	4.1
Protein, Premium, Ball, Bounce*	1 Ball/49g	209	9.0	426	30.6	40.8	18.4	2.0
Protein, Vanilla, Low Carb, Protein Plus, Power Bar*	1 Bar/35g	131	7.4	373	16.0	21.5	21.0	26.5
Raisin, Munch, Tesco*	1 Bar/30g	126	4.4	420	5.4	66.3	14.8	3.8
Raisin & Hazelnut, Weight Watchers*	1 Bar/24g	95	2.4	396	5.0	71.2	10.0	2.9
Raspberry, Baked, Asda*	1 Bar/27g	104	2.1	385	3.4	74.2	7.6	1.8
Raspberry, Yoghurt Breaks, Go Ahead, McVitie's*	1 Pack/35g	143	3.6	408	5.4	73.6	10.2	2.3
Rice Krispies, Snack, Kellogg's*	1 Bar/20g	83	2.0	415	7.0	70.0	10.0	0.5
Rice Krispies & Milk, Kellogg's*	1 Bar/20g	83	2.4	416	7.0	71.0	12.0	0.3
Rich Toffee, Weight Watchers*	1 Bar/26g	83	2.8	319	3.6	52.3	10.6	0.8
Roasted Nut, Chewy & Crisp, Sainsbury's*	1 Bar/27g	120	6.6	446	10.1	46.6	24.3	3.9
Rocky Road, Rice Krispies Squares, Kellogg's*	1 Square/34g	143	3.7	420	4.0	76.0	11.0	1.5
Sandwich, Chocolate, Rik & Rok*	1 Bar/22g	105	4.2	477	6.5	70.0	19.0	0.0

	Measure INFO/WEIGHT	per Measure KCAL	FAT	Nutrition Values per 100g / 100ml KCAL	PROT	CARB	FAT	FIBRE
BARS								
Sandwich, Chocolate Viennese, Fox's*	1 Biscuit/14g	76	4.4	542	6.9	57.4	31.6	1.6
Sandwich, Milk Chocolate Orange, Tesco*	1 Biscuit/25g	136	7.4	536	6.2	62.2	29.1	1.8
School, Apple, Fruit Bowl*	1 Bar/20g	67	0.6	337	0.7	75.0	3.0	6.0
School, Blackcurrant, Fruit Bowl*	1 Bar/20g	67	0.6	337	0.7	75.0	3.0	2.0
Sesame Snaps, Anglo-Dal*	1 Pack/30g	157	8.8	522	12.2	49.4	29.4	0.0
Sesame Snaps in Chocolate, Anglo-Dal*	1 Pack/40g	211	11.9	527	9.3	55.6	29.7	0.0
Sesame Snaps with Coconut, Anglo-Dal*	1 Pack/30g	155	8.8	517	9.7	52.9	29.5	0.0
Special Fruit Muesli, Jordans*	1 Bar/40g	140	2.4	349	5.0	68.8	6.0	5.0
Special K, Apple & Pear, Kellogg's*	1 Bar/23g	92	1.8	400	8.0	73.0	8.0	2.0
Special K, Chocolate Chip, Kellogg's*	1 Bar/22g	90	1.6	401	9.0	76.0	7.0	1.5
Special K, Fruits of the Forest, Kellogg's*	1 Bar/22g	87	1.8	397	8.0	74.0	8.0	2.5
Special K, Mint Chocolate, Bliss, Special K, Kellogg's*	1 Bar/22g	88	2.2	401	4.5	74.0	10.0	3.5
Special K, Raspberry & Chocolate, Bliss, Kellogg's*	1 Bar/22g	89	2.2	403	4.0	75.0	10.0	4.0
Special K, Red Berry, Kellogg's*	1 Bar/23g	90	1.2	383	8.0	77.0	5.0	2.0
Special Muesli, Jordans*	1 Bar/40g	152	4.8	379	6.0	61.6	12.1	5.8
Strawberry, Fruit Bakes, Go Ahead, McVitie's*	1 Bar/35g	131	3.0	375	3.5	72.0	8.5	4.0
Strawberry, Morning Shine, Atkins*	1 Bar/37g	145	8.0	392	28.9	24.9	21.6	14.1
Strawberry, Shapers, Boots*	1 Bar/22g	75	2.4	343	2.5	77.0	11.0	0.9
Supplement Cyclone, Maximuscle*	1 Bar/60g	215	4.3	358	27.2	20.4	7.2	5.3
Toffee, Nut & Raisin, Nutrition, Exante Diet*	1 Bar/59g	223	6.6	377	31.7	24.8	11.1	8.6
Totally Chocolatey, Rice Krispies Squares, Kellogg's*	1 Bar/36g	156	5.3	439	4.5	72.0	15.0	1.5
Tracker, Breakfast, Banana, Mars*	1 Bar/37g	176	8.4	476	4.7	63.3	22.6	9.4
Tracker, Chocolate Chip, Mars*	1 Bar/37g	178	8.7	480	6.8	58.0	23.6	3.8
Tracker, Forest Fruits, Mars*	1 Bar/26g	123	5.8	474	4.6	64.1	22.2	0.0
Tracker, Roasted Nut, Mars*	1 Bar/26g	127	6.6	489	8.1	55.0	25.3	4.9
Tracker, Strawberry, Mars*	1 Bar/26g	118	4.8	452	4.2	63.2	18.4	2.9
Tracker, Yoghurt, Mars*	1 Bar/27g	133	6.3	491	6.3	64.2	23.2	0.0
Triple Dazzle, Wonka*	1 Bar/39g	195	10.0	504	5.9	61.9	25.9	0.0
Wafer Biscuit, Milk Chocolate Coated, Value, Tesco*	1 Bar/24g	126	6.7	526	6.9	61.4	28.1	1.7
White Chocolate, Crispy Wafer, Tasty Little Numbers*	1 Bar/20g	100	5.2	498	7.0	59.0	26.0	3.0
White Chocolate & Hazelnuts, Porridge Oat, Stoats*	1 Bar/85g	398	26.8	468	10.1	64.8	31.5	8.0
BASA								
Tempura, Fillets, Northern Catch*	1 Fillet/160g	248	11.0	155	17.5	7.9	6.9	1.9
BASIL								
Dried, Ground	*1 Tsp/1g*	*4*	*0.1*	*251*	*14.4*	*43.2*	*4.0*	*0.0*
Fresh, Average	*1 Tbsp/5g*	*2*	*0.0*	*40*	*3.1*	*5.1*	*0.8*	*0.0*
BASKETS								
Brandy Snap, Askeys*	1 Basket/20g	98	4.3	490	1.9	72.7	21.3	0.0
BATTER MIX								
Green's*	1 Bag/125g	296	9.0	237	8.7	34.3	7.2	0.0
Pancake, Buttermilk, Krusteaz*	3 Pancakes/16g	57	0.8	352	11.3	66.0	4.7	3.4
Pancake, Sainsbury's*	1 Pancake/63g	96	1.1	152	6.5	27.4	1.8	3.1
Pancake & Yorkshire Pudding, Made Up, McDougalls*	1 Pancake/44g	84	2.6	187	6.4	27.6	5.7	0.5
Tesco*	1 Pack/130g	467	1.8	359	12.3	74.4	1.4	7.7
Yorkshire Pudding, Baked, Aunt Bessie's*	1 Pudding/13g	48	1.1	356	9.8	34.0	8.1	2.3
Yorkshire Pudding & Pancake, Morrisons*	1 Pudding/30g	43	0.8	143	6.4	23.1	2.8	4.1
Yorkshire Pudding & Pancake, Tesco*	1 Serving/17g	34	0.3	200	2.3	43.3	1.5	2.5
BAY LEAVES								
Dried, Average	*1 Tsp/0.6g*	*2*	*0.1*	*313*	*7.6*	*48.6*	*8.4*	*0.0*
BEAN MIX								
Mexican Style, Tinned, Asda*	1 Serving/81g	71	0.6	88	8.7	11.8	0.7	10.4
Wasabi, Whitworths*	1 Serving/25g	108	3.4	430	30.9	40.1	13.7	10.7

B

	Measure INFO/WEIGHT	per Measure KCAL	FAT	Nutrition Values per 100g / 100ml KCAL	PROT	CARB	FAT	FIBRE
BEAN SPROUTS								
Mung, Canned, Drained, Average	*1 Serving/90g*	*9*	*0.1*	*10*	*1.6*	*0.8*	*0.1*	*0.7*
Mung, Raw, Average	*1oz/28g*	*9*	*0.1*	*31*	*2.9*	*4.0*	*0.5*	*1.5*
Mung, Stir-Fried in Blended Oil, Average	*1 Serving/90g*	*65*	*5.5*	*72*	*1.9*	*2.5*	*6.1*	*0.9*
Raw, Average	*1 Serving/150g*	*55*	*2.6*	*37*	*2.2*	*3.2*	*1.8*	*1.2*
BEANFEAST								
Bolognese Style, Dry, Batchelors*	1 Pack/120g	362	6.7	302	23.9	39.0	5.6	13.5
Mexican Chilli, Batchelors*	1 Serving/65g	203	3.2	312	24.3	42.7	4.9	13.6
BEANS								
& Meatballs, in Tomato Sauce, Sainsbury's*	½ Can/200g	216	7.2	108	5.5	13.3	3.6	2.6
Aduki, Cooked in Unsalted Water, Average	*1 Tbsp/30g*	*37*	*0.1*	*123*	*9.3*	*22.5*	*0.2*	*5.5*
Aduki, Dried, Raw	*1 Tbsp/30g*	*82*	*0.2*	*272*	*19.9*	*50.1*	*0.5*	*11.1*
Adzuki, Dry, Love Life, Waitrose*	1 Serving/100g	340	0.5	340	19.9	62.9	0.5	12.7
Adzuki, in Water, Canned, Drained, Tesco*	½ Can/118g	118	0.5	100	6.5	13.6	0.4	6.5
Baked, & Jumbo Sausages, Asda*	1 Serving/210g	317	14.7	151	7.0	15.0	7.0	2.6
Baked, & Pork Sausages, Sainsbury's*	1 Serving/210g	248	9.2	118	5.7	13.9	4.4	3.4
Baked, & Pork Sausages, Tesco*	½ Can/210g	231	5.7	110	5.5	15.6	2.7	3.0
Baked, & Sausage, Asda*	½ Can/203g	211	4.0	104	6.7	13.0	2.0	3.5
Baked, & Sausages, Basics, Sainsbury's*	1 Serving/175g	149	2.6	85	4.8	13.1	1.5	2.6
Baked, & Sausages, Value, Tesco*	½ Can/202g	232	7.1	115	5.6	15.0	3.5	2.8
Baked, & Veggie Sausages, In Tomato Sauce, Asda*	½ Can/210g	204	4.0	97	7.4	12.5	1.9	8.4
Baked, Barbecue, Beanz, Heinz*	1 Can/390g	343	0.8	88	4.9	14.6	0.2	3.8
Baked, Basics, Sainsbury's*	1 Can/420g	206	1.3	49	4.2	7.4	0.3	4.4
Baked, Curried, Average	*½ Can/210g*	*203*	*1.9*	*96*	*4.8*	*17.2*	*0.9*	*3.6*
Baked, Curry, Beanz, Heinz*	1 Can/200g	218	3.2	109	4.8	17.0	1.6	4.0
Baked, Eat Smart, Morrisons*	1 Can/420g	294	1.7	70	5.3	11.4	0.4	5.6
Baked, Fiery Chilli, in Tomato & Chilli Sauce, Heinz*	1 Serving/100g	91	0.3	91	4.9	15.1	0.3	3.8
Baked, Five, in Tomato Sauce, Heinz*	1 Can/415g	361	0.8	87	5.4	13.6	0.2	4.3
Baked, in Barbeque Sauce, Tesco*	1 Can/220g	198	1.3	90	5.0	13.6	0.6	5.2
Baked, in Tomato Sauce, Average	*1 Can/400g*	*318*	*1.6*	*80*	*4.6*	*13.9*	*0.4*	*3.7*
Baked, in Tomato Sauce, Beanz, Heinz*	½ Can/208g	164	0.4	79	4.7	12.9	0.2	3.7
Baked, in Tomato Sauce, Corale, Aldi*	½ Can/220g	200	0.9	91	5.2	14.4	0.4	4.3
Baked, in Tomato Sauce, Everyday Value, Tesco*	½ Can/210g	185	1.0	90	3.7	14.6	0.5	4.4
Baked, in Tomato Sauce, Fridge Pack, Beanz, Heinz*	1 Serving/200g	158	0.4	79	4.5	12.9	0.2	3.5
Baked, in Tomato Sauce, Garlic & Herbs, Beanz, Heinz*	½ Can/195g	157	0.4	81	4.8	12.8	0.2	3.8
Baked, in Tomato Sauce, LC, Tesco*	½ Can/100g	80	0.5	80	4.3	12.1	0.5	3.8
Baked, in Tomato Sauce, Organic, Beanz, Heinz*	1 Can/415g	336	0.8	81	4.8	12.9	0.2	3.8
Baked, in Tomato Sauce, Reduced Sugar & Salt	*½ Can/210g*	*159*	*0.7*	*76*	*4.6*	*13.6*	*0.3*	*3.8*
Baked, in Tomato Sauce, Reduced Sugar & Salt, Asda*	½ Tin/211g	158	1.1	75	4.6	13.0	0.5	4.5
Baked, in Tomato Sauce, Smart Price, Asda*	1 Can/410g	403	1.7	96	5.0	16.4	0.4	3.5
Baked, in Tomato Sauce, Snap Pot, Beanz, Heinz*	1 Pot/200g	159	0.4	79	4.7	12.9	0.2	3.7
Baked, in Tomato Sauce, Tesco*	1 Can/220g	198	1.1	90	4.3	14.1	0.5	4.1
Baked, Jalfrezi, Mean, Beanz, Heinz*	1 Serving/195g	135	2.5	69	4.5	9.8	1.3	3.6
Baked, Mexican, Mean, Beanz, Heinz*	½ Can/208g	158	1.0	76	5.0	12.9	0.5	4.0
Baked, Reduced Sugar & Salt, Sainsbury's*	½ Can/210g	168	1.0	80	5.2	16.1	0.5	5.0
Baked, Sweet Chilli, Mean, Beanz, Heinz*	½oz/195g	142	0.6	73	4.5	13.0	0.3	3.6
Baked, Virtually Fat Free, Heinz*	½ Can/207g	164	0.4	79	4.7	12.9	0.2	3.7
Baked, with HP Sauce, Beanz, Heinz*	½ Can/208g	158	0.6	76	4.8	13.7	0.3	3.9
Baked, with Lea & Perrins Sauce, Beanz, Heinz*	1 Can/415g	303	0.8	73	4.8	13.1	0.2	3.8
Baked, with Sausages, Branston, Crosse & Blackwell*	½ Can/202g	233	6.5	115	6.9	12.2	3.2	5.0
Baked, with Vegetable Sausages, Beanz, Heinz*	1 Can/200g	210	7.2	105	6.0	12.2	3.6	2.9
Baked, with Veggie Sausages In Tomato Sauce, Tesco*	1 Can/395g	375	8.7	95	7.4	8.7	2.2	3.5
Black, Cooked, Average	*1 Cup/172g*	*227*	*0.9*	*132*	*8.8*	*23.7*	*0.5*	*8.7*
Black, Dried, Average	*1 Serving/100g*	*341*	*1.4*	*341*	*21.6*	*62.4*	*1.4*	*15.2*

BEANS

INFO/WEIGHT	Measure	per Measure KCAL	FAT	Nutrition Values per 100g / 100ml KCAL	PROT	CARB	FAT	FIBRE
Black Turtle, Dried, Love Life, Waitrose*	1 Serving/100g	351	0.9	351	21.3	63.3	0.9	24.9
Blackeye, Canned, Average	**1 Can/172g**	**206**	**1.3**	**120**	**8.4**	**19.8**	**0.8**	**3.3**
Blackeye, Dried, Raw	**1oz/28g**	**87**	**0.4**	**311**	**23.5**	**54.1**	**1.6**	**8.2**
Borlotti, Canned, Average	**1oz/28g**	**29**	**0.1**	**103**	**7.6**	**16.9**	**0.5**	**4.7**
Borlotti, Dried, Love Life, Waitrose*	1 Serving/100g	348	1.2	348	23.0	60.1	1.2	24.7
Borlotti, Dried, Raw, Average	**1 Serving/100g**	**335**	**1.2**	**335**	**23.0**	**60.0**	**1.2**	**24.7**
Broad, Canned, Drained, Average	**1 Can/195g**	**136**	**1.1**	**70**	**6.9**	**9.2**	**0.6**	**6.8**
Broad, Crispy, Wasabi Flavoured, Khao Shong*	1 Serving/30g	116	3.0	386	17.0	57.0	10.0	7.0
Broad, Dried, Raw, Average	**1oz/28g**	**69**	**0.6**	**245**	**26.1**	**32.5**	**2.1**	**27.6**
Broad, Frozen, Average	1 Serving/80g	63	0.6	79	7.6	10.8	0.7	5.3
Broad, Frozen, Sainsbury's*	1 Serving/80g	64	0.5	80	7.9	10.7	0.6	6.5
Broad, in Water, Drained, Asda*	1 Serving/98g	74	0.5	75	7.4	10.1	0.5	7.1
Broad, Weighed with Pod, Raw, Average	**1oz/28g**	**17**	**0.3**	**59**	**5.7**	**7.2**	**1.0**	**6.1**
Butter, Canned, Drained, Average	**1oz/28g**	**24**	**0.1**	**86**	**6.3**	**13.5**	**0.5**	**4.6**
Butter, Canned, Drained, Wholefoods, Tesco*	½ Can/125g	100	0.6	80	5.9	13.0	0.5	4.6
Butter, Drained Weight, M&S*	1 Serving/119g	125	0.6	105	7.2	15.3	0.5	5.6
Butter, Dried, Boiled, Average	**1oz/28g**	**30**	**0.2**	**106**	**7.2**	**18.6**	**0.6**	**5.2**
Butter, Dried, Raw, Average	**1oz/28g**	**81**	**0.5**	**290**	**19.1**	**52.9**	**1.7**	**16.0**
Cannellini, Canned, Average	**1 Can/400g**	**375**	**2.1**	**94**	**7.2**	**15.0**	**0.5**	**5.7**
Cannellini, Dried, Tesco*	1 Serving/32g	83	0.3	260	24.8	37.4	0.8	20.9
Cannellini, in Water, Canned, Drained, Asda*	½ Can/87g	86	0.3	99	7.0	14.0	0.3	6.0
Cannellini with Chorizo & Red Peppers, Morrisons*	½ Pack/100g	155	10.0	155	6.9	9.2	10.0	2.8
Chilli, Canned, Average	**1 Can/420g**	**381**	**3.1**	**91**	**5.2**	**15.8**	**0.7**	**4.4**
Curried, Mixed, Morrisons*	1 Can/420g	420	16.4	100	4.2	12.1	3.9	5.6
Edamame, Sainsbury's*	1 Serving/150g	212	9.6	141	12.3	6.8	6.4	4.2
Flageolet, Canned, Average	**1 Can/265g**	**235**	**1.6**	**89**	**6.8**	**14.0**	**0.6**	**3.5**
Flageolet, Dried, Love Life, Waitrose*	1 Serving/50g	125	3.1	250	30.4	19.8	6.2	40.4
French, Boiled, Average	**1 Serving/150g**	**38**	**0.0**	**25**	**2.3**	**3.8**	**0.0**	**3.7**
French, Canned, Average	**1oz/28g**	**6**	**0.1**	**22**	**1.6**	**3.5**	**0.3**	**2.5**
French, Raw	**1oz/28g**	**7**	**0.1**	**24**	**1.9**	**3.2**	**0.5**	**2.2**
Green, Cut, Average	**1oz/28g**	**7**	**0.1**	**24**	**1.7**	**3.6**	**0.2**	**2.7**
Green, Extra Fine, in Salted Water, Lidl*	1 Serving/220g	37	0.4	17	1.3	2.5	0.2	3.5
Green, Fine, Average	**1 Serving/75g**	**18**	**0.3**	**24**	**1.8**	**3.2**	**0.4**	**2.9**
Green, Fresh, Value, Tesco*	1 Pack/100g	27	0.1	27	1.9	3.2	0.1	4.1
Green, Sliced, Average	**1oz/28g**	**6**	**0.1**	**23**	**1.9**	**3.5**	**0.2**	**2.1**
Green, Sliced, Frozen, Average	**1 Serving/50g**	**13**	**0.0**	**26**	**1.8**	**4.4**	**0.1**	**4.1**
Green, Very Fine, Field Fresh, Birds Eye*	1 Serving/80g	20	0.4	25	1.8	2.9	0.5	2.4
Green, Whole, Average	**1oz/28g**	**6**	**0.1**	**22**	**1.6**	**3.0**	**0.4**	**1.7**
Green, Whole, Frozen, Boiled, CBY, Asda*	1 Portion/80g	28	0.1	35	1.7	4.7	0.1	4.1
Haricot, Canned, Average	1 Can/400g	77	0.5	77	6.2	10.7	0.5	5.9
Haricot, Dried, Boiled in Unsalted Water	**1oz/28g**	**27**	**0.1**	**95**	**6.6**	**17.2**	**0.5**	**6.1**
Haricot, Dried, Raw	**1oz/28g**	**80**	**0.4**	**286**	**21.4**	**49.7**	**1.6**	**17.0**
Haricot, in Water, Canned, Drained, Tesco*	½ Can/118g	76	0.6	65	5.7	9.0	0.5	7.8
Keen Bean, Mix, Graze*	1 Punnet/31g	153	10.2	486	30.5	27.6	32.5	7.1
Kidney, Curried, Rajmah, Sohna *	½ Can/225g	217	1.1	97	3.7	17.6	0.5	1.4
Kidney, Red, Canned, Drained, Average	**½ Can/90g**	**88**	**0.5**	**98**	**7.6**	**21.2**	**0.6**	**5.7**
Kidney, Red, Drained, Savers, Morrisons*	½ Can/120g	125	0.8	104	7.7	12.9	0.7	7.8
Kidney, Red, Dried, Boiled in Unsalted Water	**1oz/28g**	**29**	**0.1**	**103**	**8.4**	**17.4**	**0.5**	**6.7**
Kidney, Red, Dried, Raw	**1oz/28g**	**74**	**0.4**	**266**	**22.1**	**44.1**	**1.4**	**15.7**
Kidney, Red, in Chilli Sauce, Sainsbury's*	1 Can/420g	365	1.7	87	5.3	15.6	0.4	4.5
Kidney, Red, Value, Tesco*	1 Serving/65g	60	0.4	93	6.9	15.0	0.6	6.2
Kidney, White, Dry, Raw, Unico*	½ Cup/80g	270	0.9	338	22.5	61.2	1.1	21.2
Mix, Dry Roasted, The Food Doctor*	1 Portion/25g	98	3.3	392	34.0	23.6	13.2	21.2

	Measure INFO/WEIGHT	per Measure KCAL	FAT	Nutrition Values per 100g / 100ml KCAL	PROT	CARB	FAT	FIBRE
BEANS								
Mixed, Canned, Average	**1 Can/300g**	**300**	**3.5**	**100**	**6.8**	**15.6**	**1.2**	**4.1**
Mixed, in Mild Chilli Sauce, Sainsbury's*	1 Can/420g	328	1.3	78	4.9	13.8	0.3	3.7
Mixed, in Tomato Sauce, CBY, Asda*	½ Can/203g	196	1.0	97	5.0	15.8	0.5	4.6
Mixed, Spicy, Average	**1 Serving/140g**	**108**	**0.7**	**78**	**4.8**	**13.4**	**0.5**	**3.9**
Mung, Whole, Dried, Boiled in Unsalted Water	**1oz/28g**	**25**	**0.1**	**91**	**7.6**	**15.3**	**0.4**	**3.0**
Mung, Whole, Dried, Raw	**1oz/28g**	**78**	**0.3**	**279**	**23.9**	**46.3**	**1.1**	**10.0**
Pinto, Dried, Boiled in Unsalted Water	**1oz/28g**	**38**	**0.2**	**137**	**8.9**	**23.9**	**0.7**	**0.0**
Pinto, Dried, Love Life, Waitrose*	1 Serving/80g	288	1.0	360	21.4	62.6	1.2	15.5
Pinto, Dried, Raw	**1oz/28g**	**92**	**0.4**	**327**	**21.1**	**57.1**	**1.6**	**14.0**
Refried, Average	**1 Serving/215g**	**162**	**1.5**	**76**	**4.6**	**12.7**	**0.7**	**1.8**
Runner, Average	**1 Serving/80g**	**16**	**0.3**	**20**	**1.4**	**2.8**	**0.4**	**2.2**
Soya, Dried, Average	**1oz/28g**	**104**	**5.1**	**370**	**34.2**	**15.4**	**18.3**	**19.6**
Soya, Dried, Boiled in Unsalted Water	**1oz/28g**	**39**	**2.0**	**141**	**14.0**	**5.1**	**7.3**	**6.1**
Soya, Frozen, Birds Eye*	1 Serving/80g	98	5.1	123	12.4	4.0	6.4	4.2
Soya, in Water, Salt Added, Sainsbury's*	1 Serving/100g	102	7.3	102	4.0	5.1	7.3	6.1
Soya, Shelled, Frozen, Raw, Average	**1 Serving/80g**	**99**	**4.3**	**124**	**12.2**	**6.9**	**5.3**	**4.4**
Soya, Tesco*	1 Pack/200g	240	11.6	120	10.2	6.7	5.8	2.0
White, Campo Largo, Lidl*	½ Jar/200g	180	1.0	90	7.1	11.2	0.5	0.0
Wholesome, 10 Mix, Dried, Love Life, Waitrose*	1 Pack/500g	1850	17.0	370	13.3	71.5	3.4	10.0
BEEF								
Brisket, Boiled, Lean	1 Serving/100g	225	11.0	225	31.4	0.0	11.0	0.0
Brisket, Boiled, Lean & Fat	1 Serving/100g	268	17.4	268	27.8	0.0	17.4	0.0
Brisket, Braised, Lean	1 Serving/100g	280	17.4	280	29.0	0.0	17.4	0.0
Brisket, Raw, Lean	**1oz/28g**	**39**	**1.7**	**139**	**21.1**	**0.0**	**6.1**	**0.0**
Brisket, Raw, Lean & Fat	**1oz/28g**	**61**	**4.5**	**218**	**18.4**	**0.0**	**16.0**	**0.0**
British, Diced, Fresh, Value, Tesco*	1 Serving/125g	175	7.8	140	20.8	0.0	6.2	0.0
Cooked, Sliced, From Supermarket, Average	**1 Slice/35g**	**47**	**1.2**	**135**	**23.6**	**2.0**	**3.5**	**0.5**
Escalope, Healthy Range, Average	**1 Serving/170g**	**233**	**6.7**	**137**	**24.2**	**1.2**	**4.0**	**0.4**
Flank, Pot-Roasted, Lean	**1oz/28g**	**71**	**3.9**	**253**	**31.8**	**0.0**	**14.0**	**0.0**
Flank, Pot-Roasted, Lean & Fat	**1oz/28g**	**87**	**6.2**	**309**	**27.1**	**0.0**	**22.3**	**0.0**
Flank, Raw, Lean	**1oz/28g**	**49**	**2.6**	**175**	**22.7**	**0.0**	**9.3**	**0.0**
Flank, Raw, Lean & Fat	**1oz/28g**	**74**	**5.8**	**266**	**19.7**	**0.0**	**20.8**	**0.0**
for Casserole, Lean, Diced, Average	**1oz/28g**	**35**	**1.1**	**126**	**23.0**	**0.0**	**3.8**	**0.0**
Fore Rib, Lean & Fat, Average	**1oz/28g**	**40**	**1.8**	**144**	**21.7**	**0.0**	**6.2**	**0.2**
Fore Rib, Raw, Lean	**1oz/28g**	**41**	**1.8**	**145**	**21.5**	**0.0**	**6.5**	**0.0**
Fore Rib, Roasted, Lean	**1oz/28g**	**66**	**3.2**	**236**	**33.3**	**0.0**	**11.4**	**0.0**
Fore Rib, Roasted, Lean & Fat	**1oz/28g**	**84**	**5.7**	**300**	**29.1**	**0.0**	**20.4**	**0.0**
Grill Steak, Average	**1 Steak/170g**	**501**	**39.5**	**295**	**19.3**	**2.1**	**23.2**	**0.1**
Grill Steak, Peppered, Average	**1 Serving/172g**	**419**	**24.4**	**244**	**23.6**	**5.2**	**14.2**	**0.3**
Grillsteaks, Aberdeen Angus, Extra Special, Asda*	1 Steak/170g	403	23.3	237	23.8	4.3	13.7	0.0
Joint, for Roasting, Average	**1oz/28g**	**38**	**1.0**	**134**	**24.5**	**1.4**	**3.4**	**0.2**
Joint, Sirloin, Roasted, Lean	**1oz/28g**	**53**	**1.8**	**188**	**32.4**	**0.0**	**6.5**	**0.0**
Joint, Sirloin, Roasted, Lean & Fat	**1oz/28g**	**65**	**3.5**	**233**	**29.8**	**0.0**	**12.6**	**0.0**
Mince, Cooked, Average	**1 Serving/75g**	**214**	**15.3**	**286**	**24.0**	**0.0**	**20.3**	**0.0**
Mince, Extra Lean, Raw, Average	**1 Serving/100g**	**124**	**5.0**	**124**	**21.2**	**0.1**	**5.0**	**0.0**
Mince, Extra Lean, Stewed	**1oz/28g**	**50**	**2.4**	**177**	**24.7**	**0.0**	**8.7**	**0.0**
Mince, Lean, Raw, Average	**1oz/28g**	**48**	**2.8**	**172**	**20.8**	**0.0**	**10.0**	**0.1**
Mince, Raw, Average	**1oz/28g**	**68**	**5.1**	**242**	**19.6**	**0.2**	**18.1**	**0.0**
Mince, Raw, Frozen, Average	**1 Serving/100g**	**176**	**10.0**	**176**	**20.4**	**0.0**	**10.0**	**0.0**
Mince, Steak, Extra Lean, Average	**1oz/28g**	**37**	**1.6**	**131**	**20.5**	**0.4**	**5.6**	**0.0**
Mince, Steak, Extra Lean, Sainsbury's*	1 Pack/600g	738	27.0	123	20.5	0.0	4.5	0.0
Mince, Steak, Frozen, As Sold, LC, Tesco*	1 Serving/100g	153	7.4	153	21.5	0.0	7.4	0.0
Mince, Steak, Lean, Morrisons*	1 Pack/500g	950	59.0	190	20.9	0.0	11.8	0.0

BEEF

	Measure INFO/WEIGHT	per Measure		Nutrition Values per 100g / 100ml				
		KCAL	FAT	KCAL	PROT	CARB	FAT	FIBRE
Mince, Steak, Raw, Average	1 Serving/125g	318	25.0	254	17.2	0.0	20.0	0.0
Mince, Stewed	1oz/28g	59	3.8	209	21.8	0.0	13.5	0.0
Peppered, Sliced, Average	1 Slice/20g	26	1.1	129	18.2	1.3	5.6	1.0
Provencal, Bistro, TTD, Sainsbury's*	½ Pack/400g	411	9.4	105	7.6	11.3	2.4	4.0
Roast, Finely Sliced, TTD, Sainsbury's*	1 Slice/18g	27	0.7	148	28.0	0.3	3.9	0.0
Roast, Sliced, Average	1 Slice/35g	48	1.3	136	26.1	0.4	3.6	0.2
Roast, Traditional, Sliced, TTD, Sainsbury's*	1 Slice/33g	49	1.3	148	28.0	0.3	3.9	1.0
Salt, Average	1 Serving/70g	80	1.7	114	21.7	1.0	2.5	0.1
Salted, Dried, Raw	1oz/28g	70	0.4	250	55.4	0.0	1.5	0.0
Silverside, Pot-Roasted, Lean	1oz/28g	54	1.8	193	34.0	0.0	6.3	0.0
Silverside, Pot-Roasted, Lean & Fat	1oz/28g	69	3.8	247	31.0	0.0	13.7	0.0
Silverside, Raw, Lean	1oz/28g	38	1.2	134	23.8	0.0	4.3	0.0
Silverside, Raw, Lean & Fat	1oz/28g	60	4.1	215	20.4	0.0	14.8	0.0
Silverside, Salted, Boiled, Lean	1oz/28g	52	1.9	184	30.4	0.0	6.9	0.0
Silverside, Salted, Boiled, Lean & Fat	1oz/28g	63	3.5	224	27.9	0.0	12.5	0.0
Silverside, Salted, Raw, Lean	1oz/28g	39	2.0	140	19.2	0.0	7.0	0.0
Silverside, Salted, Raw, Lean & Fat	1oz/28g	64	5.0	227	16.3	0.0	18.0	0.0
Steak, Braising, Braised, Lean	1oz/28g	63	2.7	225	34.4	0.0	9.7	0.0
Steak, Braising, Braised, Lean & Fat	1oz/28g	69	3.6	246	32.9	0.0	12.7	0.0
Steak, Braising, Lean, Raw, Average	1oz/28g	40	1.4	144	24.8	0.0	5.0	0.0
Steak, Braising, Raw, Lean & Fat	1oz/28g	45	2.4	160	20.7	0.0	8.6	0.0
Steak, Diced, Lean, Casserole, Sainsbury's*	1 Pack/250g	400	5.0	160	34.9	0.5	2.0	0.0
Steak, Economy, Average	1oz/28g	53	2.4	190	26.9	1.2	8.7	0.4
Steak, Fillet, Cooked, Average	1oz/28g	54	2.4	191	28.6	0.0	8.5	0.0
Steak, Fillet, Lean, Average	1oz/28g	42	2.0	150	21.0	0.0	7.3	0.0
Steak, Fillet, Lean, Cooked, Average	1oz/28g	52	2.2	186	28.6	0.0	8.0	0.0
Steak, Frying, Average	1 Steak/110g	128	2.7	116	23.7	0.0	2.5	0.0
Steak, Rump, 8oz, & Chips	1 Serving/466g	870	41.1	187	10.7	16.2	8.8	0.0
Steak, Rump, Cooked, Average	1oz/28g	69	4.0	246	29.1	0.5	14.1	0.0
Steak, Rump, Grilled, Rare, Lean	1 Steak/227g	381	15.6	168	26.5	0.0	6.9	0.0
Steak, Rump, Lean, Cooked, Average	1oz/28g	50	1.7	179	31.0	0.0	6.1	0.0
Steak, Rump, Raw, Lean	1oz/28g	35	1.1	125	22.0	0.0	4.1	0.0
Steak, Rump, Raw, Lean & Fat	1oz/28g	49	2.8	174	20.7	0.0	10.1	0.0
Steak, Sirloin, Fried, Rare, Lean	1oz/28g	53	2.3	189	28.8	0.0	8.2	0.0
Steak, Sirloin, Fried, Rare, Lean & Fat	1oz/28g	65	3.9	233	26.8	0.0	14.0	0.0
Steak, Sirloin, Grilled, Medium-Rare, Lean	1oz/28g	49	2.2	176	26.6	0.0	7.7	0.0
Steak, Sirloin, Grilled, Medium-Rare, Lean & Fat	1oz/28g	60	3.5	213	24.8	0.0	12.6	0.0
Steak, Sirloin, Grilled, Rare, Lean	1oz/28g	46	1.9	166	26.4	0.0	6.7	0.0
Steak, Sirloin, Grilled, Rare, Lean & Fat	1oz/28g	60	3.6	216	25.1	0.0	12.8	0.0
Steak, Sirloin, Grilled, Well-Done, Lean	1oz/28g	63	2.8	225	33.9	0.0	9.9	0.0
Steak, Sirloin, Grilled, Well-Done, Lean & Fat	1oz/28g	72	4.0	257	31.8	0.0	14.4	0.0
Steak, Sirloin, Raw, Lean, Average	1 Steak/150g	202	6.8	135	23.5	0.0	4.5	0.0
Steak, Sirloin, Raw, Lean & Fat	1oz/28g	56	3.6	201	21.6	0.0	12.7	0.0
Steaklet, Meal, 210, Oakhouse Foods Ltd*	1 Meal/290g	435	26.4	150	5.2	12.5	9.1	2.1
Stewed Steak, Average	1 Serving/220g	258	10.1	117	15.8	3.3	4.6	0.0
Stewing Steak, Raw, Lean	1oz/28g	34	1.0	122	22.6	0.0	3.5	0.0
Stewing Steak, Stewed, Lean	1oz/28g	52	1.8	185	32.0	0.0	6.3	0.0
Stewing Steak, Stewed, Lean & Fat	1oz/28g	57	2.7	203	29.2	0.0	9.6	0.0
Strips, Stir Fry, Raw, Average	1 Serving/125g	149	3.8	119	23.0	0.0	3.0	0.2
Topside, Lean & Fat, Raw, Average	1oz/28g	55	3.6	198	20.4	0.0	12.9	0.0
Topside, Raw, Lean	1oz/28g	32	0.8	116	23.0	0.0	2.7	0.0
Wafer Thin, Cooked, Asda*	1 Serving/70g	63	1.1	90	18.2	0.7	1.6	0.0
Wafer Thin, Sliced, Cooked, Average	1 Slice/10g	13	0.3	129	24.5	0.5	3.2	0.2

	Measure INFO/WEIGHT	per Measure		Nutrition Values per 100g / 100ml				
		KCAL	FAT	KCAL	PROT	CARB	FAT	FIBRE
BEEF &								
Black Bean, Sizzling, Oriental Express*	1 Pack/400g	420	8.4	105	7.2	14.0	2.1	2.1
Black Bean, with Rice, Weight Watchers*	1 Pack/320g	288	4.2	90	5.0	14.6	1.3	0.1
Mashed Potato, Braised, Sainsbury's*	1 Pack/434g	425	14.3	98	7.6	9.4	3.3	0.8
Onions, Minced, Asda*	½ Can/196g	314	19.6	160	13.0	4.6	10.0	0.1
Onions, with Gravy, Minced, Lean, Sainsbury's*	1 Can/198g	285	13.9	144	17.0	3.1	7.0	0.2
Potatoes, Minced, LC, Tesco*	1 Pack/450g	400	9.5	80	4.3	10.3	1.9	2.3
BEEF BOURGUIGNON								
Extra Special, Asda*	1 Serving/300g	279	11.0	93	9.3	5.7	3.7	0.7
Finest, Tesco*	½ Pack/300g	247	7.8	82	9.9	4.8	2.6	0.5
BEEF BRAISED								
& Cabbage, Steak, COU, M&S*	1 Pack/380g	323	9.9	85	8.3	6.7	2.6	1.9
& Mash, Steak,,Classic, CBY, Asda*	1 Pack/453g	358	11.3	79	7.6	5.7	2.5	1.8
& Mash, Steak, M Kitchen, Morrisons*	1 Meal/250g	209	6.0	87	6.4	9.1	2.5	1.1
in Ale, with Mash & Baby Onions, COU, M&S*	1 Pack/400g	380	9.2	95	7.4	11.0	2.3	1.4
Tender, Pub Specials, Birds Eye*	1 Pack/450g	243	3.6	54	5.5	6.1	0.8	1.8
BEEF CANTONESE								
Sainsbury's*	½ Pack/175g	200	2.3	114	5.5	20.1	1.3	0.5
BEEF CHASSEUR								
Somerfield*	1 Serving/275g	287	7.4	104	14.8	5.2	2.7	2.1
BEEF CHILLI								
Crispy, Cantonese, Chilled, Sainsbury's*	1 Pack/250g	682	38.8	273	11.4	22.1	15.5	1.9
Crispy, Tesco*	1 Pack/250g	472	17.2	189	10.8	21.0	6.9	0.5
Sweet, Asda*	1 Pack/400g	356	3.6	89	7.8	12.3	0.9	1.9
BEEF DINNER								
Roast, 102, Oakhouse Foods Ltd*	1 Dinner/400g	444	18.4	111	6.8	10.6	4.6	1.3
Roast, Iceland*	1 Serving/340g	354	12.6	104	8.5	9.1	3.7	1.6
Roast, Sainsbury's*	1 Pack/400g	356	6.8	89	6.5	12.0	1.7	1.9
Roast with Trimmings	1 Dinner/840g	1310	63.0	156	6.1	17.7	7.5	2.3
BEEF HOT & SOUR								
Chef's Selection, M&S*	1 Pack/329g	395	17.4	120	9.2	8.4	5.3	1.3
BEEF IN								
Ale, Diet Chef Ltd*	1 Meal/300g	201	3.6	67	8.2	6.0	1.2	2.1
Ale Gravy, Chunky, Birds Eye*	1 Pack/340g	272	6.8	80	7.4	8.3	2.0	1.5
Black Bean Sauce, Chinese, Tesco*	1 Pack/400g	396	12.4	99	9.1	8.7	3.1	0.5
Black Bean Sauce, M&S*	1 Pack/350g	402	22.4	115	8.9	5.7	6.4	1.1
Black Bean Sauce, with Egg Noodles, M&S*	1 Pack/400g	460	6.0	115	8.6	16.7	1.5	1.8
Black Pepper Sauce, & Egg Fried Rice, Tesco*	1 Pack/451g	622	24.8	138	7.0	15.2	5.5	1.2
Chilli Sauce, Strips, Tesco*	1 Pack/166g	290	7.8	175	23.2	9.6	4.7	0.0
Gravy, Roast, Birds Eye*	1 Pack/227g	177	3.9	78	13.4	2.2	1.7	0.0
Gravy, Sliced, Iceland*	1 Pack/200g	172	3.2	86	12.1	5.9	1.6	0.3
Gravy, Sliced, Tesco*	1 Serving/200g	152	4.2	76	11.3	3.1	2.1	0.2
Oyster Sauce, Asda*	1 Serving/100g	82	4.0	82	7.0	4.4	4.0	1.7
Peppercorn Crust, Pink, Easy, Steak, Waitrose*	1 Steak/125g	195	6.6	156	18.4	8.6	5.3	1.1
Peppercorn Sauce, Creamy, Steak, Tesco*	1 Steak/150g	189	8.2	126	16.5	2.6	5.5	0.1
Peppercorn Sauce, Rump, Waitrose*	½ Pack/180g	189	5.9	105	17.9	0.9	3.3	0.2
Red Wine, Burgundy, GFY, Asda*	1 Pack/405g	348	8.1	86	8.0	9.0	2.0	1.1
Red Wine Sauce, Milson's Kitchen, Aldi*	1 Pack/400g	256	6.0	64	5.6	9.6	1.5	2.1
BEEF SZECHUAN								
Spicy, Sizzling Hot, Oriental Express*	1 Pack/400g	380	7.6	95	6.4	13.2	1.9	2.0
BEEF TERIYAKI								
Incredibly Tender, Charlie Bigham's*	½ Pack/300g	477	26.7	159	5.0	10.9	8.9	0.9
with Noodles, BGTY, Sainsbury's*	1 Pack/400g	320	4.0	80	7.7	10.1	1.0	1.0

	Measure INFO/WEIGHT	per Measure		Nutrition Values per 100g / 100ml				
		KCAL	FAT	KCAL	PROT	CARB	FAT	FIBRE
BEEF WELLINGTON								
Average	1 Serving/200g	530	33.3	265	12.4	17.0	16.6	1.0
Finest, Tesco*	1/3 Pack/216g	525	33.9	243	13.0	12.3	15.7	1.5
BEEF WITH								
Black Bean Sauce, Chilli, Sainsbury's*	1 Pack/300g	336	14.4	112	8.7	8.6	4.8	1.0
Black Bean Sauce, Rice Bowl, Uncle Ben's*	1 Pack/350g	368	4.9	105	5.6	17.4	1.4	0.0
Diane Sauce, Rump Steak, Tesco*	1 Steak/165g	182	8.1	110	15.1	1.1	4.9	0.3
Onion & Gravy, Minced, Princes*	1 Serving/200g	342	24.4	171	9.9	5.5	12.2	0.0
Onions & Gravy, Minced, Tesco*	1 Can/198g	224	10.1	113	14.0	2.8	5.1	0.8
Oyster Sauce, Ooodles of Noodles, Oriental Express*	1 Pack/425g	378	5.5	89	4.9	14.2	1.3	1.5
Peppercorn Sauce, Rib Eye Joint, Sainsbury's*	1 Serving/181g	299	12.7	165	22.2	3.4	7.0	0.1
Peppercorn Sauce, Steak, Fried, Simply Cook, Tesco*	½ Pack/125g	215	9.1	172	24.8	1.7	7.3	0.4
Peppercorn Sauce, Steak, Just Cook, Sainsbury's*	½ Pack/128g	174	7.3	136	17.7	3.4	5.7	1.2
Red Wine Sauce, Rump Steak, Tesco*	1 Serving/150g	180	8.6	120	17.2	0.1	5.7	3.3
Rigatoni Pasta, Chianti Ragu, Fuller Longer, M&S*	1 Pack/400g	440	14.4	110	8.5	11.0	3.6	1.8
Shiraz Wine Sauce, Pot Roast, Finest, Tesco*	1 Pack/350g	350	9.1	100	14.1	5.1	2.6	0.9
Vegetables & Gravy, Minced, Birds Eye*	1 Pack/178g	155	6.1	87	9.1	5.1	3.4	0.6
BEER								
Ale, Bottled, Old Speckled Hen*	1 Bottle/330ml	124	0.3	38	0.2	1.8	0.1	0.2
Ale, Hopping Hare, Hall & Woodhouse Ltd*	1 Bottle/500ml	188	0.0	38	0.4	3.0	0.0	0.0
Bitter, Average	**1 Can/440ml**	**141**	**0.0**	**32**	**0.3**	**2.3**	**0.0**	**0.0**
Bitter, Cask, Draught, London Pride, Fullers*	1 Pint/568ml	201	0.0	35	0.0	0.0	0.0	0.0
Bitter, Draught, Average	**1 Pint/568ml**	**182**	**0.0**	**32**	**0.3**	**2.3**	**0.0**	**0.0**
Bitter, Keg, Average	**1 Pint/568ml**	**176**	**0.0**	**31**	**0.3**	**2.3**	**0.0**	**0.0**
Bitter, Low Alcohol, Average	**1 Pint/568ml**	**74**	**0.0**	**13**	**0.2**	**2.1**	**0.0**	**0.0**
Bitter, Original, Tetley's*	1 Can/440ml	140	0.0	32	0.2	4.6	0.0	0.0
Bitter, Victoria, Carlton United Breweries*	1 Bottle/375ml	142	0.0	38	0.0	2.9	0.0	0.0
Brown Ale, Bottled, Average	**1 Bottle/330ml**	**99**	**0.0**	**30**	**0.3**	**3.0**	**0.0**	**0.0**
Especial, Modelo*	1 Bottle/355ml	145	0.0	41	0.0	1.1	0.0	0.0
Gingerbeard, Ale, Wychwood, Marstons PLC*	1 Bottle/500ml	304	0.0	61	0.3	3.0	0.0	0.0
Guinness*, Draught	**1 Can/440ml**	**158**	**0.2**	**36**	**0.3**	**3.0**	**0.0**	**0.0**
Guinness*, Stout	**1 Pint/568ml**	**205**	**0.0**	**36**	**0.3**	**3.0**	**0.0**	**0.0**
Guinness* Extra Stout, Bottled	**1 Bottle/500ml**	**215**	**0.0**	**43**	**4.0**	**0.0**	**0.0**	**0.0**
Honey Dew, Ale, Fullers*	1 Bottle/500ml	232	0.0	46	0.0	4.6	0.0	0.0
Kilkenny, Diageo*	1 Pint/568ml	210	0.0	37	0.3	3.0	0.0	0.0
Low Calorie, Low Carb, Cobra*	1 Bottle/330ml	96	0.0	29	0.1	1.3	0.0	0.0
Mackeson, Stout	**1 Pint/568ml**	**205**	**0.0**	**36**	**0.4**	**4.6**	**0.0**	**0.0**
Mild, Draught, Average	**1 Pint/568ml**	**136**	**0.0**	**24**	**0.2**	**1.6**	**0.0**	**0.0**
Non Alcoholic, Cobra*	1 Bottle/330ml	79	0.0	24	0.8	2.0	0.0	0.0
Oak Aged, Innis & Gunn*	1 Bottle/330ml	120	0.0	36	0.0	3.6	0.0	0.0
Old Peculiar Ale, Theakstons*	1 Serving/500ml	250	0.0	50	0.0	4.6	0.0	0.0
Pale Ale, IPA, Greene King*	1 Pint/570ml	158	0.1	28	0.3	1.6	0.0	0.3
Pale Ale, Sierra Nevada*	1 Bottle/350g	175	0.0	50	0.4	4.0	0.0	0.0
Premium, Lager, San Miguel*	1 Bottle/330ml	148	0.0	45	0.3	3.7	0.0	0.0
Raspberry, Framboise, Lindemans*	1 Serving/355ml	185	0.0	52	0.0	8.8	0.0	0.0
Scarecrow, Ale, Wychwood, Marstons PLC*	1 Bottle/500ml	214	0.0	43	0.4	4.3	0.0	0.0
Ultra, Michelob*	1 Bottle/275ml	88	0.0	32	0.0	0.9	0.0	0.0
Weissbier, Alcohol Free, Erdinger*	1 Bottle/500ml	125	0.0	25	0.4	5.3	0.0	0.0
Wheat, Tesco*	1 Bottle/500ml	155	0.0	31	0.5	0.4	0.0	0.0
Wychcraft, Ale, Wychwood, Marstons PLC*	1 Bottle/500ml	210	0.0	42	0.3	4.2	0.0	0.0
BEETROOT								
& Roasted Red Onion, M&S*	1 Serving/125g	94	2.6	75	1.5	12.6	2.1	2.5
Baby, Pickled, Average	**1 Beetroot/13g**	**5**	**0.0**	**37**	**1.7**	**7.2**	**0.1**	**1.2**
Cocktail, TTD, Sainsbury's*	½ Pack/100g	87	0.1	87	0.9	20.7	0.1	1.5

	Measure INFO/WEIGHT	per Measure		Nutrition Values per 100g / 100ml				
		KCAL	FAT	KCAL	PROT	CARB	FAT	FIBRE
BEETROOT								
Cooked, Boiled, Drained, Average	*1 Serving/100g*	*44*	*0.2*	*44*	*1.7*	*10.0*	*0.2*	*2.0*
Cooked, Morrisons*	1 Serving/100g	37	0.3	37	1.6	5.8	0.3	2.2
Crinkle Cut, Drained, Baxters*	1 Slice/10g	3	0.0	26	1.2	5.1	0.1	1.2
in Sweet Vinegar, Shredded, Drained, Sainsbury's*	1 Serving/49g	28	0.0	57	1.1	11.4	0.1	1.3
Pickled, in Sweet Vinegar, Average	*1oz/28g*	*16*	*0.0*	*57*	*1.2*	*12.8*	*0.1*	*1.5*
Pickled, in Vinegar, Average	*1 Serving/50g*	*19*	*0.0*	*37*	*1.6*	*7.5*	*0.1*	*1.2*
Raw, Average	*1oz/28g*	*9*	*0.0*	*32*	*1.6*	*6.0*	*0.1*	*1.8*
Rosebud, M&S*	½ Pack/90g	45	0.3	50	1.9	8.9	0.3	3.2
Salad, Essential, Waitrose*	1 Pack/250g	198	5.2	79	1.2	12.6	2.1	2.5
with Balsamic Vinaigrette, Side Salad, M&S*	1 Pack/225g	146	2.9	65	0.7	12.4	1.3	2.2
BHAJI								
Aubergine, & Potato, Fried in Vegetable Oil, Average	1oz/28g	36	2.5	130	2.0	12.0	8.8	1.7
Cabbage, & Pea, Fried in Vegetable Oil, Average	1oz/28g	50	4.1	178	3.3	9.2	14.7	3.4
Cauliflower, Fried in Vegetable Oil, Average	1oz/28g	60	5.7	214	4.0	4.0	20.5	2.0
Cauliflower, from 8 Snack Pack, Takeaway, Tesco*	1 Bhaji/18g	30	1.1	170	7.1	20.6	6.3	4.7
Mushroom, Fried in Vegetable Oil, Average	1oz/28g	46	4.5	166	1.7	4.4	16.1	1.3
Okra, Bangladeshi, Fried in Butter Ghee, Average	1oz/28g	27	1.8	95	2.5	7.6	6.4	3.2
Onion, Asda*	1 Bhaji/49g	96	4.9	196	6.0	20.0	10.0	2.0
Onion, Indian, Mini, Asda*	1 Bhaji/18g	33	1.8	186	4.9	19.0	10.0	6.0
Onion, Indian Starter Selection, M&S*	1 Bhaji/22g	65	5.1	295	5.7	15.8	23.3	2.8
Onion, Mini, Asda*	1 Bhaji/35g	63	2.8	179	4.8	22.0	8.0	4.4
Onion, Mini, Snack Selection, Sainsbury's*	1 Bhaji/22g	49	3.4	226	4.1	17.4	15.5	3.5
Onion, Mini, Tesco*	1 Bhaji/23g	48	1.9	210	7.3	26.7	8.2	1.3
Onion, Mini Indian Selection, Tesco*	1 Bhaji/23g	40	2.2	172	6.1	15.4	9.5	4.6
Onion, Sainsbury's*	1 Bhaji/38g	93	5.1	245	6.5	24.7	13.4	6.4
Onion, Tesco*	1 Bhaji/47g	85	4.9	181	5.7	16.2	10.4	4.3
Onion, Waitrose*	1 Bhaji/45g	124	9.4	276	4.7	17.5	20.8	2.5
Onion with Tomato & Chilli Dip, M&S*	1 Bhaji/54g	111	6.3	205	4.1	21.1	11.7	3.6
Potato, Onion & Mushroom, Fried, Average	1oz/28g	58	4.9	208	2.0	12.0	17.5	1.5
Potato, Spinach & Cauliflower, Fried, Average	1oz/28g	47	4.2	169	2.2	7.1	15.1	1.4
Potato & Onion, Fried in Vegetable Oil, Average	1oz/28g	45	2.8	160	2.1	16.6	10.1	1.6
Spinach, Fried in Vegetable Oil, Average	1oz/28g	23	1.9	83	3.3	2.6	6.8	2.4
Spinach & Potato, Fried in Vegetable Oil, Average	1oz/28g	53	3.9	191	3.7	13.4	14.1	2.3
Vegetable, Fried in Vegetable Oil, Average	1oz/28g	59	5.2	212	2.1	10.1	18.5	2.4
BHUNA								
Chicken, Curry, Tesco*	1 Serving/300g	396	22.8	132	11.4	4.5	7.6	0.5
Chicken, Indian Takeaway, Tesco*	1 Pack/350g	438	27.6	125	8.3	4.6	7.9	2.2
Chicken, with Naan Bread, Sharwood's*	1 Pack/375g	465	19.1	124	6.8	12.8	5.1	2.8
Chicken, with Rice, Ready Meal, Average	1 Pack/350g	444	20.8	127	9.4	8.9	5.9	1.4
Chicken Tikka, Tesco*	1 Pack/350g	438	23.4	125	11.3	5.0	6.7	0.9
Lamb, & Rice, Sainsbury's*	1 Pack/500g	619	26.5	124	7.4	11.6	5.3	2.0
Prawn, King, CBY, Asda*	1 Pack/375g	296	17.2	79	4.4	4.3	4.6	1.4
Prawn, King, M&S*	1 Pack/350g	262	13.3	75	6.7	3.3	3.8	1.5
Prawn, King, Morrisons*	1 Pack/350g	301	20.6	86	6.5	1.8	5.9	0.5
Prawn, Tandoori, Indian, Sainsbury's*	½ Pack/200g	152	8.0	76	5.5	4.5	4.0	1.7
BIERWURST								
Average	*1 Slice/10g*	*25*	*2.1*	*252*	*14.4*	*1.0*	*21.2*	*0.0*
BILBERRIES								
Fresh, Raw	*1oz/28g*	*8*	*0.1*	*30*	*0.6*	*6.9*	*0.2*	*1.8*
BILTONG								
Average	*1 Serving/25g*	*64*	*1.0*	*256*	*50.0*	*0.0*	*4.0*	*0.0*
BIRYANI								
Chicken, COU, M&S*	1 Pack/400g	360	8.4	90	6.9	10.8	2.1	1.9

	Measure INFO/WEIGHT	per Measure		Nutrition Values per 100g / 100ml				
		KCAL	FAT	KCAL	PROT	CARB	FAT	FIBRE
BIRYANI								
Chicken, Indian, Asda*	1 Pack/450g	778	22.5	173	9.0	23.0	5.0	0.7
Chicken, Ready Meal, Average	1 Pack/400g	521	17.1	130	7.5	15.2	4.3	1.6
Chicken, Ready Meal, Healthy Range, Average	1 Pack/400g	369	5.5	92	7.4	12.6	1.4	0.9
Chicken, Tikka, Ready Meal, Average	1 Pack/400g	460	11.5	115	7.3	14.8	2.9	1.5
Chicken, Weight Watchers*	1 Pack/330g	308	3.7	93	6.2	14.6	1.1	0.6
Chicken Tikka, & Lentil Pilau, Fuller Longer, M&S*	1 Pack/400g	440	11.6	110	9.5	12.0	2.9	2.3
Chicken Tikka, BGTY, Sainsbury's*	1 Pack/400g	316	3.8	84	6.8	10.7	1.0	2.9
Chicken Tikka, Northern Indian, Sainsbury's*	1 Pack/450g	698	25.6	155	9.4	16.5	5.7	1.2
Lamb, Average	1 Serving/200g	390	19.4	195	7.3	20.9	9.7	0.0
Lamb, Ready Meal, Average	1 Pack/400g	535	18.9	134	6.0	16.6	4.7	2.2
Seafood, M&S*	1 Pack/450g	619	25.7	138	7.1	14.4	5.7	1.7
Vegetable, & Rice, Sainsbury's*	½ Pack/125g	229	5.0	183	4.4	32.4	4.0	0.7
Vegetable, Sainsbury's*	1 Serving/225g	328	17.8	146	2.4	16.3	7.9	1.1
Vegetable, Waitrose*	1 Pack/450g	521	19.8	116	2.4	14.9	4.4	3.6
Vegetable with Rice, Patak's*	½ Pack/125g	194	1.9	155	3.6	32.9	1.5	1.2
BISCOTTI								
Almond, Kate's Cakes Ltd*	1 Biscotti/36g	137	5.5	381	8.8	51.7	15.4	3.1
Almond, Pan Ducale*	1 Serving/30g	130	5.0	433	10.0	60.0	16.7	3.3
Chocolate, Heinz*	1 Biscuit/20g	80	1.7	398	8.5	72.0	8.7	5.8
Chocolate Chip, Kate's Cakes Ltd*	1 Biscotti/36g	134	4.6	372	6.5	57.9	12.7	2.7
BISCUITS								
Abbey Crunch, McVitie's*	1 Biscuit/9g	43	1.6	477	6.0	72.8	17.9	2.5
Abernethy, Simmers*	1 Biscuit/12g	61	2.7	490	5.7	69.2	21.9	0.0
Ace Milk Chocolate, McVitie's*	1 Biscuit/24g	122	5.9	510	6.1	66.2	24.5	1.6
Aero, Nestle*	1 Bar/19g	99	5.5	534	6.4	59.4	29.4	2.1
Aero, Orange, Aero, Nestle*	1 Biscuit/19g	101	5.6	534	6.0	60.6	29.3	1.7
After Eight, Nestle*	1 Biscuit/5g	26	1.4	525	6.5	62.6	27.7	1.5
All Butter, Tesco*	1 Biscuit/9g	44	2.1	486	6.3	63.5	23.0	1.9
Almond, Artisan Bakery, Extra Special, Asda*	1 Biscuit/19g	103	6.1	548	7.9	54.3	32.3	4.2
Almond, Butter, Thins, Extra Special, Asda*	1 Biscuit/4g	15	0.5	375	5.0	60.0	12.5	2.5
Almond, Fingers, Tesco*	1 Finger/46g	180	6.8	391	6.2	58.4	14.7	1.0
Almond, Thins, Continental, Tesco*	1 Biscuit/3g	15	0.5	450	6.7	72.8	14.7	3.1
Almond, Thins, Sainsbury's*	1 Biscuit/3g	13	0.3	430	7.0	80.3	9.0	1.0
Almond, Thins, TTD, Sainsbury's*	1 Biscuit/4g	16	0.5	450	6.7	72.8	14.7	3.1
Almond & Chocolate, Biscotti, TTD, Sainsbury's*	1 Biscuit/30g	132	4.8	440	8.4	65.6	16.0	3.1
Amaretti, Doria*	1 Biscuit/4g	17	0.3	433	6.0	84.8	7.8	0.0
Amaretti, M&S*	1 Biscuit/6g	30	1.1	480	9.6	71.3	17.2	3.8
Amaretti, Sainsbury's*	1 Biscuit/6g	27	0.7	450	6.5	80.5	11.3	1.1
Apple & Blackberry, Oat Squares, Go Ahead, McVitie's*	1 Bar/40g	137	3.8	343	4.5	63.8	9.5	4.2
Apple & Cinnamon Thins, Finest, Tesco*	1 Biscuit/5g	22	0.8	470	5.9	71.7	17.5	1.5
Apple Crumble, Officially Low Fat, Fox's*	1 Biscuit/23g	85	0.6	365	5.4	80.4	2.4	2.5
Apricot, Low Fat, M&S*	1 Biscuit/23g	79	1.0	343	6.1	69.6	4.4	7.8
Arrowroot, Thin, Crawfords*	1 Biscuit/7g	35	1.2	450	6.9	71.4	15.2	2.8
Berry GI, Diet Chef Ltd*	1 Biscuit/20g	87	3.2	435	7.0	65.2	16.1	7.2
Bisc & M&M's, Master Foods*	1 Biscuit/17g	90	5.0	527	5.8	59.2	29.6	0.0
Bisc & Twix, Master Foods*	1 Bar/27g	140	7.6	520	5.2	61.1	28.3	0.0
Biscbits, Honeycomb Crunch, Cadbury*	7 Pieces/25g	120	5.2	480	6.0	67.3	20.9	1.4
Blueberry, Biscuit Moments, Special K, Kellogg's*	2 Biscuits/25g	99	2.3	394	4.5	73.0	9.0	1.5
Blueberry & Vanilla, Oaty, Weight Watchers*	1 Biscuit/19g	86	3.3	452	7.3	62.1	17.6	8.0
Bn, Chocolate Flavour, McVitie's*	1 Biscuit/18g	83	3.0	460	6.6	71.0	16.7	2.6
Bn, Strawberry Flavour, McVitie's*	1 Biscuit/18g	71	1.2	395	5.6	78.0	6.8	0.0
Bn, Vanilla Flavour, McVitie's*	1 Biscuit/18g	85	3.0	470	5.9	74.0	16.6	1.2
Bourbon, Average	1 Biscuit/13g	63	2.8	488	5.7	68.2	21.3	2.1

BISCUITS

	Measure INFO/WEIGHT	per Measure KCAL	per Measure FAT	Nutrition Values per 100g / 100ml KCAL	PROT	CARB	FAT	FIBRE
Bourbon, Trufree*	1 Biscuit/13g	61	2.8	486	7.5	62.6	22.6	1.1
Bourbon Creams, Asda*	1 Biscuit/14g	67	3.1	482	5.0	66.0	22.0	3.4
Bourbon Creams, Sainsbury's*	1 Biscuit/13g	60	2.4	476	5.7	70.4	19.1	1.7
Bourbon Creams, Tesco*	1 Biscuit/14g	68	3.0	485	5.4	66.2	21.6	3.4
Bourbon Creams, Value, Multipack, Tesco*	1 Biscuit/13g	62	2.9	494	5.9	68.0	22.8	1.7
Bournville, Cadbury*	1 Biscuit/16g	85	5.0	520	6.0	54.9	30.7	1.4
Brandy Snaps, Average	1 Biscuit/15g	69	2.2	460	2.7	79.8	14.4	0.5
Breakfast, Average	4 Biscuits/56g	249	8.8	445	11.8	61.7	15.7	7.0
Breakfast, Cranberry, Belvita, Nabisco*	4 Biscuits/50g	220	6.9	435	8.3	67.5	13.7	5.7
Breakfast, Forest Fruits, Belvita, Nabisco*	1 Biscuit/13g	60	2.1	460	8.5	67.0	16.0	5.3
Breakfast, Honey & Nuts, Belvita, Nabisco*	1 Biscuit/13g	58	2.1	464	8.0	68.0	17.0	3.5
Breakfast, Honey & Yoghurt Crunch, Belvita, Kraft*	2 Biscuits/51g	230	8.6	455	7.6	66.0	17.0	4.0
Breakfast, Muesli, Belvita, Nabisco*	1 Biscuit/13g	59	2.1	455	8.2	67.0	16.0	4.1
Breakfast, Oats, Apple, Sultana & Cinnamon, McVitie's*	4 Biscuits/50g	224	6.6	447	9.2	70.0	13.3	5.3
Breakfast, Original, All Bran, Kellogg's*	1 Pack/40g	176	8.0	440	8.0	49.0	20.0	16.0
Breakfast, Porridge Oats, with Oats & Honey, McVitie's*	4 Biscuits/50g	226	7.0	452	9.6	69.5	14.0	4.6
Breakfast, Porridge Oats, with Red Berries, McVitie's*	4 Biscuits/50g	226	6.9	452	9.6	71.0	13.8	5.1
Breakfast, Strawberry & Yoghurt, Duo Crunch, Belvita*	1 Biscuit/25g	109	3.8	435	72.0	66.5	15.0	3.2
Breakfast, Yogurt Crunch, Belvita, Nabisco*	2 Biscuits/50g	230	8.6	455	7.6	66.0	17.0	4.0
Butter, Chocolate Covered, Dark 70%, Green & Black's*	1 Biscuit/12g	62	3.5	520	7.1	5.6	29.4	0.1
Butter, Crinkle Crunch, Fox's*	1 Biscuit/11g	50	1.9	460	5.8	69.8	17.5	2.4
Butter, Milk Chocolate, Wilko*	1 Biscuit/14g	72	3.6	511	7.0	61.0	26.0	2.6
Cafe Noir, McVitie's*	1 Biscuit/9g	39	0.5	420	4.5	87.0	5.5	1.1
Cantucci with Honey, Loyd Grossman*	1 Biscuit/7g	32	1.1	450	9.5	66.3	16.3	0.9
Cantuccini, Sainsbury's*	1 Biscotti/8g	35	1.3	440	10.4	63.1	16.2	4.4
Cantuccini, with Almonds, Average	1 Biscotti/30g	130	5.0	433	10.0	60.0	16.7	3.3
Caramel & Honeycomb Cream, Velverty, Fox's*	1 Biscuit/19g	104	6.3	546	6.7	55.0	32.9	1.4
Caramel Crunch, Go Ahead, McVitie's*	1 Bar/24g	106	3.3	440	4.7	76.6	13.8	0.8
Caramelised, Lotus*	1 Biscuit/9g	43	1.7	483	4.9	72.7	18.9	1.3
Caramels, Milk Chocolate, McVitie's*	1 Serving/17g	81	3.6	478	5.6	65.8	21.4	1.8
Cheddars, Real Cheddar Cheese, Jacob's*	1 Biscuit/4g	20	1.2	526	11.0	48.6	32.1	3.0
Cheese, & Chutney, Delicious, Boots*	1 Pack/134g	290	14.7	217	9.0	19.0	11.0	2.3
Cheese Melts, Carr's*	1 Biscuit/4g	20	0.9	483	11.2	57.0	22.5	3.9
Cheese Sandwich, Ritz*	1 Biscuit/9g	50	2.8	530	9.5	55.0	30.2	2.0
Cheese Savouries, Sainsbury's*	1 Serving/50g	268	15.3	536	11.6	53.3	30.6	2.5
Cherry Bakewell, Handfinished, M&S*	1 Biscuit/40g	200	9.7	495	5.9	62.1	24.0	0.5
Choc Chip, Double, Trufree*	1 Biscuit/11g	58	3.0	523	3.0	67.0	27.0	1.8
Choc Chip, Paterson's*	1 Biscuit/17g	79	3.6	474	5.6	64.0	21.6	3.1
Chockas, Original, Fox's*	1 Biscuit/24g	85	1.0	355	1.1	10.4	4.2	0.4
Choco Leibniz, Dark Chocolate, Bahlsen*	1 Biscuit/14g	69	3.6	493	6.8	59.0	26.0	5.1
Choco Leibniz, Milk, Bahlsen*	1 Biscuit/14g	72	3.6	515	7.9	63.4	25.5	2.4
Choco Leibniz, Orange Flavour, Bahlsen*	1 Biscuit/14g	70	3.7	504	7.9	58.5	26.4	0.0
Chocolate, & Coconut, Duchy Originals*	1 Biscuit/13g	68	4.3	543	6.3	52.1	34.4	2.6
Chocolate, & Hazelnut, Quirks, McVitie's*	1 Biscuit/13g	66	3.6	511	5.0	58.4	28.0	2.6
Chocolate, Belgian, Selection, Finest, Tesco*	1 Biscuit/10g	52	2.7	515	6.0	62.0	27.0	3.0
Chocolate, Belgian, Thins, Extra Special, Asda*	1 Biscuit/9g	44	2.0	503	7.0	67.0	23.0	0.2
Chocolate, Belgian Chocolate, Weight Watchers*	1 Biscuit/18g	87	4.1	481	7.1	61.8	22.8	4.5
Chocolate, Breakaway, Nestle*	1 Bar/19g	99	4.9	509	6.0	62.7	25.2	3.7
Chocolate, Dark, All Butter, M&S*	1 Biscuit/15g	72	4.1	480	6.9	52.4	27.2	11.4
Chocolate, Double, Quirks, McVitie's*	1 Biscuit/13g	66	3.6	505	5.0	57.2	27.8	3.2
Chocolate, Extremely Chocolatey, Orange, M&S*	1 Biscuit/24g	120	6.2	510	7.5	59.9	26.5	2.7
Chocolate, Extremely Chocolatey, Rounds, M&S*	1 Biscuit/19g	97	5.6	510	6.2	55.7	29.3	6.3
Chocolate, Fingers, Average	1 Biscuit/6g	31	1.6	514	6.7	61.4	26.8	1.5

BISCUITS

	Measure INFO/WEIGHT	per Measure KCAL	FAT	Nutrition Values per 100g / 100ml KCAL	PROT	CARB	FAT	FIBRE
Chocolate, Golden Crunch, Free From Milk, Tesco*	1 Biscuit/17g	85	4.9	510	4.2	57.2	29.4	4.6
Chocolate, Milk, Belgian, M&S*	1 Biscuit/12g	60	2.5	490	6.2	70.1	20.3	2.5
Chocolate, Plain, Break, Tesco*	1 Biscuit/21g	112	6.1	535	6.7	61.2	29.2	3.8
Chocolate, Quirks, McVitie's*	1 Biscuit/13g	66	3.6	509	5.0	58.7	27.7	2.5
Chocolate, Seville, Thorntons*	1 Biscuit/19g	97	5.3	512	5.7	59.0	28.1	0.0
Chocolate, Teddy, Arnotts*	1 Biscuit/17g	80	3.2	478	6.6	69.3	19.2	2.0
Chocolate, Triple, Fox's*	1 Biscuit/21g	100	5.2	478	5.7	57.3	25.1	2.5
Chocolate, Viennese, Fox's*	1 Biscuit/16g	85	4.9	530	6.7	56.6	30.7	1.7
Chocolate Chip, Belgian, Walkers Shortbread Ltd*	2 Biscuits/25g	124	6.1	494	5.1	63.3	24.5	2.2
Chocolate Chip & Peanut, Trufree*	1 Biscuit/11g	55	2.6	496	4.0	66.0	24.0	2.0
Chocolate Chip GI, Diet Chef Ltd*	1 Pack/20g	90	3.6	450	7.4	64.4	17.9	6.4
Chocolate Fingers, Caramel, Cadbury*	1 Finger/8g	39	1.9	490	5.8	63.2	23.8	0.0
Chocolate Fingers, Milk, Cadbury*	1 Biscuit/6g	31	1.6	515	6.8	60.8	27.1	1.7
Chocolate Fingers, Milk, Extra Crunchy, Cadbury*	1 Biscuit/5g	25	1.2	505	6.6	66.2	23.6	0.0
Chocolate Fingers, Plain, Cadbury*	1 Biscuit/6g	30	1.6	508	6.2	60.6	26.8	0.0
Chocolate Florentine, M&S*	1 Serving/39g	195	9.7	500	7.4	64.5	24.9	1.7
Chocolate Ginger, Dark, Border*	1 Biscuit/17g	74	3.4	445	4.4	61.4	20.1	2.9
Chocolate Ginger, Dark, M&S*	1 Biscuit/21g	105	5.7	505	5.0	58.8	27.6	4.2
Chocolate Ginger, Organic, Duchy Originals*	1 Biscuit/12g	64	3.6	518	4.6	59.7	29.0	2.1
Chocolate Ginger, Thorntons*	1 Biscuit/19g	96	5.3	512	5.9	58.2	28.4	0.0
Chocolate Kimberley, Jacob's*	1 Biscuit/20g	86	3.4	428	3.9	64.4	17.2	1.1
Chocolate Mousse Meringue, Occasions, Sainsbury's*	1 Biscuit/47g	245	14.4	522	5.6	55.7	30.7	3.2
Chocolinis, Milk Chocolate, Go Ahead, McVitie's*	1 Biscuit/12g	56	1.7	466	7.7	77.2	14.0	2.0
Chocolinis, Plain Chocolate, McVitie's*	1 Biscuit/12g	56	1.8	468	6.9	77.0	14.7	2.6
Christmas Shapes, Assorted, Sainsbury's*	1 Biscuit/15g	77	4.3	525	5.2	59.0	29.8	1.7
Classic, Chocolate, Milk, Fox's*	1 Biscuit/13g	67	3.1	517	6.1	64.9	24.0	1.6
Coconut Crinkle, Fox's*	1 Biscuit/11g	53	2.5	487	5.2	63.8	22.6	3.7
Coconut Crinkle, Sainsbury's*	1 Biscuit/11g	54	2.8	500	6.4	59.6	26.2	3.7
Coconut Rings, Asda*	1 Biscuit/8g	37	1.7	486	6.0	66.0	22.0	2.6
Coconut Rings, Tesco*	1 Biscuit/9g	44	2.0	485	6.2	66.1	21.7	2.6
Cranberry, Crispy Slices, LC, Tesco*	1 Biscuit/15g	54	0.6	370	6.0	76.0	3.9	5.5
Cranberry & Pumpkin Seed, BGTY, Sainsbury's*	1 Biscuit/17g	68	2.8	410	7.2	56.6	17.1	13.9
Cranberry & Sunflower Seed, Oaty, Weight Watchers*	1 Biscuit/19g	87	3.7	457	7.9	58.0	19.3	10.0
Creams, Classic, Fox's*	1 Biscuit/14g	72	3.6	516	4.4	65.2	25.8	1.7
Crinkles, Classics, Milk Chocolate, Fox's*	1 Biscuit/14g	67	3.1	487	5.7	65.2	22.7	2.7
Crispy Slices, Apple, Sultana, Go Ahead, McVitie's*	1 Slice/13g	50	0.9	388	5.4	74.0	7.1	2.9
Crispy Slices, Forest Fruit, Go Ahead, McVitie's*	1 Biscuit/13g	49	0.9	380	5.4	73.7	7.0	3.0
Crispy Slices, Orange Sultana, Go Ahead, McVitie's*	1 Biscuit/13g	49	0.9	377	5.7	73.4	6.7	2.9
Crispy Slices, Raspberry, Go Ahead, McVitie's*	1 Slice/13g	50	0.9	385	5.3	74.0	7.0	2.8
Crispy Slices, Red Cherry, Go Ahead, McVitie's*	3 Slices/39g	147	2.7	380	5.5	73.9	7.0	2.9
Crunchers, Salted, Savoury, Crackers, Sainsbury's*	1 Cracker/5g	22	1.0	448	6.1	59.4	20.4	1.4
Crunchy Caramel, Tesco*	1 Bar/21g	98	5.2	467	4.6	56.0	25.0	1.4
Crunchy Oats, Breakfast, Belvita, Nabisco*	1 Biscuit/13g	59	2.1	455	8.0	67.0	16.0	5.5
Custard Cream, Gluten & Wheat Free, Lovemore*	1 Biscuit/15g	71	2.5	475	0.0	33.0	16.8	0.0
Custard Creams, 25% Less Fat, Asda*	1 Biscuit/10g	47	1.8	474	6.0	72.0	18.0	1.2
Custard Creams, 25% Less Fat, Sainsbury's*	1 Biscuit/13g	59	2.2	469	5.8	72.7	17.3	1.3
Custard Creams, 25% Less Fat, Tesco*	1 Biscuit/13g	59	2.2	473	5.8	72.2	17.9	1.2
Custard Creams, Asda*	1 Biscuit/12g	59	2.7	495	5.0	67.0	23.0	2.0
Custard Creams, BGTY, Sainsbury's*	1 Biscuit/12g	56	2.1	473	5.8	72.2	17.9	1.2
Custard Creams, Crawfords*	1 Biscuit/11g	57	2.7	517	5.9	69.2	24.1	1.5
Custard Creams, Everyday Value, Tesco*	1 Biscuit/13g	62	2.6	495	5.6	69.7	20.9	1.7
Custard Creams, Jacob's*	1 Biscuit/16g	77	3.3	481	5.3	68.0	20.9	1.6
Custard Creams, Sainsbury's*	1 Biscuit/13g	67	3.0	514	5.5	70.4	23.4	1.6

BISCUITS

Measure INFO/WEIGHT	per Measure KCAL	FAT	Nutrition Values per 100g / 100ml KCAL	PROT	CARB	FAT	FIBRE
BISCUITS							
Custard Creams, Smart Price, Asda* — 1 Biscuit/13g	61	2.6	486	6.0	69.0	21.0	1.6
Custard Creams, Tesco* — 1 Biscuit/13g	65	3.1	510	5.7	65.7	24.7	1.5
Custard Creams, Trufree* — 1 Biscuit/12g	60	2.8	504	8.7	65.0	23.0	1.0
Custard Creams, Value, Tesco* — 1 Biscuit/11g	51	1.6	450	7.2	72.5	14.3	3.0
Diet Fibre, Gullon* — 2 Biscuits/16g	65	2.6	405	6.5	48.7	16.4	23.0
Digestive, 25% Less Fat, Asda* — 1 Biscuit/16g	73	2.6	455	7.3	69.8	16.3	2.6
Digestive, 25% Less Fat, Tesco* — 1 Biscuit/14g	65	2.3	462	7.3	71.0	16.5	3.8
Digestive, BGTY, Sainsbury's* — 1 Biscuit/15g	70	2.6	468	7.4	71.0	17.2	3.8
Digestive, Caramels, Chocolate, Milk, McVitie's* — 1 Biscuit/17g	81	3.7	478	5.6	65.1	21.7	2.3
Digestive, Caramels, Chocolate, Plain, McVitie's* — 1 Biscuit/17g	82	3.8	481	5.7	65.5	22.1	2.1
Digestive, Chocolate — 1 Biscuit/17g	84	4.1	493	6.8	66.5	24.1	2.2
Digestive, Chocolate, Cadbury* — 1 Biscuit/17g	85	4.2	495	6.8	62.3	24.4	0.0
Digestive, Chocolate, Dark, McVitie's* — 1 Biscuit/17g	82	4.0	487	6.0	61.6	24.0	4.0
Digestive, Chocolate, Double, McVitie's* — 1 Biscuit/17g	83	4.0	496	6.5	60.8	24.2	3.6
Digestive, Chocolate, Milk, 25% Reduced Fat, McVitie's* — 1 Biscuit/17g	78	2.9	459	7.2	68.6	17.3	3.2
Digestive, Chocolate, Milk, Basics, Sainsbury's* — 1 Biscuit/14g	71	3.4	496	6.5	62.9	23.7	2.9
Digestive, Chocolate, Milk, GFY, Asda* — 1 Biscuit/17g	78	2.9	457	7.0	69.0	17.0	3.2
Digestive, Chocolate, Milk, Homewheat, McVitie's* — 1 Biscuit/17g	83	4.1	486	6.0	61.5	24.0	4.0
Digestive, Chocolate, Milk, M&S* — 1 Biscuit/17g	85	4.4	505	6.1	62.2	26.0	2.6
Digestive, Chocolate, Milk, McVitie's* — 1 Biscuit/17g	84	4.0	488	6.7	62.7	23.4	2.9
Digestive, Chocolate, Milk, Mini, McVitie's* — 1 Bag/25g	124	6.2	496	6.6	61.9	24.7	2.9
Digestive, Chocolate, Milk, Mini, Tesco* — 1 Pack/30g	153	8.1	510	6.6	59.8	27.1	1.8
Digestive, Chocolate, Milk, Mint, McVitie's* — 1 Biscuit/17g	81	3.9	487	6.7	62.6	23.4	2.9
Digestive, Chocolate, Milk, Sainsbury's* — 1 Biscuit/17g	87	6.3	511	6.9	65.9	36.8	2.5
Digestive, Chocolate, Milk, Tesco* — 1 Biscuit/17g	84	4.2	497	6.8	62.4	24.5	2.7
Digestive, Chocolate, Milk, Trufree* — 1 Biscuit/12g	63	3.0	521	4.0	70.0	25.0	2.0
Digestive, Chocolate, Plain, Asda* — 1 Biscuit/17g	84	4.0	500	7.0	64.0	24.0	3.2
Digestive, Chocolate, Plain, Tesco* — 1 Biscuit/17g	85	4.1	499	6.2	63.5	24.4	2.8
Digestive, Chocolate Chip, Asda* — 1 Biscuit/14g	68	3.2	491	6.0	65.0	23.0	2.9
Digestive, Cracker Selection, Tesco* — 1 Biscuit/12g	56	2.3	464	7.1	65.2	19.4	4.3
Digestive, Crawfords* — 1 Biscuit/12g	58	2.4	484	7.1	68.8	20.0	3.4
Digestive, Creams, McVitie's* — 1 Biscuit/12g	60	2.8	502	5.6	68.2	23.0	2.1
Digestive, Economy, Sainsbury's* — 1 Biscuit/13g	65	3.0	498	6.8	66.3	22.8	3.3
Digestive, Everyday Value, Tesco* — 1 Biscuit/16g	80	3.4	490	6.7	66.5	21.0	3.0
Digestive, GF, Barkat* — 1 Biscuit/15g	56	2.7	378	3.4	49.3	18.5	18.4
Digestive, Gluten & Wheat Free, Lovemore* — 1 Biscuit/15g	55	2.7	378	3.4	49.3	18.5	18.4
Digestive, Happy Shopper* — 1 Biscuit/13g	64	2.9	498	6.8	66.3	22.8	3.3
Digestive, High Fibre, Reduced Sugar, M&S* — 1 Biscuit/13g	60	2.8	460	6.5	59.3	21.7	9.4
Digestive, Hovis* — 1 Biscuit/6g	27	1.1	447	10.2	60.0	18.5	4.4
Digestive, Jacob's* — 1 Biscuit/14g	67	3.0	479	6.6	65.7	21.1	3.4
Digestive, Lemon & Ginger, McVitie's* — 1 Biscuit/15g	72	3.1	480	6.7	66.7	20.7	2.7
Digestive, Light, McVitie's* — 1 Biscuit/15g	65	2.1	437	7.3	69.5	14.4	3.6
Digestive, McVitie's* — 1 Biscuit/15g	70	3.2	470	7.2	62.7	21.5	3.6
Digestive, Oat, Weight Watchers* — 1 Biscuit/11g	50	2.1	457	6.0	66.3	18.6	6.9
Digestive, Organic, Sainsbury's* — 1 Biscuit/12g	60	2.9	483	6.6	60.9	23.7	5.8
Digestive, Plain, Average — 1 Biscuit/14g	67	2.9	480	7.1	65.6	20.5	3.5
Digestive, Plain, M&S* — 1 Biscuit/16g	80	3.9	490	6.5	62.7	23.8	3.3
Digestive, Reduced Fat, McVitie's* — 1 Biscuit/15g	70	2.4	467	7.1	72.8	16.3	3.4
Digestive, Reduced Fat, Tesco* — 1 Biscuit/16g	70	2.6	453	7.0	69.1	16.6	3.4
Digestive, Smart Price, Asda* — 1 Biscuit/14g	67	2.9	465	6.0	65.3	20.0	3.1
Digestive, Sweetmeal, Asda* — 1 Biscuit/14g	68	3.1	499	7.0	66.0	23.0	3.5
Digestive, Sweetmeal, Sainsbury's* — 1 Biscuit/14g	72	3.3	498	6.0	66.4	23.1	3.3
Digestive, Sweetmeal, Tesco* — 1 Biscuit/18g	80	2.6	444	8.4	70.0	14.5	3.1

BISCUITS

	Measure INFO/WEIGHT	per Measure KCAL	FAT	Nutrition Values per 100g / 100ml KCAL	PROT	CARB	FAT	FIBRE
Digestive, Trufree*	1 Biscuit/10g	48	2.2	485	6.1	62.4	22.1	6.2
Digestive, Value, Tesco*	1 Biscuit/15g	74	3.4	490	6.9	64.0	22.4	3.3
Digestive, Whole Wheat, Organic, Dove's Farm*	1 Biscuit/13g	56	2.4	446	5.9	61.6	19.5	7.8
Digestive, with Wheatgerm, Hovis*	1 Biscuit/12g	37	2.2	306	6.2	66.8	18.5	5.8
Florentines, Sainsbury's*	1 Florentine/8g	40	2.5	506	10.0	47.2	30.8	7.0
Fruit, All Butter, Sainsbury's*	1 Biscuit/9g	45	2.0	477	5.6	66.0	21.2	1.9
Fruit, Oat, GI, Diet Chef Ltd*	1 Biscuit/20g	85	2.9	425	7.8	65.3	14.7	7.6
Fruit & Fibre, Breakfast, Belvita, Nabisco*	1 Biscuit/13g	56	2.1	430	7.5	64.0	16.0	7.8
Fruit & Spice, Oat, Diet Chef Ltd*	2 Biscuits/20g	85	2.9	425	7.8	65.3	14.7	7.6
Fruit Bake, Organic, Tesco*	1 Biscuit/12g	53	2.1	453	7.5	65.1	18.1	5.6
Fruit Shortcake, McVitie's*	1 Biscuit/8g	37	1.6	464	5.7	65.1	20.1	2.7
Fruit Shortcake, Sainsbury's*	1 Biscuit/8g	39	1.6	483	5.9	69.6	20.1	2.1
Fruit Shortcake, Tesco*	1 Biscuit/9g	43	1.7	473	5.8	70.1	18.8	1.9
Fruit Shrewsbury, Mini Pack, Paterson's*	1 Biscuit/17g	81	3.8	484	4.9	64.9	22.7	1.9
Fruity, Oat, Organic, Dove's Farm*	1 Biscuit/12g	53	2.1	453	7.5	65.1	18.1	5.6
Fruity Iced, Blue Parrot Cafe, Sainsbury's*	1 Pack/20g	83	1.4	415	6.0	82.0	7.0	1.1
Galettes, Bonne Maman*	1 Serving/90g	460	22.5	511	6.0	65.7	25.0	0.0
Garibaldi, Asda*	1 Biscuit/10g	39	0.9	375	4.7	68.5	9.1	2.2
Garibaldi, Sainsbury's*	1 Biscuit/9g	35	1.0	389	5.7	67.1	10.9	3.3
Garibaldi, Tesco*	1 Biscuit/10g	40	0.9	400	4.7	74.0	9.1	2.2
Ginger, Belgian Dark Chocolate, Thins, Waitrose*	1 Biscuit/10g	48	2.2	481	6.2	61.2	22.5	4.6
Ginger, Crinkle, Sainsbury's*	1 Biscuit/11g	53	2.5	486	6.2	63.8	22.9	2.9
Ginger, Crinkle Crunch, Fox's*	1 Biscuit/12g	50	1.4	435	4.7	75.3	12.5	1.6
Ginger, Crunch, Hand Baked, Border*	1 Biscuit/12g	54	2.3	470	4.7	71.4	20.4	0.0
Ginger, Crunch, Organic, Against the Grain*	1 Biscuit/15g	71	3.4	474	2.8	65.6	23.0	1.2
Ginger, Crunch Creams, Fox's*	1 Biscuit/14g	73	3.7	518	4.6	64.8	26.7	0.0
Ginger, GI, Diet Chef Ltd*	1 Biscuit/20g	87	3.0	435	8.8	65.6	15.2	6.1
Ginger, Traditional, Fox's*	1 Biscuit/8g	33	1.0	404	4.4	70.1	11.7	1.4
Ginger, Value, Morrisons*	1 Biscuit/12g	55	1.9	459	5.3	74.0	15.8	1.7
Ginger Nuts, Asda*	1 Biscuit/10g	45	1.5	447	5.0	73.0	15.0	0.0
Ginger Nuts, McVitie's*	1 Biscuit/10g	47	1.7	459	5.5	71.1	16.6	2.3
Ginger Nuts, Milk Chocolate, McVitie's*	1 Biscuit/14g	68	2.8	489	5.8	71.8	19.9	1.5
Ginger Nuts, Tesco*	1 Biscuit/10g	46	1.5	450	5.3	73.2	14.7	2.2
Ginger Nuts, Value, Tesco*	1 Biscuit/12g	55	1.9	460	5.2	74.2	15.8	1.6
Ginger Snap, BGTY, Sainsbury's*	1 Biscuit/12g	51	1.2	427	6.5	78.2	9.8	1.8
Ginger Snap, Fox's*	1 Biscuit/8g	35	1.0	443	4.6	77.1	12.8	1.5
Ginger Snap, Less Than 10% Fat, Sainsbury's*	1 Biscuit/12g	51	1.1	424	6.5	78.9	9.1	1.9
Ginger Snap, Sainsbury's*	1 Biscuit/11g	47	1.6	445	5.3	73.0	14.7	2.2
Ginger Snap, Trufree*	1 Biscuit/11g	51	1.9	467	2.5	76.0	17.0	1.5
Ginger Thins, Anna's*	1 Biscuit/5g	24	1.0	480	6.0	70.0	20.0	2.0
Ginger Thins, Asda*	1 Biscuit/5g	23	0.8	462	6.0	73.0	16.0	1.9
Gingernut	1 Biscuit/11g	50	1.7	456	5.6	79.1	15.2	1.4
Golden Crunch, Bronte*	1 Biscuit/15g	69	3.3	474	5.1	62.5	22.6	0.0
Golden Crunch, Go Ahead, McVitie's*	1 Biscuit/9g	38	0.9	419	7.7	75.2	9.7	2.1
Golden Crunch, Paterson's*	1 Biscuit/15g	69	3.3	474	5.1	62.5	22.6	4.8
Golden Crunch Creams, Fox's*	1 Biscuit/15g	75	3.8	515	4.7	64.8	26.3	1.2
Golden Syrup, McVitie's*	1 Biscuit/12g	63	3.0	508	5.1	67.3	24.2	2.2
Gruyere, & Spinach, Twists, Savoury, Ardens*	1 Twist/7g	33	1.4	466	13.0	56.0	20.0	5.0
Happy Faces, Jacob's*	1 Biscuit/16g	78	3.6	485	4.8	66.1	22.3	1.6
Hazelnut, Crispies, Occasions, Sainsbury's*	1 Biscuit/7g	36	1.8	518	6.0	64.3	26.3	0.0
Hazelnut, Meringue, Sainsbury's*	1 Biscuit/6g	24	1.4	404	5.0	43.0	23.5	1.1
Hob Nobs, Chocolate, Milk, McVitie's*	1 Biscuit/19g	92	4.5	479	6.8	60.7	23.3	4.5
Hob Nobs, Chocolate, Mini, Milk, McVitie's*	1 Pack/25g	121	5.9	483	6.6	61.3	23.5	4.4

	Measure INFO/WEIGHT	per Measure KCAL	FAT	Nutrition Values per 100g / 100ml KCAL	PROT	CARB	FAT	FIBRE
BISCUITS								
Hob Nobs, Chocolate, Plain, McVitie's*	1 Biscuit/16g	81	3.9	498	6.7	63.3	24.3	4.2
Hob Nobs, Chocolate Creams, McVitie's*	1 Biscuit/12g	60	3.1	503	6.7	60.3	26.1	4.0
Hob Nobs, Light, 25% Reduced Fat, McVitie's*	1 Biscuit/14g	62	2.3	435	8.1	64.6	16.1	6.2
Hob Nobs, McVitie's*	1 Biscuit/15g	72	3.2	473	7.0	61.8	20.7	5.4
Hob Nobs, Munch Bites, McVitie's*	1 Pack/40g	203	10.1	508	6.8	63.4	25.2	2.8
Hob Nobs, Vanilla Creams, McVitie's*	1 Biscuit/12g	60	3.0	501	6.1	62.3	25.2	3.6
Iced Gems, Jacob's*	1 Serving/30g	118	0.9	393	5.0	86.3	3.1	2.0
Jaffa Cakes, Asda*	1 Cake/12g	43	1.0	368	4.7	67.5	8.8	1.9
Jaffa Cakes, Basics, Sainsbury's*	1 Jaffa Cake/11g	43	1.0	377	4.5	69.5	9.0	2.0
Jaffa Cakes, Blackcurrant, McVitie's*	1 Cake/12g	45	1.0	371	4.8	69.7	8.1	2.3
Jaffa Cakes, Chocolate, Dark, M&S*	1 Cake/11g	45	1.5	395	3.7	64.9	13.2	2.8
Jaffa Cakes, Chocolate, Dark, Mini, M&S*	1 Cake/5g	20	0.8	410	3.9	62.8	15.8	1.9
Jaffa Cakes, Chocolate, Plain, Sainsbury's*	1 Cake/13g	50	1.1	384	4.4	73.3	8.1	1.3
Jaffa Cakes, Free From, Asda*	1 Cake/12g	42	0.9	340	5.8	62.6	7.4	8.0
Jaffa Cakes, Lemon & Lime, McVitie's*	1 Cake/12g	45	1.0	370	4.7	69.5	8.1	2.1
Jaffa Cakes, Lunch Box, McVitie's*	1 Cake/7g	26	0.6	395	4.2	74.3	9.0	1.4
Jaffa Cakes, McVitie's*	1 Cake/12g	45	1.0	374	4.8	70.6	8.0	2.1
Jaffa Cakes, Mini, Asda*	1 Cake/5g	21	0.8	412	3.9	63.0	16.0	1.9
Jaffa Cakes, Mini, Bags, McVitie's*	1 Cake/5g	20	0.7	396	4.2	65.0	13.1	3.5
Jaffa Cakes, Mini, Tesco*	1 Cake/5g	19	0.6	380	4.0	64.0	12.0	2.0
Jaffa Cakes, Mini Roll, McVitie's*	1 Cake/30g	108	3.5	407	4.2	66.9	13.3	2.9
Jaffa Cakes, Mini Roll Xl, McVitie's*	1 Cake/44g	169	5.0	384	3.5	66.9	11.4	0.0
Jaffa Cakes, Sainsbury's*	1 Cake/11g	41	1.0	373	4.3	69.3	8.8	2.0
Jaffa Cakes, Smart Price, Asda*	1 Cake/12g	43	1.0	374	4.3	69.0	9.0	2.0
Jaffa Cakes, Value, Tesco*	1 Cake/11g	42	1.0	370	4.8	67.6	8.8	1.9
Jam Creams, Jacob's*	1 Biscuit/15g	75	3.4	486	5.0	67.4	21.8	1.6
Jam Rings, Crawfords*	1 Biscuit/12g	56	2.1	470	5.5	73.0	17.2	1.9
Jam Sandwich Creams, M&S*	1 Biscuit/17g	80	3.7	485	5.7	64.5	22.6	1.8
Jam Sandwich Creams, Sainsbury's*	1 Biscuit/16g	77	3.4	486	5.0	67.0	21.8	1.6
Jammie Dodgers, Minis, Lunchbox, Burton's*	1 Pack/20g	90	2.9	452	5.5	72.7	14.7	2.5
Jammie Dodgers, Original, Burton's*	1 Biscuit/19g	83	3.0	437	5.1	69.5	15.9	1.9
Kimberley, Bolands*	1 Biscuit/16g	72	1.7	449	5.1	82.6	10.9	1.4
Lebkuchen, Sainsbury's*	1 Biscuit/10g	39	0.8	400	5.7	76.1	8.0	1.3
Lemon, All Butter, Half Coated, Finest, Tesco*	1 Biscuit/17g	84	4.5	505	5.6	60.4	26.9	3.6
Lemon Butter, Thins, Sainsbury's*	1 Biscuit/13g	65	3.5	515	5.3	60.7	27.9	2.2
Lemon Puff, Jacob's*	1 Biscuit/13g	69	4.1	533	4.3	58.8	31.2	2.8
Lemon Thins, Sainsbury's*	1 Biscuit/10g	47	1.7	468	5.6	72.3	17.3	1.7
Malt, Basics, Sainsbury's*	1 Biscuit/8g	36	1.2	470	7.1	73.6	15.7	0.0
Malted Milk, Asda*	1 Biscuit/8g	39	1.8	490	7.0	66.0	22.0	2.0
Malted Milk, Average	1 Biscuit/9g	42	1.9	490	7.0	65.6	22.2	1.8
Malted Milk, Chocolate, Tesco*	1 Biscuit/10g	52	2.5	500	6.7	64.4	24.0	1.9
Malted Milk, Milk Chocolate, Asda*	1 Biscuit/11g	56	2.8	509	7.0	64.0	25.0	1.7
Malted Milk, Sainsbury's*	1 Biscuit/8g	40	1.8	488	7.1	65.5	21.9	2.0
Malted Milk, Tesco*	1 Biscuit/9g	43	1.9	490	6.6	66.7	21.8	2.0
Maple Leaf, M&S*	1 Biscuit/13g	50	1.9	395	5.1	59.8	14.8	2.0
Marie, Crawfords*	1 Biscuit/7g	33	1.1	475	7.5	76.3	15.5	2.3
Melts, Carr's*	1 Biscuit/4g	20	0.9	468	11.0	58.3	21.2	4.9
Melts, Sesame with Chive, Carr's*	1 Biscuit/5g	23	1.2	498	8.2	57.4	26.2	3.5
Mikado, Jacob's*	1 Biscuit/13g	53	1.6	397	4.2	67.7	12.1	2.5
Milk & Cereals, Breakfast, Belvita, Nabisco*	1 Biscuit/13g	56	1.9	445	8.7	69.0	15.0	3.6
Milk Chocolate, All Butter, M&S*	1 Biscuit/14g	70	3.6	490	7.9	57.4	25.5	1.4
Milk Chocolate, Assortment, Cadbury*	1 Serving/10g	51	2.6	510	6.8	61.0	26.4	0.0
Milk Chocolate, Tesco*	1 Biscuit/25g	135	7.3	535	6.4	62.1	29.0	1.8

BISCUITS

	Measure INFO/WEIGHT	per Measure KCAL	FAT	Nutrition Values per 100g / 100ml KCAL	PROT	CARB	FAT	FIBRE
Milk Chocolate Digestive, Value, Tesco*	1 Biscuit/17g	85	3.8	490	7.1	65.4	22.2	2.6
Mini Assortment, M&S*	1 Biscuit/3g	12	0.6	480	6.1	63.9	22.5	2.8
Mini Clotted Cream, Fosters Traditional Foods*	1 Biscuit/13g	66	3.6	507	5.4	59.5	27.4	0.0
Mint, Viscount*	1 Biscuit/13g	73	3.8	552	5.1	60.6	28.8	1.3
Morning Coffee, Asda*	1 Biscuit/5g	22	0.7	455	8.0	72.0	15.0	2.4
Morning Coffee, Tesco*	1 Biscuit/5g	22	0.7	450	7.6	72.3	14.5	2.4
Nice, Asda*	1 Biscuit/8g	38	1.7	480	6.0	68.0	21.0	2.4
Nice, Average	1 Biscuit/8g	36	1.6	484	6.3	67.3	21.0	2.5
Nice, Belmont, Aldi*	1 Biscuit/8g	39	1.6	489	6.2	68.9	20.4	2.3
Nice, Cream, Tesco*	1 Serving/10g	50	2.4	503	5.3	66.2	24.1	1.9
Nice, Fox's*	1 Biscuit/9g	39	1.7	450	6.3	62.4	19.4	5.0
Nice, Jacob's*	1 Biscuit/7g	33	1.3	471	6.1	68.5	19.2	1.8
Nice, Sainsbury's*	1 Biscuit/8g	40	1.7	486	5.9	68.3	20.9	2.7
Nice, Value, Multipack, Tesco*	1 Biscuit/8g	39	1.7	485	6.5	68.0	20.8	2.4
Nice, Value, Tesco*	1 Biscuit/5g	24	1.1	489	6.9	64.6	22.6	2.4
Oat, Fruit & Spice, Nairn's*	1 Biscuit/10g	43	1.5	425	7.8	65.3	14.7	7.6
Oat, Mixed Berries, Nairn's*	1 Biscuit/10g	43	1.5	427	7.5	64.8	15.3	7.1
Oat, Savoury, with Thyme, Rick Stein*	1 Biscuit/10g	46	2.1	460	9.8	66.9	21.4	10.4
Oat, Stem Ginger, Nairn's*	1 Biscuit/10g	43	1.5	434	8.8	65.6	15.2	6.1
Oat & Chocolate Chip, Cadbury*	1 Biscuit/17g	80	3.9	485	6.9	60.2	23.9	4.2
Oat & Wholemeal, Crawfords*	1 Biscuit/14g	67	3.0	482	7.7	64.2	21.6	4.8
Oat & Wholemeal, Dbc Foodservice*	1 Biscuit/14g	67	3.1	466	7.1	60.8	21.7	5.5
Oat Bites, Caramelised Onion, Diet Chef Ltd*	1 Pack/23g	99	3.9	430	7.5	64.2	16.8	6.0
Oat Bites, Cheese, Diet Chef Ltd*	1 Pack/23g	99	3.6	430	15.0	57.4	15.8	4.9
Oat Bites, Chilli, Diet Chef Ltd*	1 Pack/23g	128	3.1	556	8.1	68.4	13.3	7.2
Oat Crumbles, Border*	1 Biscuit/15g	66	3.1	443	5.3	58.9	20.7	1.8
Oat Crunch, M&S*	1 Biscuit/14g	65	2.7	450	7.8	62.0	18.7	6.1
Oat Crunch, Weight Watchers*	1 Biscuit/12g	52	2.1	448	7.4	65.2	17.8	6.1
Oat Digestives, Nairn's*	1 Biscuit/11g	50	2.0	437	12.0	57.8	17.5	7.8
Oat Digestives, TTD, Sainsbury's*	1 Biscuit/13g	56	2.3	448	9.8	56.4	18.5	8.5
Oaten, Organic, Duchy Originals*	1 Biscuit/16g	71	2.7	441	9.8	62.3	16.9	5.3
Oatie, Sweet, Scottish, Organic, Daylesford Organic*	1 Biscuit/23g	119	7.1	516	6.1	53.9	30.7	4.7
Oaties, Oatland, Tesco*	1 Biscuit/15g	70	3.1	470	6.5	64.9	20.5	4.5
Oatmeal, Asda*	1 Biscuit/12g	54	2.5	470	6.0	62.0	22.0	6.0
Oatmeal Crunch, Jacob's*	1 Biscuit/8g	37	1.5	458	6.8	65.9	18.6	3.6
Oaty Thins, Rude Health*	1 Thin/6g	23	0.3	380	11.5	68.5	4.7	8.7
Orange Chocolate, Organic, Duchy Originals*	1 Biscuit/13g	64	3.5	509	5.5	60.0	28.0	3.0
Orange Munchy Bites, Blue Riband, Nestle*	1 Box/125g	652	34.9	522	5.2	61.4	27.9	2.0
Orange Sultana, Go Ahead, McVitie's*	1 Biscuit/15g	58	1.2	400	5.1	75.7	8.1	3.0
Parmesan Cheese, Sainsbury's*	1 Biscuit/3g	18	1.0	553	14.7	56.4	29.9	1.8
Party Rings, Iced, Fox's*	1 Biscuit/6g	29	0.9	459	5.1	75.8	15.0	0.0
Peanut Butter, American Style, Sainsbury's*	1 Biscuit/13g	63	2.9	504	5.2	68.7	23.1	2.2
Peanut Butter Cups, Mini, Hershey*	1 Cup/8g	44	2.4	564	10.3	56.4	30.8	2.6
Petit Beurre, Stella Artois*	1 Biscuit/6g	26	0.9	440	9.0	73.0	15.0	0.0
Pink Wafers, Crawfords*	1 Biscuit/7g	36	1.9	521	2.5	68.6	26.5	1.1
Pink Wafers, Sainsbury's*	1 Biscuit/8g	36	1.8	486	4.6	64.2	23.4	1.7
Puffin, Chocolate, Asda*	1 Biscuit/25g	133	7.2	533	5.0	63.0	29.0	1.2
Raspberry & Cream Viennese, Melts, Fox's*	1 Biscuit/16g	84	4.5	521	4.0	62.1	28.1	1.7
Redcurrant Puffs, Eat Well, M&S*	1 Biscuit/7g	32	1.4	470	5.6	67.7	19.8	2.0
Rich Shorties, Asda*	1 Biscuit/10g	50	2.3	486	6.0	66.0	22.0	2.0
Rich Tea, 25% Less Fat, Tesco*	1 Biscuit/10g	44	1.1	435	7.1	77.0	11.0	1.3
Rich Tea, Average	1 Biscuit/10g	45	1.5	451	6.8	72.8	14.5	2.5
Rich Tea, Basics, Sainsbury's*	1 Biscuit/8g	35	1.2	450	7.1	71.3	15.2	2.9

BISCUITS

INFO/WEIGHT	per Measure KCAL	per Measure FAT	KCAL	PROT	CARB	FAT	FIBRE
Rich Tea, BGTY, Sainsbury's*	1 Biscuit/10g	43	1.1	430	7.8	75.9	10.6	2.4
Rich Tea, CBY, Asda*	1 Biscuit/8g	34	1.0	447	7.2	72.9	13.4	3.0
Rich Tea, Chocolate, Milk, Covered, Cadbury*	1 Biscuit/12g	60	2.6	490	6.6	67.6	21.4	0.0
Rich Tea, Chocolate, Milk, Sainsbury's*	1 Biscuit/13g	66	3.0	504	6.3	68.5	22.7	2.1
Rich Tea, Classic, McVitie's*	1 Biscuit/8g	38	1.3	453	7.1	71.2	15.5	2.9
Rich Tea, Essential, Waitrose*	1 Biscuit/8g	36	1.2	452	7.1	71.1	15.2	2.9
Rich Tea, Finger, Essential, Waitrose*	1 Biscuit/5g	22	0.7	450	7.2	72.5	14.3	3.0
Rich Tea, Finger, Tesco*	1 Finger/5g	23	0.7	451	7.4	72.9	14.4	2.3
Rich Tea, Fingers, Morrisons*	1 Finger/4g	22	0.7	550	10.0	90.0	17.5	5.0
Rich Tea, Light, McVitie's*	1 Biscuit/8g	36	0.9	431	7.5	75.0	11.3	3.1
Rich Tea, Low Fat, M&S*	1 Biscuit/9g	40	1.0	435	8.3	76.7	10.5	2.4
Rich Tea, Sainsbury's*	1 Biscuit/8g	34	1.0	440	7.2	72.7	13.4	3.0
Rich Tea, Tesco*	1 Biscuit/8g	36	1.2	460	7.3	72.4	15.2	2.3
Rich Tea, Value, Tesco*	1 Biscuit/8g	35	1.2	453	7.2	72.4	15.0	2.3
Rocky, Caramel, Rounds, Fox's*	1 Biscuit/15g	72	3.4	480	6.2	62.3	22.9	1.1
Rocky, Chocolate, & Caramel, Fox's*	1 Biscuit/21g	107	4.1	507	6.9	60.3	19.3	15.5
Rocky, Chocolate, Fox's*	1 Biscuit/21g	106	5.4	505	5.7	62.4	25.7	2.4
Rocky, Chocolate, Rounds, Fox's*	1 Biscuit/6g	31	1.7	517	7.2	58.5	28.3	1.6
Rocky, Funki Fudge, Fox's*	1 Biscuit/24g	125	6.6	520	6.9	60.3	27.7	1.1
Rolo, Nestle*	1 Biscuit/18g	95	4.7	507	4.4	64.2	25.2	0.6
Savoury, Organic, M&S*	1 Biscuit/7g	28	1.0	395	7.0	58.4	14.6	8.7
Shortbread, Fingers, Kate's Cakes Ltd*	2 Fingers/30g	141	8.0	471	4.6	52.8	26.8	1.6
Shortcake, Asda*	1 Biscuit/14g	73	3.6	518	5.0	66.0	26.0	2.0
Shortcake, Average	1 Biscuit/11g	55	3.0	501	6.3	66.1	27.1	2.1
Shortcake, Caramel, Average	1 Biscuit/37g	183	10.5	494	4.8	54.7	28.3	0.8
Shortcake, Caramel, Handmade Flapjack Company*	1 Biscuit/75g	383	23.0	511	4.6	54.3	30.6	0.0
Shortcake, Caramel, Mini, Finest, Tesco*	1 Biscuit/15g	74	4.2	493	4.3	56.3	27.8	1.0
Shortcake, Caramel, Mini, Thorntons*	1 Biscuit/15g	71	4.6	492	4.8	46.3	31.9	0.6
Shortcake, Caramel, Mr Kipling*	1 Biscuit/36g	182	10.4	506	4.2	57.6	28.8	1.3
Shortcake, Caramel, Squares, M&S*	1 Square/40g	190	9.6	475	5.5	59.7	23.9	1.0
Shortcake, Caramel, Squares, Tesco*	1 Square/54g	274	16.4	507	4.6	54.1	30.4	0.4
Shortcake, Chocolate, Dairy Milk, Cadbury*	1 Bar/49g	252	13.5	515	7.5	59.2	27.5	0.0
Shortcake, Crawfords*	1 Biscuit/10g	52	2.5	504	6.2	63.5	24.4	2.6
Shortcake, Dutch, M&S*	1 Biscuit/17g	90	5.2	530	5.7	58.2	30.6	0.9
Shortcake, Fruit, Crawfords*	1 Biscuit/8g	34	1.5	419	5.4	55.9	19.3	2.4
Shortcake, Jacob's*	1 Biscuit/10g	48	2.2	485	6.7	65.6	21.8	2.0
Shortcake, Mini Pack, Paterson's*	1 Biscuit/17g	82	4.2	490	5.5	60.8	25.0	3.2
Shortcake, Organic, Waitrose*	1 Biscuit/13g	64	3.2	495	5.8	63.0	24.4	1.8
Shortcake, Ring, Creations, Fox's*	1 Biscuit/20g	105	5.6	515	7.8	59.1	27.4	1.0
Shortcake, Sainsbury's*	1 Biscuit/11g	53	5.2	479	6.1	65.3	47.2	2.5
Shortcake, Snack, Cadbury*	2 Biscuits/15g	70	3.7	475	7.0	54.5	25.0	1.7
Shortcake, Value, Tesco*	1 Biscuit/10g	49	2.1	486	7.1	66.5	21.2	2.1
Shortcake, with Real Milk Chocolate, Cadbury*	1 Biscuit/15g	75	3.5	500	6.3	65.8	23.5	0.0
Shorties, Cadbury*	1 Biscuit/15g	77	3.6	511	6.5	67.3	24.0	0.0
Shorties, Chocolate, Mini, McVitie's*	1 Pack/25g	131	7.1	524	6.0	61.2	28.3	2.0
Shorties, Fruit, Value, Tesco*	1 Serving/10g	46	1.7	457	5.7	69.3	17.4	3.0
Shorties, Rich, Tesco*	1 Biscuit/10g	48	2.2	484	6.4	65.6	21.8	2.0
Shorties, Rich Highland, Tesco*	1 Biscuit/10g	48	2.2	485	6.1	65.3	21.7	2.6
Shorties, Sainsbury's*	1 Biscuit/10g	50	2.2	500	6.4	69.8	21.8	2.0
Signature Collection, Cadbury*	1 Biscuit/15g	80	4.4	530	6.2	60.1	29.5	0.0
Spiced, Whole Wheat, Prodia*	1 Biscuit/5g	17	1.0	339	7.1	41.4	19.4	8.5
Sports, Fox's*	1 Biscuit/9g	41	1.7	483	6.7	67.0	20.0	2.0
Stem Ginger, Brakes*	1 Biscuit/13g	62	3.1	495	5.6	62.6	24.7	0.0

BISCUITS

	Measure INFO/WEIGHT	per Measure KCAL	FAT	Nutrition Values per 100g / 100ml KCAL	PROT	CARB	FAT	FIBRE
Strawberry, Biscuit Moments, Special K, Kellogg's*	2 Biscuits/25g	98	2.0	391	5.0	74.0	8.0	1.5
Strawberry, Cream Tease, McVitie's*	1 Biscuit/19g	97	4.8	510	4.8	65.9	25.2	1.2
Sugar Wafers, Vanilla, Flavoured, Triunfo*	1 Biscuit/10g	53	2.5	511	4.1	70.1	24.3	0.6
Sultana, & Cinnamon, Weight Watchers*	1 Biscuit/12g	51	1.7	441	4.3	72.3	15.0	3.0
Summer Fruits, Big Softies, Fox's*	1 Bar/25g	89	0.6	356	5.9	77.8	2.6	0.0
Tangy Jaffa Viennese, Creations, Fox's*	1 Biscuit/17g	76	3.3	447	5.0	63.5	19.2	0.9
Taxi, McVitie's*	1 Biscuit/27g	134	6.9	504	4.2	63.3	26.0	0.7
Teddy Bear, Mini, M&S*	1 Biscuit/17g	80	3.8	475	5.4	62.6	22.7	3.2
Toffee Apple, Crumbles, Border Biscuits Ltd*	1 Biscuit/18g	77	3.7	427	5.0	56.7	20.4	2.3
Toffee Chip, Crinkle Crunch, Fox's*	1 Biscuit/11g	51	2.0	460	4.6	69.6	18.2	0.0
Toffee Dodgers, Burton's*	1 Biscuit/18g	84	3.2	468	5.7	71.4	17.5	1.1
Turkish Delight, Cadbury*	1 Biscuit/16g	70	3.1	445	5.5	62.0	20.0	0.9
Twix, Caramel Slice, McVitie's*	1 Slice/29g	142	7.8	491	4.5	57.3	26.8	1.4
Vanilla, Ser*	1 Biscuit/4g	14	0.3	408	8.5	77.0	8.2	3.0
Viennese, Bronte*	1 Biscuit/25g	106	6.2	424	4.4	45.6	24.8	0.0
Viennese, Chocolate, Melts, Fox's*	1 Biscuit/12g	64	3.4	526	6.1	60.5	28.3	2.4
Viennese, Jaffa, M&S*	1 Biscuit/17g	80	3.7	465	5.9	61.1	21.7	0.9
Viennese, Mini Pack, Paterson's*	1 Biscuit/20g	106	6.2	527	5.4	67.1	30.8	1.6
Viennese Creams, Raspberry, M&S*	1 Biscuit/17g	90	4.9	520	4.6	60.4	28.6	1.3
Viennese Creams, Strawberry, M&S*	1 Biscuit/17g	80	3.7	485	6.4	63.0	22.2	1.7
Viennese Finger, Mr Kipling*	1 Finger/32g	167	10.2	523	4.3	54.9	31.8	0.0
Viennese Sandwich, Chocolate, M&S*	1 Biscuit/15g	80	4.6	535	7.2	58.0	30.6	1.7
Viennese Whirl, Chocolate, Border*	1 Biscuit/19g	96	4.3	512	6.5	61.9	23.2	0.0
Viennese Whirl, Fox's*	1 Biscuit/25g	130	7.0	518	6.7	60.1	27.8	0.0
Wafer, Vanilla, Loacker*	1 Pack/45g	231	12.6	514	7.5	58.0	28.0	0.0
Water, Asda*	1 Biscuit/6g	25	0.5	412	10.0	75.0	8.0	3.3
Water, Average	1 Biscuit/6g	24	0.7	440	10.8	75.8	12.5	3.1
Water, High Bake, Jacob's*	1 Biscuit/5g	22	0.4	414	10.5	76.4	7.4	3.0
Water, High Bake, Sainsbury's*	1 Biscuit/5g	21	0.4	412	9.8	76.3	7.5	3.2
Water, High Baked, Tesco*	1 Biscuit/5g	20	0.4	405	10.1	75.0	7.1	4.2
Water, Table, Large, Carr's*	1 Biscuit/8g	30	0.6	400	9.9	73.1	7.5	4.1
Water, Table, Small, Carr's*	1 Biscuit/3g	14	0.3	406	10.1	80.0	7.6	4.2
Wholemeal Brans, Fox's*	1 Biscuit/20g	90	4.0	451	8.5	58.8	20.2	7.5
Yorkie, Nestle*	1 Biscuit/25g	128	6.7	510	6.7	60.4	26.8	1.3

BISON

	Measure INFO/WEIGHT	per Measure KCAL	FAT	Nutrition Values per 100g / 100ml KCAL	PROT	CARB	FAT	FIBRE
Raw	1oz/28g	31	0.5	109	21.6	0.0	1.8	0.0

BITES

	Measure INFO/WEIGHT	per Measure KCAL	FAT	Nutrition Values per 100g / 100ml KCAL	PROT	CARB	FAT	FIBRE
All Butter, Chocolate, M&S*	1 Biscuit/10g	55	3.1	530	7.9	57.0	30.1	3.5
Cheese & Garlic, M&S*	1 Bite/11g	40	3.1	350	8.3	17.2	27.3	5.8
Ciabatta, Garlic & Herb, Occasions, Sainsbury's*	1 Bite/12g	48	2.6	398	8.9	42.2	21.5	3.2
Corn Flake, Chocolate, Mini, Tesco*	1 Bite/14g	62	2.5	446	7.1	64.1	17.9	5.9
Crispy Potato, Salt & Vinegar, BGTY, Sainsbury's*	1 Bag/20g	71	0.5	356	5.9	77.4	2.5	4.4
Egg & Bacon, Mini, Savoury, Tesco*	1 Bite/18g	55	3.8	305	8.8	20.2	21.0	2.7
Milk Chocolate, Mini, Luxury, Holly Lane*	1 Bite/15g	72	3.9	479	5.1	55.5	26.3	2.5

BITTER LEMON

	Measure INFO/WEIGHT	per Measure KCAL	FAT	Nutrition Values per 100g / 100ml KCAL	PROT	CARB	FAT	FIBRE
Low Calorie, Tesco*	1 Glass/200ml	6	0.2	3	0.1	0.3	0.1	0.1
Sainsbury's*	1 Glass/250ml	45	0.2	18	0.1	4.4	0.1	0.1
Schweppes*	1 Glass/250ml	85	0.0	34	0.0	8.2	0.0	0.0

BLACK GRAM

	Measure INFO/WEIGHT	per Measure KCAL	FAT	Nutrition Values per 100g / 100ml KCAL	PROT	CARB	FAT	FIBRE
Urad Gram, Dried, Raw	1oz/28g	77	0.4	275	24.9	40.8	1.4	0.0

BLACK PUDDING

	Measure INFO/WEIGHT	per Measure KCAL	FAT	Nutrition Values per 100g / 100ml KCAL	PROT	CARB	FAT	FIBRE
Average, Uncooked	1 Serving/40g	101	6.0	252	10.2	19.0	14.9	0.6
Slices, Grilled, Asda*	1 Slice/36g	150	10.7	417	13.3	23.2	29.7	1.9

	Measure INFO/WEIGHT	per Measure KCAL	FAT	Nutrition Values per 100g / 100ml KCAL	PROT	CARB	FAT	FIBRE
BLACK PUDDING								
VLH Kitchens	1 Serving/40g	105	39.0	262	11.0	20.3	15.6	0.4
BLACKBERRIES								
Fresh, Raw, Average	*1oz/28g*	*7*	*0.1*	*25*	*0.9*	*5.1*	*0.2*	*3.1*
Frozen, Average	1 Serving/80g	37	0.1	46	0.9	9.6	0.2	2.9
in Fruit Juice, Average	*½ Can/145g*	*52*	*0.3*	*36*	*0.6*	*7.9*	*0.2*	*1.3*
BLACKCURRANTS								
Dried, Graze*	1 Pack/30g	95	0.3	317	3.3	79.0	1.0	0.0
Fresh, Raw	*1oz/28g*	*8*	*0.0*	*28*	*0.9*	*6.6*	*0.0*	*3.6*
in Fruit Juice, Average	*1 Serving/30g*	*11*	*0.0*	*38*	*0.6*	*8.6*	*0.2*	*2.4*
Stewed with Sugar	*1oz/28g*	*16*	*0.0*	*58*	*0.7*	*15.0*	*0.0*	*2.8*
Stewed without Sugar	*1oz/28g*	*7*	*0.0*	*24*	*0.8*	*5.6*	*0.0*	*3.1*
BLINIS								
Cocktail, M&S*	½ Pack/81g	154	1.9	190	6.3	35.9	2.3	2.0
Sausage, Cocktail, Waitrose*	1 Blini/16g	30	0.4	190	6.3	35.9	2.3	2.0
BLUEBERRIES								
Chocolate Covered, Waitrose*	1 Serving/25g	120	5.6	481	4.0	65.6	22.4	3.0
Dried, Graze*	1 Pack/27g	82	0.1	302	1.4	73.0	0.5	0.0
Dried, Love Life, Waitrose*	1 Serving/30g	107	0.2	358	1.1	80.1	0.8	3.6
Dried, Whitworths*	1 Pack/75g	226	0.1	301	0.9	74.2	0.1	11.4
Dried, Wholefoods, Tesco*	1 Serving/20g	66	0.2	329	2.0	77.9	1.0	3.2
Freshly Frozen, Asda*	1 Portion/100g	35	0.2	35	0.6	6.9	0.2	1.8
Frozen, Average	1 Serving/80g	41	0.2	51	0.6	13.8	0.2	4.4
Frozen, Essential, Waitrose*	1 Serving/80g	26	0.2	32	0.6	6.9	0.2	2.4
Frozen, Sainsbury's*	1 Serving/80g	28	0.2	35	0.6	6.9	0.2	1.8
Organic, Tesco*	1 Punnet/150g	102	0.4	68	0.7	14.5	0.3	2.4
Shearway*	1 Serving/80g	41	0.5	51	0.4	12.2	0.6	0.0
BOAR								
Wild, Raw, Average	*1 Serving/200g*	*244*	*6.7*	*122*	*21.5*	*0.0*	*3.3*	*0.0*
BOILED SWEETS								
Average	1 Sweet/7g	21	0.0	327	0.0	87.1	0.0	0.0
Blackcurrant & Liquorice, Co-Op*	1 Sweet/8g	32	0.4	405	0.9	91.0	5.0	0.0
Cherry Drops, Bassett's*	1 Sweet/5g	18	0.0	390	0.0	98.1	0.0	0.0
Clear Fruits, Sainsbury's*	1 Sweet/7g	26	0.0	372	0.1	92.9	0.0	0.0
Fruit Drops, Co-Op*	1 Sweet/6g	24	0.0	395	0.2	98.0	0.0	0.0
Fruit Sherbets, Assorted, M&S*	1 Sweet/9g	35	0.4	405	0.3	91.6	4.3	0.1
Lockets, Mars*	1 Pack/43g	165	0.0	383	0.0	95.8	0.0	0.0
Mentho-Lyptus, Cherry, Sugar Free, Hall's*	1 Lozenge/4g	8	0.0	234	0.0	62.4	0.0	0.0
Mentho-Lyptus, Extra Strong, Hall's*	1 Lozenge/4g	14	0.0	389	0.0	96.9	0.0	0.0
Pear Drops, Bassett's*	1 Sweet/4g	16	0.0	390	0.0	96.4	0.0	0.0
Soothers, Blackcurrant, Hall's*	1 Lozenge/5g	16	0.0	365	0.0	91.4	0.0	0.0
Soothers, Cherry, Hall's*	1 Pack/45g	165	0.0	365	0.0	91.3	0.0	0.0
Soothers, Strawberry Flavour, Hall's*	1 Sweet/5g	19	0.0	385	0.0	96.0	0.0	0.0
BOK CHOY								
Tesco*	1 Serving/100g	11	0.2	11	1.0	1.4	0.2	1.2
BOLOGNESE								
Al Forno, Weight Watchers*	1 Pack/354g	312	6.7	88	6.6	10.3	1.9	1.8
Beef, Asda*	1 Pack/392g	412	19.6	105	8.0	7.0	5.0	0.0
Pasta, Goodness, Tesco*	1 Pack/280g	324	8.4	116	7.1	15.1	3.0	1.8
Penne, Heinz*	1 Pack/300g	213	2.7	71	3.8	11.8	0.9	0.6
Tagliatelle, Weight Watchers*	1 Serving/300g	300	5.4	100	5.5	15.4	1.8	0.1
BOMBAY MIX								
Average	1oz/28g	141	9.2	503	18.8	35.1	32.9	6.2
Suma*	½ Pack/125g	595	35.6	476	13.6	41.2	28.5	10.1

	Measure INFO/WEIGHT	per Measure KCAL	FAT	Nutrition Values per 100g / 100ml KCAL	PROT	CARB	FAT	FIBRE
BON BONS								
Apple, Lemon & Strawberry, Co-Op*	¼ Bag/50g	202	2.5	405	1.0	88.0	5.0	0.0
Bassett's*	1 Sweet/7g	28	0.5	417	1.1	85.4	7.5	0.0
Fruit, Bassett's*	1 Serving/7g	25	0.0	380	0.1	94.2	0.0	0.0
Lemon, Bassett's*	1 Sweet/7g	30	0.7	425	0.0	83.7	9.8	0.0
BOOST								
Standard Bar, Cadbury*	1 Bar/61g	305	17.0	510	5.8	57.0	28.5	0.9
Treat Size, Cadbury*	1 Bar/24g	130	7.4	535	5.3	59.6	30.5	0.0
with Glucose, Cadbury*	1 Bar/61g	315	17.8	521	5.6	58.0	29.4	4.0
with Glucose & Guarana, Cadbury*	1 Bar/61g	314	18.0	515	5.5	56.7	29.5	0.0
BOUILLABAISSE								
Average	1 Serving/400g	556	38.8	139	11.2	2.0	9.7	0.4
BOUILLON								
Beef, Benedicta*	1 fl oz/30ml	22	0.2	73	7.5	9.5	0.5	0.0
Chicken, Benedicta*	1 fl oz/30ml	22	0.9	75	4.0	8.0	3.0	5.6
Powder, Miso, Marigold*	1 Tsp/5g	12	0.5	248	7.0	34.0	9.3	1.4
Powder, Swiss Vegetable, Green Tub, Marigold*	1 Tsp/5g	12	0.4	243	10.5	29.4	8.1	0.7
Vegetable, Benedicta*	1 fl oz/30ml	30	0.1	101	7.5	17.0	0.3	0.0
BOUNTY								
Calapuno, Mars*	1 Pack/175g	919	55.0	525	6.3	54.3	31.4	0.0
Dark, Mars*	1 Funsize/29g	142	8.0	488	3.7	55.7	27.6	0.0
Milk, Mars*	1 Funsize/29g	137	7.4	471	3.7	56.4	25.6	0.0
BOURNVITA								
Powder, Made Up with Semi-Skimmed Milk	1 Mug/227ml	132	3.6	58	3.5	7.8	1.6	0.0
Powder, Made Up with Whole Milk	1 Mug/227ml	173	8.6	76	3.4	7.6	3.8	0.0
BOVRIL								
Beef Extract, Drink, Made Up with Water, Bovril*	1 Serving/12g	22	0.1	184	38.9	4.6	1.2	0.0
Chicken Savoury Drink, Bovril*	1 Serving/13g	16	0.2	129	9.7	19.4	1.4	2.1
BRANDY								
37.5% Volume, Average	*1 Pub Shot/35ml*	*72*	*0.0*	*207*	*0.0*	*0.0*	*0.0*	*0.0*
40% Volume, Average	*1 Pub Shot/35ml*	*78*	*0.0*	*222*	*0.0*	*0.0*	*0.0*	*0.0*
Cherry, Average	*1 Pub Shot/35ml*	*89*	*0.0*	*255*	*0.0*	*32.6*	*0.0*	*0.0*
BRAZIL NUTS								
Average	*6 Whole/20g*	*136*	*13.7*	*682*	*15.3*	*2.8*	*68.4*	*5.4*
Milk Chocolate, Tesco*	1 Nut/8g	47	3.5	585	9.9	38.0	43.7	1.9
Shelled, Whole, Love Life, Waitrose*	1 Serving/30g	205	20.5	683	14.1	3.1	68.2	7.5
Wholefoods, Tesco*	1 Serving/25g	173	17.0	691	14.1	3.1	68.2	4.3
BREAD								
50/50, Wholemeal & White, Medium Sliced, Kingsmill*	1 Slice/40g	94	0.9	235	9.9	41.2	2.3	4.9
Apple Sourdough, Gail's*	1 Slice/50g	118	0.4	236	7.5	43.9	0.7	4.3
Arabic, El Amar Bakery*	1 Serving/110g	318	1.3	289	11.6	57.9	1.2	0.0
Bagel, 4 Everything, Finest, Tesco*	1 Bagel/100g	268	1.8	268	11.1	51.9	1.8	2.5
Bagel, Blueberry, Sara Lee*	1 Bagel/104g	290	1.5	279	9.6	58.6	1.4	1.9
Bagel, Caramelised Onion & Poppy Seed, Tesco*	1 Bagel/85g	221	2.1	260	10.9	47.6	2.5	3.8
Bagel, Cinnamon & Raisin, Morrisons*	1 Bagel/85g	215	1.7	253	7.7	51.1	2.0	4.5
Bagel, Cinnamon & Raisin, New York Bagel Co*	1 Bagel/90g	231	1.0	257	10.1	49.9	1.1	3.6
Bagel, Cinnamon & Raisin, Tesco*	1 Bagel/85g	230	1.4	270	10.4	51.3	1.7	3.8
Bagel, Fruit & Fibre, Kingsmill*	1 Bagel/85g	225	1.2	265	9.8	50.8	1.4	5.2
Bagel, Fruit & Spice, Sainsbury's*	1 Bagel/85g	234	1.8	275	9.7	54.3	2.1	3.8
Bagel, Granary, Bagel Factory*	1 Bagel/100g	288	2.1	288	11.9	57.4	2.1	4.5
Bagel, High Bran, Seed, & Cranberry, The Food Doctor*	1 Bagel/85g	212	1.6	250	10.8	47.4	1.9	6.7
Bagel, Mini, Sainsbury's*	1 Bagel/25g	67	0.4	268	11.2	52.4	1.6	2.8
Bagel, Multi Seed, New York Bagel Co*	1 Bagel/90g	244	4.3	271	12.4	41.6	4.8	5.8
Bagel, Multigrain, Sainsbury's*	1 Bagel/113g	293	3.5	259	10.0	49.6	3.1	2.0

BREAD

INFO/WEIGHT	Measure	per Measure KCAL	FAT	Nutrition Values per 100g / 100ml KCAL	PROT	CARB	FAT	FIBRE
Bagel, Onion, New York Bagel Co*	1 Bagel/85g	222	1.6	261	10.6	50.4	1.9	3.1
Bagel, Onion, Tesco*	1 Bagel/85g	233	2.0	274	10.5	52.4	2.4	1.9
Bagel, Onion & Poppy Seed, Average	1 Bagel/85g	225	2.8	264	9.0	50.5	3.3	3.2
Bagel, Original, Organic, New York Bagel Co*	1 Bagel/85g	220	1.2	259	9.3	52.2	1.4	4.1
Bagel, Plain, Asda*	1 Bagel/85g	226	2.0	265	15.0	46.0	2.3	2.9
Bagel, Plain, Average	**1 Bagel/78g**	**202**	**1.5**	**259**	**10.1**	**50.4**	**1.9**	**3.1**
Bagel, Plain, Bagel Factory*	1 Bagel/150g	318	1.3	212	9.4	41.6	0.9	2.1
Bagel, Plain, Free From, Tesco*	1 Bagel/80g	215	5.5	270	3.4	47.7	6.9	4.7
Bagel, Plain, GFY, Asda*	1 Bagel/84g	218	1.8	259	10.0	50.0	2.1	1.8
Bagel, Plain, New York Bagel Co*	1 Bagel/85g	216	1.6	255	9.1	50.4	1.9	2.9
Bagel, Plain, So Organic, Sainsbury's*	1 Bagel/85g	216	2.3	254	9.0	48.4	2.7	3.6
Bagel, Plain, Tesco*	1 Bagel/85g	220	1.8	259	9.8	50.2	2.1	1.8
Bagel, Plain, Value, Tesco*	1 Bagel/71g	181	0.6	255	10.3	51.7	0.8	3.7
Bagel, Poppy Seed, New York Bagel Co*	1 Bagel/85g	233	2.4	274	11.4	50.8	2.8	3.2
Bagel, Red Onion & Chive, New York Bakery Co.*	1 Bagel/90g	225	1.2	250	10.4	47.2	1.3	3.8
Bagel, Sesame, M&S*	1 Bagel/87g	240	2.8	275	10.2	51.2	3.2	2.1
Bagel, Sesame, New York Bagel Co*	1 Bagel/85g	226	2.6	266	10.3	49.2	3.1	4.0
Bagel, Sesame Seed, Essential, Waitrose*	1 Bagel/85g	243	2.7	286	9.6	54.6	3.2	3.6
Bagel, Sesame Seed, GFY, Asda*	1 Bagel/84g	227	2.1	271	11.0	51.0	2.5	2.6
Bagel, Wee Soda, Genesis Crafty*	1 Bagel/65g	148	2.5	227	6.9	41.3	3.9	2.9
Bagel, White, Asda*	1 Bagel/86g	227	2.7	264	10.0	49.0	3.1	0.0
Bagel, White, Original, Weight Watchers*	1 Bagel/67g	158	0.5	236	9.5	42.4	0.8	10.7
Bagel, Wholemeal, Average	1 Bagel/90g	235	2.7	261	12.7	44.6	3.0	7.7
Bagel, Wholemeal, Multiseed, M&S*	1 Bagel/84g	215	5.6	255	13.1	35.4	6.6	8.3
Bagel, Wholemeal, New York Bagel Co*	1 Bagel/90g	223	2.1	248	11.4	41.5	2.3	7.5
Baguette, Budgens*	1 Baguette/125g	335	1.5	268	8.5	55.7	1.2	2.3
Baguette, Crusty Brown, M&S*	½ Loaf/71g	160	1.1	225	9.8	42.7	1.6	6.3
Baguette, French, Tesco*	1 Serving/60g	144	0.7	240	7.8	49.5	1.2	3.4
Baguette, Granary, Average	1 Serving/100g	250	2.8	250	20.0	46.0	2.8	6.0
Baguette, Granary, Co-Op*	1 Serving/60g	150	1.5	250	20.0	46.0	2.5	6.0
Baguette, Harvester, French Style, Somerfield*	1 Serving/110g	276	2.1	251	10.6	47.9	1.9	3.7
Baguette, Homebake, Half, Tesco*	1 Serving/60g	141	0.5	235	7.8	49.1	0.8	1.2
Baguette, Mediterranean Herb, Sainsbury's*	1 Serving/60g	203	9.4	339	8.5	40.8	15.7	2.3
Baguette, Part Baked, Classique, Delifrance*	1 Pack/250g	745	3.0	298	9.8	54.8	1.2	2.7
Baguette, Part Baked, Half, Tesco*	½ Baguette/75g	180	0.9	240	7.8	49.5	1.2	3.4
Baguette, Paysanne, Stonebaked, Asda*	1/6 Loaf/46g	119	1.4	259	10.0	48.0	3.0	3.3
Baguette, Ready to Bake, Sainsbury's*	½ Baguette/62g	150	0.8	242	7.8	49.7	1.3	2.8
Baguette, Soft Bake, Somerfield*	1 Serving/60g	170	0.9	284	10.3	57.3	1.5	1.9
Baguette, Sourdough, la Brea Bakery*	1 Serving/60g	160	0.4	266	8.8	56.1	0.7	1.8
Baguette, White, Half, Crusty, M&S*	1 Baguette/162g	420	1.8	260	8.4	53.5	1.1	2.3
Baguette, White, Homebake, Tesco*	1 Baguette/135g	331	1.8	245	7.8	49.7	1.3	2.5
Baguette, White, Ready to Bake, Asda*	1 Serving/60g	168	1.1	280	10.0	56.0	1.8	2.6
Baguette, White, Sainsbury's*	1 Serving/50g	132	0.8	263	9.3	53.1	1.5	2.7
Baguette, White, Sandwich, Somerfield*	1 Serving/60g	155	0.8	259	9.4	52.1	1.4	1.7
Baguette, Wholemeal, Part Baked, Asda*	½ Baguette/75g	176	1.0	235	8.2	47.7	1.3	3.0
Baguette, Wholemeal, Part Baked, Mini, Landgut*	½ Baguette/25g	56	0.2	223	7.5	46.0	1.0	0.0
Bap, Brown, Large, G H Sheldon*	1 Bap/64g	169	4.3	264	5.3	47.5	6.7	4.0
Baps, Brown, Large, Asda*	1 Bap/58g	140	0.9	242	10.0	47.0	1.6	0.0
Baps, Brown, Malted Grain, Large, Tesco*	1 Bap/93g	228	3.1	245	9.9	42.7	3.3	5.3
Baps, Cheese Topped, Baker's Soft, Tesco*	1 Bap/65g	180	3.7	275	10.2	45.8	5.6	2.2
Baps, Cheese Topped, Sainsbury's*	1 Bap/75g	218	6.4	291	12.1	41.6	8.5	2.0
Baps, Cheese Topped, White, Tesco*	1 Bap/65g	179	3.6	275	10.2	45.8	5.6	0.7
Baps, Floured, M&S*	1 Bap/60g	168	3.7	280	11.5	46.8	6.2	2.0

BREAD

INFO/WEIGHT	Measure	per Measure KCAL	FAT	Nutrition Values per 100g / 100ml KCAL	PROT	CARB	FAT	FIBRE
Baps, Malted, Giant, Sainsbury's*	1 Bap/109g	282	5.2	260	8.6	45.7	4.8	5.7
Baps, Malted, Large, Co-Op*	1 Bap/85g	208	2.6	245	10.2	44.3	3.1	5.0
Baps, Multigrain, Tesco*	1 Bap/98g	238	3.1	244	8.7	45.1	3.2	1.9
Baps, White, Average	1 Bap/65g	167	2.3	257	9.5	47.0	3.5	1.9
Baps, White, Floured, Soft, M&S*	1 Bap/61g	175	3.4	285	11.5	46.6	5.5	2.8
Baps, White, Floured, Waitrose*	1 Bap/60g	147	1.2	244	8.0	48.6	2.0	1.1
Baps, White, Giant, Sainsbury's*	1 Bap/86g	235	3.2	273	8.3	51.7	3.7	3.4
Baps, White, Giant, Waitrose*	1 Bap/104g	260	3.7	250	9.5	45.0	3.6	4.8
Baps, White, Large, Tesco*	1 Bap/95g	252	4.3	265	8.7	46.2	4.5	2.4
Baps, White, Sandwich, Kingsmill*	1 Bap/80g	209	3.2	261	10.1	46.2	4.0	2.2
Baps, White, Sliced, Large, Asda*	1 Bap/58g	148	1.0	255	10.0	50.0	1.7	0.0
Baps, White, Soft, Giant, Somerfield*	1 Bap/105g	262	4.0	249	9.1	44.7	3.8	2.3
Baps, White, Warburton's*	1 Bap/57g	144	2.5	252	9.8	43.4	4.3	2.7
Baps, Wholemeal, Brace's*	1 Bap/59g	137	2.6	234	10.5	42.5	4.4	4.3
Baps, Wholemeal, Country Oven*	1 Bap/40g	92	1.3	231	9.5	41.0	3.3	4.1
Baps, Wholemeal, Giant, Rathbones*	1 Bap/110g	230	2.1	209	9.4	39.0	1.9	8.0
Baps, Wholemeal, Giant, Sainsbury's*	1 Bap/86g	230	3.5	268	9.7	48.1	4.1	7.7
Baps, Wholemeal, Large, Tesco*	1 Bap/95g	223	3.9	235	10.5	39.1	4.1	7.6
Baps, Wholemeal, Tesco*	1 Bap/46g	104	2.4	227	9.6	41.4	5.3	5.6
Baps, Wholemeal, Village Green*	1 Bap/65g	151	2.3	232	10.0	40.0	3.5	3.8
Baps, Wholemeal, Waitrose*	1 Bap/63g	148	3.3	235	11.0	35.9	5.3	7.7
Baton, L'ancienne Olive, Bakery, Morrisons*	1 Serving/100g	291	9.3	291	0.0	2.9	9.3	3.4
Best of Both, Farmhouse, Hovis*	1 Slice/44g	99	1.4	226	9.5	40.0	3.1	4.9
Best of Both, Medium, Hovis*	1 Slice/40g	91	0.9	227	9.0	40.4	2.2	4.7
Best of Both, Thick Sliced, Hovis*	1 Slice/50g	113	0.9	224	9.0	40.4	1.8	5.0
Black Olive, Finest, Tesco*	1 Serving/72g	184	4.6	255	9.7	39.7	6.4	2.9
Blackpool Milk Roll, Warburton's*	1 Slice/18g	47	0.5	254	11.0	45.0	2.8	2.8
Bloomer, COU, M&S*	1 Slice/33g	78	0.5	235	9.5	45.5	1.5	3.6
Bloomer, Multiseed, Average	1 Slice/50g	120	2.4	240	11.8	37.2	4.9	7.7
Bloomer, Multiseed, Finest, Tesco*	1 Slice/50g	100	1.9	200	12.8	28.4	3.8	11.1
Bloomer, Multiseed, Organic, Sainsbury's*	1 Serving/60g	160	4.1	266	10.9	40.3	6.8	8.8
Bloomer, Multiseed, Sliced, M&S*	1 Slice/54g	150	3.9	280	10.5	43.6	7.2	3.1
Bloomer, Multiseed, TTD, Sainsbury's*	1 Slice/50g	119	1.8	239	12.0	39.7	3.6	8.8
Bloomer, Sliced, Heyford, Waitrose*	1 Slice/50g	104	1.6	208	10.1	35.0	3.1	6.6
Bloomer, Soft Grain, M&S*	1 Slice/34g	80	0.5	235	9.5	45.5	1.5	3.6
Bloomer, Spelt & Sunflower, Bakery, Tesco*	1 Serving/100g	297	9.7	297	8.5	41.5	9.7	6.3
Bloomer, White, Sliced, Waitrose*	1 Slice/50g	130	0.9	259	8.5	52.1	1.8	2.6
Bloomer, Wholemeal, Organic, M&S*	1 Slice/50g	110	2.1	220	10.2	35.5	4.2	6.4
Both in One, Village Bakery, Aldi*	1 Slice/40g	123	0.9	307	10.4	42.6	2.2	5.2
Breadcakes, Big Brown, Morrisons*	1 Cake/63g	154	2.1	245	9.0	44.6	3.4	4.3
Brioche, Loaf, Butter, Sainsbury's*	1/8 Loaf/50g	174	5.2	347	8.0	55.0	10.5	2.2
Brown, Danish, Weight Watchers*	1 Slice/20g	47	0.4	235	9.8	40.7	2.0	7.4
Brown, Farmhouse, Linwoods*	1 Slice/25g	56	0.4	225	7.3	44.4	1.7	5.8
Brown, Free From, Sliced, Tesco*	1 Slice/45g	121	3.7	268	5.4	43.2	8.2	3.6
Brown, GF, Genius*	1 Slice/35g	97	4.7	277	6.7	42.2	13.3	9.5
Brown, Gluten & Wheat Free, Sliced	1 Slice/25g	56	1.3	224	3.4	41.0	5.2	9.4
Brown, Good Health, Warburton's*	1 Slice/35g	79	1.0	226	10.3	39.6	2.9	7.2
Brown, Granary Malted, Thick Sliced, Waitrose*	1 Slice/40g	95	0.9	238	9.4	44.8	2.3	5.1
Brown, High Fibre, Ormo*	1 Slice/24g	57	0.6	239	9.2	42.9	2.6	7.5
Brown, Honey & Oat Bran, Vogel*	1 Serving/100g	220	4.5	220	7.9	39.2	4.5	5.7
Brown, Irwin's Bakery*	1 Slice/64g	137	0.4	214	10.4	41.8	0.6	6.1
Brown, Malted, Average	1 Slice/25g	60	0.6	242	9.4	45.5	2.4	4.2
Brown, Malted, Farmhouse, Gold, Morrisons*	1 Slice/38g	94	0.5	248	8.2	49.6	1.4	3.0

BRED

Measure INFO/WEIGHT		per Measure		Nutrition Values per 100g / 100ml				
		KCAL	FAT	KCAL	PROT	CARB	FAT	FIBRE
Brown, Medium Sliced	*1 Slice/34g*	**74**	**0.7**	**218**	**8.5**	**44.3**	**2.0**	**3.5**
Brown, Medium Sliced, Asda*	1 Slice/36g	78	0.6	216	8.0	42.0	1.8	4.1
Brown, Medium Sliced, Bettabuy, Morrisons*	1 Slice/31g	66	0.4	212	8.6	42.0	1.3	3.6
Brown, Medium Sliced, Premium, Warburton's*	1 Slice/24g	59	0.9	249	10.5	43.2	3.7	4.3
Brown, Medium Sliced, Sainsbury's*	1 Slice/36g	81	0.7	225	8.2	43.8	1.9	3.9
Brown, Medium Sliced, Smart Price, Asda*	1 Slice/37g	77	0.6	210	8.0	41.0	1.6	6.0
Brown, Medium Sliced, Tesco*	1 Slice/36g	78	0.8	218	8.0	41.6	2.2	4.5
Brown, Mixed Grain, Original, Vogel*	1 Slice/45g	102	0.6	227	9.8	47.1	1.2	6.4
Brown, Multi Grain, Wheat Free, Gluten Free	1 Slice/33g	76	1.7	229	5.1	40.8	5.1	5.6
Brown, Sainsbury's*	1 Slice/34g	81	0.7	239	8.4	46.8	2.1	4.2
Brown, Seeded Batch, Large Loaf, 800g, Warburton's*	1 Slice/46g	132	4.1	288	12.3	39.7	8.9	6.0
Brown, Seeds & Oats, Gold, Kingsmill*	1 Slice/45g	126	4.4	280	12.2	35.6	9.8	4.9
Brown, Sliced, By Brennans, Weight Watchers*	1 Slice/20g	51	0.4	257	9.5	45.4	2.1	6.8
Brown, Soda, Irish, Tesco*	1 Serving/50g	110	1.9	219	9.2	36.2	3.8	6.4
Brown, Soda, M&S*	1 Slice/40g	92	1.4	229	9.2	43.6	3.6	4.9
Brown, Sunflower & Barley, Vogel*	1 Slice/42g	100	1.9	239	9.4	40.3	4.5	6.7
Brown, Thick, Warburton's*	1 Slice/38g	80	0.7	211	9.4	39.2	1.8	6.2
Brown, Thick Sliced, Tesco*	1 Serving/50g	110	1.2	219	10.3	38.9	2.5	5.3
Brown, Thin Sliced, Sainsbury's*	1 Slice/29g	65	0.5	225	8.2	43.8	1.9	3.9
Brown, Toasted, Medium Sliced, Average	*1 Slice/24g*	**65**	**0.5**	**272**	**10.4**	**56.5**	**2.1**	**4.5**
Brown, Toastie, Thick Sliced, Kingsmill*	1 Slice/44g	101	1.4	230	9.5	40.5	3.3	4.7
Brown, Very Dark, Albert Heijn*	1 Slice/35g	84	1.4	240	12.0	35.0	4.0	7.4
Brown, Wholemeal, Healthy Choice, Warburton's*	1 Slice/40g	98	1.0	244	10.4	40.7	2.5	6.5
Bruschettine, Italian, Toasted, Crosta And Mollica*	1 Portion/11g	41	1.9	382	10.1	66.2	17.6	0.0
Buckwheat, Artisan*	1 Loaf/400g	736	7.0	184	6.1	38.1	1.8	4.3
Buns, Burger, American Style, Sainsbury's*	1 Bun/50g	131	2.1	261	10.5	45.6	4.1	3.6
Buns, Burger, Cheese & Onion, Topped, Finest, Tesco*	1 Serving/105g	309	10.0	294	10.2	41.9	9.5	2.8
Buns, Burger, Giant, Sainsbury's*	1 Bun/95g	249	4.9	262	8.7	45.2	5.2	2.9
Buns, Burger, Sainsbury's*	1 Bun/56g	154	2.9	275	9.2	47.8	5.2	4.1
Buns, Burger, Sesame, American Style, Sainsbury's*	1 Bun/60g	162	3.8	270	7.3	46.2	6.3	2.2
Buns, Burger, Sesame, Sliced, Tesco*	1 Bun/60g	168	4.0	280	7.9	47.3	6.6	2.1
Buns, Burger, Warburton's*	1 Roll/60g	147	3.9	245	9.0	37.5	6.5	2.0
Buns, Burger, White, Waitrose*	1 Serving/64g	169	2.5	264	10.0	47.2	3.9	2.7
Buns, White, Stay Fresh, Tesco*	1 Bun/56g	152	3.7	271	7.5	45.5	6.6	0.0
Carrot & Raisin, Sprouted, Sunnyvale*	1 Loaf/400g	800	2.2	200	9.5	48.1	0.6	7.9
Challah, Average	*1 Slice/50g*	**143**	**3.6**	**286**	**8.9**	**53.6**	**7.1**	**3.6**
Cheese, Morrisons*	1 Serving/96g	297	13.6	311	9.9	35.9	14.2	3.0
Cheese, Onion & Garlic, Tear & Share, Waitrose*	¼ Bread/112g	326	14.6	290	9.4	33.9	13.0	2.1
Cheese, Onion Mustard Seed, Cluster, Sainsbury's*	1 Cluster/100g	276	8.1	276	10.0	40.6	8.1	3.1
Cheese, Tear & Share, Tesco*	¼ Loaf/73g	225	7.8	310	8.8	44.0	10.7	0.8
Cheese & Garlic, Pizza Style, Sainsbury's*	¼ Bread/63g	199	8.1	318	10.7	39.7	13.0	2.2
Cheese & Garlic, Stonebaked, Morrisons*	¼ Bread/69g	228	9.9	331	10.9	39.5	14.4	1.9
Cheese & Onion, Tear & Share, Sainsbury's*	¼ Bread/71g	202	6.6	285	9.8	40.6	9.3	1.9
Cheese & Onion, Toastie, Warburton's*	1 Slice/42g	120	5.8	286	7.5	33.1	13.7	0.0
Cheese & Tomato, Tear & Share, Sainsbury's*	¼ Bread/72g	211	9.5	293	8.0	35.7	13.2	1.5
Cholla, Average	*1/10 Loaf/154g*	**421**	**14.3**	**274**	**6.9**	**40.8**	**9.3**	**1.0**
Ciabatta, Black Olive, Part Baked, Sainsbury's*	¼ Ciabatta/67g	172	2.5	257	8.8	46.8	3.8	2.4
Ciabatta, Finest, Tesco*	1/6 Ciabatta/45g	124	2.7	275	10.4	44.8	5.9	2.7
Ciabatta, Gluten & Wheat Free, Average	1 Slice/55g	136	1.6	248	2.0	52.4	2.9	4.2
Ciabatta, Green Olive, Tesco*	¼ Ciabatta/70g	155	3.1	222	7.4	38.2	4.4	1.9
Ciabatta, Half, M&S*	1 Ciabatta/135g	354	5.5	262	10.3	48.1	4.1	2.1
Ciabatta, Half, Organic, Sainsbury's*	½ Ciabatta/63g	152	0.6	241	9.1	48.7	1.0	2.3
Ciabatta, Half, Part Baked, TTD, Sainsbury's*	¼ Pack/67g	173	3.3	257	8.6	44.6	4.9	3.5

BREAD

	Measure INFO/WEIGHT	per Measure KCAL	per Measure FAT	Nutrition Values per 100g / 100ml KCAL	PROT	CARB	FAT	FIBRE
Ciabatta, Half, Tesco*	1 Ciabatta/135g	351	4.7	260	8.9	47.7	3.5	2.2
Ciabatta, Italian Style, Waitrose*	1 Ciabatta/89g	231	1.2	260	10.7	51.2	1.4	2.2
Ciabatta, Olive & Rosemary, Mini, Tesco*	1 Pack/75g	319	8.2	425	17.8	63.0	10.9	3.6
Ciabatta, Organic, Tesco*	1/3 Ciabatta/100g	240	3.6	240	8.7	43.2	3.6	2.4
Ciabatta, Part Baked, Half, Sainsbury's*	½ Ciabbatta/67g	174	2.5	260	8.9	47.7	3.7	2.2
Ciabatta, Plain, Half, Two, Waitrose*	1 Roll/80g	248	5.8	310	10.0	51.3	7.2	2.2
Ciabatta, Plain, Tesco*	¼ Ciabatta/73g	174	2.8	240	9.8	41.5	3.9	2.4
Ciabatta, Ready to Bake, M&S*	1 Serving/150g	393	6.2	262	10.3	48.1	4.1	2.1
Ciabatta, Ready to Bake, Sainsbury's*	½ Ciabatta/66g	172	2.4	260	8.9	47.7	3.7	2.2
Ciabatta, Spicy Topped, Finest, Tesco*	1 Serving/73g	163	4.0	223	9.2	34.0	5.5	1.7
Ciabatta, Square, Bake at Home, Part Baked, Asda*	1 Roll/60g	157	2.1	262	8.4	49.1	3.5	2.1
Ciabatta, Tomato & Basil, GFY, Asda*	1 Serving/55g	143	1.2	260	9.0	51.0	2.2	0.0
Ciabatta, Tomato & Basil, Sun Dried, Tesco*	¼ Ciabatta/75g	193	4.3	257	8.9	42.4	5.7	2.4
Ciabatta, Tomato & Mozzarella, Iceland*	1 Ciabatta/150g	374	15.2	249	10.0	29.6	10.1	3.3
Ciabatta, TTD, Sainsbury's*	¼ Pack/68g	185	4.0	274	10.4	44.8	5.9	2.7
Ciabatta Stick, Organic, M&S*	1 Stick/140g	315	2.0	225	8.9	48.5	1.4	4.2
Cinnamon Swirl, Asda*	1 Serving/25g	87	3.2	349	6.0	52.0	13.0	1.6
Cottage Loaf, Stonebaked, Asda*	1 Serving/67g	155	0.9	232	10.0	45.0	1.3	3.2
Crostini, Olive Oil, TTD, Sainsbury's*	1 Crostini/4g	16	0.3	409	11.4	72.2	8.3	3.3
Danish, Brown, Sliced, Weight Watchers*	1 Slice/20g	48	0.4	233	9.9	40.7	1.8	7.6
Danish, Lighter, White, Warburton's*	1 Slice/26g	62	0.3	238	10.5	45.8	1.2	2.6
Danish, Malted, Sliced, Weight Watchers*	1 Slice/20g	51	0.3	249	11.8	45.1	1.5	4.2
Danish, White, Medium Sliced, Tesco*	1 Slice/20g	47	0.3	234	9.4	45.4	1.7	3.3
Danish, White, Thick Sliced, Tesco*	1 Slice/24g	60	0.6	250	9.7	47.4	2.3	2.9
Farl, Irish Soda, Irwin's Bakery*	1 Farl/150g	334	5.1	223	4.0	44.0	3.4	2.3
Farmhouse, Batch, Multiseed, Love Life, Waitrose*	1 Slice/50g	130	3.5	259	9.9	39.2	7.0	7.2
Farmhouse, Poppy Seed, Crusty, Loaf, M&S*	1 Slice/40g	104	1.3	260	9.4	47.6	3.3	2.3
Farmhouse Soft Grained, Sliced, Warburton's*	1 Slice/42g	109	1.7	258	10.2	44.6	4.0	5.0
Farmhouse with Oatmeal, Batch, Finest, Tesco*	1 Slice/44g	110	1.4	240	9.8	43.2	3.1	5.2
Fig & Almond, Bröderna Cartwright*	4 Slices/100g	267	7.5	267	9.2	39.7	7.5	0.0
Fig & Hazelnut, Loaf, M&S*	1 Serving/100g	285	8.2	285	11.0	38.9	8.2	5.4
Flatbread, Rosemary & Parsley, CBY, Asda*	1 Bread/89g	294	11.2	331	8.8	44.1	12.6	2.9
Focaccia, Onion & Herb, Tesco*	½ Pack/190g	547	23.8	288	8.7	35.2	12.5	3.7
Focaccia, Roast Cherry Tomato & Olive, GFY, Asda*	½ Pack/148g	350	6.0	237	9.0	41.0	4.1	2.8
Focaccia, Roasted Onion & Cheese, M&S*	1 Serving/89g	240	4.1	270	10.4	45.7	4.6	2.8
French	1½" Slice/45g	110	0.0	244	8.9	53.3	0.0	2.2
French, Sliced, Parisian*	2 Slices/39g	100	1.0	256	5.1	48.7	2.6	0.0
French Stick, Average	**1 Serving/60g**	**147**	**0.2**	**245**	**8.7**	**52.2**	**0.4**	**2.1**
Fruit, Continental, Schneider Brot*	1 Slice/65g	198	3.5	305	5.4	57.0	5.4	0.0
Fruit, Raisin Swirl, Sun-Maid*	1 Slice/33g	95	1.9	287	8.3	50.4	5.8	2.6
Fruit & Cinnamon Loaf, Finest, Tesco*	1 Slice/37g	134	4.9	363	6.4	54.6	13.2	1.5
Fruit Loaf, Apple, M&S*	1 Slice/39g	100	0.6	255	8.5	51.9	1.5	3.3
Fruit Loaf, Apple & Cinnamon, Soreen*	1 Serving/10g	31	0.4	307	6.9	60.5	4.2	0.0
Fruit Loaf, Banana, Lunchbox, Soreen*	1 Bar/30g	100	1.3	332	8.2	63.3	4.4	2.9
Fruit Loaf, Banana, Soreen*	1 Slice/25g	78	1.2	313	6.8	60.9	4.7	0.0
Fruit Loaf, Cinnamon & Raisin, Soreen*	1/8 Loaf/25g	77	1.0	308	7.7	54.1	4.0	4.1
Fruit Loaf, Fresh, Free From, Sainsbury's*	1 Slice/33g	93	2.5	279	3.2	45.5	7.5	8.1
Fruit Loaf, Fruity Five, Snack Pack, Soreen*	1 Pack/61g	200	5.5	329	7.1	54.9	9.0	2.7
Fruit Loaf, Luxury, Christmas, Soreen*	1 Serving/28g	85	0.6	303	4.5	66.6	2.1	0.0
Fruit Loaf, Malt, Weight Watchers*	1 Serving/23g	68	0.4	294	8.9	60.2	1.9	3.6
Fruit Loaf, Mixed Berry, Weight Watchers*	1 Slice/34g	79	0.9	231	7.6	44.3	2.6	7.7
Fruit Loaf, Plum, Lincolnshire, Soreen*	1 Slice/25g	65	0.8	261	8.4	49.3	3.4	2.1
Fruit Loaf, Sliced, Asda*	1 Serving/33g	89	1.2	269	8.0	51.0	3.7	2.9

BREAD

	Measure INFO/WEIGHT	per Measure KCAL	FAT	Nutrition Values per 100g / 100ml KCAL	PROT	CARB	FAT	FIBRE
Fruit Loaf, Sliced, Sainsbury's*	1 Slice/40g	104	1.4	260	8.9	47.9	3.6	2.4
Fruit Loaf, Sliced, Tesco*	1 Slice/36g	100	1.8	278	6.9	51.2	5.1	3.7
Fruit Loaf, Sultana & Cherry, Sainsbury's*	1 Slice/50g	178	6.1	357	2.7	59.0	12.2	1.7
Fruit Loaf, Toasted, Cafe Instore, Asda*	1 Slice/33g	89	1.2	269	8.0	51.0	3.7	2.9
Garlic, & Cheese, Slices, Tesco*	1 Slice/31g	118	5.2	380	11.7	43.9	16.8	2.0
Garlic, & Cheese, Tesco*	1 Serving/143g	490	24.0	343	9.4	38.5	16.8	2.0
Garlic, & Gruyere, Fougasse, TTD, Sainsbury's*	¼ Bread/76g	219	6.8	288	9.5	42.6	8.9	2.9
Garlic, & Herb, Ciabatta, GFY, Asda*	¼ Ciabatta/60g	137	1.4	230	8.8	43.2	2.4	1.0
Garlic, & Herb, Flatbread, Tear & Share, Sainsbury's*	¼ Bread/68g	201	6.3	297	10.9	42.5	9.3	3.7
Garlic, & Herb, Giant Feast, Sainsbury's*	1 Serving/50g	158	6.4	317	8.0	42.1	12.9	2.6
Garlic, & Herb, Tear & Share, CBY, Asda*	¼ Portion/63g	185	6.7	295	9.2	39.0	10.7	2.7
Garlic, & Herb, Tear & Share, Tesco*	1 Serving/73g	218	9.2	300	6.3	40.0	12.7	1.7
Garlic, & Parsley, Tesco*	1 Loaf/230g	699	26.7	304	9.0	41.0	11.6	2.7
Garlic, & Red Onion, Somerfield*	1 Serving/60g	177	6.7	295	9.6	38.9	11.1	2.1
Garlic, & Tomato, Pizza, Italiano, Tesco*	½ Bread/140g	405	15.1	289	7.5	40.5	10.8	2.5
Garlic, 30% Less Fat, Morrisons*	1 Serving/80g	231	7.4	289	7.9	43.8	9.2	2.7
Garlic, Average	1 Serving/100g	327	13.8	327	8.1	43.7	13.8	1.4
Garlic, Baguette, 25% Less Fat, Tesco*	1 Serving/100g	292	11.3	292	7.0	40.7	11.3	1.8
Garlic, Baguette, 50% Less Fat, Asda*	¼ Baguette/43g	123	3.0	287	10.0	46.0	7.0	2.5
Garlic, Baguette, Average	1 Slice/20g	66	2.8	330	7.8	43.1	14.2	1.8
Garlic, Baguette, Extra Strong, Italiano, Tesco*	¼ Baguette/53g	178	8.7	340	7.9	39.8	16.6	2.8
Garlic, Baguette, Extra Strong, Sainsbury's*	½ Baguette/85g	278	12.6	327	8.4	40.0	14.8	3.4
Garlic, Baguette, Frozen, GFY, Asda*	¼ Baguette/48g	132	4.3	277	7.0	42.0	9.0	2.7
Garlic, Baguette, GFY, Asda*	¼ Baguette/43g	106	2.7	249	8.1	39.9	6.3	2.1
Garlic, Baguette, Good Choice, Iceland*	1/3 Baguette/54g	158	4.6	292	8.7	45.1	8.5	2.9
Garlic, Baguette, Italian, Asda*	¼ Baguette/48g	173	9.5	364	7.0	39.0	20.0	3.4
Garlic, Baguette, Italiano, Tesco*	¼ Baguette/53g	186	9.9	355	6.9	39.2	18.8	2.4
Garlic, Baguette, LC, Tesco*	¼ Baguette/52g	130	2.9	250	7.0	42.2	5.5	2.4
Garlic, Baguette, Mediterranean Herb, Tesco*	¼ Baguette/54g	181	8.8	335	6.9	40.3	16.3	2.3
Garlic, Baguette, Morrisons*	½ Baguette/95g	295	14.2	311	6.3	37.8	15.0	1.5
Garlic, Baguette, Reduced Fat, Average	¼ Baguette/40g	102	2.6	256	7.9	41.6	6.4	2.6
Garlic, Baguette, Reduced Fat, Waitrose*	½ Baguette/85g	230	6.8	270	8.1	41.5	8.0	2.7
Garlic, Baguette, Sainsbury's*	½ Baguette/85g	342	16.3	403	8.9	48.6	19.2	2.3
Garlic, Baguette, Slices, Tesco*	1 Serving/60g	187	9.2	312	9.8	33.8	15.3	1.7
Garlic, Baguette, Value, Tesco*	½ Baguette/85g	270	11.1	318	8.1	42.0	13.1	2.3
Garlic, Baguette, Waitrose*	½ Baguette/85g	290	15.2	341	7.1	37.8	17.9	0.0
Garlic, Baguette, White, Homebake, Tesco*	1/3 Baguette/55g	160	5.5	290	7.0	43.1	10.0	1.9
Garlic, Ciabatta, & Herb Butter, Sainsbury's*	½ Ciabatta/105g	345	16.3	329	8.5	38.8	15.5	0.0
Garlic, Ciabatta, Finest, Tesco*	1 Serving/65g	205	8.9	316	8.1	40.1	13.7	2.4
Garlic, Ciabatta, Hand Stretched, Sainsbury's*	¼ Pack/75g	244	10.6	325	8.4	41.0	14.1	2.9
Garlic, Ciabatta, Italian, Sainsbury's*	1 Serving/145g	454	17.1	313	10.0	41.6	11.8	2.9
Garlic, Ciabatta, Italiano, Tesco*	1 Ciabatta/65g	211	9.4	324	7.7	40.9	14.4	2.2
Garlic, Ciabatta, Mini, Italiano, Tesco*	½ Ciabatta/47g	150	6.9	320	8.2	38.5	14.6	2.8
Garlic, Ciabatta with Herbs, Weight Watchers*	1 Pack/88g	216	3.5	245	9.2	43.0	4.0	2.9
Garlic, Finest, Tesco*	¼ Loaf/60g	187	7.9	311	7.7	40.3	13.2	1.8
Garlic, Flatbread, BGTY, Sainsbury's*	¼ Bread/56g	177	5.7	316	9.6	46.6	10.1	2.7
Garlic, Flatbread, Tesco*	1 Serving/83g	249	8.6	302	6.7	45.3	10.4	3.0
Garlic, Focaccia, & Herb, Italian Style, Morrisons*	1/6 Focaccia/76g	259	10.9	341	8.5	44.7	14.3	2.5
Garlic, Focaccia, & Onion, GFY, Asda*	¼ Focaccia/55g	150	2.2	272	12.0	47.0	4.0	0.0
Garlic, Focaccia, & Rosemary, Sainsbury's*	¼ Focaccia/75g	219	7.4	292	8.0	43.0	9.8	2.8
Garlic, Foccacia, & Rosemary, Tesco*	¼ Loaf/73g	193	4.9	266	9.0	42.1	6.8	3.7
Garlic, GFY, Asda*	1 Slice/31g	108	1.4	350	12.0	65.0	4.5	4.0
Garlic, Homebake, Tesco*	1 Serving/60g	209	12.3	348	7.1	33.7	20.5	1.5

BREAD

	Measure INFO/WEIGHT	per Measure KCAL	FAT	Nutrition Values per 100g / 100ml KCAL	PROT	CARB	FAT	FIBRE
Garlic, Italian Style Stone Baked, Morrisons*	½ Pack/115g	420	22.0	365	7.9	40.4	19.1	1.9
Garlic, Pizza Bread, Co-Op*	1 Pizza/240g	756	31.2	315	8.0	41.0	13.0	2.0
Garlic, Reduced Fat, Waitrose*	1 Pack/170g	551	18.7	324	6.9	49.4	11.0	0.9
Garlic, Slices, 50 % Less Fat, Asda*	1 Slice/29g	75	1.1	262	7.9	47.1	3.9	3.2
Garlic, Slices, Asda*	1 Slice/27g	88	3.3	328	8.0	46.2	12.4	2.8
Garlic, Slices, BGTY, Sainsbury's*	1 Slice/27g	82	2.2	305	9.4	48.9	8.0	2.9
Garlic, Slices, Chilled, Sainsbury's*	1 Pack/368g	1369	60.0	372	9.1	47.3	16.3	3.2
Garlic, Slices, GFY, Asda*	1 Slice/31g	80	1.0	259	8.9	48.1	3.3	3.0
Garlic, Slices, Italian, Chilled, Tesco*	1 Slice/27g	110	6.0	415	6.2	46.8	22.4	2.7
Garlic, Slices, LC, Tesco*	1 Slice/30g	75	1.7	250	7.3	42.3	5.7	2.9
Garlic, Slices, Morrisons*	1 Slice/30g	82	2.7	272	7.3	40.2	9.1	2.6
Garlic, Stonebaked, M&S*	1 Loaf/85g	264	10.1	310	9.3	41.4	11.9	3.1
Garlic, with Cheese, Asda*	1 Slice/34g	130	6.1	382	11.0	44.0	18.0	0.0
GF, Loaf, Unsliced, Wellfoods*	2 Slices/100g	216	2.3	216	1.6	47.1	2.3	1.5
GF, Rolls, Wellfoods*	1 Roll/70g	157	1.5	224	1.9	48.8	2.2	1.5
Granary, Baps, Large, Asda*	1 Bap/64g	143	1.4	224	10.0	41.0	2.2	4.3
Granary, Country, Multiseeded, Hovis*	1 Slice/44g	96	1.3	218	11.1	37.0	2.9	6.5
Granary, M&S*	1 Slice/30g	75	0.9	250	9.5	46.4	3.1	3.2
Granary, Malted, Medium Brown, Asda*	1 Slice/35g	81	0.9	231	9.0	43.0	2.6	3.3
Granary, Medium Sliced, Average	**1 Slice/35g**	**85**	**1.0**	**242**	**9.8**	**44.0**	**2.8**	**4.8**
Granary, Oatmeal, Hovis*	1 Slice/44g	104	0.9	236	9.2	45.3	2.1	3.1
Granary, Original, All Sizes, Hovis*	1 Slice/33g	85	0.8	256	10.6	46.4	2.4	3.7
Granary, Original, Thick Sliced, Hovis*	1 Slice/44g	112	1.0	256	10.3	46.4	2.4	3.7
Granary, Seeded, Sunflower, Hovis*	1 Slice/44g	119	2.5	271	10.1	44.9	5.7	2.9
Granary, Thick Slice, COU, M&S*	1 Slice/25g	60	0.6	240	10.5	44.1	2.2	6.0
Granary, Waitrose*	1 Slice/40g	88	1.0	220	9.4	39.9	2.5	4.3
Granary, White, Seeded, Medium Sliced, Hovis*	1 Slice/44g	109	1.8	248	10.9	41.7	4.2	3.8
Granary, Wholemeal, Hovis*	1 Slice/44g	104	1.1	237	10.6	39.8	2.4	6.8
Granary, Wholemeal, Medium Sliced, Average	1 Slice/35g	80	0.9	228	10.8	38.4	2.6	6.6
Granary, Wholemeal, Seeded, Medium Sliced, Hovis*	1 Slice/44g	104	1.1	237	10.6	39.8	2.4	6.8
Granary White, Hovis*	1 Slice/44g	102	1.5	233	9.7	40.8	3.5	5.6
Half Wheat Rye, The Polish Bakery, Tesco*	1 Slice/44g	140	0.7	319	8.0	38.3	1.7	0.0
Hi Bran, M&S*	1 Slice/26g	55	0.8	210	12.6	32.5	3.0	6.3
High Bran, M&S*	1 Slice/26g	60	0.8	230	13.4	34.2	3.0	7.4
Hot Cross Bun, Loaf, Warburton's*	1 Slice/35g	94	1.3	269	8.3	50.4	3.7	2.9
Irish Barm Brack, Tesco*	1 Serving/75g	232	5.2	310	16.0	47.6	6.9	3.0
Irish Cottage Wheaten, Tesco*	1 Serving/40g	79	0.8	198	9.1	35.4	1.9	6.1
Juvela*	1 Slice/25g	60	0.8	240	3.3	50.0	3.0	1.7
Khobez, Flatbread, White, Dina Foods Ltd*	1 Bread/56g	158	0.6	282	10.5	57.5	1.1	3.0
Lavash, Flax, Oat Bran, Whole Flour, Wrap, Joseph's*	1 Serving/32g	50	2.0	156	15.6	21.9	6.2	9.4
Low GI, Multiseed, Medium Sliced, Percy Ingle*	1 Slice/35g	99	3.1	283	0.0	0.0	8.9	6.0
Malt Loaf, Chocolatey, Soreen*	1/8 Loaf/28g	95	1.7	344	8.0	58.7	6.3	5.1
Malt Loaf, Fruity, Sliced, Soreen*	1 Slice/33g	101	0.7	303	7.6	62.1	2.2	3.8
Malt Loaf, Sticky, M&S*	1 Slice/16g	47	0.4	295	6.9	64.9	2.3	3.1
Malt Loaf, Value, Tesco*	1 Slice/25g	72	0.4	289	8.9	60.2	1.4	3.3
Malt Loaf, Weight Watchers*	1 Slice/23g	68	0.4	294	8.9	60.2	1.9	3.6
Malted, & Seeded, Batch, Organic, Waitrose*	1 Slice/50g	118	2.0	236	10.9	39.5	3.9	6.2
Malted, Crusty, Sainsbury's*	1 Slice/42g	109	1.4	259	8.6	48.6	3.3	4.4
Malted, Wheat Loaf, Crusty, Finest, Tesco*	1 Slice/50g	115	0.8	230	9.8	44.2	1.5	4.4
Malted Brown, Slice, BGTY, Sainsbury's*	1 Slice/22g	53	0.6	239	12.1	41.4	2.8	5.8
Malted Brown, Thick Sliced, Organic, Tesco*	1 Slice/44g	111	0.9	249	8.9	48.8	2.0	3.5
Malted Danish, Weight Watchers*	1 Slice/20g	49	0.3	241	12.3	44.5	1.7	4.3
Malted Grain, Co-Op*	1 Slice/43g	99	0.9	230	8.0	46.0	2.0	3.0

BREAD

INFO/WEIGHT	Measure	per Measure KCAL	per Measure FAT	Nutrition Values per 100g / 100ml KCAL	PROT	CARB	FAT	FIBRE
Malted Grain, Good As Gold, Kingsmill*	1 Slice/47g	114	1.2	243	9.5	45.4	2.6	4.2
Malted Wheatgrain, Roberts Bakery*	1 Slice/30g	80	1.0	265	11.0	48.0	3.3	3.6
Mediterranean Olive, Waitrose*	1 Slice/30g	82	2.8	273	7.4	40.1	9.2	4.9
Mediterranean Style, M&S*	1/6 Loaf/48g	150	5.3	315	10.9	42.5	11.1	1.2
Multigrain, Batch, Finest, Tesco*	1 Slice/50g	117	1.4	235	10.8	40.4	2.9	5.5
Multigrain, Brennans*	1 Slice/40g	110	1.3	275	8.8	48.0	3.3	6.3
Multigrain, Brown, Farmhouse Baker's, M&S*	1 Slice/51g	115	2.8	225	13.0	31.2	5.4	5.1
Multigrain, Crusty, Finest, Tesco*	1 Slice/40g	98	1.4	245	9.0	44.7	3.4	5.0
Multigrain, Sliced, Fresh And Easy*	1 Slice/40g	110	1.0	275	10.0	52.5	2.5	5.0
Multigrain, Soft Batch, Sainsbury's*	1 Slice/44g	106	2.9	242	11.3	34.5	6.5	5.6
Multigrain, Sub Rolls, Asda*	1 Sub/150g	357	6.3	238	0.0	0.0	4.2	0.0
Multigrain, Sunblest*	1 Slice/30g	76	0.8	254	9.0	47.0	2.5	4.5
Multigrain, Tesco*	1 Slice/31g	66	1.0	214	11.1	36.8	3.2	8.9
Multigrain, Thick Sliced, Tesco*	1 Slice/50g	112	1.2	225	8.4	42.2	2.5	3.9
Multiseed, Farmhouse, Batch, Finest, Tesco*	1 Slice/44g	108	1.9	245	9.9	40.4	4.4	7.5
Multiseed, Farmhouse, Finest, Tesco*	1 Slice/50g	135	3.8	270	12.5	37.0	7.7	5.8
Multiseed, Gluten & Wheat Free, Loaf, Lovemore*	1 Serving/35g	102	4.3	291	0.0	3.0	12.3	0.0
Multiseed, Organic, Duchy Originals*	1 Slice/43g	114	3.4	269	10.9	39.1	8.1	5.3
Multiseed, Somerfield*	1 Slice/45g	105	1.7	235	11.0	38.2	3.7	8.1
Naan, Asda*	1 Naan/130g	308	2.3	237	7.7	47.4	1.8	2.2
Naan, Average	**1 Naan/130g**	**344**	**5.6**	**264**	**8.3**	**48.5**	**4.3**	**2.0**
Naan, Bombay Brassiere, Sainsbury's*	1 Naan/140g	372	4.3	266	9.8	49.6	3.1	2.9
Naan, Chilli & Mango, Finest, Tesco*	½ Naan/90g	230	5.1	255	8.4	41.9	5.7	3.2
Naan, Fresh, BGTY, Sainsbury's*	1 Serving/150g	368	4.6	245	9.4	44.9	3.1	2.2
Naan, Fresh, Sharwood's*	1oz/28g	70	0.9	251	7.3	48.0	3.3	2.0
Naan, Garlic & Coriander, Free From, Tesco*	1 Naan/90g	215	6.0	240	5.1	38.7	6.7	4.9
Naan, Garlic & Coriander, Fresh, Sharwood's*	1oz/28g	71	0.9	252	7.7	47.8	3.3	2.2
Naan, Garlic & Coriander, Large, TTD, Sainsbury's*	¼ Pack/70g	194	3.8	277	9.4	47.7	5.4	2.2
Naan, Garlic & Coriander, M&S*	1 Naan/150g	375	2.1	250	9.8	50.1	1.4	2.0
Naan, Garlic & Coriander, Mild, Patak's*	1 Naan/140g	452	15.1	323	9.0	47.5	10.8	0.0
Naan, Garlic & Coriander, Mini, Asda*	1 Naan/110g	320	12.5	291	6.9	40.2	11.4	2.5
Naan, Garlic & Coriander, Mini, Finest, Tesco*	1 Naan/50g	160	6.8	320	6.7	42.4	13.5	0.8
Naan, Garlic & Coriander, Mini, Long Life, Sharwood's*	1oz/28g	76	2.1	272	6.5	42.9	7.4	2.4
Naan, Garlic & Coriander, Mini, Sainsbury's*	1 Naan/50g	140	2.0	280	8.2	51.2	4.1	2.6
Naan, Garlic & Coriander, Mini, Sharwood's*	1 Naan/59g	144	2.0	244	7.1	46.2	3.4	2.0
Naan, Garlic & Coriander, Mini, Tesco*	1 Naan/65g	185	5.0	285	7.6	45.6	7.7	2.6
Naan, Garlic & Coriander, Mini, Weight Watchers*	1 Naan/40g	100	1.0	250	9.3	47.6	2.5	4.2
Naan, Garlic & Coriander, Sainsbury's*	1 Serving/130g	373	10.0	287	8.7	45.8	7.7	2.4
Naan, Garlic & Coriander, Tesco*	½ Naan/83g	235	6.4	285	7.6	45.6	7.7	2.6
Naan, Garlic & Coriander, TTD, Sainsbury's*	1 Serving/70g	215	8.1	307	7.0	43.9	11.5	2.9
Naan, Garlic & Coriander, Weight Watchers*	1 Naan/60g	155	2.6	259	8.9	46.0	4.3	3.4
Naan, Indian Meal for Two, Sainsbury's*	1 Naan/125g	357	9.3	285	8.7	45.9	7.4	1.9
Naan, LC, Tesco*	1 Naan/71g	181	1.6	255	7.5	50.7	2.2	2.3
Naan, Mini, LC, Tesco*	1 Naan/65g	150	1.8	230	8.1	42.5	2.8	2.9
Naan, Onion Bhaji, M&S*	1 Naan/140g	400	17.0	285	9.5	34.2	12.1	2.0
Naan, Peshwari, Apple & Coconut, Mini, Sharwood's*	1 Naan/40g	112	2.7	281	6.9	46.6	6.7	3.1
Naan, Peshwari, Finest, Tesco*	1 Naan/130g	338	7.3	260	8.6	43.7	5.6	4.9
Naan, Peshwari, Fresh, Sharwood's*	1oz/28g	67	1.4	240	6.8	41.9	5.0	2.5
Naan, Peshwari, Long Life, Sharwood's*	1oz/28g	71	1.8	252	6.2	42.0	6.6	2.6
Naan, Peshwari, M&S*	1 Serving/127g	394	12.8	310	9.2	45.8	10.1	1.9
Naan, Peshwari, Mega, Asda*	1 Naan/220g	680	26.4	309	7.1	43.1	12.0	2.7
Naan, Peshwari, Sainsbury's*	1 Naan/166g	511	18.3	308	7.1	45.1	11.0	4.7
Naan, Peshwari, Sharwood's*	1 Naan/130g	334	6.9	257	7.2	45.1	5.3	2.5

BREAD

INFO/WEIGHT	Measure	per Measure		Nutrition Values per 100g / 100ml				
		KCAL	FAT	KCAL	PROT	CARB	FAT	FIBRE
Naan, Peshwari, Tesco*	1 Naan/215g	684	26.7	318	7.5	48.9	12.4	4.8
Naan, Peshwari, TTD, Sainsbury's*	1 Serving/80g	247	10.1	309	6.3	42.5	12.6	4.4
Naan, Plain, Average	1 Naan/160g	437	10.5	273	8.0	45.7	6.5	2.1
Naan, Plain, GFY, Asda*	1 Naan/130g	307	2.7	236	8.4	45.9	2.1	2.4
Naan, Plain, Indian, Mini, Asda*	1 Naan/110g	329	12.6	299	6.6	42.2	11.5	2.1
Naan, Plain, Large, Sainsbury's*	½ Naan/70g	191	4.6	273	7.1	46.2	6.6	3.0
Naan, Plain, Large, TTD, Sainsbury's*	¼ Pack/70g	202	4.1	288	9.5	49.3	5.9	2.5
Naan, Plain, Mega, Indian Takeaway, Asda*	1 Naan/222g	572	8.4	258	7.0	49.0	3.8	2.5
Naan, Plain, Mini, Asda*	1 Naan/58g	156	2.7	269	8.0	49.0	4.6	2.3
Naan, Plain, Mini, BGTY, Sainsbury's*	1 Naan/50g	113	1.1	226	8.2	43.2	2.2	3.3
Naan, Plain, Mini, Fresh, Sharwood's*	1oz/28g	70	0.9	251	7.3	48.0	3.3	2.0
Naan, Plain, Mini, Weight Watchers*	1 Naan/44g	108	1.1	245	9.1	46.5	2.5	4.9
Naan, Plain, Sharwood's*	1 Naan/120g	326	8.9	272	8.5	42.9	7.4	2.4
Naan, Plain, Tesco*	1 Naan/150g	392	6.9	261	8.4	46.4	4.6	2.3
Naan, Plain, Value, Tesco*	1 Naan/135g	363	9.7	269	8.1	42.9	7.2	1.6
Naan, Smart Price, Asda*	1 Naan/100g	233	1.9	233	8.7	45.3	1.9	2.8
Naan, Take Away, Tesco*	1 Naan/39g	97	1.3	248	8.7	45.6	3.4	1.7
Naan, Tandoori, Sharwood's*	1 Naan/130g	330	6.5	254	7.3	45.0	5.0	2.0
Naan, Tandoori Baked, Waitrose*	1 Naan/140g	372	4.3	266	9.8	49.6	3.1	2.9
Oatmeal, Farmhouse, Extra Special, Asda*	1 Slice/44g	102	1.1	231	11.0	41.0	2.6	6.0
Oatmeal, Farmhouse, Soft, M&S*	1 Slice/45g	110	2.0	245	11.1	39.5	4.4	5.2
Oatmeal, Sliced Loaf, Tesco*	1 Slice/50g	111	1.7	222	7.4	40.5	3.4	2.8
Olive, Waitrose*	1 Slice/28g	86	3.0	306	9.0	43.6	10.6	2.0
Pain Au Raisin, Loaf, M&S*	1 Pain/74g	215	9.5	290	5.3	38.7	12.8	1.2
Pave, Walnut, Sainsbury's*	1 Serving/50g	140	4.8	280	9.0	40.0	9.5	3.5
Petit Pain, Homebake, Mini, Tesco*	1 Roll/50g	120	0.6	240	7.8	48.5	1.2	3.4
Petit Pain, Mini, Homebake, Tesco*	1 Roll/45g	110	0.6	245	7.8	49.7	1.3	2.5
Petit Pain, Organic, Tesco*	1 Roll/100g	235	0.8	235	7.8	49.1	0.8	1.2
Petit Pain, Part Bake, Weight Watchers*	1 Roll/50g	111	0.4	223	6.8	43.5	0.9	6.8
Petit Pain, White, Ready to Bake, Sainsbury's*	1 Roll/50g	122	0.7	242	7.8	49.7	1.3	2.8
Petit Pain, White, Soft, Somerfield*	1 Roll/68g	186	1.2	274	8.5	56.1	1.7	2.1
Pitta, 159, Pride Valley*	1 Pitta/63g	159	1.2	252	10.1	51.2	1.9	2.6
Pitta, Bakersfield*	1 Pitta/67g	167	0.7	250	7.0	52.0	1.0	1.5
Pitta, Brown, Organic, Waitrose*	1 Pitta/60g	137	0.8	228	6.4	47.5	1.4	6.6
Pitta, Free From, Sainsbury's*	1 Pitta/65g	164	2.5	252	4.1	50.0	3.9	2.9
Pitta, Garlic, Morrisons*	1 Pitta/60g	149	1.1	249	9.7	51.1	1.8	0.0
Pitta, Garlic, Sainsbury's*	1 Pitta/60g	153	0.6	255	9.5	52.0	1.0	2.5
Pitta, Garlic & Coriander, Asda*	1 Pitta/55g	116	0.5	212	7.0	44.0	0.9	1.8
Pitta, Garlic & Herb, Tesco*	1 Pitta/60g	134	1.2	223	9.6	44.6	2.0	3.0
Pitta, Mexican, Santa Maria*	1 Pitta/66g	165	0.7	250	7.5	52.0	1.0	0.0
Pitta, Multi Seed, & Cereal, The Food Doctor*	1 Pitta/70g	157	1.9	224	10.1	39.9	2.7	10.2
Pitta, Organic, Tesco*	1 Pitta/60g	124	0.8	206	8.3	40.2	1.4	5.7
Pitta, Pockets, Pride Valley*	1 Pitta/63g	151	0.6	239	9.3	48.4	0.9	3.2
Pitta, Pockets, Sainsbury's*	1 Pitta/75g	188	0.8	250	8.5	52.0	1.0	3.5
Pitta, White, Average	**1 Pitta/75g**	**191**	**1.1**	**255**	**9.2**	**50.8**	**1.5**	**2.7**
Pitta, White, Basics, Sainsbury's*	1 Pitta/48g	124	0.6	261	8.8	52.7	1.2	2.0
Pitta, White, Free From, Tesco*	1 Pitta/55g	140	1.2	255	6.5	52.6	2.1	5.5
Pitta, White, Greek Style, Asda*	1 Pitta/50g	126	1.0	253	8.0	51.0	1.9	0.0
Pitta, White, Large, Tesco*	1 Pitta/90g	252	1.9	280	9.8	55.1	2.1	3.4
Pitta, White, M&S*	1 Pitta/61g	146	1.2	240	9.3	46.9	2.0	3.6
Pitta, White, Mini, Sainsbury's*	1 Pitta/20g	54	0.2	268	8.8	54.6	1.2	2.0
Pitta, White, Mini, Tesco*	1 Pitta/30g	84	0.6	280	9.8	55.1	2.1	3.4
Pitta, White, Organic, Sainsbury's*	1 Pitta/59g	150	0.6	254	10.3	50.7	1.1	2.5

BREAD

Measure INFO/WEIGHT	per Measure KCAL	FAT	Nutrition Values per 100g / 100ml KCAL	PROT	CARB	FAT	FIBRE
BREAD							
Pitta, White, Sainsbury's* — 1 Pitta/60g	161	0.8	269	9.0	54.1	1.3	2.5
Pitta, White, Soft, Sandwich, Warburton's* — ½ Pitta/36g	81	0.9	228	9.8	41.4	2.6	1.8
Pitta, White, Speciality Breads, Waitrose* — 1 Pitta/60g	149	0.7	249	10.3	49.3	1.2	3.5
Pitta, White, Tesco* — 1 Pitta/60g	170	1.3	283	9.8	55.2	2.2	3.3
Pitta, White, Weight Watchers* — 1 Pitta/45g	106	0.3	238	8.7	45.9	0.7	6.7
Pitta, White Picnic, Waitrose* — 1 Pitta/30g	75	0.4	249	10.3	49.3	1.2	3.5
Pitta, Wholemeal, Acropolis, Lidl* — 1 Pitta/57g	136	0.9	238	12.0	44.0	1.6	6.0
Pitta, Wholemeal, Asda* — 1 Pitta/56g	133	0.9	238	12.0	44.0	1.6	6.0
Pitta, Wholemeal, Average — 1 Pitta/64g	**154**	**1.1**	**241**	**11.0**	**45.8**	**1.7**	**6.4**
Pitta, Wholemeal, Essential, Waitrose* — 1 Pitta/60g	145	0.5	242	12.4	46.0	0.9	6.0
Pitta, Wholemeal, Healthy Eating, Co-Op* — 1 Pitta/63g	135	1.3	215	12.0	37.0	2.0	9.0
Pitta, Wholemeal, Hollyland Bakery* — 1 Pitta/20g	48	0.3	242	13.1	43.7	1.6	6.0
Pitta, Wholemeal, Lemon Black Pepper, Finest, Tesco* — 1 Pitta/80g	215	4.8	270	10.8	42.4	6.0	6.0
Pitta, Wholemeal, M&S* — 1 Pitta/60g	155	1.6	255	10.0	45.0	2.6	5.5
Pitta, Wholemeal, Mini, M&S* — 1 Pitta/18g	44	0.4	247	10.3	45.8	2.5	5.6
Pitta, Wholemeal, Mini, Sainsbury's* — 1 Pitta/30g	69	0.5	231	10.0	43.8	1.7	6.2
Pitta, Wholemeal, Mini, Tesco* — 1 Pitta/30g	76	0.5	255	11.8	48.2	1.7	4.2
Pitta, Wholemeal, Round, SuperValu* — 1 Pitta/48g	57	0.4	118	4.9	20.7	0.8	2.9
Pitta, Wholemeal, Sainsbury's* — 1 Pitta/60g	154	1.0	257	9.8	47.8	1.7	5.8
Pitta, Wholemeal, Tesco* — 1 Pitta/60g	147	1.5	245	11.2	43.6	2.5	8.7
Pitta, Wholemeal, Waitrose* — 1 Pitta/60g	145	0.5	242	12.4	46.0	0.9	3.1
Pitta, Wholemeal, Weight Watchers* — 1 Pitta/46g	106	0.6	229	8.7	44.5	1.2	7.6
Pitta, Wholemeal with Extra Virgin Olive Oil, Tesco* — 1 Pitta/60g	135	1.6	225	8.3	41.5	2.6	5.5
Potato Farls, Irish, Rankin Selection, Irwin's Bakery* — 1 Farl/60g	110	2.2	184	2.3	34.4	3.6	2.5
Potato Farls, M&S* — 1 Farl/55g	79	0.2	144	4.2	33.8	0.4	4.7
Potato Farls, Sunblest* — 1 Farl/100g	156	0.9	156	3.8	33.2	0.9	1.9
Pumpernickel, Organic, Bavarian Pumpernickel* — 1 Slice/50g	90	0.5	180	6.0	38.0	1.0	10.0
Pumpernickel Rye, Kelderman* — 1 Slice/50g	92	0.5	185	6.0	38.0	1.0	0.0
Pumpkin Seed, Raisin & Sunflower Seed, Sainsbury's* — 1 Slice/30g	76	0.8	255	11.6	45.9	2.8	3.4
Raisin, & Pumpkin Seed, Organic, Tesco* — 1 Slice/30g	76	1.7	253	9.7	40.6	5.8	3.8
Raisin, with Cinnamon, Warburton's* — 1 Slice/36g	96	1.3	267	7.2	51.1	3.7	3.2
Roasted Onion, M&S* — 1 Slice/50g	125	1.6	250	9.0	46.7	3.3	2.1
Rolls, 3 Seeded, Sandwich, Warburton's* — 1 Roll/77g	242	6.7	314	13.3	41.2	8.7	6.0
Rolls, American Style Deli, Tesco* — 1 Roll/65g	162	2.2	249	7.8	46.8	3.4	1.6
Rolls, Batched Sandwich, Warburton's* — 1 Roll/60g	148	2.5	246	9.6	42.7	4.1	0.0
Rolls, Best of Both, Hovis* — 1 Roll/62g	148	2.9	239	9.8	39.7	4.6	5.0
Rolls, Brioche — 1 Roll/53g	191	7.5	361	8.8	50.1	14.1	1.5
Rolls, Brioche, Average — 1 Roll/49g	177	6.9	361	8.8	50.1	14.1	1.5
Rolls, Brioche, Brialys* — 1 Roll/35g	121	3.9	347	8.8	52.8	11.2	1.5
Rolls, Brioche, Butter, Tesco* — 1 Serving/35g	126	4.5	360	8.8	51.3	12.8	2.0
Rolls, Brioche, Chocolate Chip, Milk, CBY, Asda* — 1 Roll/25g	91	3.6	363	8.0	50.0	14.5	1.8
Rolls, Brioche, Chocolate Chip, Plain, Sainsbury's* — 1 Roll/35g	131	5.6	374	8.5	49.0	16.0	5.9
Rolls, Brioche, Chocolate Chip, Tesco* — 1 Serving/35g	131	5.6	374	8.6	49.1	16.0	6.0
Rolls, Brioche, Continental Classics* — 1 Roll/35g	122	3.3	349	8.2	58.3	9.3	0.0
Rolls, Brioche, Finest, Tesco* — 1 Roll/52g	207	11.6	398	10.8	38.3	22.4	2.0
Rolls, Brioche, Sainsbury's* — 1 Roll/32g	116	3.7	362	8.5	56.0	11.5	3.6
Rolls, Brioche, Tesco* — 1 Roll/26g	92	2.9	349	8.5	54.0	11.0	0.0
Rolls, Brown, Crusty — 1 Roll/50g	**128**	**1.4**	**255**	**10.3**	**50.4**	**2.8**	**3.5**
Rolls, Brown, Free From, Tesco* — 1 Roll/65g	174	5.3	268	5.4	43.2	8.2	3.6
Rolls, Brown, Large, Asda* — 1 Roll/57g	138	0.9	242	10.0	47.0	1.6	0.0
Rolls, Brown, M&S* — 1 Roll/105g	242	6.4	230	9.2	37.3	6.1	4.4
Rolls, Brown, Malted Grain, Tesco* — 1 Roll/58g	144	1.9	248	8.7	46.2	3.2	1.9
Rolls, Brown, Mini, M&S* — 1 Roll/33g	80	2.5	245	9.8	35.5	7.6	3.8

BREAD

	Measure INFO/WEIGHT	per Measure KCAL	FAT	Nutrition Values per 100g / 100ml KCAL	PROT	CARB	FAT	FIBRE
Rolls, Brown, Morning, Farmfoods*	1 Roll/50g	134	1.8	269	12.0	47.0	3.7	4.2
Rolls, Brown, Old Fashioned, Waitrose*	1 Roll/63g	152	2.6	241	9.6	41.3	4.1	4.7
Rolls, Brown, Seeded, Organic, Sainsbury's*	1 Roll/70g	166	3.2	237	9.9	39.1	4.6	6.5
Rolls, Brown, Snack, Allinson*	1 Roll/44g	119	2.9	270	10.8	41.6	6.7	5.6
Rolls, Brown, Soft, Average	1 Roll/50g	134	1.9	268	10.0	51.8	3.8	3.5
Rolls, Brown, Soft, Organic, Sainsbury's*	1 Roll/70g	166	3.2	237	9.9	39.1	4.6	6.6
Rolls, Brown, Soft, Tesco*	1 Roll/50g	118	1.8	235	9.0	41.6	3.6	4.5
Rolls, Brown, Square, M&S*	1 Roll/105g	242	6.4	230	9.2	37.3	6.1	4.4
Rolls, Cheese & Tomato, Seeded, White, M&S*	1 Pack/160g	480	25.0	300	13.7	26.1	15.6	2.1
Rolls, Cheese Topped, Sandwich, Warburton's*	1 Roll/62g	168	4.0	270	12.1	40.7	6.5	2.6
Rolls, Cheese Topped, Village Green*	1 Roll/56g	159	4.1	284	13.1	41.2	7.4	4.8
Rolls, Ciabatta, Brown, GF, Dietary Specials*	1 Roll/50g	137	4.0	274	5.8	36.9	8.1	8.9
Rolls, Ciabatta, Cheese Topped, Mini, Finest, Tesco*	1 Roll/30g	85	2.4	282	11.5	40.9	8.1	3.8
Rolls, Ciabatta, Garlic, Asda*	1 Roll/93g	333	16.7	358	9.0	40.0	18.0	2.3
Rolls, Ciabatta, M&S*	1 Roll/80g	210	3.3	262	10.3	48.1	4.1	2.1
Rolls, Ciabatta, Mini, Finest, Tesco*	1 Roll/30g	89	2.0	297	9.9	49.1	6.8	4.1
Rolls, Ciabatta, Sun Dried Tomato, Mini, Finest, Tesco*	1 Roll/30g	79	1.9	262	8.7	42.3	6.4	2.6
Rolls, Ciabatta, Tesco*	1 Roll/80g	208	2.5	260	8.6	48.2	3.1	3.3
Rolls, Country Grain, Mini, M&S*	1 Roll/31g	85	3.0	275	10.2	38.9	9.7	3.8
Rolls, Crusty, Booths*	1 Roll/50g	124	0.6	247	8.7	50.3	1.2	2.6
Rolls, Crusty, French, M&S*	1 Roll/65g	159	0.8	245	8.1	50.5	1.2	3.3
Rolls, Crusty, Part-Baked, Budgens*	1 Roll/50g	148	0.7	296	9.4	61.4	1.4	2.5
Rolls, Finger, Morrisons*	1 Roll/46g	119	0.8	259	10.7	50.0	1.8	2.3
Rolls, Finger, White, Sainsbury's*	1 Roll/40g	96	1.0	240	9.0	45.2	2.6	3.2
Rolls, Focaccia, Tesco*	1 Roll/75g	226	7.0	302	8.7	45.6	9.4	3.8
Rolls, GF, Antoinette Savill*	1 Roll/70g	157	1.5	224	1.9	48.8	2.2	1.5
Rolls, Granary, Average	1 Roll/70g	176	2.7	251	9.6	45.2	3.9	3.3
Rolls, Granary, Bakers Premium, Tesco*	1 Roll/65g	158	0.8	243	9.9	47.8	1.3	2.3
Rolls, Granary, Homebake, Hovis*	1 Roll/75g	194	1.6	259	10.2	47.7	2.2	3.6
Rolls, Granary, Mini, Tesco*	1 Roll/34g	92	2.2	271	10.0	43.5	6.5	3.8
Rolls, Granary, Original, Hovis*	1 Roll/70g	180	2.9	257	10.7	44.3	4.1	5.3
Rolls, Granary, Waitrose*	1 Roll/59g	160	3.8	271	10.0	47.2	6.4	3.8
Rolls, Granary Malted Wheatgrain, Soft, M&S*	1 Roll/80g	208	3.1	260	9.3	47.2	3.9	2.3
Rolls, Green Olive, M&S*	1 Roll/75g	210	4.5	280	11.2	44.0	6.0	1.8
Rolls, Hot Dog, Sliced, Asda*	1 Roll/84g	197	2.8	234	7.0	44.0	3.3	0.0
Rolls, Hot Dog, Tesco*	1 Roll/85g	200	2.8	235	7.3	44.0	3.3	1.9
Rolls, Hot Dog, Value, Tesco*	1 Roll/40g	93	0.8	232	8.7	45.0	1.9	2.2
Rolls, Hot Dog, Warburton's*	1 Roll/60g	137	2.8	228	8.7	37.8	4.7	1.7
Rolls, Hot Dog, White, Jumbo, Sainsbury's*	1 Roll/85g	239	5.2	281	7.5	49.1	6.1	2.9
Rolls, Hot Dog, White, Tesco*	1 Roll/65g	169	2.4	260	9.6	46.1	3.7	3.2
Rolls, Malted, Wholegrain, Batched, Soft, M&S*	1 Roll/80g	180	3.6	225	7.8	38.5	4.5	3.1
Rolls, Malted Grain, Sainsbury's*	1 Roll/68g	190	2.9	280	8.7	51.6	4.3	4.2
Rolls, Malted Grain, Soft, Weight Watchers*	1 Roll/57g	142	1.0	251	11.7	47.1	1.8	4.2
Rolls, Malted Grain, Submarine, M&S*	1 Roll/109g	300	4.7	275	8.9	53.6	4.3	3.0
Rolls, Milk, Warburton's*	1 Slice/18g	46	0.5	253	11.0	45.1	2.7	2.7
Rolls, Morning, Scottish, Morrisons*	1 Roll/60g	157	1.3	261	11.3	51.4	2.2	2.4
Rolls, Morning, Tesco*	1 Roll/48g	117	1.2	243	10.4	44.8	2.5	4.7
Rolls, Multi Seed, Free From, Tesco*	1 Roll/70g	214	8.3	305	5.4	44.2	11.8	6.3
Rolls, Multigrain, Pain Rustique, Finest, Tesco*	1 Roll/60g	162	4.3	270	12.7	38.4	7.1	9.6
Rolls, Multigrain, Torpedo, Sainsbury's*	1 Roll/112g	328	7.5	293	10.5	47.7	6.7	6.3
Rolls, Nut & Raisin, Bakery, Tesco*	1 Serving/120g	426	11.2	355	9.0	56.8	9.3	4.0
Rolls, Oatmeal, Co-Op*	1 Roll/70g	175	3.2	250	10.1	42.6	4.6	5.6
Rolls, Oatmeal, Ploughmans, GFY, Asda*	1 Roll/72g	181	3.2	252	10.0	43.0	4.4	3.9

B

BREAD

INFO/WEIGHT	per Measure KCAL	FAT	Nutrition Values per 100g / 100ml KCAL	PROT	CARB	FAT	FIBRE
Rolls, Oatmeal, Soft, M&S*	1 Roll/83g	224	3.9	270	12.3	43.4	4.7	3.4
Rolls, Panini, Sainsbury's*	1 Roll/90g	249	5.6	276	11.0	44.1	6.2	3.0
Rolls, Panini, White, Tesco*	1 Roll/75g	210	4.6	280	10.1	45.2	6.1	2.7
Rolls, Part Baked, Mini, Tesco*	1 Roll/50g	120	0.6	240	7.8	49.5	1.2	3.4
Rolls, Poppy Seeded, Knot, Waitrose*	1 Roll/60g	169	3.2	282	10.3	48.3	5.3	2.2
Rolls, Premium Seeded, Four, Aldi, Village Bakery*	1 Roll/82g	196	3.6	239	9.4	40.5	4.4	7.3
Rolls, Rye, Toasting, Good & Hot*	1 Roll/65g	143	0.7	220	7.3	44.6	1.1	7.1
Rolls, Seed Sensations, Deli, Hovis*	1 Roll/70g	184	6.0	263	10.3	36.5	8.5	10.6
Rolls, Seeded, Genius*	1 Roll/80g	228	9.0	285	6.6	32.8	11.2	13.0
Rolls, Seeded, Mixed Mini Loaf Pack, M&S*	1 Roll/76g	220	7.3	290	10.6	39.7	9.6	4.0
Rolls, Seeded, Sandwich, Warburton's*	1 Roll/77g	242	6.7	314	13.3	41.2	8.7	6.0
Rolls, Snack, Mini, Tesco*	1 Roll/35g	95	2.1	271	19.0	43.0	6.0	4.0
Rolls, Sub, Brown, Deli, Asda*	1 Roll/60g	142	1.9	236	0.0	35.0	3.2	0.0
Rolls, Submarine, Mini, M&S*	1 Roll/23g	63	1.1	275	11.4	47.7	4.9	1.1
Rolls, Submarine, Sainsbury's*	1 Roll/117g	305	4.6	261	9.1	47.4	3.9	2.4
Rolls, Submarine, White, Mini, M&S*	1 Roll/30g	86	1.5	285	11.4	47.7	4.9	1.1
Rolls, Sunflower Seed, Toasting, Good & Hot*	1 Roll/65g	162	3.2	250	8.5	41.0	5.0	8.0
Rolls, Tiger, Crusty, Baked by Us, Morrisons*	1 Roll/63g	143	1.8	227	6.3	46.0	2.9	2.5
Rolls, Tomato, Sun Dried, Homebake, Tesco*	1 Roll/50g	123	1.5	246	11.3	44.0	3.0	0.0
Rolls, White, 50/50, Soft, Kingsmill*	1 Roll/63g	154	2.4	245	9.3	41.2	3.8	4.4
Rolls, White, Basics, Somerfield*	1 Roll/44g	107	0.7	243	8.9	48.2	1.6	2.1
Rolls, White, BGTY, Sainsbury's*	1 Roll/50g	114	0.5	227	9.1	45.3	1.0	3.0
Rolls, White, Cheese Topped, Asda*	1 Roll/46g	121	2.0	264	10.0	46.0	4.4	2.0
Rolls, White, Cheese Topped, Sainsbury's*	1 Roll/75g	218	6.4	291	12.1	41.6	8.5	2.0
Rolls, White, Chunky, Hovis*	1 Roll/73g	173	2.4	237	9.4	41.7	3.3	2.5
Rolls, White, Crusty, Average	*1 Roll/50g*	*140*	*1.2*	*280*	*10.9*	*57.6*	*2.3*	*1.5*
Rolls, White, Crusty, Home Bake, Tesco*	1 Roll/69g	185	1.0	270	9.3	54.2	1.4	2.9
Rolls, White, Crusty, Morning, M&S*	1 Roll/65g	176	0.8	270	8.8	53.8	1.3	2.7
Rolls, White, Finger, Smart Price, Asda*	1 Roll/50g	121	0.8	242	9.0	48.0	1.6	2.1
Rolls, White, Finger, Tesco*	1 Roll/68g	170	2.4	250	8.5	45.8	3.5	2.1
Rolls, White, Finger, Value, Tesco*	1 Roll/50g	116	1.0	232	8.7	45.0	1.9	2.2
Rolls, White, Floured, Batch, Tesco*	1 Roll/76g	193	2.5	254	8.8	47.3	3.3	2.2
Rolls, White, Floured, Warburton's*	1 Roll/50g	124	1.9	247	9.8	43.3	3.8	2.7
Rolls, White, Floury, Roberts Bakery*	1 Roll/63g	160	1.6	254	8.4	49.5	2.5	2.0
Rolls, White, Floury Batch, Sainsbury's*	1 Roll/68g	168	1.9	247	8.3	47.2	2.8	2.2
Rolls, White, Free From, Livwell*	1 Roll/60g	170	4.7	283	3.8	47.7	7.8	4.2
Rolls, White, Large, Sliced, Warburton's*	1 Roll/89g	230	4.0	258	10.1	44.4	4.5	2.7
Rolls, White, Low Price, Sainsbury's*	1 Roll/44g	107	0.7	243	8.9	48.2	1.6	2.1
Rolls, White, Morning, Co-Op*	1 Roll/47g	134	1.4	285	12.0	53.0	3.0	2.0
Rolls, White, Old Fashioned, Waitrose*	1 Roll/64g	176	2.9	275	8.8	49.8	4.5	2.8
Rolls, White, Organic, Sainsbury's*	1 Roll/65g	170	2.0	262	8.7	49.9	3.0	1.0
Rolls, White, Part Baked, Morrisons*	1 Roll/75g	227	1.0	303	9.6	63.0	1.4	2.6
Rolls, White, Ploughman's, Sainsbury's*	1 Roll/65g	185	2.5	285	8.6	54.1	3.8	2.3
Rolls, White, Premium, Hovis*	1 Roll/70g	180	3.1	257	9.5	44.8	4.4	3.0
Rolls, White, Premium Soft, Rathbones*	1 Roll/65g	190	3.9	293	9.3	50.3	6.0	2.7
Rolls, White, Sandwich, Large, Warburton's*	1 Roll/88g	224	3.5	254	10.2	44.3	4.0	2.5
Rolls, White, Sandwich, Regular, Warburton's*	1 Roll/58g	143	2.5	249	9.7	42.6	4.4	2.4
Rolls, White, Scottish, Tesco*	1 Roll/48g	117	1.2	243	10.4	44.8	2.5	4.7
Rolls, White, Seeded, Sainsbury's*	1 Roll/80g	217	4.7	271	10.9	43.4	5.9	4.8
Rolls, White, Seeded, Soft, M&S*	1 Roll/75g	214	4.3	285	11.7	46.2	5.7	2.8
Rolls, White, Snack, Sainsbury's*	1 Roll/67g	159	0.7	237	7.9	49.2	1.0	2.3
Rolls, White, Soft, Average	*1 Roll/45g*	*114*	*1.5*	*253*	*9.2*	*46.5*	*3.3*	*2.2*
Rolls, White, Soft, COU, M&S*	1 Roll/37g	94	1.0	255	10.7	47.1	2.7	1.5

BREAD

INFO/WEIGHT	Measure	per Measure		Nutrition Values per 100g / 100ml				
		KCAL	FAT	KCAL	PROT	CARB	FAT	FIBRE
Rolls, White, Soft, Dietary Specials*	1 Roll/75g	130	2.9	172	2.2	29.8	3.8	4.7
Rolls, White, Soft, Farmhouse, TTD, Sainsbury's*	1 Slice/47g	111	0.8	235	8.1	45.4	1.7	2.9
Rolls, White, Soft, Farmhouse, Warburton's*	1 Roll/59g	148	2.6	250	9.7	43.0	4.4	2.5
Rolls, White, Soft, Hovis*	1 Roll/70g	180	3.1	257	9.5	44.8	4.4	3.0
Rolls, White, Soft, Kingsmill*	1 Roll/62g	156	1.7	252	8.9	46.7	2.8	2.4
Rolls, White, Soft, M&S*	1 Roll/60g	150	1.9	250	10.3	45.2	3.1	2.7
Rolls, White, Soft, Morrisons*	1 Roll/42g	100	0.8	238	9.1	46.4	1.9	2.4
Rolls, White, Soft, Tesco*	1 Roll/72g	175	1.8	243	7.6	46.7	2.5	2.8
Rolls, White, Softgrain, GFY, Asda*	1 Roll/54g	128	1.0	237	9.0	46.0	1.9	2.9
Rolls, White, Split, Asda*	1 Roll/45g	113	1.5	251	10.0	45.0	3.4	2.8
Rolls, White, Sub, Tesco*	1 Roll/100g	258	4.0	258	11.1	44.4	4.0	2.8
Rolls, White, Submarine, M&S*	1 Roll/109g	300	5.4	275	11.0	47.0	5.0	1.0
Rolls, White, Tesco*	1 Roll/30g	79	0.7	262	9.7	50.5	2.3	2.9
Rolls, White, Warburton's*	1 Roll/57g	141	2.4	248	9.7	42.8	4.2	0.0
Rolls, Wholemeal	*1 Roll/45g*	*108*	*1.3*	*241*	*9.0*	*48.3*	*2.9*	*5.9*
Rolls, Wholemeal, Asda*	1 Roll/58g	130	1.6	225	11.0	39.0	2.8	6.0
Rolls, Wholemeal, COU, M&S*	1 Roll/110g	226	3.1	205	11.3	33.4	2.8	7.1
Rolls, Wholemeal, Deli, Tesco*	1 Serving/65g	156	3.1	240	9.0	40.2	4.8	5.7
Rolls, Wholemeal, Finger, Soft, M&S*	1 Roll/66g	145	1.3	220	12.6	38.0	2.0	5.8
Rolls, Wholemeal, Floury Batch, Sainsbury's*	1 Roll/68g	152	2.3	223	9.7	37.8	3.4	6.5
Rolls, Wholemeal, Golden, Hovis*	1 Roll/50g	112	2.0	223	10.5	36.5	3.9	6.8
Rolls, Wholemeal, Kingsmill*	1 Roll/68g	167	2.7	245	10.7	41.5	4.0	5.1
Rolls, Wholemeal, Mini, Assorted, Waitrose*	1 Roll/35g	86	2.1	244	9.7	37.9	6.0	7.3
Rolls, Wholemeal, Mini, Tesco*	1 Roll/34g	82	1.9	240	10.9	36.4	5.6	5.8
Rolls, Wholemeal, Mini Loaves, Hovis*	1 Loaf/70g	175	4.1	250	10.6	38.7	5.9	6.8
Rolls, Wholemeal, Morrisons*	1 Roll/67g	155	2.7	231	10.2	38.6	4.0	6.3
Rolls, Wholemeal, Oat Topped, Deli, Tesco*	1 Roll/65g	170	3.5	260	10.9	38.3	5.3	6.7
Rolls, Wholemeal, Oat Topped, Tesco*	1 Roll/65g	166	2.9	255	11.3	42.2	4.5	5.1
Rolls, Wholemeal, Old Fashioned, Waitrose*	1 Roll/57g	135	2.7	236	11.1	37.2	4.8	6.6
Rolls, Wholemeal, Organic, Sainsbury's*	1 Roll/66g	152	1.8	230	10.7	41.0	2.7	6.6
Rolls, Wholemeal, Organic, Tesco*	1 Roll/65g	177	4.0	273	10.3	44.1	6.2	5.5
Rolls, Wholemeal, Ploughman's, Sainsbury's*	1 Roll/67g	153	2.1	229	10.7	39.3	3.2	8.6
Rolls, Wholemeal, Sainsbury's*	1 Roll/65g	153	2.1	236	10.7	40.8	3.3	7.4
Rolls, Wholemeal, Seeded, The Country Miller, Waitrose*	1 Roll/75g	190	7.7	255	13.6	26.9	10.3	7.6
Rolls, Wholemeal, Sliced, Hovis*	1 Roll/60g	150	3.5	250	10.6	38.7	5.9	6.8
Rolls, Wholemeal, Soft, Average	*1 Roll/65g*	*151*	*2.7*	*233*	*10.8*	*37.3*	*4.1*	*6.3*
Rolls, Wholemeal, Soft, Sainsbury's*	1 Roll/60g	133	2.0	221	9.9	37.8	3.4	6.5
Rolls, Wholemeal, Soft, Seeded, Sainsbury's*	1 Roll/75g	193	5.6	257	11.8	35.6	7.4	6.2
Rolls, Wholemeal, Submarine, Warburton's*	1 Roll/94g	231	4.1	246	10.9	40.6	4.4	6.3
Rolls, Wholemeal, Submarine, Wheatfield Bakery*	1 Roll/100g	230	3.4	230	10.4	39.0	3.4	6.2
Rolls, Wholemeal, Sunflower & Honey, Sainsbury's*	1 Roll/85g	225	4.3	265	9.2	45.4	5.1	4.5
Rolls, Wholemeal, Tasty, Great Everyday, Kingsmill*	1 Roll/68g	158	2.6	232	10.6	38.8	3.8	6.5
Rolls, Wholemeal, Tesco*	1 Roll/46g	115	1.8	250	10.9	41.8	4.0	7.5
Rolls, Wholemeal, Warburton's*	1 Roll/58g	124	2.1	214	10.2	35.1	3.7	6.6
Rolls, Wholemeal, with Cracked Wheat, Allinson*	1 Roll/58g	134	2.3	231	11.0	38.0	3.9	7.0
Rolls, Wholemeal & White, Kingsmill*	1 Roll/60g	151	2.5	251	9.5	43.7	4.2	3.5
Rolls, Wholmeal, Deli, Tesco*	1 Roll/65g	156	3.1	240	9.0	40.2	4.8	5.7
Rosemary, Olive Oil, Round, la Brea Bakery*	1 Serving/100g	250	3.5	250	7.0	47.5	3.5	1.6
Roti, Tesco*	1 Bread/95g	256	5.2	269	8.4	46.4	5.5	3.2
Rye, Artisan, Organic*	1 Slice/50g	80	0.7	160	5.0	28.4	1.4	7.1
Rye, Average	*1 Slice/25g*	*55*	*0.4*	*219*	*8.3*	*45.8*	*1.7*	*4.4*
Rye, Dark, Sliced, Trianon*	1 Slice/41g	74	0.6	180	6.5	35.0	1.5	0.0
Rye, German Style, Bolletje*	1 Slice/60g	114	1.2	190	6.0	35.0	2.0	9.5

BREAD

Measure INFO/WEIGHT	per Measure KCAL	per Measure FAT	Nutrition Values per 100g / 100ml KCAL	PROT	CARB	FAT	FIBRE

Food	Measure INFO/WEIGHT	KCAL	FAT	KCAL	PROT	CARB	FAT	FIBRE
Rye, German Style, Kelderman*	1 Slice/64g	122	1.3	190	6.0	35.0	2.0	9.5
Rye, German Style, Loaf, Bakery in Store, M&S*	2 Slices/50g	112	0.6	225	9.5	40.8	1.1	6.3
Rye, Light, Finest, Tesco*	1 Slice/20g	47	0.4	237	10.4	44.3	2.0	3.7
Rye, Organic, Waitrose*	1 Serving/100g	207	1.2	207	6.4	42.7	1.2	5.1
Rye, Organic, with Coriander, Village Bakery*	1 Slice/30g	63	0.8	209	4.9	49.9	2.7	8.5
Rye, Swedish Style, Kelderman*	1 Slice/50g	92	1.6	185	7.2	31.5	3.2	4.3
Rye, Wholemeal, Wheat, Goldaehren, Aldi*	1 Slice/30g	68	1.2	226	8.0	36.0	4.0	7.0
Rye, Wholemeal, with Sunflower Seeds, Organic, Biona*	1 Slice/72g	150	2.9	210	7.0	36.0	4.0	6.0
Rye, with Seeds, Organic, The Village Bakery Melmerby*	1 Slice/42g	80	1.0	190	6.9	35.6	2.3	9.4
Rye, with Sunflower Seeds, Organic, Schneider Brot*	1 Slice/72g	138	2.6	191	6.2	33.4	3.6	7.9
Rye, with Sunflower Seeds, Organic, Sunnyvale*	1 Slice/25g	50	1.6	198	5.1	30.3	6.3	7.9
Sandwich Thins, White, CBY, Asda*	1 Thin/55g	141	2.2	257	9.3	44.3	4.0	3.1
Seeded, Batch, Finest, Tesco*	1 Slice/65g	168	4.0	259	9.3	41.8	6.1	6.1
Seeded, Farmhouse, Loaf, Extra Special, Asda*	1 Slice/44g	92	0.5	207	11.0	38.0	1.2	8.0
Seeded, Farmhouse, Roberts Bakery*	1 Slice/37g	89	1.1	240	10.6	49.0	2.9	6.7
Seeded, Grains & Seeds, Loaf, Tasty, Warburton's*	1 Slice/38g	100	1.6	264	10.6	45.6	4.3	5.2
Seeded, Medium Sliced, Average	1 Slice/44g	116	2.9	262	11.3	38.6	6.5	5.6
Seeded, Rye, Loaf, la Brea Bakery*	1 Slice/55g	120	0.6	218	7.0	42.5	1.0	5.7
Seeded Batch, Toasted Seeds, 800g, Warburton's*	1 Slice/50g	137	3.7	270	11.4	35.1	7.3	10.2
Seeded Farmhouse, Organic, Cranks*	2 Slices/94g	232	3.5	247	10.1	39.9	3.7	6.9
Seriously Seeded, Gold, Kingsmill*	1 Slice/50g	136	3.4	272	10.9	41.6	6.9	6.4
Sesame Seed, la Brea Bakery*	1 Slice/35g	85	0.8	244	8.8	47.1	2.3	2.0
Sliced Fruited Malt Loaf, Weight Watchers*	1 Slice/23g	68	0.4	294	8.9	60.2	1.9	3.6
Soda	**1oz/28g**	**72**	**0.7**	**258**	**7.7**	**54.6**	**2.5**	**2.1**
Soda, Brown, Irish, Sainsbury's*	1 Serving/100g	208	3.0	208	8.8	36.4	3.0	5.3
Soda, Fruit, M&S*	1 Slice/40g	105	1.9	260	5.9	51.3	4.6	2.5
Soda, Fruit, Sliced, Irish, Irwin's Bakery*	2 Slices/80g	218	4.2	273	2.4	53.8	5.3	2.5
Soda, M&S*	1 Slice/40g	82	0.6	205	8.7	39.2	1.6	4.2
Soda Farls, M&S*	1 Farl/110g	267	3.0	243	9.6	50.1	2.7	2.3
Soda Farls, Tesco*	1 Farl/142g	325	4.5	229	7.1	42.2	3.2	2.6
Softgrain, Medium Sliced, GFY, Asda*	1 Slice/35g	79	0.5	226	7.0	46.0	1.5	3.7
Softgrain, Mighty White*	1 Slice/36g	81	0.5	224	7.2	45.5	1.5	3.7
Sourdough, Average	1 Slice/50g	144	0.9	289	11.8	56.4	1.8	2.4
Sourdough, White, Country, Oval, la Brea Bakery*	1 Slice/60g	143	0.4	239	8.8	49.4	0.6	1.6
Soya & Linseed, Burgen*	1 Slice/43g	124	4.4	288	15.9	29.8	10.1	6.8
Soya & Linseed, Vogel*	1 Slice/42g	95	2.1	227	11.7	34.1	4.9	6.8
Spelt & Seed, Sliced, Lifefibre*	1 Slice/42g	141	5.8	335	11.6	32.2	13.7	9.2
Sprouted Grain, Ezekiel *	1 Slice/34g	80	0.5	235	11.8	44.1	1.5	0.9
Sprouted Spelt with Raisins, Everfresh Bakery*	¼ Loaf/100g	230	1.9	230	9.2	43.9	1.9	6.6
Stoneground, Small Loaf, Organic, Sainsbury's*	1 Slice/24g	50	0.5	208	10.0	37.9	2.1	7.9
Sunflower, Multi-Grain, Allinson*	1 Slice/47g	113	2.2	240	9.8	39.6	4.7	3.9
Sunflower & Honey, M&S*	1 Serving/67g	206	9.0	308	12.9	34.0	13.4	5.6
Sunflower & Honey, Organic, Cranks*	1 Slice/30g	64	0.9	215	11.6	37.2	3.0	8.3
Sunflower & Pumpkin Seed, Batched, Organic, Tesco*	1 Slice/30g	73	2.2	243	11.0	33.1	7.4	5.2
Sunflower & Pumpkin Seed, So Organic, Sainsbury's*	1 Slice/30g	76	1.6	254	11.4	40.0	5.4	12.9
Sunflower Seed, Organic, Natural, Mestemacher*	1 Slice/75g	162	3.0	216	5.6	34.7	4.0	9.4
Ten Seed, Organic, The Village Bakery*	1 Slice/25g	66	1.4	263	9.0	43.8	5.7	3.8
The Really Seeded One, Kingsmill *	1 Slice/44g	118	3.2	268	10.4	37.3	7.3	5.5
Three Grain, Organic, Schneider Brot*	1 Slice/72g	142	1.6	199	5.3	34.5	2.3	9.3
Tiger Loaf, Tesco*	1 Slice/40g	96	0.8	239	8.7	46.6	2.0	2.6
Toaster, White, Rathbones*	1 Slice/38g	92	0.5	243	9.1	48.6	1.3	2.3
Tomato & Garlic, Flatbread, Italian Style, Iceland*	1 Serving/75g	195	8.8	260	6.3	32.3	11.8	2.4
Tomato & Garlic, Italian Style, Morrisons*	½ Pack/155g	355	12.4	229	5.8	33.4	8.0	2.5

BREAD

BREAD	Measure INFO/WEIGHT	per Measure KCAL	FAT	Nutrition Values per 100g / 100ml KCAL	PROT	CARB	FAT	FIBRE
Tomato & Herb, Tear & Share, Tesco*	¼ Pack/73g	164	3.2	226	6.3	40.2	4.4	2.1
Veda Malt, St Michael*	1 Serving/45g	99	0.5	219	7.1	45.3	1.1	2.2
Walnut, Waitrose*	1/8 Loaf/50g	170	7.6	339	10.0	40.6	15.2	5.9
Wheat	**1 Slice/25g**	**65**	**1.0**	**260**	**9.1**	**47.2**	**4.1**	**4.3**
Wheat, Tasty, Kingsmill*	1 Serving/38g	84	1.3	221	10.1	37.6	3.4	6.8
Wheaten, Big Slice	1 Slice/65g	139	1.7	214	7.5	40.2	2.6	3.6
Wheaten, Loaf, Sliced, Genesis*	1 Slice/40g	86	1.0	214	7.5	40.2	2.6	3.6
Wheaten, M&S*	1 Slice/33g	74	1.2	225	9.3	42.9	3.5	3.9
Wheaten, Sliced, Healthy, Irwin's Bakery*	1 Slice/40g	76	0.8	190	9.0	40.5	1.9	6.2
Wheatgerm, Hovis, Soft, Sliced, M&S*	1 Slice/23g	50	0.7	220	10.1	38.5	3.0	4.6
Wheatgrain, Robertson*	1 Slice/30g	90	1.2	300	9.3	57.3	4.0	4.0
White, Average	**1 Slice/40g**	**94**	**0.8**	**235**	**8.4**	**49.3**	**1.9**	**1.5**
White, Batch, Warburton's*	1 Slice/42g	98	0.9	233	9.8	43.6	2.1	2.7
White, Batch Loaf, Extra Special, Asda*	1 Slice/47g	109	0.9	233	9.0	45.0	1.9	2.2
White, Bloomer, Loaf, Greggs*	1 Serving/56g	138	1.0	247	10.2	46.2	1.7	3.0
White, Ciabatta, Roll, GF, Dietary Specials*	1 Roll/50g	106	0.9	213	4.1	40.9	1.8	8.3
White, Classic, Medium Sliced, Hovis*	1 Slice/38g	91	0.9	240	11.4	40.3	2.3	2.5
White, Classic, Thick Sliced, Hovis*	1 Slice/50g	120	2.2	240	9.2	40.5	4.5	3.1
White, Commercially Prepared, Average	1oz/28g	74	0.9	266	7.6	50.6	3.3	2.4
White, Commercially Prepared, Toasted, Average	1oz/28g	82	1.1	293	9.0	54.4	4.0	2.5
White, Crusty, Fresh, Finest, Tesco*	1 Slice/52g	130	1.0	250	8.6	48.5	1.9	2.4
White, Crusty, Gold, Kingsmill*	1 Slice/27g	70	0.8	258	9.4	48.5	2.9	2.7
White, Crusty, Hovis*	1 Slice/44g	103	1.0	233	8.8	44.3	2.2	2.1
White, Crusty, Sliced, Premium, Budgens*	1 Slice/50g	121	1.1	242	8.8	46.9	2.2	2.2
White, Crusty, Sliced Loaf, Tesco*	1 Slice/50g	116	1.0	233	7.4	46.0	2.1	2.0
White, Danish, Medium Sliced, Soft, Somerfield*	1 Slice/21g	48	0.3	229	8.6	44.8	1.4	2.4
White, Danish, Sliced, Weight Watchers*	1 Slice/21g	50	0.3	243	9.8	46.5	1.3	2.9
White, Danish, Soft & Light, Thick Cut, Asda*	1 Slice/26g	60	0.4	230	9.0	45.0	1.6	2.1
White, Danish Style, Thick Sliced, Light, Tesco*	1 Slice/22g	55	0.6	255	9.4	47.3	2.9	2.7
White, Extra Thick Sliced, Kingsmill*	1 Slice/58g	135	1.4	232	8.8	43.8	2.4	2.8
White, Farmhouse, Seeded, Waitrose*	1 Serving/75g	192	4.1	256	10.8	40.9	5.5	5.6
White, Farmhouse, Thick, Hovis*	1 Slice/44g	103	1.0	234	8.7	44.6	2.3	2.4
White, Farmhouse Crusty, M&S*	1 Slice/34g	82	0.7	240	8.9	46.6	2.2	3.0
White, Farmhouse Gold Premium, Morrisons*	1 Slice/38g	90	0.5	236	8.9	47.4	1.2	2.2
White, Fried in Blended Oil	**1 Slice/28g**	**141**	**9.0**	**503**	**7.9**	**48.5**	**32.2**	**1.6**
White, GF, Bakers Delight*	1 Serving/28g	64	2.4	227	1.9	35.5	8.6	1.0
White, GF, Genius*	1 Slice/40g	124	5.5	311	7.7	42.3	13.8	13.8
White, Gluten & Wheat Free, Free From, Sainsbury's*	1 Slice/33g	75	2.8	227	1.9	35.5	8.6	1.0
White, Gold Seeded, Kingsmill*	1 Slice/44g	108	2.5	245	9.7	38.8	5.7	3.5
White, Good Health, Warburton's*	1 Slice/38g	84	0.7	220	9.4	41.6	1.8	4.1
White, Harvest Crust Premium, Ormo*	1 Slice/40g	92	0.6	229	9.4	47.4	1.5	2.7
White, Invisible Crust, Hovis*	1 Slice/40g	90	0.6	226	8.8	44.1	1.6	2.4
White, Loaf, Crusty, Premium, Warburton's*	1 Slice/31g	76	0.7	249	10.6	46.5	2.3	2.6
White, Loaf, Danish, Asda*	1 Serving/23g	53	0.5	236	9.0	45.0	2.2	2.0
White, Medium, Round Top, Kingsmill*	1 Slice/42g	97	1.0	232	8.8	43.8	2.4	2.8
White, Medium, Stayfresh, Tesco*	1 Slice/45g	108	0.7	240	8.2	47.8	1.5	3.0
White, Medium Sliced, Asda*	1 Slice/37g	80	0.6	218	8.0	43.0	1.5	3.3
White, Medium Sliced, Average	1 Slice/39g	93	0.6	238	7.5	48.5	1.6	1.8
White, Medium Sliced, Basics, Sainsbury's*	1 Slice/36g	83	0.5	231	8.0	46.4	1.5	2.1
White, Medium Sliced, Brace's*	1 Slice/32g	75	0.4	235	9.5	46.6	1.2	2.6
White, Medium Sliced, Great Everyday, Kingsmill*	1 Slice/40g	93	0.8	232	9.0	44.6	2.0	2.7
White, Medium Sliced, Long Life, Asda*	1 Slice/36g	82	0.6	228	8.0	45.0	1.8	2.7
White, Medium Sliced, Makes Sense, Somerfield*	1 Slice/36g	82	0.4	226	7.5	46.4	1.2	2.4

	Measure INFO/WEIGHT	per Measure KCAL	per Measure FAT	Nutrition Values per 100g / 100ml KCAL	PROT	CARB	FAT	FIBRE
BREAD								
White, Medium Sliced, Mother's Pride*	1 Slice/36g	82	0.6	229	8.0	45.6	1.6	3.0
White, Medium Sliced, Sainsbury's*	1 Slice/36g	78	0.7	216	8.7	41.1	1.9	7.1
White, Medium Sliced, Smart Price, Asda*	1 Slice/36g	81	0.5	226	7.0	46.0	1.5	2.8
White, Medium Sliced, Stay Fresh, Tesco*	1 Slice/35g	85	0.7	246	8.9	48.1	2.0	0.8
White, Medium Sliced, Superlife, Morrisons*	1 Slice/30g	79	1.2	263	9.6	47.4	3.9	2.5
White, Medium Sliced, Tesco*	1 Slice/36g	86	0.5	240	8.2	47.8	1.5	3.0
White, Medium Sliced, Value, Tesco*	1 Slice/36g	81	0.4	225	7.9	46.1	1.0	2.1
White, Medium Sliced, Warburton's*	1 Slice/40g	94	0.8	234	9.9	43.8	2.0	2.6
White, Medium Sliced, Weight Watchers*	1 Slice/12g	30	0.2	247	12.5	45.2	1.9	3.2
White, Medium VLH Kitchens	1 Serving/30g	72	6.3	241	8.4	49.3	1.9	1.5
White, Oaten, Rolls, Love Life, Waitrose*	1 Roll/70g	183	3.4	261	8.1	46.4	4.8	3.2
White, Oatmeal, Allinson*	1 Slice/47g	111	1.4	237	9.0	43.5	3.0	2.7
White, Organic, Hovis*	1 Slice/44g	108	1.4	246	8.6	45.8	3.2	2.3
White, Organic, Sainsbury's*	1 Slice/36g	84	0.6	234	8.9	45.5	1.8	2.3
White, Plain, Medium Sliced, Scottish, Mother's Pride*	1 Slice/50g	114	0.8	227	8.7	44.6	1.5	3.0
White, Plain, Scottish, Sunblest*	1 Slice/57g	133	1.5	233	10.1	42.3	2.6	2.8
White, Premium Farmhouse, Lidl*	1 Slice/44g	99	0.7	225	7.4	45.4	1.5	2.5
White, Sandwich, Bakery, Sainsbury's*	1 Slice/50g	121	0.3	242	10.3	49.0	0.6	2.9
White, Sandwich, Kingsmill*	1 Slice/42g	97	1.0	232	8.8	43.8	2.4	2.8
White, Sandwich Thins, Warburton's*	1 Thin/42g	100	1.0	239	9.2	47.1	2.5	3.8
White, Seeded, Batch, Loaf, Truly Irresistible, Co-Op*	1 Slice/47g	129	3.4	275	11.6	41.1	7.2	4.3
White, Sliced, Roberts Bakery*	1 Slice/35g	87	0.7	249	10.0	48.0	2.1	2.5
White, Small Loaf, Classic, Hovis*	1 Slice/33g	75	0.8	228	11.4	40.3	2.3	6.5
White, Soft, Batch Loaf, Sliced, Tesco*	1 Slice/50g	116	1.0	233	7.5	46.1	2.1	2.1
White, Soft, Farmhouse, M&S*	1 Slice/25g	60	0.8	239	9.8	42.6	3.3	2.5
White, Soft, Gold, Kingsmill*	1 Slice/47g	112	1.5	239	8.2	44.5	3.1	2.7
White, Soft, Great Everyday, Thick Sliced, Kingsmill*	1 Slice/44g	102	0.9	232	9.0	44.6	2.0	2.7
White, Soft, Hovis*	1 Slice/40g	94	0.9	234	8.7	44.6	2.3	2.4
White, Soft, M&S*	1 Slice/47g	105	0.8	225	7.3	46.1	1.7	2.4
White, Soft, Milk Roll, Warburton's*	1 Slice/18g	46	0.5	251	10.8	45.3	3.0	2.8
White, Soft, Sliced, Hovis*	1 Slice/25g	58	0.6	234	8.7	44.6	2.3	2.4
White, Soft Batch, Sliced, Sainsbury's*	1 Slice/44g	102	0.8	232	8.2	45.4	1.9	2.3
White, Soft Crusty, M&S*	1 Slice/25g	64	0.6	256	9.3	49.0	2.5	2.4
White, Square, Extra Thick Sliced, Hovis*	1 Slice/67g	155	1.3	231	8.5	44.7	2.0	2.6
White, Square, Medium Sliced, Hovis*	1 Slice/40g	92	0.8	231	8.5	44.7	2.0	2.6
White, Square, Thick Sliced, Hovis*	1 Slice/50g	116	1.0	231	8.5	44.7	2.0	2.6
White, Stay Fresh, Tesco*	1 Slice/40g	100	1.0	249	8.6	48.3	2.4	1.5
White, Super Toastie, Warburton's*	1 Slice/57g	134	1.0	235	10.1	44.6	1.8	2.7
White, Thick, So Organic, Sainsbury's*	1 Slice/44g	102	1.0	231	8.2	44.6	2.2	3.1
White, Thick, Super Soft, M&S*	1 Slice/48g	115	1.2	240	8.7	45.3	2.6	2.5
White, Thick, Toastie, 800g Loaf, Warburton's*	1 Slice/47g	111	0.9	234	9.9	43.9	1.9	2.5
White, Thick Sliced, Bakers Gold, Asda*	1 Slice/44g	101	0.8	229	8.0	45.0	1.9	2.3
White, Thick Sliced, Brace's*	1 Slice/38g	90	0.5	235	9.5	46.6	1.2	2.6
White, Thick Sliced, Healthy, Warburton's*	1 Slice/38g	84	0.7	222	10.3	41.2	1.8	4.1
White, Thick Sliced, M&S*	1 Slice/42g	96	0.5	228	7.3	46.7	1.3	2.8
White, Thick Sliced, Organic, Tesco*	1 Slice/44g	108	0.9	245	8.5	46.8	2.1	3.1
White, Thick Sliced, Premium, Tesco*	1 Slice/44g	99	0.3	222	8.7	45.2	0.7	1.5
White, Thick Sliced, Sainsbury's*	1 Slice/44g	95	0.8	216	8.7	41.1	1.9	7.1
White, Thick Sliced, Square Cut, Asda*	1 Slice/44g	101	0.7	230	8.0	46.0	1.5	2.1
White, Thick Sliced, Staysoft, Rathbones*	1 Slice/38g	87	0.5	228	8.5	45.5	1.3	2.7
White, Thick Sliced, Sunblest*	1 Slice/40g	91	0.6	228	8.0	45.7	1.5	2.8
White, Thick Sliced, Super Toastie, Morrisons*	1 Slice/50g	128	1.5	257	8.7	48.9	3.0	2.1
White, Thick Sliced, Tesco*	1 Slice/44g	106	0.7	240	8.2	47.8	1.5	3.0

BREAD

	Measure INFO/WEIGHT	per Measure KCAL	FAT	Nutrition Values per 100g / 100ml KCAL	PROT	CARB	FAT	FIBRE
White, Thick Sliced, Warburton's, Weight Watchers*	1 Slice/29g	69	0.2	237	10.4	48.6	0.8	2.0
White, Thick Sliced, Warburton's*	1 Slice/28g	65	0.6	233	9.8	43.6	2.1	2.7
White, Thin Sliced, Sainsbury's*	1 Slice/29g	66	0.4	228	7.1	46.4	1.5	2.8
White, Thin Sliced, Tesco*	1 Slice/30g	68	0.4	228	9.5	44.5	1.3	3.4
White, Toast, Gamle Mølle*	1 Slice/32g	83	0.6	260	8.0	52.0	2.0	3.0
White, Toasted, Average	**1 Slice/33g**	**87**	**0.5**	**265**	**9.3**	**57.1**	**1.6**	**1.8**
White, Toastie, Thick, Love to Toast, Kingsmill*	1 Slice/50g	116	1.0	232	9.0	44.6	2.0	2.7
White, Toastie, Thick Cut, Hovis*	1 Slice/50g	115	1.0	230	8.5	44.8	2.0	2.5
White, Whole, Extra Thick, Kingsmill*	1 Slice/57g	130	1.4	228	9.0	42.3	2.5	4.0
White, Whole, Kingsmill*	1 Slice/38g	87	1.0	230	9.0	42.9	2.5	3.4
White, Wholesome, Loaf, Sainsbury's*	1 Serving/36g	81	0.7	224	9.4	42.5	1.8	4.4
White, Wholesome, Medium Sliced, Premium, Tesco*	1 Slice/37g	85	0.8	232	8.9	43.9	2.3	4.2
Whole Grain, & Rye, Schneider Brot*	1 Slice/50g	98	0.6	197	5.9	36.6	1.2	8.2
Whole Grain, Batch, Finest, Tesco*	1 Slice/44g	112	1.2	254	9.8	47.7	2.7	4.2
Whole Grain, Brennans*	1 Slice/39g	79	0.6	203	9.0	40.0	1.5	4.9
Whole Grain, with Sunflower Seeds, Landgut*	1 Slice/83g	183	4.2	221	7.0	37.0	5.0	29.0
Whole Wheat, 100%, Soft, Farmhouse, Ocean Spray*	1 Slice/43g	110	2.0	256	11.6	44.2	4.7	7.0
Whole Wheat, 100%, Stoneground, Maxwell House*	1 Slice/27g	60	0.5	222	11.1	44.4	1.9	7.4
Whole Wheat, Harvest	1 Serving/42g	90	1.0	214	7.1	45.2	2.4	7.1
Whole Wheat, Nature's Own*	1 Slice/28g	66	1.0	236	14.3	39.3	3.6	10.7
Wholegrain, Average	1 Slice/44g	117	1.9	265	13.4	43.3	4.2	7.4
Wholegrain, Medium Sliced, Irish Pride*	1 Slice/38g	90	0.8	237	9.2	46.6	2.1	7.6
Wholegrain, Soft, M&S*	1 Slice/51g	115	2.8	225	13.0	31.2	5.4	8.2
Wholegrain, Toasted, Average	1 Slice/40g	117	1.9	288	14.5	47.1	4.6	8.1
Wholemeal, & Oat, Loaf, Vogel*	1 Slice/42g	86	0.6	205	8.7	34.3	1.5	9.7
Wholemeal, & Oat Flakes, Gold, Kingsmill*	1 Slice/47g	103	1.6	220	10.0	37.3	3.4	7.0
Wholemeal, & Seeds, Medium, Love Life, Waitrose*	1 Slice/27g	65	2.2	244	12.6	29.7	8.3	9.4
Wholemeal, 7 Seeded, Irwin's Bakery*	1 Slice/38g	90	2.0	237	9.5	33.4	5.2	9.4
Wholemeal, American Sandwich, Harry's*	1 Slice/43g	110	2.1	259	9.0	45.0	5.0	5.0
Wholemeal, Average	**1 Slice/40g**	**88**	**1.0**	**215**	**9.2**	**41.6**	**2.5**	**5.8**
Wholemeal, Baker's Soft, Medium, Tesco*	1 Slice/40g	94	1.1	235	10.8	37.8	2.8	6.9
Wholemeal, Batch, Organic, Waitrose*	1 Slice/40g	88	1.0	219	10.0	38.8	2.6	7.2
Wholemeal, BGTY, Sainsbury's*	1 Slice/20g	41	0.2	207	12.6	36.8	1.0	7.3
Wholemeal, Brennans*	1 Slice/33g	78	1.4	236	11.2	38.4	4.2	7.7
Wholemeal, Brown, Medium Sliced, 400g, Hovis*	1 Slice/25g	55	0.7	221	10.0	37.8	2.8	6.8
Wholemeal, Brown, Unsliced, Loaf, Little, Hovis*	1 Slice/40g	86	1.1	216	10.0	37.8	2.7	6.8
Wholemeal, COU, M&S*	1 Slice/21g	45	0.5	213	13.6	33.7	2.6	7.0
Wholemeal, Crusty, Finest, Tesco*	1 Slice/50g	103	0.8	206	10.8	37.0	1.7	6.9
Wholemeal, Crusty, Kingsmill*	1 Slice/42g	104	1.8	247	11.2	41.1	4.2	7.0
Wholemeal, Danish, BFY, Morrisons*	1 Slice/17g	39	0.3	228	11.2	47.9	1.8	6.2
Wholemeal, Danish, Warburton's*	1 Slice/25g	57	0.6	229	13.3	38.5	2.4	7.2
Wholemeal, Economy, Sainsbury's*	1 Slice/28g	61	0.7	217	10.3	38.4	2.5	6.5
Wholemeal, Farmhouse, Average	1 Slice/43g	94	1.4	219	10.7	36.2	3.3	7.3
Wholemeal, Farmhouse, Hovis*	1 Slice/44g	91	1.0	207	11.0	36.0	2.2	7.1
Wholemeal, Farmhouse Batch, Love Life, Waitrose*	1 Slice/48g	102	1.2	212	10.4	36.2	2.6	7.6
Wholemeal, Farmhouse Soft Golden, M&S*	1 Slice/30g	64	0.9	215	11.0	35.1	3.1	7.4
Wholemeal, Fh, Stoneground, Batch, Finest, Tesco*	1 Slice/50g	108	1.4	215	10.3	36.1	2.8	6.9
Wholemeal, Fresher for Longer, Sainsbury's*	1 Slice/44g	98	1.6	222	10.9	36.2	3.7	6.5
Wholemeal, Gold, Kingsmill*	1 Slice/44g	95	1.3	217	10.9	36.8	2.9	7.0
Wholemeal, Golden, M&S*	1 Slice/30g	69	1.4	230	10.8	36.6	4.5	7.7
Wholemeal, Golden Crust, Ormo*	1 Slice/38g	83	0.8	218	10.4	36.1	2.0	7.0
Wholemeal, Golden Wheat, Kingsmill*	1 Slice/44g	97	1.3	221	10.9	37.8	2.9	6.0
Wholemeal, Light, Irish Pride*	1 Slice/28g	68	0.4	241	13.3	44.1	1.3	4.5

BREAD

INFO/WEIGHT	per Measure		Nutrition Values per 100g / 100ml				
Measure	KCAL	FAT	KCAL	PROT	CARB	FAT	FIBRE
Wholemeal, Loaf, British Farmers, Hovis* — 1 Slice/47g	108	1.3	229	10.0	37.9	2.8	6.8
Wholemeal, Loaf, Sliced, Medium, 800g, Hovis* — 1 Slice/40g	88	1.1	221	10.0	37.8	2.7	6.8
Wholemeal, Loaf, Sliced, Thick, 800g, Hovis* — 1 Slice/50g	115	1.4	229	10.0	37.8	2.7	6.8
Wholemeal, Longer Life, Medium Sliced, Sainsbury's* — 1 Slice/35g	78	1.3	222	10.9	36.2	3.7	6.5
Wholemeal, Longer Life, Thick Slice, Sainsbury's* — 1 Slice/45g	101	1.6	224	10.6	37.4	3.6	5.9
Wholemeal, Makes Sense, Somerfield* — 1 Slice/36g	78	0.8	217	10.7	38.6	2.2	6.6
Wholemeal, Medium, 800g Loaf, Warburton's* — 1 Slice/40g	93	1.0	231	10.2	39.6	2.5	6.5
Wholemeal, Medium Sliced, Great Everyday, Kingsmill* — 1 Slice/40g	91	1.5	227	10.5	37.7	3.8	6.2
Wholemeal, Medium Sliced, Little Big Loaf, Kingsmill* — 1 Slice/39g	93	1.5	239	10.5	37.7	3.8	6.2
Wholemeal, Medium Sliced, M&S* — 1 Slice/40g	80	1.2	200	10.5	32.7	3.1	6.7
Wholemeal, Medium Sliced, Morrisons* — 1 Slice/32g	68	0.8	214	9.9	38.0	2.5	5.8
Wholemeal, Medium Sliced, Organic, Tesco* — 1 Slice/27g	55	0.7	209	9.2	37.2	2.8	6.0
Wholemeal, Medium Sliced, Premium, Tesco* — 1 Slice/36g	71	0.2	196	9.8	37.8	0.6	7.2
Wholemeal, Medium Sliced, Roberts Bakery* — 1 Slice/37g	86	0.6	233	10.9	38.1	1.5	6.6
Wholemeal, Medium Sliced, Sainsbury's* — 1 Slice/36g	77	0.9	214	10.3	37.8	2.4	7.4
Wholemeal, Medium Sliced, The Village Bakery* — 1 Slice/33g	69	0.7	209	9.8	38.0	2.0	6.0
Wholemeal, Medium Sliced, Waitrose* — 1 Slice/36g	76	0.9	213	10.1	37.6	2.4	7.0
Wholemeal, Multigrain, Sliced, Finest, Tesco* — 1 Slice/50g	123	2.0	246	10.1	42.1	4.1	6.5
Wholemeal, Multigrain, Soft Batch, Sainsbury's* — 1 Slice/44g	106	2.9	242	11.3	34.5	6.5	5.6
Wholemeal, Multiseed, Organic, Sainsbury's* — 1 Slice/26g	75	2.5	289	13.8	36.6	9.7	6.0
Wholemeal, Multiseed, TTD, Sainsbury's* — 1 Slice/47g	110	3.4	234	11.7	30.7	7.2	8.1
Wholemeal, Oat Topped, TTD, Sainsbury's* — 1 Slice/47g	109	1.3	232	10.0	38.5	2.8	0.3
Wholemeal, Oatbran, Sliced, Tesco* — 1 Slice/45g	90	0.7	200	10.1	35.3	1.6	7.4
Wholemeal, Organic, 400g Loaf, Warburton's* — 1 Slice/28g	63	0.9	223	10.3	37.9	3.2	6.7
Wholemeal, Organic, Hovis* — 1 Slice/44g	92	1.3	209	10.2	35.6	2.9	7.6
Wholemeal, Premium, Medium Slice, M&S* — 1 Slice/33g	65	1.0	200	10.5	32.9	3.1	6.7
Wholemeal, Premium, Thick Slice, M&S* — 1 Slice/50g	95	1.5	190	9.8	30.8	3.0	6.4
Wholemeal, Pumpkin & Poppy Seed, Brennans* — 1 Slice/33g	79	1.4	236	11.2	38.4	4.2	7.7
Wholemeal, Rustic, Tin, Tesco* — 1 Slice/37g	92	1.3	249	12.2	44.0	3.5	3.1
Wholemeal, Sandwich Loaf, Brennans* — 1 Slice/40g	88	0.7	221	9.8	38.5	1.7	8.0
Wholemeal, Seed Sensation, Hovis* — 1 Slice/44g	109	2.5	249	11.9	31.4	5.6	12.4
Wholemeal, Seeded, Roll, Love Life, Waitrose* — 1 Roll/72g	192	6.3	266	12.6	34.1	8.8	6.4
Wholemeal, Seeded Batch, Truly Irresistible, Co-Op* — 1 Slice/47g	99	1.7	210	12.0	33.0	3.6	8.5
Wholemeal, Sliced, GF, Glutano* — 1 Slice/56g	107	1.7	191	7.0	34.0	3.0	0.0
Wholemeal, Sliced, McCambridge* — 1 Slice/38g	90	0.7	237	7.9	44.7	1.8	0.0
Wholemeal, Sliced, Medium, Tesco* — 1 Slice/36g	79	0.8	220	11.0	39.1	2.2	6.6
Wholemeal, Small Loaf, Sliced, 400g, Hovis* — 1 Slice/25g	57	0.7	229	10.0	37.8	2.7	6.8
Wholemeal, Square Cut, Thick Sliced, Asda* — 1 Slice/44g	91	1.0	208	10.0	37.0	2.2	6.0
Wholemeal, Stayfresh, Tesco* — 1 Slice/36g	81	0.8	225	11.0	39.1	2.2	6.0
Wholemeal, Stoneground, 800g Loaf, Warburton's* — 1 Slice/45g	95	1.2	210	10.4	35.8	2.6	6.8
Wholemeal, Stoneground, Organic, Waitrose* — 1 Slice/25g	57	0.9	228	10.8	38.2	3.6	7.1
Wholemeal, Stoneground, Thick, Love Life, Waitrose* — 1 Slice/40g	86	1.1	214	10.1	36.5	2.8	7.9
Wholemeal, Stoneground, Thick Sliced, Sainsbury's* — 1 Slice/44g	92	0.8	210	10.2	37.9	1.9	7.8
Wholemeal, Supersoft, Eat Well, M&S* — 1 Slice/33g	81	1.1	245	10.9	40.0	3.3	6.7
Wholemeal, Tasty, Medium, Kingsmill* — 1 Slice/40g	96	1.5	239	10.5	37.7	3.8	6.2
Wholemeal, Tasty, Thick, Kingsmill* — 1 Slice/44g	105	1.7	239	10.5	37.7	3.8	6.2
Wholemeal, Thick Slice, Brennans* — 1 Slice/27g	69	0.6	257	9.2	45.4	2.1	6.8
Wholemeal, Thick Sliced, Bakers Gold, Asda* — 1 Slice/44g	99	1.4	225	12.0	37.0	3.2	6.0
Wholemeal, Thick Sliced, COU, M&S* — 1 Slice/26g	56	0.7	215	13.6	33.7	2.6	7.0
Wholemeal, Thick Sliced, Great Everyday, Kingsmill* — 1 Slice/44g	100	1.7	227	10.5	37.7	3.8	6.2
Wholemeal, Thick Sliced, Healthy Living, Co-Op* — 1 Slice/44g	95	0.9	215	11.0	38.0	2.0	7.0
Wholemeal, Thick Sliced, Organic, Tesco* — 1 Slice/44g	98	1.2	220	8.8	38.8	2.8	5.9
Wholemeal, Thick Sliced, Sainsbury's* — 1 Slice/48g	102	1.2	213	10.1	37.4	2.6	8.5

	Measure INFO/WEIGHT	per Measure KCAL	FAT	Nutrition Values per 100g / 100ml KCAL	PROT	CARB	FAT	FIBRE
BREAD								
Wholemeal, Thick Sliced, Stephenson's Bakery*	1 Slice/40g	84	0.8	209	10.7	37.3	1.9	6.2
Wholemeal, Thick Sliced, Tesco*	1 Slice/40g	96	1.1	240	9.5	40.9	2.7	6.8
Wholemeal, Thick Sliced, Waitrose*	1 Slice/44g	94	1.1	213	10.1	37.6	2.4	7.0
Wholemeal, Thick Sliced, with Mustard Seed, Lozzas	1 Slice/26g	56	0.7	215	13.6	33.7	2.6	7.0
Wholemeal, Toasted, Medium Sliced, Average	*1 Slice/26g*	*58*	*0.6*	*224*	*8.6*	*42.3*	*2.2*	*5.8*
Wholemeal, Toastie, 800g Loaf, Warburton's*	1 Slice/45g	101	1.1	224	9.7	39.3	2.4	6.6
Wholemeal, with Rye, M&S*	1 Slice/33g	79	1.2	240	10.5	37.2	3.5	7.8
Wholemeal, with Seeds, Thick, Love Life, Waitrose*	1 Slice/54g	131	4.5	243	12.7	28.8	8.4	9.7
Wraps, White, Square, Warburton's*	1 Wrap/65g	159	2.9	245	12.5	38.6	4.5	2.2
BREAD & BUTTER PUDDING								
5% Fat, M&S*	1 Pudding/237g	367	10.0	155	4.4	24.8	4.2	0.4
Average	1 Serving/250g	400	19.5	160	6.2	17.5	7.8	0.3
BGTY, Sainsbury's*	1 Serving/125g	126	2.9	101	6.3	13.4	2.3	5.4
Chilled, CBY, Asda*	¼ Pack/125g	267	13.9	213	5.1	22.0	11.1	2.4
COU, M&S*	1 Pot/140g	161	2.8	115	6.1	18.4	2.0	0.8
Finest, Tesco*	1 Serving/153g	379	22.0	248	4.9	24.6	14.4	0.9
Individual, M&S*	1 Pudding/130g	280	16.4	215	4.4	21.4	12.6	0.5
Low Fat, Individual, BGTY, Sainsbury's*	1 Pack/125g	125	2.9	100	6.3	13.4	2.3	5.4
Sainsbury's*	½ Pudding/115g	223	11.2	194	4.8	21.9	9.7	0.4
BREAD MIX								
Brown, Sunflower, Sainsbury's*	1 Serving/60g	151	3.7	251	10.0	38.9	6.1	4.0
Ciabatta, Italian, Sainsbury's*	1 Slice/45g	96	0.9	213	8.7	40.0	2.0	2.4
Ciabatta, Made Up with Water & Olive Oil, Wrights*	1 Slice/45g	113	1.8	251	10.0	43.6	4.0	1.8
Crusty White, Made Up, Tesco*	1 Slice/126g	316	2.3	251	9.4	49.3	1.8	2.5
Focaccia, Garlic & Herb, Asda*	1 Serving/125g	385	10.0	308	11.0	48.0	8.0	3.3
Mixed Grain, Sainsbury's*	1 Serving/45g	103	0.7	228	7.7	46.0	1.5	4.4
Multiseed, Baked, Sainsbury's*	1 Slice/44g	112	4.3	252	10.8	30.5	9.6	6.8
Tomato & Parmesan, Italian Sun Dried, Sainsbury's*	1 Serving/100g	247	1.7	247	8.1	50.1	1.7	2.5
Tomato & Parmesan, Sun Dried, Made Up, Wrights*	1 Slice/45g	103	0.6	229	9.3	46.0	1.3	2.4
White Loaf, Asda*	1 Slice/60g	150	0.9	250	10.0	49.0	1.5	3.1
Wholemeal, Hovis*	1 Serving/65g	148	3.1	227	10.0	35.8	4.8	6.8
Wholemeal, Made Up, M&S*	1 Loaf/600g	1410	14.4	235	11.0	42.0	2.4	5.3
BREADCRUMBS								
Average	*1oz/28g*	*98*	*0.5*	*350*	*10.8*	*74.8*	*1.9*	*2.6*
Cooks' Ingredients, Waitrose*	1 Serving/50g	174	0.7	349	9.8	74.6	1.4	3.2
Golden, Paxo*	1 Serving/70g	248	1.1	354	11.5	73.5	1.6	3.4
Rusk, GF, Dove's Farm*	1 Serving/100g	342	4.5	342	12.6	62.7	4.5	9.7
BREADFRUIT								
Raw	*1oz/28g*	*27*	*0.1*	*95*	*1.3*	*23.1*	*0.3*	*0.0*
BREADSTICKS								
Asda*	1 Serving/5g	21	0.4	412	12.0	73.0	8.0	2.9
Bruschetta, Olive & Rosemary, Graze*	1 Punnet/29g	138	7.5	480	13.4	53.0	26.0	4.1
Cheese, Italian, Tesco*	4 Breadsticks/21g	84	1.7	399	14.2	67.5	8.0	3.4
Chive & Onion Twists, Tesco*	3 Twists/24g	115	5.3	480	11.6	57.6	22.1	2.2
Classic, Somerfield*	1 Breadstick/6g	24	0.2	396	10.0	82.5	2.9	1.0
Grissini, Italian, Sainsbury's*	1 Breadstick/5g	20	0.4	408	11.6	72.9	7.8	2.9
Grissini, Sesame Seed, Sainsbury's*	1 Breadstick/5g	21	0.6	419	12.7	65.5	11.8	3.2
Grissini, Waitrose*	1 Breadstick/6g	25	0.4	397	12.0	72.5	6.2	3.1
Grissini, with Olive Oil, Thin, Forno Bianco*	1 Stick/5g	21	0.4	420	11.0	77.0	7.5	0.0
Italian Original, Tesco*	1 Stick/6g	23	0.4	410	11.6	72.9	7.8	2.9
Mini, Sainsbury's*	4 Breadsticks/5g	20	0.4	404	15.6	68.7	7.4	4.8
Mini, Wheat & GF, Free From, Tesco*	1 Stick/3g	11	0.3	414	4.0	72.1	12.2	2.2
Olive, Italian, Finest, Tesco*	1 Stick/40g	170	5.4	424	10.5	65.0	13.6	4.8

INFO/WEIGHT	Measure	per Measure		Nutrition Values per 100g / 100ml				
		KCAL	FAT	KCAL	PROT	CARB	FAT	FIBRE

BREADSTICKS

	INFO/WEIGHT	KCAL	FAT	KCAL	PROT	CARB	FAT	FIBRE
Olive Oil, & Rosemary, Finest, Tesco*	2 Sticks/10g	42	1.2	427	13.9	64.4	12.6	4.1
Onion, M&S*	1 Serving/40g	166	5.6	415	12.6	59.6	14.1	4.8
Original, Italian, Tesco*	1 Stick/6g	23	0.4	410	11.6	72.9	7.8	2.9
Original, Organic, Kallo*	1 Breadstick/6g	24	0.5	393	11.8	69.5	7.6	4.7
PB, Waitrose*	1 Breadstick/5g	20	0.1	378	13.7	77.3	1.6	3.8
Plain, Asda*	1 Stick/5g	21	0.4	412	12.0	73.0	8.0	2.9
Plain, You Count, Love Life, Waitrose*	1 Breadstick/5g	17	0.1	349	13.4	70.1	1.7	5.6
Rosemary, Asda*	1 Breadstick/7g	29	1.0	439	12.0	64.0	15.0	3.5
Thin, Healthy Eating, D'oro, Primo*	1 Breadstick/3g	11	0.2	400	10.0	75.0	6.5	1.1

BREAKFAST CEREAL

	INFO/WEIGHT	KCAL	FAT	KCAL	PROT	CARB	FAT	FIBRE
Advantage, Weetabix*	1 Serving/30g	105	0.7	350	10.2	72.0	2.4	9.0
All Bran, Asda*	1 Serving/40g	110	1.4	276	15.0	46.0	3.5	27.0
All Bran, Bran Flakes, & Fruit, Kellogg's*	1 Serving/40g	143	2.4	358	8.0	68.0	6.0	9.0
All Bran, Bran Flakes, Chocolate, Kellogg's*	1 Serving/30g	106	1.8	354	10.0	65.0	6.0	13.0
All Bran, Bran Flakes, Kellogg's*	1 Serving/30g	106	0.6	355	10.0	67.0	2.0	15.0
All Bran, Fruit 'n' Fibre, Kellogg's*	1 Serving/30g	114	1.8	380	8.0	69.0	6.0	9.0
All Bran, Golden Crunch, Kellogg's*	1 Serving/45g	182	5.0	405	8.0	62.0	11.0	13.0
All Bran, High Fibre, Morrisons*	1 Serving/40g	109	1.4	272	14.8	45.5	3.5	27.0
All Bran, Original, High Fibre, Kellogg's*	1 Serving/40g	134	1.4	334	14.0	48.0	3.5	27.0
All Bran, Yoghurty Flakes, As Sold, Kellogg's*	1 Serving/30g	112	1.2	372	10.0	68.0	4.0	12.0
Almond, Low Carb, Atkins*	1 Serving/30g	100	1.5	333	50.0	26.7	5.0	0.0
Almond, Oats & More, Nestle*	1 Serving/30g	119	2.7	398	10.7	68.7	8.9	5.5
Almond, Pecan & Cashew Muesli, Kellogg's*	1 Serving/45g	188	6.3	418	11.0	62.0	14.0	8.0
Alpen*, Crunchy Bran*	1 Serving/40g	120	1.9	299	11.8	52.3	4.7	24.8
Apple, Blackberry & Raspberry Flakes, GFY, Asda*	1 Serving/30g	103	0.5	344	9.0	73.0	1.8	11.0
Apple & Cinnamon, 7 Grain Granola, Rude Health*	1 Bowl/45g	197	5.8	437	10.0	64.0	13.0	7.0
Apple & Cinnamon, Crisp, Sainsbury's*	1 Serving/50g	216	7.4	433	6.2	69.1	14.7	3.4
Apple & Cinnamon, Quaker Oats*	1 Sachet/38g	136	2.1	358	8.0	68.0	5.5	2.5
Apple & Cinnamon Flakes, M&S*	1 Serving/30g	111	0.6	370	6.0	82.7	1.9	3.4
Apricot Wheats, Whole Grain, Tesco*	1 Serving/40g	130	0.6	326	7.6	70.6	1.4	8.0
Balance, Sainsbury's*	1 Serving/30g	111	0.4	370	11.4	77.7	1.5	3.2
Banana, Papaya & Honey Oat, Crunchy, Waitrose*	1 Serving/40g	170	4.8	426	9.6	69.8	12.0	5.5
Banana & Toffee, Oat So Easy, Jungle*	1 Pack/50g	187	4.6	374	1.8	74.7	9.2	5.1
Barley Flakes, Organic, Infinity Foods*	1 Serving/45g	140	0.8	311	10.0	57.0	1.8	4.0
Benefit Flakes, Aldi*	1 Serving/40g	148	0.6	370	11.4	77.7	1.5	3.2
Berry Burst, Oat So Simple, Quaker Oats*	1 Serving/39g	144	2.3	370	8.0	70.0	6.0	6.5
Berry Crunchy, Sainsbury's*	1 Serving/30g	122	3.6	408	7.7	67.3	12.0	4.8
Berry Granola, Rude Health*	1 Serving/40g	178	6.4	446	10.0	61.0	16.0	7.0
Bircher Muesli, Love Life, Waitrose*	1 Serving/45g	153	3.5	341	8.8	57.7	7.7	6.8
Biscuit, Baked with Golden Syrup, Weetabix*	2 Biscuits/44g	158	0.8	363	10.3	72.0	1.9	8.2
Bitesize, Weetabix*	1 Serving/40g	135	0.8	338	11.5	68.4	2.0	10.0
Blackberry & Apple, Alpen*	1 Serving/40g	140	1.5	349	9.2	69.4	3.8	8.3
Blueberry Wheats, Tesco*	1 Serving/50g	165	0.8	330	7.5	71.6	1.5	8.5
Bran Crunch, Raisin, Kellogg's*	1 Pack/80g	280	1.5	350	6.2	83.8	1.9	7.5
Bran Flakes, Asda*	1 Serving/47g	157	1.5	333	11.0	65.0	3.2	14.0
Bran Flakes, Crunchy Nut, Sainsbury's*	1 Serving/40g	203	3.8	508	19.8	85.8	9.5	11.0
Bran Flakes, Honey Nut, Asda*	1 Serving/50g	180	2.2	360	10.0	70.0	4.4	11.0
Bran Flakes, Honey Nut, Sainsbury's*	1 Serving/40g	143	1.8	358	9.6	70.0	4.4	11.0
Bran Flakes, Kellogg's*	1 Serving/50g	163	1.0	326	10.0	67.0	2.0	15.0
Bran Flakes, Sainsbury's*	1 Serving/30g	100	0.8	333	10.3	67.5	2.5	14.3
Bran Flakes, Sultana, Dry, Sainsbury's*	1 Serving/30g	98	0.6	325	8.3	68.6	1.9	12.1
Bran Flakes, Sultana Bran, Kellogg's*	1 Serving/40g	138	0.8	344	8.0	67.0	2.0	13.0
Bran Flakes, Wholegrain, Sainsbury's*	1 Serving/30g	110	0.6	365	10.5	69.4	2.0	13.8

BREAKFAST CEREAL

INFO/WEIGHT	Measure KCAL	FAT	Nutrition Values per 100g / 100ml KCAL	PROT	CARB	FAT	FIBRE
Breakfast Biscuits, Aldi*	4 Biscuits/60g	213	1.5	355	13.7	69.5	2.5	7.5
Caribbean Crunch, Alpen*	1 Serving/40g	155	3.6	388	8.8	67.9	9.0	4.6
Cheerios, Chocolate, Dry, Nestle*	1 Serving/30g	115	1.0	384	8.0	73.4	3.5	2.2
Cheerios, Honey, Nestle*	1 Serving/50g	184	1.4	369	6.6	79.2	2.8	5.8
Cheerios, Honey Nut, Nestle*	1 Serving/30g	112	1.1	374	7.0	78.3	3.7	5.2
Cheerios, Nestle*	1 Serving/30g	114	1.1	381	8.6	74.5	3.8	7.1
Choc & Nut Crisp, Tesco*	1 Serving/40g	185	8.0	462	8.3	62.5	19.9	4.8
Choco Flakes, Asda*	1 Serving/50g	187	0.4	374	6.0	86.0	0.7	2.6
Choco Flakes, Kellogg's*	1 Serving/30g	114	0.9	380	5.0	84.0	3.0	2.5
Choco Flakes, Sainsbury's*	1 Serving/30g	111	0.2	370	5.5	85.4	0.7	3.0
Choco Flakes, Tesco*	1 Serving/30g	112	0.2	374	5.6	86.3	0.7	2.6
Choco Hoops, Aldi*	1 Serving/30g	116	1.4	385	7.0	79.1	4.5	0.0
Choco Hoops, Asda*	1 Serving/40g	154	1.8	385	7.0	79.0	4.5	4.0
Choco Snaps, Asda*	1 Serving/30g	115	0.7	382	5.0	85.0	2.4	1.9
Choco Snaps, Sainsbury's*	1 Serving/30g	115	0.7	383	5.5	84.8	2.4	1.9
Choco Squares, Asda*	1 Serving/30g	130	4.2	434	10.0	67.0	14.0	4.0
Chocolate, Granola, Diet Chef Ltd*	1 Serving/40g	195	11.5	488	10.7	45.0	28.7	13.0
Chocolate, Tesco*	1 Serving/40g	169	5.6	423	8.0	66.3	14.0	6.0
Chocolate Crisp, Minis, Weetabix*	1 Serving/36g	134	1.9	371	9.0	71.7	5.3	8.5
Chocolate Hoops, Average	1 Serving/30g	116	1.3	386	7.2	79.3	4.4	3.4
Chocolate Rice, Puffed, Average	1 Serving/30g	117	1.2	389	5.7	81.0	4.1	3.2
Cinnamon Grahams, Nestle*	1 Serving/40g	164	3.9	411	4.7	76.1	9.8	4.2
Clusters, Nestle*	1 Serving/30g	111	1.4	371	9.3	72.6	4.8	7.4
Coco Pops, Crunchers, Kellogg's*	1 Serving/30g	114	1.0	380	7.0	81.0	3.5	3.0
Coco Pops, Kellogg's*	1 Serving/30g	116	0.8	387	5.0	85.0	2.5	2.0
Coco Pops, Mega Munchers, Kellogg's*	1 Serving/30g	112	0.8	375	8.0	80.0	2.5	4.5
Coco Snaps, Value, Tesco*	1 Serving/30g	117	0.7	390	7.0	84.1	2.4	2.4
Cookie Crunch, Nestle*	1 Serving/40g	154	1.1	385	4.6	85.3	2.8	1.8
Corn Flakes, Asda*	1 Serving/30g	111	0.2	370	7.0	84.0	0.7	3.0
Corn Flakes, Crispy Nut, Asda*	1 Serving/30g	117	1.3	390	7.0	81.0	4.2	2.5
Corn Flakes, Harvest Home, Nestle*	1 Serving/25g	92	0.2	367	7.3	82.7	0.8	3.6
Corn Flakes, Hint of Honey, Kellogg's*	1 Serving/30g	113	0.2	377	6.0	87.0	0.6	2.5
Corn Flakes, Honey Nut, Average	1 Serving/30g	118	1.3	393	7.0	81.4	4.3	2.4
Corn Flakes, Kellogg's*	1 Serving/30g	112	0.3	372	7.0	84.0	0.9	3.0
Corn Flakes, Organic, Whole Earth*	1 Serving/40g	154	0.4	386	8.6	84.2	1.0	3.0
Corn Flakes, Sainsbury's*	1 Serving/25g	93	0.2	371	7.3	83.8	0.7	3.0
Corn Flakes, Tesco*	1 Serving/25g	93	0.2	371	7.3	83.8	0.7	3.0
Corn Flakes, Value, Tesco*	1 Serving/30g	111	0.4	370	7.3	82.4	1.2	3.5
Country Crisp, & Flakes, Red Berry, Jordans*	1 Serving/50g	204	5.8	407	7.1	68.5	11.6	7.3
Country Crisp, Four Nut Combo, Jordans*	1 Serving/50g	240	12.4	480	8.9	55.4	24.7	6.9
Country Crisp with Real Raspberries, Jordans*	1 Serving/50g	214	7.9	429	7.5	64.1	15.8	7.1
Country Crisp with Real Strawberries, Jordans*	1 Serving/50g	214	7.8	428	7.5	64.1	15.7	7.1
Country Honey, Oat So Simple, Quaker Oats*	1 Serving/36g	134	2.3	373	8.5	69.0	6.5	6.0
Cranberry Wheats, Tesco*	1 Serving/50g	160	0.8	320	7.6	72.0	1.5	8.0
Cranberry Wheats, Whole Grain, Sainsbury's*	1 Serving/50g	162	0.7	325	7.3	70.9	1.4	7.7
Crispy Minis, Strawberry, Weetabix*	1 Serving/40g	150	0.9	375	9.4	74.1	2.3	10.0
Crispy Rice, Raisins, Almonds, & Seeds, Eat Natural*	1 Serving/50g	216	9.8	431	14.4	49.0	19.7	3.8
Crunchy Bran, Weetabix*	1 Serving/40g	140	1.4	350	11.9	57.6	3.6	20.0
Crunchy Bran Muesli, Diet Chef Ltd*	1 Serving/40g	164	3.8	409	8.1	68.4	9.5	8.9
Crunchy Nut, Clusters, Honey & Nut, Kellogg's*	1 Serving/40g	161	2.0	402	6.0	82.0	5.0	2.5
Crunchy Nut, Clusters, Milk Chocolate Curls, Kellogg's*	1 Serving/40g	183	7.2	458	8.0	66.0	18.0	4.0
Crunchy Nut, Clusters, Summer Berries, Kellogg's*	1 Serving/40g	176	6.0	439	8.0	68.0	15.0	5.0
Crunchy Nut, Corn Flakes, Kellogg's*	1 Serving/30g	118	1.2	392	6.0	83.0	4.0	2.5

B

BREAKFAST CEREAL

	Measure INFO/WEIGHT	per Measure KCAL	FAT	Nutrition Values per 100g / 100ml KCAL	PROT	CARB	FAT	FIBRE
Crunchy Nut, Red, Kellogg's*	1 Serving/40g	138	0.8	346	10.0	72.0	2.0	9.0
Crunchy Oat, with Raisins, Almonds & Fruit, Tesco*	1 Serving/50g	202	6.3	403	8.5	63.8	12.6	6.6
Crunchy Oat, with Tropical Fruits, Tesco*	1 Serving/35g	146	4.8	417	7.8	65.3	13.8	6.1
Crunchy Oats, with Tropical Fruits, Jordans*	1 Serving/75g	319	11.0	425	8.1	65.4	14.6	6.7
Crunchy Rice, & Wheat Flakes, Co-Op*	1 Serving/30g	111	0.6	370	11.0	78.0	2.0	3.0
Curiously Cinnamon, Nestle*	1 Serving/30g	124	3.0	412	4.9	75.9	9.9	4.1
Fibre 1, Nestle*	1 Serving/40g	107	1.0	267	10.8	50.2	2.6	30.5
Fibre Flakes, GF, Organic, Dove's Farm*	1 Serving/30g	105	0.4	351	7.1	69.7	1.5	15.0
Fitnesse & Fruits, Nestle*	1 Serving/40g	148	0.4	370	6.6	83.4	1.1	3.4
Flakes & Grains, Exotic Fruit, BGTY, Sainsbury's*	1 Serving/30g	113	1.5	377	6.8	76.4	4.9	5.9
Force, Nestle*	1 Serving/40g	138	0.9	344	10.6	70.3	2.3	9.2
Four Berry Crisp, Organic, Jordans*	1 Serving/50g	221	7.9	442	7.7	67.1	15.8	5.4
Frosted Flakes, Sainsbury's*	1 Serving/30g	114	0.2	381	4.9	88.0	0.6	2.0
Frosted Flakes, Tesco*	1 Serving/30g	112	0.1	374	4.9	87.8	0.4	2.4
Frosted Wheats, Kellogg's*	1 Serving/30g	104	0.6	346	10.0	72.0	2.0	9.0
Frosties, Chocolate, Kellogg's*	1 Serving/40g	158	2.4	394	5.0	80.0	6.0	3.5
Frosties, Kellogg's*	1 Serving/30g	112	0.2	375	4.5	87.0	0.6	2.0
Frosties, Reduced Sugar, Kellogg's*	1 Serving/30g	111	0.2	369	6.0	85.0	0.6	2.5
Fruit, Nuts & Flakes, M&S*	1 Serving/30g	117	2.6	391	9.1	69.6	8.5	3.5
Fruit & Fibre, Asda*	1 Serving/40g	146	2.6	366	8.2	68.4	6.6	8.5
Fruit & Fibre, Flakes, Waitrose*	1 Serving/40g	143	2.5	357	8.2	67.2	6.2	9.9
Fruit & Fibre, Harvest Morn, Aldi*	1 Serving/30g	105	1.5	349	8.5	67.6	4.9	10.1
Fruit & Fibre, Lidl*	1 Serving/25g	91	1.2	363	8.8	70.9	4.9	8.0
Fruit & Fibre, Morrisons*	1 Serving/30g	110	2.2	366	8.8	66.5	7.2	8.5
Fruit & Fibre, Organic, Sainsbury's*	1 Serving/40g	147	1.6	367	10.0	72.4	4.1	7.8
Fruit & Fibre, Somerfield*	1 Serving/40g	144	2.4	361	8.1	68.7	6.0	8.9
Fruit & Fibre, Tesco*	1 Serving/30g	111	2.0	370	8.0	69.1	6.6	7.7
Fruit & Fibre, Value, Tesco*	1 Serving/40g	144	2.2	359	11.4	65.7	5.6	8.0
Fruit & Fibre, Whole Grain, Sainsbury's*	1 Serving/30g	108	1.8	361	8.1	68.7	6.0	8.9
Fruit & Nut Crisp, Minis, Weetabix*	1 Serving/40g	144	1.8	359	9.3	70.0	4.6	8.9
Fruit 'n' Fibre, Kellogg's*	1 Serving/40g	152	2.4	380	8.0	69.0	6.0	9.0
Golden Balls, Asda*	1 Serving/30g	112	0.4	374	5.0	85.0	1.5	1.5
Golden Grahams, Nestle*	1 Serving/30g	112	0.9	375	6.0	81.0	3.0	3.4
Golden Honey Puffs, Tesco*	1 Serving/30g	115	0.4	382	6.6	86.3	1.2	3.0
Golden Nuggets, Nestle*	1 Serving/40g	152	0.3	381	6.2	87.4	0.7	1.5
Granola	1 Serving/45g	194	8.7	430	17.5	48.8	19.4	16.8
Granola, & Strawberries with Bio Yoghurt, Rumblers*	1 Pot/168g	267	9.7	159	4.3	22.4	5.8	1.1
Granola, Chocolate, Dorset Cereals*	1 Serving/40g	206	12.0	515	8.8	47.2	30.0	10.5
Granola, Honey, Dorset Cereals*	1 Serving/40g	194	10.2	484	12.6	51.2	25.4	5.6
Granola, Low Fat, Home Farm*	1 Serving/55g	180	3.0	328	7.3	69.0	5.4	9.0
Granola, Oat, Quaker Oats*	1 Serving/50g	206	4.4	411	8.6	73.0	8.8	5.2
Granola, Organic, Lizi's, The GoodCarb Food Company*	1 Serving/50g	246	14.0	493	11.3	48.6	28.1	7.4
Granola, Original, Diet Chef Ltd*	1 Pack/50g	248	14.6	496	10.9	46.2	29.3	10.6
Granola, Original, Lizi's, The GoodCarb Food Company*	1 Serving/50g	248	14.6	496	10.9	46.2	29.3	10.6
Granola, Perfekt, Ultimate, Organic, GranoVita*	1 Serving/40g	190	6.6	474	13.3	40.6	16.4	11.8
Granola, Quaker Oats*	1 Serving/48g	210	7.0	438	10.4	72.9	14.6	6.2
Granola, Superfoods, Jordans*	1 Serving/50g	208	6.7	415	9.0	64.7	13.4	8.6
Granola, Treacle & Pecan, Diet Chef Ltd*	1 Pack/40g	196	11.3	490	9.7	47.6	28.3	11.3
Grape Nuts, Kraft*	1 Serving/45g	158	0.9	350	10.9	81.9	2.0	11.9
Harvest Crunch, Nut, Quaker Oats*	1 Serving/40g	184	7.8	459	8.0	62.5	19.5	6.0
Harvest Crunch, Soft Juicy Raisins, Quaker Oats*	1 Serving/50g	221	8.0	442	6.0	67.0	16.0	4.0
Hawaiian Crunch, Asda*	1 Serving/50g	224	7.6	448	8.0	69.6	15.3	7.0
Hawaiian Crunch, Mornflake*	1 Serving/60g	247	7.4	411	8.1	66.8	12.4	6.8

BREAKFAST CEREAL

	Measure INFO/WEIGHT	per Measure KCAL	FAT	Nutrition Values per 100g / 100ml KCAL	PROT	CARB	FAT	FIBRE
High Bran, CBY, Asda*	1 Serving/40g	136	1.5	341	13.6	49.5	3.8	27.1
High Fibre, Alpen*	1 Serving/45g	154	3.2	343	7.7	62.1	7.1	14.1
High Fibre Bran, Sainsbury's*	1 Serving/40g	134	1.5	335	14.3	48.4	3.7	25.4
High Fruit Muesli, BGTY, Sainsbury's*	1 Serving/50g	164	1.0	328	6.7	71.0	1.9	6.6
Honey & Nut Crisp, Mini, Weetabix*	1 Serving/40g	150	0.8	375	9.4	75.1	2.0	9.3
Honey Loops, Kellogg's*	1 Serving/30g	110	0.9	367	8.0	77.0	3.0	6.0
Honey Raisin & Almond, Crunchy, Waitrose*	1 Serving/40g	170	4.8	425	10.5	68.8	12.0	5.7
Hoops, Multigrain, Asda*	1 Serving/30g	113	1.2	376	6.5	78.4	4.0	4.6
Hoops, Multigrain, Tesco*	1 Serving/30g	112	1.1	375	6.5	78.6	3.8	4.6
Hot Oat, Aldi*	1 Serving/40g	142	3.3	356	11.6	58.8	8.3	8.9
Hot Oats, Instant, Tesco*	1 Serving/30g	108	2.6	360	11.8	58.4	8.7	7.9
Instant Oats, Dry Weight	1 Sachet/36g	129	3.1	359	11.5	59.1	8.5	8.3
Just Right, Kellogg's*	1 Serving/40g	145	1.2	362	7.0	77.0	3.0	4.5
Krave, Chocolate & Hazelnut, Kellogg's*	1 Serving/30g	132	4.8	440	8.0	66.0	16.0	4.0
Lion, Nestle*	1 Serving/40g	166	3.1	415	7.2	76.9	7.7	4.3
Luxury Muesli, Diet Chef Ltd*	1 Pack/40g	166	4.7	414	10.6	61.0	11.8	10.9
Malted Wheaties, Asda*	1 Serving/50g	171	1.4	342	10.0	69.0	2.9	10.0
Malted Wheats, Waitrose*	1 Serving/32g	110	0.6	343	9.7	71.7	1.9	9.9
Malties, Sainsbury's*	1 Serving/40g	137	1.2	343	10.0	69.2	2.9	10.0
Malty Flakes, Tesco*	1 Serving/40g	148	0.6	371	11.0	78.4	1.5	4.3
Maple & Pecan, Crisp, Asda*	1 Serving/30g	135	5.7	451	8.0	62.0	19.0	6.0
Maple & Pecan, Crunchy, Special, Luxury, Jordans*	1 Serving/50g	220	8.6	440	9.5	61.6	17.3	7.2
Maple & Pecan, Sainsbury's*	1 Serving/60g	318	13.2	530	13.3	69.7	22.0	5.3
Maple & Pecan Crisp, Sainsbury's*	1 Serving/50g	226	9.8	452	7.9	61.3	19.5	5.4
Maple & Pecan Crisp, Tesco*	1 Serving/50g	215	7.6	430	10.5	62.5	15.2	10.2
Maple Frosted Flakes, Whole Earth*	1 Serving/30g	112	0.3	375	6.2	85.6	1.0	1.6
Millet Rice Oatbran Flakes, Nature's Path*	1 Serving/56g	204	3.2	365	11.3	67.0	5.8	10.0
Mini Wheats, Sainsbury's*	1 Serving/45g	157	1.0	348	11.8	69.9	2.3	11.8
Minibix, Weetabix*	1 Serving/40g	134	1.5	335	8.8	71.2	3.8	8.1
Muesli, Apricot, Traidcraft*	1 Serving/30g	103	1.8	344	8.0	68.0	6.0	5.0
Muesli, Base, Nature's Harvest*	1 Serving/50g	179	2.6	358	11.0	71.2	5.1	7.4
Muesli, Basics, Sainsbury's*	1 Serving/50g	172	3.2	344	11.2	60.6	6.3	10.1
Muesli, Berries & Cherries, Dorset Cereals*	1 Serving/70g	225	1.5	321	6.5	68.8	2.2	6.3
Muesli, Carb Control, Tesco*	1 Serving/35g	154	9.3	439	25.0	25.0	26.6	13.8
Muesli, COU, M&S*	1 Serving/60g	201	1.5	335	7.6	70.2	2.5	8.1
Muesli, Cranberry & Blueberry, Love Life, Waitrose*	1 Serving/50g	164	1.8	329	8.5	65.3	3.7	7.5
Muesli, Creamy Tropical Fruit, Finest, Tesco*	1 Serving/80g	283	4.5	354	7.2	68.8	5.6	6.9
Muesli, Crunchy, Organic, Sainsbury's*	1 Serving/40g	168	5.8	420	11.6	62.0	14.4	9.2
Muesli, De Luxe, No Added Salt or Sugar, Sainsbury's*	1 Serving/40g	161	5.6	403	11.9	57.6	13.9	8.4
Muesli, Flahavans*	1 Serving/52g	187	2.8	360	10.4	72.1	5.3	5.5
Muesli, Fruit, 55%, Asda*	1 Serving/35g	111	1.0	318	6.0	67.0	2.9	7.0
Muesli, Fruit, GFY, Asda*	1 Serving/50g	152	0.9	304	8.0	64.0	1.8	10.0
Muesli, Fruit, Nuts & Seeds, Dorset Cereals*	1 Serving/70g	265	8.0	379	10.6	58.4	11.4	6.1
Muesli, Fruit, Sainsbury's*	1 Serving/40g	132	1.8	330	8.1	64.3	4.5	9.6
Muesli, Fruit, Somerfield*	1 Serving/50g	164	2.0	329	6.4	66.5	4.1	4.8
Muesli, Fruit, Waitrose*	1 Serving/30g	101	1.4	338	7.2	66.8	4.7	6.8
Muesli, Fruit & Nut, 55%, Asda*	1 Serving/40g	151	5.6	378	9.0	54.0	14.0	7.0
Muesli, Fruit & Nut, COU, M&S*	1 Serving/40g	128	1.1	320	7.4	74.5	2.8	7.4
Muesli, Fruit & Nut, Jordans*	1 Serving/50g	180	4.7	361	8.0	61.2	9.4	7.5
Muesli, Fruit & Nut, Luxury, Co-Op*	1 Serving/40g	150	4.0	375	8.0	64.0	10.0	6.0
Muesli, Fruit & Nut, Luxury, Lidl*	1 Serving/57g	205	5.6	360	8.0	60.0	9.8	7.5
Muesli, Fruit & Nut, Luxury, Sainsbury's*	1 Serving/50g	178	4.6	355	10.3	57.9	9.1	11.3
Muesli, Fruit & Nut, Luxury, Waitrose*	1 Serving/40g	145	3.8	363	9.0	60.3	9.5	6.5

BREAKFAST CEREAL

Measure INFO/WEIGHT	per Measure KCAL	per Measure FAT	Nutrition Values per 100g / 100ml KCAL	PROT	CARB	FAT	FIBRE
Muesli, Fruit & Nut, M&S*	1 Serving/40g	128	1.1	320	7.4	74.5	2.8	7.4
Muesli, Fruit & Nut, Organic, M&S*	1 Serving/50g	166	3.0	333	8.2	61.6	6.0	7.6
Muesli, Fruit & Nut, Sainsbury's*	1 Serving/30g	121	5.2	402	10.4	51.3	17.2	9.2
Muesli, Fruit & Nut, Tesco*	1 Serving/50g	190	5.6	380	8.4	60.3	11.3	5.3
Muesli, Fruit & Nut, Whole Wheat, Organic, Asda*	1 Serving/50g	172	3.5	343	10.0	60.0	7.0	7.0
Muesli, Fruit & Seeds, Organic, Pertwood Farm*	1 Serving/50g	164	3.4	328	11.4	55.5	6.7	12.6
Muesli, Fruit Nut & Seed, Love Life, Waitrose*	1 Serving/45g	159	6.7	392	12.2	48.5	16.6	8.0
Muesli, Fruit Nut & Seed, Organic, Dorset Cereals*	1 Serving/70g	251	6.9	358	10.8	56.6	9.8	8.4
Muesli, Fruit Sensation, M&S*	1 Serving/50g	158	1.5	315	6.0	66.0	3.0	7.4
Muesli, Fruity, Roast & Toast, Dorset Cereals*	1 Bowl/60g	251	10.1	418	11.9	54.7	16.8	7.4
Muesli, Fruity Fibre, Jordans*	1 Serving/50g	172	3.2	344	7.7	64.2	6.3	8.5
Muesli, GF, Nature's Harvest, Holland & Barrett*	1 Serving/60g	234	7.8	390	14.1	54.1	13.0	3.3
Muesli, Golden Sun*	1 Serving/40g	144	3.9	360	8.0	60.0	9.8	7.5
Muesli, High Fibre, Neal's Yard*	1 Serving/50g	182	1.0	364	7.6	72.7	1.9	12.9
Muesli, High Fibre, You Count, Love Life, Waitrose*	1 Serving/45g	155	1.3	344	7.7	67.4	2.9	8.8
Muesli, Luscious Berries & Cherries, Dorset Cereals*	1 Serving/50g	164	1.1	327	6.5	66.2	2.2	8.4
Muesli, Luxury, Finest, Tesco*	1 Serving/50g	197	6.6	394	8.3	60.8	13.1	5.4
Muesli, Luxury, Jordans*	1 Serving/40g	154	5.0	384	9.6	58.4	12.5	8.2
Muesli, Luxury, Sainsbury's*	1 Serving/40g	144	4.3	359	8.5	57.1	10.7	7.7
Muesli, Luxury Fruit, Harvest Morn, Aldi*	1 Serving/50g	158	1.6	315	6.8	64.5	3.3	6.9
Muesli, Luxury Fruit, PB, Waitrose*	1 Serving/50g	162	1.6	324	7.1	66.4	3.3	7.0
Muesli, Natural, No Added Sugar Or Salt, Jordans*	1 Serving/50g	210	4.1	420	16.0	70.4	8.2	8.4
Muesli, No Added Sugar, Morrisons*	1 Serving/50g	166	2.6	331	11.2	64.7	5.1	6.3
Muesli, No Added Sugar, Waitrose*	1 Serving/40g	146	2.5	364	12.0	64.9	6.3	6.7
Muesli, No Added Sugar Or Salt, Organic, Jordans*	1 Serving/50g	175	4.4	350	9.2	58.4	8.8	9.3
Muesli, Organic, Waitrose*	1 Serving/50g	188	0.8	375	10.3	59.6	1.6	8.3
Muesli, Original, Holland & Barrett*	1 Serving/30g	105	2.5	351	11.1	61.2	8.4	7.1
Muesli, Original, Sainsbury's*	1 Serving/60g	226	5.0	376	9.3	65.7	8.4	7.1
Muesli, Original, Simply, Hubbards*	1 Serving/50g	212	6.7	424	11.8	59.4	13.4	9.2
Muesli, Really Nutty, Dorset Cereals*	1 Serving/70g	253	6.1	362	9.8	61.1	8.7	6.3
Muesli, Rich, Nature's Harvest*	1 Serving/40g	143	3.7	358	10.0	60.5	9.2	7.6
Muesli, Simply Delicious, Dorset Cereals*	1 Serving/70g	256	6.6	366	10.8	59.2	9.5	7.4
Muesli, Simply Fruity, As Sold, Dorset Cereals*	1 Serving/45g	150	1.2	334	7.4	66.4	2.6	7.7
Muesli, Simply Sumptuous, Luxury Fruit, Lidl*	1 Serving/45g	154	1.5	343	6.5	68.7	3.3	6.2
Muesli, Special, Fruit, Jordans*	1 Serving/50g	162	1.4	323	6.6	68.0	2.7	8.4
Muesli, Special, Jordans*	1 Serving/50g	183	5.4	366	7.9	59.5	10.7	8.5
Muesli, Spelt, Barley & Oat Flakes, Dorset Cereals*	1 Serving/40g	148	4.5	371	9.5	57.9	11.3	7.4
Muesli, Super Berry, Jordans*	1 Serving/50g	174	3.8	348	9.0	60.8	7.6	8.1
Muesli, Super High Fibre, Dorset Cereals*	1 Serving/70g	250	6.6	357	8.0	60.1	9.4	8.4
Muesli, Swiss Style, Aldi*	1 Serving/50g	180	3.2	359	9.8	65.3	6.5	8.3
Muesli, Swiss Style, Apple & Raisin, M&S*	1 Serving/200g	250	2.4	125	3.3	25.3	1.2	3.3
Muesli, Swiss Style, Bettabuy, Morrisons*	1 Serving/50g	170	2.5	340	11.0	62.8	5.0	9.4
Muesli, Swiss Style, Co-Op*	1 Serving/40g	148	2.4	370	11.0	67.0	6.0	6.0
Muesli, Swiss Style, No Added Salt Or Sugar, Tesco*	1 Serving/50g	182	3.2	364	11.0	61.0	6.4	9.6
Muesli, Swiss Style, No Added Sugar Or Salt, Asda*	1 Serving/50g	182	3.5	363	11.0	64.0	7.0	8.0
Muesli, Swiss Style, Organic, Whole Earth*	1 Serving/50g	172	3.6	344	9.2	60.8	7.1	11.3
Muesli, Swiss Style, Smart Price, Asda*	1 Serving/60g	222	3.6	370	9.0	70.0	6.0	10.0
Muesli, Swiss Style with Fruit, Tesco*	1 Serving/40g	144	2.1	360	10.4	67.4	5.3	7.4
Muesli, Swiss, with Berries, Dry, Love Life, Waitrose*	1 Serving/45g	172	4.3	383	13.5	55.7	9.6	9.8
Muesli, The Ultimate, Organic, Rude Health*	1 Serving/50g	163	4.5	326	10.8	50.5	9.0	12.3
Muesli, Tropical, Sainsbury's*	1 Serving/50g	182	3.4	365	6.5	69.4	6.8	6.4
Muesli, Tropical Fruits, Jordans*	1 Serving/50g	164	1.4	329	6.9	68.7	2.9	7.1
Muesli, Unsweetened, M&S*	1 Serving/40g	129	1.1	322	8.1	68.0	2.7	9.4

BREAKFAST CEREAL

	Measure INFO/WEIGHT	per Measure KCAL	per Measure FAT	Nutrition Values per 100g / 100ml KCAL	PROT	CARB	FAT	FIBRE
Muesli, Value, Tesco*	1 Serving/50g	177	2.6	354	10.3	60.9	5.2	11.3
Muesli, Whole Wheat, No Added Sugar & Salt, Tesco*	1 Serving/40g	154	5.0	386	9.5	59.1	12.4	7.4
Muesli, Whole Wheat, Organic, Asda*	1 Serving/50g	197	3.0	394	10.0	75.0	6.0	9.0
Muesli, Wholewheat, Asda*	1 Serving/45g	150	3.5	333	8.0	57.9	7.7	9.7
Muesli, with Buckwheat, Toasted, GF, Eat Natural*	1 Serving/50g	230	11.4	461	11.7	53.2	22.8	2.0
Muesli Base, Wholesome, Waitrose*	1 Portion/50g	125	4.2	250	11.5	31.8	8.4	5.0
Muesli Mix, Perfect Start, Organic, The Food Doctor*	1 Serving/50g	196	7.1	392	12.1	55.5	14.2	7.1
Multigrain, Balanced Lifestyle, Aldi*	1 Serving/30g	108	0.7	360	7.5	77.1	2.4	4.5
Multigrain, Fitnesse, Nestle*	1 Serving/30g	109	0.4	363	8.0	79.8	1.3	5.1
Multigrain, Flakes with Fruit & Nuts, Aldi*	1 Serving/30g	108	0.7	360	7.5	77.1	2.4	4.5
Multigrain, Hoops, Average	1 Serving/30g	112	1.1	374	6.6	77.4	3.6	6.1
Multigrain Boulders, Tesco*	1 Serving/30g	112	0.4	375	8.2	82.3	1.3	3.6
Nesquik, Chocolatey Corn & Rice, Nestle*	1 Serving/30g	114	1.2	380	7.2	79.1	3.9	5.1
Nutty Crunch, Deliciously, M&S*	1 Serving/50g	238	11.2	476	8.8	59.6	22.5	4.4
Oat, Blueberry & Cranberry, Crunchy, Waitrose*	1 Serving/60g	259	9.1	432	8.0	65.9	15.2	8.5
Oat, Crunchy, Sainsbury's*	1 Serving/50g	226	10.2	453	8.2	59.3	20.3	6.6
Oat, Raisin, Nut & Honey, Crunchy, Dry, Sainsbury's*	1 Serving/50g	201	7.0	402	8.5	60.2	14.1	7.6
Oat & Bran Flakes, Sainsbury's*	1 Serving/30g	97	1.7	324	12.2	56.0	5.7	17.7
Oat Bran, Crispies, Quaker Oats*	1 Serving/40g	153	2.6	383	11.0	69.0	6.5	9.0
Oat Bran, Hodgson Mill*	1 Serving/40g	48	1.2	120	6.0	23.0	3.0	6.0
Oat Krunchies, Quaker Oats*	1 Serving/30g	118	2.1	393	9.5	72.0	7.0	5.5
Oat Meal, Medium, Heart's Content, Mornflake*	1 Serving/30g	108	2.4	359	11.0	60.4	8.1	8.5
Oatbran 100%, Mornflake*	1 Serving/40g	146	3.8	364	13.4	47.3	9.4	18.2
Oatbran Flakes, Nature's Path*	1 Serving/30g	124	1.4	414	8.7	83.0	4.7	6.7
Oatbran Flakes, Original, Mornflake*	1 Serving/40g	149	2.1	372	11.9	63.2	5.2	12.4
Oatbran Sprinkles, Mornflake*	1 Serving/40g	146	3.8	364	13.4	47.3	9.4	18.2
Oatibix, Bites, Cranberry, Weetabix*	1 Serving/40g	155	3.2	388	9.4	63.5	8.0	11.9
Oatibix, Bitesize, Original, Weetabix*	1 Serving/36g	133	2.4	370	10.6	66.5	6.8	10.1
Oatibix, Flakes, Weetabix*	1 Serving/50g	190	2.8	381	9.5	73.2	5.6	3.5
Oatibix, Weetabix*	2 Biscuits/48g	189	3.8	394	12.5	64.3	8.0	7.3
Oatiflakes, with Raisin, Cranberry & Apple, Weetabix*	1 Serving/40g	135	0.5	338	6.7	75.0	1.2	8.6
Oatmeal, Cinnamon, Weight Control, Quaker Oats*	1 Pack/45g	160	3.0	356	15.6	64.4	6.7	13.3
Oatmeal, Quick Oats, Dry, Quaker Oats*	1 Serving/30g	114	2.0	380	14.0	66.7	6.7	10.0
Oatmeal, Scottish, Hamlyns of Scotland*	1 Portion/40g	157	3.7	392	11.2	66.0	9.2	7.1
Oats, Crunch, Quaker Oats*	1 Serving/40g	146	2.0	366	9.1	71.1	5.0	7.4
Oats, Free From, Sainsbury's*	1 Serving/40g	155	3.2	388	14.9	64.0	8.0	11.0
Oats, Ginger Bread, Bench Press, Instant, Oomf*	1 Pot/75g	296	3.4	395	28.3	57.1	4.5	6.7
Oats, Golden Syrup, Dry, Micro, Tesco*	1 Sachet/39g	144	2.2	370	7.8	71.6	5.7	6.4
Oats, Golden Syrup Flavour, Instant, Hot, Waitrose*	1 Serving/39g	153	2.3	393	7.8	77.4	5.8	6.0
Oats, Jumbo, Organic, Waitrose*	1 Serving/50g	180	4.0	361	11.0	61.1	8.1	7.8
Oats, Superfast, Mornflake*	1 Serving/40g	144	3.2	359	11.0	60.4	8.1	8.5
Oats, Tesco*	1 Serving/40g	142	3.2	356	11.0	60.0	8.0	8.0
Oats, Wholegrain, Organic, Quaker Oats*	1 Serving/25g	89	2.0	356	11.0	60.0	8.0	9.0
Optivita, Berry Oat Crisp, Kellogg's*	1 Serving/30g	107	1.5	357	10.0	68.0	5.0	9.0
Organic, Spelt Flakes, Queenswood*	1 Tbsp/10g	33	0.3	331	11.0	60.0	3.0	9.0
Organic, Weetabix*	2 Biscuits/38g	134	0.7	358	11.5	68.6	2.0	10.0
Original, Crunchy, Raisins & Almonds, Jordans*	1 Serving/50g	204	6.4	407	8.7	64.0	12.9	6.6
Original, Crunchy, Tropical Fruits, Jordans*	1 Serving/50g	212	7.2	423	8.1	65.1	14.5	6.7
Original, Dry, Micro Oats, Tesco*	1 Sachet/27g	97	2.2	360	11.0	60.4	8.1	8.5
Original, with Raisins, Hazelnuts & Almonds, Alpen*	1 Serving/40g	144	2.3	359	10.5	66.6	5.8	7.3
Pink Apple & Cinnamon, Granola, Diet Chef Ltd*	1 Pack/40g	193	10.7	483	10.1	49.3	26.8	11.2
Pomegranate & Raspberry Wheats, Tesco*	1 Serving/45g	151	0.6	335	7.5	71.8	1.4	8.2
Porridge, Apple, Sultana & Cinnamon, M&S*	1 Sachet/40g	144	3.0	360	10.3	62.3	7.5	8.6

BREAKFAST CEREAL

	Measure INFO/WEIGHT	per Measure KCAL	FAT	Nutrition Values per 100g / 100ml KCAL	PROT	CARB	FAT	FIBRE
Porridge, Apple & Cinnamon, without Milk, Graze*	1 Punnet/43g	143	1.6	336	5.7	68.4	3.8	6.2
Porridge, Apple & Raspberry, Seriously Oaty, Weetabix*	1 Serving/40g	142	2.4	354	8.3	63.7	6.0	7.8
Porridge, Blackcurrant & Cranberry, without Milk, Graze*	1 Punnet/42g	147	1.6	349	5.4	70.8	3.8	5.5
Porridge, Blueberries, Cranberries & Nuts, Micro, Alpen*	1 Sachet/40g	154	3.4	385	10.8	62.6	8.5	7.3
Porridge, Blueberry & Lingonberry, without Milk, Graze*	1 Punnet/42g	143	2.5	345	8.0	63.0	6.0	10.0
Porridge, Cherry & Almond, without Milk, Graze*	1 Punnet/48g	174	3.3	364	7.0	68.0	7.0	6.0
Porridge, Chocolate, Oatibix, Weetabix*	1 Pack/40g	149	3.9	372	9.9	61.3	9.7	6.2
Porridge, Express, Apple & Cinnamon, Dry, Sainsbury's*	1 Sachet/36g	138	2.1	383	8.6	70.3	5.9	7.2
Porridge, Fig & Blueberry, without Milk, Graze*	1 Punnet/45g	149	2.3	331	8.0	62.0	5.0	9.0
Porridge, Flakes, Organic, Barkat*	1 Serving/30g	109	0.9	362	8.5	74.1	3.0	0.0
Porridge, Free From, Sainsbury's*	1 Serving/50g	174	1.5	348	8.6	72.0	3.0	3.4
Porridge, Fruitful, Traditional, Hubbards*	1 Bowl/50g	180	3.8	360	13.4	51.6	7.7	13.3
Porridge, Fruity, Apple & Raisin, Dorset Cereals*	1 Serving/70g	233	3.4	333	9.7	62.7	4.8	8.9
Porridge, Fruity, Cranberry & Raspberry, Dorset Cereals*	1 Sachet/30g	99	1.8	330	10.2	58.7	6.0	12.3
Porridge, Fruity, Fruit & Nut, Dorset Cereals*	1 Serving/70g	242	5.6	346	9.4	59.0	8.0	8.2
Porridge, Fruity, Mixed Berries, Dorset Cereals*	1 Serving/70g	243	4.2	347	10.8	62.6	6.0	7.9
Porridge, Golden Honey, Oatibix, Weetabix*	1 Serving/40g	145	2.6	363	9.2	66.7	6.6	7.0
Porridge, Golden Syrup, Oat So Simple, Quaker Oats*	1 Sachet/36g	137	2.2	380	8.4	68.7	6.2	6.8
Porridge, Hazelnut & Flame Raisin, without Milk, Graze*	1 Punnet/45g	178	6.3	397	9.0	56.0	14.0	7.0
Porridge, Instant, Quaker Oats*	1 Serving/34g	124	2.9	364	11.0	60.0	8.5	9.0
Porridge, Made with Semi Skimmed Milk, Waitrose*	1 Serving/50g	277	7.5	554	24.6	80.4	15.0	8.6
Porridge, Multigrain, Jordans*	1 Serving/40g	134	2.2	335	10.4	60.9	5.5	10.0
Porridge, Oats, Golden Syrup, Sainsbury's*	1 Sachet/39g	143	2.1	367	6.3	73.6	5.3	6.7
Porridge, Original, As Sold, Moma Foods*	1 Pot/70g	257	4.2	367	15.6	59.0	6.0	7.6
Porridge, Original, Diet Chef Ltd*	1 Sachet/40g	157	2.5	392	12.0	67.0	6.3	9.8
Porridge, Original, Dry, Oat So Simple, Quaker Oats*	1 Serving/27g	100	2.1	370	11.0	58.9	7.7	10.5
Porridge, Original, Express, Sainsbury's*	1 Pack/27g	100	2.2	370	11.0	58.0	8.0	10.8
Porridge, Original, Simply Porridge, Asda*	1 Sachet/27g	96	2.2	356	11.0	60.0	8.0	8.0
Porridge, Perfectly, Dorset Cereals*	1 Sachet/30g	107	2.5	356	11.8	58.2	8.4	11.0
Porridge, Porage Oats, Old Fashioned, Dry, Scotts*	1 Serving/40g	142	3.2	355	11.0	60.0	8.0	9.0
Porridge, Porage Oats, Original, Dry, Scotts*	1 Serving/40g	142	3.2	356	11.0	60.0	8.0	9.0
Porridge, Porage Oats, Original, So-Easy, Dry, Scotts*	1 Serving/30g	109	2.6	364	11.0	60.0	8.5	9.0
Porridge, Porage Oats, Syrup Swirl, So-Easy, Dry, Scotts*	1 Sachet/37g	135	2.2	366	8.0	70.0	6.0	6.5
Porridge, Spelt, Sharpham Park*	1 Serving/50g	159	1.6	318	11.3	7.0	3.3	9.5
Porridge, Toffee Flavour, Oat So Simple, Quaker Oats*	1 Serving/30g	122	3.9	407	6.5	66.0	13.0	5.0
Porridge, Walnut & Pecan, without Milk, Graze*	1 Punnet/39g	162	6.6	419	8.0	57.0	17.0	6.0
Porridge, with Apple & Cinnamon, Diet Chef Ltd*	1 Pack/40g	150	1.9	375	8.9	69.5	4.7	9.0
Porridge Oats, & Bran, Somerfield*	1 Serving/40g	154	2.8	385	12.0	68.0	7.0	0.0
Porridge Oats, Blueberry, Paw Ridge, Quaker Oats*	1 Sachet/28g	107	2.0	376	9.7	64.4	7.0	8.1
Porridge Oats, Co-Op*	1 Serving/40g	144	3.2	360	12.0	61.0	8.0	9.0
Porridge Oats, Dry Weight, Value, Tesco*	1 Serving/50g	180	4.0	359	11.0	60.4	8.1	8.5
Porridge Oats, Mornflake*	1 Serving/50g	180	4.0	359	11.0	60.4	8.1	8.5
Porridge Oats, Organic, As Sold, Jordans*	1 Serving/40g	146	3.7	364	11.7	58.4	9.3	9.0
Porridge Oats, Organic, Tesco*	1 Serving/28g	100	2.3	358	11.0	60.4	8.1	8.5
Porridge Oats, Original, Paw Ridge, Quaker Oats*	1 Sachet/25g	89	2.0	356	11.0	60.0	8.0	9.0
Porridge Oats, Quaker Oats*	1 Serving/45g	160	3.6	356	11.0	60.0	8.0	4.0
Porridge Oats, Rolled, Tesco*	1 Serving/50g	180	4.0	359	11.0	60.4	8.1	8.5
Porridge Oats, Scottish, Organic, Sainsbury's*	1 Serving/45g	172	2.2	383	10.0	74.4	5.0	7.9
Porridge Oats, Scottish, Tesco*	1 Serving/50g	180	4.0	359	11.0	60.4	8.1	8.5
Porridge Oats, Smart Price, Asda*	1 Serving/50g	178	4.0	356	11.0	60.0	8.0	8.0
Porridge Oats, Whole Oats, Jordans*	1 Serving/40g	146	3.7	364	11.7	58.4	9.3	9.0
Porridge Oats, with Bran, Scottish, Sainsbury's*	1 Serving/50g	190	2.5	380	9.6	74.1	5.0	10.3
Porridge Oats, with Wheat Bran, Tesco*	1 Serving/50g	167	3.6	334	12.3	55.0	7.2	13.0

BREAKFAST CEREAL

	Measure INFO/WEIGHT	per Measure KCAL	FAT	Nutrition Values per 100g / 100ml KCAL	PROT	CARB	FAT	FIBRE
Porridge Oats, with Wheatbran, Essential, Waitrose*	1 Serving/50g	168	3.8	336	11.2	55.8	7.6	13.0
Puffed Rice, Average	1 Serving/30g	115	0.8	382	7.1	82.2	2.8	3.0
Puffed Rice, Organic, Natural, Kallo*	1 Bowl/25g	92	0.5	370	7.0	81.0	2.0	3.0
Puffed Rice, Wholegrain, Original, Organic, Kallo*	1 Serving/25g	95	0.8	380	8.0	80.0	3.0	9.0
Puffed Rice Cereal, Honey, Organic, Kallo*	1 Serving/25g	98	0.9	392	5.0	85.0	3.5	2.1
Puffed Wheat, Quaker Oats*	1 Serving/15g	49	0.2	328	15.3	62.4	1.3	5.6
Puffed Wheat, Tesco*	1 Serving/28g	104	0.9	373	13.9	72.2	3.2	5.7
Raisin, & Almond, Crunchy, Jordans*	1 Serving/56g	230	7.0	411	8.4	66.0	12.5	5.0
Raisin, Oats & More, Nestle*	1 Serving/30g	112	1.4	373	8.9	73.7	4.7	5.8
Raisin Wheats, Kellogg's*	1 Serving/30g	99	0.6	330	9.0	70.0	2.0	8.0
Raisin Wheats, Sainsbury's*	1 Serving/50g	166	0.8	332	8.2	71.5	1.5	8.0
Ready Brek, Chocolate, Porridge Oats, Weetabix*	1 Serving/30g	114	2.4	380	10.0	63.6	8.0	7.0
Ready Brek, Original, Weetabix*	1 Serving/40g	149	3.5	373	11.7	57.9	8.7	7.9
Red Berry & Almond Luxury Crunch, Jordans*	1 Serving/40g	176	7.4	441	8.2	60.5	18.5	6.6
Rice Krispies, Kellogg's*	1 Serving/30g	115	0.3	383	6.0	87.0	1.0	1.0
Rice Krispies, Multi-Grain Shapes, Kellogg's*	1 Serving/30g	111	0.8	370	8.0	77.0	2.5	8.0
Rice Pops, Blue Parrot Cafe, Sainsbury's*	1 Serving/30g	111	0.4	370	7.2	82.3	1.3	2.2
Rice Pops, Sainsbury's*	1 Serving/25g	98	0.4	391	6.7	87.1	1.4	1.7
Rice Snaps, Asda*	1 Serving/28g	105	0.4	376	7.0	84.0	1.3	1.5
Rice Snaps, Everyday Value, Tesco*	1 Serving/30g	115	0.3	380	7.5	84.5	0.9	1.4
Ricicles, Kellogg's*	1 Serving/30g	114	0.2	381	4.5	89.0	0.8	0.8
Right Balance, Morrisons*	1 Serving/50g	181	1.1	362	6.9	78.6	2.2	5.3
Rye Flakes, Organic, Infinity Foods*	1 Serving/100g	318	2.1	318	8.0	65.8	2.1	9.6
Shredded Wheat, Average	2 Biscuits/45g	157	0.8	348	9.0	77.0	1.8	10.0
Shredded Wheat, Bitesize, Nestle*	1 Serving/45g	166	1.0	369	11.8	69.6	2.2	11.8
Shredded Wheat, Fruitful, No Added Salt, Nestle*	1 Serving/40g	142	2.0	354	8.3	68.7	5.1	8.9
Shredded Wheat, Honey Nut, Nestle*	1 Serving/40g	151	2.6	378	11.2	68.8	6.5	9.4
Shredded Wheat, Triple Berry, Nestle*	1 Serving/40g	138	0.8	344	10.6	70.6	2.1	11.1
Shreddies, Coco, Nestle*	1 Serving/45g	161	0.9	358	8.4	76.5	2.0	8.6
Shreddies, Coco Orange Flavoured, Nestle*	1 Serving/40g	150	0.8	374	8.5	76.2	2.0	8.6
Shreddies, Frosted, Kellogg's*	1 Serving/50g	162	0.9	323	0.7	78.5	1.8	4.7
Shreddies, Frosted, Nestle*	1 Serving/45g	164	0.7	365	7.4	80.7	1.5	6.4
Shreddies, Honey, Nestle*	1 Serving/45g	169	0.7	375	8.2	78.1	1.5	8.1
Shreddies, Honey with 125ml Skimmed Milk, Nestle*	1 Serving/40g	210	2.7	525	17.8	91.8	6.8	8.0
Shreddies, Malt Wheats, Tesco*	1 Serving/45g	169	0.9	375	10.3	73.8	2.0	8.2
Shreddies, Nestle*	1 Serving/45g	186	1.0	371	10.0	73.7	1.9	9.9
Special Flakes, Tesco*	1 Serving/20g	74	0.3	371	11.0	78.4	1.5	4.3
Special K, Bliss, Creamy Berry Crunch, Kellogg's*	1 Serving/30g	114	0.8	379	13.0	76.0	2.5	2.5
Special K, Bliss, Strawberry & Chocolate, Kellogg's*	1 Serving/30g	115	0.9	383	13.0	76.0	3.0	2.5
Special K, Choco, Kellogg's*	1 Serving/40g	160	2.8	400	14.0	70.0	7.0	3.5
Special K, Clusters, Honey, Kellogg's*	1 Serving/45g	175	1.4	389	9.0	80.0	3.0	3.5
Special K, Kellogg's*	1 Serving/30g	114	0.4	379	14.0	76.0	1.5	2.5
Special K, Oats & Honey, Kellogg's*	1 Serving/50g	192	1.2	383	13.0	77.0	2.5	3.0
Special K, Peach & Apricot, Kellogg's*	1 Serving/30g	112	0.3	373	14.0	77.0	1.0	2.5
Special K, Protein Plus, Kellogg's*	1 Serving/29g	100	3.0	345	34.5	31.0	10.3	17.2
Special K, Purple Berries, Kellogg's*	1 Serving/30g	112	0.3	374	13.0	77.0	1.0	3.5
Special K, Red Berries, Kellogg's*	1 Serving/30g	112	0.4	374	14.0	76.0	1.5	3.0
Special K, Yoghurty, Kellogg's*	1 Serving/30g	115	0.9	383	14.0	75.0	3.0	2.5
Start, Kellogg's*	1 Serving/30g	112	0.8	375	8.0	80.0	2.5	5.0
Start Right, Asda*	1 Serving/40g	150	2.4	376	8.0	74.0	6.0	5.0
Strawberry, Alpen*	1 Serving/40g	144	1.9	359	9.4	69.5	4.8	7.9
Strawberry & Almond Crunch, M&S*	1 Serving/40g	186	7.4	465	8.0	66.0	18.6	4.9
Strawberry Crisp, Asda*	1 Serving/45g	194	7.0	431	8.1	64.7	15.5	5.9

	Measure INFO/WEIGHT	per Measure KCAL	FAT	Nutrition Values per 100g / 100ml KCAL	PROT	CARB	FAT	FIBRE
BREAKFAST CEREAL								
Sugar Puffs, Quaker Oats*	1 Serving/30g	114	0.5	379	5.3	85.8	1.6	3.7
Sultana Bran, Co-Op*	1 Serving/40g	130	1.2	325	9.0	66.0	3.0	11.0
Sultana Bran, Morrisons*	1 Serving/30g	98	0.9	325	8.8	65.8	3.0	11.4
Sultana Bran, Sainsbury's*	1 Serving/30g	97	0.6	324	8.2	68.6	1.9	11.6
Sultana Bran, Waitrose*	1 Serving/30g	97	0.6	324	8.2	68.6	1.9	11.6
Toasted Coconut & Wheat Flakes, Dorset Cereals*	1 Serving/45g	171	3.6	381	8.2	54.0	8.0	8.0
Vitality, Asda*	1 Serving/30g	111	0.4	370	11.0	78.0	1.5	3.2
Vitality with Red Fruit, Asda*	1 Serving/30g	110	0.5	366	11.0	77.0	1.6	3.8
Weet Bix, Sanitarium*	2 Biscuits/30g	106	0.4	352	12.0	67.0	1.4	10.5
Weetabix, Chocolate, Weetabix*	2 Biscuits/45g	166	1.8	368	10.1	67.9	4.0	10.0
Weetabix*	1 Biscuit/19g	67	0.4	358	11.5	68.6	2.0	10.0
Weetaflakes, Weetabix*	1 Serving/30g	102	0.4	340	8.9	72.9	1.4	11.0
Weetos, Chocolate, Weetabix*	1 Serving/30g	113	1.5	378	8.4	75.1	4.9	5.8
Wheat Biscuits, Average	2 Biscuits/38g	130	0.8	347	11.7	68.4	2.2	9.9
Wheat Bisks, Harvest Morn, Aldi*	2 Biscuits/38g	136	0.8	358	11.5	68.6	2.0	10.0
Wheat Pillows, Wholegrain, Tesco*	1 Biscuit/45g	151	0.9	335	10.6	67.6	2.1	11.3
Wholegrain, Apricot, Wheats, Sainsbury's*	1 Serving/50g	160	0.8	320	7.9	71.6	1.5	8.2
Wholegrain, Fruit & Fibre, Sainsbury's*	1 Serving/30g	109	1.8	363	8.1	69.1	6.0	8.9
Wholegrain, Mini Wheats, Sainsbury's*	1 Serving/40g	139	0.9	348	11.8	69.9	2.3	11.9
Wholegrain, Minis, Weetabix*	1 Serving/40g	149	0.8	372	10.2	73.2	2.0	10.0
Wholegrain, Sultana Bran, Sainsbury's*	1 Serving/30g	98	0.6	325	8.3	68.6	1.9	12.1
Yoghurt & Raspberry, Crisp, Sainsbury's*	1 Serving/45g	191	6.7	424	7.5	65.2	14.8	6.4
BRESAOLA								
Della Valtellina, Sainsbury's*	1 Slice/14g	23	0.4	163	34.7	0.1	2.6	0.1
Finest, Tesco*	1 Serving/35g	64	1.4	182	36.0	0.5	4.0	0.0
BROCCOLI								
& Cauliflower, Crowns, TTD, Sainsbury's*	1 Serving/100g	33	0.9	33	4.4	1.8	0.9	2.6
& Cauliflower, Floret Mix, Fresh, Tesco*	1 Serving/80g	27	0.7	34	3.9	2.5	0.9	2.7
& Cauliflower, Floret Mix, Iceland*	1 Serving/100g	26	0.7	26	2.6	2.2	0.7	2.4
& Cheese, Morrisons*	1 Pack/350g	406	24.8	116	6.2	6.6	7.1	0.8
Bellaverde, TTD, Sainsbury's*	1 Serving/100g	33	0.9	33	4.4	1.8	0.9	2.6
Cauliflower & Carrots, Frozen, Great Value, Asda*	1 Serving/100g	25	0.6	25	2.2	2.6	0.6	5.0
Chinese, Kai Lan, Cooked	1 Serving/80g	18	0.6	22	1.4	3.8	0.7	2.5
Green, Boiled, Average	**1 Serving/80g**	**19**	**0.6**	**24**	**3.1**	**1.1**	**0.8**	**2.3**
Green, Raw, Average	**1 Serving/80g**	**25**	**0.7**	**31**	**3.9**	**1.7**	**0.9**	**2.6**
Purple Sprouting, Boiled, Average	**1 Serving/80g**	**15**	**0.5**	**19**	**2.1**	**1.3**	**0.6**	**2.3**
Purple Sprouting, Raw	**1oz/28g**	**10**	**0.3**	**35**	**3.9**	**2.6**	**1.1**	**3.5**
Purple Sprouting, Raw, Spears, TTD, Sainsbury's*	1 Serving/100g	36	1.1	36	3.9	2.6	1.1	3.5
Steamed, Average	1 Serving/100g	24	0.8	24	3.1	1.1	0.8	2.3
Tenderstem, Finest, Tesco*	½ Pack/100g	31	0.2	31	4.2	3.2	0.2	3.1
Tenderstem, Ready Prepared, Raw, M&S*	1 Pack/200g	80	0.4	40	4.1	4.9	0.2	1.7
with a Cheese Sauce, Mash Direct*	½ Pack/150g	115	6.6	77	4.9	4.4	4.4	3.0
BROWNIES								
Average	1 Brownie/60g	243	10.1	405	4.6	0.0	16.8	0.0
Chocolate, Average	1 Serving/100g	446	22.3	446	5.9	55.6	22.3	2.2
Chocolate, Bites, Mini, Weight Watchers*	1 Brownie/9g	29	0.5	325	5.3	63.7	5.5	2.2
Chocolate, Cadbury*	1 Brownie/36g	145	5.7	403	6.1	59.7	15.8	0.0
Chocolate, Chewy, M&S*	1 Brownie/29g	130	6.0	455	6.5	59.8	21.1	2.0
Chocolate, Chunky, Belgian, M&S*	1 Brownie/55g	242	11.2	440	6.2	57.7	20.3	2.5
Chocolate, Devondale*	1 Cake/60g	246	12.9	410	4.4	51.0	21.5	2.1
Chocolate, Double, Bites, Mini, Sainsbury's*	1 Brownie/15g	49	2.5	326	5.8	38.9	16.4	1.6
Chocolate, Double, Iced, Otis Spunkmeyer*	1 Brownie/57g	250	6.8	439	3.5	61.4	12.0	1.8
Chocolate, Fudge, Entenmann's*	1/8 Cake/55g	168	2.4	306	4.0	62.7	4.4	1.5

	Measure INFO/WEIGHT	per Measure KCAL	FAT	Nutrition Values per 100g / 100ml KCAL	PROT	CARB	FAT	FIBRE
BROWNIES								
Chocolate, Fudgy, M&S*	1 Brownie/87g	400	21.9	460	4.8	56.9	25.2	3.0
Chocolate, Gluten & Wheat Free, Lovemore*	1 Slice/36g	127	4.6	352	3.7	56.1	12.8	0.2
Chocolate, Mini Bites, Asda*	1 Brownie/15g	62	3.0	420	5.0	55.0	20.0	1.4
Chocolate, Sainsbury's*	1 Brownie/60g	265	13.6	442	4.6	55.0	22.6	1.6
Chocolate, Slices, M&S*	1 Brownie/36g	158	8.7	440	5.3	51.1	24.1	1.3
Chocolate, Tray Bake, Tesco*	1 Brownie/37g	155	6.8	420	5.5	57.1	18.4	5.7
Chocolate, Waitrose*	1 Brownie/45g	192	8.9	426	6.3	55.6	19.8	2.7
Chocolate, Weight Watchers*	1 Brownie/47g	143	1.8	304	4.8	62.5	3.8	3.2
Chocolate, Wheat & GF, Mrs Crimble's*	1 Slice/48g	180	9.6	379	4.2	47.9	20.3	1.5
Chocolate & Pecan, Gu*	1 Brownie/40g	188	11.6	471	7.2	47.6	29.1	2.5
Chocolate Orange, Organic, The Village Bakery*	1 Brownie/30g	126	6.7	421	5.0	50.5	22.2	0.9
Fudge, The Handmade Flapjack Company*	1 Cake/75g	286	9.2	381	4.9	62.8	12.3	0.0
Praline, Mini, Finest, Tesco*	1 Brownie/12g	59	3.1	492	4.2	60.0	25.8	0.8
The Graze Brownie, Graze*	1 Portion/35g	129	6.3	368	7.1	50.5	17.9	3.8
BRUSCHETTA								
Cheese & Tomato, Asda*	1 Bruschetta/38g	68	1.7	180	8.6	26.0	4.6	2.9
Olive Oil & Sea Salt, Toasted, Tesco*	1 Serving/30g	126	4.6	420	11.5	58.7	15.5	4.5
Pane Italia*	1 Serving/75g	367	18.8	489	12.4	53.6	25.1	1.4
Ploughman's Relish, Brunchetta, Golden Vale*	1 Pack/90g	261	15.5	290	14.2	20.2	17.2	1.6
Red Pepper & Onion, Brunchetta, Golden Vale*	1 Pack/90g	266	17.1	296	14.6	17.0	19.0	1.3
Soft Cheese, & Cranberry, Brunchetta, Golden Vale*	1 Pack/95g	200	8.6	211	8.2	24.8	9.0	1.3
BRUSSELS SPROUTS								
& Sweet Chestnuts, Asda*	1 Serving/100g	73	1.7	73	3.1	11.0	1.7	4.2
Baby, Sainsbury's*	1 Serving/80g	34	1.1	42	3.5	3.9	1.4	4.1
Boiled, Average	*1 Serving/90g*	*32*	*1.2*	*35*	*3.1*	*3.2*	*1.3*	*3.5*
Button, & Chestnuts, Tesco*	1 Serving/100g	80	1.8	80	3.1	12.8	1.8	4.1
Button, Raw, Average	*1 Serving/80g*	*30*	*1.1*	*37*	*3.5*	*2.9*	*1.3*	*3.2*
Canned, Drained	*1oz/28g*	*8*	*0.3*	*28*	*2.6*	*2.4*	*1.0*	*2.6*
Frozen, Morrisons*	1 Serving/200g	70	2.6	35	3.5	2.5	1.3	4.3
Raw, Average	*1 Serving/80g*	*29*	*0.9*	*37*	*3.5*	*3.3*	*1.1*	*3.0*
Steamed, Average	1 Serving/100g	35	1.3	35	3.1	3.2	1.3	3.5
BUBBLE & SQUEAK								
Fried in Vegetable Oil	1oz/28g	35	2.5	124	1.4	9.8	9.1	1.5
Morrisons*	1 Serving/110g	168	9.6	153	2.2	16.3	8.7	0.7
Tesco*	½ Pack/325g	292	12.7	90	1.6	11.3	3.9	0.9
Waitrose*	½ Pack/225g	166	5.2	74	1.4	11.9	2.3	2.2
BUCKWHEAT								
Average	*1oz/28g*	*102*	*0.4*	*364*	*8.1*	*84.9*	*1.5*	*2.1*
BUFFALO								
Mince, Raw, Lean, Abel & Cole*	1 Serving/100g	95	0.7	95	21.7	0.4	0.7	0.0
BULGAR WHEAT								
Dry Weight, Average	*1oz/28g*	*99*	*0.5*	*353*	*9.7*	*76.3*	*1.7*	*8.0*
Wholefoods, Tesco*	1 Serving/50g	180	0.8	360	9.7	76.3	1.7	9.1
BUNS								
Belgian, Asda*	1 Bun/133g	464	19.9	350	4.8	49.0	15.0	2.2
Belgian, Co-Op*	1 Bun/118g	413	15.3	350	5.0	54.0	13.0	2.0
Belgian, Dairy Cream, Somerfield*	1 Serving/121g	400	13.4	331	5.2	52.6	11.1	2.0
Belgian, Iced, CBY, Asda*	1 Bun/115g	375	6.8	327	6.1	62.3	5.9	2.9
Belgian, Sainsbury's*	1 Bun/110g	398	11.3	362	6.1	61.3	10.3	1.9
Belgian, Tesco*	1 Bun/123g	438	15.7	356	5.2	54.9	12.8	2.2
Chelsea	1 Bun/78g	285	10.8	366	7.8	56.1	13.8	1.7
Chelsea, Sainsbury's*	1 Bun/85g	239	4.4	281	6.9	51.6	5.2	2.9
Chelsea, Tesco*	1 Bun/85g	269	6.5	316	7.9	53.9	7.6	2.3

	Measure INFO/WEIGHT	per Measure		Nutrition Values per 100g / 100ml				
		KCAL	FAT	KCAL	PROT	CARB	FAT	FIBRE
BUNS								
Choux, Caramel, Asda*	1 Bun/189g	745	51.0	394	4.3	33.5	27.0	1.3
Choux, Custard, M&S*	1 Bun/85g	234	18.7	275	4.2	15.0	22.0	0.3
Choux, Fresh Cream, Tesco*	1 Bun/95g	340	23.7	358	4.9	28.5	24.9	0.9
Currant	1 Bun/60g	178	4.5	296	7.6	52.7	7.5	0.0
Currant, Sainsbury's*	1 Bun/72g	197	3.7	274	7.0	50.0	5.1	2.8
Fingers, Sticky, Iced, CBY, Asda*	1 Finger/40g	132	2.4	330	7.1	62.0	5.9	2.7
Fruit, Waitrose*	1 Bun/54g	155	2.3	287	8.1	54.0	4.3	1.6
Hot Cross	1 Bun/50g	156	3.5	312	7.4	58.5	7.0	1.7
Hot Cross, 25% Reduced Fat, Asda*	1 Bun/61g	153	1.4	253	9.0	49.0	2.3	3.0
Hot Cross, Apple & Cinnamon, Large, Finest, Tesco*	1 Bun/117g	342	8.2	292	7.3	49.9	7.0	3.6
Hot Cross, Asda*	1 Bun/60g	190	3.8	317	10.0	55.0	6.3	3.3
Hot Cross, Best of Both, Hovis*	1 Bun/65g	185	4.3	285	9.1	47.3	6.6	4.4
Hot Cross, BGTY, Sainsbury's*	1 Bun/70g	160	1.6	229	7.6	44.4	2.3	2.7
Hot Cross, Chocolate, Mini, Sainsbury's*	1 Bun/39g	127	4.4	325	7.7	48.1	11.3	2.5
Hot Cross, Chocolate & Raisin, Mini, Tesco*	1 Bun/40g	127	4.4	318	8.1	47.0	10.9	2.8
Hot Cross, Classics, M&S*	1 Bun/65g	159	1.2	245	8.5	49.1	1.8	2.2
Hot Cross, Co-Op*	1 Bun/60g	165	3.6	275	8.0	47.0	6.0	3.0
Hot Cross, Finest, Tesco*	1 Bun/75g	210	4.0	280	7.8	49.5	5.4	2.8
Hot Cross, Lightly Fruited, M&S*	1 Bun/64g	165	3.4	260	8.1	45.1	5.4	4.7
Hot Cross, Low Fat, Co-Op*	1 Bun/60g	156	1.8	260	9.0	50.0	3.0	3.0
Hot Cross, Low Fat, Good Intentions, Somerfield*	1 Bun/50g	135	1.3	270	10.0	51.8	2.6	2.8
Hot Cross, Luxury, Cafe, M&S*	1 Bun/78g	199	3.1	255	8.6	46.2	4.0	2.1
Hot Cross, Luxury, M&S*	1 Bun/79g	201	3.2	255	8.6	46.2	4.0	2.1
Hot Cross, Mini, M&S*	1 Bun/41g	110	1.4	265	7.8	51.4	3.4	3.7
Hot Cross, Mini, Tesco*	1 Bun/36g	99	2.0	274	7.9	48.1	5.5	2.7
Hot Cross, Morrisons*	1 Bun/729g	178	1.4	247	7.4	49.9	2.0	3.3
Hot Cross, Reduced Fat, GFY, Asda*	1 Bun/63g	156	1.6	248	8.4	47.9	2.5	3.7
Hot Cross, Reduced Fat, Waitrose*	1 Bun/67g	171	1.4	255	8.1	54.3	2.1	3.3
Hot Cross, Tesco*	1 Bun/70g	186	1.9	265	7.4	51.8	2.7	3.6
Hot Cross, TTD, Sainsbury's*	1 Bun/75g	200	4.2	267	7.2	47.0	5.6	3.8
Hot Cross, White, Kingsmill*	1 Bun/25g	71	1.5	286	7.0	51.1	6.0	3.0
Hot Cross, White, LC, Tesco*	1 Bun/70g	185	1.4	260	8.3	50.3	1.9	3.8
Hot Cross, White, Waitrose*	1 Bun/68g	174	2.1	258	8.1	49.5	3.1	3.9
Hot Cross, Wholemeal, Asda*	1 Bun/70g	182	4.2	262	9.0	43.0	6.0	6.0
Hot Cross, Wholemeal, Golden, 3% Fat, M&S*	1 Bun/67g	144	1.5	215	8.9	39.6	2.2	6.7
Hot Cross, Wholemeal, Golden, Sainsbury's*	1 Bun/65g	180	4.0	277	9.9	45.4	6.2	4.3
Hot Cross, Wholemeal, Organic, Tesco*	1 Bun/55g	140	2.7	254	7.6	44.8	4.9	4.5
Hot Cross, Wholemeal, Waitrose*	1 Bun/64g	177	4.3	276	8.8	45.2	6.7	4.9
Hot Cross, You Count, Love Life, Waitrose*	1 Bun/70g	195	3.2	278	6.8	51.5	4.5	2.3
Iced, Filled with Raspberry Jam, M&S*	1 Bun/48g	155	3.2	320	6.4	58.9	6.6	1.9
Iced, Finger, Average	1 Bun/40g	130	3.1	325	7.2	57.0	7.7	2.3
Iced, Fingers, Coconut, Genesis Crafty*	1 Bun/64g	210	6.9	328	7.7	52.4	10.8	2.4
Iced, Spiced Fruit, M&S*	1 Bun/90g	270	3.3	300	7.0	60.3	3.7	1.5
Iced, Tesco*	1 Bun/35g	117	3.4	334	7.0	54.8	9.6	2.5
Iced Finger, Tesco*	1 Bun/41g	115	1.4	280	7.1	54.7	3.4	2.9
Iced Lemon, Tesco*	1 Bun/48g	156	4.2	325	5.2	56.5	8.7	1.9
Marlborough, M&S*	1 Bun/71g	215	6.3	305	6.2	43.4	8.9	2.2
Saffron, Somerfield*	1 Bun/70g	266	11.7	380	6.4	50.9	16.7	1.9
Spiced, PB, Waitrose*	1 Bun/65g	177	2.2	272	8.0	52.3	3.4	2.9
Vanilla Iced, Soft, M&S*	1 Bun/39g	125	3.1	320	7.6	54.9	8.0	2.9
White Hot Cross, Sainsbury's*	1 Bun/70g	199	3.4	284	7.9	50.6	4.8	3.4
BURGERS								
American Style, Tesco*	1 Burger/125g	250	9.1	200	13.0	20.4	7.3	3.9

BURGERS

	Measure INFO/WEIGHT	per Measure KCAL	FAT	Nutrition Values per 100g / 100ml KCAL	PROT	CARB	FAT	FIBRE
Bean, Mexican, & Tomato Salsa, Love Life, Waitrose*	1 Burger/163g	173	4.6	106	4.1	16.2	2.8	3.8
Beef, & Mature Cheddar, Asda*	1 Burger/80g	178	10.0	223	21.5	6.2	12.5	0.5
Beef, & Onion, Grilled, Asda*	1 Burger/81g	201	11.5	248	23.1	6.9	14.2	0.5
Beef, 100%, Average	1 Burger/52g	148	11.6	286	20.5	0.6	22.3	0.1
Beef, 100%, Birds Eye*	1 Burger/41g	120	10.2	292	17.3	0.0	24.8	0.0
Beef, 100%, Half Pounders, Sainsbury's*	1 Burger/148g	462	33.1	313	26.0	1.7	22.4	0.2
Beef, 100%, Mega, Birds Eye*	1 Burger/96g	280	23.8	293	17.3	0.0	24.9	0.0
Beef, 100%, Organic, Waitrose*	1 Burger/57g	140	9.6	247	23.6	0.0	16.9	0.0
Beef, 100%, Quarter Pounders, Aldi*	1 Burger/114g	320	23.3	282	24.3	0.1	20.5	1.3
Beef, 100%, Quarter Pounders, Ross*	1 Burger/74g	222	18.8	301	16.8	1.1	25.5	0.0
Beef, 100%, Sainsbury's*	1 Burger/44g	133	10.4	302	21.4	0.9	23.6	0.9
Beef, 100%, Somerfield*	1 Burger/114g	328	27.2	289	17.0	1.0	24.0	0.0
Beef, 100%, without Onion, Sainsbury's*	1 Burger/43g	133	10.4	308	21.9	0.8	24.1	0.8
Beef, 100% Pure, Ross*	1 Burger/56g	128	9.6	229	17.1	1.4	17.1	0.0
Beef, 100% with Seasoning, No Onion, Birds Eye*	1 Burger/41g	134	11.9	326	16.1	0.2	29.0	0.0
Beef, Aberdeen Angus, ¼ Pounders, TTD, Sainsbury's*	1 Serving/91g	258	15.6	284	29.9	2.4	17.2	0.5
Beef, Aberdeen Angus, Asda*	1 Burger/112g	249	13.3	222	22.2	6.7	11.8	0.9
Beef, Aberdeen Angus, Fresh, Waitrose*	1 Burger/113g	269	21.0	238	16.4	1.2	18.6	0.0
Beef, Aberdeen Angus, Frozen, Waitrose*	1 Serving/57g	145	11.6	255	18.1	0.0	20.3	1.1
Beef, Aberdeen Angus, Gourmet, Finest, Tesco*	1 Burger/118g	225	13.4	190	18.9	2.0	11.3	1.0
Beef, Aberdeen Angus, M&S*	1 Burger/142g	298	18.9	210	18.3	4.1	13.3	0.1
Beef, Aberdeen Angus, Mega, Birds Eye*	1 Burger/101g	279	22.6	276	16.3	2.4	22.4	0.1
Beef, Asda*	1 Burger/114g	304	18.6	267	26.8	3.2	16.3	0.7
Beef, Barbecue, Tesco*	1 Burger/114g	295	22.7	260	15.6	3.5	20.0	0.5
Beef, BGTY, Sainsbury's*	1 Burger/110g	177	6.0	161	20.8	7.1	5.5	1.1
Beef, British, Finest, Tesco*	1 Burger/95g	185	11.8	195	17.2	3.3	12.4	0.9
Beef, British, Organic, Waitrose*	1 Burger/85g	226	16.6	266	19.0	3.5	19.5	1.0
Beef, British, Waitrose*	1 Burger/113g	279	21.0	247	18.6	1.2	18.6	0.0
Beef, Chargrill, Tesco*	1 Burger/114g	246	18.4	217	17.0	0.8	16.2	2.5
Beef, Cheese & Caramelised Onion Topped, Waitrose*	1 Burger/165g	378	26.6	229	14.2	6.9	16.1	0.5
Beef, Farmfoods*	1 Burger/50g	128	9.8	255	14.4	5.4	19.6	0.1
Beef, Flame Grilled, Dalepak*	1 Burger/44g	134	11.4	304	15.3	2.1	26.0	0.4
Beef, Morrisons*	1 Burger/57g	169	14.3	298	12.3	5.5	25.2	0.6
Beef, New York Style, Grilled, Tesco*	1 Burger/35g	80	5.2	229	18.6	5.7	14.9	0.6
Beef, Organic, M&S*	1 Burger/110g	239	17.6	217	18.2	0.0	16.0	0.2
Beef, Original, & Best, Birds Eye*	1 Burger/46g	115	8.9	252	14.1	5.1	19.5	0.4
Beef, Original, with Onion, Grilled, Birds Eye*	1 Burger/38g	110	9.5	287	13.4	2.6	24.8	0.3
Beef, Quarter Pounders, Chilled, Morrisons*	1 Burger/115g	228	13.9	198	17.2	4.4	12.1	0.2
Beef, Quarter Pounders, Farmfoods*	1 Burger/113g	289	22.1	256	14.4	5.4	19.6	0.1
Beef, Quarter Pounders, Flame Grilled, Rustlers*	1 Burger/190g	557	28.7	293	14.9	24.3	15.1	0.0
Beef, Quarter Pounders, Flame Grilled, Tesco*	1 Burger/88g	246	20.4	280	13.1	4.8	23.2	0.8
Beef, Quarter Pounders, Grilled, The Best, Morrisons*	1 Burger/97g	223	13.9	230	21.0	4.0	14.3	0.5
Beef, Quarter Pounders, Morrisons*	1 Burger/114g	338	28.6	298	12.3	5.5	25.2	0.6
Beef, Quarter Pounders, Reduced Fat, Tesco*	1 Burger/95g	171	12.4	180	14.0	1.8	13.0	0.8
Beef, Quarter Pounders, Scotch, Sainsbury's*	1 Burger/114g	255	15.4	225	22.2	3.5	13.6	0.5
Beef, Quarter Pounders, Somerfield*	1 Burger/114g	295	20.6	259	20.9	3.0	18.1	0.0
Beef, Quarter Pounders, Steak Country*	1 Burger/68g	188	15.1	276	16.3	2.4	22.2	0.1
Beef, Quarter Pounders, Tesco*	1 Burger/113g	292	23.1	258	17.8	0.7	20.4	1.3
Beef, Quarter Pounders, with Onion, BGTY, Sainsbury's*	1 Burger/83g	171	7.8	205	26.6	3.8	9.3	0.9
Beef, Quarter Pounders, with Onion, Birds Eye*	1 Burger/114g	286	22.1	252	14.1	5.1	19.5	0.4
Beef, Quarter Pounders, with Onion, Cooked, Birds Eye*	1 Burger/100g	230	16.0	230	16.0	5.9	16.0	0.4
Beef, Quarter Pounders, with Onion, Sainsbury's*	1 Burger/113g	306	22.4	271	18.0	5.1	19.8	1.5
Beef, Sainsbury's*	1 Burger/57g	152	9.1	267	29.6	1.3	15.9	1.5

BURGERS

	Measure INFO/WEIGHT	per Measure KCAL	FAT	Nutrition Values per 100g / 100ml KCAL	PROT	CARB	FAT	FIBRE
Beef, Scotch, Quarter Pounders, Moordale*	1 Burger/114g	277	21.2	243	0.0	0.8	18.6	0.0
Beef, Scotch, Ultimate, TTD, Sainsbury's*	1 Burger/142g	284	12.2	200	26.0	4.7	8.6	1.0
Beef, Steak, British, Cooked, TTD, Sainsbury's*	1 Burger/93g	191	11.9	205	21.0	1.5	12.8	0.5
Beef, Steak, Rump, The Grill, M&S*	1 Burger/169g	330	20.6	195	18.7	2.6	12.2	1.1
Beef, Steak, Ultimate, TTD, Sainsbury's*	1 Burger/136g	355	24.1	261	25.3	0.1	17.7	0.5
Beef, with Cheese Melt, COOK!, M&S*	1 Burger/182g	400	28.9	220	17.9	1.3	15.9	1.2
Beef, with Fresh Garden Herbs, Raw, TTD, Sainsbury's*	1 Burger/142g	280	14.8	197	21.5	4.4	10.4	1.3
Beef, with Herbs, Finest, Tesco*	1 Burger/105g	200	11.8	190	17.3	4.5	11.2	0.7
Beef, with Jalapeno Chilli, Finest, Tesco*	1 Burger/205g	379	22.3	185	17.0	3.4	10.9	0.4
Beef, with Mediterranean Tomato & Basil, M&S*	1 Burger/169g	304	18.6	180	15.7	5.1	11.0	1.4
Beef, with Onion, Cooked, Ross*	1 Burger/41g	117	9.8	284	14.7	2.8	23.8	0.4
Beef, with Onion, Sainsbury's*	1 Burger/42g	102	6.2	243	20.7	6.9	14.8	1.0
Beef, with Red Onion & Mustard, Finest, Tesco*	1 Burger/130g	308	24.2	237	17.2	0.2	18.6	2.6
Beef, with Shallots, Finest, Tesco*	1 Burger/84g	175	9.5	208	20.2	6.4	11.3	0.5
Beef, with West Country Cheddar, TTD, Sainsbury's*	1 Burger/112g	252	13.7	225	26.4	2.3	12.2	0.0
Cheeseburger	1 Serving/275g	706	29.0	257	13.7	25.6	10.6	1.8
Cheeseburger, American, Tesco*	1 Burger/275g	660	26.3	240	13.6	24.9	9.6	1.6
Cheeseburger, Bacon, with Bun, Chargrilled, Tesco*	1 Burger/265g	726	42.1	274	13.0	19.6	15.9	1.0
Cheeseburger, with Sesame Seed Bun, Tesco*	1 Burger/275g	644	32.2	234	12.2	20.1	11.7	2.0
Chicken, Average	1 Burger/46g	111	5.6	242	14.9	18.7	12.1	1.0
Chicken, Breaded, Value, Tesco*	1 Burger/57g	165	10.8	290	10.5	19.2	19.0	1.4
Chicken, Cooked, Birds Eye*	1 Burger/90g	126	4.1	140	20.0	5.1	4.6	0.2
Chicken, Crunch Crumb, Tesco*	1 Burger/57g	161	10.8	282	12.3	15.6	18.9	0.0
Chicken, Fresh, Non Coated, Waitrose*	1 Burger/100g	141	4.0	141	16.0	10.4	4.0	0.9
Chicken, Golden Breadcrumbs, Frozen, Birds Eye*	1 Burger/56g	130	6.9	232	13.8	16.4	12.4	0.3
Chicken, in Bun, Morrisons*	1 Burger/110g	250	4.7	228	12.7	38.1	4.3	3.8
Chicken, Quarter Pounders, Birds Eye*	1 Burger/117g	280	16.1	239	13.5	15.2	13.8	0.6
Chicken, Sainsbury's*	1 Burger/46g	115	7.0	247	15.6	12.2	15.1	1.3
Chicken, Southern Fried, Sainsbury's*	1 Burger/52g	154	10.3	297	12.6	17.2	19.8	1.3
Chicken, Spar*	1 Burger/67g	163	7.5	244	16.1	20.8	11.2	1.5
Chilli, Quarter Pounders, Asda*	1 Burger/88g	221	14.0	252	25.0	2.0	16.0	0.0
Chilli, Quarter Pounders, Farmfoods*	1 Burger/115g	285	23.3	248	13.5	2.9	20.3	0.9
Classic, Eddie Rockets*	1 Burger/295g	620	35.0	210	10.8	14.9	11.9	0.0
Lamb, Minted, Average	1 Burger/56g	125	7.4	223	20.6	5.5	13.2	0.2
Lamb, Quarter Pounders, Average	1 Burger/113g	283	19.3	250	17.4	5.2	17.1	0.8
Lamb, Waitrose*	1 Burger/67g	99	4.7	148	15.7	5.4	7.0	0.9
Meat Free, Sainsbury's*	1 Burger/57g	86	2.8	151	22.0	4.4	5.0	3.4
Mushroom & Spinach, Cooked, Love Veg, Sainsbury's*	1 Burger/76g	192	11.0	254	5.2	22.7	14.6	5.6
Ostrich, Quarter Pounder, Oslinc*	1 Burger/113g	132	1.5	117	22.9	3.5	1.3	1.1
Pork, & Apple, Quarter Pounder, Grilled, Asda*	1 Burger/80g	147	6.4	184	23.9	4.1	8.0	0.5
Pork, Free Range, Waitrose*	1 Burger/115g	306	19.9	266	19.3	7.7	17.3	1.0
Pork, Quarter Pounder, Birds Eye*	1 Burger/122g	292	23.2	239	13.9	3.2	19.0	0.2
Quarter Pounders, Beef, BGTY, Sainsbury's*	1 Burger/114g	188	9.3	166	16.9	6.1	8.2	1.0
Quarter Pounders, Big Country*	1 Burger/90g	271	20.8	301	22.1	1.8	23.1	0.0
Quarter Pounders, Iceland*	1 Burger/83g	253	18.8	305	20.4	5.1	22.6	0.6
Quarter Pounders, with Cheese, Flame Grilled, Feasters*	1 Burger/200g	550	19.8	275	17.2	22.1	9.9	0.9
Quarter Pounders, with Cheese & Buns, Sainsbury's*	1 Burger/198g	471	22.8	238	15.6	19.1	11.5	1.4
Salmon, Quarters Pounder, Morrisons*	1 Burger/110g	235	13.0	214	21.4	5.5	11.8	1.7
Spicy Bean, Ainsley Harriott*	1 Burger/200g	302	7.5	151	7.2	23.5	3.8	5.2
Spicy Bean, in Herby Nacho Crumb, Morrisons*	1 Burger/102g	185	8.1	181	5.2	19.5	7.9	5.5
Spicy Bean, Sainsbury's*	1 Burger/110g	262	13.5	240	5.0	27.1	12.4	2.0
Steak with Cheese Melt, COOK!, M&S*	1 Burger/196g	480	35.7	245	18.4	2.3	18.2	0.2
Turkey, Cheeseburgers, Tesco*	1 Burger/105g	252	14.8	240	15.4	12.8	14.1	1.3

	Measure INFO/WEIGHT	per Measure KCAL	FAT	Nutrition Values per 100g / 100ml KCAL	PROT	CARB	FAT	FIBRE
BURGERS								
Turkey, Crispy Crumb, Bernard Matthews*	1 Burger/60g	158	9.5	263	12.6	17.5	15.8	1.8
Turkey, Grilled, Cranberry Foods Ltd*	1 Serving/100g	173	5.9	173	21.1	8.8	5.9	1.4
Turkey, Harvestland*	1 Burger/112g	179	9.0	160	23.0	1.0	8.0	0.0
Value, Farmfoods*	1 Burger/49g	138	10.8	282	11.4	9.6	22.1	0.9
Venison, Finnebrougue Estate*	1 Burger/142g	170	7.0	120	19.9	4.2	4.9	0.5
Venison, TTD, Sainsbury's*	1 Burger/150g	224	6.3	149	20.4	6.5	4.2	3.2
Venison & Sweet Onion, M&S*	1 Burger/142g	163	5.0	115	19.3	1.4	3.5	0.5
BURGERS VEGETARIAN								
Bean, Tesco*	1 Burger/90g	192	10.9	213	4.4	21.6	12.1	5.0
Black Bean, Organic, Cauldron Foods*	1 Burger/88g	169	10.1	193	9.2	13.1	11.5	8.5
Cheese & Spring Onion, Tesco*	1 Burger/87g	178	10.3	204	4.4	20.0	11.8	3.2
Chilli, Cauldron Foods*	1 Burger/88g	148	8.1	169	11.5	8.5	9.3	3.3
Flame Grilled, Linda McCartney*	1 Burger/60g	104	3.1	174	17.9	13.8	5.2	3.3
Meat Free, Asda*	1 Burger/60g	138	6.0	230	24.0	11.0	10.0	0.3
Meat Free, Average	1 Burger/113g	195	8.8	172	17.5	7.9	7.8	3.0
Meat Free, Sainsbury's*	1 Burger/57g	92	4.2	161	19.6	3.9	7.4	4.8
Meat Free, Spicy, Bean & Nacho, Cooked, Asda*	1 Burger/113g	247	9.6	218	5.3	27.7	8.5	4.7
Mexican Style, Bean, Meat Free, Tesco*	1 Burger/94g	206	8.7	220	4.9	28.2	9.3	3.9
Mozzarella, ¼ Pound, Linda McCartney*	1 Burger/114g	233	15.5	205	16.5	7.7	13.6	3.3
Mushroom, Cauldron Foods*	1 Burger/88g	125	5.5	143	5.5	16.1	6.3	2.6
Mushroom, Meat Free, Tesco*	1 Burger/87g	151	9.5	173	3.6	15.3	10.8	3.7
Mushroom, Organic, Cauldron Foods*	1 Burger/88g	136	7.3	156	7.1	18.2	8.3	2.3
Peri Peri, Frozen, Linda McCartney*	1 Burger/113g	251	9.7	222	20.8	14.7	8.6	4.1
Quarter Pounder, Average	1 Burger/113g	210	9.8	186	9.1	17.7	8.6	3.2
Quarter Pounders, Beef Style, Sainsbury's*	1 Burger/114g	216	10.8	190	20.0	6.0	9.5	2.5
Quarter Pounders, Chargrilled, Tesco*	1 Burger/114g	186	9.1	164	16.0	7.0	8.0	2.5
Quarter Pounders, Linda McCartney*	1 Burger/114g	187	11.3	165	14.4	4.4	10.0	4.2
Spicy Bean, Average	1 Burger/56g	125	6.8	223	5.6	24.3	12.2	4.8
Spicy Bean, BGTY, Sainsbury's*	1 Burger/85g	123	2.3	145	6.9	23.3	2.7	3.1
Spicy Bean, Cauldron Foods*	1 Burger/88g	203	9.8	232	5.4	27.4	11.2	6.2
Spicy Bean, Linda McCartney*	1 Burger/85g	190	9.5	223	4.3	26.2	11.2	2.9
Spicy Bean, Quarter Pounder, Dalepak*	1 Burger/115g	237	12.5	206	4.6	22.3	10.9	2.6
Tesco*	1 Burger/56g	92	4.5	164	16.0	7.0	8.0	2.5
Traditional, Fry's Special Vegetarian*	1 Burger/75g	175	9.0	233	19.2	13.0	12.0	0.2
Vegeburger, Linda McCartney*	1 Burger/50g	62	1.4	124	15.8	10.7	2.9	5.8
Vegetable, Average	1 Burger/56g	100	4.5	179	4.4	22.4	8.0	2.3
Vegetable, Captains, Birds Eye*	1 Burger/48g	96	4.2	200	4.7	25.5	8.8	2.0
Vegetable, Organic, Goodlife*	1 Burger/67g	114	3.9	170	3.2	26.3	5.8	2.6
Vegetable, Organic, Tesco*	1 Burger/90g	108	3.9	120	2.6	17.6	4.3	2.1
Vegetable, Quarter Pounders, Crunchy, Birds Eye*	1 Burger/114g	240	11.6	211	4.8	24.9	10.2	1.8
Vegetable, Quarter Pounders, Dalepak*	1 Burger/114g	227	9.6	200	4.8	26.3	8.5	1.8
Vegetable, Quarter Pounders, Tesco*	1 Burger/108g	227	13.1	211	4.4	20.8	12.2	2.7
Vegetable, Spicy, Asda*	1 Burger/56g	108	6.2	193	3.4	20.0	11.0	0.0
with Tofu, Organic, Evernat*	1oz/28g	52	2.3	186	7.9	16.9	8.3	0.0
BURRITO								
Beef	1 Serving/225g	430	19.0	191	9.6	18.7	8.5	2.2
BUTTER								
Brandy, Average	1 Serving/10g	56	3.8	556	0.2	46.2	38.4	0.1
Brandy, Tesco*	1oz/28g	152	10.8	543	0.3	48.3	38.7	0.5
Coconut, Artisana*	2 Tbsp/32g	186	18.0	574	6.2	21.6	55.5	15.4
Creamery, Average	*1 Serving/10g*	*74*	*8.1*	*736*	*0.5*	*0.4*	*81.4*	*0.0*
Fresh, Average	*1 Thin Spread/7g*	*51*	*5.7*	*735*	*0.6*	*0.4*	*81.3*	*0.0*
Garlic, Somerfield*	1oz/28g	192	21.0	686	1.0	2.0	75.0	0.0

INFO/WEIGHT	Measure	per Measure KCAL	FAT	Nutrition Values per 100g / 100ml KCAL	PROT	CARB	FAT	FIBRE

BUTTER

	Measure INFO/WEIGHT	KCAL	FAT	KCAL	PROT	CARB	FAT	FIBRE
Goats, St Helen's Farm*	1 Serving/10g	79	8.8	794	0.5	0.0	88.0	0.0
Granules, Butter Buds*	1 Tsp/1g	5	0.1	368	1.8	77.9	6.5	2.3
Jersey, TTD, Sainsbury's*	1 Thin Spread/7g	52	5.8	744	0.5	0.6	82.2	0.0
Reduced Fat, Fresh, Average	*1 Thin Spread/7g*	*26*	*2.8*	*368*	*2.3*	*1.2*	*39.4*	*0.2*
Salted, Average	*1 Thin Spread/7g*	*51*	*5.7*	*729*	*0.4*	*0.3*	*81.1*	*0.0*
Spreadable, Butterpak, Lighter, Tesco*	1 Serving/10g	54	5.6	545	0.5	0.5	56.0	0.0
Spreadable, Fresh, Average	*1 Thin Spread/7g*	*51*	*5.7*	*730*	*0.4*	*0.3*	*80.8*	*0.0*
Spreadable, Lighter, Norpak, Aldi*	1 Serving/10g	51	5.6	510	0.6	0.9	56.0	0.0
Spreadable, Lightest, Lurpak*	1oz/28g	106	11.2	377	3.3	0.9	40.0	0.0
Spreadable, Organic, Lighter, Yeo Valley*	1 Serving/12g	66	7.3	550	0.7	0.9	60.7	0.0
Spreadable, Reduced Fat, Average	*1 Thin Spread/7g*	*38*	*4.2*	*540*	*0.5*	*0.5*	*60.0*	*0.0*
Spreadable, Slightly Salted, Lurpak*	1 Serving/10g	72	8.0	724	0.5	0.6	80.0	0.0
with Crushed Garlic, Lurpak*	1 Serving/10g	70	7.5	700	1.0	4.0	75.0	0.0

BUTTERMILK

	Measure INFO/WEIGHT	KCAL	FAT	KCAL	PROT	CARB	FAT	FIBRE
Average	*1 Mug/400ml*	*177*	*1.3*	*44*	*4.2*	*5.9*	*0.3*	*0.0*

BUTTONS

	Measure INFO/WEIGHT	KCAL	FAT	KCAL	PROT	CARB	FAT	FIBRE
Chocolate, Giant, Dairy Milk, Cadbury*	1 Button/3g	15	0.9	525	7.7	56.7	29.9	0.7
Dairy Milk, Cadbury*	1 Pack/32g	170	9.7	525	7.7	56.7	29.9	0.7
Milk Chocolate, Asda*	1 Bag/70g	368	21.0	526	7.0	57.0	30.0	1.5
Milk Chocolate, M&S*	1 Pack/75g	375	19.0	500	8.6	59.8	25.3	1.9
Milk Chocolate, Somerfield*	1 Pack/75g	390	21.0	520	8.0	58.0	28.0	0.0
Milk Chocolate, Tesco*	1 Bag/70g	359	19.3	513	7.1	59.1	27.6	2.1
White Chocolate, Cadbury*	1 Pack/32g	180	11.0	555	4.5	58.4	33.8	0.0
White Chocolate, Co-Op*	½ Pack/35g	186	9.8	530	7.0	64.0	28.0	0.0
White Chocolate, Milkybar, Nestle*	1 Bag/30g	164	9.5	546	7.5	58.1	31.6	0.0
White Chocolate, Tesco*	1 Bag/70g	388	23.4	554	5.1	58.0	33.5	0.0

	Measure INFO/WEIGHT	per Measure KCAL	per Measure FAT	Nutrition Values per 100g / 100ml KCAL	PROT	CARB	FAT	FIBRE
CABBAGE								
& Leek, Crunchy Mix, Ready to Cook, Sainsbury's*	1 Serving/125g	34	0.6	27	1.9	3.7	0.5	2.6
& Leek, Ready Sliced, Sainsbury's*	1 Pack/240g	53	1.2	22	1.1	2.2	0.5	2.1
& Leek, Sliced, Tesco*	1/3 Pack/100g	32	0.6	32	2.1	3.4	0.6	2.6
Boiled, Average	*1 Serving/90g*	*14*	*0.3*	*15*	*1.0*	*2.2*	*0.3*	*1.7*
Creamed, Sainsbury's*	½ Pack/150g	88	6.3	59	1.5	3.9	4.2	2.3
Greens, Trimmed, Average	*1oz/28g*	*8*	*0.1*	*28*	*2.9*	*3.0*	*0.5*	*3.4*
Medley, Red, Spring & Savoy, Pre Packed, Sainsbury's*	½ Pack/80g	26	0.5	32	2.0	3.4	0.6	2.3
Medley, Washed, Ready to Cook, Tesco*	1 Pack/200g	60	1.2	30	2.3	3.7	0.6	2.8
Raw, Average	*1 Serving/100g*	*21*	*0.4*	*21*	*1.3*	*3.2*	*0.4*	*1.8*
Red, Average	*1 Serving/90g*	*19*	*0.2*	*21*	*1.0*	*3.7*	*0.3*	*2.2*
Red, Braised with Red Wine, M&S*	½ Pack/150g	180	7.2	120	1.4	17.1	4.8	1.0
Red, Pickled, Average	*1 Serving/100g*	*26*	*0.2*	*26*	*0.9*	*4.6*	*0.2*	*1.6*
Red, Spiced, Steamer, Sainsbury's*	½ Pack/150g	105	3.3	70	1.0	10.5	2.2	2.9
Red, with Apple, Finest, Tesco*	½ Pack/150g	177	8.8	118	1.6	14.7	5.9	4.6
Red, with Apple, Frozen, Sainsbury's*	1 Serving/75g	38	0.0	50	1.8	10.8	0.0	2.2
Red, with Apples, Onions & Redcurrant Jelly, M&S*	½ Pack/150g	112	3.3	75	0.9	12.4	2.2	2.0
Red, with Bramley Apple, Aunt Bessie's*	1 Serving/125g	72	1.1	58	0.9	10.0	0.9	2.7
Red, with Bramley Apple, Braised, Sainsbury's*	½ Pack/150g	146	7.2	97	0.9	12.6	4.8	1.7
Savoy, Boiled in Salted Water, Average	*1 Serving/90g*	*15*	*0.4*	*17*	*1.1*	*2.2*	*0.5*	*2.0*
Savoy, Raw, Average	*1 Serving/90g*	*24*	*0.4*	*27*	*2.1*	*3.9*	*0.5*	*3.1*
Steamed, Average	1 Serving/100g	15	0.3	15	1.0	2.2	0.3	1.7
Sweetheart, Raw	*1 Serving/100g*	*26*	*0.6*	*26*	*2.1*	*3.2*	*0.6*	*2.8*
White, Raw, Average	*1oz/28g*	*8*	*0.1*	*27*	*1.4*	*5.0*	*0.2*	*2.1*
CAKE								
Action Man, Birthday, Memory Lane Cakes*	1/12 Cake/83g	322	13.6	388	3.0	57.0	16.4	0.8
Aero, Mint, Celebration, Nestle*	1 Slice/58g	232	11.8	400	4.0	49.7	20.3	1.7
Alabama Chocolate Fudge, Farmfoods*	1/6 Cake/61g	201	5.9	329	4.7	55.7	9.7	2.7
Alabama Chocolate Fudge, Morrisons*	1/6 Cake/58g	195	6.4	337	4.5	55.1	11.0	2.3
Almond Flavoured Rounds, Country Garden Cakes*	1 Cake/45g	183	6.7	403	4.3	62.4	14.7	2.3
Almond Slices, Lyons*	1 Slice/27g	114	6.9	426	7.1	41.3	25.8	1.6
Almond Slices, Mr Kipling*	1 Slice/33g	131	4.6	403	6.3	63.4	14.0	2.0
Almond Slices, Sainsbury's*	1 Serving/27g	120	7.1	444	5.9	45.9	26.3	1.5
Almond Slices, Weight Watchers*	1 Slice/26g	95	2.6	365	5.2	63.8	9.9	2.4
Angel, Asda*	1 Serving/46g	184	7.8	399	4.5	57.0	17.0	0.9
Angel, Average	1 Slice/44g	175	7.9	397	4.5	54.9	17.9	0.8
Angel, Co-Op*	1/8 Cake/35g	131	6.0	375	4.0	52.0	17.0	0.7
Angel, Sainsbury's*	1/8 Cake/41g	171	8.1	417	4.1	55.7	19.8	0.8
Angel Layer, Somerfield*	1 Serving/37g	146	7.0	395	4.1	51.9	19.0	0.6
Angel Layer, Tesco*	1 Serving/25g	101	4.3	403	4.5	57.4	17.3	0.9
Angel Slices, Mr Kipling*	1 Slice/34g	140	6.2	417	2.8	59.4	18.5	0.6
Angel Slices, Snap Packs, Mr Kipling*	1 Slice/34g	148	6.6	417	2.7	60.1	18.5	0.6
Apple, & Blackcurrant, Crumble, Graze*	1 Punnet/33g	121	7.5	365	6.1	34.5	22.7	3.1
Apple, & Cinnamon, Oat Break, Go Ahead, McVitie's*	1 Serving/35g	122	2.3	349	5.2	67.2	6.6	2.6
Apple, Bramley, & Blackberry Crumble, M&S*	1/8 Cake/56g	221	10.0	395	4.4	54.1	17.9	1.5
Apple, Home Style, M&S*	1 Cake/54g	189	7.9	350	5.3	49.4	14.7	1.5
Apple, Slice, Delightful, Mr Kipling*	1 Slice/29g	92	1.1	317	4.4	66.2	3.9	1.3
Apple, Spicy, Tray Bake, Kate's Cakes Ltd*	1 Serving/100g	363	20.6	363	4.4	40.0	20.6	2.4
Apple Bakes, Go Ahead, McVitie's*	1 Cake/35g	126	2.7	361	2.6	70.0	7.8	2.0
Apple Crumble, Slices, Weight Watchers*	1 Slice/26g	90	2.0	346	4.5	64.8	7.7	2.3
Bakewell, Lemon, Average	1 Cake/42g	173	6.4	411	3.7	64.6	15.2	1.3
Bakewell, Slice, Kate's Cakes Ltd*	1 Serving/100g	425	23.3	425	7.5	45.9	23.3	2.7
Bakewell, Slice, Weight Watchers*	1 Slice/26g	84	0.6	324	3.7	71.0	2.4	2.0
Bakewell, Slices, Mr Kipling*	1 Slice/36g	163	7.3	454	4.2	63.4	20.4	1.2

CAKE

INFO/WEIGHT	Measure KCAL	FAT	KCAL	PROT	CARB	FAT	FIBRE
Bakewell, Toffee, Tesco*	1 Cake/49g	203	7.9	414	3.9	63.5	16.1	1.4
Bakewell, Tray Bake, Kate's Cakes Ltd*	1 Serving/100g	475	28.3	475	6.6	46.3	28.3	2.8
Bakewells, Trifle, Mr Kipling*	1 Tart/45g	193	8.0	423	3.7	62.2	17.5	1.1
Banana, Iced, Waitrose*	1/6 Cake/55g	190	5.9	345	4.2	58.0	10.7	2.7
Banana, Organic, Loaf, Respect Organics*	¼ Pack/65g	254	13.6	391	3.9	48.6	21.0	1.5
Banana Bread, Brilliant, Graze*	1 Cake/23g	72	3.6	312	5.2	40.4	15.6	3.0
Banana Loaf, Waitrose*	1 Slice/70g	236	7.5	337	5.0	55.2	10.7	1.7
Banoffee, Slice, Kate's Cakes Ltd*	1 Serving/100g	445	23.6	445	7.9	48.0	23.6	2.5
Banoffee, Slices, Dessert Classics, Mr Kipling*	1 Slice/34g	140	6.2	414	2.9	59.0	18.4	0.6
Battenberg, Asda*	1 Slice/25g	104	3.0	418	6.0	71.1	12.2	0.8
Battenberg, Mini, Mr Kipling*	1 Cake/35g	144	3.8	410	4.6	76.2	11.0	1.3
Battenberg, Mr Kipling*	1 Serving/38g	161	4.6	421	5.0	73.3	12.0	1.6
Battenburg, Mini, Mr Kipling*	1 Cake/32g	147	3.9	450	4.9	81.2	11.8	1.5
Battenburg, Mr Kipling*	1 Slice/38g	164	4.8	428	6.1	73.0	12.5	1.4
Birthday, Chocolate, Tesco*	1 Serving/54g	229	13.2	425	5.9	45.5	24.4	2.1
Birthday, M&S*	1 Serving/60g	240	7.1	400	2.3	70.9	11.9	0.8
Birthday, Piece of Cake, M&S*	1 Serving/85g	395	24.4	465	4.3	39.7	28.7	0.9
Birthday, Shrek, Tesco*	1/16 Cake/72g	248	8.8	344	3.3	64.0	12.2	0.5
Birthday, Spooky, Memory Lane Cakes*	1 Slice/75g	295	14.6	393	3.5	50.8	19.5	0.7
Birthday, Winnie the Pooh, Disney, Nestle*	1 Serving/100g	361	10.9	361	2.4	63.3	10.9	0.5
Birthday Present, Tesco*	1 Serving/79g	347	13.9	439	3.5	66.6	17.6	0.4
Bites, Caramel, Mr Kipling*	1 Cake/14g	68	3.8	492	5.9	55.3	27.4	0.8
Bites, Chocolate Roll, Mini, Tesco*	1 Bite/18g	78	3.6	435	6.0	58.0	19.8	1.9
Bites, Coconut, Sainsbury's*	1 Bite/80g	339	16.9	424	5.3	53.0	21.2	4.2
Butterfly, Mr Kipling*	1 Cake/29g	114	6.4	392	4.4	43.4	22.2	0.6
Buttons, Happy Birthday, Cadbury*	1 Slice/50g	235	13.6	470	4.1	52.8	27.1	0.0
Caramel Shortbread, Devondale*	1 Cake/75g	356	18.6	474	3.0	57.0	24.8	0.8
Caramel Shortbread, Tray Bake, Kate's Cakes Ltd*	1 Serving/100g	471	27.3	471	3.0	53.3	27.3	1.2
Caramel Shortcake, Slices, McVitie's*	1 Slice/32g	146	7.7	463	4.3	56.5	24.4	1.6
Caramel Slice, M&S*	1 Slice/64g	304	16.1	475	4.9	60.4	25.2	2.6
Carrot, Average	1 Slice/56g	211	10.4	377	4.6	47.6	18.6	1.4
Carrot, Handmade, Delicious, Boots*	1 Slice/75g	292	13.5	389	4.1	53.0	18.0	1.4
Carrot, Iced, Tesco*	1 Serving/61g	246	12.0	404	3.1	53.7	19.6	1.6
Carrot, Mini, Weight Watchers*	1 Cake/31g	120	3.3	388	3.7	68.9	10.8	2.7
Carrot, Organic, Respect Organics*	1 Slice/45g	179	10.1	398	3.1	47.4	22.4	1.5
Carrot, Slices, Asda*	1 Slice/80g	302	13.2	377	3.4	53.8	16.5	1.7
Carrot, Slices, Eat Smart, Morrisons*	1 Cake/27g	84	0.6	312	3.0	70.0	2.2	2.3
Carrot, Slices, Inspirations, Mr Kipling*	1 Slice/34g	139	6.3	411	3.5	57.7	18.5	1.3
Carrot, Super, Graze*	1 Punnet/31g	102	4.9	330	4.1	46.5	15.7	3.5
Carrot, The Handmade Flapjack Company*	1 Cake/75g	295	13.0	393	6.4	53.0	17.3	0.0
Carrot, The Ultimate Passion, Entenmann's*	1 Slice/52g	210	12.6	403	4.6	42.4	24.3	1.0
Carrot & Orange, Extra Special, Asda*	1/6 Cake/65g	240	11.7	369	4.7	47.0	18.0	0.9
Carrot & Orange, Finest, Tesco*	1/8 Cake/50g	205	10.2	410	4.6	51.2	20.5	2.1
Carrot & Orange, Slices, LC, Tesco*	1 Slice/30g	93	0.7	310	3.2	68.5	2.2	1.9
Carrot & Orange, Waitrose*	1/6 Cake/47g	164	7.4	350	5.3	46.8	15.7	1.8
Carrot & Pecan, M&S*	1 Slice/90g	330	14.6	365	6.4	48.7	16.2	2.3
Carrot & Walnut, Layered, Asda*	1 Serving/42g	172	8.0	409	4.6	55.0	19.0	1.0
Carrot & Walnut, Mini Classics, Mr Kipling*	1 Cake/39g	172	9.8	440	4.5	48.6	25.2	1.0
Carrot Slices, GFY, Asda*	1 Slice/28g	83	0.6	298	2.8	66.4	2.3	2.1
Carrot Slices, Less Than 3% Fat, BGTY, Sainsbury's*	1 Slice/30g	94	0.8	313	3.4	68.7	2.7	2.4
Carrot Slices, Weight Watchers*	1 Slice/27g	84	0.2	311	2.8	73.0	0.8	0.9
Carrot Wedge, Tesco*	1 Pack/175g	532	27.6	304	3.9	36.6	15.8	1.5
Celebration, Sainsbury's*	1/12 Cake/100g	265	9.2	265	2.1	43.6	9.2	0.3

CAKE

	Measure INFO/WEIGHT	per Measure KCAL	FAT	Nutrition Values per 100g / 100ml KCAL	PROT	CARB	FAT	FIBRE
Cherry, Asda*	1 Slice/37g	131	4.5	351	4.7	56.0	12.0	0.6
Cherry, Co-Op*	1/8 Cake/47g	190	8.5	405	4.0	57.0	18.0	0.8
Cherry, M&S*	1 Serving/75g	285	9.5	380	5.0	60.6	12.7	0.8
Cherry Bakewell, Co-Op*	1 Cake/47g	205	8.0	435	3.7	67.2	16.9	1.8
Cherry Bakewell, Layer, Asda*	1/8 Cake/50g	210	11.0	420	4.4	51.0	22.0	0.6
Cherry Bakewell, Mini, Sainsbury's*	1 Cake/27g	101	3.3	370	3.4	62.2	12.0	0.4
Cherry Bakewell, Sainsbury's*	1 Cake/46g	200	8.1	436	3.1	66.3	17.6	1.4
Cherry Bakewell, Slices, GFY, Asda*	1 Slice/29g	98	0.7	337	3.4	75.4	2.4	0.7
Cherry Bakewell, Tesco*	1 Cake/39g	171	7.5	439	3.2	63.3	19.2	1.1
Cherry Bakewells, Delightful, Mr Kipling*	1 Cake/45g	176	5.8	390	3.9	66.4	12.9	1.2
Cherry Bakewells, Mr Kipling*	1 Cake/45g	193	8.3	428	3.9	61.3	18.5	1.4
Cherry Shortbread, Devondale*	1 Cake/75g	340	18.0	453	3.9	52.0	24.0	1.3
Choc Cherry Crunchy, Devondale*	1 Cake/80g	346	16.8	432	3.6	58.8	21.0	2.4
Choc Chip Shortbread, Devondale*	1 Cake/75g	356	19.5	474	4.3	50.0	26.0	1.9
Chocolate	1oz/28g	128	7.4	456	7.4	50.4	26.4	0.0
Chocolate, & Beetroot, Sweetest, Battle Bakehouse*	1/6 Cake/49g	185	8.7	379	5.2	48.6	17.9	4.0
Chocolate, & Brandy Butter, Entenmann's*	1 Serving/39g	144	6.7	374	3.4	53.5	17.5	2.8
Chocolate, & Caramel Tiffin Bites, Gu*	1 Tiffin/35g	168	9.9	480	3.8	51.9	28.3	2.8
Chocolate, & Madeira, Marble Loaf, M&S*	1/6 Cake/88g	380	20.4	430	5.0	50.0	23.1	1.0
Chocolate, & Orange Rolls, M&S*	1 Cake/60g	228	17.0	380	3.6	27.0	28.4	1.3
Chocolate, Belgian, Choux Bun, Sainsbury's*	1 Bun/90g	347	35.3	386	6.2	22.0	39.2	1.4
Chocolate, Belgian, Slices, Weight Watchers*	1 Slice/25g	86	2.4	344	6.5	57.6	9.8	2.9
Chocolate, Belgian, Waitrose*	1 Slice/47g	223	12.6	474	4.8	53.1	26.9	1.9
Chocolate, Caterpillar, Tesco*	1 Serving/53g	248	13.2	468	5.7	55.3	24.9	1.1
Chocolate, Cup, Mini, Weight Watchers*	1 Cake/17g	72	3.6	422	6.1	52.0	21.1	1.8
Chocolate, Double, Ganache, M&S*	1/12 Cake/61g	281	16.8	460	5.9	46.1	27.6	2.5
Chocolate, Double, Wedge, Tesco*	1 Piece/100g	416	20.3	416	5.0	53.4	20.3	0.9
Chocolate, Fudge, The Cake Shop*	1 Cake/37g	178	10.8	480	3.7	50.5	29.2	1.3
Chocolate, Happy Birthday, Tesco*	1 Serving/58g	241	13.2	415	4.7	46.9	22.7	2.9
Chocolate, Iced, Tesco*	1 Serving/40g	158	6.3	395	4.7	58.5	15.8	1.8
Chocolate, Individual with Mini Eggs, Cadbury*	1 Cake/26g	119	6.1	455	4.6	57.5	23.1	1.3
Chocolate, Large, Happy Birthday, Tesco*	1/18 Cake/63g	249	12.2	396	6.2	49.3	19.3	1.8
Chocolate, Loaf, Moist, McVitie's*	1 Slice/30g	119	6.1	398	4.8	49.0	20.3	1.9
Chocolate, Mini Rolls, Weight Watchers*	1 Roll/22g	86	2.8	397	5.0	61.2	12.7	8.0
Chocolate, Morrisons*	1 Serving/32g	159	10.2	505	5.3	48.0	32.4	1.2
Chocolate, Part of Tea Time Selection, Iceland*	1 Cake/31g	144	7.9	464	4.5	54.1	25.5	2.0
Chocolate, Party, Tesco*	1 Slice/62g	244	13.1	394	4.6	46.3	21.2	0.9
Chocolate, Sainsbury's*	1 Serving/30g	118	5.6	395	4.1	52.6	18.5	1.3
Chocolate, Sara Lee*	1/4 Cake/88g	339	14.8	385	4.1	54.3	16.8	0.0
Chocolate, Smarties, Celebration, Large, Nestle*	1/16 Cake/71g	308	17.4	432	5.4	48.9	24.4	1.2
Chocolate, The Handmade Flapjack Company*	1 Cake/75g	303	16.2	404	12.5	39.8	21.6	0.0
Chocolate, Thorntons*	1 Serving/87g	408	25.1	469	5.2	47.1	28.8	0.6
Chocolate, Triple, Roll, Cadbury*	1 Serving/40g	165	6.7	410	4.3	60.1	16.6	1.5
Chocolate, Triple Layer, Celebration, Tesco*	1 Slice/100g	385	18.4	385	5.4	49.0	18.4	6.4
Chocolate, with Butter Icing, Average	1oz/28g	135	8.3	481	5.7	50.9	29.7	0.0
Chocolate, with White Chocolate, The Cake Shop*	1 Cake/29g	146	9.3	503	4.6	49.2	32.0	1.2
Chocolate Box, Asda*	1 Serving/60g	263	13.8	439	5.0	53.0	23.0	0.7
Chocolate Button, Cakes for the Connoisseur*	1 Cake/30g	145	9.8	485	5.2	42.1	32.8	2.3
Chocolate Chip, Co-Op*	1/6 Cake/63g	275	16.9	440	5.0	44.0	27.0	0.5
Chocolate Chip, The Cake Shop*	1 Cake/35g	178	11.0	508	4.7	50.2	31.5	1.1
Chocolate Crunch, Tray Bake, Kate's Cakes Ltd*	1 Serving/80g	400	23.0	500	4.8	53.4	28.8	3.7
Chocolate Flavour Slices, GFY, Asda*	1 Slice/28g	71	0.7	257	4.3	54.0	2.6	1.4
Chocolate Fudge	1 Serving/110g	415	19.1	377	4.4	50.4	17.4	1.4

CAKE

INFO/WEIGHT	Measure	per Measure		Nutrition Values per 100g / 100ml				
		KCAL	FAT	KCAL	PROT	CARB	FAT	FIBRE
Chocolate Fudge, & Vanilla Cream, M&S*	1/6 Cake/69g	310	17.9	450	5.2	49.8	26.0	1.3
Chocolate Fudge, Belgian, TTD, Sainsbury's*	1 Slice/66g	278	14.3	423	4.4	52.5	21.7	2.5
Chocolate Fudge, Classics, M&S*	1 Serving/71g	195	7.5	275	2.8	42.8	10.6	1.1
Chocolate Fudge, Entenmann's*	1 Serving/48g	173	7.2	361	4.4	51.8	15.1	0.9
Chocolate Fudge, Sainsbury's*	1/8 Cake/98g	402	21.9	410	5.5	47.3	22.3	1.9
Chocolate Fudge, Slice, Waitrose*	1 Slice/60g	230	9.7	383	4.7	54.6	16.2	1.5
Chocolate Fudge, Tea Time Treats, Asda*	1 Cake/37g	157	8.1	424	3.6	53.0	22.0	1.7
Chocolate Fudge, Tray Bake, Kate's Cakes Ltd*	1 Serving/100g	360	16.9	360	4.8	46.8	16.9	1.1
Chocolate Heaven, Extra Special, Asda*	1/6 Cake/66g	255	13.1	388	4.0	48.0	20.0	1.0
Chocolate Indulgence, Finest, Tesco*	1 Slice/51g	207	9.1	405	4.8	55.9	17.9	1.2
Chocolate Log, Fresh Cream, Finest, Tesco*	1 Slice/85g	301	15.4	354	4.5	43.2	18.1	1.4
Chocolate Orange, Slices, Weight Watchers*	1 Slice/82g	249	2.2	304	4.9	64.9	2.7	2.6
Chocolate Orange, Sponge, Asda*	1 Serving/70g	298	18.2	425	4.9	42.9	26.0	3.0
Chocolate Party, M&S*	1 Serving/61g	240	12.6	395	4.6	46.9	20.8	1.1
Chocolate Rice Crispy, Knightsbridge*	1 Cake/24g	88	4.2	368	3.9	48.7	17.5	0.1
Chocolate Roll, Sainsbury's*	1 Slice/50g	210	10.2	420	5.0	54.0	20.4	3.3
Chocolate Sensation, Sainsbury's*	1 Serving/92g	320	17.7	348	3.7	40.0	19.2	2.3
Chocolate Slices, Mr Kipling*	1 Slice/33g	132	6.7	406	5.6	50.4	20.6	2.7
Chocolate Sponge, Budgens*	1/6 Cake/76g	297	13.6	392	3.8	55.9	18.0	2.1
Chocolate Sponge, Less Than 5% Fat, Asda*	1 Sponge/110g	198	4.2	180	4.4	32.0	3.8	1.1
Chocolate Sponge, Morrisons*	1 Serving/59g	179	7.6	303	4.4	42.5	12.8	0.7
Chocolate Sponge, Tesco*	1 Serving/35g	129	5.1	373	5.3	54.4	14.9	1.5
Chocolate Truffle, Extra Special, Asda*	1 Serving/103g	402	26.8	390	5.0	34.0	26.0	1.8
Chocolate Truffle, Mini, Finest, Tesco*	1 Cake/28g	125	6.6	448	5.9	52.9	23.7	0.3
Chocolate Victoria Sponge, Co-Op*	1 Slice/61g	201	9.8	330	5.0	42.0	16.0	1.0
Chorley, Asda*	1 Cake/60g	269	12.6	449	6.0	59.0	21.0	2.2
Christmas, Connoisseur, M&S*	1 Slice/60g	216	5.5	360	4.1	64.7	9.2	3.3
Christmas, GF, Costa*	1 Portion/98g	403	12.0	411	3.9	70.3	12.2	1.2
Christmas, Iced, Slices, Tesco*	1 Slice/45g	168	4.4	369	2.9	67.6	9.6	1.2
Christmas, Iced Rich Fruit, Finest, Tesco*	1 Serving/100g	345	7.7	345	3.1	65.3	7.7	3.7
Christmas, Rich Fruit, All Iced, Sainsbury's*	1/16 Cake/85g	307	7.6	361	4.0	66.4	8.9	1.5
Christmas, Rich Fruit, Free From, Tesco*	1 Serving/100g	340	3.6	340	2.6	73.6	3.6	2.7
Christmas, Rich Fruit, Organic, Tesco*	1 Serving/76g	282	7.6	374	3.9	67.1	10.0	2.0
Christmas, Rich Fruit, Tesco*	1 Serving/75g	256	5.6	342	3.9	64.3	7.4	3.1
Christmas, Royal Iced, Waitrose*	1/6 Cake/75g	270	4.6	360	3.7	71.3	6.2	2.0
Christmas, Slice, Devondale*	1 Cake/70g	245	6.9	350	3.6	65.9	9.8	1.3
Christmas Pudding, Slices, Mr Kipling*	1 Slice/51g	173	3.6	339	3.6	62.1	7.1	1.3
Christmas Slices, Mr Kipling*	1 Slice/43g	157	3.8	363	2.9	67.5	8.8	0.9
Christmas Slices, Weight Watchers*	1 Slice/40g	136	2.6	339	4.4	66.0	6.4	3.0
Classic Lemon Drizzle, M&S*	1/6 Cake/68g	253	10.3	375	4.7	55.0	15.3	0.6
Coconut	1 Slice/70g	304	16.7	434	6.7	51.2	23.8	2.5
Coconut & Raspberry, M&S*	1 Serving/52g	231	13.9	445	5.0	45.5	26.8	2.3
Coconut Snowball, Bobby's*	1 Cake/18g	80	4.0	436	2.2	57.3	22.1	0.0
Coconut Snowballs, Tunnock's*	1 Cake/30g	134	6.2	446	4.2	56.7	20.8	3.6
Coconut Sponge, Memory Lane*	1/6 Cake/42g	172	7.5	406	4.1	57.1	17.6	1.5
Coconut Sponge, Mini Classics, Mr Kipling*	1 Cake/38g	155	8.7	409	3.7	47.0	22.9	0.9
Coffee, Iced, M&S*	1 Slice/33g	135	6.5	410	4.4	54.5	19.6	1.6
Coffee, TTD, Sainsbury's*	1 Slice/68g	294	16.4	430	4.3	49.1	24.0	2.6
Coffee & Walnut, Mrs Beeton's*	1 Slice/54g	219	13.5	405	3.7	41.4	25.0	0.3
Coffee Sponge Roll, M&S*	1/6 Roll/42g	160	7.4	385	3.1	53.1	17.8	1.4
Colin the Caterpillar, M&S*	1 Slice/60g	234	12.8	390	5.3	57.2	21.3	1.3
Cornflake, Average	1 Cake/18g	83	3.7	464	5.2	64.6	20.4	2.0
Cornflake, Chocolate Clusters, Asda*	1 Cake/14g	64	2.6	460	8.2	65.2	18.5	2.7

CAKE

	Measure INFO/WEIGHT	per Measure KCAL	FAT	Nutrition Values per 100g / 100ml KCAL	PROT	CARB	FAT	FIBRE
Country Farmhouse, Waitrose*	1 Serving/80g	308	12.1	385	4.7	57.5	15.1	1.4
Country Slices, Good Intentions, Somerfield*	1 Cake/22g	70	0.4	318	5.5	70.0	1.8	1.8
Country Slices, Mr Kipling*	1 Slice/32g	121	4.8	380	4.4	56.7	15.0	1.2
Cream Oysters, M&S*	1 Cake/72g	227	15.3	315	3.6	27.5	21.2	3.0
Cream Slices, M&S*	1 Slice/80g	310	18.3	387	2.3	45.7	22.9	0.6
Crispy Chocolate Clusters, Mini, Tesco*	1 Cluster/8g	37	1.5	470	7.0	67.8	18.7	2.5
Date, Linda Kearns*	1 Serving/100g	269	16.8	269	12.7	24.4	16.8	4.4
Date & Walnut, Sainsbury's*	1/10 Slice/40g	148	8.2	371	6.7	40.1	20.4	1.0
Eccles, All Butter, M&S*	1 Cake/86g	345	14.8	400	4.5	57.4	17.2	3.2
Eccles, Fresh Baked	1 Cake/45g	171	7.6	381	4.3	56.3	17.0	1.5
Fairy, Average	1 Cake/23g	96	4.6	416	5.1	53.0	20.2	1.5
Fairy, Holly Lane*	1 Cake/26g	118	6.7	460	3.7	52.5	26.1	3.5
Fairy, Iced, Average	1 Cake/23g	91	3.4	394	4.2	60.8	14.8	0.9
Fairy, Lemon Iced, Average	1 Cake/23g	90	3.1	393	4.4	63.2	13.6	1.1
Fairy, Mini, Kids, Tesco*	1 Cake/12g	54	2.8	435	5.3	53.3	22.3	1.1
Fairy, Mini, Tesco*	1 Cake/13g	53	2.5	424	6.1	54.6	20.1	1.3
Fairy, Plain, Average	1 Cake/23g	95	4.6	413	5.5	51.1	20.2	1.5
Fairy, Plain, Sainsbury's*	1 Cake/20g	84	4.3	422	4.9	46.4	21.5	1.2
Fairy, Plain, Value, Tesco*	1 Cake/15g	52	1.3	348	5.3	62.4	8.6	0.9
Fairy, Strawberry Iced, Tesco*	1 Cake/24g	94	3.2	392	4.9	62.9	13.4	1.4
Fairy, Vanilla Iced, Average, Tesco*	1 Cake/23g	89	2.8	388	4.4	65.1	12.2	1.2
Flake, Cadbury*	1 Cake/20g	90	4.5	445	6.3	54.5	22.3	0.0
Fondant, Dark Chocolate, Graze*	1 Pack/40g	157	5.8	393	3.5	66.2	14.5	0.0
Fondant Fancies, Lemon, Waitrose*	1 Cake/40g	176	7.1	441	2.5	67.9	17.7	0.6
Fondant Fancies, Sainsbury's*	1 Cake/27g	95	2.4	353	2.4	65.7	9.0	0.4
Fondants with Chocolate, Mini, Delhaize*	1 Cake/20g	88	6.2	440	4.6	36.3	30.8	3.8
French Fancies, Average	1 Cake/27g	100	2.5	371	2.7	69.6	9.1	0.8
French Fancies, Lemon, Mr Kipling*	1 Cake/28g	106	2.7	378	2.5	69.9	9.8	0.5
French Fancies, Mr Kipling*	1 Cake/28g	106	2.8	378	2.6	69.7	9.9	0.6
French Fancies, Strawberry, Mr Kipling*	1 Cake/28g	106	2.7	379	2.5	70.6	9.6	0.4
Fruit, Iced, Smart Price, Asda*	1 Serving/100g	371	8.2	371	4.0	70.2	8.2	3.0
Fruit, Luxury, Fully Iced Slice, The Best, Morrisons*	1 Serving/50g	178	3.8	356	3.7	66.6	7.6	3.1
Fruit, Plain, Average	1 Slice/90g	319	11.6	354	5.1	57.9	12.9	0.0
Fruit, Rich, Average	1 Slice/70g	225	8.8	322	4.9	50.7	12.5	1.7
Fruit, Rich, Iced	1 Slice/70g	249	8.0	356	4.1	62.7	11.4	1.7
Fruit, Rich, M&S*	1 Serving/50g	158	3.2	315	3.1	60.9	6.5	4.3
Fruit, Rich, Sainsbury's*	1 Serving/100g	321	8.5	321	3.9	57.3	8.5	2.1
Fruit, Rich, Slices, Free From, Sainsbury's*	1 Slice/40g	144	5.0	361	4.5	57.4	12.6	3.7
Fruit, Rich, Truly Irresistible, Co-Op*	1/6 Cake/70g	235	6.0	335	3.9	59.9	8.6	2.0
Fruit, Slices, Gluten & Wheat Free, Lovemore*	1 Slice/40g	122	3.8	304	2.3	51.1	9.4	1.5
Fruit, Slices, Rich, Iced, Finest, Tesco*	1 Slice/41g	152	3.4	370	3.2	69.4	8.3	2.1
Fruit, Slices, Value, Tesco*	1 Slice/23g	84	4.0	372	4.0	48.7	17.7	1.3
Fruit, with Marzipan & Icing, Asda*	1/12 Slice/76g	280	6.8	369	3.9	68.0	9.0	0.0
Fruit & Nut Cluster, Finest, Tesco*	1 Slice/77g	262	10.3	338	4.5	50.1	13.3	2.7
Fruit & Nut Cluster, TTD, Sainsbury's*	1 Slice/62g	239	9.2	383	5.7	56.8	14.8	4.2
Genoa, Tesco*	1 Serving/44g	150	3.9	340	3.7	59.1	8.8	3.1
Ginger Drizzle, Iced, Co-Op*	1/6 Cake/65g	226	7.7	350	3.0	58.0	12.0	1.0
Ginger Orange, The Handmade Flapjack Company*	1 Cake/75g	289	15.2	385	4.3	46.3	20.3	0.0
Glitzy Bag, Birthday, Tesco*	1 Serving/81g	314	6.9	388	2.1	75.9	8.5	0.6
Happy Birthday, Sainsbury's*	1 Slice/50g	207	8.0	414	2.8	64.5	16.1	0.6
Hot Chocolate Fudge, Sainsbury's*	1/8 Cake/91g	343	15.6	376	5.1	50.3	17.1	3.5
Iced Cupcake, Gluten & Wheat Free, Lovemore*	1 Cake/33g	138	6.3	418	2.1	54.5	19.0	0.4
Iced Madeira, Sainsbury's*	1/8 Cake/47g	182	6.6	388	3.6	61.6	14.1	0.7

C

CAKE

INFO/WEIGHT	Measure	per Measure		Nutrition Values per 100g / 100ml				
		KCAL	FAT	KCAL	PROT	CARB	FAT	FIBRE
Jamaica Ginger, McVitie's*	1 Cake/291g	1056	30.6	363	3.7	63.4	10.5	1.6
La Madeleine, Bonne Maman*	1 Cake/113g	512	30.3	453	6.3	46.2	26.8	0.8
Lardy, Warings The Bakers*	1 Slice/120g	379	14.8	316	0.0	48.0	12.3	0.0
Lemon, Average	1 Slice/81g	320	14.5	396	4.1	54.8	18.0	0.6
Lemon, Half Moon, Bobby's*	1/6 Cake/60g	244	11.0	406	4.1	55.7	18.4	0.0
Lemon, Mini, Weight Watchers*	1 Cake/27g	90	3.0	333	3.7	66.7	11.1	11.1
Lemon, Slices, Eat Smart, Morrisons*	1 Slice/26g	81	0.7	312	3.8	68.1	2.7	1.9
Lemon, Slices, Low Fat, Weight Watchers*	1 Slice/26g	79	0.5	303	3.1	68.1	2.0	2.2
Lemon, Slices, Mr Kipling*	1 Slice/27g	109	4.5	405	4.1	59.4	16.7	0.7
Lemon & Orange, Finest, Tesco*	1 Serving/53g	216	10.7	410	4.5	52.4	20.3	1.1
Lemon Bakewell, Mr Kipling*	1 Cake/48g	195	7.3	407	2.6	65.0	15.2	0.7
Lemon Buttercream, & Lemon Curd, The Cake Shop*	1 Cake/28g	124	7.8	444	3.5	43.4	27.8	0.6
Lemon Crunchy, Devondale*	1 Cake/80g	346	17.6	432	3.3	57.0	22.0	2.4
Lemon Drizzle, Cake, Asda*	1 Serving/50g	150	6.0	299	2.8	45.0	12.0	0.4
Lemon Drizzle, M&S*	1/6 Cake/63g	230	8.8	365	4.2	55.8	13.9	1.4
Lemon Drizzle, Slices, LC, Tesco*	1 Slice/23g	67	0.5	290	4.8	62.7	2.0	2.8
Lemon Drizzle, Tray Bake, Kate's Cakes Ltd*	1 Serving/100g	324	14.4	324	4.5	44.2	14.4	1.1
Leo the Lion, Birthday, Asda*	1 Slice/81g	325	12.9	402	2.6	62.0	16.0	0.5
Madeira	1 Slice/40g	157	6.8	393	5.4	58.4	16.9	0.9
Madeira, All Butter, Sainsbury's*	1 Serving/30g	116	5.9	388	5.2	47.4	19.7	0.8
Madeira, Cherry, Tesco*	1/4 Cake/100g	342	11.2	342	4.3	55.9	11.2	2.6
Madeira, Iced, Tesco*	1/16 Cake/56g	218	6.8	389	2.6	67.2	12.2	0.4
Madeira, Lemon, Half Moon, Dan Cake*	1 Slice/50g	215	10.0	430	3.5	59.0	20.0	0.0
Madeira, Lemon Iced, Co-Op*	1 Cake/290g	1131	52.2	390	4.0	53.0	18.0	0.6
Madeira, Lemon Iced, Tesco*	1 Slice/30g	122	5.2	407	4.5	57.8	17.5	0.9
Madeira, Tesco*	1 Serving/50g	197	7.8	394	5.5	57.9	15.6	1.2
Manor House, Mr Kipling*	1 Serving/69g	277	13.8	400	5.3	49.7	20.0	1.4
Marble, Tesco*	1/8 Cake/45g	184	8.4	410	4.4	55.9	18.7	1.5
Mini Rolls, Cadbury*	1 Roll/27g	120	6.1	445	4.4	56.4	22.5	1.3
Mini Rolls, Chocolate, Average	1 Cake/27g	122	6.2	453	4.8	56.9	22.9	0.9
Mini Rolls, Chocolate, Tesco*	1 Roll/29g	135	6.7	465	5.5	58.1	23.1	1.3
Mini Rolls, Jaffa, Average	1 Cake/29g	111	3.3	382	3.5	67.2	11.2	1.4
Mini Rolls, Jam, Average	1 Cake/29g	115	4.5	395	3.8	59.8	15.6	1.8
Mini Rolls, Jammy Strawberry, Cadbury*	1 Cake/29g	119	4.8	411	4.9	59.8	16.5	0.5
Mini Rolls, Lemon, Average	1 Cake/29g	125	5.8	430	4.8	58.6	19.9	0.9
Mini Rolls, Milk Chocolate, Cadbury*	1 Roll/27g	120	6.0	445	4.4	56.5	22.2	0.0
Orange & Ginger, Oat Break, Go Ahead, McVitie's*	1 Cake/35g	121	2.2	347	5.2	67.1	6.4	2.6
Orange Marmalade, Loaf, Aldi*	1 Slice/33g	88	0.7	267	4.5	57.4	2.2	1.8
Orange Marmalade, M&S*	1 Slice/50g	195	9.2	390	3.6	53.2	18.3	1.8
Panettone, Average	1 Portion/90g	345	15.3	383	8.0	52.0	17.0	0.0
Panettone, Bauli*	1 Serving/75g	314	15.1	418	5.9	53.5	20.1	0.0
Panettone, M&S*	1/8 Loaf/51g	184	6.7	360	6.5	53.4	13.2	2.0
Party Bake, M&S*	1/15 Cake/60g	230	12.1	385	4.0	46.6	20.2	0.9
Plum & Ginger, Crumble, Graze*	1 Punnet/33g	119	9.1	361	6.2	35.1	27.6	3.3
Pumpkin & Ginger, Perfect, Graze*	1 Punnet/34g	101	5.1	298	6.1	38.6	15.0	4.0
Rice Pop & Chocolate, Chewy, Dove's Farm*	1 Bar/35g	156	7.1	447	3.9	69.9	20.2	2.3
Rock	1 Cake/40g	158	6.6	396	5.4	60.5	16.4	1.5
Rock, Tesco*	1 Serving/87g	311	8.4	357	7.4	60.1	9.7	1.6
Simnel, Slices, Mr Kipling*	1 Slice/47g	177	5.9	379	2.9	63.4	12.6	1.2
Snowballs, Sainsbury's*	1 Snowball/18g	80	4.1	445	2.5	55.6	23.0	3.6
Snowballs, Tesco*	1 Snowball/18g	79	4.0	432	2.5	55.8	22.1	5.4
Sponge	1 Slice/53g	243	13.9	459	6.4	52.4	26.3	0.9
Sponge, Apple, Bramley, Fresh Cream, Tesco*	1/6 Slice/43g	130	7.0	303	3.6	35.4	16.3	1.0

CAKE

	Measure INFO/WEIGHT	per Measure KCAL	FAT	Nutrition Values per 100g / 100ml KCAL	PROT	CARB	FAT	FIBRE
Sponge, Fatless	1 Slice/53g	156	3.2	294	10.1	53.0	6.1	0.9
Sponge, Fresh Cream, & Strawberry, Asda*	1/12 Cake/60g	170	6.0	284	4.6	44.0	10.0	1.1
Sponge, Iced, M&S*	1 Serving/100g	400	17.0	400	3.4	58.4	17.0	1.3
Sponge, Jam Filled	1 Slice/65g	196	3.2	302	4.2	64.2	4.9	1.8
Sponge, Roll, Chocolate, M&S*	¼ Cake/66g	251	12.1	380	3.9	50.5	18.4	1.8
Sponge, Strawberry, Roll, M&S*	1/6 Cake/49g	160	4.6	330	2.8	58.0	9.5	0.8
Sponge, Vanilla, Fresh Cream, Sainsbury's*	1 Slice/50g	152	5.1	304	7.5	45.6	10.2	0.4
Sponge, with Butter Icing	1 Slice/65g	318	19.9	490	4.5	52.4	30.6	0.6
Stem Ginger, Mrs Crimble's*	1 Slice/48g	158	1.1	329	2.7	73.3	2.2	2.7
Stollen, Bites, Finest, Tesco*	1 Piece/22g	81	3.2	370	6.5	52.7	14.4	4.4
Stollen, Kuchenmeister*	1 Serving/80g	357	16.0	446	5.0	61.2	20.0	2.5
Stollen, Rich Fruit, & Brandy, Christmas, Finest, Tesco*	1 Slice/70g	248	8.2	355	5.6	56.4	11.7	3.1
Stollen, Slices, Finest, Tesco*	1 Slice/45g	164	5.2	365	6.9	57.3	11.6	4.2
Sultana, Apple & Cranberry, 99% Fat Free, Trimlyne*	1/6 Cake/67g	130	0.6	195	4.6	45.5	0.9	3.3
Sultana, Fair Trade, Co-Op*	1/8 Cake/45g	155	4.0	345	5.0	60.0	9.0	1.0
Sultana & Cherry, Tesco*	1 Cake/37g	124	4.0	334	4.7	54.4	10.8	2.5
Summer Fruit Cream, GFY, Asda*	1 Serving/74g	165	3.6	223	3.6	41.0	4.9	2.5
Swiss Roll, Average	1oz/28g	77	1.2	276	7.2	55.5	4.4	0.8
Swiss Roll, Chocolate, Individual	1 Roll/26g	88	2.9	337	4.3	58.1	11.3	0.0
Swiss Roll, Chocolate, Lyons*	1 Serving/50g	190	9.6	379	4.3	47.0	19.3	0.9
Swiss Roll, Chocolate, M&S*	1 Serving/46g	168	11.1	365	4.6	32.6	24.2	1.2
Swiss Roll, Chocolate, Morrisons*	1/6 Roll/26g	103	4.9	401	4.4	56.4	18.9	3.1
Swiss Roll, Chocolate, Somerfield*	¼ Roll/44g	167	7.0	384	6.0	55.0	16.0	0.0
Swiss Roll, Chocolate, Value, Tesco*	1 Serving/20g	81	3.7	404	5.0	54.1	18.7	2.1
Swiss Roll, Chocolate Flavour, Value, Tesco*	1 Slice/20g	79	3.9	394	5.5	49.2	19.5	1.4
Swiss Roll, Raspberry, Average	1 Slice/35g	107	1.2	305	3.8	64.8	3.5	0.6
Swiss Roll, Raspberry, Lyons*	1 Roll/175g	485	2.4	277	5.2	60.6	1.4	0.0
Swiss Roll, Raspberry & Vanilla, Morrisons*	1 Serving/28g	98	2.7	350	4.2	61.8	9.5	0.0
Swiss Roll, Raspberry Jam, Mr Kipling*	1/6 Cake/52g	184	5.3	355	2.8	63.0	10.2	1.0
Syrup & Ginger, Tesco*	1 Serving/32g	134	7.0	420	4.5	51.4	21.8	0.7
The Big Frosty Fancy, Mr Kipling*	1/12 Cake/82g	321	10.6	389	2.5	65.7	12.9	1.8
Tiffin, Chocolate, Sainsbury's*	1 Cake/61g	184	11.6	301	2.7	29.8	19.0	1.3
Toffee, Slices, BGTY, Sainsbury's*	1 Slice/27g	88	0.7	327	4.3	71.7	2.5	1.8
Toffee, Slices, Low Fat, Weight Watchers*	1 Slice/27g	80	0.7	297	4.2	63.9	2.6	3.2
Toffee, Temptation, Finest, Tesco*	1 Serving/50g	212	11.6	423	4.7	49.0	23.1	0.6
Toffee, Thorntons*	1/6 Cake/70g	302	16.8	431	4.6	49.2	24.0	0.8
Toffee & Pecan Slices, M&S*	1 Slice/36g	160	8.5	445	4.7	54.0	23.7	1.3
Toffee Apple, McVitie's*	1 Slice/29g	104	3.2	354	3.5	60.2	11.0	1.5
Very Berry, Kate's Cakes Ltd*	1 Serving/100g	346	14.6	346	3.4	50.3	14.6	1.4
Victoria Sandwich, Average	1 Slice/68g	267	12.9	392	4.4	50.9	19.0	1.0
Victoria Slices, Mr Kipling*	1 Slice/28g	122	4.4	432	3.9	68.8	15.7	0.4
Victoria Sponge, Fresh Cream, Value, Tesco*	1 Serving/50g	168	8.7	337	4.4	40.7	17.4	0.6
Victoria Sponge, Kate's Cakes Ltd*	1 Serving/100g	410	19.7	410	4.0	52.8	19.7	0.9
Victoria Sponge, Lemon, Co-Op*	1 Slice/42g	151	8.0	360	4.0	44.0	19.0	0.7
Victoria Sponge, Mini, Bobby's*	1 Cake/35g	164	9.6	469	4.0	51.3	27.5	0.2
Victoria Sponge, Mini, Mr Kipling*	1 Cake/36g	152	6.9	420	3.9	58.5	19.0	0.8
Victoria Sponge, Mini, Weight Watchers*	1 Cake/30g	103	2.5	343	5.7	57.2	8.3	8.4
Victoria Sponge, TTD, Sainsbury's*	1 Slice/57g	229	11.0	401	5.0	51.8	19.3	1.4
Viennese Whirl, Average	1 Cake/28g	131	6.9	467	4.1	56.7	24.8	1.1
Viennese Whirl, Chocolate, Mr Kipling*	1 Whirl/28g	134	7.8	484	4.6	53.1	28.0	2.1
Viennese Whirl, Lemon, Mr Kipling*	1 Cake/28g	115	4.5	409	4.2	62.2	15.9	0.7
Viennese Whirl, Mr Kipling*	1 Cake/28g	141	7.8	504	3.9	59.1	28.0	1.4
Walnut, Sandwich, Sainsbury's*	1/8 Cake/48g	182	8.3	379	5.4	53.8	17.3	1.3

	Measure INFO/WEIGHT	per Measure KCAL	FAT	Nutrition Values per 100g / 100ml KCAL	PROT	CARB	FAT	FIBRE
CAKE								
Walnut Layer, Somerfield*	¼ Cake/78g	295	15.5	381	6.0	45.0	20.0	0.0
Welsh, Average	1oz/28g	121	5.5	431	5.6	61.8	19.6	1.5
Xmas Pudding, Tesco*	1 Cake/17g	58	1.6	349	3.3	60.5	9.3	1.4
CAKE BAR								
Boost, Cadbury*	1 Bar/40g	190	10.8	475	5.3	52.8	26.9	1.1
Caramel, Cadbury*	1 Bar/26g	107	4.4	411	6.4	57.0	16.8	0.0
Caramel, Weight Watchers*	1 Bar/23g	89	3.0	381	5.3	56.2	12.8	9.9
Carrot, Gu*	1 Slice/38g	135	6.6	354	1.4	17.2	17.5	0.9
Carrot, Tesco*	1 Bar/68g	239	12.6	351	4.7	41.4	18.5	2.4
Carrot with Cheese Cream Icing, Kate's Cakes Ltd*	1 Serving/100g	345	15.6	345	3.3	48.3	15.6	1.5
Chocolate, Average	1 Cake/28g	125	6.2	446	5.6	56.3	22.1	1.9
Chocolate, Double, Free From, Sainsbury's*	1 Cake/50g	196	7.9	391	4.2	58.2	15.7	1.0
Chocolate, Double, Free From, Tesco*	1 Serving/45g	190	9.1	425	4.2	55.6	20.3	4.1
Chocolate, Milk, Cadbury*	1 Bar/35g	150	7.6	430	5.6	53.3	21.7	1.2
Chocolate, Rich, Trimlyne*	1 Serving/40g	115	1.7	288	5.2	59.2	4.2	2.2
Chocolate, Snack Cakes, Penguin, McVitie's*	1 Bar/24g	122	7.2	510	4.8	54.6	30.2	1.6
Chocolate Brownie, Slice, Kate's Cakes Ltd*	1 Bar/60g	258	13.0	430	4.9	52.9	21.7	1.5
Chocolate Chip, Average	1 Cake/28g	428	21.6	428	6.3	51.9	21.6	1.6
Chocolate Chip, Mr Kipling*	1 Bar/32g	151	8.4	472	5.3	53.5	26.3	1.2
Chocolate Chip, Sainsbury's*	1 Cake/25g	108	5.6	430	6.1	51.2	22.3	0.6
Chocolate Chip, Tesco*	1 Cake/30g	124	5.9	415	7.0	51.4	19.7	2.3
Chocolate Chip, Value, Tesco*	1 Cake/28g	115	5.5	410	6.3	52.2	19.5	1.7
Chocolate Orange, Milk, Sandwich Bar, Lyons*	1 Bar/28g	142	8.0	516	5.0	62.0	29.0	0.0
Cinder Toffee, Cadbury*	1 Bar/32g	149	8.4	465	4.2	53.4	26.2	0.9
Flake, Cadbury*	1 Cake/22g	97	5.1	442	6.5	51.8	23.3	0.5
Fudge, Cadbury*	1 Pack/52g	220	9.2	420	5.7	60.3	17.6	0.0
Galaxy Caramel, McVitie's*	1 Cake/31g	137	6.5	441	5.5	57.4	21.1	0.0
Golden Syrup, McVitie's*	1 Cake/33g	127	4.8	385	3.6	60.2	14.4	1.2
Iced Rich Fruit, Finest, Tesco*	1 Serving/100g	360	10.7	360	3.8	61.3	10.7	4.2
Jaffa, McVitie's*	1 Bar/25g	94	3.5	385	3.2	61.1	14.2	2.4
Jaffa Cakes, Spooky, McVitie's*	1 Bar/25g	96	3.5	390	3.2	62.1	14.2	2.7
Jamaica Ginger, McVitie's*	1 Cake/33g	128	4.9	388	3.5	60.2	14.7	1.2
Lemon Meringue, Indulgence, Weight Watchers*	1 Bar/24g	21	0.3	86	1.1	7.1	1.3	0.0
Lemon with Sugar Pearls, Kate's Cakes Ltd*	1 Serving/100g	325	15.8	325	4.2	43.4	15.8	0.9
Milky Way, McVitie's*	1 Cake/26g	124	6.2	476	5.1	58.5	23.6	1.2
Pecan Brownie, Slice, Kate's Cakes Ltd*	1 Serving/100g	460	25.3	460	5.2	51.4	25.3	3.1
CAKE MIX								
Brownie, Chocolate Chips, Weight Watchers*	1 Pack/190g	568	13.5	299	3.2	55.6	7.1	2.1
Carrot, Betty Crocker*	¼ Pack/125g	504	8.4	403	5.8	78.9	6.7	1.4
Cheesecake, Original, Made Up, Asda*	1/6 Cake/85g	228	10.2	268	4.1	36.0	12.0	1.4
Cheesecake, Tesco*	1 Serving/76g	199	7.9	262	4.1	38.0	10.4	1.6
Chocolate, GF, Organic, Classic, Hale & Hearty*	1 Serving/100g	378	5.3	378	3.9	78.2	5.3	3.7
Sponge, Value, Tesco*	1 Slice/55g	181	4.8	329	4.6	57.9	8.8	1.4
Sponge, Vanilla, GF, Organic, Classic, Hale & Hearty*	1 Serving/100g	368	1.0	368	2.7	87.1	1.0	1.2
CALLALOO								
Leaves, Raw, Unprepared	1oz/28g	6	0.1	23	2.5	4.0	0.3	0.0
CALZONE								
Bolognese, Weight Watchers*	1 Calzone/88g	178	3.0	202	11.7	31.2	3.4	4.3
Cheese & Tomato, Weight Watchers*	1 Calzone/88g	191	3.8	217	11.3	33.4	4.3	3.4
Ham & Gruyere, Asda*	1 Serving/280g	661	22.4	236	10.0	31.0	8.0	2.7
CANNELLONI								
Beef, & Red Wine, TTD, Sainsbury's*	½ Pack/180g	448	11.5	249	14.8	32.1	6.4	1.8
Beef, & Red Wine, Waitrose*	½ Pack/170g	355	16.0	209	17.5	13.8	9.4	1.0

	Measure INFO/WEIGHT	per Measure KCAL	FAT	Nutrition Values per 100g / 100ml KCAL	PROT	CARB	FAT	FIBRE
CANNELLONI								
Beef, Great Value, Asda*	1 Pack/400g	384	10.8	96	6.0	12.0	2.7	1.6
Beef, Italian, Sainsbury's*	1 Pack/400g	498	26.2	124	5.9	10.5	6.6	1.6
Beef, Italian, Tesco*	1 Pack/400g	520	26.8	130	5.3	11.6	6.7	0.9
Beef, Ready Meal	1 Serving/335g	501	21.8	149	8.4	14.1	6.5	1.4
Beef, Ready Meal, Healthy Range, Average	1 Serving/300g	267	7.0	89	6.0	11.0	2.4	1.6
Parmesan & Basil, M&S*	1 Pack/360g	504	28.4	140	5.9	11.4	7.9	0.8
Spinach & Cheese, Finest, Tesco*	1 Pack/350g	532	31.8	152	5.4	12.1	9.1	1.5
Spinach & Ricotta, Fresh, Ready Meal, Average	1 Serving/300g	393	22.0	131	5.0	10.8	7.4	1.2
Spinach & Ricotta, Italian Style, Co-Op*	1 Pack/450g	540	27.0	120	5.0	12.0	6.0	2.0
Spinach & Ricotta, Ready Meal, Average	1 Serving/300g	426	22.0	142	5.6	13.3	7.3	1.4
Spinach & Ricotta, Ready Meal, Healthy Range	1 Serving/300g	251	7.3	84	4.2	11.1	2.4	1.4
Spinach & Wild Mushroom, Linda McCartney*	1 Pack/340g	381	13.6	112	4.9	14.1	4.0	1.7
Tubes, Dry, Average	*1oz/28g*	*101*	*1.0*	*361*	*12.5*	*69.1*	*3.6*	*1.2*
Vegetarian, Tesco*	1 Pack/400g	552	34.4	138	5.3	9.8	8.6	1.5
CANTONESE								
with Long Grain Rice, Rice Time, Uncle Ben's*	1 Pot/300g	378	2.7	126	2.1	27.0	0.9	0.7
CAPERS								
Caperberries, Spanish, Waitrose*	1 Serving/55g	9	0.3	17	1.1	2.1	0.5	2.5
Capucines, Sainsbury's*	1 Tsp/6g	1	0.0	14	1.4	1.3	0.3	2.2
in Brine, Tesco*	1 Tsp/2g	1	0.0	29	2.4	3.5	0.6	2.7
in Vinegar, Average	1 Tsp/5g	2	0.0	34	1.7	3.0	0.6	0.0
CAPPELLETTI								
Goats Cheese & Red Pesto, Waitrose*	½ Pack/125g	374	10.9	299	11.6	43.5	8.7	2.2
Meat, Italian, Somerfield*	½ Pack/125g	331	7.9	265	13.6	38.5	6.3	2.4
Parma Ham, Fresh, Waitrose*	½ Pack/125g	368	11.5	294	14.1	38.6	9.2	2.2
CAPRI SUN								
Orange	1 Pouch/200ml	90	0.0	45	0.0	11.0	0.0	0.0
Orange, 100%, Juice	1 Pouch/200ml	75	0.0	38	0.5	9.2	0.0	0.1
CARAMAC								
Nestle*	1 Bar/30g	173	11.0	567	5.7	54.7	36.1	0.0
CARAMBOLA								
Average	*1oz/28g*	*9*	*0.1*	*32*	*0.5*	*7.3*	*0.3*	*1.3*
CARAMEL								
Egg, Cadbury*	1 Egg/40g	195	10.2	485	4.8	59.3	25.3	0.4
CARAWAY								
Seeds, Schwartz*	1 Pack/38g	170	8.1	448	23.3	40.9	21.2	0.0
CARDAMOM								
Black, Ground, Average	*1 Tsp/2g*	*6*	*0.1*	*311*	*10.8*	*68.5*	*6.7*	*28.0*
Ground, Average	*1 Tsp/2g*	*6*	*0.1*	*314*	*10.7*	*53.6*	*7.1*	*28.6*
CAROB POWDER								
Average	*1 Tsp/2g*	*3*	*0.0*	*159*	*4.9*	*37.0*	*0.1*	*0.0*
CARP								
Fillet, Raw, Average	1 Fillet/218g	244	10.2	112	17.5	0.0	4.7	0.0
CARROT & SWEDE								
Diced, for Mashing, Average	*½ Pack/250g*	*58*	*0.7*	*23*	*0.6*	*4.7*	*0.3*	*1.9*
Mash, From Supermarket, Average	1 Serving/150g	138	7.5	92	1.3	10.4	5.0	1.3
Mash, Healthy Range, Average	1 Serving/150g	98	4.2	66	1.3	8.6	2.8	2.1
CARROTS								
& Peas, Sainsbury's*	1 Serving/200g	100	1.0	50	3.3	8.3	0.5	3.8
Baby, & Green Beans, in Honey & Mustard, McCain*	1 Pack/128g	59	2.4	46	1.3	6.2	1.9	1.7
Baby, Canned, Average	*1 Can/195g*	*40*	*0.5*	*21*	*0.5*	*4.2*	*0.3*	*2.1*
Baby, Fresh, Average	*1 Serving/80g*	*28*	*0.1*	*35*	*0.6*	*8.2*	*0.1*	*2.9*
Baby, with Fine Beans, Tesco*	1 Pack/200g	58	1.0	29	1.3	4.7	0.5	2.3

	Measure INFO/WEIGHT	per Measure KCAL	FAT	Nutrition Values per 100g / 100ml KCAL	PROT	CARB	FAT	FIBRE
CARROTS								
Batons, & Sliced Runner Beans, Sainsbury's*	1 Serving/200g	40	1.0	20	1.0	3.2	0.5	3.2
Batons, Broccoli & Cauliflower, Freshly Frozen, Asda*	1 Bag/156g	39	0.9	25	1.9	2.9	0.6	2.4
Batons, Fresh, Average	*½ Pack/150g*	*41*	*0.4*	*28*	*0.6*	*5.7*	*0.3*	*2.6*
Boiled, Average	*1oz/28g*	*6*	*0.1*	*22*	*0.6*	*4.4*	*0.4*	*2.3*
Canned, Average	*1oz/28g*	*6*	*0.1*	*22*	*0.6*	*4.4*	*0.2*	*2.1*
Chantenay, Frozen, Morrisons*	1 Serving/80g	28	0.3	35	0.4	6.7	0.4	3.2
Chantenay, Steamer, Sainsbury's*	½ Pack/125g	60	2.1	48	0.5	7.7	1.7	2.2
Crunchies, Shapers, Boots*	1 Bag/80g	28	0.2	35	0.6	7.5	0.3	3.0
Raw, Scrubbed, Average	1 Serving/80g	24	0.4	30	0.7	6.0	0.5	2.4
Sliced, Canned, Average	*1 Serving/180g*	*36*	*0.2*	*20*	*0.7*	*4.1*	*0.1*	*1.5*
Sliced, Fresh, Average	*1 Serving/60g*	*17*	*0.2*	*28*	*0.7*	*5.7*	*0.3*	*2.0*
Sweetcorn, & Broccoli, Steam & Serve, Morrisons*	1 Pack/120g	54	1.3	45	2.3	8.9	1.1	2.6
Whole, Raw, Peeled, Average	*1 Carrot/75g*	*21*	*0.2*	*29*	*0.6*	*6.4*	*0.3*	*2.2*
with Parsley, & English Butter, M&S*	½ Pack/100g	65	3.9	65	0.6	7.1	3.9	2.4
CASHEW NUTS								
Plain, Average	*½ Pack/25g*	*146*	*12.2*	*584*	*15.7*	*18.8*	*48.9*	*3.4*
Roasted & Salted, Average	*1 Serving/50g*	*306*	*25.6*	*612*	*18.8*	*19.6*	*51.1*	*3.1*
CASHEWS & PEANUTS								
Honey Roasted, Average	*1 Serving/50g*	*290*	*21.4*	*579*	*21.6*	*26.6*	*42.9*	*4.2*
CASSAVA								
Baked, Average	*1oz/28g*	*43*	*0.1*	*155*	*0.7*	*40.1*	*0.2*	*1.7*
Boiled in Unsalted Water, Average	*1oz/28g*	*36*	*0.1*	*130*	*0.5*	*33.5*	*0.2*	*1.4*
Gari, Average	*1oz/28g*	*100*	*0.1*	*358*	*1.3*	*92.9*	*0.5*	*0.0*
Raw, Average	*1oz/28g*	*40*	*0.1*	*142*	*0.6*	*36.8*	*0.2*	*1.6*
Steamed, Average	*1oz/28g*	*40*	*0.1*	*142*	*0.6*	*36.8*	*0.2*	*1.6*
CASSEROLE								
Bean, & Lentil, Morrisons*	1 Can/410g	287	1.6	70	4.1	12.5	0.4	0.0
Bean, Cassoulet, Organic, Free & Easy*	1 Tin/400g	256	1.2	64	3.4	11.9	0.3	2.3
Bean, Spicy, BGTY, Sainsbury's*	1 Pack/300g	171	2.7	57	3.0	9.1	0.9	4.2
Beef	1 Serving/336g	490	23.0	146	16.3	4.6	6.8	0.6
Beef, & Ale, Average	1 Serving/300g	251	6.8	84	9.4	6.5	2.2	1.3
Beef, & Ale, Finest, Tesco*	½ Pack/300g	234	4.2	78	11.5	5.0	1.4	1.1
Beef, & Dumplings, M Kitchen, Morrisons*	1 Pack/450g	596	28.0	132	7.3	11.0	6.2	1.7
Beef, & Red Wine, Average	1 Serving/350g	290	7.3	83	7.2	8.2	2.1	1.5
Beef, & Red Wine, BGTY, Sainsbury's*	1 Pack/300g	192	1.8	64	8.0	6.7	0.6	0.9
Beef, & Red Wine, Fuller Longer, M&S*	1 Pack/420g	355	11.7	85	7.2	6.9	2.8	1.7
Beef, & Red Wine, Weight Watchers*	1 Pack/330g	254	9.2	77	4.3	8.6	2.8	0.3
Beef, & Red Wine, You Count, Love Life, Waitrose*	1 Pack/381g	297	5.2	78	6.5	9.5	1.4	0.9
Beef, Diet Chef Ltd*	1 Pack/300g	177	3.0	59	7.8	4.7	1.0	2.4
Beef, Meal for One, Tesco*	1 Pack/450g	425	18.9	94	3.6	10.6	4.2	1.7
Beef, Mini Favourites, M&S*	1 Pack/200g	210	8.4	105	7.1	9.3	4.2	1.4
Beef, with Dumplings, Ready Meal, Average	1 Serving/350g	464	21.1	132	9.5	10.1	6.0	1.5
Beef, with Herb Potatoes, Tesco*	1 Serving/475g	504	17.1	106	6.8	11.5	3.6	1.6
Chicken, & Asparagus in White Wine, Finest, Tesco*	1 Pack/350g	683	42.4	195	10.0	11.6	12.1	0.3
Chicken, & Asparagus in White Wine, Tesco*	½ Pack/300g	444	23.7	148	11.5	7.7	7.9	0.8
Chicken, & Dumplings, M&S*	½ Pack/227g	261	10.0	115	9.7	9.0	4.4	0.9
Chicken, & Dumplings, Morrisons*	1 Pack/300g	291	12.6	97	3.4	11.4	4.2	1.3
Chicken, & Dumplings, Sainsbury's*	1 Serving/450g	612	32.4	136	6.8	11.0	7.2	0.6
Chicken, & Dumplings, with Veg, Fuller Longer, M&S*	1 Pack/445g	477	32.7	105	9.4	10.8	7.2	1.1
Chicken, & Red Wine, Duchy Originals*	½ Pack/175g	187	7.5	107	14.0	5.1	4.3	1.6
Chicken, & Tomato, Asda*	¼ Pack/273g	569	41.0	208	16.0	2.2	15.0	0.5
Chicken, & Vegetable, Apetito*	1 Pack/330g	286	9.9	87	6.3	9.4	3.0	1.6
Chicken, & Vegetable, Ready Meal, Healthy Range	1 Serving/330g	265	11.9	80	4.7	7.6	3.6	1.1

CASEROLE

Measure INFO/WEIGHT		per Measure KCAL	FAT	Nutrition Values per 100g / 100ml KCAL	PROT	CARB	FAT	FIBRE
CASSEROLE								
Chicken, & White Wine, Ready Meal, Healthy Range	1 Serving/300g	234	7.4	78	7.7	6.3	2.4	1.2
Chicken, Carrots, Peas & Potatoes, Weight Watchers*	1 Serving/302g	193	4.2	64	4.3	8.6	1.4	0.5
Chicken, Chorizo, & Three Bean, Fuller Longer, M&S*	1 Pack/420g	336	11.3	80	8.0	5.3	2.7	5.9
Chicken, Green Isle*	1 Pack/400g	300	6.8	75	5.7	9.2	1.7	1.0
Chicken, Leek & Mushroom, Tesco*	1 Pack/350g	382	22.0	109	4.5	8.6	6.3	1.0
Chicken, Mediterranean, Tesco*	1 Pack/400g	260	9.2	65	6.7	4.5	2.3	0.9
Chicken, PB, Waitrose*	1 Pack/400g	392	14.4	98	6.6	9.8	3.6	1.2
Chicken, You Count, Love Life, Waitrose*	1 Pack/400g	297	4.8	74	7.4	7.9	1.2	1.2
Lamb, & Dumpling, with Vegetables, Minced, M&S*	1 Pack/200g	260	12.8	130	7.0	11.6	6.4	1.2
Lamb, & Rosemary, Eat Well, M&S*	1 Pack/380g	325	11.0	86	7.6	7.0	2.9	2.2
Lamb, BGTY, Sainsbury's*	1 Serving/200g	242	8.6	121	20.7	0.1	4.3	0.1
Lamb, Braised, British Classics, Tesco*	1 Pack/350g	332	18.2	95	7.5	4.6	5.2	1.2
Lamb, COU, M&S*	1 Pack/390g	254	6.6	65	5.9	6.7	1.7	1.6
Lamb, Ready Meal, Healthy Range, Average	1 Serving/220g	200	7.3	91	10.5	4.9	3.3	1.0
Lamb, with Mint Dumplings, Minced, Sainsbury's*	1 Pack/450g	558	30.6	124	5.4	10.4	6.8	1.1
Mushroom, & Onion, Iceland*	1 Pack/400g	272	12.4	68	1.3	8.8	3.1	1.9
Pork, & Apple, with Boiled Potatoes, & Veg, Apetito*	1 Pack/350g	251	3.9	72	5.1	8.5	1.1	1.1
Pork, Normandy Style, Finest, Tesco*	1 Pack/450g	405	21.6	90	7.6	4.1	4.8	2.3
Rabbit, Average	1oz/28g	29	1.4	102	11.6	2.6	5.1	0.4
Sausage, & Potato, M&S*	1 Serving/200g	190	11.8	95	3.3	7.5	5.9	0.9
Sausage, 328, Wiltshire Farm Foods*	1 Pack/420g	394	20.4	94	3.0	9.7	4.9	1.4
Sausage, CBY, Asda*	1 Pot/400g	240	15.2	60	3.6	1.9	3.8	2.1
Sausage, Pork & Leek, 387, Wiltshire Farm Foods*	1 Serving/280g	307	17.3	110	4.6	7.8	6.2	1.0
Sausage, Solo Slim, Rosemary Conley*	1 Pack/300g	312	15.0	104	5.7	9.0	5.0	3.1
Steak, & Ale, Average	1 Serving/275g	324	14.4	118	9.0	8.8	5.2	1.0
Steak, & Ale, British Classics, Tesco*	1 Serving/100g	93	3.4	93	11.2	4.5	3.4	1.1
Steak, & Ale, Sainsbury's*	1 Pack/300g	288	10.5	96	10.6	5.6	3.5	0.4
Steak, & Mushroom, Average	1 Serving/275g	274	15.5	100	6.2	6.0	5.6	1.0
Steak, & Mushroom with Mustard Mash, Finest, Tesco*	1 Pack/550g	522	21.4	95	5.9	9.0	3.9	1.1
Vegetable, & Lentil, Canned, Granose*	1 Can/400g	272	8.0	68	3.5	9.0	2.0	3.0
Vegetable, Average	1 Serving/275g	77	0.8	28	0.8	5.5	0.3	1.5
Vegetable, Country, Sainsbury's*	1 Can/400g	300	10.0	75	2.2	11.0	2.5	1.1
Vegetable, Tesco*	1 Serving/220g	66	0.7	30	0.8	6.1	0.3	1.5
Vegetable, with Dumplings, Ready Meal, Average	1 Serving/400g	376	13.8	94	2.1	13.0	3.5	2.7
Venison, Scottish Wild, & Beaujolais, Tesco*	1 Pack/425g	366	8.9	86	11.9	4.9	2.1	0.6
CASSEROLE MIX								
Beef, Colman's*	1 Pack/40g	123	0.6	308	7.5	66.0	1.5	2.5
Beef, Recipe, Colman's*	1 Pack/42g	142	0.5	338	9.1	13.1	1.1	4.0
Beef, Recipe, Schwartz*	1 Pack/43g	123	0.9	287	7.0	56.6	2.1	6.6
Beef & Ale, Colman's*	1 Pack/45g	144	0.9	320	9.2	66.3	2.0	2.3
Chicken, Authentic, Schwartz*	1 Pack/36g	131	1.5	363	10.4	70.7	4.3	2.0
Chicken, Traditional, Colman's*	1 Pack/40g	124	0.5	311	5.7	69.4	1.3	1.5
Chicken Chasseur, Asda*	1 Pack/80g	273	0.8	341	9.0	74.0	1.0	1.4
Chicken Chasseur, Morrisons*	1 Pack/40g	115	0.5	288	9.2	59.8	1.2	0.0
Farmhouse Sausage, Schwartz*	1 Pack/39g	124	1.1	317	8.1	64.6	2.9	0.5
Honey Chicken, Colman's*	1 Pack/50g	128	0.6	257	3.4	58.3	1.1	1.8
Lamb, Authentic, Schwartz*	1 Pack/35g	116	1.2	332	7.7	68.0	3.3	1.3
Moroccan Lamb, Schwartz*	1 Pack/35g	124	2.0	354	6.2	74.1	5.7	4.5
Peppered Beef, Schwartz*	1 Pack/40g	129	2.0	323	7.0	62.9	4.9	7.3
Pork, Colman's*	1 Pack/40g	131	0.6	328	6.7	72.0	1.4	2.8
Pork, Somerset, Schwartz*	1 Pack/36g	115	1.4	320	9.4	61.9	3.8	7.7
Sausage, & Onion, Colman's*	1 Pack/45g	143	1.2	318	9.6	64.2	2.6	2.6
Sausage, Asda*	¼ Pack/25g	80	1.0	321	6.0	65.0	4.1	3.0

	Measure INFO/WEIGHT	per Measure KCAL	FAT	Nutrition Values per 100g / 100ml KCAL	PROT	CARB	FAT	FIBRE
CASEROLE MIX								
Sausage, Classic, Schwartz*	1 Pack/35g	96	0.9	275	12.4	50.1	2.7	14.9
Sausage, Colman's*	1 Pack/40g	144	0.6	361	8.9	77.7	1.6	1.6
Turkey, Colman's*	1 Pack/50g	156	1.0	313	5.9	68.0	1.9	3.5
CATFISH								
Cooked, Steamed, Weighed with Bone, Average	*1 Serving/100g*	*101*	*3.1*	*101*	*18.2*	*0.0*	*3.1*	*0.7*
Raw, Average	*1oz/28g*	*27*	*0.8*	*96*	*17.6*	*0.0*	*2.8*	*0.0*
CAULIFLOWER								
Boiled, Average	*1 Serving/80g*	*22*	*0.7*	*28*	*2.9*	*2.1*	*0.9*	*1.6*
Florets, Peas & Carrots, Frozen, Asda*	1 Serving/100g	37	0.6	37	3.0	5.0	0.6	2.8
Raw, Average	*1 Serving/80g*	*25*	*0.7*	*31*	*3.2*	*2.7*	*0.8*	*1.6*
Steamed, Average	1 Serving/100g	28	0.9	28	2.9	2.1	0.9	1.6
CAULIFLOWER CHEESE								
& Bacon, Gastropub, M&S*	1 Pack/300g	318	21.0	106	6.3	4.5	7.0	1.0
& Broccoli, Average	1 Serving/200g	127	6.4	64	3.8	4.6	3.2	2.0
Grills, Meat Free, Tesco*	1 Grill/91g	160	7.4	175	5.3	20.0	8.1	2.9
Grills, Tesco*	1 Grill/92g	207	10.9	225	6.5	22.2	11.9	4.0
Made with Semi-Skimmed Milk	1oz/28g	28	1.8	100	6.0	5.2	6.4	1.3
Made with Skimmed Milk	1oz/28g	27	1.7	97	6.0	5.2	6.0	1.3
Made with Whole Milk	1oz/28g	29	1.9	105	6.0	5.2	6.9	1.3
Pre Packed, Average	1 Meal/400g	362	23.3	90	4.5	4.6	5.8	1.3
Pre Packed, Healthy Range, Average	1 Serving/200g	123	4.9	61	4.4	4.9	2.4	1.3
CAVATELLI								
Egg, Fresh, Asda*	1 Serving/100g	203	3.4	203	9.0	34.0	3.4	3.0
CAVIAR								
Average	*1oz/28g*	*26*	*1.3*	*92*	*12.0*	*0.5*	*4.7*	*0.0*
CELERIAC								
Boiled in Salted Water, Average	*1oz/28g*	*4*	*0.1*	*15*	*0.9*	*1.9*	*0.5*	*3.2*
Raw, Average	*1 Serving/100g*	*42*	*0.3*	*42*	*1.5*	*9.2*	*0.3*	*1.8*
CELERY								
Boiled in Salted Water	*1 Serving/50g*	*4*	*0.2*	*8*	*0.5*	*0.8*	*0.3*	*1.2*
Raw, Trimmed	*1 Stalk/40g*	*3*	*0.1*	*7*	*0.5*	*0.9*	*0.2*	*1.1*
CHAMPAGNE								
Average	*1 Sm Glass/125ml*	*95*	*0.0*	*76*	*0.3*	*1.4*	*0.0*	*0.0*
CHANNA MASALA								
Indian, Sainsbury's*	1 Serving/149g	165	7.3	111	4.2	12.4	4.9	3.3
M & S*	1 Pack/225g	360	23.7	160	5.6	11.2	10.5	8.2
Waitrose*	1 Pack/300g	300	18.3	100	3.7	7.4	6.1	7.9
CHAPATIS								
Brown Wheat Flour, Waitrose*	1 Chapati/42g	128	3.4	305	8.6	49.4	8.0	4.6
Elephant Atta*	1 Chapati/45g	129	2.9	287	7.5	53.1	6.4	3.2
Indian Style, Asda*	1 Chapati/43g	95	0.4	221	8.0	45.0	1.0	2.9
Made with Fat	1 Chapati/60g	197	7.7	328	8.1	48.3	12.8	0.0
Made without Fat	1 Chapati/55g	111	0.6	202	7.3	43.7	1.0	0.0
Morrisons*	1 Chapati/40g	108	2.8	269	8.6	49.8	6.9	0.0
Plain, Wraps, Original, Patak's*	1 Chapati/42g	115	3.2	273	9.4	48.8	7.5	0.0
Wholemeal, Patak's*	1 Chapati/42g	130	4.0	310	11.2	44.9	9.5	9.0
CHAR								
Arctic, Whole, Raw	1 Serving/100g	137	6.0	137	20.8	0.0	6.0	0.0
CHARD								
Average	1 Serving/80g	15	0.2	19	1.4	3.3	0.2	0.8
Swiss, Boiled in Unsalted Water	*1oz/28g*	*6*	*0.0*	*20*	*1.9*	*4.1*	*0.1*	*2.1*
Swiss, Raw	*1oz/28g*	*5*	*0.1*	*19*	*1.8*	*3.7*	*0.2*	*1.6*

	Measure INFO/WEIGHT	per Measure KCAL	FAT	Nutrition Values per 100g / 100ml KCAL	PROT	CARB	FAT	FIBRE
CHEDDARS								
Baked, Mini, Cheese & Ham Flavour, McVitie's*	1 Bag/30g	160	8.9	534	11.0	55.5	29.8	2.0
Baked, Mini, Original, Cheddar Cheese, McVitie's*	1 Bag/26g	130	7.5	522	10.6	51.4	29.9	2.5
Baked, Mini, Peperami, McVitie's*	1 Bag/30g	160	9.1	532	9.7	55.2	30.2	2.0
Baked, Mini, Tangy Salsa, McVitie's*	1 Bag/50g	266	15.0	532	11.0	54.7	29.9	2.1
McVitie's*	1 Cracker/4g	22	1.3	543	10.0	55.1	31.3	2.6
Smokey BBQ, McVitie's*	1 Pack/30g	155	8.9	516	9.3	52.8	29.8	2.6
CHEESE								
Ail & Fines Herbes, Boursin*	1oz/28g	116	11.8	414	7.0	2.0	42.0	0.0
Appenzellar, Sainsbury's*	1 Serving/25g	96	7.9	386	25.4	0.0	31.6	0.0
Babybel, Cheddar Variety, Mini, Fromageries Bel*	1 Cheese/20g	75	6.2	375	24.0	0.0	31.0	0.0
Babybel, Emmental, Fromageries Bel*	1 Serving/20g	63	4.9	316	23.0	1.0	24.5	0.0
Babybel, Goat's Variety, Mini, Fromageries Bel*	1 Cheese/20g	65	5.4	327	21.0	0.0	27.0	0.0
Babybel, Gouda Variety, Mini, Fromageries Bel*	1 Cheese/20g	68	5.6	340	4.8	0.0	28.0	0.0
Babybel, Light, Mini, Fromageries Bel*	1 Cheese/20g	40	2.3	208	25.0	0.0	12.0	0.0
Babybel, Original, Mini, Fromageries Bel*	1 Cheese/20g	61	4.8	304	22.0	0.1	24.0	0.0
Bavarian, Smoked, Slices, Asda*	1 Slice/18g	50	4.1	277	17.0	0.4	23.0	0.0
Bavarian, Smoked with Ham, Sainsbury's*	1 Serving/30g	89	7.2	298	19.4	0.8	24.1	0.0
Bleu D' Auvergne, Sainsbury's*	1 Serving/25g	84	6.6	335	22.0	2.0	26.5	0.0
Bleu d'Auvergne, TTD, Sainsbury's*	1 Serving/100g	322	26.0	322	22.0	0.0	26.0	0.0
Blue, Basics, Sainsbury's*	1 Serving/100g	410	35.0	410	23.7	0.1	35.0	0.0
Blue, Castello, Soft, Castello*	¼ Pack/38g	162	15.6	432	14.0	0.5	41.5	0.0
Blue, Saint Agur*	1 Serving/30g	109	9.9	363	16.0	0.2	33.0	0.0
Brie, Average	*1 Serving/25g*	*74*	*6.0*	*296*	*19.7*	*0.3*	*24.0*	*0.0*
Brie, Reduced Fat, Average	*1 Serving/50g*	*99*	*5.7*	*198*	*23.0*	*0.8*	*11.4*	*0.0*
Caerphilly, Average	*1 Serving/50g*	*187*	*15.6*	*374*	*23.0*	*0.1*	*31.3*	*0.0*
Cambazola, Tesco*	1 Serving/30g	128	12.3	425	13.5	0.5	41.0	0.0
Camembert, Average	*1 Serving/50g*	*141*	*11.1*	*283*	*20.5*	*0.1*	*22.2*	*0.0*
Camembert, Breaded, Average	1 Serving/90g	307	20.9	342	16.6	14.2	23.2	0.4
Cantal, French, Sainsbury's*	1 Serving/30g	106	8.7	353	23.0	0.1	29.0	0.0
Cheddar, & Mozzarella, Spicy, Grated, Tesco*	1 Serving/40g	140	10.5	350	26.0	2.5	26.2	0.0
Cheddar, Average	*1 Serving/30g*	*123*	*10.3*	*410*	*25.0*	*0.1*	*34.4*	*0.0*
Cheddar, Canadian, Average	*1 Serving/30g*	*123*	*10.3*	*409*	*25.0*	*0.1*	*34.3*	*0.0*
Cheddar, Davidstow, Mature, Average	*1 Serving/28g*	*115*	*9.6*	*410*	*25.0*	*0.1*	*34.4*	*0.0*
Cheddar, Extra Mature, Average	*1 Serving/30g*	*123*	*10.3*	*410*	*25.1*	*0.1*	*34.4*	*0.0*
Cheddar, Grated, Average	*1 Serving/50g*	*206*	*17.2*	*413*	*24.4*	*1.5*	*34.3*	*0.0*
Cheddar, Mature, Average	*1 Serving/30g*	*123*	*10.3*	*410*	*25.0*	*0.1*	*34.4*	*0.0*
Cheddar, Mature, Grated, Average	*1 Serving/28g*	*113*	*9.3*	*404*	*24.7*	*1.6*	*33.2*	*0.0*
Cheddar, Mature, Reduced Fat, Average	*1 Serving/25g*	*68*	*4.2*	*271*	*30.0*	*0.1*	*16.7*	*0.0*
Cheddar, Medium, Average	*1 Serving/30g*	*123*	*10.4*	*411*	*24.9*	*0.2*	*34.5*	*0.0*
Cheddar, Mild, Average	*1 Serving/30g*	*123*	*10.3*	*409*	*25.0*	*0.1*	*34.3*	*0.0*
Cheddar, Reduced Fat, Average	*1 Serving/30g*	*76*	*4.2*	*255*	*32.2*	*0.1*	*14.0*	*0.0*
Cheddar, Smoked, Average	*1 Serving/30g*	*123*	*10.3*	*411*	*25.2*	*0.1*	*34.4*	*0.0*
Cheddar, West Country Farmhouse, Average	*1 Serving/28g*	*115*	*9.6*	*410*	*25.0*	*0.1*	*34.4*	*0.0*
Cheddar, Wexford, Average	*1 Serving/20g*	*82*	*6.9*	*410*	*25.0*	*0.1*	*34.4*	*0.0*
Cheddar, with Caramelised Onion, Sainsbury's*	1 Serving/28g	109	8.7	391	22.8	5.1	31.0	0.0
Cheddar, with Caramelised Onion, Tesco*	1 Serving/50g	183	14.0	366	21.4	7.1	28.0	0.4
Cheddar, with Onion & Chives, Davidson*	1 Serving/25g	100	8.3	400	24.3	0.6	33.3	0.0
Cheddar, with Pickled Onion Relish, Christmas, Tesco*	¼ Cheese/50g	191	15.5	382	23.0	2.7	31.0	0.1
Chedds, Bricks, Cathedral City*	1 Brick/18g	75	6.3	416	25.4	0.1	34.9	0.0
Chedds, Cheese & Toasties, Cathedral*	1 Pack/33g	137	8.0	414	20.0	28.0	24.3	0.0
Chedds, Nibbles, Cathedral City*	1 Bag/18g	75	6.3	416	25.4	0.1	34.9	0.0
Cheestrings, Cheddar, Original, Golden Vale*	1 Stick/21g	69	5.0	328	28.0	0.0	24.0	0.0
Cheestrings, Double Cheese Flavour, Golden Vale*	1 Stick/21g	69	5.0	328	28.0	0.0	24.0	0.0

CHEESE

	Measure INFO/WEIGHT	per Measure KCAL	FAT	Nutrition Values per 100g / 100ml KCAL	PROT	CARB	FAT	FIBRE
Cheshire	**1oz/28g**	**106**	**8.8**	**379**	**24.0**	**0.1**	**31.4**	**0.0**
Chevre Pave D'affinois, Finest, Tesco*	1 Pack/150g	404	32.6	269	18.5	0.0	21.7	0.0
Cottage, Low Fat, 2% Fat, Natural, Average	1 Serving/75g	68	1.4	90	13.7	3.6	1.9	0.0
Cottage, Natural, Plain, Average	**1oz/28g**	**27**	**1.1**	**98**	**11.8**	**3.9**	**3.8**	**0.1**
Cottage, Onion & Chive, 1.4% Fat, Love Life, Waitrose*	1 Serving/60g	42	0.8	70	9.5	4.6	1.4	0.5
Cottage, Onion & Chive, 2% Fat, BGTY, Sainsbury's*	1 Pot/250g	180	2.5	72	10.9	4.5	1.0	0.5
Cottage, Onion & Chive, Waitrose*	1 Serving/20g	18	0.6	91	10.8	4.9	3.1	0.3
Cottage, Onion & Chives, LC, Tesco*	1 Serving/60g	51	0.9	85	11.4	4.8	1.5	0.1
Cottage, Pineapple, LC, Tesco*	1 Serving/60g	54	0.8	90	9.8	8.5	1.3	0.4
Cottage, Pineapple, PB, Waitrose*	½ Pot/125g	106	1.8	85	8.4	9.7	1.4	0.5
Cottage, Plain, Average	**1 Tbsp/20g**	**19**	**0.7**	**93**	**12.0**	**3.3**	**3.5**	**0.1**
Cottage, Plain, Reduced Fat, Average	**1oz/28g**	**24**	**0.5**	**85**	**12.3**	**4.4**	**1.9**	**0.1**
Cottage, Red Pepper, GFY, Asda*	¼ Pot/75g	66	1.9	88	11.1	4.3	2.5	0.1
Cottage, Virtually Fat Free, Average	1 Tbsp/20g	16	0.2	79	13.0	4.5	1.0	0.0
Cottage, West Country, Low Fat 1.5%, Waitrose*	1 Serving/100g	77	1.5	77	11.8	4.4	1.5	0.0
Cottage, West Country, Waitrose*	1 Serving/100g	113	6.1	113	6.1	3.3	6.1	0.0
Cottage, Whole Milk, Natural, Average	1 Serving/75g	77	3.4	103	12.5	2.7	4.5	0.0
Cottage, with Chives, Good Intentions, Somerfield*	1 Pot/125g	101	3.5	81	10.8	3.2	2.8	0.0
Cottage, with Chives, Low Fat, Westacre*	1 Pot/100g	81	1.4	81	13.7	3.5	1.4	1.2
Cottage, with Chives, Virtually Fat free, Longley Farm*	½ Pot/125g	88	0.1	70	14.3	2.9	0.1	0.0
Cottage, with Cucumber & Mint, COU, M&S*	1 Pot/113g	85	1.7	75	11.6	3.1	1.5	0.2
Cottage, with Grilled Pepper & Pesto, LC, Tesco*	1 Portion/60g	45	0.9	75	10.2	4.3	1.5	0.5
Cottage, with Mango & Pineapple, BGTY, Sainsbury's*	½ Pot/125g	112	0.9	90	10.7	10.4	0.7	0.2
Cottage, with Mango & Pineapple, Morrisons*	1 Pot/125g	112	0.9	90	10.7	10.4	0.7	0.0
Cottage, with Onion & Chive, GFY, Asda*	¼ Tub/75g	50	1.0	66	9.3	3.8	1.4	0.5
Cottage, with Onion & Chive, Good Choice, Iceland*	1 Serving/100g	74	1.6	74	11.1	3.8	1.6	0.3
Cottage, with Onion & Chive, M&S*	¼ Pot/65g	88	5.5	135	10.4	4.0	8.5	0.1
Cottage, with Onion & Chives, Everyday, Value, Tesco*	1 Portion/60g	45	0.9	75	10.2	5.0	1.5	0.5
Cottage, with Pineapple, BGTY, Sainsbury's*	1 Serving/125g	105	0.9	84	10.5	8.9	0.7	0.1
Cottage, with Pineapple, GFY, Asda*	1 Pot/227g	193	2.3	85	9.0	10.0	1.0	0.5
Cottage, with Pineapple, Less Than 5% Fat, Sainsbury's*	½ Pot/125g	122	4.2	98	10.0	6.8	3.4	0.1
Cottage, with Tomato & Cracked Black Pepper, Asda*	½ Pot/113g	86	2.4	76	10.0	3.1	2.1	1.3
Cottage, with Tuna & Pesto, Asda*	1 Serving/170g	184	10.2	108	10.0	3.5	6.0	0.7
Cream, Average	**1 Portion/30g**	**132**	**14.2**	**439**	**3.1**	**0.0**	**47.4**	**0.0**
Cream, Garlic & Herbs, Light, Boursin*	1 Portion/20g	28	1.8	140	12.0	2.5	9.0	0.0
Cream, Reduced Fat, Average	**1 Serving/20g**	**23**	**1.1**	**117**	**13.0**	**4.0**	**5.3**	**0.1**
Cream, with Onion & Chives, Morrisons*	1 Serving/20g	38	3.0	190	11.0	3.0	15.0	0.0
Cream, with Pineapple, Asda*	1 Serving/40g	77	5.2	193	8.0	11.0	13.0	0.0
Creme de Saint Agur, Saint Agur*	1 Serving/10g	28	2.5	285	13.5	2.3	24.7	0.0
Dairylea, Light, Slices, Kraft*	1 Slice/25g	51	2.6	205	17.0	8.6	10.5	0.0
Dairylea, Rippers, Straight, Kraft*	1 Ripper/21g	60	3.9	285	28.0	1.0	18.5	0.0
Dairylea, Slices, Kraft*	1 Slice/25g	69	5.1	275	13.0	8.6	20.5	0.0
Danish Blue, Average	**1 Serving/30g**	**106**	**8.7**	**352**	**20.8**	**0.0**	**29.1**	**0.0**
Demi Pont L'eveque, Finest, Tesco*	1 Serving/46g	138	10.6	301	21.1	0.4	23.0	0.0
Dolcelatte, Average	**1 Serving/30g**	**110**	**9.7**	**366**	**17.8**	**0.4**	**32.3**	**0.4**
Double Gloucester, Average	**1 Serving/30g**	**121**	**10.2**	**404**	**24.5**	**0.1**	**34.0**	**0.0**
Double Gloucester, with Onion & Chives, Sainsbury's*	1 Serving/30g	110	8.5	365	22.2	5.5	28.2	0.0
Doux De Montagne, Average	**1 Serving/25g**	**88**	**7.1**	**352**	**22.9**	**1.5**	**28.3**	**0.0**
Edam, Average	**1 Serving/10g**	**33**	**2.5**	**326**	**25.3**	**0.0**	**24.9**	**0.0**
Edam, Dutch, Garlic & Herb Wedge, Asda*	1 Serving/60g	197	15.0	329	26.0	0.0	25.0	0.0
Edam, Reduced Fat, Average	**1 Serving/30g**	**69**	**3.3**	**230**	**32.4**	**0.1**	**11.1**	**0.0**
Edam, Slices, Average	**1 Slice/30g**	**96**	**7.2**	**320**	**25.0**	**0.4**	**24.1**	**0.0**
Emmental, Average	**1 Serving/10g**	**37**	**2.8**	**368**	**28.4**	**0.0**	**28.4**	**0.0**

CHEESE

	Measure INFO/WEIGHT	per Measure KCAL	FAT	Nutrition Values per 100g / 100ml KCAL	PROT	CARB	FAT	FIBRE
Emmental, Light, Slices, President*	1 Slice/20g	60	3.6	298	34.0	0.0	18.0	0.0
Farmhouse, Reduced Fat, Healthy Range, Average	**1 Serving/30g**	**78**	**4.6**	**260**	**30.4**	**0.0**	**15.4**	**0.0**
Feta, Apetina, Light, 10 % Fat, Arla*	1 Serving/30g	52	3.0	173	18.4	0.6	10.1	0.0
Feta, Average	**1 Serving/30g**	**79**	**6.4**	**262**	**16.3**	**1.0**	**21.5**	**0.0**
Feta, Barrel Aged, TTD, Sainsbury's*	1 Serving/30g	83	6.9	276	16.5	0.7	23.0	0.2
Feta, Lemon, Asda*	1 Serving/25g	76	6.8	302	13.2	1.0	27.2	0.6
Feta, Light, Greek, Salad, 40% Reduced Fat, Attis*	1 Portion/30g	51	3.6	170	20.0	0.6	12.0	0.0
Fondue, Original, Fromalp*	1 Pack/400g	888	68.0	222	15.0	2.5	17.0	0.0
Fondue, Swiss, Easy Cook, Tesco*	¼ Pack/100g	235	17.0	235	15.5	4.0	17.0	0.0
Fondue, Traditionnelle, Co-Op*	1 Serving/100g	409	34.0	409	26.0	0.9	34.0	0.0
Fontina, Average	**1 Serving/28g**	**109**	**9.0**	**389**	**25.0**	**0.0**	**32.1**	**0.0**
for Pizza, Grated	**1 Serving/50g**	**163**	**12.2**	**326**	**25.0**	**1.6**	**24.4**	**0.0**
Goats, Average	**1 Tsp/10g**	**26**	**2.1**	**262**	**13.8**	**3.8**	**21.2**	**0.0**
Goats, Breaded, Bites, Sainsbury's*	1 Bite/25g	84	6.2	337	13.0	15.1	25.0	0.8
Goats, French, Mild, Average	**1 Serving/30g**	**49**	**3.5**	**163**	**11.2**	**3.0**	**11.8**	**0.0**
Goats, Premium, Average	**1 Serving/30g**	**98**	**7.8**	**327**	**20.5**	**0.6**	**26.1**	**0.0**
Goats, Soft, Average	**1 Serving/30g**	**79**	**6.3**	**262**	**16.7**	**1.8**	**20.8**	**0.5**
Gorgonzola, Average	**1 Serving/30g**	**100**	**8.1**	**334**	**20.0**	**0.0**	**27.0**	**0.0**
Gouda, Average	**1 Serving/30g**	**113**	**9.4**	**376**	**24.0**	**0.0**	**31.5**	**0.0**
Grana Padano, Italian Cheese, Waitrose*	1 Serving/14g	54	4.0	388	33.0	0.0	28.4	0.0
Gruyere	**1oz/28g**	**115**	**9.3**	**409**	**27.2**	**0.0**	**33.3**	**0.0**
Halloumi, Average	**1 Serving/80g**	**253**	**19.7**	**316**	**20.8**	**1.6**	**24.7**	**0.0**
Halloumi, Light Average	1 Serving/100g	245	15.3	245	24.7	1.7	15.3	0.0
Italian, Grated, Average	**1 Serving/30g**	**144**	**10.0**	**481**	**44.0**	**1.1**	**33.4**	**0.0**
Jarlsberg, Slices, Average	**1 Slice/15g**	**54**	**4.0**	**360**	**27.0**	**0.0**	**27.0**	**0.0**
Lactose Free, Arla*	1 Serving/30g	103	8.1	344	25.3	1.0	27.0	0.0
Lactose Free, Semi Hard, Lactofree, Arla*	1 Serving/30g	103	8.1	344	25.3	1.0	27.0	0.0
Lancashire	**1oz/28g**	**104**	**8.7**	**373**	**23.3**	**0.1**	**31.0**	**0.0**
Light Salad, Discover*	1oz/28g	61	3.6	216	24.0	1.0	13.0	0.0
Manchego	**1 Serving/70g**	**340**	**30.8**	**485**	**22.2**	**0.1**	**44.0**	**0.0**
Marscapone, Lighter, Tesco*	½ Tub/125g	306	26.9	245	9.5	3.0	21.5	0.0
Mascarpone, 25% Less Fat, Sainsbury's*	1 Portion/30g	95	9.0	316	6.7	4.8	30.0	0.0
Mascarpone, Average	**1 Serving/30g**	**131**	**13.1**	**437**	**5.6**	**4.1**	**43.6**	**0.0**
Mature, Full Flavoured, LowLow, Kerry*	1 Serving/30g	91	6.6	302	26.0	0.2	22.0	0.0
Mature, Half Fat, Average	1 Serving/25g	66	3.9	265	29.9	0.4	15.6	0.1
Mature Cheddar, Spread, Low Low, Kerry Group*	1 Serving/20g	41	3.0	205	13.0	5.0	15.0	0.0
Mild, Reduced Fat, Grated, Average	**1 Serving/30g**	**70**	**3.3**	**235**	**31.5**	**2.2**	**11.1**	**0.0**
Monterey Jack, Iga*	1 Serving/28g	110	9.0	393	25.0	0.0	32.1	0.0
Monterey Jack, Shredded, Kraft*	¼ Cup/28g	101	8.1	360	22.0	3.6	28.8	0.0
Morbier, Sainsbury's*	1 Serving/10g	33	2.4	330	28.0	0.1	24.2	0.0
Mozza-Cheddar, Light, Shredded, Kraft*	1/3 of a Cup/30g	80	6.0	267	26.7	3.3	20.0	0.0
Mozzarella, Average	**½ Ball/63g**	**172**	**12.9**	**275**	**21.2**	**1.2**	**20.6**	**0.0**
Mozzarella, Reduced Fat, Average	**½ Ball/63g**	**115**	**6.4**	**184**	**21.2**	**1.0**	**10.2**	**0.0**
Norvegia, Sliced Light, Tine*	1 Slice/10g	27	1.6	272	32.0	0.0	16.0	0.0
Ossau-Iraty, Average	**1 Serving/30g**	**120**	**10.2**	**400**	**22.3**	**0.2**	**34.0**	**0.0**
Parlick Fell, Hard, Sheeps, Sainsbury's*	1 Serving/30g	109	9.1	364	22.6	0.0	30.4	0.0
Parmesan, Average	**1 Tbsp/10g**	**40**	**2.9**	**401**	**35.2**	**0.0**	**29.4**	**0.0**
Pastrami Flavour, Sandwich, Swiss Processed, Gerber*	1 Slice/13g	44	3.5	348	24.0	0.0	28.0	0.0
Pecorino, Italian, Tesco*	1 Serving/30g	119	9.9	397	22.0	0.0	33.0	0.0
Philadelphia, for Salad, Kraft*	1 Pot/50g	158	15.2	315	6.6	2.6	30.5	0.5
Poivre, Boursin*	1oz/28g	116	11.8	414	7.0	2.0	42.0	0.0
Quark, Average	**1 Serving/20g**	**13**	**0.0**	**66**	**11.9**	**4.0**	**0.2**	**0.0**
Raclette, Richsmonts*	1 Slice/28g	100	8.0	357	25.0	0.0	28.6	0.0

CHEESE

INFO/WEIGHT	Measure	per Measure KCAL	FAT	Nutrition Values per 100g / 100ml KCAL	PROT	CARB	FAT	FIBRE
Reblochon	1 Serving/30g	95	8.0	318	19.7	0.0	26.6	0.0
Red Leicester, Average	1 Serving/30g	120	10.1	400	23.8	0.1	33.7	0.0
Red Leicester, Reduced Fat, Average	1 Serving/30g	78	4.6	261	30.2	0.1	15.4	0.0
Ricotta, Average	1 Serving/50g	67	4.8	134	9.3	2.9	9.5	0.0
Roquefort, Average	1oz/28g	105	9.2	375	19.7	0.0	32.9	0.0
Roule, French, Sainsbury's*	1 Serving/30g	96	9.2	321	8.5	3.0	30.5	0.0
Roule, Garlic & Parsley, Light, BGTY, Sainsbury's*	1 Serving/30g	51	3.2	171	16.4	2.6	10.6	0.0
Sage Derby	1oz/28g	113	9.5	402	24.2	0.1	33.9	0.0
Shropshire, Blue, Average	1 Serving/50g	196	17.1	391	21.0	0.0	34.2	0.0
Slices, Cheddar, Mexican Spices & Jalapeno, Tesco*	1 Slice/28g	105	8.4	375	22.7	2.5	30.1	0.8
Slices, Smoked with Ham, Aldi*	1 Slice/21g	66	5.2	313	21.0	1.0	25.0	0.1
Soft, 75 % Reduced Fat, BGTY, Sainsbury's*	1 Serving/30g	29	1.2	98	12.0	3.5	4.0	0.0
Soft, Cracked Pepper, Less Than 5% Fat, M&S*	1 Serving/30g	30	1.4	100	11.0	4.2	4.5	0.3
Soft, Extra Light, Average	1 Serving/20g	25	1.2	125	14.3	3.6	5.9	0.1
Soft, Full Fat, Average	1 Serving/50g	156	15.2	312	8.2	1.7	30.3	0.0
Soft, Garlic & Herb, Extra Light, LC, Tesco*	1 Serving/38g	49	2.4	130	12.3	5.1	6.3	0.3
Soft, Garlic & Herb, Roulade, M&S*	1 Portion/100g	295	27.3	295	7.8	4.1	27.3	1.3
Soft, Herbs & Garlic, Creamery, Light, Sainsbury's*	1 Serving/30g	54	4.6	180	7.2	3.4	15.5	0.3
Soft, Light, Average	1 Tbsp/30g	54	3.9	179	12.1	3.2	13.1	0.0
Soft, Medium Fat, Average	1 Serving/30g	62	5.4	207	8.4	3.0	17.9	0.0
Soft, Onion & Chives, Extra Light, LC, Tesco*	1 Serving/30g	38	1.8	125	11.7	5.6	6.0	0.2
Soft, Philadelphia, Basil, Light, Kraft*	1 Serving/35g	51	3.7	146	8.0	4.0	10.5	0.5
Soft, Philadelphia, Blue, Kraft*	1 Serving/28g	76	7.1	270	6.8	3.4	25.5	0.2
Soft, Philadelphia, Cadbury Chocolate, Mini Tubs, Kraft*	1 Mini Tub/30g	86	4.0	287	6.5	34.0	13.3	1.7
Soft, Philadelphia, Extra Light, Kraft*	1 Serving/30g	33	1.4	110	11.7	5.0	4.7	0.3
Soft, Philadelphia, Garlic & Herb, Light, Kraft*	1 Serving/30g	46	3.3	154	7.8	5.4	11.0	0.3
Soft, Philadelphia, Light, Kraft*	1 Serving/30g	47	3.5	157	8.7	4.0	11.7	0.3
Soft, Philadelphia, Mini Tubs, Cracked Pepper, Kraft*	1 Tub/35g	56	4.6	161	7.7	2.5	13.0	0.4
Soft, Philadelphia, Mini Tubs, Extra Light, Kraft*	1 Tub/35g	38	1.8	108	11.0	4.2	5.0	0.6
Soft, Philadelphia, Mini Tubs, Light, Kraft*	1 Tub/35g	55	4.0	158	8.7	4.0	11.5	0.4
Soft, Philadelphia, Original, Full Fat, Kraft*	1 Serving/30g	76	7.2	253	6.0	3.3	24.0	0.3
Soft, Philadelphia, with Chives, Light, Kraft*	1 Serving/30g	48	3.6	160	8.3	4.3	12.0	0.7
Soft, Pineapple Halo, Discover*	1 Serving/25g	101	8.2	404	7.2	16.6	32.6	1.2
Soft, Tomato & Basil, Sun Dried, Light, Kraft*	1/8 Pack/25g	39	2.8	157	8.3	4.8	11.0	0.4
Soft, White, Lactofree, Arla*	1 Serving/30g	59	5.0	197	8.6	3.0	16.5	0.0
Soft, with Black Pepper, Light, Sainsbury's*	½ Pack/100g	205	16.5	205	11.0	3.0	16.5	0.0
Soft, with Garlic & Herbs, Full Fat, Deli, Boursin*	1 Serving/28g	84	8.3	299	3.5	5.0	29.5	0.0
Soft, with Garlic & Herbs, Lighter, Asda*	½ Pack/100g	106	4.4	106	11.8	4.3	4.4	0.1
Soft, with Garlic & Herbs, Medium Fat, Westacre*	1 Serving/30g	56	4.8	188	8.0	3.0	16.0	0.1
Soft, with Garlic & Herbs, Sainsbury's*	1 Serving/33g	89	8.6	269	6.1	2.7	26.0	0.0
Soft, with Onion & Chives, Lighter, Asda*	1 Serving/30g	32	1.3	105	11.6	4.5	4.3	0.2
Soft, with Roasted Onion & Chive, Weight Watchers*	¼ Pack/50g	46	1.4	92	12.4	4.5	2.7	2.5
Soft & Creamy, with Pineapple, Asda*	1 Serving/32g	62	4.2	193	8.0	11.0	13.0	0.0
Stilton, Average	1 Serving/30g	123	10.6	410	22.4	0.1	35.5	0.0
Stilton, Blue, Average	1 Serving/30g	124	10.7	412	22.8	0.1	35.7	0.0
Stilton, White, & Apricot, M&S*	1oz/28g	94	6.5	337	13.8	18.5	23.1	0.0
Stilton, White, Average	1oz/28g	101	8.8	362	19.9	0.1	31.3	0.0
Stilton, White, with Apricot, Somerfield*	1oz/28g	103	8.4	369	16.0	8.0	30.0	0.0
Stilton, White, with Cranberries, Tesco*	1 Serving/50g	184	14.8	368	15.8	9.5	29.7	0.7
Stilton, White, with Mango & Ginger, Tesco*	1/3 Pack/65g	228	14.0	350	13.1	25.8	21.6	0.6
Stilton White, & Cranberry, M&S*	1oz/28g	101	7.1	362	18.2	15.5	25.3	0.0
Taleggio D.o.p., Finest, Tesco*	1 Serving/30g	89	7.5	297	18.0	0.0	25.0	0.0
Wedge, Leerdammer*	1 Serving/30g	112	8.6	373	28.3	0.0	28.6	0.0

CHEESE	Measure INFO/WEIGHT	per Measure KCAL	FAT	Nutrition Values per 100g / 100ml KCAL	PROT	CARB	FAT	FIBRE
Wedges, Camembert, Breaded, Morrisons*	1 Wedge/25g	88	5.6	352	15.1	22.9	22.2	2.0
Wensleydale, & Ginger, Truckle, Morrisons*	1 Truckle/90g	330	23.7	367	18.0	14.0	26.3	1.1
Wensleydale, Average	*1 Serving/25g*	*92*	*7.8*	*369*	*22.4*	*0.1*	*31.0*	*0.0*
Wensleydale, Cranberry & Mustard, Lozzas	1 Block/50g	179	13.9	359	20.7	6.4	27.8	0.0
Wensleydale, with Blueberries, M&S*	1 Portion/30g	111	7.9	370	18.7	13.4	26.4	0.9
Wensleydale, with Cranberries, Sainsbury's*	1 Serving/50g	180	13.9	359	20.7	6.4	27.8	0.0
CHEESE ALTERNATIVE								
Cheezly, Cheddar, Garlic & Herb, The Redwood Co*	1 Serving/25g	62	4.4	249	3.6	19.4	17.4	0.0
Cheezly, Cream, Garlic & Herb, The Redwood Co*	1 Pack/113g	360	34.5	319	5.8	5.4	30.5	0.0
Cheezly, Cream, Original, The Redwood Co*	1 Pack/113g	357	34.5	316	5.6	4.8	30.5	0.0
Cheezly, Feta Style in Oil, The Redwood Co*	1 Serving/25g	119	11.8	475	2.5	10.6	47.0	0.0
Cheezly, Grated Cheddar Style, The Redwood Co*	1 Pack/150g	242	11.2	161	3.1	21.5	7.5	0.0
Cheezly, Mature Cheddar, Cranberry, The Redwood Co*	1 Serving/25g	60	3.6	239	3.2	24.3	14.3	0.0
Cheezly, Mozzarella Style, The Redwood Co*	1 Portion/25g	69	6.4	274	5.4	5.9	25.4	1.0
Cheezly, Nacho Style, The Redwood Co*	1 Serving/25g	42	2.0	169	3.3	21.1	7.9	0.0
Mozzarella, Slices, Dairy Free	1 Slice/19g	80	6.0	420	10.5	10.5	31.5	0.0
Vegetarian, Average	1 Serving/30g	110	8.4	368	28.2	0.0	28.1	0.0
CHEESE DIPPERS								
Original, The Laughing Cow, Fromageries Bel*	1 Pack/35g	101	6.0	288	11.0	25.0	17.0	0.0
CHEESE HEADS								
Cheese & Onion, Walkers*	1 Bag/27g	128	6.0	475	10.8	58.0	22.3	2.8
CHEESE ON TOAST								
Average	1 Slice/130g	494	34.2	380	13.8	23.8	26.3	0.7
CHEESE PUFFS								
Average	1 Bag/25g	129	7.4	517	7.8	54.8	29.5	1.5
Cheeky, Tesco*	1 Bag/20g	108	7.0	542	6.7	50.2	34.9	0.0
Healthy Range, Average	1 Bag/25g	113	3.8	454	7.6	71.2	15.0	2.2
Morrisons*	1 Bag/25g	136	8.7	542	6.7	50.2	34.9	1.1
Sainsbury's*	1 Pack/100g	530	32.0	530	9.1	51.4	32.0	1.9
Shapers, Boots*	1 Bag/16g	80	3.8	500	7.1	64.0	24.0	0.9
Value, Tesco*	1 Pack/16g	84	4.6	525	6.2	60.0	28.8	0.6
CHEESE SINGLES								
Healthy Range, Average	1 Slice/20g	39	2.1	197	20.6	5.2	10.4	0.0
Kraft*	1 Single/20g	52	3.7	260	13.5	7.6	18.5	0.0
CHEESE SLICES								
Average	1 Slice/23g	82	6.6	358	24.0	0.8	28.6	0.0
Cheddar, Mild, Value, Tesco*	1 Slice/24g	100	8.4	410	25.0	0.1	34.4	0.0
Gouda, Tesco*	1 Slice/25g	94	7.5	375	23.0	0.1	30.0	0.0
Havarti, Tesco*	1 Slice/25g	85	6.5	340	24.0	1.4	26.0	0.0
Healthy Range, Average	1 Slice/25g	45	2.2	180	19.5	5.4	9.0	0.0
Jarlsberg, Tesco*	1 Slice/25g	91	7.0	365	27.5	0.0	28.0	0.0
Leerdammer*	1 Slice/25g	90	7.0	358	27.0	0.1	28.0	0.0
Light, The Laughing Cow, Fromageries Bel*	1 Slice/20g	41	2.1	203	21.0	6.0	10.5	0.0
Red Leicester, Tesco*	1 Slice/30g	120	10.1	400	23.7	0.0	33.7	0.0
CHEESE SPREAD								
60% Less Fat, Asda*	1 Serving/30g	52	2.7	174	16.0	7.3	9.0	0.0
Asda*	1 Serving/33g	92	7.9	280	9.0	7.0	24.0	0.0
Average	1 Serving/30g	76	6.4	254	9.4	5.9	21.4	0.1
Cheese & Garlic, Primula*	1 Serving/20g	49	3.7	247	15.7	4.3	18.6	0.0
Cheese & Ham, Primula*	1 Serving/20g	40	3.0	200	12.3	3.1	15.0	4.9
Cheese & Salmon, with Dill, Primula*	1 Serving/30g	78	5.8	261	17.6	3.8	19.5	0.0
Cheez Whiz, Original, Light, 41% Less Fat, Kraft*	1 Tbsp/15g	32	1.7	210	15.7	11.7	11.3	0.0
Cream, Light, Sainsbury's*	1 Serving/50g	94	7.8	187	7.8	4.1	15.5	0.3

INFO/WEIGHT	Measure	per Measure		Nutrition Values per 100g / 100ml				
		KCAL	FAT	KCAL	PROT	CARB	FAT	FIBRE
CHEESE SPREAD								
Creamery, Light, Sainsbury's*	1 Serving/25g	46	3.8	185	9.0	3.5	15.0	0.0
Dairylea, Light, Tub, Kraft*	1 Serving/30g	44	2.1	147	14.5	6.1	7.0	0.0
Dairylea, Tub, Kraft*	1 Serving/25g	60	4.9	240	11.0	5.3	19.5	0.0
Flavoured	1oz/28g	72	5.7	258	14.2	4.4	20.5	0.0
Garlic & Herbs, Light, Benecol*	1 Serving/20g	35	2.8	174	7.8	4.2	14.0	0.7
Healthy Range, Average	1 Serving/30g	31	1.0	102	14.3	3.8	3.2	0.9
Light, Primula*	1 Serving/20g	30	1.8	149	15.2	3.0	8.9	3.6
Low Fat, Weight Watchers*	1 Serving/50g	56	1.4	112	18.1	3.4	2.9	1.2
Mediterranean Soft & Creamy, Extra Light, Asda*	1 Serving/32g	42	1.9	130	13.0	6.0	6.0	0.0
Plain, Original, Primula*	1 Serving/30g	60	4.6	200	12.1	3.3	15.3	4.4
Soft, Low Fat, M&S*	1 Pack/100g	111	4.5	111	13.0	4.2	4.5	0.3
Squeeze, Light, The Laughing Cow*	1 Portion/30g	42	2.1	139	12.0	7.0	7.0	5.0
Squeeze, Original, The Laughing Cow*	1 Portion/30g	71	6.0	236	9.0	5.0	20.0	0.0
Triangles, 50% Less Fat, Morrisons*	1 Portion/18g	29	1.4	166	15.0	8.5	8.0	0.0
with Chives, Primula*	1 Serving/30g	57	4.3	190	12.5	2.9	14.2	4.5
with Prawn, Primula*	1 Squeeze/25g	48	3.6	190	12.5	3.3	14.4	3.6
CHEESE STRAWS								
& Bacon, Party, Tesco*	1 Straw/13g	40	2.6	321	10.5	23.8	20.4	2.1
Cheddar, M&S*	1 Straw/11g	59	3.8	535	14.9	40.1	34.9	2.4
Cheese Twists, Tesco*	1 Serving/20g	99	5.6	494	14.0	46.4	28.0	4.2
Finest, Tesco*	1 Straw/7g	39	2.6	558	13.3	41.5	37.6	1.5
Fudges*	1 Serving/10g	53	3.5	534	14.9	40.1	34.9	0.0
Homemade or Bakery, Average	1 Straw/41g	173	12.6	422	12.0	24.2	30.7	0.7
Selection, Sainsbury's*	1 Straw/7g	41	2.9	558	16.6	34.5	39.3	2.8
CHEESE TRIANGLES								
Average	1 Triangle/14g	33	2.2	238	10.3	14.2	15.6	0.2
Dairylea, Light, Kraft*	1 Triangle/18g	36	2.2	205	15.5	6.3	12.5	0.0
Emmental, Light, The Laughing Cow*	1 Triangle/16g	25	1.5	155	12.0	6.0	9.0	0.0
Extra Light, The Laughing Cow, Fromageries Bel*	1 Triangle/18g	20	0.5	116	15.0	6.5	3.0	0.0
Light, Creamy Swiss, The Laughing Cow *	1 Triangle/18g	25	1.2	143	13.7	6.8	6.8	0.0
Light Choices, Tesco*	1 Triangle/18g	30	1.2	170	17.5	8.5	7.0	0.0
Original, The Laughing Cow, Fromageries Bel*	1 Triangle/18g	42	3.3	239	11.0	6.0	19.0	0.0
Reduced Fat, Average	1 Triangle/18g	27	1.2	154	15.4	7.0	7.0	0.0
Tri-Bites, Dairylea, Kraft*	1 Triangle/20g	60	4.6	300	20.0	3.2	23.0	0.0
CHEESE TWISTS								
All Butter, M&S*	1 Pack/125g	625	33.4	500	14.2	50.2	26.7	3.2
Asda*	1 Twist/8g	42	2.4	500	14.0	48.0	28.0	5.0
Gruyere & Poppy Seed, Truly Irresistible, Co-Op*	1 Twist/8g	42	2.4	520	13.2	48.8	30.1	2.5
Pre Packed, Average	1 Twist/8g	41	2.2	515	13.7	47.9	27.7	2.3
CHEESECAKE								
After Noon, Mango & Passionfruit, 3 Pack, Gu*	1 Portion/45g	155	11.3	345	3.4	26.5	25.2	0.4
American, Red White & Blueberry, Sainsbury's*	1/6 Cake/83g	264	15.4	318	3.8	35.1	18.5	0.4
Apple & Cinnamon, Baked, M&S*	1 Serving/116g	390	22.0	335	3.7	39.7	18.9	2.1
Apricot, Co-Op*	1 Cake/100g	230	11.0	230	4.0	29.0	11.0	0.9
Autumn Berry, Waitrose*	1 Slice/92g	316	20.3	343	4.4	31.5	22.1	2.0
Average	1 Slice/115g	490	40.8	426	3.7	24.6	35.5	0.4
Blackcurrant, Average	1 Serving/90g	237	11.9	263	3.6	32.3	13.2	2.4
Blackcurrant, Healthy Range, Average	1 Serving/90g	182	4.7	203	4.7	33.6	5.3	2.1
Blackcurrant, PB, Waitrose*	1/6 Cake/99g	212	3.6	214	4.0	39.6	3.6	2.4
Blackcurrant, Sainsbury's*	1 Serving/100g	238	9.3	238	3.9	34.6	9.3	1.3
Blackcurrant, Value, Tesco*	1 Serving/70g	174	8.6	248	2.8	31.4	12.3	1.0
Blackcurrant, VLH Kitchens	1 Serving/120g	341	13.7	285	3.4	32.0	16.4	0.9
Blackcurrant, Weight Watchers*	1 Cake/103g	191	2.9	185	4.6	35.4	2.8	3.5

CHEESECAKE

	Measure INFO/WEIGHT	per Measure KCAL	FAT	Nutrition Values per 100g / 100ml KCAL	PROT	CARB	FAT	FIBRE
Blueberry, & Lemon Flavour Wedges, Sainsbury's*	1 Serving/80g	262	16.9	327	5.1	29.2	21.1	1.2
Blueberry, & Vanilla, TTD, Sainsbury's*	1 Serving/95g	353	24.8	372	5.4	28.9	26.1	2.1
Blueberry, Gorgeous, Cooked, Aunt Bessie's*	1 Portion/75g	225	6.2	300	3.9	33.5	8.2	0.9
Caramel Swirl, Cadbury*	1 Slice/91g	373	23.5	410	6.0	40.1	25.8	0.0
Cherry, BGTY, Sainsbury's*	1 Serving/91g	181	3.9	199	4.6	35.5	4.3	0.5
Cherry, Healthy Range, Average	1 Serving/90g	172	3.0	191	3.7	36.4	3.3	1.1
Chocolate, & Hazelnut, Sara Lee*	1 Serving/65g	224	13.9	345	6.5	31.2	21.4	1.2
Chocolate, & Irish Cream Liqueur, Tesco*	1 Serving/93g	385	28.0	414	5.0	30.7	30.1	0.8
Chocolate, & Vanilla, Gu*	1 Pot/90g	379	27.1	421	4.1	34.6	30.1	1.6
Chocolate, & Vanilla, Tesco*	1 Serving/90g	330	19.4	365	5.2	37.1	21.5	1.6
Chocolate, Average	1 Serving/75g	265	15.7	353	5.7	35.6	20.9	1.9
Chocolate, Baked, Ultimate, Entenmann's*	1 Serving/100g	331	19.0	331	5.7	34.2	19.0	2.8
Chocolate, Belgian, M&S*	1 Slice/100g	385	23.9	385	5.3	39.2	23.9	2.5
Chocolate, Double, Wedge, Sainsbury's*	1 Serving/75g	327	24.8	436	5.7	29.0	33.0	1.7
Chocolate, Pure Indulgence, Thorntons*	1 Serving/75g	308	17.6	410	5.6	44.3	23.4	0.6
Chocolate, Swirl, Deeply Delicious, Heinz*	1/5 Cake/82g	221	9.4	271	4.6	37.4	11.5	4.7
Chocolate, Tesco*	1 Serving/91g	317	17.4	348	6.2	37.8	19.1	1.5
Chocolate, Weight Watchers*	1 Cake/95g	143	3.8	151	7.5	20.7	4.0	0.7
Citrus, Good Choice, Mini, Iceland*	1 Cake/111g	198	4.7	178	3.5	31.6	4.2	0.4
Commercially Prepared	1/6 Cake/80g	257	18.0	321	5.5	25.5	22.5	0.4
Fruit, Average	1 Serving/75g	207	10.9	276	5.3	32.3	14.5	1.6
Fudge, Tesco*	1 Serving/102g	384	23.6	376	4.6	37.5	23.1	0.5
Indulgent with Liqueur, Average	1 Serving/90g	366	23.4	406	5.0	38.2	26.0	0.8
Lemon, Asda*	1 Slice/90g	319	21.2	354	4.3	31.2	23.5	1.1
Lemon, Average	1 Serving/90g	307	19.5	341	4.1	33.0	21.6	1.8
Lemon, BGTY, Sainsbury's*	1/6 Cake/71g	142	2.7	200	4.4	37.0	3.8	0.5
Lemon, Healthy Range, Average	1 Serving/90g	185	4.0	205	5.4	33.6	4.4	1.2
Lemon, Sainsbury's*	1 Serving/180g	650	37.1	361	4.0	39.9	20.6	1.3
Lemon, Swirl, Asda*	1 Pack/125g	445	29.9	356	3.1	32.1	23.9	1.8
Lemon, Tesco*	1 Slice/93g	315	21.0	339	5.2	28.6	22.6	0.3
Lemon, Value, Tesco*	1 Serving/79g	221	11.8	281	4.3	32.2	15.0	4.2
Lemon, Weight Watchers*	1 Serving/100g	211	5.0	211	6.3	30.1	5.0	1.8
Lemon Creamy & Light, M&S*	1/6 Cake/68g	236	13.8	350	3.5	32.3	20.4	0.4
Lemon Meringue, Tesco*	1 Slice/94g	352	25.0	375	3.8	30.1	26.6	0.3
Mandarin, Morrisons*	1 Serving/135g	335	16.9	248	3.8	32.2	12.5	0.8
Millionaires, Belgian Chocolate, Bistro, Morrisons*	1 Pot/128g	469	27.2	366	2.8	40.4	21.2	1.4
Raspberry, BGTY, Sainsbury's*	1 Pot/95g	154	2.5	163	6.6	28.2	2.6	2.8
Raspberry, Creamy, Tesco*	1 Serving/100g	365	23.4	365	5.9	32.1	23.4	0.9
Raspberry, LC, Tesco*	1 Cake/95g	185	4.1	195	4.3	34.7	4.3	1.3
Raspberry, M&S*	1 Slice/105g	331	21.5	315	5.0	32.2	20.5	1.0
Raspberry, PB, Waitrose*	1 Serving/106g	212	3.7	200	4.0	36.2	3.5	1.7
Raspberry, Weight Watchers*	1 Serving/100g	213	4.3	213	5.9	29.7	4.3	1.9
Raspberry & Mascarpone, Best, Morrisons*	1 Cake/84g	257	14.0	306	3.9	34.8	16.7	1.0
Raspberry & Strawberry, M&S*	1 Slice/105g	340	21.1	325	3.9	33.4	20.2	1.2
Raspberry Brulee, M&S*	1 Serving/100g	255	12.9	255	5.7	29.7	12.9	2.1
Raspberry Rapture, Slices, Tesco*	1 Slice/110g	341	20.4	310	4.2	30.8	18.5	1.8
Raspberry Swirl, Heinz*	1 Serving/100g	266	14.5	266	3.9	30.1	14.5	2.8
Rhubarb Crumble, Sainsbury's*	1 Serving/114g	268	10.6	235	3.1	34.8	9.3	2.4
Sticky Toffee, Tesco*	1 Slice/66g	248	16.0	375	4.0	35.3	24.2	0.5
Strawberry, & Cream, Finest, Tesco*	1 Serving/104g	325	22.4	312	4.3	25.3	21.5	0.5
Strawberry, & Devonshire Cream, Heinz*	1/6 Cake/66g	184	10.1	279	3.9	31.4	15.3	3.7
Strawberry, Baked New York, Sara Lee*	1 Serving/100g	248	9.9	248	4.7	34.9	9.9	0.7
Strawberry, Creamy, Weight Watchers*	1 Cake/105g	187	2.6	178	4.7	34.2	2.5	2.2

	Measure INFO/WEIGHT	per Measure KCAL	FAT	Nutrition Values per 100g / 100ml KCAL	PROT	CARB	FAT	FIBRE
CHEESECAKE								
Strawberry, Devonshire, McVitie's*	1/6 Cake/66g	192	10.7	291	4.4	31.8	16.2	3.6
Strawberry, Finest, Tesco*	1 Slice/113g	383	25.1	339	4.8	30.1	22.2	0.9
Strawberry, Fresh, M&S*	¼ Cake/125g	300	19.2	240	2.8	23.1	15.4	1.1
Strawberry, Frozen, Sainsbury's*	1/6 Cake/84g	277	14.2	332	4.3	40.4	17.0	2.3
Strawberry, Shortcake, Sara Lee*	1/6 Slice/68g	230	15.7	337	4.9	27.6	23.0	0.5
Strawberry, Swirl, CBY, Asda*	1 Serving/100g	329	15.9	329	4.5	41.5	15.9	1.0
Strawberry, Tesco*	1 Serving/100g	254	12.0	254	3.9	32.5	12.0	0.0
The Ultimate New York Baked, Entenmann's*	1 Cake/100g	347	21.3	347	4.2	35.7	21.3	0.9
Toffee, American Style, Asda*	1 Serving/75g	269	15.8	359	4.5	38.0	21.0	3.8
Toffee, Asda*	1 Cake/87g	295	19.1	339	4.3	31.0	22.0	3.5
Toffee, M&S*	1 Serving/105g	357	22.6	340	5.2	37.2	21.5	0.9
Toffee, Morrisons*	1 Serving/100g	341	17.4	341	5.5	40.4	17.4	0.0
Toffee, Tesco*	1 Serving/100g	265	12.9	265	4.3	33.1	12.9	0.8
Toffee & Pecan, Wedge, Sainsbury's*	1 Serving/75g	296	21.8	395	5.4	28.1	29.0	3.1
Vanilla	1 Serving/100g	395	26.2	395	5.3	42.8	26.2	1.1
Vanilla, Creamy, New York, Slices, Tesco*	1 Slice/106g	371	26.7	350	4.6	25.9	25.2	2.2
Vanilla, Tesco*	1 Serving/115g	417	28.4	363	5.7	29.4	24.7	0.6
Vanilla Chocolate, Baked, Slice, Sainsbury's*	1 Slice/90g	349	23.0	388	5.7	33.8	25.6	2.7
Zesty Lemon, M&S*	1/6 Cake/97g	325	18.9	335	4.0	38.7	19.5	2.6
CHERRIES								
Black, Fresh, Average	*1 Serving/80g*	*41*	*0.1*	*51*	*0.9*	*11.5*	*0.1*	*1.6*
Black in Syrup, Average	*1 Serving/242g*	*160*	*0.0*	*66*	*0.6*	*16.0*	*0.0*	*0.7*
Dried, Love Life, Waitrose*	1 Portion/10g	35	0.1	348	0.2	84.3	1.1	2.1
Dried, Sainsbury's*	1 Tbsp/14g	45	0.2	319	3.8	72.4	1.5	6.2
Dried, Sweetened, Sour, Love Life, Waitrose*	1 Bag/80g	293	1.0	366	1.3	86.0	1.2	2.7
Dried, Wholefoods, Tesco*	1 Serving/25g	86	0.2	345	1.9	81.6	0.8	4.6
Glace, Average	*1oz/28g*	*79*	*0.0*	*280*	*0.4*	*71.2*	*0.2*	*1.1*
Picota, Average	1 Serving/80g	42	0.1	52	0.9	11.4	0.1	1.2
Raw, Average	*1oz/28g*	*14*	*0.0*	*49*	*0.9*	*11.2*	*0.1*	*1.4*
Stewed, with Sugar, Average	*1oz/28g*	*23*	*0.0*	*82*	*0.7*	*21.0*	*0.1*	*0.7*
Stewed, without Sugar, Average	*1oz/28g*	*12*	*0.0*	*42*	*0.8*	*10.1*	*0.1*	*0.8*
CHESTNUTS								
Roasted, Peeled, Average	*1 Nut/10g*	*17*	*0.3*	*170*	*2.0*	*36.6*	*2.7*	*4.1*
CHEWING GUM								
Airwaves, Sugar Free, Wrigleys*	1 Pack/15g	23	0.0	155	0.0	62.0	0.0	0.0
Extra, Cool Breeze, Wrigleys*	1 Piece/2g	3	0.0	153	0.0	64.0	0.0	0.0
Extra, Peppermint, Sugar Free, Wrigleys*	1 Piece/2g	3	0.0	155	0.0	39.0	0.0	0.0
Peppermint, Soft, Sugar Free, Trident*	1 Stick/3g	4	0.0	155	0.4	62.3	0.4	0.0
Spearmint, Extra, Wrigleys*	1 Piece/1g	1	0.0	143	0.0	64.3	0.0	0.0
Spearmint, Wrigleys*	1 Piece/3g	9	0.0	295	0.0	73.0	0.0	0.0
Splash, Raspberry & Peach, Trident*	1 Piece/2g	4	0.0	180	1.6	68.5	0.5	0.0
Sugar Free, Pulse, Crisp Tropical Flavour, Wrigleys*	1 Stick/1g	2	0.0	161	0.0	65.0	0.0	0.0
CHICK PEAS								
Bombay Firecracker Flavour, Dry Roasted, Garbanzo*	1 Bag/65g	88	1.3	135	10.2	23.8	2.0	7.4
Canned, Drained, Average	1 Can/240g	276	6.0	115	7.4	15.2	2.5	4.6
Dried, Average	*1 Serving/100g*	*319*	*5.4*	*319*	*21.7*	*47.4*	*5.4*	*8.0*
Dried, Boiled, Average	*1 Serving/75g*	*85*	*1.7*	*114*	*7.3*	*16.4*	*2.2*	*2.6*
in Salted Water, Canned, Average	*1 Can/179g*	*204*	*5.2*	*114*	*7.2*	*14.9*	*2.9*	*4.1*
in Water, Canned, Average	*1 Can/250g*	*282*	*6.6*	*113*	*7.2*	*15.3*	*2.6*	*4.8*
Thai Sweet Chilli Flavour, Dry Roasted, Garbanzo*	1 Bag/65g	88	1.3	135	10.2	23.8	2.0	7.4
Tomato, Garlic & Herb Flavour, Dry Roasted, Garbanzo*	1 Pack/65g	88	1.3	135	10.2	23.8	2.0	7.4
CHICKEN								
BBQ Slices, Morrisons*	½ Pack/75g	101	0.8	135	23.9	7.5	1.1	0.0

CHICKEN

	Measure INFO/WEIGHT	per Measure		Nutrition Values per 100g / 100ml				
		KCAL	FAT	KCAL	PROT	CARB	FAT	FIBRE
Bites, Battered, Tesco*	1 Pack/200g	440	28.6	220	15.2	7.6	14.3	2.0
Bites, Hot & Spicy, Tesco*	1 Pack/110g	143	1.8	130	18.9	9.6	1.6	2.5
Bites, in Light Batter, Captain Birds Eye, Birds Eye*	1 Piece/15g	32	1.9	210	18.6	5.8	12.5	0.2
Bites, Southern Fried, Tesco*	1 Pack/300g	720	33.3	240	18.1	16.9	11.1	2.1
Bites, Tikka, Average	1 Serving/50g	96	5.3	193	20.7	3.8	10.5	1.9
Breast, Basil Pesto & Parmesan Crust, COOK!, M&S*	½ Pack/150g	240	11.0	160	20.9	1.8	7.3	0.8
Breast, Chargrill Style, Slices, Asda*	1 Slice/28g	31	0.6	112	22.7	0.8	2.0	0.0
Breast, Chargrilled, Lime & Coriander, Asda*	1 Breast/160g	260	11.2	163	25.0	0.1	7.0	1.5
Breast, Chargrilled, Premium, Average	1 Piece/10g	20	1.1	197	21.6	1.5	11.2	0.3
Breast, Chargrilled, Sliced, Average	1 Slice/19g	24	0.5	124	24.4	0.5	2.7	0.4
Breast, Chinese Style, Cooked, Sliced, Sainsbury's*	½ Pack/65g	96	1.2	148	28.3	4.7	1.8	0.1
Breast, Diced, Average	**1 Serving/188g**	**242**	**4.4**	**129**	**26.9**	**0.1**	**2.4**	**0.1**
Breast, Escalope, Pesto Chargrilled, M&S*	1 Serving/100g	135	6.2	135	19.6	0.7	6.2	0.6
Breast, Escalope, Plain, Average	**1 Serving/100g**	**110**	**2.2**	**110**	**22.3**	**0.7**	**2.2**	**0.5**
Breast, Fillets, Breaded, Average	1 Fillet/112g	246	11.6	220	17.6	14.0	10.4	1.3
Breast, Fillets, Breaded, Lemon & Pepper, Average	1 Fillet/89g	133	2.0	150	22.0	10.1	2.3	1.3
Breast, Fillets, Cajun, Average	1 Fillet/93g	124	2.6	134	23.6	3.5	2.8	0.3
Breast, Fillets, Chargrilled, Average	1 Serving/100g	120	1.1	120	27.3	0.3	1.1	0.3
Breast, Fillets, Frozen, Value, Tesco*	1 Breast/125g	125	2.1	100	20.4	0.7	1.7	0.0
Breast, Fillets, Garlic & Herb, Tesco*	1 Fillet/135g	290	12.2	215	18.9	14.4	9.0	1.3
Breast, Fillets, Garlic & Herb Marinated, Mini, Morrisons*	1 Pack/300g	336	3.0	112	20.2	4.9	1.0	0.5
Breast, Fillets, Korma Style, Average	1 Serving/100g	132	2.8	132	27.4	0.8	2.8	0.6
Breast, Fillets, Lemon Parsley, M&S*	½ Pack/145g	232	3.5	160	14.3	20.7	2.4	4.3
Breast, Fillets, Lime & Coriander, Just Add, M&S*	1 Pack/140g	182	2.4	130	26.1	2.7	1.7	0.1
Breast, Fillets, Mexican Style, Ready to Eat, Asda*	½ Pack/100g	147	1.5	147	27.8	5.5	1.5	0.1
Breast, Fillets, Mini, Raw, Average	**1oz/28g**	**34**	**0.4**	**121**	**26.9**	**0.2**	**1.5**	**0.1**
Breast, Fillets, Mini, Smoky BBQ Marinade, CBY, Asda*	3 Fillets/150g	144	1.5	96	18.5	3.3	1.0	0.0
Breast, Fillets, Organic, Average	**1 Serving/150g**	**153**	**1.1**	**102**	**24.0**	**0.0**	**0.8**	**0.0**
Breast, Fillets, Skinless & Boneless, Raw, Average	**1 Breast/100g**	**129**	**2.0**	**129**	**27.8**	**0.0**	**2.0**	**0.0**
Breast, Fillets, Slices, Red Thai, Mini, Tesco*	2 Slices/65g	81	0.6	125	25.8	2.4	0.9	0.5
Breast, Fillets, Sundried Tomato & Basil, M&S*	½ Pack/110g	165	4.5	150	22.5	4.7	4.1	1.1
Breast, Fillets, Tikka, Mini, Ready to Eat, Tesco*	½ Pack/95g	120	1.8	125	22.4	4.2	1.9	0.2
Breast, Grilled, Average	**1 Breast/130g**	**174**	**2.8**	**134**	**29.0**	**0.1**	**2.2**	**0.0**
Breast, in Breadcrumbs, Southern Fried, Birds Eye*	1 Breast/88g	240	12.0	273	15.9	20.4	13.6	1.2
Breast, Joint, Ready to Roast, CBY, Asda*	1 Serving/100g	141	5.4	141	22.7	0.1	5.4	0.5
Breast, Joint, with Sage & Onion Stuffing, CBY, Asda*	1 Serving/150g	213	6.9	142	21.1	3.7	4.6	0.5
Breast, Meat & Skin, Raw, Average	**1 Serving/145g**	**249**	**13.4**	**172**	**20.8**	**0.0**	**9.2**	**0.0**
Breast, Meat & Skin, Weighed with Bone, Raw, Average	**1oz/28g**	**48**	**2.6**	**172**	**20.8**	**0.0**	**9.2**	**0.0**
Breast, Pieces, Tikka, Average	1 Serving/100g	154	3.4	154	28.2	2.8	3.4	0.4
Breast, Piri Piri Marinade, Simply Cook, Tesco*	½ Pack/150g	235	9.0	157	23.8	1.9	6.0	0.1
Breast, Roast, Sliced, From Supermarket, Average	**1 Slice/13g**	**17**	**0.4**	**139**	**25.0**	**1.8**	**3.5**	**0.2**
Breast, Roast, without Skin, Average	**1oz/28g**	**42**	**1.3**	**149**	**25.4**	**1.0**	**4.7**	**0.2**
Breast, Roll, Average	**1 Slice/10g**	**17**	**1.0**	**167**	**16.1**	**3.2**	**10.0**	**0.2**
Breast, Short Sliced, Mexican, Sainsbury's*	1 Pack/130g	177	2.9	136	26.4	2.5	2.2	0.1
Breast, Sliced, in Sweet Chilli, Cooked, Sainsbury's*	1/6 Pack/50g	69	0.8	138	26.4	4.4	1.5	0.7
Breast, Sliced, Mexican Style, Cooked, Asda*	1 Pack/234g	307	5.1	131	25.5	4.3	2.2	0.1
Breast, Slices, Roast, Hot 'n' Spicy, Sainsbury's*	½ Pack/65g	91	1.0	139	27.1	3.9	1.6	0.1
Breast, Smoked, Sliced, Average	**1 Slice/20g**	**22**	**0.5**	**110**	**20.7**	**0.9**	**2.6**	**0.1**
Breast, Southern Fried, Premium, Bernard Matthews*	1 Serving/60g	70	1.7	117	19.6	3.1	2.9	0.6
Breast, Strips, Raw, Average	**1 Serving/280g**	**358**	**5.7**	**128**	**27.1**	**0.4**	**2.0**	**0.3**
Breast, Strips, with Garlic & Rosemary, Sainsbury's*	1 Serving/58g	87	2.9	150	25.9	0.3	5.0	0.0
Breast, Tandoori Style, Average	1 Serving/180g	237	6.8	132	22.3	2.3	3.8	1.0
Breast, Tikka, Sliced, Average	1oz/28g	34	0.5	120	24.9	2.0	1.7	0.6

CHICKEN

INFO/WEIGHT	Measure	per Measure KCAL	per Measure FAT	Nutrition Values per 100g / 100ml KCAL	PROT	CARB	FAT	FIBRE
Breast, with Cheese & Breadcrumbs, Elmwood, Co-Op*	½ Pack/170g	306	141.1	180	193.0	69.0	83.0	8.0
Breasts, Chilli & Ginger, COU, M&S*	1 Breast/120g	156	2.4	130	19.5	8.6	2.0	1.7
Butter Basted, TTD, Sainsbury's*	1 Slice/30g	44	1.9	147	22.8	0.0	6.2	0.6
Chargrilled, Fine Sliced, CBY, Asda*	1 Slice/21g	24	0.4	112	22.7	0.8	2.0	0.0
Chargrills, Garlic, Weight After Cooking, Birds Eye*	1 Chargrill/95g	182	10.4	192	19.0	4.0	11.0	0.1
Chargrills, Garlic, Weight Before Cooking, Birds Eye*	1 Chargrill/95g	190	10.7	200	20.3	4.2	11.3	0.1
Chargrills, Original, Weight Before Cooking, Birds Eye*	1 Chargrill/95g	156	8.6	164	17.5	3.2	9.0	0.1
Chargrills, Weight After Cooking, Baked, Birds Eye*	1 Chargrill/90g	160	8.7	178	18.9	3.4	9.7	0.1
Cooked, Sliced, Average	*1 Slice/15g*	*18*	*0.4*	*118*	*22.4*	*1.6*	*2.4*	*0.1*
Diced, Market Value, Value, Tesco*	1 Pack/410g	574	25.0	140	20.5	0.2	6.1	0.0
Dippers, Crispy, Average	5 Dippers/93g	231	14.3	249	13.2	14.4	15.4	0.6
Drumsticks, & Thighs, Garlic & Herb, Sainsbury's*	1 Serving/120g	184	10.7	153	16.6	1.5	8.9	0.1
Drumsticks, BBQ Flavour, Average	1 Serving/200g	348	16.0	174	22.6	3.1	8.0	0.4
Drumsticks, Breaded, Fried, Average	1oz/28g	70	4.1	248	19.6	9.9	14.6	0.6
Drumsticks, Chinese Style, Average	1 Drumstick/100g	178	8.1	178	22.6	3.6	8.1	0.7
Drumsticks, Raw, Meat & Skin, Weighed with Bone	1 Drumstick/133g	281	16.4	211	23.4	0.2	12.4	0.0
Drumsticks, Raw, Meat Only, Weighed with Bone	1 Drumstick/122g	237	13.8	194	21.5	0.1	11.3	0.0
Drumsticks, Roast, Meat Only, Weighed with Bone	*1 Serving/100g*	*163*	*7.8*	*163*	*22.6*	*0.5*	*7.8*	*0.2*
Drumsticks, Southern Fried, Sainsbury's*	1 Serving/87g	190	8.6	218	20.8	11.2	9.9	0.7
Drumsticks with Skin, Average	*1 Piece/125g*	*268*	*16.6*	*215*	*22.1*	*1.8*	*13.3*	*0.3*
Escalope, Breaded, Average	1 Escalope/128g	361	21.6	282	13.4	19.1	16.9	0.7
Fillets, Battered, Average	1 Fillet/90g	199	10.4	221	16.1	13.3	11.5	0.5
Fillets, Breaded, Average	1 Piece/98g	214	10.5	219	14.2	15.9	10.7	1.9
Fillets, Chilli & Mango, Tesco*	1 Serving/100g	130	0.7	130	27.1	3.7	0.7	1.0
Fillets, Chinese Style, Average	1oz/28g	37	0.5	132	24.4	4.6	1.8	0.5
Fillets, Coronation, BGTY, Sainsbury's*	1 Fillet/100g	136	2.6	136	27.1	2.4	2.6	1.0
Fillets, Green Thai Marinated, Mini, Love Life, Waitrose*	½ Pack/138g	153	3.3	111	21.2	1.2	2.4	0.6
Fillets, Honey & Mustard, Average	1 Serving/100g	138	3.7	138	18.4	7.5	3.7	0.8
Fillets, Hot & Spicy, Average	1oz/28g	58	3.1	206	16.4	10.5	11.0	1.1
Fillets, Lime & Coriander, Mini, Average	1 Fillet/42g	49	0.5	118	24.3	2.6	1.3	0.6
Fillets, Piri Piri Style, Mini, Ready to Eat, Tesco*	1 Pack/190g	256	2.1	135	22.7	7.6	1.1	0.8
Fillets, Red Thai, Mini, Average	1oz/28g	36	0.6	128	21.7	5.4	2.0	0.6
Fillets, Skewers, Sticky Sweet Soy Marinade, M&S*	½ Pack/124g	155	1.4	125	20.7	7.6	1.1	0.3
Fillets, Southern Fried, Meat Only, Average	1 Piece/100g	222	12.0	222	16.4	12.2	12.0	1.1
Fillets, Strips, Barbeque, Birds Eye*	4 Strips/101g	180	8.7	179	18.9	6.5	8.6	0.2
Fillets, Sweet Chilli, Mini, Sainsbury's*	½ Pack/100g	119	1.1	119	21.8	5.4	1.1	0.9
Fillets, Sweet Chilli, Roast, Mini, Waitrose*	1 Pack/200g	314	1.0	157	29.4	8.8	0.5	1.0
Fillets, Sweet Chilli & Lime, Mini, M&S*	1 Serving/50g	78	1.1	155	28.3	5.1	2.2	0.0
Fillets, Tandoori Style, Mini, Average	1 Serving/100g	128	2.0	128	24.7	2.6	2.0	0.4
Fillets, Tikka, Average	1 Serving/100g	141	5.0	141	22.4	1.7	5.0	1.1
Fillets, Tikka, Mini, Average	1oz/28g	35	0.6	124	25.1	1.3	2.2	1.2
Fillets, Tomato & Basil, Mini, Average	1oz/28g	34	0.6	123	23.4	2.5	2.1	0.4
Fingers, Average	1 Serving/75g	188	9.9	250	13.7	18.8	13.2	1.2
Garlic, Frozen, Tesco*	1 Serving/95g	182	8.3	192	15.6	12.9	8.7	1.0
Goujons, Breaded, Average	1 Serving/114g	293	17.1	258	15.8	15.2	15.0	1.0
Goujons, Breaded, BBQ, Tesco*	3 Goujons/92g	250	14.0	270	11.6	20.9	15.1	0.8
Goujons, Breast, Fresh, Average	1oz/28g	36	0.5	127	28.0	0.0	1.6	0.0
Honey Roast, Sliced, Average	1 Slice/13g	15	0.3	117	21.6	2.2	2.4	0.1
Leg, Meat Only, Raw, Average	*1oz/28g*	*34*	*1.1*	*120*	*20.1*	*0.0*	*3.8*	*0.0*
Leg, Meat Only, Raw, Weighed with Skin & Bone	*1oz/28g*	*38*	*1.2*	*134*	*22.5*	*0.0*	*4.3*	*0.0*
Leg, Meat Only, Stewed with Bone & Skin, Average	*1oz/28g*	*52*	*2.3*	*185*	*26.3*	*0.0*	*8.1*	*0.0*
Leg or Thigh, Hot & Spicy, Average	1oz/28g	50	3.0	179	19.4	1.0	10.8	0.4
Leg Portion, Roast, Weighed with Bone, without Skin	1 Portion/114g	246	15.5	216	43.5	0.0	13.6	0.0

CHICKEN

INFO/WEIGHT	Measure	per Measure		Nutrition Values per 100g / 100ml				
		KCAL	FAT	KCAL	PROT	CARB	FAT	FIBRE
Leg Portion, with Skin, no Bone, Roasted, Average	1 Portion/120g	244	15.3	203	21.6	0.3	12.7	0.2
Leg with Skin, Raw, Average	1oz/28g	48	2.9	172	19.1	0.0	10.4	0.0
Leg with Skin, Roasted, Weighed with Bone, Average	1oz/28g	66	4.6	234	21.5	0.1	16.4	0.0
Light Meat, Raw	1oz/28g	30	0.3	106	24.0	0.0	1.1	0.0
Light Meat, Roasted	1oz/28g	43	1.0	153	30.2	0.0	3.6	0.0
Meat, Roasted, Average	1oz/28g	50	2.1	177	27.3	0.0	7.5	0.0
Meat & Skin, Roasted, Average	1oz/28g	60	3.9	216	22.6	0.0	14.0	0.0
Mexican, Simply Add, Tesco*	1 Pack/600g	570	19.8	95	8.1	7.0	3.3	2.0
Mexican Chilli, Sliced, Eat Well, M&S*	1 Pack/130g	169	3.4	130	25.9	0.8	2.6	0.5
Mince, Average	1oz/28g	39	1.7	140	20.9	0.1	6.0	0.2
Nuggets, Battered, Average	1 Nugget/20g	50	2.9	251	13.5	16.9	14.4	0.9
Nuggets, Breaded, Average	1 Nugget/14g	37	2.0	263	14.8	19.8	13.8	1.9
Pieces, Barbeque, Chunky, Ready to Eat, Tesco*	1 Pack/200g	290	4.0	145	25.4	5.3	2.0	0.5
Pieces, Breaded, Boneless, Fried, From Restaurant	1 Piece/17g	51	3.3	301	17.0	14.4	19.4	0.0
Pieces, Hot & Spicy, Chunky, Tesco*	½ Pack/100g	135	1.1	135	27.0	4.2	1.1	0.5
Pops, Southern Fried, Frozen, Tesco*	1 Pack/225g	518	25.9	230	13.1	18.1	11.5	1.9
Portions, Meat & Skin, Deep Fried, Average	1oz/28g	73	4.7	259	26.9	0.0	16.8	0.0
Skewers, BBQ, George Foreman's Lean Mean Grillers*	1 Skewer/60g	68	0.8	114	20.0	5.5	1.4	0.4
Skewers, Marinated, Asda*	1 Skewer/35g	50	0.4	142	24.9	8.0	1.2	0.5
Skewers, with Chorizo, Bighams*	1 Skewer/95g	129	6.5	136	17.1	1.5	6.9	0.5
Spatchcock, Poussin, Sainsbury's*	1 Serving/122g	168	6.6	138	21.1	0.1	5.4	0.2
Spatchcock, Salt & Cracked Pepper, Sainsbury's*	1 Serving/122g	168	6.6	138	21.1	0.1	5.4	0.2
Steaks, Average	1 Serving/100g	205	9.4	205	21.1	9.0	9.4	0.7
Strips, Breast, Grilled, KP Snacks*	1 Serving/84g	90	1.5	107	25.0	0.0	1.8	0.0
Strips, Mexican, Sliced, M&S*	½ Pack/70g	77	0.4	110	24.3	2.3	0.6	0.5
Strips or Tenders, Chinese Style, Average	1oz/28g	41	1.1	145	19.6	8.0	4.1	1.0
Sweet Chilli, Pieces, Morrisons*	1 Pack/200g	282	5.0	141	25.5	4.1	2.5	0.5
Tandoori, Skewers, Six, M Kitchen, Morrisons*	½ Pack/90g	158	5.0	175	28.9	2.0	5.6	0.5
Thigh, Meat & Skin, Average	1 Serving/100g	218	14.7	218	21.4	0.0	14.7	0.0
Thigh, Meat & Skin, Casseroled, Average	1oz/28g	65	4.6	233	21.5	0.0	16.3	0.0
Thigh, Meat & Skin, Weighed with Bone, Raw, Average	1 Serving/100g	219	16.6	219	16.2	0.2	16.6	0.0
Thigh, Meat Only, Diced, Casseroled	1oz/28g	50	2.4	180	25.6	0.0	8.6	0.0
Thigh, Meat Only, Raw, Average	1 Thigh/90g	113	4.9	126	19.4	0.0	5.4	0.0
Thigh, Roast, Average	1 Serving/100g	238	15.6	238	23.8	0.4	15.6	0.0
Wafer Thin, Average	1 Slice/10g	12	0.4	120	19.0	2.8	3.6	0.2
Whole, in Parmesan & Tomato Marinade, Waitrose*	¼ Pack/175g	332	22.9	190	17.8	0.1	13.1	1.0
Whole, Roast, Average	1oz/28g	59	3.7	211	21.2	1.5	13.4	0.2
Whole, Roasted, Brown Sugar Marinade, Tesco*	1 Serving/100g	195	11.3	195	22.1	0.1	11.3	0.1
Wing, Breaded, Fried, Average	1oz/28g	82	5.2	294	18.4	14.0	18.5	0.4
Wing, Meat & Skin, Cooked, Average	1oz/28g	67	4.4	241	23.3	1.9	15.6	0.3
Wing Quarter, Meat Only, Casseroled	1oz/28g	46	1.8	164	26.9	0.0	6.3	0.0
Wings, BBQ Flavour, Average	1oz/28g	61	3.5	220	20.3	6.6	12.4	0.6
Wings, Chinese Style, Average	1oz/28g	72	4.3	256	24.2	5.1	15.5	0.6
Wings, Hot & Spicy, Average	1oz/28g	65	3.8	231	21.8	5.2	13.6	0.8
Wings, Meat & Skin, Raw, Average	1oz/28g	52	3.3	184	19.0	0.5	11.8	0.2

CHICKEN &

INFO/WEIGHT	Measure	per Measure		Nutrition Values per 100g / 100ml				
Bacon, Parcels, Finest, Tesco*	1 Pack/233g	379	21.6	163	16.1	3.7	9.3	0.5
Bacon, Parcels, Sainsbury's*	½ Pack/170g	406	28.6	239	21.9	0.1	16.8	0.0
Black Bean, Chinese, Tesco*	1 Pack/350g	382	17.2	109	8.9	7.4	4.9	0.7
Black Bean, Chinese Takeaway, Tesco*	1 Serving/200g	190	6.6	95	8.3	8.0	3.3	0.5
Black Bean, with Egg Fried Rice, Ready Meal, Average	1 Serving/400g	390	6.1	97	6.5	14.5	1.5	0.8
Black Bean, with Noodles, Sainsbury's*	1 Serving/130g	155	0.9	119	4.3	23.9	0.7	0.8
Black Bean, with Noodles, Tesco*	1 Pack/475g	470	7.6	99	7.6	13.6	1.6	0.2

	Measure INFO/WEIGHT	per Measure KCAL	FAT	Nutrition Values per 100g / 100ml KCAL	PROT	CARB	FAT	FIBRE
CHICKEN &								
Butternut Squash, Curry Pot, Weight Watchers*	1 Pot/250g	232	3.5	93	6.6	12.5	1.4	1.6
Cashew Nuts, Chinese, Cantonese, Sainsbury's*	½ Pack/175g	172	8.8	98	8.4	4.9	5.0	1.3
Cashew Nuts, Chinese, Ready Meal, Average	1 Serving/400g	497	24.0	124	9.2	7.5	6.0	1.2
Cashew Nuts, Chinese, Tesco*	1 Pack/350g	378	19.6	108	9.5	4.9	5.6	0.6
Chorizo Paella, Go Cook, Asda*	½ Pack/475g	591	10.5	124	10.2	15.9	2.2	2.6
Fries, Southern Fried, Sainsbury's*	½ Pack/250g	562	21.8	225	10.5	26.2	8.7	0.8
Fries, Southern Fried Style, Tesco*	1 Pack/500g	930	40.0	186	11.5	16.0	8.0	1.4
Gravy, COU, M&S*	1 Pack/300g	216	3.9	72	7.2	7.8	1.3	1.6
King Prawn, Special Fried Rice, Finest, Tesco*	1 Pack/450g	734	32.0	163	7.7	17.0	7.1	0.7
Mushroom, Chinese, Sainsbury's*	½ Pack/175g	116	3.5	66	7.6	4.4	2.0	0.9
Mushroom, Chinese, Tesco*	1 Pack/460g	474	12.9	103	5.7	13.8	2.8	1.0
Mushroom, in White Wine Sauce, GFY, Asda*	1 Pack/400g	272	7.2	68	6.0	7.0	1.8	1.2
Mushroom, with Rice, Egg Fried, Average	1 Serving/400g	421	10.1	105	6.3	14.4	2.5	0.8
Peppers, in a Black Bean Sauce, M&S*	1 Pack/320g	256	4.8	80	9.4	7.3	1.5	1.2
Pineapple, with Egg Fried Rice, Tesco*	1 Pack/450g	450	10.8	100	7.6	12.1	2.4	1.2
Tomato & Basil, COU, M&S*	½ Pack/200g	180	4.6	90	14.3	3.4	2.3	0.8
CHICKEN ALFREDO								
Average	1 Pack/400g	416	10.0	104	12.2	8.2	2.5	0.8
CHICKEN BANG BANG								
Waitrose*	1 Pack/350g	368	17.2	105	9.4	5.9	4.9	1.2
CHICKEN BUTTER								
with Rice, Average	1 Serving/400g	561	27.6	140	10.6	8.9	6.9	1.4
CHICKEN CAJUN								
Breast, Chargrilled, Iceland*	1 Serving/80g	114	1.5	142	27.4	3.9	1.9	0.0
Breast, Morrisons*	½ Pack/180g	328	16.9	182	16.6	7.7	9.4	2.0
HE, Tesco*	1 Pack/365g	412	4.7	113	7.9	17.3	1.3	0.7
CHICKEN CANTONESE								
Breast, Fillets, Sainsbury's*	1 Serving/154g	168	2.3	109	20.3	3.6	1.5	0.6
Chinese, Tesco*	½ Pack/175g	196	6.5	112	10.3	9.4	3.7	0.4
CHICKEN CARIBBEAN								
Style, Breasts, COU, M&S*	1 Serving/205g	205	3.1	100	14.6	7.3	1.5	1.3
CHICKEN CHASSEUR								
Average	1 Serving/400g	363	9.2	91	12.2	4.9	2.3	0.9
Breast Fillets, Morrisons*	1 Pack/380g	384	11.4	101	15.7	2.9	3.0	0.8
Finest, Tesco*	½ Pack/200g	200	6.4	100	14.3	2.4	3.2	1.1
Mix, Colman's*	1 Pack/38g	120	0.4	316	8.6	68.2	1.0	3.7
CHICKEN CHILLI								
& Lemon Grass with Egg Noodles, BGTY, Sainsbury's*	1 Pack/450g	500	15.3	111	10.0	10.2	3.4	1.2
Sweet, Just Cook, Sainsbury's*	½ Pack/191g	200	1.3	105	15.2	9.4	0.7	0.5
Sweet, with Noodles, Ready Meal, Average	1 Serving/400g	404	5.8	101	6.5	15.5	1.4	1.4
with Sticky Rice, Japanese Style, CBY, Asda*	1 Tub/350g	304	2.4	87	8.1	11.0	0.7	2.0
CHICKEN CHINESE								
Balls, M&S*	1 Ball/16g	45	2.2	280	10.8	29.2	13.6	2.1
Chinese Chicken, Morrisons*	1 Pack/340g	347	15.6	102	10.3	5.0	4.6	0.8
Chinese Chicken, Oriental Express*	1 Pack/340g	286	2.0	84	4.8	16.2	0.6	0.8
Fillets, with Sweet Chilli Sauce, Tesco*	1 Serving/350g	592	22.0	169	8.8	19.2	6.3	0.7
Stir Fry, Morrisons*	1 Serving/319g	341	5.4	107	5.7	17.0	1.7	1.5
Style Sauce, Breast Fillets, Morrisons*	½ Pack/200g	162	2.0	81	13.5	4.6	1.0	1.2
with Ginger & Spring Onion, Tesco*	1 Serving/350g	299	10.1	85	7.6	7.3	2.9	0.6
CHICKEN CORDON BLEU								
Breast, Fillets, Sainsbury's*	1 Serving/150g	304	14.3	203	17.5	11.5	9.5	1.6
Waitrose*	1 Serving/160g	325	15.4	203	20.1	9.1	9.6	2.4

	Measure INFO/WEIGHT	per Measure KCAL	FAT	Nutrition Values per 100g / 100ml KCAL	PROT	CARB	FAT	FIBRE
CHICKEN CORONATION								
COU, M&S*	1oz/28g	34	0.6	120	16.3	8.6	2.2	0.7
M & S*	1 Serving/200g	420	26.4	210	12.6	10.6	13.2	1.3
CHICKEN DINNER								
Breast, with Pork, Sage & Onion Stuffing, Tesco*	1 Serving/180g	277	14.8	154	19.4	0.7	8.2	0.5
Kershaws*	1 Pack/350g	210	3.5	60	4.3	8.4	1.0	1.2
Roast, with Mash, Green Beans & Carrots, CBY, Asda*	1 Dinner/400g	280	6.8	70	6.4	6.2	1.7	2.2
Tesco*	1 Serving/400g	388	7.2	97	9.2	10.9	1.8	1.2
with Gravy, The Crafty Cook*	1 Serving/320g	330	6.7	103	5.6	15.3	2.1	1.9
CHICKEN EN CROUTE								
Breast, Tesco*	1 Serving/215g	555	33.1	258	9.4	20.4	15.4	0.6
Creamy Bacon, Cheese & Leek Sauce, Waitrose*	½ Pack/177g	479	29.8	270	11.9	17.4	16.8	2.8
Just Cook, Sainsbury's*	1 Serving/180g	481	27.2	267	16.8	15.9	15.1	0.4
with Cheddar & Ham, Oven Baked, CBY, Asda*	½ Pack/209g	568	33.4	272	16.0	15.1	16.0	1.7
CHICKEN ESCALOPE								
Lemon & Herb, Waitrose*	1 Serving/200g	242	6.4	121	22.0	1.0	3.2	0.6
Topped with Cheese, Ham & Mushrooms, Asda*	½ Pack/149g	217	9.0	145	22.0	0.8	6.0	0.4
CHICKEN FU YUNG								
Chinese Takeaway, Tesco*	1 Pack/350g	315	3.5	90	5.6	14.5	1.0	0.8
CHICKEN HARISSA								
with Cous Cous, PB, Waitrose*	1 Pack/400g	348	8.0	87	7.6	9.5	2.0	1.7
CHICKEN IN								
Bacon, Mushroom & Red Wine Sauce, Asda*	1 Serving/151g	145	3.9	96	16.0	2.2	2.6	0.5
Barbecue Sauce, COU, M&S*	1 Pack/352g	370	5.6	105	8.6	13.8	1.6	1.2
Barbeque Sauce, Breasts, COU, M&S*	1 Pack/350g	420	6.7	120	8.5	20.6	1.9	0.6
BBQ Sauce, Breast, Sainsbury's*	1 Serving/170g	199	1.2	117	14.5	13.1	0.7	1.3
BBQ Sauce, Chargrilled, Breast, GFY, Asda*	1 Serving/166g	214	6.1	129	19.0	5.0	3.7	1.0
BBQ Sauce, Weight Watchers*	1 Pack/339g	332	11.9	98	5.8	10.8	3.5	0.9
Black Bean, with Egg Fried Rice, Tesco*	1 Pack/450g	652	26.1	145	7.0	16.1	5.8	1.2
Black Bean Sauce, Budgens*	1 Pack/350g	332	14.0	95	9.9	4.9	4.0	0.9
Black Bean Sauce, Chinese Takeaway, Iceland*	1 Pack/400g	348	12.8	87	9.3	5.3	3.2	0.7
Black Bean Sauce, M&S*	1 Pack/350g	298	7.0	85	8.7	8.0	2.0	1.1
Black Bean Sauce, Sainsbury's*	1 Pack/465g	484	7.9	104	5.0	17.3	1.7	0.3
Black Bean Sauce, Waitrose*	1 Pack/300g	243	3.6	81	10.9	6.6	1.2	0.8
Black Bean Sauce, with Egg Fried Rice, Somerfield*	1 Pack/340g	384	13.6	113	7.0	13.0	4.0	0.0
Black Bean Sauce, with Noodles, Pro Cuisine*	1 Pack/600g	366	3.6	61	5.6	8.5	0.6	0.0
Black Bean Sauce, with Rice, Asda*	1 Pack/400g	500	7.6	125	7.0	20.0	1.9	0.6
Black Bean Sauce & Rice, Morrisons*	1 Pack/400g	408	9.2	102	3.9	16.4	2.3	1.2
Cheese & Bacon, Wrapped, Breast, Tesco*	1 Serving/300g	474	23.4	158	20.7	1.2	7.8	0.5
Chilli & Lemon Grass with Rice, Sainsbury's*	1 Pack/450g	526	11.2	117	6.2	17.4	2.5	0.7
Garlic & Cream Sauce, Breast Fillet, Morrisons*	1 Serving/180g	262	15.8	146	14.9	1.8	8.8	0.6
Garlic & Herbs, Breast, Sainsbury's*	1 Serving/200g	316	5.2	158	28.3	5.4	2.6	0.1
Ginger & Chilli with Veg Noodles, COU, M&S*	1 Pack/400g	300	2.4	75	6.4	10.7	0.6	1.1
Gravy, Breast, Sainsbury's*	1 Box/200g	124	1.0	62	11.8	2.9	0.5	0.2
Hunter's BBQ Sauce, Asda*	½ Pack/190g	348	14.1	183	19.1	10.3	7.4	0.0
Lemon & Garlic Marinade, Thighs, Go Cook, Asda*	½ Pack/265g	493	30.2	186	19.7	1.2	11.4	0.8
Lemon Sauce, with Rice, Sainsbury's*	1 Pack/450g	513	6.8	114	8.1	17.0	1.5	0.7
Madeira Sauce, with Mushrooms, Finest, Tesco*	½ Pack/200g	210	8.3	105	13.8	3.0	4.2	1.0
Madeira Wine, with Porcini Mushrooms, PB, Waitrose*	1 Pack/415g	378	11.2	91	8.8	7.9	2.7	2.8
Mango Ginger Marinade, Chargrilled, GFY, Asda*	½ Pack/190g	234	2.3	123	17.0	11.0	1.2	0.5
Mexican Salsa, Tesco*	1 Pack/320g	368	8.6	115	19.5	3.1	2.7	0.6
Mexican Style Sauce, Tesco*	1 Serving/180g	128	1.4	71	13.3	2.6	0.8	0.7
Mushroom, Red Wine & Brandy Sauce, Waitrose*	1 Pack/500g	650	35.5	130	14.6	1.9	7.1	4.7
Mushroom & Red Wine Sauce, Breast Fillets, Morrisons*	1 Serving/177g	184	4.4	104	15.7	4.6	2.5	0.7

	Measure INFO/WEIGHT	per Measure KCAL	FAT	Nutrition Values per 100g / 100ml KCAL	PROT	CARB	FAT	FIBRE
CHICKEN IN								
Mushroom Sauce, Creamy, Weight Watchers*	1 Pack/330g	343	9.6	104	7.0	12.5	2.9	0.6
Mushroom Sauce, Diet Chef Ltd*	1 Pack/300g	225	6.9	75	7.9	5.7	2.3	0.1
Oyster Sauce, & Mushrooms, Tesco*	1 Pack/350g	252	5.6	72	8.0	6.3	1.6	0.7
Oyster Sauce, with Mushrooms, Tesco*	1 Pack/350g	189	3.2	54	8.0	3.5	0.9	0.8
Parma Ham, with Cheese, Breast, COOK!, M&S*	½ Pack/189g	340	20.8	180	18.0	2.5	11.0	0.9
Pesto Style Dressing, Asda*	1 Serving/150g	210	10.0	140	18.7	1.3	6.7	0.0
Red Wine & Bacon Sauce, Breast, Somerfield*	1 Breast/150g	130	3.0	87	14.0	3.0	2.0	0.0
Reggae Reggae Sauce, Drumsticks, Levi Roots*	1 Serving/100g	165	7.3	165	21.5	3.4	7.3	0.0
Smoky Barbeque Sauce, Tesco*	1 Serving/185g	229	3.9	124	16.3	9.9	2.1	1.0
Spicy Chilli Sauce, Topped with Cheese, Breast, Asda*	½ Pack/190g	241	7.0	127	20.0	3.4	3.7	0.0
Sweet Chilli Sauce, Breast, Fresh Tastes, Asda*	½ Pack/180g	288	9.0	160	18.4	10.3	5.0	0.5
Tarragon Sauce, Lean Cuisine*	1 Pack/338g	270	6.8	80	4.0	11.0	2.0	1.5
Tikka Style Sauce, Creamy, Tesco*	1 Breast/190g	215	10.4	113	15.1	0.7	5.5	0.8
Tomato & Basil Sauce, Breast, Fresh Tastes, Asda*	½ Pack/130g	136	2.7	105	19.3	2.3	2.1	0.7
Tomato & Basil Sauce, Breast, GFY, Asda*	1 Pack/392g	447	13.3	114	12.0	9.0	3.4	1.5
Tomato & Basil Sauce, GFY, Asda*	½ Pack/189g	231	6.1	122	22.0	1.2	3.2	2.0
Tomato & Basil Sauce, Oven Baked, Asda*	½ Pack/143g	153	3.0	107	19.3	2.3	2.1	0.7
Tomato & Herb Sauce, Breasts, Tesco*	½ Pack/173g	155	2.4	90	15.0	3.6	1.4	0.5
White Sauce, Canned, Asda*	½ Can/400g	644	44.0	161	12.0	3.5	11.0	0.0
White Wine & Tarragon Sauce, Breasts, Finest, Tesco*	½ Pack/200g	326	20.2	163	16.8	1.3	10.1	0.0
White Wine & Tarragon Sauce, Waitrose*	½ Pack/225g	281	17.3	125	10.7	3.1	7.7	0.3
White Wine Sauce, Creamy, Sainsbury's*	1 Pack/324g	285	12.0	88	8.9	4.7	3.7	1.0
Wild Mushroom Sauce, Extra Special, Asda*	1 Serving/225g	319	19.0	142	14.2	2.2	8.4	0.3
CHICKEN KUNG PO								
Sainsbury's*	½ Pack/175g	131	4.4	75	9.2	4.0	2.5	1.0
Waitrose*	1 Pack/350g	318	3.9	91	8.2	12.1	1.1	1.2
with Egg Fried Rice, Asda*	1 Pack/450g	688	22.5	153	6.0	21.0	5.0	1.0
CHICKEN LEMON								
Battered, Cantonese, Sainsbury's*	1 Pack/350g	560	19.6	160	10.7	16.6	5.6	0.9
Battered, Chinese Meal for Two, Tesco*	½ Serving/175g	294	13.0	168	6.6	18.8	7.4	2.0
Breast, Fillets, BGTY, Sainsbury's*	1 Fillet/113g	195	2.4	173	18.4	19.9	2.1	1.9
Chinese, Tesco*	1 Serving/350g	564	11.2	161	7.0	26.0	3.2	0.3
Tesco*	½ Pack/175g	214	7.4	122	11.0	10.1	4.2	0.6
CHICKEN LUNCH								
French Style, Light, John West*	1 Pack/240g	194	6.5	81	7.2	6.9	2.7	2.1
CHICKEN MEAL								
Breast Fillets, Meal For One, Eat Well, M&S*	1 Pack/400g	340	10.4	85	7.0	7.9	2.6	1.5
Roast, M&S*	1 Pack/280g	294	9.2	105	6.6	11.6	3.3	1.9
CHICKEN MEXICAN								
Style, GFY, Asda*	½ Pack/200g	256	10.0	128	17.0	3.7	5.0	0.3
Style with Rice, Morrisons*	1 Pack/400g	360	5.2	90	5.1	14.1	1.3	0.8
CHICKEN MOROCCAN								
Style, Sainsbury's*	½ Pack/269g	334	7.0	124	14.7	10.4	2.6	3.1
Style, with Spicy Cous Cous, BGTY, Sainsbury's*	1 Serving/225g	304	3.8	135	9.2	20.6	1.7	0.0
with Cous Cous, GFY, Asda*	1 Serving/450g	414	5.8	92	8.0	12.0	1.3	0.8
with Cous Cous & Fruity Sauce, BGTY, Sainsbury's*	1 Pack/400g	440	8.0	110	10.0	13.1	2.0	2.6
CHICKEN PAPRIKA								
COU, M&S*	1 Pack/400g	380	6.4	95	9.0	11.7	1.6	2.0
with Savoury Rice & Vegetables, BGTY, Sainsbury's*	1 Pack/400g	383	2.4	96	7.2	15.5	0.6	1.1
CHICKEN PARMESAN								
Sun Dried Tomato, Fillets, BGTY, Sainsbury's*	½ Pack/100g	138	2.9	138	22.1	6.0	2.9	0.5
CHICKEN PENANG								
Waitrose*	1 Pack/400g	364	10.8	91	10.1	6.6	2.7	0.8

	Measure INFO/WEIGHT	per Measure KCAL	FAT	Nutrition Values per 100g / 100ml KCAL	PROT	CARB	FAT	FIBRE
CHICKEN PIRI PIRI								
Breast, Fillets, Mini, Tesco*	½ Pack/100g	135	1.1	135	22.7	7.6	1.1	0.0
GFY, Asda*	1 Pack/400g	406	2.8	102	5.8	18.0	0.7	1.4
M & S*	1 Pack/300g	420	23.1	140	10.0	7.3	7.7	1.3
Sainsbury's*	½ Pack/200g	248	10.8	124	14.0	4.8	5.4	0.5
CHICKEN ROAST								
in a Pot, Sainsbury's*	1 Pack/450g	477	13.0	106	9.6	10.3	2.9	0.7
Meal, Blue Parrot Cafe, Sainsbury's*	1 Pack/285g	259	9.7	91	6.9	8.1	3.4	1.5
with Lemon & Herb Stuffing, 759, Wiltshire Farm Foods*	1 Serving/410g	412	17.4	100	6.8	8.8	4.2	1.2
CHICKEN ROLL								
Value, Tesco*	1 Slice/13g	30	2.2	223	15.4	3.9	16.2	0.1
with Pork, Sage & Onion Stuffing, Value, Tesco*	1 Roll/125g	166	8.9	133	9.4	7.8	7.1	0.5
CHICKEN SIZZLER								
GFY, Asda*	1 Pack/350g	289	5.0	83	12.9	4.6	1.4	1.4
CHICKEN SPANISH								
Style, Asda*	½ Pack/275g	322	13.5	117	14.0	4.1	4.9	0.7
CHICKEN STUFFED								
with Mushrooms, Finest, Tesco*	1 Serving/150g	177	7.6	118	15.9	2.0	5.1	0.6
CHICKEN SUPREME								
Breast, Sainsbury's*	1 Serving/187g	421	29.5	225	20.6	0.3	15.8	0.6
with Rice, Asda*	1 Pack/450g	616	31.5	137	15.0	3.4	7.0	1.1
with Rice, Birds Eye*	1 Pack/376g	470	9.8	125	6.6	18.8	2.6	0.5
with Rice, Weight Watchers*	1 Pack/300g	255	4.8	85	5.6	11.9	1.6	0.5
CHICKEN SZECHUAN								
Tesco*	1 Pack/350g	385	10.5	110	7.2	13.6	3.0	0.3
with Noodles, Sainsbury's*	1 Pack/450g	423	14.0	94	6.0	10.4	3.1	0.9
CHICKEN TAGINE								
with Cous Cous, BGTY, Sainsbury's*	1 Pack/450g	626	17.6	139	10.1	15.9	3.9	1.5
CHICKEN TANDOORI								
Fresh Tastes, Asda*	1 Pack/400g	356	5.6	89	6.4	12.7	1.4	2.1
GFY, Asda*	1 Pack/400g	324	9.6	81	7.5	7.3	2.4	1.7
Masala, Asda*	1 Pack/400g	580	20.0	145	7.0	18.0	5.0	1.3
Masala, Indian, Tesco*	1 Serving/350g	430	25.9	123	10.2	4.0	7.4	1.8
Sizzler, Sainsbury's*	1 Pack/400g	536	29.2	134	12.8	4.3	7.3	1.7
Tesco*	1 Serving/175g	198	8.6	113	10.6	6.7	4.9	1.0
CHICKEN TERIYAKI								
& Noodles, Asda*	½ Pack/340g	445	8.8	131	9.0	18.0	2.6	0.9
Asda*	1 Pack/360g	299	5.0	83	9.1	8.6	1.4	0.8
Japanese with Ramen Noodles, Sainsbury's*	1 Pack/450g	482	9.4	107	6.5	15.5	2.1	0.8
CHICKEN THAI								
& Siu Mai Dumplings, M&S*	1 Dumpling/21g	35	1.6	170	16.0	9.4	7.6	0.8
Diet Chef Ltd*	1 Pouch/300g	288	9.3	96	9.1	8.0	3.1	0.5
Low Fat, Solo Slim, Rosemary Conley*	1 Pack/300g	291	12.6	97	5.8	9.0	4.2	2.4
Style Marinade, Breast, Chargrilled, GFY, Asda*	½ Pack/178g	178	5.3	100	17.0	1.3	3.0	0.5
Style with Noodles, Tesco*	1 Pack/400g	332	6.8	83	7.5	9.5	1.7	1.0
CHICKEN TIKKA								
& Coriander Rice, Weight Watchers*	1 Pack/400g	348	2.4	87	6.2	14.3	0.6	1.6
& Rice, Everyday, Value, Tesco*	1 Pack/396g	535	21.4	135	7.3	12.8	5.4	2.5
BGTY, Sainsbury's*	1 Serving/188g	265	3.0	141	10.5	21.2	1.6	0.0
Creamy, Breast, Tesco*	1 Breast/190g	215	10.4	113	15.1	0.7	5.5	0.8
Masala, & Pilau Rice, Asda*	1 Serving/500g	720	20.0	144	6.2	20.7	4.0	0.9
Masala, COU, M&S*	½ Pack/175g	245	13.0	140	12.5	5.6	7.4	1.6
Masala, Indian, Takeaway, CBY, Asda*	½ Pack/225g	256	11.0	114	8.6	8.3	4.9	1.2
Masala, M&S*	½ Pack/175g	245	13.0	140	12.5	5.6	7.4	1.6

	Measure INFO/WEIGHT	per Measure KCAL	FAT	Nutrition Values per 100g / 100ml KCAL	PROT	CARB	FAT	FIBRE
CHICKEN TIKKA								
Masala, with Pilau Rice, Hot, Tesco*	1 Pack/550g	798	31.9	145	7.4	15.0	5.8	1.4
Masala, with Rice, Ready Meal, Healthy Range, Average	1 Serving/400g	390	6.4	98	6.6	14.3	1.6	1.1
Masala, with Rice & Naan, Big Dish, Tesco*	1 Pack/600g	960	40.4	160	6.7	18.1	6.7	1.2
Masala, with Yellow Rice, LC, Tesco*	1 Pack/441g	485	8.8	110	4.9	17.4	2.0	1.0
with Pilau Rice, GFY, Asda*	1 Pack/450g	382	2.7	85	7.0	13.0	0.6	1.8
CHICKEN VINDALOO								
Average	1 Serving/410g	787	51.2	192	18.5	2.6	12.5	0.3
Sainsbury's*	1 Pack/400g	460	16.8	115	14.6	4.8	4.2	0.6
Waitrose*	1 Pack/340g	398	18.4	117	10.6	6.4	5.4	1.6
CHICKEN WITH								
Asparagus, Prosciutto Ham, Bearnaise Butter, Waitrose*	½ Pack/168g	203	6.4	121	20.6	1.1	3.8	0.5
Bacon & Leeks, & Mash Potato, BGTY, Sainsbury's*	1 Pack/450g	435	11.3	97	8.4	10.1	2.5	0.7
Black Bean Sauce, Green Peppers & Rice, Farmfoods*	1 Meal/324g	408	12.6	126	5.5	17.1	3.9	0.4
Cheddar & Bacon Filling, Just Cook, Sainsbury's*	1 Serving/180g	346	14.6	192	23.2	6.5	8.1	0.1
Cheese, Leek & Ham, Breast, Fresh Tastes, Asda*	1 Pack/430g	658	30.5	153	18.9	3.4	7.1	0.7
Cheese & Bacon, Tesco*	½ Pack/175g	262	11.9	150	18.9	2.6	6.8	0.4
Chorizo & Patatas Bravas, COU, M&S*	1 Pack/400g	380	9.2	95	7.8	10.8	2.3	1.7
Coriander & Lime, Asda*	1 Serving/105g	122	0.9	116	24.0	2.9	0.9	0.2
Cous Cous, Lemon & Herb, Finest, Tesco*	1 Pack/370g	492	18.5	133	10.5	11.5	5.0	0.9
Garlic & Chilli Balti, Tesco*	1 Pack/400g	320	7.6	80	11.0	4.4	1.9	0.8
Garlic & Herbs, Asda*	1 Slice/25g	28	0.4	114	23.9	1.1	1.5	0.0
Garlic Mushrooms, Asda*	1 Serving/320g	342	16.0	107	13.8	1.8	5.0	2.2
Garlic Mushrooms, Breast, Oven Baked, Asda*	½ Pack/160g	180	6.6	112	17.8	0.8	4.1	0.4
Garlic Mushrooms, Breast, Simply Cook, Tesco*	½ Pack/125g	170	6.6	136	22.0	0.1	5.3	0.1
Gruyere Cheese, & Parma Ham, Breast, COOK!, M&S*	1 Breast/194g	349	21.3	180	18.0	2.5	11.0	0.9
Honey & Mustard Sauce, Breasts, Simply Cook, Tesco*	½ Pack/219g	230	1.3	105	16.3	8.0	0.6	0.3
Leek, Cheese & Bacon, Simple Solutions, Tesco*	1 Serving/200g	296	16.8	148	17.6	0.5	8.4	0.3
Lime & Coriander, Chargrilled, Asda*	1 Serving/190g	352	17.1	185	24.0	2.0	9.0	1.1
Lyonnaise Potatoes, M&S*	½ Pack/260g	286	8.1	110	12.6	8.0	3.1	0.9
Madeira Wine & Porcini Mushrooms, Love Life, Waitrose*	1 Pack/380g	318	8.3	84	7.2	8.0	2.2	1.6
Mango Salsa & Potato Wedges, BGTY, Sainsbury's*	1 Pack/400g	336	6.4	84	7.0	10.4	1.6	1.5
Mozzarella, & Pancetta, Breast, Finest, Tesco*	½ Pack/225g	326	14.0	145	14.4	7.9	6.2	1.1
Mozzarella, & Pesto Melt, Breasts, COOK!, M&S*	½ Pack/165g	206	10.2	125	16.4	1.3	6.2	0.7
Mushroom, & Bacon, Fillets, M&S*	½ Pack/188g	225	11.2	120	15.5	0.5	6.0	1.7
Mushroom, & Bacon, in White Wine Sauce, M&S*	½ Pack/189g	255	13.8	135	15.7	1.1	7.3	0.6
Mushroom, & Garlic, Just Cook, Sainsbury's*	½ Pack/166g	330	17.1	199	20.0	4.6	10.3	0.1
Mushroom Risotto, M&S*	1 Pack/400g	480	11.6	120	6.9	16.7	2.9	0.8
Pork Stuffing, Breast, Roast, M&S*	1 Serving/100g	165	6.5	165	24.1	3.0	6.5	0.0
Potato Wedges, Tomato & Basil, Weight Watchers*	1 Pack/330g	254	6.6	77	4.7	9.2	2.0	1.6
Rice, Fiesta, Weight Watchers*	1 Pack/330g	307	6.6	93	6.1	12.8	2.0	0.4
Rice 'n' Peas, Sainsbury's*	1 Pack/300g	489	18.3	163	12.5	14.4	6.1	2.1
Sage & Onion Stuffing, Breast, Roast, Sliced, M&S*	1 Slice/17g	27	1.1	165	24.1	3.0	6.5	0.0
Sea Salt & Black Pepper Crust, Breast, Asda*	1 Serving/154g	186	4.3	121	19.0	5.0	2.8	0.0
Soured Cream, Cajun Spiced, Breast, COOK!, M&S*	½ Pack/200g	230	10.2	115	14.7	2.1	5.1	1.1
Spirelli, Steam Meal, Tesco*	1 Serving/400g	400	10.8	100	6.6	12.0	2.7	1.2
Spring Vegetables, Chargrilled, COU, M&S*	1 Pack/414g	290	3.7	70	8.8	7.3	0.9	1.8
Sticky Honey & Chilli Sauce, Breast, Asda*	1 Serving/175g	247	5.6	141	20.0	8.0	3.2	0.0
Stuffing, TTD, Sainsbury's*	1 Slice/34g	50	2.0	148	22.7	1.3	5.8	0.9
Sweet Chilli & Garlic, Chinese, Asda*	1 Serving/400g	436	2.4	109	8.0	18.0	0.6	2.1
Sweet Potato Mash, Jerk, Super Naturals, Sainsbury's*	1 Pack/400g	284	4.4	71	6.1	9.2	1.1	2.2
Tagine, Cous Cous, PB, Waitrose*	1 Pack/400g	516	14.0	129	8.2	16.2	3.5	1.0
CHICORY								
Fresh, Raw, Average	**1 Head/150g**	**30**	**0.9**	**20**	**0.6**	**2.8**	**0.6**	**0.9**

CHILLI

INFO/WEIGHT	Measure	per Measure KCAL	FAT	Nutrition Values per 100g / 100ml KCAL	PROT	CARB	FAT	FIBRE
& Potato Wedges, Good Choice, Iceland*	1 Pack/400g	368	13.6	92	5.5	9.8	3.4	1.2
& Potato Wedges, Sainsbury's*	1 Pack/371g	393	15.2	106	7.2	10.1	4.1	2.2
& Rice, Morrisons*	1 Serving/500g	630	15.5	126	5.7	18.9	3.1	1.1
& Spicy Wedges, Good Intentions, Somerfield*	1 Serving/400g	340	9.2	85	5.6	10.5	2.3	1.1
Beef, & Mushrooms, GFY, Asda*	1 Pack/400g	364	6.0	91	9.1	10.2	1.5	1.2
Beef, & Potato Crush, Weight Watchers*	1 Pack/400g	232	6.0	58	5.0	5.9	1.5	3.4
Beef, & Rice Pot, Shapers, Boots*	1 Pot/301g	250	4.5	83	4.0	12.0	1.5	2.1
Beef, Asda*	½ Pack/200g	190	7.8	95	7.0	8.0	3.9	1.2
Beef, with Rice, GFY, Asda*	1 Serving/402g	354	6.0	88	4.7	14.0	1.5	0.9
Beef, with Rice, Sainsbury's*	1 Serving/300g	360	5.1	120	5.6	20.6	1.7	1.1
Beef with Rice, Minced, Mini, CBY, Asda*	1 Pack/250g	308	9.8	123	5.3	15.8	3.9	1.7
Con Carne, & Potato Wedges, Weight Watchers*	1 Pack/320g	245	6.7	77	4.4	9.3	2.1	1.4
Con Carne, & Rice, Everyday, Value, Tesco*	1 Pack/400g	455	11.1	115	5.0	15.5	2.8	3.3
Con Carne, & Rice, Healthy Living, Co-Op*	1 Pack/400g	400	6.8	100	7.8	13.9	1.7	2.1
Con Carne, & Rice, Meal for One, M&S*	1 Pack/450g	495	12.2	110	6.4	13.6	2.7	1.6
Con Carne, & Rice, Somerfield*	1 Pack/500g	490	5.0	98	5.0	18.0	1.0	0.0
Con Carne, Asda*	1 Can/392g	376	13.7	96	7.0	9.0	3.5	0.0
Con Carne, Beef, Look What We Found*	1 Pack/270g	194	7.6	72	7.6	2.9	2.8	2.3
Con Carne, BGTY, Sainsbury's*	1 Serving/400g	384	8.8	96	5.3	13.8	2.2	2.8
Con Carne, Canned, Morrisons*	1 Can/392g	368	11.8	94	8.8	8.0	3.0	2.4
Con Carne, Canned, Sainsbury's*	½ Can/200g	162	4.2	81	6.6	8.9	2.1	2.5
Con Carne, Canned, Tesco*	½ Can/200g	220	11.4	110	7.8	6.4	5.7	4.7
Con Carne, Diet Chef Ltd*	1 Pack/300g	333	13.5	111	7.3	10.4	4.5	2.1
Con Carne, Dynamite Hot, Stagg*	1 Serving/250g	310	15.5	124	7.6	9.6	6.2	2.5
Con Carne, Fluffy White Rice, COU, M&S*	1 Pack/400g	360	7.6	90	5.7	12.3	1.9	1.5
Con Carne, From Restaurant, Average	1 Serving/253g	256	8.3	101	9.7	8.7	3.3	0.0
Con Carne, Frozen, Co-Op*	1 Pack/340g	306	3.4	90	6.0	15.0	1.0	1.0
Con Carne, Homepride*	1 Can/390g	234	2.3	60	2.5	11.2	0.6	0.0
Con Carne, M&S*	1 Pack/285g	285	10.5	100	8.7	7.4	3.7	2.0
Con Carne, Recipe Mix, Colman's*	1 Pack/50g	158	1.2	316	10.4	62.9	2.5	6.8
Con Carne, Restaurant, Sainsbury's*	1 Serving/100g	80	2.7	80	6.9	7.0	2.7	1.5
Con Carne, Tex Mex, Recipe Mix, Schwartz*	1 Sachet/35g	97	2.3	277	12.9	66.6	6.6	24.6
Con Carne, with Rice, Birds Eye*	1 Pack/285g	291	7.1	102	3.3	16.6	2.5	0.8
Con Carne, with Rice, GFY, Asda*	1 Serving/400g	456	6.4	114	6.0	19.0	1.6	0.9
Con Carne, with Rice, Healthy Choice, Asda*	1 Pack/400g	412	8.4	103	6.0	15.0	2.1	0.9
Con Carne, with Rice, Morrisons*	1 Pack/400g	328	5.2	82	5.3	12.2	1.3	1.4
Con Carne, with Rice, Organic, Sainsbury's*	1 Pack/400g	472	10.8	118	5.0	18.5	2.7	1.8
Con Carne, with Rice, PB, Waitrose*	1 Pack/400g	404	7.2	101	5.8	15.3	1.8	1.7
Con Carne, with Rice, Weight Watchers*	1 Serving/301g	262	3.3	87	4.6	14.7	1.1	0.4
Medium, Uncle Ben's*	1 Jar/500g	305	4.0	61	1.8	11.1	0.8	0.0
Mexican, with Long Grain Rice, Rice Time, Uncle Ben's*	1 Pot/300g	339	3.0	113	2.5	22.8	1.0	1.3
Non Carne, with Rice, Linda McCartney*	1 Pack/400g	364	9.2	91	4.2	14.9	2.3	3.1
Peruvian, Hot in Sunflower Oil, Barts*	1 Serving/100g	62	1.5	62	1.5	10.7	1.5	0.0
Vegetable	1oz/28g	16	0.2	57	3.0	10.8	0.6	2.6
Vegetable, & Rice, BGTY, Sainsbury's*	1 Pack/450g	410	5.0	91	3.5	16.7	1.1	3.5
Vegetable, Canned, Sainsbury's*	1 Can/400g	230	1.6	58	3.1	10.4	0.4	3.2
Vegetable, Diet Chef Ltd*	1 Pack/300g	258	4.8	86	3.4	14.5	1.6	4.4
Vegetable, Mixed, Tesco*	1 Pack/400g	352	11.6	88	3.9	11.0	2.9	3.2
Vegetable, Retail	1oz/28g	20	0.6	70	4.0	9.4	2.1	0.0
Vegetable Garden, Stagg*	1 Can/410g	254	2.0	62	3.6	10.8	0.5	2.3
Vegetarian, with Rice, Ready Meal, Average	1 Serving/400g	434	6.0	108	3.8	20.0	1.5	1.3
Vegetarian, with Rice, Tesco*	1 Pack/500g	575	13.0	115	4.0	19.0	2.6	1.8

	Measure INFO/WEIGHT	per Measure KCAL	per Measure FAT	Nutrition Values per 100g / 100ml KCAL	PROT	CARB	FAT	FIBRE
CHINESE LEAF								
Fresh, Raw, Average	**1oz/28g**	**4**	**0.1**	**14**	**1.5**	**1.5**	**0.2**	**1.7**
CHINESE MEAL								
Duck, Crispy & Pancakes, Kit, Asda*	½ Pack/59g	173	12.9	294	12.0	12.0	22.0	0.5
for One, GFY, Asda*	1 Pack/570g	946	16.5	166	7.0	28.0	2.9	0.0
for Two, Tesco*	1 Pack/500g	480	8.0	96	4.4	16.0	1.6	1.1
House Special, with Egg Fried Rice, Tesco*	1 Pack/450g	562	8.6	125	7.2	19.7	1.9	0.8
CHIPS								
& Curry Sauce, Tesco*	1 Serving/400g	440	20.0	110	2.1	14.1	5.0	1.0
11mm Fresh, Deep Fried, McCain*	1oz/28g	66	3.0	235	3.2	31.8	10.6	0.0
14mm Fresh, Deep Fried, McCain*	1oz/28g	59	1.9	209	2.7	34.2	6.8	0.0
14mm Friers Choice, Deep Fried, McCain*	1oz/28g	56	2.2	199	3.5	29.3	8.0	0.0
3 Way Cook, Somerfield*	1 Serving/96g	145	4.8	151	2.5	24.0	5.0	1.6
9/16" Straight Cut Caterpack, Deep Fried, McCain*	1oz/28g	63	2.6	225	3.1	32.1	9.4	0.0
American Style, Oven, Co-Op*	1 Serving/150g	255	9.0	170	2.0	26.0	6.0	3.0
American Style, Oven, Sainsbury's*	1 Serving/165g	314	13.7	190	5.4	23.6	8.3	1.3
American Style, Thin, Oven, Tesco*	1 Serving/125g	210	8.1	168	2.7	24.6	6.5	2.1
Beefeater, Deep Fried, McCain*	1oz/28g	71	2.8	253	3.3	37.7	9.9	0.0
Beefeater, Oven Baked, McCain*	1oz/28g	55	1.6	195	4.0	32.2	5.6	0.0
Chippy, Microwave, McCain*	1oz/28g	49	2.0	176	2.6	25.2	7.2	1.7
Chunky, Baked, Organic, M&S*	1 Serving/100g	150	3.7	150	1.7	27.1	3.7	2.2
Chunky, British, Oven, Frozen, Cooked, Finest, Tesco*	1 Serving/125g	240	5.1	192	2.3	35.1	4.1	2.7
Chunky, COU, M&S*	1 Serving/150g	158	2.4	105	2.1	20.5	1.6	2.3
Chunky, Crisp & Golden, Waitrose*	½ Pack/225g	259	7.0	115	2.1	17.7	3.1	3.9
Chunky, Fresh, Chilled, Finest, Tesco*	1 Pack/450g	608	18.0	135	2.1	22.3	4.0	2.7
Chunky, Gastropub, M&S*	1 Pack/400g	520	12.4	130	2.6	22.4	3.1	2.3
Chunky, Ready to Bake, M&S*	1 Serving/200g	310	8.4	155	2.2	26.8	4.2	2.0
Crinkle Cut, Frozen, Fried in Corn Oil	1oz/28g	81	4.7	290	3.6	33.4	16.7	2.2
Crinkle Cut, M&S*	1 Serving/150g	270	8.1	180	3.3	29.5	5.4	2.4
Fat with Fluffy Centres, M&S*	1 Serving/200g	210	9.0	105	1.6	14.2	4.5	1.8
Fine Cut, Frozen, Fried in Blended Oil	1oz/28g	102	6.0	364	4.5	41.2	21.3	2.4
Fine Cut, Frozen, Fried in Corn Oil	1oz/28g	102	6.0	364	4.5	41.2	21.3	2.7
Fried, Average	1 Serving/130g	266	10.9	204	3.2	29.6	8.4	1.2
Fried, Chip Shop, Average	1 Serving/100g	239	12.4	239	3.2	30.5	12.4	2.2
Frozen, Crinkle Cut, Aunt Bessie's*	1 Serving/100g	163	7.3	163	3.1	21.3	7.3	2.2
Frying, Cooked in Sunflower Oil, Value, Tesco*	1 Portion/125g	172	4.9	138	2.5	23.1	3.9	1.6
Frying, Crinkle Cut, Tesco*	1 Serving/125g	161	4.1	129	2.6	22.2	3.3	1.9
Homefries, Chunky, Weighed Baked, McCain*	1 Serving/100g	153	3.1	153	3.2	28.0	3.1	2.3
Homefries, Chunky, Weighed Frozen, McCain*	1 Serving/100g	123	2.5	123	2.5	22.6	2.5	1.6
Homefries, Crinkle Cut, Weighed Baked, McCain*	1 Serving/100g	176	5.0	176	2.6	30.1	5.0	2.3
Homefries, Crinkle Cut, Weighed Frozen, McCain*	1 Serving/100g	142	5.1	142	1.9	22.2	5.1	1.3
Homefries, Jacket Oven, McCain*	1 Serving/100g	220	7.4	220	3.9	37.9	7.4	0.0
Homefries, Straight Cut, Weighed Baked, McCain*	1 Serving/100g	181	6.2	181	3.1	28.1	6.2	2.4
Homefries, Straight Cut, Weighed Frozen, McCain*	1 Serving/100g	134	4.6	134	2.2	21.0	4.6	1.7
Homefries, Thin & Crispy, Weighed Frozen, McCain*	1 Serving/100g	143	4.1	143	2.6	24.0	4.1	1.5
Homemade, Actify, 1000g Potatoes, 3ml Oil, Actifry*	1 Portion/250g	197	1.2	79	1.9	16.9	0.5	1.2
Homemade, Fried in Blended Oil, Average	1oz/28g	53	1.9	189	3.9	30.1	6.7	2.2
Homemade, Fried in Corn Oil, Average	1oz/28g	53	1.9	189	3.9	30.1	6.7	2.2
Homemade, Fried in Dripping, Average	1oz/28g	53	1.9	189	3.9	30.1	6.7	2.2
Homestyle, Frozen, Aunt Bessie's*	1 Serving/200g	260	11.2	130	2.2	17.6	5.6	2.7
Homestyle, Oven Cooked, Aunt Bessie's*	1 Serving/100g	191	7.8	191	3.1	27.0	7.8	2.9
Homestyle Oven, Sainsbury's*	1 Serving/125g	206	5.4	165	2.4	29.2	4.3	2.1
Just Bake, Low Fat, M&S*	1oz/28g	37	1.0	133	2.0	24.7	3.7	1.7
Micro Chips, Crinkle Cut, Cooked, McCain*	1 Pack/100g	166	4.2	166	2.9	28.9	4.2	2.4

CHIPS

Measure INFO/WEIGHT	per Measure KCAL	per Measure FAT	Nutrition Values per 100g / 100ml KCAL	PROT	CARB	FAT	FIBRE
Micro Chips, Straight Cut, Cooked, McCain*	1 Pack/100g	163	4.8	163	2.3	27.7	4.8	2.0
Microwave, Cooked	1oz/28g	62	2.7	221	3.6	32.1	9.6	2.9
Oven, 5% Fat, Frozen, McCain*	1 Serving/200g	238	6.0	119	1.9	21.0	3.0	1.6
Oven, American Style, Champion*	1 Serving/200g	372	14.4	186	2.2	28.2	7.2	2.0
Oven, Best in the World, Iceland*	1 Serving/175g	332	11.7	190	3.4	28.9	6.7	3.5
Oven, Champion*	1 Pack/133g	210	6.0	158	2.5	27.0	4.5	0.0
Oven, Chunky, Extra Special, Asda*	1 Serving/125g	238	7.0	190	3.4	31.5	5.6	3.2
Oven, Chunky, Harry Ramsden's*	1 Serving/150g	184	5.4	123	2.8	19.9	3.6	1.6
Oven, Chunky, Ross*	1 Serving/100g	177	6.5	177	3.1	26.6	6.5	3.9
Oven, Chunky, TTD, Sainsbury's*	1 Serving/166g	250	5.3	151	2.0	28.6	3.2	2.3
Oven, Cooked, Value, Tesco*	1 Serving/125g	308	9.8	246	4.5	39.5	7.8	2.9
Oven, Cooked, Weight Watchers*	1 Serving/100g	150	3.0	150	2.8	33.7	3.0	5.9
Oven, Crinkle Cut, 5% Fat, Weighed Baked, McCain*	1 Serving/100g	163	4.3	163	3.1	27.9	4.3	3.0
Oven, Crinkle Cut, 5% Fat, Weighed Frozen, McCain*	1 Serving/100g	134	3.6	134	2.4	23.2	3.6	2.4
Oven, Crinkle Cut, Asda*	1 Serving/100g	134	3.8	134	2.0	23.0	3.8	8.0
Oven, Crinkle Cut, Baked, Aunt Bessie's*	1 Serving/100g	206	9.2	206	2.9	28.0	9.2	3.2
Oven, Crinkle Cut, Co-Op*	1oz/28g	32	0.9	115	2.1	19.6	3.2	2.2
Oven, Crinkle Cut, Frozen, Essential, Waitrose*	1 Serving/165g	225	6.4	136	2.7	22.6	3.9	1.7
Oven, Crinkle Cut, Oven Baked, Tesco*	1oz/28g	50	1.5	180	3.3	29.5	5.4	2.4
Oven, Crinkle Cut, Sainsbury's*	1 Serving/165g	297	9.1	180	3.3	29.5	5.5	2.4
Oven, Family Fries, Tesco*	1 Serving/125g	164	4.6	131	2.0	22.4	3.7	1.8
Oven, Frozen, Baked	1 Portion/80g	130	3.4	162	3.2	29.8	4.2	2.0
Oven, Frozen, Basics, Sainsbury's*	1 Serving/165g	249	8.1	151	3.0	23.6	4.9	2.9
Oven, Frozen, BGTY, Sainsbury's*	1 Serving/165g	226	4.6	137	2.9	25.0	2.8	2.7
Oven, Frozen, Value, Tesco*	1 Serving/125g	189	5.8	151	2.8	24.7	4.6	1.9
Oven, Morrisons*	1 Serving/100g	134	3.9	134	2.4	22.2	3.9	0.0
Oven, Organic, Waitrose*	1 Serving/165g	233	6.3	141	1.5	25.1	3.8	1.6
Oven, Original, McCain*	1 Serving/100g	158	3.8	158	2.5	28.5	3.8	2.3
Oven, Original, Straight Cut, 5% Fat, Cooked, McCain*	1 Serving/100g	172	4.9	172	3.4	32.4	4.9	2.3
Oven, Original, Straight Cut, 5% Fat, Frozen, McCain*	1 Serving/100g	138	4.0	138	2.5	26.2	4.0	1.9
Oven, Reduced Fat, Waitrose*	1oz/28g	37	0.8	133	2.3	24.3	3.0	1.6
Oven, Rooster, Albert Bartlett & Sons Ltd*	1 Serving/125g	156	2.4	125	2.9	27.7	1.9	3.7
Oven, Steak Cut, Asda*	1 Serving/100g	153	4.1	153	2.0	27.0	4.1	2.5
Oven, Steak Cut, Sainsbury's*	1 Serving/165g	266	7.8	161	2.6	27.1	4.7	2.8
Oven, Steak Cut, Somerfield*	1 Serving/180g	265	9.0	147	2.4	23.0	5.0	1.5
Oven, Steak Cut, Waitrose*	1 Serving/165g	218	5.6	132	2.7	22.7	3.4	1.7
Oven, Steakhouse, Frozen, Tesco*	1 Serving/125g	165	4.2	132	2.7	22.7	3.4	1.7
Oven, Straight Cut, 5% Fat, Sainsbury's*	1 Serving/165g	280	8.1	170	3.4	28.0	4.9	2.5
Oven, Straight Cut, Asda*	1 Serving/100g	199	5.0	199	3.5	35.0	5.0	3.0
Oven, Straight Cut, BFY, Morrisons*	1 Serving/165g	249	5.8	151	2.8	27.1	3.5	2.1
Oven, Straight Cut, GFY, Asda*	1oz/28g	42	1.0	150	2.6	27.0	3.5	2.4
Oven, Straight Cut, Iceland*	1 Serving/100g	197	6.2	197	3.6	31.6	6.2	2.3
Oven, Straight Cut, Oven Baked, LC, Tesco*	1 Serving/125g	150	2.1	120	2.4	22.1	1.7	2.6
Oven, Straight Cut, Tesco*	1oz/28g	46	1.4	166	2.6	27.8	4.9	1.7
Oven, Straight Cut, Waitrose*	1 Serving/165g	219	6.1	133	2.0	23.0	3.7	1.7
Oven, Stringfellows, McCain*	1oz/28g	72	2.9	256	4.1	37.0	10.2	0.0
Oven, Sweet Potato, Tesco*	¼ Pack/125g	169	6.5	135	2.6	18.9	5.2	5.0
Oven, Thick Cut, Frozen, Baked	1oz/28g	44	1.2	157	3.2	27.9	4.4	1.8
Oven, Thin & Crispy, Tesco*	1 Portion/100g	205	4.9	205	2.7	37.6	4.9	5.8
Oven, Thin Cut, American Style, Asda*	1 Serving/100g	240	10.0	240	3.4	34.0	10.0	3.0
Oven, Thin Fries, Morrisons*	1 Serving/100g	161	6.1	161	2.9	23.6	6.1	1.2
Potato, Lights, Reduced Fat, Lay's*	1 Serving/25g	118	5.5	470	7.5	60.0	22.0	5.0
Rustic, TTD, Sainsbury's*	½ Pack/122g	176	2.9	144	2.8	27.9	2.4	2.8

Measure INFO/WEIGHT	per Measure KCAL	FAT	Nutrition Values per 100g / 100ml KCAL	PROT	CARB	FAT	FIBRE

CHIPS

Food	Measure INFO/WEIGHT	KCAL	FAT	KCAL	PROT	CARB	FAT	FIBRE
Steak Cut, Frying, Asda*	1 Serving/97g	181	6.8	187	2.9	28.0	7.0	2.8
Steak Cut, Oven, Tesco*	1 Serving/165g	233	6.4	141	2.0	24.4	3.9	2.0
Steakhouse, Fry, Tesco*	1 Serving/125g	278	15.1	222	3.1	25.2	12.1	2.0
Straight Cut, Frozen, Fried in Blended Oil	1oz/28g	76	3.8	273	4.1	36.0	13.5	2.4
Straight Cut, Frozen, Fried in Corn Oil	1oz/28g	76	3.8	273	4.1	36.0	13.5	2.4
Straight Cut, Low Fat, Tesco*	1 Serving/125g	159	3.8	127	2.3	22.7	3.0	2.1
Straight Cut, Oven, BGTY, Sainsbury's*	1 Portion/165g	226	3.5	137	2.7	26.8	2.1	4.1
The Big Chip, Frozen, Tesco*	1 Serving/200g	220	4.8	110	1.8	20.3	2.4	2.1
Thick Cut, Caterpack, Deep Fried, McCain*	1oz/28g	60	2.7	215	3.1	28.8	9.7	2.0
Thick Cut, Frozen, Fried in Corn Oil, Average	1oz/28g	66	2.9	234	3.6	34.0	10.2	2.4
Three Way Cook, Skinny, Co-Op*	1 Serving/100g	175	7.0	175	2.0	26.0	7.0	3.0
Waffle, Birds Eye*	1 Serving/75g	156	8.4	208	2.5	24.3	11.2	2.6

CHIVES

Food	Measure INFO/WEIGHT	KCAL	FAT	KCAL	PROT	CARB	FAT	FIBRE
Fresh, Average	1 Tsp/2g	0	0.0	23	2.8	1.7	0.6	1.9

CHOC ICES

Food	Measure INFO/WEIGHT	KCAL	FAT	KCAL	PROT	CARB	FAT	FIBRE
Chocolate, Dark, Seriously Creamy, Waitrose*	1 Ice/82g	195	12.9	238	2.6	21.6	15.7	1.7
Chocolate, Real Milk, Sainsbury's*	1 Ice/48g	151	9.5	312	3.5	30.3	19.7	0.8
Chunky, Wall's Ice Cream*	1 Ice/81g	162	10.6	200	2.6	18.9	13.1	0.0
Mini Mix, Eis Stern*	1 Ice/39g	129	8.9	334	4.2	29.0	23.0	0.0
Neapolitan Chocolate, Co-Op*	1 Ice/62g	120	8.2	194	2.0	16.9	13.2	0.4
White Chocolate, Sainsbury's*	1 Ice/48g	140	8.9	292	3.8	27.3	18.6	0.1

CHOCOLATE

Food	Measure INFO/WEIGHT	KCAL	FAT	KCAL	PROT	CARB	FAT	FIBRE
Advent Calendar, Dairy Milk, Cadbury*	1 Chocolate/4g	22	1.3	525	7.5	56.6	30.1	0.7
Advent Calendar, Magic of Christmas, Cadbury*	1 Chocolate/10g	48	2.7	510	7.0	57.7	28.0	0.7
Advent Calendar, Maltesers, Mars*	1 Chocolate/4g	21	1.2	537	6.8	57.9	30.9	0.0
Advent Calendar, Pirates of the Caribbean, Kinnerton*	1 Chocolate/4g	19	1.0	525	5.4	61.2	28.6	1.6
Advent Calendar, The Simpsons, Kinnerton*	1 Chocolate/4g	20	1.1	526	5.3	63.2	29.0	1.6
Advent Calendar, The Snowman, M&S*	1 Chocolate/4g	21	1.2	550	6.6	60.4	31.0	0.0
Baking, Belgian, Milk for Cakes, Luxury, Sainsbury's*	1 Chunk/8g	44	2.7	556	7.6	56.5	33.3	1.5
Bar, Alpini, Continental, Thorntons*	1 Bar/36g	192	11.4	538	6.9	55.3	32.0	2.7
Bar, Animal, Nestle*	1 Bar/19g	97	5.0	513	5.8	63.6	26.1	0.0
Bar, Baby Ruth, Candy, Nestle*	1 Bar/60g	296	14.1	494	6.7	63.9	23.5	1.7
Bar, Bliss, Hazelnut Truffle, Cadbury*	1 Serving/100g	565	37.9	565	7.2	47.7	37.9	2.6
Bar, Bliss Truffle, Cadbury*	1 Bar/40g	226	14.9	565	6.6	48.8	37.3	2.8
Bar, Bubbles, Galaxy, Mars*	1 Bar/31g	172	10.6	555	6.5	54.7	34.2	1.5
Bar, Cappuccino, Thorntons*	1 Bar/38g	201	13.2	529	5.2	49.7	34.7	0.5
Bar, Chocolate, Cherry, Lindt*	1 Bar/100g	470	22.8	470	4.5	61.7	22.8	0.0
Bar, Chocolate, Pistachio, Lindt*	1 Bar/100g	585	40.6	585	7.1	48.2	40.6	0.0
Bar, Chocolate, Strawberry, Lindt*	1 Bar/100g	470	22.8	470	4.5	61.6	22.8	0.0
Bar, Chocolate Cream, Fry's*	1 Piece/10g	42	1.3	415	2.8	70.8	13.2	1.2
Bar, Chocoletti, Stracciatella, Lindt*	1 Bar/6g	32	2.3	590	7.7	49.0	41.0	0.0
Bar, Dark, 60% Cocoa with Macadamia, Thorntons*	1 Bar/70g	183	12.8	523	6.5	42.3	36.5	12.6
Bar, Dark, 63%, Blueberry & Raspberry, Thorntons*	1 Bar/80g	394	27.5	492	6.4	39.3	34.4	8.1
Bar, Dark, Diabetic, Thorntons*	1 Bar/75g	345	26.8	460	5.4	28.5	35.8	8.1
Bar, Dark, Thorntons*	1 Bar/48g	250	17.7	521	7.3	39.9	36.9	10.9
Bar, Dark, with Ginger, Thorntons*	1 Bar/100g	509	35.1	509	5.8	44.3	35.1	8.8
Bar, Extra Dark, 60% Cocoa, Lindor, Lindt*	1 Bar/150g	900	73.5	600	5.0	35.0	49.0	2.0
Bar, Flake Allure, Cadbury*	1 Bar/30g	170	10.9	567	6.7	51.0	36.3	0.7
Bar, Hazel Nut & Cashew, Dairy Milk, Cadbury*	3 Chunks/18g	96	6.0	540	8.8	50.6	33.5	1.8
Bar, Jazz Orange, Thorntons*	1 Bar/56g	304	18.1	543	6.8	55.7	32.3	1.2
Bar, Lemon Mousse, Thorntons*	1oz/28g	141	8.2	503	4.1	55.3	29.3	0.0
Bar, Milk, Thorntons*	1 Bar/50g	269	16.0	538	7.5	54.8	32.0	1.0
Bar, Milk Chocolate, Diabetic, Thorntons*	½ Bar/37g	174	12.2	470	7.3	43.0	33.1	2.2

CHOCOLATE

	Measure INFO/WEIGHT	per Measure KCAL	per Measure FAT	Nutrition Values per 100g / 100ml KCAL	PROT	CARB	FAT	FIBRE
Bar, Milk Chocolate, Galaxy, Mars*	1 Bar/46g	250	15.0	544	6.6	56.3	32.5	1.5
Bar, Milk Chocolate, Gold, Lindt*	1 Bar/300g	1605	92.9	535	6.6	58.7	31.0	0.0
Bar, Milk Chocolate, Hazelnut, Gold, Lindt*	1 Bar/300g	1665	108.2	555	7.9	50.7	36.1	0.0
Bar, Milk Chocolate, Hazelnut, Lindt*	1 Bar/100g	570	38.8	570	8.5	47.0	38.8	0.0
Bar, Milk Chocolate, Lindt*	1 Bar/100g	535	31.0	535	6.6	57.6	31.0	0.0
Bar, Milk Chocolate, Raisin & Hazelnut, Gold, Lindt*	1 Bar/300g	1590	94.8	530	6.8	54.7	31.6	0.0
Bar, Milk Chocolate, Raisin & Hazelnut, Lindt*	1 Bar/100g	530	31.6	530	3.1	54.7	31.6	0.0
Bar, Mountain, Swiss, M&S*	1 Bar/100g	555	35.3	555	6.5	55.2	35.3	0.2
Bar, Strawberries & Creme, Dairy Milk, Cadbury*	1 Chunk/5g	28	1.8	560	5.7	53.5	35.5	0.5
Bar, Truffle, M&S*	1 Bar/35g	168	11.4	480	5.9	41.7	32.5	8.3
Bar, Truffle, Orange, M&S*	1 Bar/33g	177	10.5	535	6.6	55.6	31.9	1.4
Bar, Twisted, Creme Egg, Cadbury*	1 Bar/45g	210	9.4	465	5.2	64.6	20.8	0.5
Bar, Viennese, Continental, Thorntons*	1 Bar/38g	206	13.0	542	4.2	54.0	34.2	0.8
Bar, White, Thorntons*	1 Bar/50g	274	15.6	547	6.5	59.5	31.3	0.0
Bars, Milk, M&S*	1 Bar/40g	214	12.8	535	7.8	54.0	32.0	1.9
Beans, Coffee, Dark, Solid, M&S*	1 Serving/10g	53	3.8	532	4.7	42.4	37.6	11.6
Bear, Lindt*	1 Bear/11g	60	3.6	572	7.5	57.7	34.6	0.0
Belgian, Kschocolat*	4 Pieces/40g	212	12.2	530	6.0	57.5	30.5	2.3
Belgian, Milk, Mini Eggs, M&S*	1 Egg/8g	43	2.5	535	7.0	55.8	31.7	2.7
Black Magic, Nestle*	1oz/28g	128	5.8	456	4.4	62.6	20.8	1.6
Bubbly, Dairy Milk, Cadbury*	1 Bar/35g	185	10.5	525	7.7	56.9	29.7	0.7
Bubbly Santa, M&S*	1 Santa/23g	124	7.3	540	7.0	55.8	31.7	2.7
Bunny, Easter, Mars*	1 Bunny/29g	155	9.2	535	6.2	56.2	31.7	0.0
Bunny, Lindt*	1 Bunny/11g	60	3.6	572	7.5	57.5	34.6	0.0
Cappuccino, Nestle*	1 Serving/20g	109	6.6	545	6.1	56.0	32.9	0.0
Caramel, Chunk, Dairy Milk, Cadbury*	1 Chunk/33g	158	7.6	480	5.0	63.0	23.0	0.0
Caramel, Dairy Milk, Cadbury*	1 Bar/45g	215	10.4	480	4.9	62.8	23.2	0.4
Chocolat Noir, Lindt*	1/6 Bar/17g	87	5.4	510	6.0	50.0	32.0	0.0
Chocolate Favourites, Tesco*	½ Box/227g	1015	43.6	447	4.2	64.3	19.2	0.3
Chomp, Cadbury*	1 Bar/24g	112	4.8	465	3.3	67.9	20.0	0.2
Christmas Tree Decoration, Average	1 Chocolate/12g	63	3.6	522	7.6	56.4	29.9	0.4
Christmas Tree Decoration, Cadbury*	1 Piece/12g	60	3.4	525	7.6	56.2	29.9	0.0
Chunk Bar, Dairy Milk, Cadbury*	1 Chunk/7g	35	2.0	525	7.5	57.0	29.8	0.1
Chunky Hazelnut Bar, M&S*	1 Bar/52g	293	19.4	563	8.8	48.1	37.3	1.7
Coconut, White, Excellence, Lindt*	1 Square/10g	61	4.4	610	6.0	48.0	44.0	0.0
Coins, Milk, Sainsbury's*	1 Coin/5g	26	1.4	502	5.5	58.8	27.1	2.5
Counters, Galaxy, Mars*	4 Counters/10g	53	2.9	529	6.8	59.4	29.1	1.4
Creme Egg Splats, Cadbury*	¼ Pack/40g	192	9.0	480	5.7	64.5	22.5	0.5
Crispello, Double Choc, Cadbury*	1 Peice/10g	55	3.5	560	7.0	51.0	36.0	1.9
Crispies, Chunk, Dairy Milk, Cadbury*	1 Chunk/31g	158	8.5	510	7.6	58.6	27.4	0.0
Crispies, Dairy Milk, Cadbury*	1 Bar/49g	250	13.4	510	7.6	58.6	27.4	0.0
Crispy, Sainsbury's*	4 Squares/19g	99	5.4	521	9.1	56.9	28.5	2.1
Dairy Milk, Cadbury*	1 Bar/45g	236	13.4	525	7.6	57.0	29.8	0.7
Dairy Milk, King Size, Cadbury*	1 Serving/85g	446	25.2	525	7.6	56.4	29.7	0.0
Dairy Milk, Little Bars, Cadbury*	1 Bar/21g	110	6.3	530	7.7	56.6	30.1	0.7
Dairy Milk, Snack Size, Cadbury*	1 Bar/30g	159	9.0	530	7.8	57.1	29.9	0.0
Dairy Milk, Toffee Popcorn, Dairy Milk, Cadbury*	1 Bar/150g	765	39.8	510	7.0	59.5	26.5	1.7
Dairy Milk with Oreo, Dairy Milk, Cadbury*	3 Chunks/15g	85	5.4	560	6.1	53.5	35.5	0.7
Dark, 70% Cocoa Solida, Extra Fine, Lindt*	1 Square/10g	54	4.1	537	8.0	33.0	41.0	0.0
Dark, 70% Cocoa Solids, Organic, Green & Black's*	1 Bar/35g	193	14.4	551	9.3	36.0	41.1	11.5
Dark, 70% Cocoa Solids, Organic, Morrisons*	½ Bar/50g	266	20.6	531	7.9	31.6	41.1	11.0
Dark, 75% Cacao, Rausch*	1 Row/31g	163	12.9	522	8.8	28.5	41.1	15.0
Dark, 85% Cocoa, Excellence, Lindt*	1 Serving/40g	212	18.4	530	11.0	19.0	46.0	0.0

CHOCOLATE

INFO/WEIGHT	Measure	per Measure KCAL	per Measure FAT	KCAL	PROT	CARB	FAT	FIBRE
Dark, 85% Cocoa, TTD, Sainsbury's*	1 Serving/25g	142	12.8	569	9.7	17.0	51.4	14.1
Dark, 99% Cocoa, Excellence, Lindt*	1 Serving/25g	132	12.5	530	13.0	8.0	50.0	8.0
Dark, Belgian, Extra Special, Asda*	2 Squares/20g	102	8.0	508	11.0	26.0	40.0	16.0
Dark, Belgian, Luxury Continental, Sainsbury's*	1 Bar/100g	490	38.7	490	11.1	24.2	38.7	7.4
Dark, Chilli, Excellence, Lindt*	1 Serving/40g	202	12.8	506	5.4	49.0	32.0	0.0
Dark, Classic, Bourneville, Cadbury*	4 Squares/25g	125	6.8	505	4.7	58.8	27.3	2.0
Dark, Continental, Luxury, Sainsbury's*	½ Bar/50g	252	20.0	504	10.7	25.5	40.0	16.1
Dark, Continental, Luxury, Tesco*	1 Bar/100g	571	37.8	571	11.3	46.5	37.8	0.1
Dark, Co-Op*	1 Bar/50g	252	14.5	505	4.0	57.0	29.0	6.0
Dark, Espresso, Arabica, 70%, Green & Black's*	½ Bar/50g	290	20.8	580	9.0	37.2	41.7	11.0
Dark, Espresso, with Coffee, Green & Black's*	1 Bar/150g	824	62.4	549	9.8	33.8	41.6	11.7
Dark, Fair Trade, Co-Op*	1 Bar/45g	214	13.0	475	4.0	49.0	29.0	6.0
Dark, Feuilles, with Orange, Nestle*	1 Piece/8g	42	2.6	524	4.6	54.4	32.0	0.0
Dark, Hazelnuts & Currant, Organic, Green & Black's*	1 Bar/100g	513	33.5	513	7.6	45.4	33.5	9.2
Dark, Mint, Intense, Lindt*	1 Square/10g	51	3.2	510	5.0	50.0	32.0	0.0
Dark, Orange & Spices, Maya Gold, Green & Black's*	1 Bar/35g	184	11.8	526	7.3	48.2	33.8	8.2
Dark, Orange with Slivered Almonds, Excellence, Lindt*	1 Square/10g	50	3.1	500	6.0	49.0	31.0	0.0
Dark, Plain, Average	*1oz/28g*	*143*	*7.8*	*510*	*5.0*	*63.5*	*28.0*	*2.5*
Dark, Plain, Rich, Sainsbury's*	1oz/28g	144	8.3	514	3.7	65.0	29.5	0.9
Dark, Raspberry, Ruffles, Jameson's*	1oz/28g	123	5.3	441	1.9	65.9	18.9	4.4
Dark, Raw Organic, Loving Earth*	1 Serving/20g	99	7.9	495	9.3	46.4	39.5	0.0
Dark, Rich, Tesco*	1 Serving/20g	98	6.1	491	5.8	60.0	30.4	11.5
Dark, Smooth, Bar, Galaxy, Mars*	1 Bar/125g	651	42.0	521	6.2	48.0	33.6	9.3
Dark, Special, Hershey*	1 Pack/41g	180	12.0	439	4.9	61.0	29.3	7.3
Dark, Whole Nut, Tesco*	1 Serving/13g	67	4.5	539	6.1	48.3	35.7	6.5
Dark, with a Soft Mint Centre, Organic, Green & Black's*	1 Bar/100g	478	27.3	478	7.4	50.5	27.3	8.6
Dark, with Cherries, Organic, Green & Black's*	1 Bar/100g	477	28.2	477	7.9	48.0	28.2	8.7
Dark, with Chilli, Thorntons*	4 Squares/20g	107	7.9	533	7.2	36.3	39.5	10.4
Dark, with Crystallised Ginger, Organic, Green & Black's*	150g	752	43.6	501	6.8	53.0	29.1	9.6
Dark, with Dried Sweetened Cranberries, Fairtrade, Co-Op*	2 Chunks/20g	106	6.3	530	4.4	54.0	31.3	6.6
Diet, Ritter Sport*	1 Square/6g	25	1.8	412	6.0	44.0	30.0	0.0
Divine, Milk, Co-Op*	1 Bar/45g	243	14.4	540	7.0	57.0	32.0	2.0
Dream with Real Strawberries, Cadbury*	1 Bar/45g	250	14.9	555	4.5	59.6	33.1	0.0
Drops, Plain, Sainsbury's*	1 Serving/125g	638	34.5	510	5.3	60.1	27.6	4.0
Egg, Mars*	1 Egg/38g	183	9.4	482	5.3	59.7	24.7	0.0
Elves, Magical, with Popping Candy, Cadbury*	1 Elf/15g	77	4.2	515	6.9	60.0	27.7	0.0
Ferrero Rocher, Ferrero*	1 Chocolate/13g	74	5.1	593	7.0	49.0	41.0	0.0
Football, Milk Chocolate, Thorntons*	1 Football/200g	1088	67.0	544	7.6	52.9	33.5	1.0
Freddo, Caramel, Dairy Milk, Cadbury*	1 Freddo/19g	93	4.7	490	5.5	60.5	24.8	0.5
Freddo, Dairy Milk, Cadbury*	1 Freddo/18g	95	5.4	530	7.5	57.0	29.8	0.7
Fruit & Nut, Assortment, M&S*	1oz/28g	148	9.6	527	7.6	49.8	34.3	1.3
Fruit & Nut, Belgian, Waitrose*	1 Serving/50g	254	14.6	508	8.6	54.6	29.2	3.4
Fruit & Nut, Dark, Tesco*	4 Squares/25g	124	7.0	494	5.8	54.8	27.9	6.5
Ginger, Traidcraft*	1 Bar/50g	212	7.4	424	3.9	68.2	14.8	0.0
Golden Biscuit Crunch, Dairy Milk, Cadbury*	4 Chunks/25g	135	8.2	545	6.2	55.5	33.0	0.8
Golf Balls, Milk Chocolate, Lindt*	1 Pack/110g	619	39.5	563	6.5	53.6	35.9	0.0
Kinder, Bueno, Bar, White, Ferrero*	1 Piece/20g	111	7.0	571	8.8	52.6	35.9	1.0
Kinder, Bueno Bar, Milk, Ferrero*	1 Bar/22g	123	8.0	575	9.2	49.5	37.3	2.0
Kinder, Riegel, Ferrero*	1 Bar/21g	117	7.1	558	10.0	53.0	34.0	0.0
Kinder Maxi, Ferrero*	1 Bar/21g	116	7.1	550	10.0	51.0	34.0	0.0
Kinder Surprise, Ferrero*	1 Egg/20g	113	7.1	564	9.0	52.5	35.3	1.0
Lait Intense, Experiences, Cote D'or*	3 Squares/100g	575	40.0	575	7.2	44.5	40.0	5.0
Light & Whippy, Bite Sized, Sainsbury's*	1 Bar/15g	66	2.4	439	3.3	69.7	16.3	0.1

CHOCOLATE

	Measure INFO/WEIGHT	per Measure KCAL	FAT	Nutrition Values per 100g / 100ml KCAL	PROT	CARB	FAT	FIBRE
Matchmakers, Mint, Nestle*	1 Stick/4g	20	0.8	477	4.3	69.7	20.1	0.9
Milk, & Hazelnut, Bar, Swiss, M&S*	1oz/28g	156	10.1	556	6.4	51.9	36.0	3.3
Milk, Average	**1oz/28g**	**146**	**8.6**	**520**	**7.7**	**56.9**	**30.7**	**0.8**
Milk, Baking, Luxury, Tesco*	1 Pack/150g	838	54.3	559	7.0	51.4	36.2	1.7
Milk, Belgian, TTD, Sainsbury's*	1 Piece/10g	55	3.5	549	9.6	48.3	35.3	2.0
Milk, Biscuit Sticks, Mikado, Kraft*	1 Stick/2g	11	0.5	475	7.8	67.0	19.8	3.1
Milk, Bubbly, Swiss, M&S*	1 Serving/40g	218	13.7	545	8.0	52.0	34.3	2.5
Milk, Chips, Silver Spoon*	1oz/28g	148	8.4	529	6.9	58.0	30.1	0.3
Milk, Creamy, Organic, Green & Black's*	6 Pieces/20g	110	7.0	560	9.1	50.3	35.5	1.6
Milk, Darker Shade of Milk Chocolate, Green & Black's*	1 Bar/35g	183	10.4	523	9.9	54.0	29.7	3.7
Milk, Extra Au Lait, Milch Extra, Lindt*	½ Bar/50g	268	15.5	535	6.5	57.0	31.0	0.0
Milk, Extra Creamy, Excellence, Lindt*	1 Bar/100g	560	37.1	560	6.0	51.1	37.1	0.0
Milk, Extra Fine, Swiss, M&S*	1 Serving/25g	141	9.2	565	7.2	50.9	36.7	2.3
Milk, Fair Trade, Tesco*	1 Serving/45g	236	13.3	524	7.6	56.7	29.6	2.0
Milk, Figures, Hollow, Dairyfine, Aldi*	1 Serving/11g	58	3.2	523	5.5	59.9	29.0	3.1
Milk, for Baking, Value, Tesco*	½ Bar/50g	265	14.5	530	6.7	60.0	29.0	2.2
Milk, Giant Buttons, M&S*	1 Button/8g	44	2.7	550	7.1	52.3	34.2	0.4
Milk, Less Than 99 Calories, M&S*	1 Bar/16g	85	4.6	531	7.5	61.2	28.8	0.6
Milk, Lindor, Lindt*	1 Square/11g	68	5.2	615	4.7	43.0	47.0	0.0
Milk, Ryelands*	4 Squares/29g	155	8.2	520	7.3	60.7	27.6	1.7
Milk, Sainsbury's*	4 Squares/25g	133	7.7	533	9.2	54.6	30.8	2.2
Milk, Santas, Tesco*	1 Bag/90g	433	21.8	481	4.5	61.4	24.2	1.4
Milk, Shapes, Easter Friends, Tesco*	1 Chocolate/13g	68	4.3	540	8.0	52.3	34.2	2.3
Milk, Smart Price, Asda*	1 Square/6g	32	1.9	536	8.0	54.0	32.0	1.8
Milk, Swiss, Diabetic, with Fruit & Nuts, Boots*	½ Bar/21g	97	6.7	462	7.0	55.0	32.0	2.7
Milk, Swiss Made, Organic, Traidcraft*	4 Squares/17g	91	5.6	550	7.0	50.0	34.0	0.0
Milk, Tesco*	1 Serving/25g	133	7.7	533	9.5	54.7	30.7	2.2
Milk, Value, Tesco*	1/6 Bar/16g	83	4.5	520	6.8	60.0	28.0	2.3
Milk, Whole Nut, Tesco*	1 Serving/25g	129	8.4	517	8.7	53.4	33.8	9.0
Milk, with a Soft Caramel Centre, Green & Black's*	1 Bar/100g	495	26.4	495	8.3	56.2	26.4	2.8
Milk, with Crisped Rice, Dubble*	1 Bar/40g	211	11.8	528	6.4	59.6	29.4	0.0
Milk, with Crunchy Butterscotch, Organic, Green & Black's*	1 Bar/100g	810	47.1	540	9.3	52.5	31.4	2.9
Milk, with Honey & Almond Nougat, Swiss, Toblerone*	1 Piece/8g	42	2.4	525	5.4	59.0	29.5	2.2
Milk, with Peanut Butter Filling, Ghirardelli*	1 Serving/45g	250	17.0	556	8.9	48.9	37.8	2.2
Milk, with Raisins & Hazelnuts, Green & Black's*	1 Bar/100g	556	36.9	556	9.2	46.8	36.9	3.2
Milk, with Whole Almonds, Organic, Green & Black's*	1 Bar/100g	578	42.2	578	11.8	37.7	42.2	5.2
Milky Bar, Giant Buttons, Mars*	1 Sweet/2g	11	0.6	546	7.5	57.7	31.6	0.0
Mini, Toblerone*	1 Serving/6g	32	1.8	525	5.6	57.5	30.0	3.5
Mini Eggs, Cadbury*	1 Egg/3g	16	0.7	490	4.6	67.8	21.9	1.3
Mini Eggs, Caramel, Cadbury*	1 Egg/11g	55	2.9	485	5.7	59.0	25.7	0.4
Mini Eggs, Lindor, Lindt*	3 Eggs/15g	90	6.3	600	6.7	46.7	42.0	0.0
Mint, Lamb, Aero, Nestle*	1 Lamb/27g	147	8.3	543	5.3	60.2	30.7	0.0
Mint Creme, Sainsbury's*	1 Serving/20g	93	4.9	467	2.8	62.7	24.5	2.1
Mint Crisp, Cadbury*	1oz/28g	141	6.2	505	6.4	70.3	22.2	0.0
Mint Crisp, M&S*	1 Mint/8g	40	2.4	494	5.4	54.8	29.6	3.1
Mousse au Chocolat, Dark, Lindt*	1oz/28g	158	10.4	563	6.0	50.0	37.0	5.6
Natural Orange, Excellence, Lindt*	1 Bar/100g	560	37.0	560	7.0	50.0	37.0	0.0
Natural Vanilla, Excellence, Lindt*	1 Bar/100g	590	40.0	590	6.0	51.0	40.0	0.0
Neapolitans, Terry's*	1oz/28g	146	8.3	522	6.0	57.3	29.7	4.1
Nibs, Raw, Cacao, Organic, Navitas Naturals*	1 Serving/28g	130	12.0	464	14.3	35.7	42.9	32.1
NutRageous, Reese's, Hershey*	1 Bar/51g	260	16.0	510	11.8	54.9	31.4	3.9
Nuts About Caramel, Cadbury*	1 Bar/55g	272	15.1	495	5.8	56.6	27.4	0.0
Nutty Caramel, Dairy Milk, Cadbury*	4 Squares/28g	155	9.9	550	6.9	51.0	35.0	1.2

CHOCOLATE

INFO/WEIGHT	Measure	per Measure		Nutrition Values per 100g / 100ml				
		KCAL	FAT	KCAL	PROT	CARB	FAT	FIBRE
Nutty Nougat, Bite Sized, Sainsbury's*	1 Bar/23g	111	5.5	481	7.6	59.0	23.8	0.6
Old Jamaica, Bournville, Cadbury*	4 Chunks/23g	107	5.4	465	4.2	59.6	23.4	2.0
Orange, Bar, Terry's*	1 Bar/40g	210	11.7	530	7.3	58.0	29.5	2.1
Orange Cream, Fry's*	1 Bar/50g	210	6.8	420	2.8	72.3	13.7	0.0
Peanut Butter Cup, Big Cup, Reese's, Hershey*	1 Cup/39g	210	12.0	538	10.3	53.8	30.8	2.6
Peanut Butter Cup, Miniature, Reese's, Hershey*	1 Cup/9g	44	2.6	500	9.1	59.1	29.6	2.3
Peanut Butter Cup, Reese's, Hershey*	1 Cup/21g	105	6.5	500	11.9	57.1	31.0	5.9
Peanut Butter Cup, White, Mini, Reese's, Hershey*	5 Cups/39g	210	12.0	538	12.8	53.8	30.8	2.6
Peppermint, Ritter Sport*	1 Bar/100g	483	26.0	483	3.0	60.0	26.0	0.0
Peppermint Cream, Fry's*	1 Bar/51g	217	7.9	425	2.6	68.8	15.4	0.0
Peppermint Patty, Hershey*	3 Patties/41g	160	3.0	390	2.4	80.5	7.3	0.0
Plain, 50% Cocoa Solids Minimum, Tesco*	4 Squares/22g	115	6.2	523	7.4	60.0	28.1	1.8
Plain, 72% Cocoa Solids, Finest, Tesco*	1 Square/10g	60	4.4	603	7.7	44.0	44.0	3.7
Plain, Belgian, Organic, Waitrose*	1 Bar/100g	505	37.6	505	9.6	32.0	37.6	5.6
Plain, Belgian, TTD, Sainsbury's*	1 Piece/10g	57	4.7	570	7.0	29.3	47.2	10.2
Plain, Continental, Waitrose*	1 Square/4g	23	1.8	558	7.7	32.9	44.0	5.9
Plain, Dark, Fruit & Nut, Rich, Sainsbury's*	4 Squares/25g	122	7.0	489	5.2	53.9	27.9	5.7
Plain, Fair Trade, Tesco*	1 Bar/40g	200	11.8	501	4.8	53.8	29.6	6.6
Plain, Wholenut, Sainsbury's*	1 Serving/25g	142	9.0	567	5.7	54.6	36.2	2.5
Plain, with Ginger, Swiss, Waitrose*	4 Squares/17g	88	5.0	519	5.3	58.3	29.4	2.0
Plain, with Hazelnuts, Tesco*	4 Squares/25g	135	8.9	539	6.1	48.3	35.7	6.5
Planets, Mars*	1 Pack/37g	178	8.3	481	4.9	65.4	22.4	0.0
Praline, M&S*	1 Bar/34g	185	12.0	545	7.3	49.6	35.2	3.1
Probiotic, Bar, Ohso*	1 Bar/14g	72	5.0	514	5.0	47.0	36.0	15.5
Rafaello, Roche, Ferrero*	1 Sweet/10g	60	4.7	600	9.7	35.4	46.6	0.0
Reese's Pieces, Bite Size, Minis, Hershey*	11 Pieces/39g	200	12.0	513	7.7	59.0	30.8	2.6
Rocky Road, Clusters, Tesco*	1 Serving/32g	160	9.5	500	7.1	51.0	29.7	6.7
Shortcake, Snack Shots, Cadbury*	½ Bag/50g	260	14.0	520	5.8	60.4	27.9	2.0
Snack Bar, Kinder*	1 Bar/21g	116	7.1	554	10.0	52.0	34.0	0.0
Snowman, Mousse, Dairy Milk, Cadbury*	1 Snowman/29g	162	10.2	560	6.7	54.5	35.0	0.4
Speckled Eggs, M&S*	1 Egg/6g	25	1.0	440	6.6	63.1	18.2	1.5
Tasters, Dairy Milk, Cadbury*	1 Bag/45g	238	13.7	530	7.6	56.4	30.5	0.0
Taz, Cadbury*	1 Bar/25g	121	6.0	485	4.8	62.0	24.0	0.0
Teddy Bear, Milk Chocolate, Thorntons*	1 Teddy/250g	1358	83.8	543	7.6	52.6	33.5	1.0
Toffifee, Storck*	1 Sweet/6g	32	1.9	535	6.0	58.0	31.0	0.0
Treatsize, Dairy Milk, Cadbury*	1 Bar/14g	74	4.2	525	7.5	57.0	29.8	0.7
Turkish Delight, Large Bar, Dairy Milk, Cadbury*	1 Square/8g	35	1.6	470	5.6	63.2	21.4	0.5
Twirl, Bites, Cadbury*	1 Bite/2g	11	0.6	530	7.7	56.5	30.3	0.8
White, Average	*1oz/28g*	*148*	*8.7*	*529*	*8.0*	*58.3*	*30.9*	*0.0*
White, Bar, Swiss, M&S*	1oz/28g	152	8.7	543	8.0	58.3	30.9	0.0
White, Creamy, Aldi*	1 Bar/40g	220	13.2	551	5.5	58.0	33.0	0.0
White, Creamy, Tesco*	1 Serving/25g	139	8.7	557	5.1	55.7	34.9	3.3
White, Creamy Vanilla, Green & Black's*	1 Bar/35g	201	12.8	573	7.4	53.5	36.6	0.1
White, Crispy, Fair Trade, Co-Op*	½ Bar/50g	278	17.5	555	9.0	51.0	35.0	0.1
White, Nestle*	4 Pieces/40g	220	13.0	550	7.5	55.0	32.5	0.0
White, Value, Tesco*	1 Serving/10g	55	3.1	548	4.7	62.0	31.2	0.0
White, with Honey & Almond Nougat, Toblerone*	1 Serving/25g	132	7.2	530	6.2	60.5	29.0	0.2
White, with Strawberries, Divine*	1 Piece/3g	16	0.9	534	7.6	59.9	29.3	0.1
Whole Nut, Dairy Milk, Cadbury*	1 Bar/49g	270	17.4	550	8.9	49.5	35.4	1.7
Whole Nut, Sainsbury's*	4 Chunks/25g	142	9.4	566	8.5	48.5	37.6	2.6
Whole Nut, Smart Price, Asda*	½ Bar/16g	92	6.2	562	8.0	47.0	38.0	3.3
Wildlife Bar, Cadbury*	1 Bar/21g	109	6.2	520	7.8	56.8	29.3	0.0
Wispa, Bitsa Wispa, Cadbury*	¼ Bag/43g	238	14.7	550	7.3	53.0	34.0	0.9

CHOCOLATE	Measure INFO/WEIGHT	per Measure KCAL	per Measure FAT	KCAL	PROT	CARB	FAT	FIBRE
with Almonds, Dark, Organic, Evernat*	1oz/28g	169	12.1	604	16.3	37.4	43.2	0.0
with Almonds, Nestle*	1 Square/20g	109	7.0	547	9.2	48.7	35.1	0.1
with Creme Egg, Dairy Milk, Cadbury*	1 Bar/45g	210	9.3	470	5.2	64.8	20.9	0.5
with Crunchie Bits, Dairy Milk, Cadbury*	1 Bar/200g	1000	48.8	500	6.2	63.3	24.4	0.0
with Shortcake Biscuit, Dairy Milk, Cadbury*	1 Square/6g	31	1.7	520	7.5	59.0	28.0	0.0
CHOCOLATE DROPS								
Plain, Asda*	1 Serving/100g	489	29.0	489	7.0	50.0	29.0	10.0
White for Cooking & Decorating, Sainsbury's*	1oz/28g	152	8.6	544	6.5	60.3	30.8	0.0
CHOCOLATE NUTS								
Almonds, Dark Chocolate Covered, Bolero*	2 Almonds/3g	15	1.0	510	2.6	48.8	33.5	0.0
Peanuts, Belgian Coated, M&S*	1 Serving/20g	109	7.6	545	14.7	35.6	38.0	5.8
Peanuts, Co-Op*	1oz/28g	153	10.9	545	15.0	34.0	39.0	4.0
Peanuts, Milk, Tesco*	1 Bag/227g	1221	86.0	538	17.5	31.8	37.9	4.4
CHOCOLATE ORANGE								
Bar, Montana*	1 Serving/25g	131	6.8	523	7.0	62.2	27.4	0.0
Crunchball, Terry's*	1 Segment/9g	45	2.4	520	6.9	59.8	28.1	2.0
Dark, Terry's*	1 Segment/9g	45	2.6	511	4.3	57.0	29.3	6.2
Egg & Spoon, Terry's*	1 Egg/34g	195	12.9	575	5.5	51.6	38.0	1.7
Milk, Mini Segments, Minis, Terry's*	1 Segment/4g	21	1.1	525	5.4	60.5	28.5	2.1
Milk, Terry's*	1 Orange/175g	931	51.6	532	7.4	57.8	29.5	2.1
Plain, Terry's*	1 Orange/175g	889	51.4	508	3.8	56.8	29.4	6.2
Segsations, Terry's*	1 Segsation/8g	43	2.3	520	6.9	58.5	28.5	2.8
White, Terry's*	1 Segment/11g	61	3.4	535	6.3	60.9	29.4	0.0
CHOCOLATE RAISINS								
Assorted, Thorntons*	1 Bag/140g	601	27.6	429	4.2	58.8	19.7	2.9
Californian, Tesco*	½ Bag/57g	268	11.7	472	5.2	66.2	20.7	1.3
Chocolate Coated, Milk, Average	1 Serving/50g	207	7.7	415	4.4	64.6	15.4	2.0
Coated, Californian, M&S*	1 Bag/130g	520	19.1	400	4.3	63.2	14.7	1.9
Co-Op*	½ Pack/50g	205	7.5	410	4.0	64.0	15.0	1.0
M & S*	1oz/28g	116	4.1	414	4.5	66.5	14.6	1.2
Milk, Asda*	1 Serving/28g	120	4.2	430	5.1	66.4	15.1	4.2
Milk, Co-Op*	½ Bag/100g	420	17.0	420	5.0	63.0	17.0	6.0
Milk, Sainsbury's*	1oz/28g	116	3.9	413	4.1	67.7	14.0	2.8
Milk, Tesco*	1 Bag/227g	933	35.0	411	4.8	63.3	15.4	0.9
White Chocolate, Belgian, Californian, M&S*	1 Pack/100g	450	20.9	450	4.3	60.6	20.9	0.8
CHOCOLATE SPREAD								
& Caramel, CBY, Asda*	1 Serving/100g	564	34.7	564	2.5	60.1	34.7	0.8
Average	**1 Tsp/12g**	**68**	**4.5**	**569**	**4.1**	**57.1**	**37.6**	**0.0**
Hazelnut, Nutella, Ferrero*	1oz/28g	149	8.7	533	6.6	56.4	31.0	3.5
with Nuts	**1 Tsp/12g**	**66**	**4.0**	**549**	**6.2**	**60.5**	**33.0**	**0.8**
CHOCOLATES								
All Gold, Dark, Terry's*	1 Serving/30g	152	8.7	505	4.0	57.5	29.0	4.3
All Gold, Milk, Terry's*	1 Serving/30g	158	9.2	525	4.8	58.0	30.5	1.5
Almond Marzipan, Milk Chocolate, Thorntons*	1 Chocolate/13g	60	2.9	464	6.6	59.4	22.6	5.6
Almond Mocca Mousse, Thorntons*	1 Chocolate/14g	76	5.3	543	8.5	40.7	37.9	2.9
Alpini, Thorntons*	1 Chocolate/13g	70	4.2	538	7.0	54.6	32.3	2.3
Assortment, Belgian, Waitrose*	1oz/28g	127	7.6	453	6.3	45.5	27.3	3.8
Assortment, Occasions, Tesco*	1 Chocolate/15g	70	3.1	470	4.6	65.8	20.9	0.5
Bites, Galaxy, Mars*	1 Pack/40g	197	9.7	492	5.0	63.0	24.2	0.8
Bittermint, Bendicks*	1 Mint/18g	80	3.0	440	4.3	68.9	16.3	2.4
Brazil Nut Assortment, M&S*	1oz/28g	163	12.7	581	9.6	37.5	45.3	1.5
Cafe Au Lait from Continental Selection, Thorntons*	1 Chocolate/16g	77	4.0	481	5.3	58.1	25.0	0.6
Cappuccino from Continental Selection, Thorntons*	1 Chocolate/13g	70	4.7	538	5.9	48.5	36.2	0.8

CHOCOLATES

INFO/WEIGHT	Measure		Nutrition Values per 100g / 100ml				
	KCAL	FAT	KCAL	PROT	CARB	FAT	FIBRE
Caramel, Milk, Country, Thorntons*	1 Chocolate/9g	45	2.4	500	4.6	62.2	26.7	0.0
Caramels, Sainsbury's*	1 Sweet/12g	57	2.6	490	3.5	69.0	22.2	0.2
Celebrations, Mars*	1 Sweet/8g	41	2.2	512	5.7	61.5	27.0	1.7
Chocolate Mousse, Thorntons*	1 Chocolate/13g	67	4.7	515	7.5	40.0	36.2	3.1
Classic Collection, Thorntons*	1 Chocolate/12g	58	2.8	472	4.3	62.7	22.8	2.4
Coconut, Lindor, Lindt*	1 Ball/13g	79	6.0	632	5.4	42.0	48.0	0.0
Coffee Cream, Average	1 Chocolate/12g	54	2.0	446	3.3	70.4	17.0	2.4
Coffee Creme, Dark, Thorntons*	1 Chocolate/13g	52	1.4	400	3.0	71.5	10.8	0.8
Coffee Creme, Milk, Thorntons*	1 Chocolate/13g	52	1.3	400	2.8	74.6	10.0	0.8
Continental, Belgian, Thorntons*	1 Chocolate/13g	67	3.9	514	5.8	53.5	30.3	2.9
Continental, Thorntons*	1 Chocolate/15g	76	4.4	506	5.6	54.5	29.3	2.7
Dairy Box, Milk, Nestle*	1 Piece/11g	50	2.1	456	4.4	65.9	19.4	0.7
Dark, Elegant, Elizabeth Shaw*	1 Chocolate/8g	38	1.8	469	2.9	62.5	23.1	0.0
Dark, Rose & Violet Creams	1 Chocolate/13g	55	1.6	422	2.2	76.1	12.5	1.7
Dark, Swiss Thins, Lindt*	1 Pack/125g	681	46.2	545	4.8	49.2	37.0	0.0
Eclipse, Truffle, Plain, Dark, Montezuma*	1 Truffle/16g	93	8.5	581	0.6	21.9	53.1	0.0
Heroes, Cadbury*	1 Sweet/8g	38	1.8	480	4.8	65.1	22.4	0.4
Italian Collection, Amaretto, M&S*	1 Chocolate/13g	60	3.1	480	4.4	59.7	25.1	2.3
Italian Collection, Favourites, M&S*	1 Chocolate/14g	74	4.7	530	5.7	50.4	33.7	1.6
Liqueurs, Barrels, Cointreau	1 Chocolate/10g	44	1.8	435	3.5	57.0	18.0	0.0
Liqueurs, Brandy, Asda*	1 Chocolate/8g	34	1.4	409	4.0	60.0	17.0	0.8
Liqueurs, Cherry, M&S*	1 Chocolate/13g	55	2.6	435	3.2	50.6	20.2	4.1
Liqueurs, Cognac Truffle, Thorntons*	1 Chocolate/14g	65	3.8	464	7.3	40.0	27.1	2.9
Milk, Mini Eggs, Green & Black's*	1 Egg/8g	42	2.7	562	8.6	48.3	35.5	3.8
Milk, Swiss Thins, Lindt*	1 Pack/125g	688	43.3	550	5.8	53.6	34.6	0.0
Milk Tray, Cadbury*	1 Chocolate/9g	47	2.4	495	4.7	61.5	25.8	0.7
Mingles, Bendicks*	1 Chocolate/5g	27	1.6	540	6.5	56.5	31.3	0.1
Mini Eggs, with Soft White Truffle Centre, M&S*	1 Egg/6g	33	2.0	550	6.5	56.3	33.9	1.4
Mint Creams, Dark, Smooth & Fragrant, Waitrose*	1 Sweet/10g	42	0.9	410	3.0	77.9	9.1	2.4
Mint Crisp, Bendicks*	1 Mint/8g	38	2.3	494	5.2	55.0	29.9	0.0
Mint Crisp, Dark, Elizabeth Shaw*	1 Chocolate/6g	27	1.2	458	1.9	68.0	20.7	0.0
Mint Crisp, Milk, Elizabeth Shaw*	1 Chocolate/6g	30	1.3	493	4.0	70.9	21.4	0.0
Mint Crisp, Thorntons*	1 Chocolate/7g	34	2.2	486	7.7	40.0	31.4	4.3
Mints, After Eight, Dark, Nestle*	1 Sweet/7g	32	0.9	461	5.0	63.0	12.9	2.0
Mints, After Eight, Orange, Nestle*	1 Sweet/7g	29	0.9	417	2.5	72.6	12.9	1.1
Mints, After Eight, Straws, Nestle*	1 Sweet/5g	24	1.4	526	5.1	56.6	31.0	4.0
Misshapes, Assorted, Cadbury*	1 Chocolate/8g	41	2.3	515	5.2	57.5	29.1	0.0
Moments, Thorntons*	1 Chocolate/7g	37	2.0	511	5.4	59.9	27.8	1.9
Orange Cream, Average	1 Chocolate/12g	53	2.0	440	3.2	69.3	16.7	0.0
Orange Crisp, Elizabeth Shaw*	1 Chocolate/6g	29	1.3	478	2.9	68.2	21.5	0.0
Peppermint Cream, Average	1 Chocolate/12g	50	1.4	418	1.9	76.4	11.4	1.6
Praline, Coffee, Thorntons*	1 Chocolate/7g	37	2.4	529	7.0	47.1	34.3	2.9
Praline, Hazelnut, Thorntons*	1 Chocolate/5g	27	1.8	540	7.0	48.0	36.0	4.0
Praline, Marzipan, Thorntons*	1 Chocolate/14g	63	3.0	450	5.9	58.6	21.4	2.1
Praline, Roast Hazelnut, Thorntons*	1 Chocolate/13g	70	4.4	538	6.0	51.5	33.8	3.1
Quality Street, Nestle*	1 Sweet/9g	44	1.9	470	3.5	67.3	20.5	1.5
Rocher, Continental, Thorntons*	1 Chocolate/15g	76	5.0	507	6.8	45.3	33.3	2.0
Roses, Cadbury*	1 Chocolate/9g	42	2.2	495	4.8	62.6	25.3	0.7
Sea Shells, Belgian, Guylian*	1 Shell/11g	65	4.4	574	8.0	49.0	39.0	0.0
Sea Shells, Milk & White, Belgian, Waitrose*	1 Serving/15g	77	4.6	511	5.0	53.1	31.0	2.8
Stars, Mini Wishes, Truffle Centre, Cadbury*	1 Star/13g	70	4.1	540	6.9	55.6	31.8	1.3
Strawberries & Cream, Thorntons*	1 Chocolate/12g	64	3.9	533	5.1	54.2	32.5	0.8
Swiss Tradition, De Luxe, Lindt*	1 Pack/250g	1388	90.7	555	6.3	51.9	36.3	0.0

CHOCOLATES	Measure INFO/WEIGHT	per Measure KCAL	FAT	Nutrition Values per 100g / 100ml KCAL	PROT	CARB	FAT	FIBRE
Swiss Tradition, Mixed, Lindt*	1 Pack/392g	2215	149.4	565	6.1	49.8	38.1	0.0
Truffle, Amaretto, Thorntons*	1 Chocolate/14g	66	3.6	471	5.5	55.0	25.7	2.9
Truffle, Belgian, Flaked, Tesco*	1 Truffle/14g	80	5.4	575	4.4	52.7	38.5	2.3
Truffle, Belgian Milk, Waitrose*	1 Truffle/14g	74	4.8	525	5.8	52.9	34.1	1.2
Truffle, Brandy, Thorntons*	1 Chocolate/14g	68	3.8	486	6.1	52.1	27.1	0.7
Truffle, Caramel, Thorntons*	1 Chocolate/14g	67	3.6	479	4.2	57.9	25.7	2.1
Truffle, Champagne, Continental, Thorntons*	1 Chocolate/16g	78	4.5	488	6.1	51.3	28.0	0.6
Truffle, Champagne, Petit, Thorntons*	1 Chocolate/6g	31	1.9	517	7.5	48.3	31.7	3.3
Truffle, Champagne, Premier, Thorntons*	1 Chocolate/17g	88	5.6	518	6.9	45.3	32.9	2.4
Truffle, Cherry, Thorntons*	1 Chocolate/14g	58	3.0	414	4.2	50.7	21.4	1.4
Truffle, Dark, Balls, Lindor, Lindt*	1 Ball/12g	76	6.2	630	3.4	38.5	51.4	0.0
Truffle, French Cocoa, Dusted, Sainsbury's*	1 Truffle/10g	57	4.5	570	4.0	37.0	45.0	0.0
Truffle, Grand Marnier, Thorntons*	1 Chocolate/15g	77	5.1	513	7.2	40.7	34.0	4.0
Truffle, Hazelnut, Balls, Lindor, Lindt*	1 Ball/12g	76	6.1	632	5.0	39.1	50.6	0.0
Truffle, Lemon, White, Thorntons*	1 Chocolate/14g	63	3.5	450	4.6	64.3	25.0	0.7
Truffle, Milk, Balls, Lindor, Lindt*	1 Ball/12g	73	6.0	611	5.6	41.7	50.0	2.8
Truffle, Mini Milk, Balls, Lindor, Lindt*	3 Balls/15g	90	7.0	600	6.7	40.0	46.7	0.0
Truffle, Rum, Average	1 Truffle/11g	57	3.7	521	6.1	49.7	33.7	1.9
Truffle, Rum, Thorntons*	1 Chocolate/13g	63	3.2	485	4.8	58.5	24.6	4.8
Truffle, Selection, Tesco*	1 Chocolate/14g	75	4.2	539	5.1	62.0	29.8	0.5
Truffle, Seville, Thorntons*	1 Chocolate/14g	76	4.7	543	7.1	53.6	33.6	1.4
Truffle, Thorntons*	1 Chocolate/7g	33	1.9	471	6.0	48.6	27.1	1.4
Truffle, Vanilla, Thorntons*	1 Chocolate/13g	64	3.5	492	4.8	57.7	26.9	1.5
Truffle, Viennese, Dark, Thorntons*	1 Chocolate/10g	53	3.6	530	5.9	47.0	36.0	3.0
Truffle, Viennese, Milk, Thorntons*	1 Chocolate/10g	56	3.6	560	4.9	54.0	36.0	0.0
Truffle, White, Balls, Lindor, Lindt*	1 Ball/12g	78	6.2	649	5.2	40.2	51.9	0.0
Truffle Filled, Swiss, Balls, Finest, Tesco*	3 Balls/37g	240	19.0	640	5.0	40.7	50.8	1.5
Truffle Hearts, Baileys*	1 Chocolate/15g	76	4.3	506	5.2	52.6	28.9	1.3
Twilight, Dark with Mint, Terry's*	1 Chocolate/6g	33	1.9	530	3.1	59.5	30.5	4.2
Valentine, Thorntons*	1 Chocolate/11g	60	3.8	542	5.7	52.0	34.5	2.1
Winter Selection, Thorntons*	1 Chocolate/10g	51	3.1	506	6.2	51.3	30.6	3.8
CHOP SUEY								
Chicken, with Noodles, Sainsbury's*	1 Pack/300g	300	7.5	100	5.7	13.6	2.5	1.2
Chinese, Vegetable, Stir Fry, Sharwood's*	1 Pack/310g	223	3.4	72	1.5	13.9	1.1	0.6
Vegetable, M&S*	½ Pack/150g	90	6.2	60	2.0	3.1	4.1	2.9
CHORIZO								
Iberico, Bellota, TTD, Sainsbury's*	1 Slice/3g	17	1.5	498	27.0	1.0	42.9	0.0
CHOW MEIN								
Beef, Ready Meal, Average	1 Serving/400g	422	12.2	106	6.0	13.4	3.0	1.0
Beef, Sainsbury's*	1 Pack/450g	500	11.2	111	6.6	15.5	2.5	0.8
Cantonese Vegetable Stir Fry, Sainsbury's*	¼ Pack/100g	85	3.8	85	2.2	10.6	3.8	1.2
Chicken, & Vegetable, Fuller Longer, M&S*	1 Pack/380g	266	4.9	70	6.3	8.7	1.3	2.1
Chicken, Ainsley Harriott*	1 Serving/250g	447	11.8	179	14.0	21.2	4.7	2.0
Chicken, CBY, Asda*	1 Pack/400g	312	2.8	78	8.3	9.2	0.7	0.9
Chicken, Chinese, Asda*	1 Pack/400g	479	20.4	120	6.7	11.0	5.1	1.5
Chicken, Chinese Takeaway, Sainsbury's*	1 Pack/316g	338	8.5	107	9.1	11.6	2.7	0.7
Chicken, Chinese Takeaway, Tesco*	1 Serving/350g	294	8.4	84	8.1	7.5	2.4	1.1
Chicken, COOK!, M&S*	1 Pack/375g	356	7.9	95	7.9	10.5	2.1	1.7
Chicken, Co-Op*	1 Pack/300g	270	9.0	90	8.0	9.0	3.0	0.9
Chicken, COU, M&S*	1 Pack/200g	170	5.4	85	5.9	9.5	2.7	1.4
Chicken, LC, Tesco*	1 Pack/400g	380	4.0	95	8.1	12.6	1.0	1.7
Chicken, Less Than 3% Fat, BGTY, Sainsbury's*	1 Pack/400g	358	9.1	94	6.5	10.3	2.4	2.8
Chicken, Morrisons*	1 Pack/400g	368	9.2	92	5.8	13.0	2.3	1.1

	Measure INFO/WEIGHT	per Measure KCAL	FAT	Nutrition Values per 100g / 100ml KCAL	PROT	CARB	FAT	FIBRE
CHOW MEIN								
Chicken, Ready Meal, Average	1 Serving/400g	375	9.4	94	6.5	11.5	2.4	1.2
Chicken, Ready Meal, Healthy Range, Average	1 Serving/400g	329	8.5	82	5.9	9.9	2.1	1.3
Chicken, Sainsbury's*	1 Pack/450g	558	21.2	124	6.5	12.6	4.7	2.6
Chicken, Waitrose*	1 Serving/400g	384	11.6	96	6.0	11.4	2.9	1.3
Chicken, with Vegetable Spring Roll, Oriental Express*	1 Pack/300g	213	1.8	71	5.5	12.4	0.6	1.9
Pork, PB, Waitrose*	½ Pack/310g	332	2.8	107	7.6	17.2	0.9	1.6
Special, COU, M&S*	1 Pack/400g	400	15.2	100	6.6	10.3	3.8	1.4
Special, Ready Meal, Average	1 Serving/400g	383	9.7	96	6.5	12.1	2.4	1.0
Stir Fry, Tesco*	½ Pack/240g	180	3.4	75	2.8	12.0	1.4	1.6
Stir Fry, with Veg & Noodles, Somerfield*	1 Serving/200g	234	12.0	117	2.8	12.9	6.0	1.3
Vegetable, Ready Meal, Average	1 Serving/400g	337	6.7	84	4.2	12.8	1.7	2.0
Vesta*	1 Pack/433g	594	17.3	137	4.8	20.4	4.0	3.3
CHRISTMAS PUDDING								
Average	1oz/28g	81	2.7	291	4.6	49.5	9.7	1.3
Cooked, Fox's*	¼ Pudding/114g	384	11.1	338	3.6	56.0	9.8	5.7
Luxury	1 Serving/114g	416	18.8	365	2.5	48.6	16.4	1.0
Luxury, Tesco*	¼ Pudding/114g	346	11.0	305	3.7	50.8	9.7	1.3
Retail	1oz/28g	92	3.3	329	3.0	56.3	11.8	1.7
Rich Fruit, Laced with Brandy, Tesco*	1 Serving/100g	305	9.7	305	3.7	50.8	9.7	1.3
Rich Fruit, Tesco*	1 Serving/114g	331	6.7	290	2.4	55.0	5.9	0.0
Sticky Toffee, Tesco*	¼ Pudding/114g	372	7.3	326	2.5	64.5	6.4	0.8
Tesco*	1 Serving/113g	305	6.7	270	2.4	55.0	5.9	1.5
Traditional Style, Asda*	1 Pudding/100g	296	6.0	296	2.6	58.0	6.0	1.6
Vintage, M&S*	1/8 Pudding/113g	335	6.4	295	2.6	59.8	5.6	1.4
VLH Kitchens	1 Serving/114g	310	2.2	272	3.1	59.3	2.5	4.6
Wheat Free, GF, Tesco*	1oz/28g	84	2.0	295	1.9	60.4	7.1	4.5
with Cider & Sherry, Waitrose*	¼ Pudding/113g	344	7.2	303	2.5	59.0	6.3	3.2
CHUTNEY								
Albert's Victorian, Baxters*	1 Serving/25g	40	0.1	159	1.1	37.9	0.3	1.5
Apple, Tomato & Sultana, Tesco*	1 Serving/50g	88	0.1	176	1.1	42.4	0.2	1.3
Apple & Pear, TTD, Sainsbury's*	1 Serving/20g	38	0.2	190	0.6	45.2	0.8	1.7
Apple & Walnut, Waitrose*	1 Serving/20g	49	0.5	243	12.0	53.8	2.6	3.8
Apricot, Sharwood's*	1 Tsp/16g	21	0.0	131	0.6	32.0	0.1	2.3
Bengal Spice Mango, Sharwood's*	1 Tsp/5g	12	0.0	236	0.5	58.0	0.2	1.2
Fruit, Spiced, Baxters*	1 Tsp/16g	23	0.0	143	6.0	34.8	0.1	0.0
Fruit, Traditional, M&S*	1oz/28g	43	0.1	155	0.9	37.2	0.3	1.7
Indian, Appetisers, Pot, Waitrose*	1 Pot/158g	330	2.2	209	1.8	47.3	1.4	1.8
Lime & Chilli, Geeta's*	1 Serving/25g	69	0.4	277	2.0	64.0	1.4	1.9
Mango, & Apple, Sharwood's*	1oz/28g	65	0.0	233	0.4	57.6	0.1	1.1
Mango, & Chilli, Geeta's*	1 Serving/30g	74	0.0	246	0.5	60.7	0.1	0.2
Mango, & Ginger, Baxters*	1 Jar/320g	598	0.6	187	5.0	45.7	0.2	0.9
Mango, & Lime, Sharwood's*	1oz/28g	58	0.1	206	0.4	50.5	0.3	0.8
Mango, & Mint, Cofresh*	1 Tbsp/20g	31	0.1	155	1.7	36.4	0.3	2.0
Mango, Budgens*	1oz/28g	66	0.0	235	0.3	58.2	0.1	0.0
Mango, Green Label, Sharwood's*	1 Tsp/10g	24	0.0	241	0.3	59.7	0.1	0.9
Mango, Hot, Patak's*	1 Jar/340g	877	0.7	258	0.4	67.1	0.2	0.7
Mango, Hot & Spicy, Waitrose*	1 Serving/20g	46	0.1	230	0.6	51.6	0.3	1.8
Mango, Indian Takeaway, Asda*	1 Pack/70g	145	0.1	207	0.3	50.9	0.2	1.0
Mango, Major Grey, Patak's*	1 Tbsp/15g	38	0.0	255	0.4	66.0	0.2	0.7
Mango, Premium, Geeta's*	1 Serving/50g	126	0.1	253	0.8	62.0	0.2	0.8
Mango, Spicy, Sainsbury's*	1 Tbsp/15g	24	0.1	160	0.7	37.0	0.7	1.3
Mango, Sweet	**1 Tbsp/16g**	**30**	**0.0**	**189**	**0.7**	**48.3**	**0.1**	**0.0**
Mango, Sweet, M&S*	1oz/28g	67	0.1	240	0.3	58.8	0.2	1.5

	Measure INFO/WEIGHT	KCAL	FAT	KCAL	PROT	CARB	FAT	FIBRE
CHUTNEY								
Mango, Sweet, Patak's*	1 Tbsp/15g	39	0.0	259	0.3	67.4	0.1	0.7
Mango, Tesco*	1 Serving/20g	45	0.0	224	0.4	55.5	0.1	1.3
Mango, Waitrose*	1 Serving/20g	43	0.3	215	1.0	49.0	1.5	2.0
Mango, with Hint of Chilli & Ginger, Waitrose*	1 Serving/20g	52	0.0	259	0.5	64.2	0.0	0.7
Mixed Fruit	*1 Tbsp/16g*	*25*	*0.0*	*155*	*0.6*	*39.7*	*0.0*	*0.0*
Onion, Caramelised, Red, & Cranberry, Baxters*	1 Serving/20g	31	0.0	154	0.3	38.0	0.1	0.3
Onion, Caramelised, Sainsbury's*	1 Serving/25g	28	0.4	111	1.1	23.5	1.4	1.1
Onion, Caramelised, TTD, Sainsbury's*	1 Serving/20g	31	0.1	157	0.8	37.3	0.5	2.1
Onion, Red, & Sherry Vinegar, Sainsbury's*	1 Serving/10g	24	0.1	236	0.5	57.1	0.6	1.4
Onion, Red, Caramelised, Loyd Grossman*	1 Serving/10g	11	0.0	111	0.5	27.2	0.0	0.5
Onion, Spicy, Organic, The English Provender Co.*	1 Serving/10g	24	0.0	245	1.2	59.0	0.5	3.5
Peach, Spicy, Waitrose*	1 Serving/20g	43	0.3	215	1.0	49.0	1.5	1.5
Ploughman's, Plum, The English Provender Co.*	1 Tsp/10g	16	0.0	160	1.3	38.1	0.2	1.6
Spicy Fruit, Baxters*	1 Serving/15g	22	0.0	146	0.6	35.4	0.2	0.0
Tomato	*1 Tbsp/16g*	*20*	*0.0*	*128*	*1.2*	*31.0*	*0.2*	*1.3*
Tomato, & Red Pepper, Baxters*	1 Jar/312g	512	1.2	164	2.0	38.0	0.4	1.5
Tomato, Waitrose*	1 Pot/100g	195	0.3	195	1.3	46.8	0.3	0.0
Tomato & Chilli, Sweet, The English Provender Co.*	1 Tsp/10g	19	0.0	189	0.9	46.0	0.2	1.7
CIDER								
Basics, Sainsbury's*	1 Glass/250ml	200	0.0	80	0.0	0.0	0.0	0.0
Berry, Irish, Magner's*	1 Bottle/500ml	215	0.0	43	0.0	4.3	0.0	0.0
Cyder, Organic, Aspall*	1 Serving/200ml	120	0.2	60	0.1	3.1	0.1	0.0
Cyder, Perronelle's Blush, Aspall*	1 Serving/200ml	122	0.2	61	0.1	5.4	0.1	0.5
Cyder, Premier Cru, Aspall*	1 Serving/200ml	120	0.0	60	0.0	3.1	0.0	0.0
Cyder, Suffolk, Medium, Aspall*	1 Serving/200ml	134	0.0	67	0.1	4.4	0.0	0.0
Dry, Average	*1 Pint/568ml*	*205*	*0.0*	*36*	*0.0*	*2.6*	*0.0*	*0.0*
Dry, French, So Good, Somerfield*	1 Bottle/500ml	150	0.0	30	0.0	0.3	0.0	0.0
Dry, Strongbow*	1 Bottle/375ml	161	0.0	43	0.0	3.4	0.0	0.0
Frosty Jacks, Strong, Aston Manor Brewery Co Ltd*	1 Pint/568ml	250	0.0	44	0.0	0.0	0.0	0.0
Gold, Thatchers*	1 Bottle/500ml	230	0.0	46	0.0	4.5	0.0	0.0
Light, Bulmers*	1 Can/500ml	140	0.0	28	0.0	0.8	0.0	0.0
Low Alcohol	*1 Pint/568ml*	*97*	*0.0*	*17*	*0.0*	*3.6*	*0.0*	*0.0*
Low Alcohol, Sainsbury's*	1 Serving/200ml	62	0.0	31	0.0	6.4	0.0	0.0
Low Carb, Stowford*	1 Bottle/500ml	140	0.0	28	0.0	0.2	0.0	0.0
Magner's*	½ Pint/284ml	105	0.0	37	0.0	2.0	0.0	0.0
Medium Sweet, Somerfield*	1 Pint/568ml	233	0.0	41	0.0	5.0	0.0	0.0
Organic, Westons*	1 Serving/200ml	96	0.0	48	0.0	3.1	0.0	0.0
Original, Bulmers*	1 Serving/250ml	105	0.0	42	0.0	4.0	0.0	0.0
Original, Gaymers*	1 Bottle/330ml	148	0.0	45	0.0	4.7	0.0	0.0
Pear, Average	*1 Serving/200ml*	*86*	*0.0*	*43*	*0.0*	*3.6*	*0.0*	*0.0*
Pear, Bulmers*	1 Serving/200ml	86	0.0	43	0.0	3.6	0.0	0.0
Pear, Gaymers*	1 Bottle/330ml	168	0.0	51	0.0	6.2	0.0	0.0
Pear, Magner's*	1 Bottle/568ml	179	0.0	32	0.0	0.0	0.0	0.0
Pear, Non Alcoholic, Kopparberg*	1 Bottle/500ml	170	0.5	34	0.0	8.4	0.1	0.0
Pear, Organic, Westons*	1 Serving/200ml	106	0.0	53	0.0	5.1	0.0	0.0
Ritz, Perry, Bulmers*	1 Bottle/330ml	142	0.0	43	0.0	4.0	0.0	0.0
Scrumpy, Average	*1 Serving/200ml*	*93*	*0.0*	*46*	*0.0*	*2.3*	*0.0*	*0.0*
Scrumpy, Westons*	1 Serving/200ml	94	0.0	47	0.0	1.8	0.0	0.0
Sweet, Average	*1 Pint/568ml*	*239*	*0.0*	*42*	*0.0*	*4.3*	*0.0*	*0.0*
Vintage	*1 Pint/568ml*	*574*	*0.0*	*101*	*0.0*	*7.3*	*0.0*	*0.0*
CINNAMON								
Ground, Average	*1 Tsp/3g*	*8*	*0.1*	*261*	*3.9*	*55.5*	*3.2*	*0.0*
Stick, Schwartz*	1 Stick/2g	7	0.0	339	4.7	79.3	0.3	0.0

C

	Measure INFO/WEIGHT	per Measure KCAL	per Measure FAT	Nutrition Values per 100g / 100ml KCAL	PROT	CARB	FAT	FIBRE
CLAMS								
in Brine, Average	1oz/28g	22	0.2	79	16.0	2.4	0.6	0.0
Raw, Average	20 Sm/180g	133	1.7	74	12.8	2.6	1.0	0.0
CLEMENTINES								
Raw, Weighed with Peel, Average	1 Med/61g	29	0.1	47	0.8	12.0	0.2	1.7
Raw, Weighed without Peel, Average	1 Med/46g	22	0.1	47	0.8	12.0	0.2	1.7
COCKLES								
Boiled	1 Cockle/4g	2	0.0	53	12.0	0.0	0.6	0.0
Bottled in Vinegar, Drained	1oz/28g	17	0.2	60	13.3	0.0	0.7	0.0
COCKTAIL								
Alcoholic, Juice Based, Average	1 Glass/200ml	464	29.2	232	6.4	18.7	14.6	1.4
Bucks Fizz, Premixed, M&S*	1 Glass/250ml	152	0.0	61	0.0	9.0	0.0	0.0
Cosmopolitan, Canned, M&S*	1 Serving/200ml	456	0.0	228	0.0	22.0	0.0	0.0
Grenadine, Orange Juice, Pineapple Juice	1 Serving/200ml	158	0.3	79	0.5	19.2	0.1	0.2
Mai Tai, Average	1 Serving/200ml	209	0.1	105	0.2	13.9	0.1	0.1
Pina Colada	1 Glass/250ml	592	20.0	237	1.0	28.0	8.0	0.0
COCOA								
Nibs, Naturya*	1 Serving/10g	58	5.0	578	13.0	18.2	50.3	13.4
COCOA BUTTER								
Average	1oz/28g	251	27.9	896	0.0	0.0	99.5	0.0
COCOA POWDER								
Cadbury*	1 Tbsp/16g	52	3.3	322	23.1	10.5	20.8	0.0
Dry, Unsweetened, Average	1 Tbsp/5g	11	0.7	229	19.6	54.3	13.7	33.2
Organic, Green & Black's*	1 Tbsp/7g	25	1.7	345	22.5	12.5	22.6	30.5
Valrhona*	1 Tsp/5g	22	1.0	450	25.0	45.0	20.0	30.0
COCONUT								
Creamed, Average	1oz/28g	186	19.2	666	6.0	6.7	68.4	7.0
Desiccated, Average	1oz/28g	169	17.4	604	5.6	6.4	62.0	13.7
Fresh, Flesh Only, Average	1oz/28g	98	10.1	351	3.2	3.7	36.0	7.3
Ice, Average	1oz/28g	104	3.6	371	1.7	66.7	12.7	2.6
Milk, Average	1 Can/400ml	698	69.7	174	1.4	2.9	17.4	2.9
Milk, KTC*	1 Can/400g	776	73.2	194	0.9	1.2	18.3	0.0
Milk, Reduced Fat, Average	1 Serving/100g	104	10.0	104	1.0	2.4	10.0	0.4
Sliced, Dried, Forest Feast*	1oz/28g	166	17.4	593	5.6	6.4	62.0	13.7
Water with Pineapple, Vita Coco*	1 Carton/330ml	82	0.0	25	0.0	6.0	0.0	0.0
COD								
Baked, Average	1oz/28g	27	0.3	96	21.4	0.0	1.2	0.0
Beer Battered, Crispy, Finest, Tesco*	1 Portion/250g	575	35.0	230	12.0	13.4	14.0	1.3
Dried, Salted, Average	1oz/28g	82	0.7	290	62.8	0.0	2.4	0.0
Dried, Salted, Boiled, Average	1oz/28g	39	0.3	138	32.5	0.0	0.9	0.0
Fillets, Battered, Average	1 Fillet/125g	219	10.2	176	12.6	13.0	8.2	1.0
Fillets, Battered, Harry Ramsdens, Birds Eye*	1 Fillet/122g	310	18.8	254	11.4	17.2	15.4	0.6
Fillets, Battered, Lge, Frozen, Chip Shop, Youngs*	1 Fillet/120g	269	17.5	224	10.4	12.7	14.6	2.6
Fillets, Breaded, Average	1 Fillet/125g	258	12.2	206	13.0	16.7	9.8	1.0
Fillets, Breaded, Chunky, Average	1 Piece/135g	204	8.0	151	13.7	10.9	5.9	1.4
Fillets, Breaded, Light, Healthy Range, Average	1 Fillet/135g	209	6.9	154	13.6	13.3	5.1	1.2
Fillets, Breaded, Simply Fish, Birds Eye*	1 Fillet/127g	285	13.0	224	12.5	20.1	10.2	1.0
Fillets, Chunky, Average	1 Fillet/198g	267	7.3	135	17.1	8.2	3.7	0.8
Fillets, Portions, Large, Battered, Morrisons*	1 Fillet/118g	219	11.9	186	9.6	14.1	10.1	1.3
Fillets, Skinless & Boneless, Raw, Average	1 Fillet/140g	137	2.4	98	17.8	2.7	1.8	0.4
Fillets, Smoked, Average	1 Serving/150g	152	2.4	101	21.6	0.0	1.6	0.0
Fillets, with a Red Pepper Salsa, Love Life, Waitrose*	½ Pack/170g	92	1.5	54	9.0	2.5	0.9	0.5
Fillets, with Tomato & Basil Sauce, Simply Bake, Tesco*	1 Fillet/142g	170	8.1	120	15.2	1.8	5.7	0.1
Loin, Skinless, TTD, Sainsbury's*	1 Serving/100g	83	0.9	83	18.6	0.0	0.9	0.0

	Measure INFO/WEIGHT	per Measure KCAL	FAT	Nutrition Values per 100g / 100ml KCAL	PROT	CARB	FAT	FIBRE
COD								
Loins, Average	**1 Serving/145g**	**116**	**1.2**	**80**	**17.9**	**0.1**	**0.8**	**0.2**
Loins, Beer Battered, TTD, Sainsbury's*	1 Fillet/93g	182	10.8	196	14.4	8.5	11.6	2.7
Loins, Steaks, Skinless & Boneless, TTD, Sainsbury's*	1 Steak/100g	105	0.4	105	25.2	0.1	0.4	0.1
Poached, Average	**1oz/28g**	**26**	**0.3**	**94**	**20.9**	**0.0**	**1.1**	**0.0**
Smoked, Raw, Average	**1oz/28g**	**22**	**0.2**	**79**	**18.3**	**0.0**	**0.6**	**0.0**
Steaks, Battered, Chip Shop Style, Average	1 Serving/150g	321	18.0	214	12.5	14.3	12.0	1.1
Steamed, Average	**1oz/28g**	**23**	**0.3**	**83**	**18.6**	**0.0**	**0.9**	**0.0**
with Serrano Ham & Lentils, Espana, M&S*	½ Pack/210g	220	8.6	105	10.8	5.9	4.1	0.5
COD &								
Cauliflower Bake, Asda*	1 Pack/400g	492	28.0	123	9.5	5.5	7.0	1.0
Cauliflower Cheese, Fillets, Iceland*	½ Pack/176g	234	13.5	133	12.7	3.3	7.7	1.7
Parsley Sauce, Frozen, M&S*	1 Pack/184g	156	7.2	85	11.1	1.9	3.9	1.0
COD IN								
Butter Sauce, Ross*	1 Serving/150g	126	5.8	84	9.1	3.2	3.9	0.1
Butter Sauce, Sainsbury's*	1 Serving/170g	224	15.3	132	10.6	2.0	9.0	0.1
Butter Sauce, Steaks, Birds Eye*	1 Pack/170g	185	9.4	109	9.8	5.0	5.5	0.1
Butter Sauce, Steaks, Frozen, Asda*	1 Pouch/152g	163	4.0	107	16.0	5.0	2.6	0.8
Butter Sauce, Steaks, Morrisons*	1 Steak/170g	153	5.6	90	10.9	4.1	3.3	0.4
Butter Sauce, Steaks, Youngs*	1 Pack/139g	107	3.2	77	9.7	4.1	2.3	0.4
Butter Sauce, Tesco*	1 Pack/150g	123	5.4	82	9.4	2.9	3.6	0.5
Cheese Sauce, Pre Packed, Average	1 Serving/150g	136	4.4	90	11.8	4.2	3.0	0.0
Mushroom Sauce, BGTY, Sainsbury's*	1 Serving/170g	112	2.9	66	9.9	2.8	1.7	0.1
Olive Oil, Rosemary & Tomato Sauce, Simply, Birds Eye*	1 Fillet/140g	190	10.9	131	14.9	0.9	7.5	0.0
Parsley Sauce, COU, M&S*	1 Pack/185g	130	4.6	70	10.6	1.4	2.5	0.6
Parsley Sauce, Pre Packed, Average	1 Serving/150g	123	4.7	82	10.1	3.3	3.1	0.5
Parsley Sauce, Steaks, Birds Eye*	1 Steak/172g	155	4.8	90	10.5	5.6	2.8	0.1
Sweet Red Pepper Sauce, Fillets, GFY, Asda*	½ Pack/170g	143	2.7	84	15.0	2.3	1.6	0.1
COD MEDITERRANEAN								
PB, Waitrose*	1 Serving/370g	255	3.7	69	13.1	1.9	1.0	1.2
Style, Fillets, GFY, Asda*	1 Pack/397g	274	9.9	69	9.0	2.5	2.5	0.9
Style, Fillets, Herb, Tesco*	1 Serving/115g	163	11.0	142	13.8	0.1	9.6	0.1
COD WITH								
Cheddar Cheese, & Chive Sauce, Fillets, Tesco*	1 Pack/400g	520	22.0	130	14.3	4.4	5.5	0.6
Chunky Chips, M&S*	1 Serving/340g	510	20.4	150	6.5	17.5	6.0	1.5
Fish Pesto, Fillets, COOK!, M&S*	½ Pack/165g	210	5.1	127	16.4	8.4	3.1	4.2
Mediterranean Butter, Sainsbury's*	1 Pack/170g	196	8.9	115	17.0	0.1	5.2	0.1
Mediterranean Pepper Sauce, Fillets, Waitrose*	1 Pack/370g	240	4.8	65	12.2	1.1	1.3	0.9
Parma Ham, & Sardinian Chick Peas, M&S*	½ Pack/255g	268	12.5	105	9.8	5.3	4.9	0.5
Roasted Vegetables, M&S*	1 Serving/280g	238	10.6	85	8.0	4.9	3.8	1.7
Salsa & Rosemary Potatoes, BGTY, Sainsbury's*	1 Pack/450g	356	4.0	79	4.7	13.1	0.9	1.6
Sunblush Tomato Sauce, GFY, Asda*	½ Pack/177g	117	2.7	66	13.0	0.1	1.5	1.0
Sweet Chilli, COU, M&S*	1 Pack/400g	360	2.0	90	7.7	13.1	0.5	1.6
Thai Crust, PB, Waitrose*	1 Pack/280g	249	7.0	89	15.1	1.6	2.5	0.6
Tomato Sauce, Fillets, Asda*	1 Serving/181g	210	10.9	116	13.0	2.6	6.0	2.3
COFFEE								
Azera, Barista Style Instant, Nescafe*	1 Serving/200ml	2	0.0	1	0.1	0.0	0.0	0.0
Black, Average	1 Mug/270ml	5	0.0	2	0.2	0.3	0.0	0.0
Cafe Caramel, Cafe Range, Nescafe*	1 Sachet/17g	72	2.4	423	9.2	64.6	14.1	1.3
Cafe Irish Cream, Cafe Range, Nescafe*	1 Sachet/23g	98	3.2	425	8.2	65.2	14.1	1.2
Cafe Latte, Dry, Douwe Egberts*	1 Serving/12g	58	2.6	480	10.0	60.0	22.0	0.0
Cafe Latte, Instant, Maxwell House*	1 Serving/16g	67	3.0	420	17.0	45.5	18.9	0.1
Cafe Mocha, Cafe Range, Nescafe*	1 Sachet/22g	92	2.9	418	8.5	66.6	13.1	0.0
Cappuccino, Cappio, Kenco*	1 Sachet/18g	79	1.9	439	11.7	73.9	10.6	0.6

COFFEE

	Measure INFO/WEIGHT	per Measure		Nutrition Values per 100g / 100ml				
		KCAL	FAT	KCAL	PROT	CARB	FAT	FIBRE
Cappuccino, Co-Op*	1 Serving/13g	55	2.0	440	16.0	64.0	16.0	8.0
Cappuccino, Decaff, Instant, Made Up, Nescafe*	1 Mug/200ml	68	2.3	34	1.0	5.0	1.2	0.0
Cappuccino, Decaff, Nescafe*	1 Sachet/16g	68	2.3	428	11.6	62.6	14.6	0.0
Cappuccino, Decaff, Unsweetened, Nescafe*	1 Sachet/16g	70	3.1	437	14.5	51.2	19.4	4.3
Cappuccino, Dry, Waitrose*	1 Sachet/13g	58	2.3	439	15.1	56.0	17.2	4.4
Cappuccino, Instant, Aldi*	1 Sachet/13g	49	1.7	393	12.5	55.1	13.6	0.0
Cappuccino, Instant, Asda*	1 Sachet/15g	60	2.3	399	13.0	53.0	15.2	0.9
Cappuccino, Instant, Kenco*	1 Sachet/20g	80	2.8	401	13.5	55.7	13.8	0.0
Cappuccino, Instant, Made Up, Maxwell House*	1 Serving/280g	123	5.3	44	0.6	5.8	1.9	0.0
Cappuccino, Instant, Unsweetened, Douwe Egberts*	1 Serving/12g	48	1.9	400	11.0	53.0	16.0	0.0
Cappuccino, Italian, Nescafe*	1 Cup/150ml	60	2.9	40	1.2	4.4	1.9	0.0
Cappuccino, M&S*	1 Serving/164g	66	2.6	40	1.5	4.4	1.6	0.0
Cappuccino, Made Up, Dolce Gusto, Nescafe*	1 Serving/240ml	84	3.7	35	1.6	4.0	1.5	0.3
Cappuccino, Original, Sachets, Nescafe*	1 Sachet/18g	80	3.1	444	11.7	60.3	17.4	0.0
Cappuccino, Reduced Sugar, Sainsbury's*	1 Serving/12g	48	2.3	418	18.0	41.0	20.0	0.0
Cappuccino, Sainsbury's*	1 Serving/12g	49	1.9	411	14.9	52.9	15.5	0.4
Cappuccino, Semi Skimmed Milk, Average	1 Serving/200ml	63	2.3	31	2.2	3.2	1.2	0.0
Cappuccino, Swiss Chocolate, Nescafe*	1 Sachet/20g	81	2.3	404	10.5	65.3	11.5	2.9
Cappuccino, to Go, Original, Nescafe*	1 Serving/19g	84	3.3	444	11.7	60.3	17.4	0.0
Cappuccino, to Go, Unsweetened, Nescafe*	1 Serving/17g	79	4.0	464	15.0	47.3	23.8	0.0
Cappuccino, Unsweetened, Cappio, Kenco*	1 Serving/18g	73	1.8	406	12.2	66.7	10.0	0.6
Cappuccino, Unsweetened, Nescafe*	1 Sachet/16g	74	3.8	464	15.0	47.3	23.8	0.0
Cappuccino Ice, Made Up, Dolce Gusto, Nescafe*	1 Serving/240ml	111	2.8	46	1.8	7.2	1.2	0.2
Chococino, Made up, Dolce Gusto, Nescafe*	1 Serving/210g	147	5.4	70	2.3	9.4	2.6	0.7
Columbian, Nescafe*	1 Serving/2g	2	0.0	111	16.7	11.1	0.0	5.6
Compliment*	1 Serving/14ml	20	1.8	143	1.4	6.4	12.9	0.0
Dandelion, Symingtons*	1 Tsp/6g	19	0.0	320	2.8	79.3	0.0	0.0
Espresso, Double Shot, McDonald's*	1 Serving/60ml	0	0.0	0	0.0	0.0	0.0	0.0
Espresso, Made Up, Dolce Gusto, Nescafe*	1 Serving/60ml	1	0.1	2	0.1	0.0	0.2	0.3
Frappe, Iced, Nestle*	1 Sachet/24g	92	1.0	384	15.0	72.0	4.0	0.5
Gold Blend, Decaffinated, Nescafe*	1 Tsp/5g	3	0.0	63	7.0	9.0	0.2	27.0
Gold Blend, Nescafe*	1 Tsp/5g	3	0.0	63	7.0	9.0	0.2	27.0
Infusion, Average with Semi-Skimmed Milk	1 Cup/220ml	15	0.4	7	0.6	0.7	0.2	0.0
Infusion, Average with Single Cream	1 Cup/220ml	31	2.6	14	0.4	0.3	1.2	0.0
Infusion, Average with Whole Milk	1 Cup/220ml	15	0.9	7	0.5	0.5	0.4	0.0
Instant, Alta Rica, Nescafe*	1 Tsp/2g	2	0.0	98	13.8	10.0	0.3	21.0
Instant, Decaffeinated, Nescafe*	1 Tsp/2g	2	0.0	101	14.9	10.0	0.2	8.4
Instant, Fine Blend, Nescafe*	1 Tsp/2g	1	0.0	63	7.0	9.0	0.2	27.0
Instant, Made with Skimmed Milk	1 Serving/270ml	15	0.0	6	0.6	0.8	0.0	0.0
Instant, Made with Water & Semi-Skimmed Milk	1 Serving/350ml	24	1.4	7	0.4	0.5	0.4	0.0
Instant, Original, Nescafe*	1 Tsp/2g	1	0.0	63	7.0	9.0	0.2	27.0
Instant with Skimmed Milk, Costa Rican, Kenco*	1 Mug/300ml	17	0.1	6	0.6	0.8	0.0	0.0
Latte, Cafe, M&S*	1 Serving/190g	142	5.3	75	4.3	8.3	2.8	0.0
Latte, Instant, Skinny, Douwe Egberts*	1 Serving/12g	35	1.3	290	11.0	38.0	11.0	29.0
Latte, Macchiato, Tassimo*	1 Cup/275ml	135	7.7	49	2.3	3.6	2.8	0.0
Latte, Nescafe*	1 Sachet/22g	110	6.3	498	14.5	45.7	28.5	0.0
Latte, No Sugar, in Cup, From Machine, Kenco*	1 Cup/4g	17	0.9	400	7.6	44.0	22.0	0.0
Latte, Skinny, Nescafe*	1 Sachet/20g	72	1.1	359	24.1	54.3	5.3	1.1
Latte, Vanilla, afe Range, Nescafe*	1 Sachet/19g	73	1.6	395	9.2	68.3	8.5	4.1
Latte Macchiato, Made Up, Dolce Gusto, Nescafe*	1 Serving/220ml	89	4.2	40	2.0	4.1	1.9	0.3
Mocha, Cappuccino, Dry, Maxwell House*	1 Serving/23g	100	2.5	434	4.3	78.2	10.8	0.0
Mocha, Double Choca, Cafe Range, Nescafe*	1 Sachet/23g	94	2.5	408	9.2	68.0	11.0	2.8
Mocha, Iced, Nescafe, Nestle*	1 Bottle/280ml	160	3.4	57	1.1	10.5	1.2	0.0

	Measure INFO/WEIGHT	per Measure KCAL	FAT	Nutrition Values per 100g / 100ml KCAL	PROT	CARB	FAT	FIBRE
COFFEE								
Mocha, Instant, Skinny, Douwe Egberts*	1 Serving/12g	37	1.3	308	10.8	40.8	10.8	5.0
Mocha, Made Up, Dolce Gusto, Nescafe*	1 Serving/210g	117	5.1	56	2.4	6.1	2.4	0.6
Mocha, Sainsbury's*	1 Serving/22g	84	3.0	383	14.0	51.0	13.7	1.3
Regular, Ground or Instant	1 Cup/177g	6	0.0	4	0.2	0.7	0.0	0.0
Skinny Cappuccino, Made Up, Dolce Gusto, Nescafe*	1 Mug/15g	49	0.1	337	33.3	48.8	0.9	2.3
COFFEE MATE								
Creamer, Hazelnut, Fat Free, Nestle*	1 Tbsp/15ml	25	0.0	167	0.0	33.3	0.0	0.0
Original, Nestle*	1 Tsp/4g	19	1.2	547	2.4	56.7	34.4	0.0
Virtually Fat Free, Nestle*	1 Tsp/5g	10	0.2	200	1.0	42.0	3.0	0.0
COFFEE SUBSTITUTE								
Bambu, Vogel*	1 Tsp/3g	10	0.0	320	3.5	75.3	0.5	0.0
COFFEE WHITENER								
Half Fat, Co-Op*	1 Tsp/5g	22	0.6	430	0.9	78.0	13.0	0.0
Light, Asda*	1 Serving/3g	13	0.4	433	0.9	78.0	13.0	0.0
Light, Tesco*	1 Tsp/3g	13	0.4	429	0.9	77.7	12.7	0.0
Morrisons*	1 Serving/10g	54	3.3	535	2.6	57.5	32.8	0.0
Tesco*	1 Tsp/3g	16	0.9	533	1.2	61.3	31.4	0.0
COGNAC								
40% Volume	**1 Pub Shot/35ml**	**78**	**0.0**	**222**	**0.0**	**0.0**	**0.0**	**0.0**
French, All Flavours, Alize*	1 fl oz/30ml	69	0.0	230	0.0	6.7	0.0	0.0
COLA								
Average	1 Can/330ml	135	0.0	41	0.0	10.9	0.0	0.0
Coke, Cherry, Coca-Cola*	1 Bottle/500ml	225	0.0	45	0.0	11.2	0.0	0.0
Coke, Coca-Cola*	1 Can/330ml	142	0.0	43	0.0	10.7	0.0	0.0
Coke, Diet, Caffeine Free, Coca-Cola*	1 Can/330ml	1	0.0	0	0.0	0.1	0.0	0.0
Coke, Diet, Coca-Cola*	1 Can/330ml	1	0.0	0	0.0	0.0	0.0	0.0
Coke, Diet with Cherry, Coca-Cola*	1 Bottle/500ml	5	0.0	1	0.0	0.0	0.0	0.0
Coke, Vanilla, Coca-Cola*	1 Bottle/500ml	215	0.0	43	0.0	10.7	0.0	0.0
Coke with Lemon, Diet, Coca-Cola*	1 Can/330ml	5	0.0	1	0.0	0.0	0.0	0.0
Curiosity, Fentiman's*	1 Bottle/275ml	129	0.0	47	0.1	11.6	0.0	0.0
Diet, Asda*	1 Serving/200ml	0	0.0	0	0.0	0.0	0.0	0.0
Diet, Average	1 Serving/200ml	1	0.0	1	0.0	0.0	0.0	0.0
Diet, Classic, Sainsbury's*	1 Can/330ml	1	0.0	0	0.0	0.0	0.0	0.0
Diet, Just, Asda*	1 Bottle/250ml	0	0.0	0	0.0	0.0	0.0	0.0
Diet, M&S*	1 Can/330ml	3	0.0	1	0.0	0.3	0.0	0.0
Diet, Morrisons*	1 Glass/250ml	2	0.0	1	0.0	0.0	0.0	0.0
Diet, Pepsi*	1 Can/330ml	1	0.0	0	0.0	0.0	0.0	0.0
Diet, Tesco*	1 Glass/200ml	2	0.2	1	0.1	0.1	0.1	0.0
Max, Pepsi*	1 Can/330ml	2	0.0	1	0.1	0.1	0.0	0.0
Pepsi*	1 Can/330ml	145	0.0	44	0.0	11.1	0.0	0.0
Twist, Light, Pepsi*	1 Bottle/500ml	4	0.0	1	0.0	0.1	0.0	0.0
Zero, Caffeine Free, Coca-Cola*	1 Glass/200ml	0	0.0	0	0.0	0.0	0.0	0.0
Zero, Coca-Cola*	1 Can/330ml	2	0.0	0	0.0	0.0	0.0	0.0
COLESLAW								
20% Less Fat, Asda*	1 Serving/100g	88	6.0	88	1.5	7.0	6.0	1.7
99% Fat Free, Kraft*	1 Serving/40ml	50	0.4	126	1.0	28.9	1.0	0.0
Aldi*	1 Serving/100g	206	18.7	206	0.8	8.6	18.7	0.0
Apple, Raisin & Walnut, TTD, Sainsbury's*	1 Serving/75g	212	19.6	283	2.3	8.0	26.2	2.8
Asda*	1 Serving/100g	190	18.0	190	1.0	6.0	18.0	1.4
Basics, Sainsbury's*	1 Serving/25g	27	2.4	107	1.0	3.7	9.8	1.6
Budgens*	1 Serving/50g	103	9.0	206	1.2	9.5	18.1	2.0
Cheese, Asda*	1 Serving/100g	242	22.0	242	4.8	6.3	22.0	1.6
Cheese, Co-Op*	1 Serving/125g	344	31.2	275	6.0	6.0	25.0	1.0

C

	Measure INFO/WEIGHT	per Measure KCAL	FAT	Nutrition Values per 100g / 100ml KCAL	PROT	CARB	FAT	FIBRE
COLESLAW								
Cheese, M&S*	1 Serving/57g	185	19.1	325	4.2	2.0	33.5	1.7
Cheese, Sainsbury's*	1 Serving/75g	184	16.8	246	3.8	6.5	22.4	1.4
Cheese, Supreme, Waitrose*	¼ Pack/88g	197	18.2	225	4.5	5.0	20.8	1.2
Cheese, TTD, Sainsbury's*	¼ Pot/75g	213	20.4	284	5.0	4.7	27.2	2.7
Coronation, Sainsbury's*	¼ Pot/75g	145	11.6	193	1.0	11.4	15.5	1.9
COU, M&S*	½ Pack/125g	75	3.4	60	1.3	7.4	2.7	1.7
Creamy, Asda*	1 Serving/25g	62	6.0	248	0.9	7.0	24.0	1.8
Creamy, GFY, Asda*	1 Serving/100g	163	14.9	163	0.7	6.5	14.9	0.8
Creamy, LC, Tesco*	1/3 Pot/100g	105	8.8	105	1.2	4.9	8.8	1.6
Creamy, Morrisons*	1 Serving/40g	111	11.1	277	1.1	5.5	27.7	1.3
Creamy, Tesco*	1 Serving/75g	142	13.4	190	1.0	5.5	17.8	1.5
Crunchy, Premium, Millcroft*	1 Pack/400g	756	69.6	189	0.9	7.3	17.4	1.5
Deli Style, BGTY, Sainsbury's*	1 Serving/75g	75	5.6	100	1.1	6.2	7.5	1.7
Deli Style, M&S*	1 Serving/50g	110	10.6	220	1.0	4.8	21.2	1.9
Deli Style, Sainsbury's*	½ Pot/150g	267	25.5	178	0.8	5.4	17.0	1.5
Finest, Tesco*	1 Serving/51g	145	15.0	285	0.8	4.1	29.4	1.3
Fruity, M&S*	1 Serving/63g	151	14.3	240	1.1	8.3	22.7	3.1
Half Fat, Waitrose*	1 Serving/100g	64	4.5	64	1.0	4.8	4.5	2.0
Iceland*	1 Serving/110g	112	8.2	102	0.7	7.8	7.5	1.6
Less Than 5% Fat, Side Salad, M&S*	1 Serving/80g	44	3.4	55	1.0	3.4	4.2	3.9
Light, Reduced Fat, Morrisons*	1 Serving/30g	38	3.1	125	0.8	7.4	10.2	0.0
Luxury, Asda*	1 Serving/50g	108	10.5	217	0.9	6.0	21.0	0.0
Luxury, Lidl*	1 Serving/50g	102	9.7	203	0.9	5.9	19.4	0.0
Luxury, Morrisons*	1 Serving/50g	136	13.5	273	1.2	6.4	27.0	0.0
Prawn, CBY, Asda*	1 Pot/280g	490	43.1	175	2.2	6.8	15.4	1.8
Premium, Co-Op*	1 Serving/50g	160	17.0	320	1.0	3.0	34.0	2.0
Reduced Calorie, Budgens*	½ Pot/125g	124	8.6	99	1.0	8.3	6.9	2.3
Reduced Fat, Asda*	1 Pot/250g	218	15.8	87	1.5	6.0	6.3	1.6
Reduced Fat, Average	1 Tbsp/20g	23	1.9	113	1.0	6.4	9.3	2.0
Reduced Fat, Co-Op*	1 Serving/50g	45	3.5	90	0.9	6.0	7.0	2.0
Reduced Fat, Creamy, Morrisons*	1 Portion/100g	163	14.5	163	1.3	7.2	14.5	1.7
Reduced Fat, Essential, Waitrose*	1/6 Tub/50g	65	5.1	130	1.2	8.3	10.2	1.6
Reduced Fat, Healthy Living, Co-Op*	1 Serving/50g	48	3.5	95	0.8	8.0	7.0	2.0
Reduced Fat, M&S*	½ Tub/112g	230	22.4	205	1.1	5.4	20.0	2.8
Tesco*	1 Serving/50g	79	7.2	158	2.2	5.2	14.3	1.6
Three Cheese, Asda*	1 Serving/78g	203	18.7	260	5.0	6.0	24.0	1.7
Three Cheese, Finest, Tesco*	1/3 Pack/100g	255	22.7	255	6.4	5.8	22.7	1.1
TTD, Sainsbury's*	¼ Pot/75g	186	18.7	248	1.0	4.8	25.0	1.2
with Reduced Calorie Dressing, Retail	1 Serving/40g	27	1.8	67	0.9	6.1	4.5	1.4
COLESLAW MIX								
Average	*1oz/28g*	*8*	*0.2*	*30*	*0.8*	*4.9*	*0.8*	*2.0*
COLEY								
Portions, Raw, Average	*1 Serving/92g*	*75*	*0.7*	*82*	*18.4*	*0.0*	*0.7*	*0.0*
Steamed, Average	*1oz/28g*	*29*	*0.4*	*105*	*23.3*	*0.0*	*1.3*	*0.0*
CONCHIGLIE								
Cooked, Average	*1 Serving/185g*	*247*	*1.6*	*134*	*4.8*	*26.6*	*0.8*	*0.6*
Dry Weight, Average	*1 Serving/100g*	*352*	*1.7*	*352*	*12.5*	*71.6*	*1.7*	*2.6*
Whole Wheat, Dry Weight, Average	*1 Serving/75g*	*237*	*1.5*	*316*	*12.6*	*62.0*	*2.0*	*10.7*
CONCHIGLIONI								
Dry, Waitrose*	1 Serving/75g	256	1.0	341	12.5	69.8	1.3	3.7
CONSERVE								
Apricot, Average	*1 Tbsp/15g*	*37*	*0.0*	*244*	*0.5*	*59.3*	*0.2*	*1.5*
Blackcurrant, Average	*1 Tbsp/15g*	*37*	*0.0*	*245*	*0.6*	*60.0*	*0.1*	*1.9*

	Measure INFO/WEIGHT	per Measure KCAL	per Measure FAT	Nutrition Values per 100g / 100ml KCAL	PROT	CARB	FAT	FIBRE
CONSERVE								
Blueberry, M&S*	1 Tsp/8g	15	0.0	206	0.3	51.1	0.1	1.3
Hedgerow, TTD, Sainsbury's*	1 Tbsp/15g	41	0.0	276	0.5	68.2	0.1	0.5
Morello Cherry, Waitrose*	1 Tbsp/15g	39	0.0	258	0.4	64.2	0.0	1.4
Plum, TTD, Sainsbury's*	1 Tbsp/15g	44	0.0	295	0.3	73.1	0.1	0.5
Raspberry, Average	*1 Tbsp/15g*	*37*	*0.1*	*249*	*0.6*	*61.0*	*0.3*	*1.3*
Red Cherry, Finest, Tesco*	1 Tbsp/15g	42	0.0	277	0.6	67.6	0.1	0.8
Red Cherry, TTD, Sainsbury's*	1 Tbsp/15g	43	0.0	283	0.4	70.2	0.1	0.5
Strawberry, 60% Fruit, Reduced Sugar, M&S*	1 Tsp/7g	9	0.0	135	0.4	30.1	0.2	1.9
Strawberry, Average	*1 Tbsp/15g*	*37*	*0.0*	*250*	*0.4*	*61.6*	*0.1*	*0.5*
CONSOMME								
Average	*1oz/28g*	*3*	*0.0*	*12*	*2.9*	*0.1*	*0.0*	*0.0*
Beef, Canned, Sainsbury's*	1 Can/415g	46	0.0	11	2.0	0.7	0.0	0.0
Beef, Luxury, with Sherry, Baxters*	1 Can/415g	62	0.0	15	2.7	1.0	0.0	0.0
COOKIES								
All Butter, Almond, Italian Style, M&S*	1 Cookie/23g	120	6.4	515	6.7	59.4	27.6	3.6
All Butter, Ginger Bread, M&S*	1 Cookie/23g	102	5.0	445	4.3	57.5	21.8	2.4
All Butter, Italian Style Sorrento Lemon, M&S*	1 Cookie/24g	120	6.4	500	4.9	60.4	26.7	2.1
All Butter, Melting Moment, M&S*	1 Cookie/23g	110	6.4	470	4.5	51.5	27.5	3.4
All Butter, Sultana, TTD, Sainsbury's*	1 Biscuit/17g	79	3.8	476	5.4	62.7	22.6	2.6
Almond, Ose*	1 Cookie/10g	46	1.4	456	8.4	74.0	14.0	0.0
Apple & Raisin, Go Ahead, McVitie's*	1 Cookie/15g	66	1.9	443	5.3	76.8	12.7	3.4
Apple Crumble, M&S*	1 Cookie/26g	90	0.5	345	4.6	76.8	2.0	2.9
Bites, Weight Watchers*	1 Pack/21g	97	4.0	464	5.8	67.0	19.2	4.3
Blueberry & Oatmeal, M&S*	1 Cookie/100g	90	3.5	90	1.1	13.4	3.5	0.5
Brazil Nut, Organic, Traidcraft*	1 Cookie/17g	91	5.4	547	5.8	57.7	32.6	2.1
Butter & Sultana, Sainsbury's*	1 Cookie/13g	61	2.6	473	4.5	68.4	20.1	1.6
Cherry Bakewell, COU, M&S*	1 Cookie/25g	90	0.6	355	6.0	77.2	2.5	3.4
Choc Chip, & Coconut, Maryland*	1 Cookie/10g	55	2.5	512	5.1	62.9	23.7	0.0
Choc Chip, & Hazelnut, Maryland*	1 Cookie/11g	55	2.7	513	6.3	65.3	25.0	0.0
Choc Chip, Bronte*	1 Cookie/17g	79	3.6	474	5.8	64.0	21.6	0.0
Choc Chip, Cadbury*	1 Cookie/11g	55	2.8	503	5.9	62.2	25.6	0.0
Choc Chip, Giant, Paterson's*	1 Cookie/60g	296	15.2	493	0.1	61.3	25.3	3.2
Choc Chip, Lyons*	1 Cookie/11g	57	2.7	499	5.2	68.3	23.4	1.7
Choc Chip, Maryland*	1 Cookie/11g	56	2.6	511	6.2	68.0	23.9	1.3
Choc Chip, 'n' Chunk, McVitie's*	1 Cookie/11g	55	2.9	498	5.8	59.2	26.4	3.5
Choc Chip, Parkside*	1 Cookie/11g	56	2.7	495	5.3	64.5	23.7	0.0
Choc Chip, Reduced Fat, Maryland*	1 Cookie/11g	51	1.9	478	5.9	73.0	18.0	0.0
Choc Chip, Sainsbury's*	1 Cookie/11g	55	2.6	508	6.2	67.0	23.9	1.3
Choc Chunk, Finest, Tesco*	1 Cookie/80g	355	14.1	445	5.7	65.3	17.7	1.8
Chocolate, & Nut, Organic, Evernat*	1 Cookie/69g	337	15.6	489	7.2	64.1	22.6	0.0
Chocolate, Almond, & Toffee, Kate's Cakes Ltd*	1 Serving/100g	406	14.9	406	5.5	62.5	14.9	2.4
Chocolate, Belgian, Extra Special, Asda*	1 Cookie/26g	138	8.0	535	6.0	58.0	31.0	2.0
Chocolate, Chunky, Kate's Cakes Ltd*	1 Serving/100g	441	22.0	441	5.2	55.5	22.0	2.4
Chocolate, Double, Cadbury*	1 Biscuit/11g	55	2.5	485	7.3	64.3	22.2	0.0
Chocolate, Fruit & Nut, Extra Special, Asda*	1 Cookie/25g	125	7.1	509	6.0	56.0	29.0	2.0
Chocolate, Milk, Free From, Tesco*	1 Cookie/20g	100	6.1	500	5.6	50.4	30.7	4.1
Chocolate, Quadruple, Sainsbury's*	1 Cookie/20g	117	6.6	585	6.0	66.5	33.0	1.5
Chocolate, Quadruple, TTD, Sainsbury's*	1 Biscuit/20g	104	5.7	518	6.2	59.8	28.2	1.6
Chocolate, Soft, American Style, Budgens*	1 Cookie/50g	216	9.3	431	5.1	60.8	18.6	2.2
Chocolate, Triple, Half Coated, Finest, Tesco*	1 Cookie/25g	131	7.3	525	5.7	58.7	29.3	2.3
Chocolate Chip, & Hazelnut, Extra Special, Asda*	1 Cookie/25g	130	8.1	516	6.0	51.0	32.0	2.5
Chocolate Chip, Asda*	1 Cookie/12g	57	2.9	497	5.0	63.0	25.0	2.6
Chocolate Chip, Average	1 Cookie/10g	49	2.5	489	5.5	64.1	24.7	2.9

COOKIES

	Measure INFO/WEIGHT	per Measure KCAL	FAT	KCAL	PROT	CARB	FAT	FIBRE
				Nutrition Values per 100g / 100ml				
Chocolate Chip, BGTY, Sainsbury's*	1 Cookie/17g	72	2.0	428	4.5	75.6	11.9	2.5
Chocolate Chip, Chips Ahoy*	1 Cookie/11g	55	2.8	500	6.0	65.0	25.0	3.0
Chocolate Chip, Co-Op*	1 Cookie/11g	55	2.6	500	5.0	65.0	24.0	1.0
Chocolate Chip, Dough, Otis Spunkmeyer*	1 Cookie/38g	160	8.0	421	5.3	60.5	21.0	2.6
Chocolate Chip, GF, Organic, Dove's Farm*	1 Cookie/17g	77	3.1	451	4.3	66.9	18.5	0.0
Chocolate Chip, GFY, Asda*	1 Cookie/10g	48	2.0	463	5.0	68.0	19.0	3.5
Chocolate Chip, Gluten & Wheat Free, Lovemore*	1 Cookie/17g	81	4.5	483	3.8	57.8	26.8	3.5
Chocolate Chip, Handbaked, Border*	1 Cookie/15g	72	3.4	480	5.9	67.4	22.6	0.0
Chocolate Chip, Low Price, Sainsbury's*	1 Cookie/11g	54	2.3	500	7.0	70.1	21.3	2.5
Chocolate Chip, Lyons*	1 Cookie/12g	56	2.5	483	5.6	66.5	21.6	1.7
Chocolate Chip, M&S*	1 Cookie/12g	59	3.0	495	5.7	62.1	24.8	2.7
Chocolate Chip, McVitie's*	1 Cookie/11g	54	2.8	496	5.8	60.2	25.8	3.0
Chocolate Chip, Mini, McVitie's*	1 Bag/40g	196	9.2	491	5.5	65.1	23.1	2.8
Chocolate Chip, Mini, Tesco*	1 Bag/30g	148	7.1	493	5.4	64.6	23.7	1.7
Chocolate Chip, Morrisons*	1 Cookie/10g	52	2.5	502	5.0	66.2	24.1	1.3
Chocolate Chip, Organic, Sainsbury's*	1 Cookie/17g	89	4.9	530	5.0	61.8	29.2	0.3
Chocolate Chip, Tesco*	1 Cookie/11g	56	2.7	510	5.2	67.2	24.1	1.6
Chocolate Chip, The Decadent, President's Choice*	1 Cookie/16g	79	4.1	513	6.1	61.3	26.4	3.6
Chocolate Chip, Value, Tesco*	1 Cookie/11g	56	2.9	512	4.8	64.8	26.0	1.6
Chocolate Chip, Weight Watchers*	1 Cookie/11g	49	1.9	443	7.6	65.4	17.2	4.6
Chocolate Chunk, & Hazelnut, Tesco*	1 Cookie/22g	118	6.7	538	6.2	60.2	30.3	1.9
Chocolate Chunk, & Hazelnut, TTD, Sainsbury's*	1 Biscuit/17g	88	5.2	528	6.5	54.8	31.4	2.8
Chocolate Chunk, & Hazelnut, So Good, Somerfield*	1 Cookie/22g	118	7.0	530	6.3	55.7	31.3	2.4
Chocolate Chunk, All Butter, COU, M&S*	1 Cookie/24g	110	4.3	460	5.7	69.1	17.9	2.3
Chocolate Chunk, All Butter, M&S*	1 Cookie/24g	120	6.0	500	5.2	62.4	25.2	2.9
Chocolate Chunk, Big Milk, Cookie Coach*	1 Cookie/35g	174	8.8	497	6.2	61.4	25.1	0.0
Chocolate Chunk, Cadbury*	1 Cookie/22g	119	6.9	540	6.5	58.0	31.2	0.0
Chocolate Chunk, Devondale*	1 Cookie/65g	308	16.3	474	4.6	59.2	25.1	2.8
Chocolate Chunk, Milk, Greggs*	1 Serving/100g	480	25.0	480	5.7	63.2	25.0	2.8
Chocolate Chunk, Triple, Bakery, Finest, Tesco*	1 Cookie/80g	360	15.9	450	7.4	59.2	19.9	2.1
Chocolate Orange, Half Coated, Finest, Tesco*	1 Cookie/22g	107	5.6	488	4.9	59.6	25.5	1.2
Chunkie Extremely Chocolatey, Fox's*	1 Cookie/26g	130	6.8	506	6.2	61.0	26.3	2.6
Cranberry & Orange, Finest, Tesco*	1 Cookie/26g	125	5.8	490	4.1	67.4	22.6	3.2
Danish Butter, Tesco*	1 Cookie/26g	133	6.6	516	4.7	66.7	25.6	1.3
Dark Chocolate Chunk & Ginger, The Best, Morrisons*	1 Cookie/25g	126	6.4	503	4.6	63.7	25.5	2.8
Double Choc, Maryland*	1 Cookie/10g	51	2.6	510	5.2	64.4	25.7	0.0
Double Choc Chip, Giant, Paterson's*	1 Cookie/60g	293	15.2	489	0.3	61.3	25.3	3.7
Double Choc Chip, Mini, M&S*	1 Cookie/22g	108	5.2	490	5.3	63.6	23.7	1.8
Double Choc Chip, Tesco*	1 Cookie/11g	55	2.7	500	4.2	65.3	24.7	3.0
Double Choc Chip, Weight Watchers*	1 Biscuit/11g	49	1.9	443	7.6	65.4	17.2	4.6
Double Chocolate, Premium, Co-Op*	1 Cookie/17g	86	4.6	505	5.0	62.0	27.0	2.0
Double Chocolate & Walnut, Soft, Tesco*	1 Cookie/25g	116	6.4	463	5.8	52.1	25.7	4.7
Double Chocolate Chip, Co-Op*	1 Cookie/17g	87	4.6	510	5.0	63.0	27.0	2.0
Double Chocolate Chip, Organic, Waitrose*	1 Cookie/18g	96	5.6	535	5.1	58.6	31.0	1.9
Double Chocolate Chip, Somerfield*	1 Cookie/11g	56	2.8	513	5.2	64.9	25.8	1.3
Fortune, Average	1 Cookie/8g	30	0.2	378	4.2	84.0	2.7	1.6
Fruit & Oat, Soft, Diet Chef Ltd*	1 Cookie/45g	198	8.8	439	4.8	58.8	19.6	4.0
Fruit & Oat, Soft, Diet Chef Ltd*	1 Bar/45g	198	8.8	440	4.8	58.8	19.6	4.0
Fudge Brownie, Maryland*	1 Cookie/11g	56	2.8	510	5.8	63.0	25.0	0.0
Ginger, & Brazil Nut, Organic, Dove's Farm*	1 Cookie/17g	79	3.5	464	5.0	65.0	20.5	4.8
Ginger, Low Fat, M&S*	1 Cookie/23g	82	1.0	358	5.1	74.9	4.3	2.4
Glace Cherry, Border*	1 Cookie/15g	74	3.8	493	5.4	64.3	25.6	0.0
Hazelnut, & Choc Chip 'n' Chunk, McVitie's*	1 Cookie/11g	55	3.0	505	6.1	57.8	27.7	3.5

	Measure INFO/WEIGHT	per Measure KCAL	FAT	Nutrition Values per 100g / 100ml KCAL	PROT	CARB	FAT	FIBRE

COOKIES

	Measure INFO/WEIGHT	KCAL	FAT	KCAL	PROT	CARB	FAT	FIBRE
Lemon & Ginger, Weight Watchers*	1 Biscuit/11g	50	2.0	450	6.4	65.0	18.2	5.0
Lemon Meringue, COU, M&S*	1 Cookie/25g	89	0.6	355	5.6	77.6	2.6	3.0
Lemon Zest, GF, Organic, Dove's Farm*	1 Cookie/17g	80	3.1	473	3.3	73.7	18.3	0.0
Milk Chocolate, Classic, Millie's Cookies*	1 Cookie/45g	190	10.2	422	5.1	49.3	22.7	1.3
Milk Chocolate Chunk, Average	1 Cookie/25g	129	6.9	515	6.6	60.0	27.6	1.6
Oat, & Fruit, Kate's Cakes Ltd*	1 Serving/100g	418	18.2	418	4.2	59.5	18.2	3.0
Oat, Giant Jumbo, Paterson's*	1 Cookie/60g	299	16.2	499	0.4	58.4	27.0	3.2
Oat & Cranberry, BGTY, Sainsbury's*	1 Cookie/28g	126	5.0	449	6.8	65.0	18.0	5.1
Oat & Raisin, Health Matters*	1 Cookie/8g	33	0.7	414	7.0	76.6	8.8	3.3
Oat & Treacle, TTD, Sainsbury's*	1 Biscuit/25g	121	5.9	482	5.7	61.8	23.6	3.7
Oatflake & Raisin, Waitrose*	1 Cookie/17g	80	3.8	469	5.8	61.7	22.1	4.7
Oatmeal, Chocolate Chip, Chewy, Dad's*	1 Cookie/15g	70	3.0	467	6.7	66.7	20.0	3.3
Oreo, Nabisco*	1 Cookie/11g	52	2.3	471	5.9	70.6	20.6	2.9
Pecan & Maple, Mini, Bronte*	1 Pack/100g	509	27.3	509	5.4	60.3	27.3	1.6
Raisin & Cinnamon, Low Fat, M&S*	1 Cookie/22g	78	0.9	355	6.2	73.0	4.1	3.2
Rolo, Nestle*	1 Cookie/73g	242	11.1	331	3.4	46.0	15.2	0.6
Spiced Apple, M&S*	1 Cookie/25g	90	0.7	360	5.2	75.6	2.8	2.0
Stem Ginger, Free From, Sainsbury's*	1 Cookie/17g	84	4.8	489	6.5	58.0	28.0	6.8
Stem Ginger, Kate's Cakes Ltd*	1 Serving/100g	376	11.7	376	5.0	62.7	11.7	1.7
Stem Ginger, Reduced Fat, Waitrose*	1 Cookie/17g	75	2.7	448	4.5	71.0	16.2	1.6
Stem Ginger, Tesco*	1 Cookie/20g	98	4.8	489	4.2	64.0	24.0	2.0
Stem Ginger, TTD, Sainsbury's*	1 Cookie/17g	79	3.7	476	5.2	64.3	22.0	2.3
Sultana, All Butter, Reduced Fat, M&S*	1 Cookie/17g	70	2.4	420	4.9	68.6	14.2	2.6
Sultana, Soft & Chewy, Sainsbury's*	1 Cookie/25g	104	3.5	414	4.4	67.8	13.9	2.5
Sultana & Cinnamon, Weight Watchers*	1 Cookie/12g	46	1.4	398	5.0	67.1	12.1	1.8
Tennessee, American Style, Stiftung & Co*	1 Cookie/19g	96	4.6	504	6.0	66.0	24.0	0.0
Toffee, Weight Watchers*	1 Cookie/12g	52	1.9	456	5.2	71.1	16.8	2.9
White Chocolate, & Cranberry, Kate's Cakes Ltd*	1 Serving/100g	389	13.4	389	4.7	62.3	13.4	2.0
White Chocolate, Asda*	1 Cookie/54g	256	11.9	474	5.0	64.0	22.0	2.1
White Chocolate, Chunk, Average	1 Cookie/25g	124	6.2	498	5.5	62.8	24.8	1.0
White Chocolate, Maryland*	1 Cookie/10g	51	2.5	512	5.7	64.0	25.0	0.0
White Chocolate, TTD, Sainsbury's*	1 Cookie/25g	126	6.4	504	5.5	62.5	25.8	1.2
White Chocolate & Cranberry, Devondale*	1 Cookie/65g	300	15.3	462	4.7	60.7	23.5	2.1
White Chocolate & Raspberry, Finest, Tesco*	1 Cookie/76g	304	9.6	400	5.2	66.3	12.6	2.4
White Chocolate & Raspberry, McVitie's*	1 Cookie/17g	87	4.4	512	4.7	64.1	25.9	1.8

COQ AU VIN

	Measure INFO/WEIGHT	KCAL	FAT	KCAL	PROT	CARB	FAT	FIBRE
Diet Chef Ltd*	1 Pack/300g	285	13.2	95	7.7	6.1	4.4	2.2
M & S*	1 Serving/295g	398	22.7	135	14.2	1.5	7.7	1.0
Sainsbury's*	1 Pack/400g	484	17.6	121	16.8	3.5	4.4	0.2

CORDIAL

	Measure INFO/WEIGHT	KCAL	FAT	KCAL	PROT	CARB	FAT	FIBRE
Blackcurrant, New Zealand Honey Co*	1 Serving/30ml	109	0.3	363	1.0	88.0	1.0	0.0
Cox's Apple & Plum, Diluted, Bottle Green*	1 Serving/10ml	3	0.0	29	0.0	7.2	0.0	0.0
Elderflower, Made Up, Bottle Green*	1 Glass/200ml	46	0.0	23	0.0	5.6	0.0	0.0
Elderflower, Undiluted, Waitrose*	1 Serving/20ml	22	0.0	110	0.0	27.5	0.0	0.0
Lemon & Elderflower, Sicilian, Diluted, Weight Watchers*	1 Serving/250ml	3	0.1	1	0.0	0.3	0.0	0.0
Lemon & Lime, High Juice, M&S*	1 Glass/250ml	75	0.0	30	0.0	7.0	0.0	0.0
Lime, Juice, Diluted, Rose's*	1 Serving/50ml	12	0.0	24	0.0	5.7	0.0	0.0
Lime, Sainsbury's*	1 Serving/50ml	14	0.0	27	0.0	6.2	0.0	0.0
Lime, Tesco*	1 Serving/74ml	8	0.0	11	0.2	0.5	0.0	0.0
Lime, with Aromatic Bitters & Ginger, Sainsbury's*	1 Serving/40ml	12	0.1	29	0.0	6.9	0.3	0.3
Lime Juice, Concentrated	1 Serving/20ml	22	0.0	112	0.1	29.8	0.0	0.0
Lime Juice, Diluted	1 Glass/250ml	55	0.0	22	0.0	6.0	0.0	0.0
Lime Juice, Waitrose*	1 Serving/20ml	21	0.0	104	10.0	23.7	0.0	0.0

INFO/WEIGHT	Measure	per Measure KCAL	FAT	Nutrition Values per 100g / 100ml KCAL	PROT	CARB	FAT	FIBRE
CORDIAL								
Pomegranate & Elderflower, Bottle Green*	1 fl oz/30ml	7	0.0	22	0.0	5.6	0.0	0.0
Pomegreat, Original, Pomegreat*	1 Serving/50ml	16	0.0	32	0.0	7.6	0.0	0.0
CORIANDER								
Leaves, Dried, Average	*1oz/28g*	*78*	*1.3*	*279*	*21.8*	*41.7*	*4.8*	*0.0*
Leaves, Fresh, Average	*1 Bunch/20g*	*5*	*0.1*	*23*	*2.1*	*3.7*	*0.5*	*2.8*
Seeds, Ground, Schwartz*	1 Tsp/5g	22	0.9	446	14.2	54.9	18.8	0.0
CORN								
Baby, Average	*1 Serving/80g*	*21*	*0.3*	*26*	*2.5*	*3.1*	*0.4*	*1.7*
Baby & Mange Tout, Tesco*	1 Serving/100g	27	0.2	27	2.9	3.3	0.2	2.1
Cobs, Boiled, Weighed with Cob, Average	*1 Cob/200g*	*132*	*2.8*	*66*	*2.5*	*11.6*	*1.4*	*1.3*
Creamed Style, Green Giant*	1 Can/418g	238	2.1	57	1.2	11.9	0.5	3.0
CORN CAKES								
M & S*	½ Pack/85g	238	17.0	280	6.4	19.8	20.0	3.4
Organic, Kallo*	1 Cake/5g	16	0.2	340	12.7	74.3	4.1	11.2
Slightly Salted, Mrs Crimble's*	1 Pack/28g	104	0.9	380	7.9	80.0	3.4	5.4
CORN SNACKS								
Crispy, Bugles*	1 Bag/20g	102	5.6	508	4.8	60.7	28.0	1.4
Light Bites, Cheese, Special K, Kellogg's*	1 Pack/28g	116	2.2	416	9.0	77.0	8.0	1.0
Light Bites, Tomato & Basil, Special K, Kellogg's*	1 Pack/28g	116	2.2	416	7.0	79.0	8.0	1.5
Paprika, Shapers, Boots*	1 Pack/13g	64	3.5	494	8.7	54.0	27.0	2.2
Scampi, Smiths, Walkers*	1 Bag/27g	134	7.0	496	13.0	52.5	26.0	0.0
CORNED BEEF								
Average	*1 Slice/35g*	*75*	*4.3*	*214*	*25.9*	*0.7*	*12.2*	*0.0*
Lean, Healthy Range, Average	*1 Slice/30g*	*57*	*2.6*	*191*	*27.0*	*1.0*	*8.7*	*0.0*
Morrisons*	1 Can/340g	738	42.5	217	25.0	1.0	12.5	0.0
Sliced, Morrisons*	1 Slice/31g	63	3.2	203	26.0	1.3	10.3	0.0
Sliced, Premium, Average	*1 Slice/31g*	*69*	*3.9*	*222*	*26.6*	*0.5*	*12.6*	*0.0*
Slices, Value, Tesco*	1 Slice/31g	66	3.7	213	26.0	0.8	11.8	0.0
CORNFLOUR								
Average	*1 Tsp/5g*	*18*	*0.1*	*355*	*0.6*	*86.9*	*1.2*	*0.1*
COURGETTE								
Fried, Average	*1oz/28g*	*18*	*1.3*	*63*	*2.6*	*2.6*	*4.8*	*1.2*
Raw, Average	*1 Courgette/224g*	*40*	*0.9*	*18*	*1.8*	*1.8*	*0.4*	*0.9*
Stuffed, Round, Lovely Vegetables, M&S*	½ Pack/200g	110	2.6	55	1.8	7.7	1.3	1.8
COUS COUS								
& Chargrilled Vegetables, M&S*	1 Serving/200g	200	3.0	100	3.9	17.3	1.5	1.6
& Chickpeas, TTD, Sainsbury's*	¼ Pot/72g	121	6.8	167	4.7	15.8	9.4	1.4
Citrus Kick, Cooked, Ainsley Harriott*	1 Serving/130g	182	1.6	140	4.3	27.9	1.2	2.4
Citrus Kick, Dry, Ainsley Harriott*	½ Sachet/50g	184	1.2	368	11.6	77.0	2.4	9.2
Cooked, Average	*1 Tbsp/15g*	*24*	*0.3*	*158*	*4.3*	*31.4*	*1.9*	*1.3*
Coriander & Lemon, Asda*	1 Pack/110g	378	3.5	128	5.1	24.2	1.2	2.5
Coriander & Lemon, Cooked, Tesco*	1 Serving/137g	207	3.3	151	4.0	28.3	2.4	2.0
Coriander & Lemon, Dry, Tesco*	1 Pack/110g	375	3.0	341	11.0	68.2	2.7	6.1
Coriander & Lemon, Morrisons*	1 Serving/100g	159	3.4	159	4.4	27.7	3.4	1.4
Coriander & Lemon, Sainsbury's*	½ Pack/137g	206	5.9	150	4.3	23.4	4.3	2.7
Dry, Average	*1 Serving/50g*	*178*	*0.7*	*356*	*13.7*	*72.8*	*1.5*	*2.6*
Garlic & Coriander, Dry, Waitrose*	1 Serving/70g	235	2.5	336	11.7	64.2	3.6	6.2
Giant, Tesco*	1 Pack/220g	350	14.4	160	4.1	20.7	6.6	1.2
Harissa Style Savoury, Sainsbury's*	1 Serving/260g	434	12.0	167	4.7	26.8	4.6	1.3
Hot & Spicy Flavour, Dry, Amazing Grains, Haldane's*	1 Serving/50g	182	2.1	365	12.5	67.0	4.2	3.1
Mediterranean Style, Cooked, Tesco*	1 Serving/146g	215	3.8	147	4.4	26.5	2.6	1.3
Mediterranean Style, Dry, Tesco*	1 Pack/110g	368	3.3	335	11.9	65.1	3.0	5.6
Moroccan Medley, Ainsley Harriott*	½ Sachet/130g	178	2.0	137	5.4	25.4	1.5	2.2

	Measure INFO/WEIGHT	per Measure KCAL	FAT	Nutrition Values per 100g / 100ml KCAL	PROT	CARB	FAT	FIBRE
COUS COUS								
Moroccan Style, Break, GFY, Asda*	1 Pack/150g	215	2.7	143	5.6	26.1	1.8	1.8
Moroccan Style, Finest, Tesco*	1 Tub/225g	292	5.6	130	4.3	22.6	2.5	3.7
Moroccan Style, Fruity, M&S*	1 Serving/200g	370	5.4	185	3.4	36.7	2.7	3.4
Moroccan Style, Sainsbury's*	½ Pack/150g	195	4.0	130	5.0	21.5	2.7	1.0
Moroccan Style, Savoury, Sainsbury's*	½ Pack/151g	196	4.1	130	5.0	21.5	2.7	1.0
Moroccan Style, TTD, Sainsbury's*	1 Pot/200g	364	7.2	182	4.4	30.3	3.6	5.5
Morrisons*	1 Serving/100g	126	1.2	126	5.5	23.2	1.2	3.5
Pepper, Red & Yellow, Chargrilled, Tesco*	1 Pack/200g	212	3.6	106	4.6	17.8	1.8	0.5
Plain, Dry Weight, Tesco*	1 Serving/50g	182	0.6	365	15.1	73.1	1.1	0.8
Red Pepper & Chilli, Waitrose*	1 Pack/200g	344	13.8	172	4.5	23.0	6.9	1.3
Spice Sensation, Cooked, No Butter/Oil, Ainsley Harriott*	1 Serving/130g	165	2.0	127	4.3	23.9	1.5	3.4
Spice Sensation, Dry, Ainsley Harriott*	½ Sachet/50g	166	1.2	332	11.6	66.2	2.4	9.2
Spicy Moroccan Chicken & Veg, COU, M&S*	1 Pack/400g	380	6.8	95	9.1	10.3	1.7	1.9
Tangy Tomato, Dry, Ainsley Harriott*	½ Sachet/50g	166	0.8	332	12.2	67.2	1.6	8.8
Tomato & Basil, Made Up, Tesco*	1 Serving/200g	348	16.6	174	3.9	21.0	8.3	3.4
Tomato & Garlic, Sundried, Made Up, Ainsley Harriott*	1 Serving/130g	196	1.8	151	5.3	27.9	1.4	2.2
Tomato & Onion, Dry Weight, Waitrose*	1 Pack/110g	376	4.0	342	12.6	64.9	3.6	5.1
Vegetable, Chargrilled, Morrisons*	1 Serving/225g	227	5.4	101	3.3	16.5	2.4	1.3
Vegetable, Roasted, Cooked, Ainsley Harriott*	1 Serving/130g	180	2.0	138	5.6	25.5	1.5	2.6
Vegetable, Roasted, Dry, Ainsley Harriott*	½ Sachet/50g	180	2.0	360	14.6	66.4	4.0	6.8
Vegetable, Roasted, Veg Pot, Innocent*	1 Pot/400g	460	9.2	115	3.6	17.5	2.3	4.3
Vegetable, Roasted, Waitrose*	1 Serving/200g	328	13.2	164	3.9	22.0	6.6	0.9
Vegetable, Spicy, GFY, Asda*	½ Pack/55g	71	0.6	129	4.7	25.0	1.1	2.0
Vegetable, Spicy, Morrisons*	1 Pack/110g	187	5.5	170	5.1	26.2	5.0	2.9
Vegetables, & Olive Oil, Chargrilled, Delphi*	½ Pot/75g	105	2.9	140	3.8	22.5	3.9	1.9
Vegetarian, Oriental, Findus*	½ Pack/300g	510	25.5	170	4.5	19.0	8.5	0.0
Wholewheat, Tesco*	1 Serving/50g	178	1.0	355	12.0	72.0	2.0	5.0
with Balsamic Roasted Vegetables, TTD, Sainsbury's*	1/3 Pack/80g	94	4.3	117	2.8	14.3	5.4	1.1
with Sun Dried Tomato, CBY, Asda*	1 Pack/310g	515	12.1	166	4.6	26.2	3.9	4.0
CRAB								
Blue, Soft Shelled, Raw, Average	1 Crab/84g	73	0.9	87	18.1	0.0	1.1	0.0
Boiled, Meat Only, Average	*1 Tbsp/40g*	*51*	*2.2*	*128*	*19.5*	*0.0*	*5.5*	*0.0*
Brown, Cornish, Seafood & Eat It*	1 Pack/100g	171	10.7	171	17.9	1.9	10.7	0.0
Claws, Asda*	1oz/28g	25	0.3	89	11.0	9.0	1.0	0.2
Cocktail, Waitrose*	1 Serving/100g	217	17.6	217	10.8	3.8	17.6	0.4
Cornish 50/50, Seafood & Eat It*	1 Pot/100g	144	5.8	144	21.6	1.2	5.8	0.5
Cornish Potted, Seafood & Eat It*	1 Pack/100g	235	17.5	235	15.0	5.1	17.5	0.8
Dressed, Average	*1 Can/43g*	*66*	*3.4*	*154*	*16.8*	*4.1*	*7.9*	*0.2*
Dressed, Shetland Isles, TTD, Sainsbury's*	½ Pack/75g	137	8.2	183	9.9	7.4	10.9	0.8
Meat, Raw, Average	*1oz/28g*	*28*	*0.2*	*100*	*20.8*	*2.8*	*0.6*	*0.0*
Meat in Brine, Average	*½ Can/60g*	*46*	*0.3*	*76*	*17.2*	*0.9*	*0.4*	*0.1*
White Cornish, Seafood & Eat It*	1 Pack/100g	81	0.5	81	19.0	0.1	0.5	0.0
White Meat, See Food & Eat It*	1 Pack/100g	81	0.5	81	19.0	0.1	0.5	0.0
CRAB CAKES								
Goan, M&S*	1 Pack/190g	228	7.6	120	8.0	12.9	4.0	1.8
Iceland*	1 Serving/18g	52	3.2	288	7.2	25.6	18.0	1.3
Shetland Isles, Dressed, TTD, Sainsbury's*	1 Crab/75g	130	8.3	174	12.4	6.0	11.1	0.5
Tesco*	1 Serving/130g	281	16.0	216	11.0	15.4	12.3	1.1
Thai, TTD, Sainsbury's*	½ Pack/106g	201	9.5	189	9.5	17.8	8.9	1.4
CRAB STICKS								
Average	1 Stick/15g	14	0.0	94	9.1	13.9	0.3	0.0
CRACKERBREAD								
Original, Ryvita*	1 Slice/5g	19	0.1	378	10.8	75.0	2.8	4.8

	Measure INFO/WEIGHT	per Measure KCAL	FAT	Nutrition Values per 100g / 100ml KCAL	PROT	CARB	FAT	FIBRE
CRACKERBREAD								
Rice, Asda*	1 Slice/5g	19	0.1	374	9.1	79.4	2.2	1.9
Sainsbury's*	1 Slice/5g	19	0.2	380	10.0	80.0	4.0	2.0
Wholegrain, Ryvita*	1 Slice/6g	20	0.2	360	12.4	68.7	3.9	9.8
CRACKERS								
Aromatic Spices & Sweet Chilli, Phileas Fogg*	1 Serving/30g	151	7.8	503	1.7	64.7	26.0	2.0
Bath Oliver, Jacob's*	1 Cracker/12g	52	1.6	432	9.6	67.6	13.7	2.6
Bean Mix, Habas Tapas, Graze*	1 Punnet/30g	131	3.8	438	11.7	68.9	12.8	1.5
Black Olive, M&S*	1 Cracker/4g	20	1.0	485	8.3	59.4	23.5	4.3
Black Pepper, for Cheese, Ryvita*	1 Cracker/7g	27	0.2	384	13.2	72.9	2.9	6.8
Bran, Jacob's*	1 Cracker/7g	32	1.3	454	9.7	62.8	18.2	3.2
Brooklyn Bites, Graze*	1 Punnet/28g	146	10.4	521	19.0	35.0	37.0	5.5
Butter Puff, Sainsbury's*	1 Cracker/10g	54	2.7	523	10.4	60.7	26.5	2.5
Chapati Chips, Tikka, Medium Spicy, Patak's*	1 Serving/25g	127	7.0	508	8.0	56.0	28.0	4.0
Cheese, Bites, Sour Cream & Onion, Mrs Crimble's*	1 Pack/30g	125	4.6	416	15.9	54.0	15.2	2.0
Cheese, Cheddar, Crispies, TTD, Sainsbury's*	1 Thin/4g	21	1.5	576	14.2	39.0	40.4	2.2
Cheese, Crispy, M&S*	1 Cracker/4g	20	1.0	470	9.4	58.1	22.1	3.0
Cheese, Mini, Heinz*	1 Pack/25g	108	3.6	433	9.4	68.6	14.6	0.6
Cheese, Puff Pastry, Somerfield*	1 Cracker/4g	21	1.5	500	10.6	36.1	34.8	2.1
Cheese, Ritz*	1 Cracker/4g	17	0.9	486	10.1	55.9	24.7	2.2
Cheese, Thins, Asda*	1 Cracker/4g	21	1.3	532	12.0	49.0	32.0	0.0
Cheese, Thins, Cheddar, The Planet Snack Co*	1 Serving/30g	153	8.8	509	11.5	50.1	29.2	2.1
Cheese, Thins, Co-Op*	1 Cracker/4g	21	1.3	530	12.0	49.0	32.0	3.0
Cheese, Thins, Mini, Snack Rite*	1 Bag/30g	144	6.8	480	12.9	55.9	22.7	2.5
Cheese, Thins, Waitrose*	1 Cracker/4g	21	1.2	545	11.9	52.6	31.9	2.5
Cheese, Trufree*	1 Cracker/8g	42	2.6	524	9.0	50.0	32.0	0.5
Chives, Jacob's*	1 Cracker/6g	28	1.0	457	9.5	67.5	16.5	2.7
Choice Grain, Jacob's*	1 Cracker/8g	32	1.1	427	9.0	65.5	14.3	5.4
Corn, Thins, 97% Fat Free, Real Foods*	1 Cracker/6g	23	0.2	378	10.2	81.7	3.0	8.6
Corn, Thins, Real Foods*	1 Serving/6g	22	0.2	378	10.2	81.7	3.0	8.6
Cream, 45% Less Fat, Morrisons*	1 Cracker/8g	32	0.6	403	10.5	74.2	7.1	3.3
Cream, Aldi*	1 Cracker/8g	36	1.2	456	9.1	71.7	14.7	3.0
Cream, Asda*	1 Cracker/8g	35	1.2	443	10.0	67.0	15.0	0.0
Cream, Average	1 Cracker/7g	31	1.1	440	9.5	68.3	16.3	2.2
Cream, BFY, Morrisons*	1 Cracker/8g	32	0.6	406	10.9	74.4	7.2	2.8
Cream, BGTY, Sainsbury's*	1 Cracker/8g	32	0.6	400	10.9	71.7	7.7	3.1
Cream, Choice Grain, Jacob's*	1 Cracker/7g	30	0.9	400	9.0	64.5	11.8	7.0
Cream, Jacob's*	1 Cracker/8g	34	1.1	431	10.0	67.5	13.5	3.8
Cream, Light, Jacob's*	1 Cracker/8g	31	0.5	388	10.6	72.2	6.3	4.1
Cream, Lower Fat, Tesco*	1 Cracker/5g	20	0.3	393	11.0	72.4	6.6	3.1
Cream, Morrisons*	1 Cracker/8g	36	1.2	446	9.6	68.5	14.8	2.7
Cream, Reduced Fat, Tesco*	1 Cracker/8g	31	0.5	406	10.9	74.4	7.2	2.8
Cream, Sainsbury's*	1 Cracker/8g	35	1.3	422	9.5	66.7	15.2	2.8
Cream, Tesco*	1 Cracker/8g	34	1.2	447	9.0	69.0	15.0	3.0
Cruskits, Arnotts*	2 Cruskits/12g	40	0.2	331	9.0	63.7	1.5	0.0
El Picante, Graze*	1 Punnet/25g	121	6.4	481	13.5	51.7	25.4	6.1
Extra Wheatgerm, Hovis*	1 Serving/6g	27	1.1	447	10.2	60.0	18.5	4.4
Firecracker, The, Graze*	1 Punnet/24g	120	6.8	520	10.5	52.6	29.5	2.0
Garden Herbs, Jacob's*	1 Cracker/6g	28	1.0	457	9.5	67.5	16.5	2.7
Garlic, CBY, Asda*	2 Biscuits/12g	58	2.6	483	7.0	63.3	21.5	4.2
Garlic & Herb, Jacob's*	1 Cracker/100g	450	16.7	450	10.0	68.3	16.7	3.3
Glutafin*	1 Serving/11g	52	2.2	470	2.4	70.0	20.0	0.7
Golden Rye, for Cheese, Ryvita*	1 Cracker/7g	27	0.2	384	13.2	72.9	2.9	6.5
Harvest Grain, Sainsbury's*	1 Cracker/6g	27	1.1	458	8.5	64.5	18.4	4.1

CRACKERS

	Measure INFO/WEIGHT	per Measure KCAL	per Measure FAT	Nutrition Values per 100g / 100ml KCAL	PROT	CARB	FAT	FIBRE
Herb & Onion, 99% Fat Free, Rakusen's*	1 Cracker/5g	18	0.0	360	9.1	82.6	1.0	3.9
Herb & Onion, Trufree*	1 Cracker/6g	25	0.7	418	2.5	75.0	12.0	10.0
Japanese Beef Teriyaki, Sensations, Walkers*	1 Serving/24g	118	6.3	490	1.4	62.0	26.0	3.5
Japanese Style Rice Mix, Asda*	1 Serving/25g	96	0.2	385	6.8	88.0	0.6	0.5
Krackawheat, McVitie's*	1 Cracker/7g	33	1.4	446	9.7	60.0	18.6	5.8
Lightly Salted, Crispy, Sainsbury's*	1 Cracker/5g	25	1.3	533	7.8	62.6	27.9	2.1
Lightly Salted, Italian, Jacob's*	1 Cracker/6g	26	0.8	429	10.3	67.6	13.0	2.9
Mediterranean, Jacob's*	1 Cracker/6g	27	1.0	450	9.7	66.5	16.1	2.7
Mix, Yaki Soba, Graze*	1 Punnet/32g	159	9.3	498	24.0	36.0	29.0	6.0
Mixed Seed, Multi Grain, Asda*	1 Cracker/6g	28	1.1	445	11.0	62.0	17.0	4.4
Multigrain, Aldi, Savour Bakes, Aldi*	1 Cracker/5g	20	0.8	404	8.3	55.0	16.8	5.1
Multigrain, Corn Thins, Real Foods*	1 Cracker/6g	23	0.2	388	10.9	71.0	3.7	10.3
Multigrain, Morrisons*	10 Crackers/20g	76	2.2	379	8.8	61.3	11.0	5.1
Multigrain, Snack Crackers, Special K, Kellogg's*	1 Pack/30g	120	3.0	400	10.0	73.3	10.0	6.7
Multigrain, Tesco*	1 Cracker/6g	27	1.1	458	8.5	64.5	18.4	4.1
Oat & Wheat, Weight Watchers*	4 Crackers/20g	74	0.5	370	10.5	75.0	2.5	4.0
Olive Oil & Oregano, Mediterraneo, Jacob's*	1 Cracker/6g	25	0.7	412	12.4	65.5	11.2	6.0
Peanut, Wasabi, Graze*	1 Pack/26g	125	5.6	479	15.2	53.8	21.4	5.4
Peking Dynasty, Graze*	1 Punnet/26g	130	7.3	498	19.8	43.1	27.9	4.6
Peking Spare Rib & 5 Spice, Sensations, Walkers*	1 Bag/24g	116	6.2	485	1.3	62.0	26.0	3.5
Pesto, Jacob's*	1 Cracker/6g	27	1.0	450	9.7	66.5	16.1	2.7
Poppy & Sesame Seed, Sainsbury's*	1 Cracker/4g	21	1.1	530	9.6	58.9	28.4	3.4
Ritz, Mini, Kraft*	1 Bag/25g	126	6.0	504	7.9	63.0	24.0	2.0
Ritz, Original, Jacob's*	1 Cracker/3g	17	1.0	509	6.9	55.6	28.8	2.0
Rye, Organic, Dove's Farm*	1 Cracker/7g	28	1.0	393	7.0	58.4	14.6	8.7
Salt & Black Pepper, Eat Well, M&S*	1 Pack/25g	106	3.7	422	9.6	62.9	14.7	5.1
Salt & Black Pepper, Jacob's*	1 Cracker/6g	27	1.0	457	9.5	67.5	16.5	2.7
Salted, Ritz, Nabisco*	1 Cracker/3g	17	0.9	493	7.0	57.5	26.1	2.9
Selection, Finest, Tesco*	1 Serving/30g	136	4.3	452	9.6	71.0	14.4	0.0
Sesame & Poppy Thins, Tesco*	1 Cracker/4g	20	1.0	485	9.9	57.6	23.5	4.4
Sweet Chilli, Thins, Savours, Jacob's*	1 Cracker/4g	21	0.9	472	8.0	62.3	21.2	3.6
Tarallini with Fennel Seeds, Crosta & Mollica*	1 Cracker/4g	21	0.9	529	8.2	67.5	22.0	4.2
The British Barbecue, Graze*	1 Punnet/23g	117	7.4	508	17.4	36.8	32.2	7.4
Tom Yum Yum, Graze*	1 Pack/23g	90	0.6	390	7.2	84.8	2.4	1.4
Tuc, Cheese Sandwich, Jacob's*	1 Cracker/14g	72	4.3	531	8.4	53.8	31.4	0.0
Tuc, Jacob's*	1 Cracker/5g	24	1.3	522	7.0	60.5	28.0	2.9
Tuc, Mini with Sesame Seeds, Jacob's*	1 Biscuit/2g	10	0.5	523	9.7	63.1	25.8	3.9
Vegetable, Spicy Indonesian, Waitrose*	1 Pack/60g	295	16.3	492	1.2	60.6	27.2	2.2
Vegetable, Thai Spicy, Sainsbury's*	1 Pack/50g	231	10.4	462	7.2	61.5	20.8	2.6
Wasapeas, Graze*	1 Pack/32g	128	2.5	406	14.8	65.2	7.8	7.1
Waterthins, Wafers, Philemon*	1 Crackers/2g	7	0.1	392	10.6	77.9	3.6	5.0
Wheaten, M&S*	1 Cracker/4g	20	0.9	450	10.2	57.0	20.2	5.0
Whole Wheat, 100%, Oven Baked, Master Choice*	1 Cracker/4g	17	0.4	429	10.0	75.0	9.6	12.1
Wholemeal, Tesco*	1 Cracker/7g	29	1.0	414	9.4	60.6	14.9	10.4
Wholmeal, Organic, Nairn's*	1 Cracker/14g	58	2.0	413	9.0	61.4	14.6	8.7

CRANBERRIES

	Measure INFO/WEIGHT	per Measure KCAL	per Measure FAT	Nutrition Values per 100g / 100ml KCAL	PROT	CARB	FAT	FIBRE
& Raisins, Dried, Sweetened, Ocean Spray*	1 Serving/50g	163	0.2	326	0.1	80.3	0.5	4.6
Dried, Sweetened, Average	*1 Serving/10g*	*34*	*0.1*	*335*	*0.3*	*81.1*	*0.8*	*4.4*
Fresh, Raw, Average	*1oz/28g*	*4*	*0.0*	*15*	*0.4*	*3.4*	*0.1*	*3.0*

CRAYFISH

	Measure INFO/WEIGHT	per Measure KCAL	per Measure FAT	Nutrition Values per 100g / 100ml KCAL	PROT	CARB	FAT	FIBRE
Raw	*1oz/28g*	*19*	*0.2*	*67*	*14.9*	*0.0*	*0.8*	*0.0*
Tails, Chilli & Garlic, Asda*	1 Serving/140g	133	4.3	95	16.0	1.1	3.1	0.8
Tails in Brine, Luxury, The Big Prawn Co*	½ Tub/90g	46	0.6	51	10.1	1.0	0.7	0.0

	Measure INFO/WEIGHT	per Measure		Nutrition Values per 100g / 100ml				
		KCAL	FAT	KCAL	PROT	CARB	FAT	FIBRE
CREAM								
Aerosol, Average	1oz/28g	87	8.7	309	1.8	6.2	30.9	0.0
Aerosol, Reduced Fat, Average	1 Serving/55ml	33	3.0	60	0.6	2.0	5.4	0.0
Brandy, Pourable with Remy Martin*, Finest, Tesco*	½ Pot/125ml	460	35.5	368	2.7	19.8	28.4	0.0
Brandy, Really Thick, Finest, Tesco*	½ Pot/125ml	579	49.5	463	1.3	19.7	39.6	0.0
Chantilly, TTD, Sainsbury's*	2 Tbsp/30g	136	14.0	455	1.4	6.9	46.8	0.0
Clotted, Fresh, Average	1 Serving/28g	162	17.5	579	1.6	2.3	62.7	0.0
Double, Average	1 Tbsp/15ml	68	7.3	452	1.6	2.4	48.4	0.0
Double, Reduced Fat, Average	1 Serving/30g	73	7.0	243	2.7	5.6	23.3	0.1
Extra Thick, Reduced Fat, Weight Watchers*	1 Serving/30g	42	3.4	140	2.5	6.7	11.5	0.8
Extra Thick, with Baileys, Baileys*	1 fl oz/30ml	129	11.6	431	1.5	13.4	38.6	0.0
Oat Alternative, Dairy Free, Oatly*	1 Carton/250ml	375	32.5	150	1.0	6.0	13.0	0.8
Single, Average	1 Tbsp/15ml	28	2.7	188	2.6	3.9	18.0	0.1
Single, Extra Thick, Average	1 Serving/38ml	72	6.9	192	2.7	4.1	18.4	0.0
Soured, Fresh, Average	1 Tsp/5ml	10	0.9	191	2.7	3.9	18.4	0.0
Soured, Reduced Fat, Average	1 Tsp/5g	6	0.4	119	5.2	6.7	8.6	0.4
Strawberry, Light, Real Dairy, Uht, Anchor*	1 Serving/13g	25	2.1	198	2.6	8.7	17.0	0.0
Thick, Sterilised, Average	1 Tbsp/15ml	35	3.5	233	2.6	3.6	23.1	0.0
Uht, Double, Average	1 Tbsp/15g	41	3.9	274	2.2	7.4	26.3	0.0
Uht, Reduced Fat, Average	1 Serving/25ml	16	1.4	62	0.6	2.2	5.6	0.0
Uht, Single, Average	1 Tbsp/15ml	29	2.8	194	2.6	4.0	18.8	0.0
Whipping, Average	1 Tbsp/15ml	52	5.5	348	2.1	3.2	36.4	0.0
CREAM HORN								
Fresh, Tesco*	1 Horn/57g	244	15.8	428	4.1	40.3	27.8	0.3
CREAM SODA								
American with Vanilla, Tesco*	1 Glass/313ml	75	0.0	24	0.0	5.9	0.0	0.0
Diet, Sainsbury's*	1 Serving/250ml	2	0.0	1	0.0	0.0	0.0	0.0
No Added Sugar, Sainsbury's*	1 Can/330ml	2	0.3	0	0.1	0.1	0.1	0.1
Shapers, Boots*	1 Bottle/300ml	3	0.0	1	0.0	0.0	0.0	0.0
Traditional Style, Tesco*	1 Can/330ml	139	0.0	42	0.0	10.4	0.0	0.0
CREME BRULEE								
Average	1 Serving/100g	313	26.0	313	3.8	15.7	26.0	0.2
Gastropub, M&S*	1 Brulee/84g	285	24.6	340	3.1	15.7	29.3	0.7
M & S*	1 Pot/100g	360	32.6	360	3.3	13.0	32.6	0.0
CREME CARAMEL								
Asda*	1 Pot/100g	113	2.6	113	2.4	20.0	2.6	0.0
Average	1 Serving/128g	140	2.8	109	3.0	20.6	2.2	0.0
Chosen By You, Asda*	1 Pot/100g	101	1.0	101	2.0	20.8	1.0	0.0
La Laitiere*	1 Pot/100g	135	4.0	135	5.0	20.0	4.0	0.0
Morrisons*	1 Pot/100g	120	2.8	120	2.4	21.4	2.8	0.0
Tesco*	1 Pot/100g	115	1.6	115	2.8	21.8	1.6	0.0
CREME EGG								
Cadbury*	1 Egg/39g	180	6.3	462	4.1	73.0	16.1	0.5
Minis, Cadbury*	1 Egg/11g	50	1.8	445	4.1	67.5	16.4	0.4
CREME FRAICHE								
Average	1 Pot/295g	1067	112.2	362	2.2	2.6	38.0	0.0
Extra Light, President*	1 Tub/200g	182	10.0	91	2.7	8.7	5.0	0.0
Half Fat, Average	1 Serving/30g	54	4.9	181	3.1	5.5	16.2	0.0
Low Fat, Average	1 Tbsp/30ml	43	3.6	143	3.3	5.6	12.1	0.1
Low Fat, Weight Watchers*	1 Tbsp/20g	15	0.5	76	5.1	7.7	2.7	0.5
CREPES								
Chocolate Filled, Tesco*	1 Crepe/32g	140	5.8	438	5.9	62.5	18.1	1.6
CREPES								
Mushroom, M&S*	1 Pack/186g	195	4.5	105	5.7	17.1	2.4	2.5

	Measure INFO/WEIGHT	per Measure		Nutrition Values per 100g / 100ml				
		KCAL	FAT	KCAL	PROT	CARB	FAT	FIBRE

CRISPBAKES

	Measure INFO/WEIGHT	KCAL	FAT	KCAL	PROT	CARB	FAT	FIBRE
Beef, Minced, M&S*	1 Bake/113g	226	12.3	200	10.0	15.6	10.9	1.5
Bubble & Squeak, M&S*	1 Bake/47g	79	4.1	170	2.7	19.6	8.8	1.5
Cheese, Spring Onion & Chive, Sainsbury's*	1 Bake/114g	287	16.8	253	7.1	24.5	14.8	1.7
Cheese & Onion, Cooked, Dalepak*	1 Bake/86g	192	8.8	223	4.9	26.9	10.2	1.7
Cheese & Onion, M&S*	1 Bake/114g	285	18.5	250	6.4	19.4	16.2	1.7
Dutch, Asda*	1 Bake/8g	31	0.3	388	14.7	74.9	3.3	4.2
Dutch, Sainsbury's*	1 Bake/10g	38	0.5	392	14.5	72.3	5.0	5.8
Vegetable, M&S*	1 Bake/114g	200	10.3	175	2.5	19.2	9.0	2.6
Vegetable, Sainsbury's*	1 Bake/114g	246	13.0	216	2.0	26.2	11.4	2.0

CRISPBREAD

	Measure INFO/WEIGHT	KCAL	FAT	KCAL	PROT	CARB	FAT	FIBRE
3 Seed, Classic, Gourmet, Dr Karg*	1 Bread/25g	108	4.9	430	16.5	46.6	19.7	10.9
3 Seed, Organic, Gourmet	1 Bread/25g	101	4.7	405	15.8	48.8	18.8	14.6
Corn, Orgran*	1 Bread/5g	18	0.1	360	7.5	83.0	1.8	3.0
Corn, Thins, Sesame, Real Foods*	1 Thin/6g	23	0.2	384	10.7	69.9	3.4	10.2
Cracked Black Pepper, Ryvita*	1 Slice/11g	38	0.2	344	8.8	66.6	1.6	14.5
Crisp 'n' Light, Wasa*	1 Bread/7g	24	0.1	360	12.0	73.0	2.2	5.3
Dark Rye, Morrisons*	1 Bake/13g	39	0.4	300	11.5	61.5	3.1	16.9
Dark Rye, Ryvita*	1 Bread/10g	34	0.1	342	8.5	66.5	1.2	15.2
Emmental Cheese & Pumpkin Seed, Organic, Dr Karg*	1 Bread/25g	107	3.7	428	17.7	50.7	14.9	9.6
Fibre Plus, Wholegrain with Sesame, Wasa*	1 Bread/10g	35	0.7	350	13.0	47.0	7.0	24.0
Fruit Crunch, Ryvita*	1 Slice/15g	54	0.8	360	8.0	62.0	5.3	14.7
Gluten Free	1 Serving/8g	25	0.1	331	6.4	72.9	1.5	0.0
Hint of Chilli, Ryvita*	1 Slice/12g	42	0.2	349	8.6	66.6	1.9	16.8
Light Rye, Leksands Knacke*	4 Slices/50g	158	1.1	317	10.4	62.7	2.2	16.0
Mini, Sesame & Linseed, Dr Karg*	1 Crispbread/3g	13	0.4	424	12.1	57.6	12.1	9.1
Multigrain, Ryvita*	1 Slice/11g	41	0.8	370	11.2	56.0	7.2	18.3
Multigrain, Wasa*	1 Bread/13g	43	0.3	320	12.0	62.0	2.6	14.0
Original, Ryvita*	1 Bread/10g	35	0.2	350	8.5	66.9	1.7	16.5
Original Rye, Thin, Finn Crisp*	1 Slice/6g	20	0.1	360	11.0	60.0	2.4	19.0
Original Rye, Wasa*	1 Bread/11g	35	0.2	315	9.0	67.0	1.4	14.0
Provita*	1 Bread/6g	26	0.6	416	12.5	68.4	9.9	0.0
Pumpkin Seeds & Oats, Ryvita*	1 Slice/13g	46	0.9	370	11.2	56.0	7.2	18.3
Rice & Cracked Pepper, Orgran*	1 Bread/5g	18	0.1	388	8.4	81.9	1.8	2.0
Rounds, Multigrain, Finn Crisp*	1 Bread/13g	41	0.8	330	13.0	56.0	6.0	18.0
Scan Bran, Slimming World*	1 Slice/10g	31	0.5	310	14.9	29.0	5.3	42.1
Seeded, Spelt, Organic, Dr Karg*	1 Bread/25g	108	4.5	430	17.2	44.4	18.0	11.2
Sesame, Ryvita*	1 Bread/10g	37	0.7	373	10.5	58.3	7.0	17.5
Sesame, Savour Bakes, Aldi*	1 Crispbread/9g	33	0.5	366	12.3	57.2	5.2	20.6
Spelt, Cheese, Sunflower Seeds, Organic, Dr Karg*	1 Bread/25g	103	4.5	411	19.2	42.8	18.1	10.4
Spelt, Muesli, Organic, Dr Karg*	1 Bread/25g	94	2.8	375	14.2	54.4	11.2	10.6
Spelt, Sesame, Sunflower, Amisa*	1 Bread/29g	85	4.3	297	11.7	28.5	15.1	5.0
Sport, Wasa*	1 Bread/15g	46	0.2	310	9.0	64.0	1.5	16.0
Sunflower Seeds & Oats, Ryvita*	1 Bread/12g	46	1.1	384	9.7	58.4	9.0	15.3
Sweet Onion, Ryvita*	1 Crispbread/12g	43	0.2	356	9.0	70.6	1.4	12.6
Thin Crisps, Original Taste, Finn Crisp*	1 Bread/6g	20	0.2	320	11.0	63.0	2.4	19.0
Wholegrain, Classic Three Seed, Organic, Dr Karg*	1 Bread/25g	101	4.5	405	15.8	44.8	18.0	14.6
Wholegrain, Crispy, Thin, Kavli*	3 Breads/15g	50	0.3	333	10.0	70.0	1.7	12.7
Wholemeal, Light, Allinson*	1 Bread/5g	17	0.1	349	11.7	69.7	2.6	11.0
Wholemeal, Organic, Allinson*	1 Bread/5g	17	0.1	336	14.2	66.0	1.7	12.2
Wholemeal, Rye with Milk, Grafschafter*	1 Bread/9g	29	0.1	316	11.4	64.0	1.6	15.0
Wholemeal Rye, Organic, Kallo*	1 Bread/10g	31	0.2	314	9.7	65.0	1.7	15.4

CRISPS

	Measure INFO/WEIGHT	KCAL	FAT	KCAL	PROT	CARB	FAT	FIBRE
American Cheeseburger, Quarterbacks, Red Mill*	1 Pack/14g	72	4.2	512	6.7	54.2	29.8	3.7

CRISPS

INFO/WEIGHT	Measure	per Measure		Nutrition Values per 100g / 100ml				
		KCAL	FAT	KCAL	PROT	CARB	FAT	FIBRE
Bacon, Shapers, Boots*	1 Bag/23g	99	3.4	431	8.0	66.0	15.0	3.0
Bacon, Webs, Monster Munch*	1 Pack/15g	74	3.4	497	6.5	65.2	23.1	1.6
Bacon & Cheddar, Baked, Walkers*	1 Pack/38g	149	3.2	397	6.5	73.7	8.5	4.7
Bacon Crispies, Sainsbury's*	1 Bag/25g	117	5.7	468	19.9	45.8	22.8	4.8
Bacon Rashers, Blazin, Tesco*	1 Bag/25g	121	6.6	485	16.5	45.7	26.3	3.8
Bacon Rashers, COU, M&S*	1 Pack/20g	72	0.6	360	9.4	77.5	2.9	3.5
Bacon Rashers, Iceland*	1 Bag/75g	330	13.2	440	8.3	61.9	17.6	2.9
Bacon Rashers, Tesco*	1 Serving/25g	125	6.4	500	7.1	59.8	25.5	4.0
Bacon Rice Bites, Asda*	1 Bag/30g	136	4.8	452	7.0	70.0	16.0	0.4
Bacon Sizzler, Ridge Cut, McCoys*	1 Bag/32g	165	9.7	516	7.1	53.6	30.3	3.9
Baked, Average	1 Bag/25g	93	1.5	374	6.5	73.5	5.9	5.8
Barbecue, Handcooked, Tesco*	1 Bag/40g	187	10.0	468	6.6	53.8	25.1	5.2
Barbecue, Savoury Snacks, Weight Watchers*	1 Pack/22g	81	1.9	366	18.6	61.0	8.7	6.1
Barbecue, Snack Rite*	1 Bag/25g	131	8.3	524	5.1	51.3	33.2	0.0
Barbecue, Sunseed Oil, Walkers*	1 Pack/33g	171	10.7	525	6.5	50.0	33.0	4.0
Barbecue Beef, Select, Tesco*	1 Pack/25g	134	8.7	536	6.4	49.2	34.8	4.4
BBQ Rib, Sunseed, Walkers*	1 Bag/25g	131	8.2	525	6.5	50.0	33.0	4.0
Beef, Chinese Sizzling, McCoys*	1 Bag/35g	178	10.6	506	6.9	51.8	30.2	4.0
Beef, Sizzling, Spice, McCoys*	1 Bag/35g	175	10.4	501	6.4	51.7	29.8	4.0
Beef, Space Raiders, KP Snacks*	1 Pack/13g	64	2.9	495	6.5	65.3	22.8	1.0
Beef, Squares, Walkers*	1 Bag/25g	105	4.5	420	6.0	59.0	18.0	4.6
Beef & Onion, Tayto*	1 Bag/35g	184	11.9	526	7.6	47.3	34.0	4.5
Beef & Onion, Walkers*	1 Bag/33g	171	10.7	525	6.5	50.0	33.0	4.0
Beef & Onion Flavour, Average	1 Bag/25g	131	8.3	524	6.5	50.0	33.1	4.3
Beetroot, Seasoned In Salt, Glennans*	1 Bag/27g	130	8.9	480	8.2	36.0	32.8	13.2
Buffalo Mozzarella Tomato & Basil, Kettle Chips*	1 Serving/50g	238	12.8	476	6.7	54.4	25.7	4.9
Butter & Chive, COU, M&S*	1 Bag/26g	95	0.5	365	7.7	77.3	1.9	4.6
Cassava, Salt & Vinegar, 70% Less Fat, Velvet Crunch*	1 Pack/20g	84	2.0	418	0.7	80.4	9.8	2.9
Cheddar, Leek & Pink Peppercorn, Boots*	1 Pack/45g	221	11.7	492	7.8	56.0	26.0	3.8
Cheddar & Onion, Crinkles, Walkers*	1 Pack/28g	150	9.3	538	7.7	51.5	33.3	3.5
Cheddar & Onion, Hand Cooked, Aldi*	1 Pack/150g	753	41.8	502	7.7	54.9	27.9	4.0
Cheddar & Onion, Ridge Cut, McCoys*	1 Bag/32g	165	9.8	516	7.0	53.2	30.6	3.9
Cheddar & Red Onion Chutney, Sensations, Walkers*	1 Bag/40g	198	11.2	495	6.5	54.0	28.0	4.5
Cheddar & Sour Cream, Extra Crunchy, Walkers*	1 Serving/30g	143	6.8	476	6.6	59.1	22.6	4.7
Cheddar & Spring Onion, 35% Less Fat, Sainsbury's*	1 Pack/20g	93	4.2	463	6.3	62.4	20.9	0.9
Cheddar Cheese & Bacon, Temptingly, Walkers*	1 Pack/33g	169	10.0	520	6.2	52.3	30.9	4.2
Cheese, with Onion, Soulmates, Kettle Chips*	1 Pack/40g	195	11.6	488	7.7	50.2	29.0	5.4
Cheese & Chives, Walkers*	1 Bag/33g	172	10.7	530	6.5	50.0	33.0	4.1
Cheese & Onion, Asda*	1 Bag/25g	130	7.8	519	5.6	53.6	31.4	3.7
Cheese & Onion, Baked, Walkers*	1 Bag/25g	99	2.1	396	6.5	73.8	8.3	4.7
Cheese & Onion, BGTY, Sainsbury's*	1 Bag/25g	120	6.2	479	7.0	57.0	24.8	5.7
Cheese & Onion, Crinkle Cut, Love Life, Waitrose*	1 Bag/25g	115	5.2	459	6.3	60.1	20.6	3.8
Cheese & Onion, Crinkle Cut, Low Fat, Waitrose*	1 Bag/25g	122	5.8	490	7.7	62.6	23.2	4.7
Cheese & Onion, GFY, Asda*	1 Pack/26g	122	5.7	470	7.0	61.0	22.0	4.2
Cheese & Onion, Golden Wonder*	1 Bag/25g	129	7.9	516	5.8	52.4	31.5	3.8
Cheese & Onion, KP Snacks*	1 Bag/25g	134	8.7	534	6.6	48.7	34.8	4.8
Cheese & Onion, Lights, Walkers*	1 Bag/24g	113	5.0	470	7.5	62.0	21.0	5.0
Cheese & Onion, M&S*	1 Bag/25g	134	8.9	535	5.5	48.8	35.5	5.0
Cheese & Onion, Max, Walkers*	1 Pack/50g	262	16.0	525	6.8	52.0	32.0	5.2
Cheese & Onion, Oven Baked, Asda*	1 Bag/25g	95	2.0	380	5.1	72.0	8.0	3.3
Cheese & Onion, Oven Baked, Tesco*	1 Bag/25g	102	1.6	410	5.3	74.7	6.6	7.7
Cheese & Onion, Potato Chips, Popped, M&S*	1 Bag/23g	95	3.2	413	7.4	60.9	13.9	4.4
Cheese & Onion, Potato Heads, Walkers*	1 Pack/23g	108	5.3	470	6.0	60.0	23.0	5.5

CRISPS

INFO/WEIGHT	per Measure		Nutrition Values per 100g / 100ml				
Measure	KCAL	FAT	KCAL	PROT	CARB	FAT	FIBRE
Cheese & Onion, Rings, Crunchy, Shapers, Boots*							
1 Bag/15g	56	0.4	374	5.9	81.0	2.9	2.0
Cheese & Onion, Sainsbury's*							
1 Bag/25g	132	8.7	527	4.6	48.8	34.8	3.9
Cheese & Onion, Seabrook*							
1 Pack/30g	159	9.8	530	7.0	50.8	32.6	3.9
Cheese & Onion, Snack Rite*							
1 Pack/25g	132	8.4	527	5.3	51.3	33.4	0.0
Cheese & Onion, Sprinters*							
1 Bag/25g	137	9.2	549	5.4	49.4	36.6	0.0
Cheese & Onion, Squares, Walkers*							
1 Bag/25g	108	4.5	430	6.5	61.0	18.0	5.5
Cheese & Onion, Sunseed Oil, Walkers*							
1 Bag/33g	171	10.7	525	7.0	50.0	33.0	4.0
Cheese & Onion, Tayto*							
1 Bag/25g	132	8.5	526	7.6	47.3	34.0	4.5
Cheese & Onion, Tesco*							
1 Pack/25g	132	8.3	530	5.8	51.6	33.2	4.4
Cheese & Onion, Value, Tesco*							
1 Bag/20g	108	7.2	541	6.0	48.3	36.0	4.8
Cheese & Red Onion, Extra Crunchy, Walkers*							
1 Serving/30g	140	6.3	468	6.8	60.6	20.9	4.9
Cheese & Sweet Onion, Crispy Bakes, Kettle Chips*							
1 Bag/24g	91	1.9	379	10.6	66.7	7.8	4.3
Cheese Bites, Weight Watchers*							
1 Pack/18g	73	1.0	406	13.9	71.1	5.6	2.2
Cheese Curls, Morrisons*							
1 Bag/14g	71	4.5	510	4.5	51.0	32.0	2.6
Cheese Curls, Shapers, Boots*							
1 Pack/14g	68	3.8	489	4.5	57.0	27.0	2.7
Cheese Curls, Sprinters*							
1 Bag/14g	68	3.8	483	4.1	56.4	26.8	0.0
Cheese Curls, Tesco*							
1 Bag/14g	75	4.5	520	4.5	54.4	31.1	1.9
Cheese Curls, Weight Watchers*							
1 Pack/20g	78	1.7	392	5.0	73.8	8.6	3.4
Cheese Puffs, Weight Watchers*							
1 Pack/18g	80	1.9	444	7.8	77.2	10.6	3.3
Cheese Tasters, M&S*							
1 Bag/30g	154	8.8	515	8.1	55.0	29.3	1.7
Cheesy Curls, Asda*							
1 Pack/17g	87	4.9	511	3.8	59.7	28.6	1.7
Cheesy Curls, Bobby's*							
1 Bag/40g	225	14.8	563	7.6	50.1	36.9	0.0
Cheesy Curls, Tesco*							
1 Pack/17g	90	5.4	530	3.5	56.0	32.0	1.9
Cheesy Puffs, Co-Op*							
1 Bag/60g	321	20.4	535	3.0	54.0	34.0	2.0
Chicken, & Thyme, Oven Roasted, Tesco*							
1 Pack/150g	728	40.5	485	6.5	54.0	27.0	4.5
Chicken, Chargrilled, Ridge Cut, McCoys*							
1 Pack/32g	167	10.0	521	7.0	52.9	31.3	4.0
Chicken, Oven Roasted with Lemon & Thyme, Walkers*							
1 Bag/40g	200	11.2	500	6.5	55.0	28.0	4.5
Chicken, Potato Heads, Walkers*							
1 Pack/23g	106	4.8	460	8.5	58.0	21.0	6.0
Chilli & Lemon, Walkers*							
1 Pack/25g	131	8.2	525	6.3	51.0	33.0	3.8
Cider Vinegar & Sea Salt, Tyrrells*							
1 Pack/40g	192	9.8	481	7.2	60.1	24.6	2.4
Corn Chips, Fritos*							
1 Pack/43g	240	15.0	565	4.7	56.5	35.3	0.0
Crinkle Cut, Lower Fat, No Added Salt, Waitrose*							
1 Bag/40g	193	10.0	483	6.5	58.0	25.0	3.9
Crushed Natural Sea Salt, Darling Spuds*							
1 Bag/40g	195	12.0	488	5.6	53.4	30.0	4.5
D'lites, Cheddar & Red Onion Bites, The Real Crisp Co.*							
1 Pack/20g	83	2.0	414	2.1	78.8	10.0	2.7
Double Gloucester & Red Onion, Kettle Chips*							
1 Serving/40g	188	9.9	471	6.6	55.5	24.7	4.8
Extra Crunchy, Salt & Malt Vinegar, Walkers*							
1 Pack/30g	139	6.2	463	6.6	59.9	20.8	4.8
Flame Grilled Steak, Argentinean, Walkers*							
1 Bag/35g	182	11.3	520	6.5	50.7	32.4	4.2
Flame Grilled Steak, Extra Crunchy, Walkers*							
1 Bag/150g	702	31.6	468	6.9	60.0	21.1	5.0
Flame Grilled Steak, Ridge Cut, McCoys*							
1 Bag/32g	165	9.8	516	7.0	53.0	30.7	4.0
Flamed Grilled Steak, Deep Ridge, Walkers*							
1 Pack/28g	144	8.4	515	6.4	52.6	30.1	4.3
Four Cheese & Red Onion, Sensations, Walkers*							
1 Bag/40g	194	10.8	485	6.5	54.0	27.0	4.5
Garlic & Herbs Creme Fraiche, Kettle Chips*							
1 Bag/50g	248	14.2	497	6.0	54.7	28.3	4.2
Ham, Honey Roast, Hand Cooked, Finest, Tesco*							
1 Serving/25g	130	7.3	515	5.1	58.6	28.8	2.5
Ham & Mustard, Salty Dog*							
1 Pack/40g	192	10.8	480	7.5	54.5	27.1	4.2
Ham & Pickle, Smoked, Thick Cut, Brannigans*							
1 Bag/40g	203	11.9	507	7.0	52.8	29.8	3.8
Ham Flavour, Canadian, Seabrook*							
1 Pack/30g	159	9.8	531	5.7	50.9	32.7	5.1
Honey & BBQ, Wholgrain, Snacks, M&S*							
1 Serving/30g	146	7.5	485	7.8	57.6	24.9	5.2
Honey Roasted Ham, Sensations, Walkers*							
1 Bag/40g	196	10.8	490	6.5	55.0	27.0	4.0
Hoops, Ready Salted, Weight Watchers*							
1 Bag/20g	73	0.3	365	3.4	82.7	1.4	4.1
Hot & Spicy Salami, Tesco*							
1 Bag/50g	216	18.0	431	26.2	0.7	35.9	0.0
King Prawn, Sizzling, Ridge Cut, McCoys*							
1 Pack/50g	259	15.2	518	6.6	54.7	30.3	4.0
Lamb & Mint, Slow Roasted, Sensations, Walkers*							
1 Bag/35g	170	9.4	485	6.5	54.0	27.0	4.5
Lant Chips, Ikea*							
1 Serving/25g	126	6.9	505	8.3	55.9	27.6	4.5

CRISPS

Measure INFO/WEIGHT	per Measure KCAL	per Measure FAT	Nutrition Values per 100g / 100ml KCAL	PROT	CARB	FAT	FIBRE
Lightly Salted, Baked, COU, M&S*	1 Bag/25g	88	0.6	350	8.5	76.4	2.3	5.7
Lightly Salted, Crinkle Cut, Love Life, Waitrose*	1 Bag/25g	118	5.6	473	6.6	59.5	22.3	4.1
Lightly Salted, Crinkle Cut, Low Fat, Waitrose*	1 Pack/35g	163	8.0	466	5.2	60.1	22.8	5.1
Lightly Salted, Crinkles, Shapers, Boots*	1 Pack/20g	96	4.8	482	6.6	60.0	24.0	4.0
Lightly Salted, Handcooked, Finest, Tesco*	1 Bag/40g	206	11.5	515	5.1	58.6	28.8	2.5
Lightly Salted, Hoops, Mini, Weight Watchers*	1 Pack/20g	71	0.2	355	4.0	82.0	1.0	3.5
Lightly Salted, Kettle Chips*	1 Serving/50g	255	15.2	510	5.9	50.5	30.3	5.6
Lightly Salted, Low Fat, Waitrose*	1 Bag/25g	125	6.2	500	7.5	61.3	25.0	4.8
Lightly Salted, Potato Bakes, Weight Watchers*	1 Pack/20g	78	1.8	392	5.0	72.0	9.0	4.0
Lightly Salted, Potato This, LC, Tesco*	1 Pack/20g	72	0.4	360	5.1	79.5	2.0	4.2
Lightly Salted, Reduced Fat, Crinkles, Eat Well, M&S*	1 Pack/30g	140	6.6	460	6.7	59.4	21.8	4.5
Lightly Sea Salted, Jonathan Crisp*	1 Bag/35g	176	10.2	503	6.5	52.0	29.0	5.4
Lightly Sea Salted, Potato Chips, Hand Fried, Burts*	¼ Bag/50g	252	13.8	504	6.4	57.4	27.7	0.0
Lightly Sea Salted, Tyrrells*	1 Pack/40g	204	10.2	510	5.9	49.0	25.4	5.3
Lime & Thai Spices, Sensations, Walkers*	1 Pack/40g	200	11.6	500	6.5	54.0	29.0	4.0
Lincolnshire Sausage, Tyrrells*	1 Pack/100g	530	28.2	530	8.6	60.8	28.2	3.0
Mango Chilli, Kettle Chips*	1 Serving/40g	190	9.6	475	6.3	53.9	24.0	6.1
Marmite, Sunseed, Walkers*	1 Bag/33g	169	10.7	520	6.5	49.0	33.0	4.0
Marmite*	1 Pack/25g	130	7.7	519	6.2	52.6	30.7	3.7
Mature Cheddar & Chive, Kettle Chips*	1 Serving/50g	239	12.7	478	8.1	54.4	25.4	5.0
Mature Cheddar & Chive, Tyrrells*	1 Bag/40g	194	10.0	485	8.4	58.7	25.1	2.4
Mature Cheddar & Onion, Deep Ridge, Walkers*	1 Pack/28g	145	8.6	518	6.4	51.8	30.7	4.3
Mature Cheddar & Red Onion, Kettle Chips*	1 Bag/40g	202	11.6	505	7.1	51.1	28.9	6.2
Mature Cheddar & Shallot, Temptations, Tesco*	1/6 Bag/25g	131	8.6	524	6.6	47.4	34.2	4.4
Mediterranean Baked Potato, COU, M&S*	1 Pack/25g	90	0.6	360	7.6	74.0	2.4	6.8
Mexican Chilli, Ridge Cut, McCoys*	1 Bag/32g	164	9.8	514	6.9	53.0	30.5	4.5
Mexican Lime with a Hint of Chilli, Kettle Chips*	1 Serving/50g	242	13.8	484	5.0	54.1	27.5	5.4
New York Cheddar, Kettle Chips*	1 Bag/50g	242	13.4	483	6.7	53.9	26.7	4.5
Onion Rings, Corn Snacks, Average	1 Bag/25g	122	6.1	486	5.8	60.9	24.2	2.7
Onion Rings, Crunchy, Shapers, Boots*	1 Bag/12g	61	3.4	507	2.5	62.0	28.0	2.6
Onion Rings, M&S*	1 Pack/40g	186	8.6	465	5.2	62.1	21.5	4.3
Onion Rings, Tayto*	1 Pack/17g	82	4.1	484	3.0	63.4	24.0	2.4
Onion Rings, Tesco*	1 Serving/30g	148	7.6	495	8.4	57.8	25.5	2.5
Oriental Ribs, Ridge Cut, McCoys*	1 Pack/50g	256	15.0	511	7.3	52.7	30.1	4.2
Paprika, Max, Walkers*	1 Bag/50g	260	16.0	520	6.5	52.0	31.9	5.1
Peri Peri Chicken, Nando's*	½ Bag/75g	410	20.2	547	5.1	57.4	27.0	3.4
Pickled Onion, Golden Wonder*	1 Bag/25g	131	8.5	524	5.6	49.0	34.0	2.0
Pickled Onion, Monster Bites, Sainsbury's*	1 Bag/20g	107	6.7	535	5.2	53.5	33.3	1.0
Pickled Onion, Space Raiders, KP Snacks*	1 Bag/13g	64	2.9	495	6.5	65.3	22.8	1.0
Pickled Onion, Sunseed, Walkers*	1 Bag/33g	171	10.7	525	6.5	50.0	33.0	4.0
Pickled Onion Flavour, Average	1 Bag/25g	132	8.2	527	6.6	52.5	32.6	3.5
Pickled Onion Rings, COU, M&S*	1 Bag/20g	69	0.3	345	5.0	81.7	1.5	3.7
Pom Bear, Cheese & Onion, Intersnack Ltd*	1 Bag/19g	95	5.3	498	3.8	58.1	27.8	3.2
Pom Bear, Salt & Vinegar, Intersnack Ltd*	1 Pack/25g	124	6.8	494	3.0	58.8	27.4	2.7
Pom Bear, Smoky Bacon, Intersnack Ltd*	1 Bag/19g	98	5.1	515	3.9	63.8	27.0	0.7
Pom Bear, Zoo, Really Cheesy, Intersnack Ltd.*	1 Bag/19g	100	5.8	525	3.6	57.0	30.7	3.1
Potato	1oz/28g	148	9.6	530	5.7	53.3	34.2	5.3
Potato, Baked, COU, M&S*	1 Bag/25g	88	0.6	350	8.5	76.4	2.3	5.7
Potato, Low Fat	1oz/28g	128	6.0	458	6.6	63.5	21.5	5.3
Potato, Tyrrells*	1 Pack/261g	1362	72.8	522	6.1	56.5	27.9	0.0
Potato Chips, Anglesey Sea Salt, Red Sky*	1 Serving/40g	185	8.7	463	6.8	59.8	21.8	5.0
Prawn Cocktail, Boots*	1 Pack/21g	99	4.6	470	6.8	60.0	22.0	4.3
Prawn Cocktail, Golden Wonder*	1 Bag/25g	130	8.4	521	5.8	49.0	33.5	2.0

CRISPS

	Measure INFO/WEIGHT	per Measure KCAL	per Measure FAT	Nutrition Values per 100g / 100ml KCAL	PROT	CARB	FAT	FIBRE
Prawn Cocktail, KP Snacks*	1 Bag/25g	133	8.7	531	5.9	48.4	34.9	4.7
Prawn Cocktail, Lites, Advantage, Tayto*	1 Pack/21g	96	4.1	455	5.3	65.1	19.3	3.8
Prawn Cocktail, Lites, Shapers, Boots*	1 Bag/21g	92	3.8	438	5.1	64.0	18.0	4.1
Prawn Cocktail, Seabrook*	1 Bag/30g	163	10.1	544	5.7	49.2	33.7	4.5
Prawn Cocktail, Snack Rite*	1 Bag/25g	129	8.3	516	5.0	49.2	33.2	0.0
Prawn Cocktail, Sunseed Oil, Walkers*	1 Bag/33g	171	10.7	525	6.5	50.0	33.0	4.0
Prawn Cocktail, Tayto*	1 Bag/35g	185	12.3	526	7.5	46.6	35.0	4.5
Prawn Crackers, Tesco*	1 Bag/60g	316	17.5	527	3.2	62.8	29.2	0.8
Prawn Spirals, Shapers, Boots*	1 Pack/100g	468	22.0	468	3.1	64.0	22.0	2.8
Ready Salted, 30% Less Fat, Sainsbury's*	1 Serving/25g	122	5.6	486	7.3	63.7	22.4	8.2
Ready Salted, Average	1 Bag/25g	127	7.4	508	6.1	53.4	29.7	4.0
Ready Salted, Baked, Walkers*	1 Pack/38g	146	3.0	390	6.0	74.0	8.0	5.5
Ready Salted, Co-Op*	1 Bag/25g	131	8.5	525	6.0	51.0	34.0	3.0
Ready Salted, Deep Ridge, Walkers*	1 Pack/28g	148	9.0	529	6.4	51.1	32.1	4.6
Ready Salted, Golden Wonder*	1 Bag/25g	135	8.8	539	5.5	49.9	35.3	2.0
Ready Salted, Lidl*	1 Bag/25g	138	9.2	554	4.9	50.3	37.0	0.0
Ready Salted, Lower Fat, Asda*	1 Bag/25g	120	6.2	481	6.0	58.0	25.0	4.8
Ready Salted, Lower Fat, Sainsbury's*	1 Bag/25g	111	5.4	444	7.0	55.0	21.8	5.1
Ready Salted, M&S*	1 Bag/25g	136	9.2	545	5.6	47.8	36.6	4.9
Ready Salted, Morrisons*	1 Bag/25g	134	8.7	536	4.9	50.9	34.8	4.3
Ready Salted, Oven Baked, Asda*	1 Bag/25g	95	1.9	379	4.4	73.1	7.7	2.6
Ready Salted, Oven Baked, Tesco*	1 Bag/25g	95	1.9	380	4.4	73.1	7.7	8.4
Ready Salted, Potato Chips, Tesco*	1 Bag/25g	132	8.2	526	5.6	51.7	33.0	3.8
Ready Salted, Potato Squares, Sainsbury's*	1 Bag/50g	192	8.0	384	6.5	53.8	15.9	7.8
Ready Salted, Reduced Fat, Tesco*	1 Pack/25g	114	6.2	456	6.3	52.0	24.7	5.9
Ready Salted, Ridge Cut, McCoys*	1 Bag/49g	257	15.6	524	6.6	52.6	31.9	4.1
Ready Salted, Sainsbury's*	1 Bag/25g	132	8.1	530	5.0	52.5	32.5	3.7
Ready Salted, Select, Tesco*	1 Bag/25g	136	9.2	544	6.2	47.9	36.6	4.5
Ready Salted, Smart Price, Asda*	1 Bag/18g	97	6.3	538	6.5	49.3	35.0	4.2
Ready Salted, Snack Rite*	1 Bag/25g	136	9.0	545	4.9	50.3	36.0	0.0
Ready Salted, Squares, M&S*	1 Bag/35g	150	6.3	430	6.8	63.5	18.1	3.9
Ready Salted, Squares, Walkers*	1 Pack/25g	109	4.8	435	6.5	60.0	19.0	6.0
Ready Salted, Sunseed Oil, Walkers*	1 Bag/33g	175	11.1	537	5.9	49.7	34.1	4.2
Ready Salted, Value, Morrisons*	1 Pack/18g	95	6.0	528	6.7	50.0	33.3	0.6
Ready Salted, Value, Tesco*	1 Pack/18g	100	6.3	528	6.8	50.1	33.4	3.1
Red Leicester & Spring Onion, Handcooked, M&S*	1 Pack/40g	194	10.6	485	6.8	55.0	26.4	5.1
Roast Beef & Mustard, Thick Cut, Brannigans*	1 Bag/40g	203	12.0	507	7.6	51.7	30.0	3.7
Roast Chicken, Golden Wonder*	1 Bag/25g	130	8.4	522	6.2	48.6	33.6	2.0
Roast Chicken, Select, Tesco*	1 Bag/25g	134	8.8	536	6.6	48.6	35.0	4.4
Roast Chicken, Snack Rite*	1 Bag/25g	132	8.3	526	5.3	51.3	33.3	0.0
Roast Chicken, Sunseed Oil, Walkers*	1 Bag/33g	171	10.7	525	6.5	50.0	33.0	4.0
Roast Chicken, Tayto*	1 Bag/35g	184	11.9	526	7.6	47.3	34.0	4.5
Roast Chicken Flavour	1 Bag/25g	130	7.7	519	5.2	53.5	30.8	3.7
Roast Chicken Flavour, Average	1 Bag/25g	132	8.6	528	6.1	48.8	34.2	3.9
Roast Chicken Flavour, Crinkle, Weight Watchers*	1 Pack/16g	76	3.3	475	5.6	63.1	20.6	6.2
Roast Ham & Mustard, Ridge Cut, McCoys*	1 Pack/35g	181	10.7	518	7.1	53.5	30.6	3.9
Roasted Lamb, Moroccan Spices, Sensations, Walkers*	1 Bag/40g	198	11.6	495	6.0	53.0	29.0	4.5
Roasted Peanut Puffs, Ellert*	1 Serving/25g	125	6.0	500	13.0	56.0	24.0	4.1
Salt & Black Pepper, Handcooked, M&S*	1 Bag/40g	180	9.2	450	5.7	55.0	22.9	5.2
Salt & Malt Vinegar, Deep Ridge, Walkers*	1 Pack/28g	143	8.6	511	6.1	50.7	30.7	4.3
Salt & Malt Vinegar, Hunky Dorys*	1 Serving/30g	141	8.6	469	6.3	49.3	28.7	0.0
Salt & Malt Vinegar, Ridge Cut, McCoys*	1 Bag/32g	165	9.8	515	6.7	53.3	30.6	3.9
Salt & Malt Vinegar Flavour, Sainsbury's*	1 Bag/25g	134	8.8	538	4.9	50.3	35.2	2.3

CRISPS

Measure INFO/WEIGHT		per Measure		Nutrition Values per 100g / 100ml				
		KCAL	FAT	KCAL	PROT	CARB	FAT	FIBRE
Salt & Shake, Walkers*	1 Bag/30g	162	10.5	540	6.5	50.0	35.0	4.0
Salt & Vinegar, 30% Less Fat, Sainsbury's*	1 Bag/25g	114	5.4	458	7.2	58.3	21.8	5.1
Salt & Vinegar, Asda*	1 Bag/25g	130	8.5	522	6.0	48.0	34.0	4.2
Salt & Vinegar, Average	1 Bag/25g	130	8.2	519	5.5	50.3	32.9	3.4
Salt & Vinegar, Baked, Walkers*	1 Pack/38g	150	3.0	400	6.0	73.5	8.1	4.6
Salt & Vinegar, Chiplets, M&S*	1 Pack/50g	220	9.4	440	5.7	61.3	18.9	4.7
Salt & Vinegar, Crinkle, M&S*	1 Pack/25g	120	5.9	485	6.5	61.0	24.0	3.5
Salt & Vinegar, Crinkle Cut, Love Life, Waitrose*	1 Bag/25g	118	5.6	473	6.6	59.5	22.3	4.1
Salt & Vinegar, Crinkle Cut, Seabrook*	1 Bag/32g	181	11.7	569	5.4	54.4	36.7	3.9
Salt & Vinegar, Crinkles, Shapers, Boots*	1 Pack/20g	96	4.8	482	6.6	60.0	24.0	4.0
Salt & Vinegar, Crispy Discs, Shapers, Boots*	1 Bag/92g	404	17.5	439	4.8	63.0	19.0	4.9
Salt & Vinegar, Distinctively, Walkers*	1 Pack/33g	169	10.0	519	5.9	52.6	30.8	4.2
Salt & Vinegar, Everyday, Co-Op*	1 Bag/17g	77	3.4	455	6.0	62.0	20.0	2.0
Salt & Vinegar, Fish Shapes, Food Explorers, Waitrose*	1 Bag/20g	86	3.2	430	2.4	69.1	16.0	1.3
Salt & Vinegar, Fries, COU, M&S*	1 Bag/25g	85	0.4	340	5.0	80.0	1.6	4.0
Salt & Vinegar, Golden Lights, Golden Wonder*	1 Bag/21g	94	3.9	446	4.2	65.7	18.5	3.7
Salt & Vinegar, Golden Wonder*	1 Bag/25g	130	8.5	522	5.4	48.5	34.0	2.0
Salt & Vinegar, Half Fat, M&S*	1 Bag/40g	168	6.8	420	5.8	61.0	17.0	7.7
Salt & Vinegar, in Sunflower Oil, Sainsbury's*	1 Serving/25g	131	8.4	524	5.2	49.7	33.8	3.7
Salt & Vinegar, KP Snacks*	1 Bag/25g	133	8.8	532	5.5	48.7	35.0	4.7
Salt & Vinegar, Lights, Walkers*	1 Bag/28g	133	6.2	475	7.0	62.0	22.0	4.5
Salt & Vinegar, M&S*	1 Bag/25g	131	8.6	525	5.4	48.8	34.5	4.6
Salt & Vinegar, Morrisons*	1 Bag/25g	129	7.8	515	4.9	53.9	31.1	3.6
Salt & Vinegar, Potato Bakes, Weight Watchers*	1 Bag/20g	81	1.8	404	5.3	76.0	8.8	2.3
Salt & Vinegar, Rough Cuts, Tayto*	1 Bag/30g	152	9.2	506	4.6	56.8	30.8	0.0
Salt & Vinegar, Sainsbury's*	1 Bag/25g	130	8.8	522	4.1	46.9	35.3	3.9
Salt & Vinegar, Select, Tesco*	1 Bag/25g	132	8.7	529	5.9	47.8	34.9	4.3
Salt & Vinegar, Snack Rite*	1 Bag/25g	127	8.2	508	4.7	48.1	33.0	0.0
Salt & Vinegar, Space Raiders, KP Snacks*	1 Bag/17g	81	3.8	478	6.9	61.7	22.6	2.2
Salt & Vinegar, Spirals, Shapers, Boots*	1 Pack/15g	71	3.4	475	3.1	64.0	23.0	1.7
Salt & Vinegar, Squares, Walkers*	1 Bag/28g	121	4.9	441	6.5	61.0	18.0	5.5
Salt & Vinegar, Sunseed Oil, Walkers*	1 Bag/33g	171	10.7	525	6.5	50.0	33.0	4.0
Salt & Vinegar, Tayto*	1 Bag/35g	184	11.9	526	7.6	47.3	34.0	4.5
Salt & Vinegar, Value, Tesco*	1 Bag/20g	109	7.4	547	5.7	47.7	37.0	4.8
Salt & Vinegar, Waitrose*	1 Pack/25g	132	8.4	529	6.3	50.5	33.8	4.4
Salt Your Own, Excluding Salt, Aldi*	1 Pack/24g	130	8.1	536	6.0	52.6	33.5	4.5
Scotch Bonnet Flavour, Mackies*	1 Pack/150g	732	369.0	488	78.0	574.0	246.0	42.0
Sea Salt, Golden Lights, Golden Wonder*	1 Bag/21g	94	3.9	448	3.9	66.4	18.5	4.4
Sea Salt, Gourmet, TTD, Sainsbury's*	1/3 Pack/50g	249	15.0	498	5.7	51.4	30.0	6.4
Sea Salt, Handcooked, Extra Special, Asda*	1 Pack/31g	149	7.8	477	7.0	56.0	25.0	4.1
Sea Salt, Original, Crinkle Cut, Seabrook*	1 Bag/30g	155	9.3	517	5.7	53.7	31.1	4.2
Sea Salt & Balsamic Vinegar, Kettle Chips*	1 Bag/40g	201	11.4	502	5.4	53.0	28.4	6.1
Sea Salt & Balsamic Vinegar, Low Fat, Peak*	1 Serving/25g	87	0.4	348	7.4	76.6	1.4	6.7
Sea Salt & Black Pepper, GFY, Asda*	1 Bag/100g	476	24.0	476	6.0	59.0	24.0	6.0
Sea Salt & Black Pepper, Tyrrells*	1/4 Pack/38g	182	9.3	480	7.3	59.9	24.5	2.4
Sea Salt & Cider Vinegar, TTD, Sainsbury's*	1/3 Pack/50g	245	14.3	489	5.5	52.7	28.5	6.1
Sea Salt & Cracked Black Pepper, Sensations, Walkers*	1 Bag/40g	196	10.8	490	6.5	55.0	27.0	4.0
Sea Salt & Indian Black Pepper, Pipers Crisps*	1 Pack/40g	195	11.6	487	6.6	49.9	29.0	0.0
Sea Salt & Malt Vinegar, Sensations, Walkers*	1 Bag/40g	194	10.8	485	6.5	54.0	27.0	4.5
Sea Salt & Malt Vinegar Flavour, Fries, GFY, Asda*	1 Bag/15g	54	0.3	358	6.3	79.6	1.7	2.1
Sea Salt & Modena Balsamic Vivegar, Darling Spuds*	1 Bag/40g	190	11.4	475	5.4	54.3	28.5	4.2
Sea Salt with Crushed Black Peppercorns, Kettle Chips*	1 Serving/40g	201	11.4	502	5.7	52.4	28.6	7.5
Shells, Prawn Cocktail, Asda*	1 Bag/18g	90	5.3	501	4.6	54.9	29.2	6.2

CRISPS

INFO/WEIGHT Measure	per Measure KCAL	FAT	Nutrition Values per 100g / 100ml KCAL	PROT	CARB	FAT	FIBRE
CRISPS							
Simply Salted, Extra Crunchy, Walkers*	1 Bag/30g	142	6.5	473	6.8	59.8	21.8	5.0
Simply Salted, Lights, Walkers*	1 Bag/24g	113	5.3	470	7.0	61.0	22.0	5.0
Smokey Bacon, Crinkle, Shapers, Boots*	1 Pack/20g	96	4.8	482	6.6	60.0	24.0	4.0
Smokey Bacon, Select, Tesco*	1 Bag/25g	134	8.7	536	6.4	49.0	34.9	4.3
Smokey Bacon Potato Hoops, COU, M&S*	1 Pack/16g	58	0.4	360	5.6	78.7	2.7	4.5
Smoky Bacon, Golden Wonder*	1 Bag/25g	131	8.4	523	5.9	49.1	33.7	2.0
Smoky Bacon, Snack Rite*	1 Bag/25g	131	8.3	525	5.5	51.2	33.1	0.0
Smoky Bacon, Sunseed Oil, Walkers*	1 Bag/35g	183	11.4	530	6.5	51.0	33.0	4.0
Smoky Bacon, Tayto*	1 Bag/35g	184	11.9	526	7.6	47.3	34.0	4.5
Smoky Bacon Flavour, Average	1 Bag/25g	132	8.4	527	6.2	49.7	33.7	3.2
Snaps, Spicy Tomato Flavour, Walkers*	1 Bag/18g	91	4.8	508	1.5	65.5	26.8	0.0
Snax, Tayto*	1 Pack/17g	82	3.7	483	2.4	70.0	21.5	1.6
Sour Cream & Chilli Lentil Curls, M&S*	1 Pack/60g	243	5.2	405	13.6	65.3	8.7	4.3
Sour Cream & Chive, Baked, Walkers*	1 Pack/38g	148	3.2	395	7.0	73.0	8.5	5.0
Sour Cream & Chive, Crinkle, Reduced Fat, M&S*	1 Bag/40g	178	8.2	445	5.6	58.8	20.6	5.6
Sour Cream & Chive, Lights, Walkers*	1 Bag/24g	114	5.3	475	7.5	62.0	22.0	5.0
Sour Cream & Chive, Potato Bakes, Weight Watchers*	1 Bag/20g	83	1.8	417	3.8	80.7	8.8	3.6
Sour Cream & Chive Baked Potato, COU, M&S*	1 Pack/24g	84	0.7	350	7.5	73.2	2.8	7.9
Sour Cream & Chive Crispy Discs, Shapers, Boots*	1 Bag/21g	94	4.0	448	5.7	61.9	19.0	4.3
Sour Cream & Chive Flavour, Average	1 Bag/25g	127	7.7	508	6.8	50.7	30.9	4.6
Sour Cream & Onion, Golden Lights, Golden Wonder*	1 Bag/21g	93	3.8	442	4.1	66.0	17.9	4.4
Spiced Chilli, McCoys*	1 Bag/35g	175	10.1	500	6.1	54.2	28.8	4.2
Spicy Chilli, Sunseed, Walkers*	1 Pack/35g	183	11.4	530	6.5	51.0	33.0	4.0
Steak, Chargrilled, Max, Walkers*	1 Bag/55g	289	18.2	525	6.5	50.0	33.0	4.0
Steak & Onion, Walkers*	1 Pack/33g	169	10.7	520	6.5	49.0	33.0	4.0
Sunbites, Cheddar & Caramelised Onion, Walkers*	1 Bag/25g	120	5.4	480	7.6	60.8	21.6	6.4
Sunbites, Sweet Chilli, Sun Ripened, Walkers*	1 Bag/25g	120	5.4	480	7.6	60.8	21.6	6.4
Sweet Chill, Mexican, Phileas Fogg*	1 Bag/38g	193	11.0	507	6.7	54.8	29.0	4.2
Sweet Chilli, Cracker, Special K, Kellogg's*	1 Serving/23g	94	2.1	409	5.0	73.0	9.0	8.0
Sweet Chilli, Crinkle Cut, Weight Watchers*	1 Bag/20g	94	4.1	470	5.6	62.9	20.6	5.8
Sweet Chilli, Hand Cooked, Asda*	1 Pack/25g	120	7.1	479	5.7	54.5	28.3	4.5
Sweet Chilli, Thai, Sensations, Walkers*	1 Bag/40g	194	10.4	485	6.0	57.0	26.0	4.2
Sweet Chilli, Thai, Velvet Crunch, King*	1 Pack/20g	81	1.9	404	1.6	77.5	9.7	2.0
Sweet Chilli & Red Peppers, Fusion, Tayto*	1 Bag/28g	140	8.3	500	4.9	52.2	29.8	4.6
Sweet Chilli Chicken, Extra Crunchy, Walkers*	1 Bag/30g	143	6.8	477	6.5	59.9	22.5	4.8
Sweet Chilli Flavour, Average	1 Bag/25g	115	5.6	461	5.1	59.9	22.6	4.6
T Bone Steak, Roysters*	1 Pack/28g	148	9.0	530	5.2	55.3	32.0	3.0
Tangy Toms, Red Mill*	1 Bag/15g	76	4.1	507	6.0	60.0	27.3	0.7
Thai Sweet Chicken, Ridge Cut, McCoys*	1 Bag/50g	257	15.0	514	7.0	54.0	30.0	4.1
Tomato Ketchup, Heinz, Sunseed, Walkers*	1 Bag/35g	179	11.0	520	6.5	51.0	32.0	4.0
Tomato Ketchup Flavour, Golden Wonder*	1 Bag/25g	135	8.0	521	5.1	54.0	30.8	3.6
Tortillas, Nacho Cheese Flavour, Weight Watchers*	1 Pack/18g	78	2.9	433	6.1	66.7	16.1	3.9
Traditional, Hand Cooked, Finest, Tesco*	1 Bag/150g	708	39.2	472	6.4	52.9	26.1	5.1
Unsalted, Seabrook*	1 Bag/30g	163	10.7	544	5.7	47.9	35.8	4.1
Vegetable, Average	1 Bag/25g	118	7.4	470	4.1	46.5	29.6	12.1
Vegetable, Crunchy, Asda*	½ Bag/50g	251	12.0	502	1.4	70.0	24.0	6.0
Vegetable, Finest, Tesco*	1 Serving/50g	203	12.8	406	5.0	39.0	25.5	14.6
Vegetable, Waitrose*	1 Pack/100g	490	35.2	490	4.7	38.5	35.2	13.0
Wild Paprika Flavour, Croky*	1 Pack/45g	234	13.0	521	6.0	58.0	29.0	0.0
Worcester Sauce, Sunseed Oil, Walkers*	1 Bag/35g	183	11.4	530	6.5	52.0	33.0	4.0
Worcester Sauce Flavour, Hunky Dorys*	1 Bag/45g	211	12.9	469	6.3	49.3	28.7	0.0
CRISPY PANCAKE							
Beef, Minced, Findus*	1 Pancake/63g	100	2.5	160	6.5	25.0	4.0	1.0

	Measure INFO/WEIGHT	per Measure KCAL	FAT	Nutrition Values per 100g / 100ml KCAL	PROT	CARB	FAT	FIBRE
CRISPY PANCAKE								
Beef Bolognese, Findus*	1 Pancake/65g	104	2.6	160	6.5	25.0	4.0	1.0
Cheeses, Three, Findus*	1 Pancake/62g	118	4.0	190	7.0	25.0	6.5	0.9
Chicken, Bacon & Sweetcorn, Findus*	1 Pancake/63g	101	2.5	160	5.5	26.0	4.0	1.1
CROISSANT								
All Butter, BGTY, Sainsbury's*	1 Croissant/44g	151	6.5	343	9.3	42.7	14.8	1.8
All Butter, Budgens*	1 Croissant/45g	185	11.1	412	7.9	39.7	24.6	3.3
All Butter, Finest, Tesco*	1 Croissant/77g	328	18.2	426	8.6	44.9	23.6	1.9
All Butter, M&S*	1 Croissant/54g	222	12.8	415	7.4	45.2	23.8	1.6
All Butter, Mini, Sainsbury's*	1 Croissant/35g	150	8.6	428	9.2	42.6	24.5	1.2
All Butter, Mini, Tesco*	1 Croissant/35g	150	8.2	430	9.3	45.2	23.5	2.0
All Butter, Reduced Fat, Tesco*	1 Croissant/52g	164	5.5	315	7.5	47.4	10.6	1.8
All Butter, Sainsbury's*	1 Croissant/44g	188	10.8	428	9.2	42.6	24.5	1.2
All Butter, Tesco*	1 Croissant/48g	192	10.4	400	8.5	41.7	21.6	2.6
Asda*	1 Croissant/47g	190	9.9	405	9.0	45.0	21.0	0.0
Average	1 Croissant/50g	180	10.2	360	8.3	38.3	20.3	1.6
Butter, Asda*	1 Croissant/46g	191	11.0	416	8.0	42.0	24.0	1.9
Butter, GFY, Asda*	1 Croissant/44g	153	7.0	352	6.0	46.0	16.0	2.0
Butter, Morrisons*	1 Croissant/44g	196	12.5	446	9.3	38.2	28.4	2.0
Cheese & Ham, Delice de France*	1 Serving/91g	225	12.3	247	7.0	24.4	13.5	2.5
Cheese & Ham, Mini, Waitrose*	1 Croissant/17g	64	4.1	383	13.2	28.1	24.6	3.0
Continental, Mini, CBY, Asda*	1 Croissant/35g	150	8.9	427	9.2	40.6	25.3	1.6
Creme Patissiere & Raisins, Mini Chinois, Aldi*	1 Croissant/50g	133	3.4	266	0.0	20.2	6.8	0.0
Flaky Pastry with a Plain Chocolate Filling, Tesco*	1 Croissant/78g	318	19.0	408	6.5	41.0	24.3	2.0
French Butter, You Count, Love Life, Waitrose*	1 Croissant/44g	168	7.4	382	9.8	46.4	16.8	3.1
Low Fat, M&S*	1 Croissant/45g	180	9.1	400	8.2	46.0	20.2	1.8
Mini, Lidl*	1 Croissant/30g	112	5.0	373	7.8	48.0	16.6	0.0
Reduced Fat, Asda*	1 Croissant/44g	159	6.5	361	9.7	47.2	14.8	2.0
Reduced Fat, Sainsbury's*	1 Croissant/44g	173	7.7	393	9.8	49.2	17.5	2.2
TTD, Sainsbury's*	1 Croissant/70g	289	16.1	413	8.1	43.4	23.0	2.5
with Egg, Cheese & Ham from Restaurant, Average	1 Croissant/152g	474	33.6	312	12.4	15.9	22.1	0.0
CROQUETTES								
Morrisons*	1 Serving/150g	231	8.1	154	3.3	23.1	5.4	1.1
Potato, & Parsnip, Finest, Tesco*	2 Croquettes/74g	155	7.3	210	6.0	23.2	9.9	3.9
Potato, Asda*	3 Croquettes/81g	144	5.7	177	2.0	26.5	7.0	2.2
Potato, Birds Eye*	1 Croquette/29g	44	1.7	152	2.6	22.6	5.7	1.2
Potato, Chunky, Aunt Bessie's*	1 Serving/41g	62	2.5	152	2.3	22.9	6.1	1.8
Potato, Crispy, Chilled, Sainsbury's*	3 Croquettes/125g	245	11.5	196	2.5	25.7	9.2	1.9
Potato, Fried in Blended Oil, Average	1 Croquette/80g	171	10.5	214	3.7	21.6	13.1	1.3
Potato, M&S*	1 Croquette/41g	68	3.6	165	2.4	19.3	8.8	2.2
Potato, Sainsbury's*	1 Croquette/28g	50	2.4	180	2.8	22.6	8.6	2.5
Potato, Waitrose*	1 Croquette/30g	47	2.4	157	3.0	17.9	8.1	1.5
Vegetable, Sainsbury's*	1 Serving/175g	392	20.8	224	5.8	23.3	11.9	2.2
CROUTONS								
Fresh, M&S*	1 Serving/10g	53	3.3	530	11.4	50.0	32.8	3.2
Garlic, Waitrose*	1 Serving/40g	209	12.0	522	10.8	52.1	30.0	2.7
Herb, & Garlic, La Rochelle*	¼ Pack/18g	106	7.2	587	6.9	49.8	40.0	2.1
Herb, Sainsbury's*	1 Serving/15g	64	1.7	429	13.4	68.2	11.4	2.8
La Rochelle*	1 Bag/70g	400	28.0	572	7.0	49.0	40.0	0.0
Prepacked, Average	1 Serving/15g	74	3.6	495	10.8	58.7	24.0	2.6
Salad, Italian, Sainsbury's*	1 Pack/40g	204	10.0	510	8.5	62.7	25.0	2.5
Sea Salted, Lightly, Asda*	1 Serving/20g	83	1.9	414	12.9	69.7	9.3	4.3
Tomato, Sun Dried, Sainsbury's*	¼ Pack/15g	75	3.8	497	11.7	55.2	25.5	2.5

	Measure INFO/WEIGHT	per Measure KCAL	FAT	Nutrition Values per 100g / 100ml KCAL	PROT	CARB	FAT	FIBRE
CRUDITE								
Platter, Sainsbury's*	1 Pack/275g	96	0.8	35	1.4	6.6	0.3	1.6
Selection, Prepared, M&S*	1 Serving/250g	75	1.0	30	1.4	5.8	0.4	2.0
Vegetable Sticks, Average	1 Serving/100g	24	0.2	24	0.7	4.5	0.2	1.9
CRUMBLE								
Almond & Apricot, Devondale*	1 Cake/80g	314	13.2	392	3.6	57.0	16.5	9.8
Apple, & Custard, Asda*	1 Serving/125g	250	8.8	200	2.3	32.0	7.0	0.0
Apple, & Toffee, Weight Watchers*	1 Pot/98g	190	4.5	194	1.6	36.6	4.6	0.0
Apple, Average	1 Serving/240g	497	12.0	207	0.9	40.5	5.0	1.1
Apple, Basics, Sainsbury's*	¼ Crumble/125g	235	4.9	188	1.7	36.5	3.9	1.2
Apple, Bramley, & Blackberry, BGTY, Sainsbury's*	1 Crumble/120g	196	2.9	163	1.7	32.3	2.4	2.9
Apple, Bramley, Favourites, M&S*	1 Serving/140g	390	13.8	279	4.6	43.2	9.9	1.2
Apple, Bramley, M&S*	1 Serving/149g	387	13.7	260	4.3	40.3	9.2	1.1
Apple, Bramley, Tesco*	1/3 Pack/155g	378	14.9	244	2.8	36.7	9.6	1.8
Apple, Co-Op*	¼ Crumble/110g	270	7.7	245	2.0	43.0	7.0	2.0
Apple, Farmfoods*	½ Pack/185g	411	10.9	222	2.9	39.3	5.9	2.3
Apple, Fresh, Chilled, Tesco*	¼ Pack/150g	368	13.4	245	2.8	38.0	8.9	1.4
Apple, Frozen, Tesco*	¼ Pack/150g	345	16.3	230	2.1	30.7	10.9	3.9
Apple, Sainsbury's*	1 Crumble/565g	1034	32.8	183	2.3	30.5	5.8	2.9
Apple, Sara Lee*	1 Serving/200g	606	18.0	303	2.3	53.3	9.0	1.2
Apple, Somerfield*	1 Serving/195g	454	16.4	233	2.5	36.8	8.4	1.1
Apple, Waitrose*	1 Serving/125g	310	2.9	248	2.2	54.5	2.3	1.2
Apple, with Custard, Green's*	1 Serving/79g	171	5.3	216	1.9	37.0	6.7	1.2
Apple, with Custard, Individual, Sainsbury's*	1 Pudding/120g	286	13.9	238	2.0	31.4	11.6	2.4
Apple, with Sultanas, Weight Watchers*	1 Dessert/110g	196	4.3	178	1.4	34.2	3.9	1.3
Apple & Blackberry, Asda*	1 Serving/175g	427	15.8	244	2.7	38.0	9.0	1.2
Apple & Blackberry, Budgens*	1 Serving/240g	821	31.2	342	3.7	54.0	13.0	0.6
Apple & Blackberry, M&S*	1 Serving/135g	398	15.1	295	3.5	44.9	11.2	1.6
Apple & Blackberry, Sainsbury's*	1 Serving/110g	232	6.2	211	3.0	37.1	5.6	2.1
Apple & Blackberry, Somerfield*	1 Serving/125g	315	11.2	252	3.4	39.4	9.0	2.4
Apple & Blackberry, Tesco*	1 Crumble/335g	737	32.2	220	2.8	30.7	9.6	2.0
Apple & Blackberry with Custard, Somerfield*	1 Serving/120g	324	15.0	270	2.3	36.3	12.5	1.1
Fruit	1 Portion/170g	337	11.7	198	2.0	34.0	6.9	1.7
Fruit, with Custard	1 Serving/270g	463	17.6	171	2.4	27.0	6.5	1.3
Gooseberry, M&S*	1 Serving/133g	379	14.2	285	3.5	43.3	10.7	1.7
Rhubarb, Asda*	½ Crumble/200g	460	24.0	230	2.4	28.0	12.0	5.0
Rhubarb, Average	1 Portion/150g	330	11.1	220	2.7	35.5	7.4	1.9
Rhubarb, Co-Op*	¼ Crumble/110g	270	7.7	245	2.0	42.0	7.0	1.0
Rhubarb, M&S*	1 Serving/133g	366	13.2	275	3.4	42.6	9.9	1.4
Rhubarb, Tesco*	1/6 Crumble/117g	228	9.7	195	2.8	27.3	8.3	1.7
Rhubarb with Custard, Sainsbury's*	1 Serving/120g	288	13.9	240	2.4	31.4	11.6	2.3
Salmon, Youngs*	1 Pie/360g	367	14.4	102	5.4	11.1	4.0	1.0
CRUMBLE MIX								
Luxury, Tesco*	¼ Pack/55g	243	9.0	441	5.7	67.9	16.3	3.2
Luxury, Wholegrain, GF, Hale & Hearty*	1 Serving/100g	447	17.0	447	2.5	71.0	17.0	3.6
CRUMBLE TOPPING								
Morrisons*	1 Serving/40g	179	6.6	448	5.4	69.5	16.5	2.8
Sainsbury's*	1 Serving/47g	188	9.2	401	5.9	50.3	19.6	5.3
CRUMPETS								
Asda*	1 Crumpet/45g	85	0.4	188	6.0	39.0	0.9	2.1
Basics, Sainsbury's*	1 Crumpet/35g	69	0.4	198	5.9	41.0	1.1	1.6
Co-Op*	1 Crumpet/40g	70	0.3	175	7.0	35.0	0.7	2.0
Essential, Waitrose*	1 Crumpet/52g	94	0.6	182	6.5	35.1	1.1	2.6
Everyday, Value, Tesco*	1 Crumpet/40g	75	0.4	190	6.0	37.5	0.9	2.9

	Measure INFO/WEIGHT	per Measure KCAL	FAT	Nutrition Values per 100g / 100ml KCAL	PROT	CARB	FAT	FIBRE
CRUMPETS								
Fruit from Bakery, Tesco*	1 Crumpet/73g	161	1.7	220	6.2	43.2	2.3	1.1
Gluten, Wheat & Milk Free, Free From, Livwell*	1 Crumpet/55g	83	1.7	151	3.6	26.9	3.1	2.0
Golden Sun*	1 Crumpet/43g	83	0.7	193	7.8	37.1	1.6	1.6
Kingsmill*	1 Crumpet/55g	99	0.4	180	5.8	37.5	0.8	1.7
Less Than 2% Fat, M&S*	1 Crumpet/61g	116	0.8	190	8.0	36.9	1.3	2.1
Morrisons*	1 Crumpet/40g	70	0.3	174	6.6	35.3	0.7	1.8
Mother's Pride*	1 Crumpet/43g	80	0.4	185	5.6	38.3	1.0	2.3
PB, Waitrose*	1 Crumpet/55g	94	0.2	171	6.1	36.1	0.3	4.4
Sainsbury's*	1 Crumpet/46g	92	0.6	199	6.0	39.7	1.3	2.4
Scottish, Nick Nairn's*	1 Serving/100g	186	9.6	186	5.3	43.0	9.6	1.5
Smart Price, Asda*	1 Crumpet/36g	67	0.3	188	6.0	39.0	0.9	2.1
Soldier, Mother's Pride*	1 Crumpet/30g	58	0.5	193	7.8	37.1	1.6	1.6
Square, Tesco*	1 Crumpet/60g	101	0.5	168	6.3	33.8	0.8	2.7
Toasted, Average	1 Crumpet/40g	80	0.4	199	6.7	43.4	1.0	2.0
Toasted, Tesco*	1 Crumpet/65g	120	0.6	185	5.2	37.9	0.9	3.7
TTD, Sainsbury's*	1 Crumpet/65g	124	1.0	191	5.9	38.5	1.5	2.3
Waitrose*	1 Crumpet/62g	116	0.7	188	6.3	37.9	1.2	2.1
Warburton's*	1 Crumpet/55g	98	0.4	178	5.6	36.1	0.7	2.3
CRUNCHIE								
Blast, Cadbury*	1 Serving/42g	199	8.3	480	4.7	69.6	20.1	0.7
Cadbury*	1 Bar/40g	185	7.5	465	4.0	69.5	18.9	0.5
Nuggets, Cadbury*	1 Bag/125g	569	20.5	455	3.8	73.1	16.4	0.0
Treat Size, Cadbury*	1 Bar/17g	80	3.1	470	4.0	71.5	18.4	0.0
CRUNCHY CURLS								
Cheeky Chutney, Snack-A-Jacks, Quaker Oats*	1 Pack/22g	88	1.6	402	2.1	81.0	7.4	0.8
Sweet Chilli Kick, Snack-A-Jacks, Quaker Oats*	1 Pack/18g	72	1.3	402	2.1	81.0	7.4	0.8
CRUNCHY STICKS								
Salt & Vinegar, Sainsbury's*	1 Bag/25g	118	6.1	474	5.9	58.0	24.3	2.4
Salt & Vinegar, Shapers, Boots*	1 Pack/21g	96	3.8	457	5.7	66.7	18.1	2.4
Salt & Vinegar, Tesco*	1 Serving/25g	118	6.1	470	6.9	55.7	24.4	2.7
Salt & Vinegar, Value, Tesco*	1 Bag/22g	113	5.9	512	5.7	62.1	26.8	0.7
CUCUMBER								
Average	*1 Serving/80g*	*8*	*0.1*	*10*	*0.7*	*1.5*	*0.1*	*0.6*
CUMIN								
Seeds, Ground, Schwartz*	1 Tsp/5g	22	1.2	446	19.0	40.3	23.2	0.0
Seeds, Whole, Average	*1 Tsp/2g*	*8*	*0.5*	*375*	*17.8*	*44.2*	*22.7*	*10.5*
CURACAO								
Average	*1 Pub Shot/35ml*	*109*	*0.0*	*311*	*0.0*	*28.3*	*0.0*	*0.0*
CURLY WURLY								
Cadbury*	1 Bar/26g	115	4.5	442	3.5	69.2	17.3	0.8
Squirlies, Cadbury*	1 Squirl/3g	13	0.5	442	3.5	69.2	17.3	0.8
CURRANTS								
Average	*1oz/28g*	*75*	*0.1*	*267*	*2.3*	*67.8*	*0.4*	*1.9*
CURRY								
& Chips, Curry Sauce, Chipped Potatoes, Kershaws*	1 Serving/330g	391	8.2	118	10.0	14.0	2.5	2.0
Aubergine	1oz/28g	33	2.8	118	1.4	6.2	10.1	1.5
Beef, & Rice, CBY, Asda*	1 Pack/400g	452	7.6	113	4.6	18.6	1.9	1.6
Beef, Hot, Canned, M&S*	1 Can/425g	446	21.7	105	12.2	2.8	5.1	1.0
Beef, Sainsbury's*	1 Serving/400g	552	32.8	138	10.7	5.4	8.2	0.9
Beef, Thai, Finest, Tesco*	1 Serving/500g	770	29.0	154	9.0	16.5	5.8	1.2
Beef, with Rice, Asda*	1 Pack/400g	476	10.4	119	6.0	18.0	2.6	0.9
Beef, with Rice, Birds Eye*	1 Pack/388g	524	10.9	135	6.9	20.8	2.8	0.8
Beef, with Rice, Morrisons*	1 Serving/400g	480	20.0	120	6.0	12.6	5.0	0.6

CURRY

	Measure INFO/WEIGHT	per Measure KCAL	per Measure FAT	Nutrition Values per 100g / 100ml KCAL	PROT	CARB	FAT	FIBRE
Beef, with Rice, Tesco*	1 Pack/400g	595	18.0	149	2.8	23.1	4.5	1.9
Blackeye Bean, Gujerati	1oz/28g	36	1.2	127	7.2	16.1	4.4	2.8
Bombay Butternut Squash, Veg Pot, Innocent*	1 Pot/380g	296	4.2	78	2.6	12.5	1.1	4.1
Cabbage	1oz/28g	23	1.4	82	1.9	8.1	5.0	2.1
Cauliflower & Chickpea, Lovely Vegetables, M&S*	1 Serving/390g	351	13.6	90	2.9	11.2	3.5	3.7
Cauliflower & Potato	1oz/28g	17	0.7	59	3.4	6.6	2.4	1.8
Chana Dahl, Curry Special*	1 Pack/350g	434	22.8	124	6.0	10.5	6.5	5.9
Chick Pea, Whole, Average	1oz/28g	50	2.1	179	9.6	21.3	7.5	4.5
Chick Pea, Whole, Basic, Average	1oz/28g	30	1.0	108	6.0	14.2	3.6	3.3
Chicken, Asda*	1 Can/200g	210	10.0	105	10.0	5.0	5.0	0.0
Chicken, Canned, Sainsbury's*	1 Serving/100g	136	6.1	136	11.1	9.1	6.1	1.0
Chicken, Chinese, with Rice, Ready Meal, Average	1 Serving/450g	490	11.5	109	7.2	14.1	2.6	1.3
Chicken, Green Thai, & Rice, Fuller Longer, M&S*	1 Pack/395g	375	5.9	95	7.8	12.7	1.5	0.9
Chicken, Green Thai, BGTY, Sainsbury's*	1 Pack/400g	316	10.4	79	10.6	3.4	2.6	1.9
Chicken, Green Thai, Birds Eye*	1 Pack/450g	536	19.8	119	4.7	15.2	4.4	0.3
Chicken, Green Thai, Breasts, Finest, Tesco*	1 Serving/200g	292	16.0	146	16.5	2.0	8.0	0.7
Chicken, Green Thai, Jasmine Rice, Weight Watchers*	1 Pack/320g	291	3.2	91	6.1	14.3	1.0	0.5
Chicken, Green Thai, no Rice, Average	1 Serving/200g	174	7.0	87	8.2	5.0	3.5	1.4
Chicken, Green Thai, Nutritionally Balanced, M&S*	1 Pack/400g	400	5.2	100	9.2	12.4	1.3	1.4
Chicken, Green Thai, Sainsbury's*	½ Pack/200g	264	13.6	132	13.0	4.8	6.8	0.9
Chicken, Green Thai, with Jasmine Rice, Ready Meal	1 Serving/450g	520	17.2	116	7.7	12.6	3.8	1.1
Chicken, Green Thai Style & Sticky Rice, Asda*	1 Pack/450g	585	10.8	130	7.0	20.0	2.4	0.1
Chicken, Hot, Can, Tesco*	1 Can/418g	514	26.3	123	9.7	6.9	6.3	0.9
Chicken, Kashmiri, Waitrose*	1 Serving/400g	640	36.4	160	14.5	5.0	9.1	0.6
Chicken, Malaysian, CBY, Asda*	1 Serving/375g	390	9.8	104	6.1	13.3	2.6	1.5
Chicken, Malaysian, Finest, Tesco*	1 Pack/375g	375	8.3	100	7.4	12.2	2.2	0.8
Chicken, Mild, Asda*	½ Can/190g	239	11.4	126	11.0	7.0	6.0	0.5
Chicken, Mild, BGTY, Sainsbury's*	1 Serving/200g	184	5.2	92	10.0	7.2	2.6	0.5
Chicken, Red Thai, & Rice, Ready Meal, Healthy Range	1 Serving/400g	400	7.8	100	6.4	14.0	2.0	1.0
Chicken, Red Thai, & Sticky Rice, Ready Meal	1 Serving/450g	527	15.7	117	6.7	14.2	3.5	1.7
Chicken, Red Thai, 97% Fat Free, Birds Eye*	1 Pack/366g	425	7.0	116	5.7	19.0	1.9	0.5
Chicken, Red Thai, Asda*	1 Pack/360g	461	27.7	128	9.1	5.5	7.7	1.0
Chicken, Red Thai, COU, M&S*	1 Pack/400g	420	9.2	105	7.1	13.4	2.3	1.4
Chicken, Red Thai, GFY, Asda*	1 Serving/400g	364	8.4	91	6.0	12.0	2.1	1.6
Chicken, Red Thai, No Rice, Average	1 Serving/200g	194	6.9	97	7.2	9.0	3.4	1.4
Chicken, Red Thai, Tesco*	1 Serving/175g	215	11.6	123	10.5	5.5	6.6	1.4
Chicken, Red Thai, with Jasmine Rice, Ready Meal	1 Serving/450g	500	15.3	111	7.5	12.6	3.4	1.0
Chicken, Red Thai with Fragrant Rice, Somerfield*	1 Pack/340g	503	17.0	148	8.0	18.0	5.0	0.0
Chicken, Red Thai with Jasmine Rice, Weight Watchers*	1 Pack/400g	344	3.2	86	6.5	12.9	0.8	0.8
Chicken, Red Thai with Rice, Tesco*	1 Serving/475g	746	32.3	157	7.2	16.8	6.8	1.1
Chicken, Thai Green, Charlie Bigham's*	½ Pack/300g	402	26.7	134	9.9	3.6	8.9	0.8
Chicken, Thai Mango, Sainsbury's*	½ Pack/200g	288	17.8	144	11.2	4.8	8.9	1.9
Chicken, with Potatoes, Diet Chef Ltd*	1 Pack/300g	291	13.2	97	7.5	6.9	4.4	2.8
Chicken, with Rice, Average	1 Serving/400g	465	11.0	116	5.1	17.8	2.8	0.8
Chicken, with Rice, Birds Eye*	1 Pack/400g	468	11.2	117	4.5	18.4	2.8	0.6
Chicken, with Rice, Frozen, Tesco*	1 Pack/400g	488	15.6	122	4.6	17.2	3.9	0.7
Chicken, with Rice, Malaysian, Bernard Matthews*	1 Pack/400g	512	15.6	128	6.1	17.0	3.9	0.0
Chicken, with Rice, Ready Meal, Average	1 Serving/400g	446	10.5	112	5.2	16.8	2.6	1.0
Chicken, with White Rice, Weight Watchers*	1 Pack/320g	306	4.8	96	5.3	15.4	1.5	0.1
Chicken & Rice, International Cuisine*	1 Serving/400g	420	11.6	105	3.3	16.4	2.9	0.8
Chicken Katsu, City Kitchen, Tesco*	1 Pack/385g	465	13.2	121	6.0	16.3	3.4	1.3
Cod, Red Thai with Rice, PB, Waitrose*	1 Pack/400g	360	7.2	90	7.5	11.0	1.8	1.0
Courgette, & Potato	1oz/28g	24	1.5	86	1.9	8.7	5.2	1.2

CURRY

	Measure INFO/WEIGHT	per Measure KCAL	FAT	Nutrition Values per 100g / 100ml KCAL	PROT	CARB	FAT	FIBRE
Fish, Bangladeshi, Average	1oz/28g	35	2.2	124	12.2	1.5	7.9	0.3
Fish, Red Thai, Waitrose*	1 Pack/500g	275	11.0	55	5.2	3.7	2.2	1.0
Fish & Vegetable, Bangladeshi, Average	1oz/28g	33	2.4	117	9.1	1.4	8.4	0.5
Gobi Aloo Sag, Retail	1oz/28g	27	1.9	95	2.2	7.1	6.9	1.4
Green Thai & Rice, GFY, Asda*	1 Pack/400g	356	7.6	89	7.0	11.0	1.9	1.6
Indian Daal, Tasty Veg Pot, Innocent*	1 Pot/380g	319	9.9	84	2.8	9.7	2.6	5.3
King Prawn, Coconut & Lime, Sainsbury's*	½ Pack/351g	207	8.8	59	3.7	5.4	2.5	1.0
King Prawn, Goan, M&S*	1 Pack/400g	680	44.4	170	5.1	11.6	11.1	1.5
King Prawn, Malay with Rice, Sainsbury's*	1 Pack/400g	608	20.4	152	5.0	21.5	5.1	1.4
King Prawn, Red Thai, City Kitchen, Tesco*	1 Pack/385g	460	14.4	119	4.5	16.7	3.7	1.0
King Prawn Malay, Waitrose*	1 Pack/350g	364	19.2	104	6.6	7.1	5.5	0.9
Lamb, Hot, M&S*	½ Can/213g	320	19.6	150	14.9	6.0	9.2	2.3
Lamb, Kefthedes, Waitrose*	½ Pack/200g	294	17.6	147	9.0	8.0	8.8	2.1
Lamb & Potato, 385, Wiltshire Farm Foods*	1 Serving/210g	334	23.0	159	8.9	6.2	11.0	1.7
Masala, Aubergine, TTD, Sainsbury's*	½ Pack/115g	135	11.4	117	2.9	4.1	9.9	5.8
Masala, Indian, Veg Pot, Innocent*	1 Pot/380g	331	10.3	87	2.9	11.6	2.7	3.6
Matar Paneer, Peas & Cheese, Ashoka*	½ Pack/150g	183	10.0	122	5.3	10.0	6.7	2.0
Medium, with Long Grain Rice, Rice Time, Uncle Ben's*	1 Pot/300g	396	9.0	132	2.3	23.2	3.0	1.2
Mild Chicken Tikka Masala, Diet Chef Ltd*	1 Meal/300g	291	6.6	97	10.4	9.0	2.2	0.6
Mushroom & Pea, Masala, Indian, Sainsbury's*	1 Pack/300g	264	14.7	88	3.3	5.2	4.9	5.1
Potato & Pea	1oz/28g	26	1.1	92	2.9	13.0	3.8	2.4
Prawn, & Mushroom	1oz/28g	47	4.0	168	7.3	2.5	14.4	1.0
Prawn, Red Thai, Sainsbury's*	1 Pack/300g	546	39.6	182	6.3	9.4	13.2	1.7
Prawn, Thai, with Jasmine Rice, BGTY, Sainsbury's*	1 Serving/401g	353	6.0	88	4.2	14.5	1.5	2.0
Prawn, with Rice, Asda*	1 Pack/400g	420	10.4	105	3.5	17.0	2.6	1.1
Red Kidney Bean, Punjabi	1oz/28g	30	1.6	106	4.7	10.1	5.6	3.8
Spicy Paneer, Lovely Vegetables, M&S*	1 Pot/300g	330	12.0	110	4.3	11.9	4.0	4.0
Thai Coconut, Veg Pot, Innocent*	1 Pot/390g	316	9.4	81	3.2	10.3	2.4	2.5
Vegetable, & Rice, Microwaveable, M&S*	1 Pot/325g	390	7.2	120	2.3	22.3	2.2	2.2
Vegetable, Asda*	1 Pack/350g	329	21.0	94	1.9	8.0	6.0	1.9
Vegetable, Canned, Sainsbury's*	½ Can/200g	200	12.2	100	1.4	9.8	6.1	1.8
Vegetable, Canned, Savers, Morrisons*	1 Can/400g	208	1.2	52	2.2	9.3	0.3	1.9
Vegetable, in a Mild & Creamy Curry Sauce, Waitrose*	1 Pack/400g	388	26.4	97	2.6	6.9	6.6	1.5
Vegetable, in Sweet Sauce, Average	1 Serving/330g	162	6.9	49	1.4	6.7	2.1	1.3
Vegetable, Indian, Sainsbury's*	½ Pack/200g	206	14.6	103	2.5	6.8	7.3	4.6
Vegetable, Indian, Tesco*	1 Serving/225g	257	17.8	114	2.1	8.6	7.9	1.6
Vegetable, Indian Meal for One, Tesco*	1 Serving/200g	218	14.4	109	2.0	9.0	7.2	1.2
Vegetable, LC, Tesco*	1 Pack/350g	350	4.2	100	2.3	19.4	1.2	1.5
Vegetable, Masala, LC, Tesco*	1 Pack/350g	298	6.0	85	3.8	13.6	1.7	3.4
Vegetable, Mixed Vegetables, Frozen, Average	1oz/28g	25	1.7	88	2.5	6.9	6.1	0.4
Vegetable, Pakistani, Average	1oz/28g	17	0.7	60	2.2	8.7	2.6	2.2
Vegetable, Sabzi Tarkari, Patak's*	1 Pack/400g	500	31.2	125	2.5	11.1	7.8	2.2
Vegetable, Solo Slim, Rosemary Conley*	1 Pack/300g	153	3.6	51	2.0	8.0	1.2	2.1
Vegetable, Takeaway, Average	1 Serving/330g	346	24.4	105	2.5	7.6	7.4	0.0
Vegetable, with Rice, Healthy Range, Average	1 Serving/400g	351	4.6	88	2.3	16.8	1.1	1.9
Vegetable, with Rice, Ready Meal, Average	1 Serving/330g	337	9.9	102	3.3	16.4	3.0	0.0
Vegetable, with Rice, Tesco*	1 Pack/400g	440	12.0	110	2.1	18.7	3.0	1.0
Vegetable, with Yoghurt, Average	1oz/28g	17	1.1	62	2.6	4.6	4.1	1.4
Vegetable, Yellow Thai, Sainsbury's*	1 Pack/400g	624	48.8	156	2.2	9.4	12.2	1.1

CURRY LEAVES

	Measure INFO/WEIGHT	per Measure KCAL	FAT	Nutrition Values per 100g / 100ml KCAL	PROT	CARB	FAT	FIBRE
Fresh	**1oz/28g**	**27**	**0.4**	**97**	**7.9**	**13.3**	**1.3**	**0.0**

CURRY PASTE

	Measure INFO/WEIGHT	per Measure KCAL	FAT	Nutrition Values per 100g / 100ml KCAL	PROT	CARB	FAT	FIBRE
Balti, Sharwood's*	¼ Pack/73g	328	28.7	453	5.0	19.2	39.6	3.1

CURRY PASTE

	Measure INFO/WEIGHT	per Measure KCAL	FAT	Nutrition Values per 100g / 100ml KCAL	PROT	CARB	FAT	FIBRE
Balti, Tomato & Coriander, Original, Patak's*	1 Tbsp/15g	58	5.1	388	4.0	14.6	34.0	3.7
Bhuna, Tomato & Tamarind, Patak's*	1 Serving/10g	40	5.6	397	4.3	17.5	56.2	6.3
Green Thai, Average	1 Tsp/5g	6	0.4	128	2.1	11.7	7.9	3.1
Hot, Sharwood's*	1oz/28g	123	10.7	439	5.1	18.6	38.3	2.6
Jalfrezi, Patak's*	1 Serving/30g	96	8.1	320	3.7	14.2	26.9	5.6
Korma, Coconut & Coriander, Original, Patak's*	1 Serving/30g	124	11.7	415	3.5	11.6	39.0	5.2
Madras, Cumin & Chilli, Hot, Patak's*	¼ Jar/70g	202	18.1	289	4.7	7.6	25.9	10.8
Mild, Coriander & Cumin, Original, Patak's*	1 Serving/35g	99	8.6	283	4.8	9.1	24.6	10.7
Red Thai, Average	1 Tsp/5g	7	0.5	132	2.3	9.5	9.1	3.0
Rogan Josh, Tomato & Paprika, Patak's*	1 Serving/30g	119	11.0	397	4.1	12.7	36.7	5.9
Tandoori, Sharwood's*	1oz/28g	64	4.4	228	5.9	15.5	15.8	1.9
Tandoori, Tamarind & Ginger, Patak's*	1 Serving/30g	33	0.5	110	3.1	20.4	1.8	2.6
Tikka Masala, Coriander & Lemon, Medium, Patak's*	1 Serving/30g	111	9.5	369	3.8	16.9	31.8	2.9
Tikka Masala, Sharwood's*	1oz/28g	53	4.3	191	3.2	9.9	15.4	2.6
Tom Yum, Thai Taste*	1 Tsp/13g	35	2.0	269	5.4	30.8	15.4	7.7

CURRY POWDER

	Measure INFO/WEIGHT	per Measure KCAL	FAT	Nutrition Values per 100g / 100ml KCAL	PROT	CARB	FAT	FIBRE
Average	**1 Tsp/2g**	**6**	**0.3**	**325**	**12.7**	**41.8**	**13.8**	**0.0**

CURRY SAUCE

	Measure INFO/WEIGHT	per Measure KCAL	FAT	Nutrition Values per 100g / 100ml KCAL	PROT	CARB	FAT	FIBRE
Asda*	1 Tbsp/15g	62	2.1	414	13.0	59.0	14.0	1.3
Balti, Asda*	¼ Jar/125g	155	12.5	124	1.6	7.0	10.0	1.7
Balti, Loyd Grossman*	½ Jar/175g	180	11.7	103	1.3	8.4	6.7	1.7
Basics, Sainsbury's*	¼ Jar/110g	70	2.8	64	0.7	9.7	2.5	0.9
Biryani, Medium & Aromatic, Oven Bake, Patak's*	½ Jar/175g	135	9.3	77	1.1	6.1	5.3	1.7
Chinese Style, Cooking, Asda*	1 Jar/560g	465	24.1	83	1.5	9.6	4.3	1.7
Dopiaza, Finest, Tesco*	1 Jar/350g	234	10.5	67	1.3	8.5	3.0	3.7
Green Thai, Asda*	1 Jar/340g	309	27.2	91	0.5	4.3	8.0	0.2
Jalfrezi, Average	1 Jar/350g	326	23.7	93	1.3	6.7	6.8	1.6
Jalfrezi, Loyd Grossman*	½ Jar/175g	159	10.3	91	1.4	7.3	5.9	1.6
Jalfrezi, Piri Piri, Finest, Tesco*	1 Serving/175g	145	10.8	83	1.2	5.7	6.2	1.5
Jalfrezi, Tesco*	1 Jar/500g	450	32.5	90	1.3	6.6	6.5	2.4
Korma, Average	1 Jar/350g	584	42.3	167	2.3	11.7	12.1	1.3
Korma, Loyd Grossman*	½ Jar/175g	224	14.5	128	1.5	11.3	8.3	0.8
Korma, Uncle Ben's*	1 Jar/500g	630	42.0	126	1.4	11.1	8.4	0.0
Madras, Aldi*	1 Serving/113g	68	2.3	60	1.5	9.0	2.0	0.0
Madras, Average	1 Jar/350g	355	24.2	102	1.7	8.0	6.9	1.7
Madras, Cooking, Sharwood's*	1 Tsp/2g	2	0.1	86	1.5	6.9	5.8	1.3
Madras, Cooking, Tesco*	1/3 Jar/161g	145	9.2	90	1.9	6.9	5.7	2.5
Madras, Cumin & Chilli, Original, in Glass Jar, Patak's*	1 Jar/540g	648	38.3	120	2.1	11.9	7.1	1.8
Madras, Indian, Sharwood's*	1 Jar/420g	433	26.5	103	1.8	9.7	6.3	1.9
Madras, Sharwood's*	1 Jar/420g	466	28.1	111	1.8	10.9	6.7	2.5
Madras, Tesco*	½ Jar/200g	168	13.0	84	1.1	5.2	6.5	1.3
Makhani, Sharwood's*	1 Jar/420g	399	29.0	95	0.9	7.2	6.9	0.4
Malaysian Rendang, Loyd Grossman*	1 Serving/100g	143	10.1	143	2.6	10.4	10.1	1.4
Medium, Uncle Ben's*	1 Jar/500g	330	10.0	66	0.9	10.9	2.0	0.0
Red Curry, Thai, Stir Fry, Blue Dragon*	1 Sachet/120g	112	9.6	93	0.9	4.4	8.0	0.5
Rogan Josh, Loyd Grossman*	1 Serving/106g	206	16.7	194	2.4	10.5	15.8	1.5
Rogan Josh, Worldwide Sauces*	1 Jar/500g	255	1.5	51	1.1	11.0	0.3	0.0
Smart Price, Asda*	¼ Jar/110g	73	2.0	66	1.4	11.0	1.8	0.6
Sri Lankan Devil Curry, Sharwood's*	1 Jar/380g	220	11.4	58	0.5	7.2	3.0	2.1
Thai Green Curry, Stir Fry, Blue Dragon*	1 Sachet/120g	74	4.8	62	0.9	5.7	4.0	0.5
Tikka, Cooking, Tesco*	1 Jar/500g	617	42.2	123	1.7	10.1	8.4	2.0
Tikka Masala, COU, M&S*	½ Pack/100g	80	2.6	80	4.5	9.9	2.6	1.7
Tikka Masala, Ready Made, Average	1 Jar/350g	422	28.8	121	2.0	9.6	8.2	1.2

	Measure INFO/WEIGHT	per Measure KCAL	per Measure FAT	Nutrition Values per 100g / 100ml KCAL	PROT	CARB	FAT	FIBRE
CURRY SAUCE								
Vindaloo, Cooking, CBY, Asda*	½ Jar/160g	128	5.4	80	1.5	10.4	3.4	1.0
Vindaloo, Hot, Patak's*	1 Jar/540g	643	46.4	119	1.7	8.5	8.6	2.1
CUSTARD								
Banana Flavour, Ambrosia*	1 Pot/135g	139	3.9	103	2.9	16.1	2.9	0.0
Banana Flavour, Pot, Average	1 Pot/135g	138	3.9	102	2.9	16.0	2.9	0.0
Chocolate, COU, M&S*	1 Pot/140g	147	3.1	105	3.1	18.6	2.2	1.0
Chocolate Flavour, Ambrosia*	1 Pot/150g	177	4.4	118	3.0	20.0	2.9	0.7
Chocolate Flavour, Pot, Average	1 Pot/125g	138	3.4	111	3.1	18.2	2.7	0.6
Creamy, No Added Sugar, Made Up, Aunt Bessie's*	1 Serving/23g	97	2.7	425	6.3	71.6	11.9	1.7
Instant, Just Add Water, Made Up, Weight Watchers*	1 Serving/145g	93	0.6	64	1.2	13.9	0.4	0.9
Low Fat, Average	***1/3 Pot/141g***	***116***	***1.6***	***82***	***2.9***	***15.0***	***1.2***	***0.0***
Powder	***1 Tsp/5g***	***18***	***0.0***	***354***	***0.6***	***92.0***	***0.7***	***0.1***
Ready to Eat, Chocolate, Tesco*	1 Pot/150g	150	3.4	100	3.2	16.2	2.3	0.3
Ready to Serve, Average	***1 Serving/50g***	***59***	***2.3***	***118***	***3.3***	***16.1***	***4.6***	***0.2***
Ready to Serve, Tinned, Value, Tesco*	1 Serving/99g	75	0.7	76	3.1	14.4	0.7	0.0
Strawberry Flavour, Pot, Average	1 Pot/125g	130	3.3	104	2.7	17.3	2.7	0.0
Strawberry Flavoured, Ambrosia*	1 Serving/135g	139	3.8	103	2.8	16.7	2.8	0.0
Summer, Ambrosia*	1 Pack/500g	490	15.0	98	2.7	15.0	3.0	0.0
Vanilla, COU, M&S*	1 Pot/140g	147	3.5	105	4.3	16.6	2.5	0.6
Vanilla, Madagascan, Simply Creamy, Fresh, Waitrose*	1/5 Pot/100g	208	14.4	208	3.4	16.3	14.4	1.1
Vanilla, TTD, Sainsbury's*	1 Pot/150g	312	23.2	208	2.5	14.7	15.5	0.1
Vanilla Flavour, Pot, Average	1 Pot/125g	128	3.5	102	2.8	16.4	2.8	0.0
CUSTARD APPLE								
Cherimoya, Weighed without Skin & Seeds, Average	1 Cherimoya/312g	234	2.1	75	1.6	17.7	0.7	3.0
CUTLETS								
Nut, Goodlife*	1 Cutlet/88g	283	19.4	322	9.1	21.8	22.0	3.4
Nut, Meat Free, Tesco*	1 Cutlet/70g	235	16.4	330	8.0	22.7	23.0	3.8
Nut, Retail, Grilled, Average	1 Cutlet/90g	191	11.7	212	5.1	19.9	13.0	1.8
CUTTLEFISH								
Raw	***1oz/28g***	***20***	***0.2***	***71***	***16.1***	***0.0***	***0.7***	***0.0***

	Measure INFO/WEIGHT	per Measure KCAL	FAT	Nutrition Values per 100g / 100ml KCAL	PROT	CARB	FAT	FIBRE
DAB								
Raw	1oz/28g	21	0.3	74	15.7	0.0	1.2	0.0
DAIRYLEA DUNKERS								
Jumbo Munch, Dairylea, Kraft*	1 Serving/50g	150	9.2	300	7.2	26.5	18.5	1.2
Salt & Vinegar, Dairylea, Kraft*	1 Tub/42g	116	8.2	275	6.7	17.5	19.5	0.3
with Jumbo Tubes, Kraft*	1 Pack/43g	108	5.1	255	9.1	27.0	12.0	0.9
with Ritz Crackers, Dairylea, Kraft*	1 Tub/46g	122	6.4	265	9.6	25.0	13.9	0.6
DAIRYLEA LUNCHABLES								
Ham & Cheese Pizza, Dairylea, Kraft*	1 Pack/97g	247	10.7	255	11.5	26.0	11.0	1.6
Harvest Ham, Dairylea, Kraft*	1 Pack/110g	314	18.7	285	16.5	16.5	17.0	0.3
Tasty Chicken, Dairylea, Kraft*	1 Pack/110g	314	18.2	285	17.0	17.5	16.5	0.3
DAMSONS								
Raw, Weighed with Stones, Average	1oz/28g	10	0.0	34	0.5	8.6	0.0	1.6
Raw, Weighed without Stones, Average	1oz/28g	11	0.0	38	0.5	9.6	0.0	1.8
DANDELION & BURDOCK								
Barr*	1 Bottle/250ml	40	0.0	16	0.0	4.0	0.0	0.0
Original, Ben Shaws*	1 Can/440ml	128	0.0	29	0.0	7.0	0.0	0.0
Sparkling, Diet, Morrisons*	1 Glass/200ml	2	0.0	1	0.0	0.3	0.0	0.0
DANISH PASTRY								
Apple, Bakery, Waitrose*	1 Pastry/123g	400	22.2	325	5.1	35.7	18.0	2.4
Apple, Fresh Cream, Sainsbury's*	1 Pastry/67g	248	14.6	368	3.1	40.2	21.6	0.4
Apple, Iceland*	¼ Pastry/95g	223	5.0	235	5.3	41.5	5.3	2.3
Apple & Cinnamon, Danish Twist, Entenmann's*	1 Serving/52g	150	1.0	288	5.6	62.0	1.9	1.5
Apple & Sultana, Tesco*	1 Pastry/72g	293	16.4	407	5.4	45.0	22.8	1.4
Average	1 Pastry/110g	411	19.4	374	5.8	51.3	17.6	1.6
Cherry, & Custard, Bar, Tesco*	1 Bar/350g	910	49.0	260	3.5	29.9	14.0	7.7
Cherry, Bar, Sainsbury's*	¼ Bar/88g	220	10.0	252	4.2	33.2	11.4	1.7
Custard, Bar, Sara Lee*	¼ Bar/100g	228	6.4	228	6.6	36.1	6.4	0.8
Fruit Filled, Average	1 Pastry/94g	335	15.9	356	5.1	47.9	17.0	0.0
Pecan, M&S*	1 Serving/67g	287	17.4	428	6.2	45.0	26.0	1.3
Toasted Pecan, Danish Twist, Entenmann's*	1 Slice/48g	171	7.6	351	7.0	47.2	15.6	1.4
DATES								
Bite Size, Snack Pack, Whitworths*	1 Pack/35g	119	0.6	340	2.0	74.7	1.8	8.2
Deglet Nour, Graze*	1 Pack/60g	181	0.3	301	2.1	72.0	0.5	0.0
Deglet Nour, Love Life, Waitrose*	1 Portion/50g	144	0.1	287	3.3	68.0	0.2	8.0
Dried, Average	1 Date/20g	54	0.1	272	2.8	65.4	0.4	4.2
Dried, Medjool, Average	1 Date/20g	56	0.1	279	2.2	69.3	0.3	4.3
Fresh, Raw, Yellow, Average	1 Date/20g	23	0.0	116	1.4	29.1	0.1	1.6
Hadrawi, Love Life, Waitrose*	5 Dates/50g	144	0.1	288	3.4	68.0	0.2	8.0
Halawi, Tesco*	6 Dates/60g	165	0.1	275	2.3	65.5	0.2	4.3
Medjool, Love Life, Waitrose*	1 Date/20g	58	0.0	291	3.3	68.0	0.2	6.7
Medjool, Stuffed with Walnuts, Tesco*	2 Dates/40g	98	2.3	245	4.4	44.0	5.7	3.4
Medjool, TTD, Sainsbury's*	1 Serving/50g	148	0.0	296	1.9	72.0	0.1	6.7
Milk Chocolate Coated, Julian Graves*	1 Pack/200g	768	22.6	384	4.5	66.0	11.3	2.6
Organic, Medjool, Pitted, Love Life, Waitrose*	1 Date/18g	52	0.0	292	3.3	68.0	0.2	6.7
Soft, Dried, Whitworths*	1 Serving/25g	85	0.4	340	2.0	74.7	1.8	8.2
DELI FILLER								
Cheese & Onion, Sainsbury's*	1 Pack/170g	673	62.7	396	10.8	4.8	36.9	0.9
Chicken, Caesar Style, Sainsbury's*	1 Pack/80g	212	18.2	265	14.0	1.0	22.7	2.6
Chicken & Bacon, Co-Op*	1 Pack/200g	420	29.6	210	17.6	1.0	14.8	2.6
Prawn Cocktail, Eat Well, M&S*	½ Pot/85g	119	7.3	140	9.1	6.4	8.6	0.6
Salmon, Smoked, & Soft Cheese, M&S*	1 Serving/85g	208	17.3	245	11.7	3.3	20.4	0.5
DELIGHT								
Butterscotch Flavour, No Added Sugar, Tesco*	1 Pack/49g	225	10.0	460	4.8	63.3	20.5	0.0

D

	Measure INFO/WEIGHT	per Measure KCAL	FAT	Nutrition Values per 100g / 100ml KCAL	PROT	CARB	FAT	FIBRE
DELIGHT								
Chocolate Flavour, Dry, Tesco*	1 Pack/49g	220	9.0	450	6.2	64.2	18.4	2.3
Vanilla, No Added Sugar, Dry, Tesco*	1 Pack/49g	51	1.8	105	3.4	13.7	3.7	0.1
DESSERT								
Baked Lemon, COU, M&S*	1 Serving/100g	140	2.5	140	6.8	22.0	2.5	0.8
Banana Split	1 Serving/175g	368	25.5	210	2.2	18.0	14.6	0.2
Banoffee, Layered, Sainsbury's*	1 Pot/115g	270	14.7	235	2.2	27.8	12.8	1.0
Banoffee, Weight Watchers*	1 Dessert/81g	170	3.6	210	4.9	37.7	4.4	1.4
Black Forest, Tesco*	1 Pot/100g	287	14.4	287	3.5	35.8	14.4	2.4
Black Forest Gateaux, After Dark, Gu*	1 Pot/85g	258	18.5	303	3.0	24.7	21.8	1.3
Blueberry Muffin, Tesco*	1 Pot/91g	265	18.7	291	2.0	24.5	20.6	3.0
Buttons, Milk Chocolate, Cadbury*	1 Pot/100g	280	14.9	280	6.2	30.8	14.9	0.0
Caramel, Delights, Shape, Danone*	1 Pot/110g	109	2.5	99	3.3	16.3	2.3	0.1
Caramel, Pots Of Joy, Dairy Milk, Cadbury*	1 Pot/70g	150	7.3	215	2.5	27.1	10.5	0.1
Caramel Crunch, Weight Watchers*	1 Serving/89g	174	2.6	196	4.6	37.9	2.9	1.7
Caramel Flavour, Soya, Dairy Free, Organic, Provamel*	1 Pot/125g	125	2.2	100	3.0	17.8	1.8	0.5
Cheeky & Saucy Little Pots Au Chocolat, Gu*	1 Pot/45g	199	16.6	443	3.3	24.1	36.9	2.3
Chocolate, Campina*	1 Pot/125g	186	8.6	149	3.2	18.5	6.9	0.0
Chocolate, Delights, Shape, Danone*	1 Pot/110g	109	2.4	99	3.3	16.3	2.2	0.6
Chocolate, Frappe, Skinny, COU, M&S*	1 Pot/100g	115	2.0	115	5.7	18.3	2.0	0.5
Chocolate, M&S*	1 Serving/120g	168	2.5	140	5.6	26.4	2.1	1.1
Chocolate, Soya, Dairy Free, Organic, Provamel*	1 Pot/125g	111	3.0	89	3.0	13.6	2.4	1.0
Chocolate, Weight Watchers*	1 Serving/82g	145	2.5	177	5.2	32.3	3.0	2.9
Chocolate Banoffee, Gu*	1 Pot/85g	325	21.5	382	3.9	35.0	25.3	1.0
Chocolate Brownie, M&S*	¼ Pack/144g	610	39.5	425	4.7	39.6	27.5	1.0
Chocolate Buttons, Cadbury*	1 Pack/100g	275	14.5	275	5.0	30.5	14.5	0.0
Chocolate Desire, Magnum, Wall's Ice Cream*	1 Dessert/85g	374	24.0	440	5.3	40.0	28.2	0.0
Chocolate Duetto, Weight Watchers*	1 Pot/85g	99	2.4	117	4.4	18.4	2.8	0.0
Chocolate Fudge Brownie, Tesco*	1 Pot/125g	374	16.6	299	4.6	40.2	13.3	1.3
Chocolate Honeycomb Crisp, COU, M&S*	1 Serving/71g	110	2.1	155	4.6	27.6	2.9	1.0
Chocolate Mousse Cake, Weight Watchers*	1 Dessert/75g	148	2.2	198	5.9	37.1	2.9	1.0
Chocolate Muffin, COU, M&S*	1 Pot/110g	154	2.8	140	6.1	26.1	2.5	1.5
Chocolate Muffin, Tesco*	1 Serving/104g	354	21.2	340	3.5	35.5	20.4	2.1
Chocolate Profiterole, Weight Watchers*	1 Dessert/88g	186	5.4	211	4.8	34.1	6.1	3.7
Creme Caramel, Sainsbury's*	1 Pot/100g	116	1.6	116	2.6	22.9	1.6	0.0
Double Chocolate Brownie, Weight Watchers*	1 Pot/86g	167	3.3	194	5.1	33.7	3.8	2.4
Flake, Milk Chocolate, Cadbury*	1 Pot/90g	216	11.3	240	4.4	26.6	12.6	0.0
Fruit & Nut, Cadbury*	1 Pot/100g	285	12.5	285	6.4	36.3	12.5	0.0
Fudge, Cadbury*	1 Pot/90g	216	11.2	240	4.1	28.5	12.4	0.0
Galaxy, Mars*	1 Pot/75g	166	9.2	221	4.9	22.7	12.3	0.0
Hot Chocolate & Raspberry Truffle Bakes, M&S*	1 Truffle/92g	363	15.5	395	3.2	30.9	16.9	2.0
Key Lime Pie	1 Serving/125g	431	25.0	344	4.1	37.9	20.0	1.4
Lemon Meringue, Weight Watchers*	1 Pot/85g	161	0.4	189	2.4	43.1	0.5	0.6
Lemon Mousse Cake, Weight Watchers*	1 Serving/90g	130	2.4	144	3.2	26.7	2.7	0.5
Mandarin, COU, M&S*	1 Serving/150g	195	5.7	130	1.0	22.0	3.8	0.1
Millionaire's Shortbread, M&S*	1 Dessert/120g	425	25.7	355	2.6	38.3	21.5	1.4
Mississippi Mud Pie	1 Serving/125g	480	32.0	384	5.3	33.1	25.6	1.8
Pots Of Joy, Dairy Milk, Cadbury*	1 Pot/70g	158	8.2	225	4.2	25.6	11.7	0.1
Raspberry, Frappe, Skinny, COU, M&S*	1 Pot/95g	109	1.3	115	3.1	22.0	1.4	0.5
Raspberry Royale, Finest, Tesco*	½ Pack/170g	314	15.8	185	1.7	22.8	9.3	1.4
Rice, Vanilla, Creamed, Weight Watchers*	1 Pot/130g	112	0.6	86	3.2	16.9	0.5	0.4
Rich Chocolate, Weight Watchers*	1 Pot/70g	62	1.7	89	3.5	13.4	2.4	1.4
Rocky Road, Sainsbury's*	1 Pot/110g	328	21.6	298	3.6	26.8	19.6	2.1
Rolo, Nestle*	1 Pot/70g	170	8.3	243	3.3	30.8	11.9	0.5

	Measure INFO/WEIGHT	per Measure		Nutrition Values per 100g / 100ml				
		KCAL	FAT	KCAL	PROT	CARB	FAT	FIBRE
DESSERT								
Strawberry & Rhubarb, COU, M&S*	1 Pot/110g	104	0.8	95	1.5	20.1	0.7	0.9
Strawberry Meringue, Iced, Luxury, Weight Watchers*	1 Pot/100ml	86	0.7	162	2.4	34.2	1.4	1.0
Strawberry Mousse Cake, Weight Watchers*	1 Serving/90g	124	2.4	138	3.0	25.5	2.7	0.5
Tart, Millionaire, Tesco*	1 Pot/105g	420	26.3	405	3.5	38.7	25.4	1.6
Tiramisu	1 Serving/150g	420	20.8	280	4.4	34.0	13.9	0.8
Toffee, with Biscuit Pieces, Iced, Weight Watchers*	1 Pot/57g	93	2.7	163	2.7	26.2	4.8	0.2
Toffee & Vanilla, Weight Watchers*	1 Pot/67g	107	0.5	159	3.1	34.8	0.8	3.9
Toffee Chocolate, Weight Watchers*	1 Pot/100g	197	4.5	197	4.3	34.9	4.5	2.2
Toffee Muffin, COU, M&S*	1 Serving/100g	180	2.2	180	3.7	35.8	2.2	0.3
Trifle, Chocolate, Cadbury*	1 Pot/90g	234	13.8	260	4.8	22.5	15.3	0.0
Trifle, Chocolate, Light, Cadbury*	1 Pot/93g	130	4.0	140	4.6	20.4	4.3	0.0
Triple Chocolate, Delice, Sainsbury's*	1 Serving/105g	399	27.4	380	3.8	32.4	26.1	0.7
Triple Chocolate Layered, BGTY, Sainsbury's*	1 Pot/105g	147	2.9	140	4.2	24.4	2.8	0.5
Vanilla, & Caramel, Little Desserts, Petits Filous, Yoplait*	1 Pot/50g	75	2.6	150	4.7	21.0	5.3	0.2
Vanilla, & Raspberry Swirl, Weight Watchers*	1 Serving/100ml	81	2.2	81	1.5	13.3	2.2	0.2
Vanilla, Iced, Madagascan, Love Life, Waitrose*	1/8 Tub/65g	75	1.0	115	4.1	21.2	1.6	4.1
Vanilla, Soya, Dairy Free, Organic, Provamel*	1 Pot/125g	105	2.2	84	3.2	13.4	1.8	0.5
White Buttons, Pots of Joy, Cadbury*	1 Pot/70g	158	6.6	225	4.8	30.4	9.4	0.0
White Chocolate, Delights, Shape, Danone*	1 Pot/110g	109	2.6	99	3.5	15.9	2.4	0.1
DESSERT SAUCE								
Chocolate, M&S*	1 Dtsp/11g	35	1.0	330	2.1	59.3	9.4	1.9
Raspberry, M&S*	1 Serving/20g	24	0.1	120	0.5	28.7	0.3	2.6
Toffee, Old English, Asda*	1 Serving/28g	99	1.7	355	2.3	73.0	6.0	0.0
DHAL								
Black Gram, Average	1oz/28g	21	1.0	74	4.2	7.0	3.4	1.7
Chick Pea	1oz/28g	42	1.7	149	7.4	17.7	6.1	3.8
Chickpea, Mazadar*	1 Tin/400g	360	11.2	90	4.5	11.6	2.8	4.5
Lentil, Patak's*	1 Can/283g	156	2.8	55	2.8	9.3	1.0	1.0
Lentil, Red, WTF Sainsbury's*	½ Pack/273g	254	4.1	93	5.5	14.4	1.5	1.4
Lentil, Red Masoor, Punjabi, Average	1oz/28g	39	1.3	139	7.2	19.2	4.6	2.0
Lentil, Red Masoor & Tomato with Butter, Average	1oz/28g	26	1.4	94	4.0	9.7	4.9	0.9
Lentil, Red Masoor & Vegetable, Average	1oz/28g	31	1.1	110	5.8	14.7	3.8	1.8
Lentil, Red Masoor with Vegetable Oil, Average	1oz/28g	48	2.2	172	7.6	19.2	7.9	1.8
Lentil, Red Masoorl & Mung Bean, Average	1oz/28g	32	1.9	114	4.8	9.9	6.7	1.6
Lentil, Tesco*	1 Serving/200g	248	13.2	124	5.1	10.6	6.6	2.5
Makhani, Curry Collection, Veetee*	1 Pack/300g	306	17.4	102	4.2	11.1	5.8	2.8
Mung Bean, Bengali	1oz/28g	20	0.9	73	4.2	7.4	3.3	1.7
Mung Beans, Dried, Boiled in Unsalted Water	1oz/28g	26	0.1	92	7.8	15.3	0.4	0.0
Mung Beans, Dried, Raw	1oz/28g	81	0.3	291	26.8	46.3	1.1	0.0
Split Peas, Yellow, Chana, Asda*	1 Serving/275g	300	19.2	109	2.6	9.0	7.0	1.8
Tarka, Asda*	½ Pack/150g	216	12.0	144	6.0	12.0	8.0	6.0
DHANSAK								
Chicken with Bagara Rice, Waitrose*	1 Pack/450g	549	8.1	122	8.2	18.2	1.8	1.2
Vegetable, Sainsbury's*	1 Serving/200g	148	5.6	74	3.1	8.9	2.8	2.8
DILL								
Dried, Average	*1 Tsp/1g*	*3*	*0.0*	*253*	*19.9*	*42.2*	*4.4*	*13.6*
Fresh, Average	*1 Tbsp/3g*	*1*	*0.0*	*25*	*3.7*	*0.9*	*0.8*	*2.5*
DIM SUM								
Dumplings, Chicken, Spicy, Zao, Taiko Foods*	1 Dumpling/18g	31	0.4	166	14.1	21.4	2.1	1.5
From Restaurant, Average	1 Piece/12g	50	2.4	433	28.9	31.3	20.4	0.0
Steamed, Prawn, M&S*	6 Dim Sum/120g	222	3.2	185	1.1	39.0	2.7	1.5
DIME								
Terry's*	1oz/28g	154	9.5	550	4.6	68.5	33.8	0.6

DIP

	Measure INFO/WEIGHT	per Measure KCAL	FAT	Nutrition Values per 100g / 100ml KCAL	PROT	CARB	FAT	FIBRE
Aubergine, Fresh, Waitrose*	1 Serving/85g	159	12.8	187	2.5	10.5	15.0	1.7
Bean & Cheese, Asda*	1 Serving/50g	78	4.5	157	7.0	12.0	9.0	1.7
Beetroot & Sesame, Sainsbury's*	¼ Pot/45g	65	3.7	145	4.2	11.8	8.3	3.1
Blue Cheese, Fresh, Sainsbury's*	1/5 Pot/34g	115	11.7	337	3.6	3.1	34.5	0.1
Cheese, Nacho, Average	1 Serving/50g	175	17.2	350	6.3	3.4	34.4	0.9
Cheese, Nacho, Doritos, Walkers*	1 Serving/40g	92	8.1	231	3.4	8.5	20.2	0.6
Cheese, Nacho, From Tex-Mex Multipack, Tesco*	1 Tub/125g	619	62.0	495	5.9	5.8	49.6	0.0
Cheese, Nacho, Sainsbury's*	1 Serving/50g	244	25.1	487	4.8	3.9	50.2	0.0
Cheese & Chive, 50% Less Fat, Asda*	1 Pot/125g	261	21.5	209	4.5	9.0	17.2	0.0
Cheese & Chive, Asda*	1 Serving/43g	190	19.6	447	4.9	3.4	46.0	0.0
Cheese & Chive, Mature Cheddar, Fresh, Waitrose*	½ Pot/85g	393	40.5	462	5.8	2.4	47.7	1.7
Cheese & Chive, Tesco*	¼ Pack/50g	268	27.6	535	4.3	4.3	55.1	0.1
Chilli Cheese, Asda*	1 Serving/50g	131	11.0	262	8.0	8.0	22.0	1.1
Chillimole, Tesco*	1 Serving/50g	142	11.9	285	4.2	13.0	23.8	3.9
Cool Flavour, Tortilla Chips, Big, Morrisons*	½ Pack/100g	453	22.0	453	6.4	57.4	22.0	8.1
Frijolemole, Cannellini Bean & Chick Pea, Waitrose*	¼ Pot/50g	104	7.6	208	4.3	12.2	15.2	2.6
Garlic & Herb	1 Serving/100g	584	62.4	584	1.4	4.1	62.4	0.2
Guacamole, Reduced Fat, BGTY, Sainsbury's*	¼ Pot/43g	62	5.7	146	1.3	2.9	13.5	4.0
Guacamole, Supreme, Waitrose*	½ Pot/85g	105	10.3	124	1.6	2.1	12.1	4.3
Guacamole Style, Topping, Discovery*	1 Serving/37g	29	2.1	79	1.2	6.0	5.6	1.2
Hot Salsa, Doritos, Walkers*	1 Jar/300g	99	0.3	33	1.1	6.4	0.1	0.9
Hummus, Black Olive, Wild Garden*	2 Tbsp/30g	35	2.0	117	6.7	13.3	6.7	3.3
Hummus, Red Pepper, Wild Garden*	2 Tbsp/30g	35	2.0	117	6.7	13.3	6.7	3.3
Hummus, Roasted Garlic, Wild Garden*	2 Tbsp/30g	35	2.0	117	6.7	13.3	6.7	3.3
Hummus, Traditional, Wild Garden*	2 Tbsp/30g	35	2.0	117	6.7	13.3	6.7	4.3
Moroccan, Spicy, BGTY, Sainsbury's*	½ Pot/85g	56	1.7	66	2.1	10.0	2.0	1.7
Onion & Garlic, Average	1 Tbsp/15g	62	6.4	410	1.7	4.8	42.7	0.4
Onion & Garlic, Classic, Tesco*	1 Serving/30g	133	13.9	442	1.7	4.6	46.3	0.2
Pea, Yogurt & Mint, Sainsbury's*	¼ Pack/50g	119	10.8	238	3.4	7.5	21.6	2.1
Pecorino, Basil & Pine Nut, Fresh, Waitrose*	½ Pot/85g	338	33.7	398	5.1	5.1	39.7	0.0
Pepper, Red, Nando's*	1 Serving/260g	490	7.2	188	5.2	35.2	2.8	1.6
Pepper, Red, Sainsbury's*	1 Pot/100g	103	4.0	103	2.3	14.6	4.0	0.0
Pepper, Smoky Red, Gazpacho, Graze*	1 Punnet/23g	54	1.3	242	5.7	40.1	5.9	3.7
Raita, Indian, Asda*	1 Pot/70g	120	11.5	172	2.6	3.6	16.4	0.5
Salmon & Dill, Smoked, Fresh, Waitrose*	½ Pot/85g	373	38.0	439	5.1	4.1	44.7	0.1
Salsa, Chunky, Fresh, Sainsbury's*	1 Serving/100g	51	1.7	51	1.1	7.8	1.7	1.2
Salsa, Chunky Tomato, Tesco*	1 Pot/170g	68	2.2	40	1.1	5.9	1.3	1.1
Salsa, Mild, Asda*	1 Portion/100g	47	0.3	47	1.4	8.7	0.3	1.8
Salsa, Mild, Doritos, Walkers*	1 Tbsp/30g	9	0.1	30	0.8	6.0	0.3	1.5
Sour Cream, Tesco*	1 Serving/38g	111	11.2	297	3.4	3.9	29.8	0.2
Sour Cream & Chive, Average	1 Tbsp/15g	48	4.8	317	3.2	4.0	32.0	0.3
Sour Cream & Chive, BGTY, Sainsbury's*	1 Serving/170g	253	17.5	149	4.2	9.9	10.3	0.1
Sour Cream & Chive, Classic, Tesco*	1 Serving/25g	81	8.4	323	1.7	3.2	33.7	0.2
Sour Cream & Chive, Doritos, Walkers*	1 Tbsp/20g	52	4.9	258	1.9	6.9	24.7	1.9
Sour Cream & Chive, Fresh, Tesco*	½ Pot/75g	305	31.8	407	2.1	4.1	42.4	0.0
Sour Cream & Chive, Half Fat, Waitrose*	½ Pot/85g	133	9.9	157	5.5	7.6	11.6	0.1
Sour Cream & Chive, Morrisons*	1 Serving/100g	317	32.6	317	2.6	3.3	32.6	0.0
Sour Cream & Chive, Sainsbury's*	1 Serving/50g	141	13.8	282	3.1	5.4	27.5	0.1
Sour Cream & Chives, Mexican Style, Morrisons*	¼ Pack/25g	68	7.0	274	2.2	3.4	27.9	0.4
Sweet Chilli, Chinese Snack Selection, Morrisons*	½ Pot/20g	64	0.0	320	0.1	79.4	0.2	0.6
Sweet Chilli, Oriental Selection, Waitrose*	½ Pot/35g	88	0.3	250	1.3	59.4	0.8	0.4
Sweet Chilli, Thai, Primula*	1 Serving/57g	126	0.1	221	0.6	54.4	0.1	0.2
Tomato Ketchup, Asda*	1 Pack/25g	18	0.0	71	1.6	16.0	0.1	1.0

	Measure INFO/WEIGHT	per Measure		Nutrition Values per 100g / 100ml				
		KCAL	FAT	KCAL	PROT	CARB	FAT	FIBRE
DISCOS								
Beef, KP Snacks*	1 Pack/28g	145	8.2	518	5.1	58.7	29.3	2.4
Cheese & Onion, KP Snacks*	1 Pack/28g	146	8.2	520	5.1	59.1	29.3	2.5
Salt & Vinegar, KP Snacks*	1 Bag/28g	145	8.3	517	4.7	58.3	29.5	2.3
DOLLY MIXTURES								
M & S*	1 Pack/115g	431	1.6	375	1.8	89.2	1.4	0.0
Sainsbury's*	1 Serving/10g	40	0.2	401	1.4	94.4	1.9	0.1
Smart Price, Asda*	1 Sweet/3g	11	0.0	380	0.5	91.0	1.6	0.0
Tesco*	1 Pack/100g	376	1.5	376	1.6	88.9	1.5	0.0
DOPIAZA								
Chicken, M&S*	1 Pack/350g	402	21.4	115	11.5	3.7	6.1	2.5
Chicken, Sainsbury's*	½ Pack/200g	272	15.8	136	13.2	3.1	7.9	0.8
Chicken, Tesco*	1 Pack/350g	448	24.8	128	10.8	5.3	7.1	0.6
Chicken, with Pilau Rice, Sharwood's*	1 Pack/375g	472	17.2	126	5.3	15.8	4.6	0.8
Mushroom, Retail	1oz/28g	19	1.6	69	1.3	3.7	5.7	1.1
Mushroom, Waitrose*	½ Pack/150g	81	4.6	54	2.2	4.3	3.1	2.3
DORADA								
Whole	1 Serving/100g	92	5.9	92	18.0	1.0	5.9	0.0
DORITOS								
Chargrilled BBQ, Walkers*	1 Bag/35g	170	8.8	485	5.5	59.0	25.0	3.5
Cheesy 3d's, Doritos, Walkers*	1 Pack/20g	89	3.2	445	7.0	68.0	16.0	3.0
Chilli Heatwave, Walkers*	1 Bag/30g	150	7.8	500	7.0	60.0	26.0	3.0
Cool, Ranch Chips, Walkers*	1 Pack/50g	250	13.0	504	8.1	64.5	26.2	4.0
Cool Original, Walkers*	1 Bag/40g	200	10.8	500	7.5	58.0	27.0	3.0
Cool Spice 3ds, Walkers*	1 Bag/24g	108	4.3	450	8.0	64.0	18.0	4.4
Dippas, Hint of Chilli, Dipping Chips, Walkers*	1 Bag/35g	173	8.8	495	7.0	61.0	25.0	3.5
Dippas, Hint of Garlic, Dipping Chips, Walkers*	1 Serving/35g	175	8.8	500	7.0	61.0	25.0	3.5
Dippas, Hint of Lime, Walkers*	1 Bag/35g	173	8.8	495	7.0	60.0	25.0	3.5
Dippas, Lightly Salted, Dipping Chips, Walkers*	1 Serving/35g	178	9.4	510	6.5	60.0	27.0	3.0
Latinos, Chargrilled BBQ, Walkers*	1 Serving/35g	170	8.8	485	5.5	59.0	25.0	3.5
Lighly Salted, Corn Chips, Doritos*	1 Bag/30g	149	7.1	497	6.9	62.9	23.6	3.3
Mexican Hot, Walkers*	1 Bag/40g	202	10.8	505	8.0	57.0	27.0	3.5
Tangy Cheese, Walkers*	1 Bag/40g	200	10.8	500	7.0	57.0	27.0	3.0
DOUBLE DECKER								
Cadbury*	1 Bar/55g	251	10.3	460	4.4	68.4	18.9	0.6
Snack Size, Cadbury*	1 Bar/36g	165	7.4	465	4.8	64.5	20.9	0.0
DOUGH BALLS								
Cheese & Garlic, Occasions, Sainsbury's*	1 Ball/12g	41	2.2	341	10.3	33.4	18.5	2.1
Garlic, GFY, Asda*	1 Ball/8g	21	0.2	250	9.0	49.0	2.0	2.0
Garlic, Tesco*	1 Serving/10g	40	2.3	400	7.0	40.0	23.0	1.0
Garlic, Waitrose*	1 Ball/11g	38	1.8	347	8.5	41.4	16.4	3.3
Garlic & Herb, Asda*	4 Balls/48g	173	8.5	361	9.2	40.9	17.8	3.6
Garlic & Herb, Occasions, Sainsbury's*	1 Ball/12g	41	2.1	343	8.4	38.7	17.2	2.2
Sainsbury's*	1 Ball/12g	41	2.1	343	8.4	38.7	17.2	2.2
Supermarket, Pizza Express*	8 Balls/100g	363	1.7	363	14.3	72.9	1.7	3.3
with Garlic & Herb Butter, Aldi*	1 Ball/12g	45	2.2	365	7.7	46.7	18.2	1.8
DOUGHNUTS								
Apple & Custard, Finger, Sainsbury's*	1 Serving/65g	136	6.0	210	4.4	27.5	9.2	1.9
Chocolate, Somerfield*	1 Doughnut/57g	203	9.5	356	7.8	43.8	16.6	1.7
Cream & Jam, Assorted Box, Sainsbury's*	1 Doughnut/71g	229	12.7	322	6.2	34.2	17.9	2.2
Cream & Jam, Tesco*	1 Doughnut/90g	288	14.1	320	5.4	39.4	15.7	2.0
Custard, & Bramley Apple, Sainsbury's*	1 Doughnut/91g	256	12.6	282	4.5	34.6	13.9	1.0
Custard, Sainsbury's*	1 Doughnut/70g	172	7.5	246	5.1	32.3	10.7	2.3
Custard, Tesco*	1 Doughnut/91g	266	14.4	292	4.1	33.4	15.8	1.1

	Measure INFO/WEIGHT	per Measure		Nutrition Values per 100g / 100ml				
		KCAL	FAT	KCAL	PROT	CARB	FAT	FIBRE

DOUGHNUTS

Custard Filled, Average	1 Doughnut/75g	268	14.2	358	6.2	43.3	19.0	0.0
Jam, American Style, Sainsbury's*	1 Doughnut/65g	220	20.6	339	4.9	49.6	31.8	3.5
Jam, Fresh Cream, Sweet Fresh, Tesco*	1 Doughnut/74g	248	12.1	335	5.5	40.7	16.4	1.9
Jam, M&S*	1 Doughnut/49g	141	2.0	287	5.0	57.6	4.0	1.3
Jam, Mini, Frozen, Party, Tesco*	2 Doughnuts/25g	101	5.5	405	5.3	45.0	22.1	2.0
Jam & Cream, Strawberry, Sainsbury's*	1 Doughnut/80g	299	18.5	374	5.3	36.2	23.2	1.3
Jam Filled, Average	1 Doughnut/75g	252	10.9	336	5.7	48.8	14.5	0.0
Mini, Chocolate Topped, CBY, Asda*	1 Serving/100g	393	19.5	393	5.2	49.1	19.5	2.0
Mini, Sainsbury's*	1 Doughnut/14g	53	2.7	379	5.2	47.9	18.9	2.1
Plain, Ring, Average	1 Doughnut/60g	238	13.0	397	6.1	47.2	21.7	0.0
Raspberry Jam, Sainsbury's*	1 Doughnut/70g	241	10.4	344	5.3	47.4	14.8	2.5
Ring, Co-Op*	1 Doughnut/106g	392	21.2	370	4.0	44.0	20.0	1.0
Ring, Iced, Average	1 Doughnut/70g	268	12.2	383	4.8	55.1	17.5	0.0
Ring, Waitrose*	1 Doughnut/107g	396	21.3	370	4.2	43.5	19.9	0.7
Toffee, Tesco*	1 Doughnut/75g	235	8.7	313	8.0	44.2	11.6	1.6
Yum Yums, Glazed, Sweet, Waitrose*	1 Doughnut/45g	172	10.0	382	4.0	41.6	22.2	2.0
Yum Yums, M&S*	1 Doughnut/37g	155	8.9	420	4.9	45.7	23.9	1.6
Yum Yums, Tesco*	1 Doughnut/50g	220	13.2	440	4.7	43.7	26.4	3.1

DOVER SOLE

Fillet, Raw, Average	*1oz/28g*	*25*	*0.5*	*89*	*18.1*	*0.0*	*1.8*	*0.0*

DR PEPPER*

Coca-Cola*	1 Bottle/500ml	210	0.0	42	0.0	10.9	0.0	0.0
Z, Coca-Cola*	1 Glass/250ml	10	0.0	4	0.0	0.0	0.0	0.0
Zero, Coca-Cola*	1 Can/330ml	2	0.0	0	0.0	0.0	0.0	0.0

DRAGON FRUIT

Raw, Edible Portion, Average	1 Serving/100g	41	0.5	41	0.7	9.6	0.5	3.6

DRAMBUIE

39% Volume	*1 Pub Shot/35ml*	*95*	*0.0*	*272*	*0.0*	*23.0*	*0.0*	*0.0*

DREAM TOPPING

Dry, Bird's*	1oz/28g	193	16.4	690	6.7	32.5	58.5	0.5
Made Up, Skimmed Milk, Bird's*	1oz/28g	21	1.5	75	2.0	4.8	5.3	0.0
Sugar Free, Dry, Bird's*	1oz/28g	195	16.9	695	7.3	30.5	60.5	0.5
White Chocolate, Cadbury*	1 Piece/8g	44	2.7	555	4.5	59.7	33.3	0.0

DRESSING

Balsamic, Bliss, Ainsley Harriott*	1 Tbsp/15g	41	3.2	272	0.8	19.3	21.1	0.0
Balsamic, Fresh Olive Co*	1 Tbsp/15g	42	0.1	282	1.5	67.8	0.5	0.6
Balsamic, LC, Tesco*	1 Tbsp/14g	12	0.2	85	0.3	16.7	1.5	0.2
Balsamic, M&S*	1 Tbsp/15g	74	7.2	490	0.3	9.7	48.0	0.5
Balsamic, New, Sainsbury's*	1 Tbsp/15g	58	5.2	389	0.6	18.3	34.8	0.8
Balsamic, Raspberry, The English Provender Co.*	1 Serving/50g	34	0.0	67	0.4	15.7	0.1	0.6
Balsamic, Schwartz*	1 Tbsp/15ml	12	0.3	77	0.5	14.2	2.0	0.0
Balsamic, Sweet, Finest, Tesco*	1 Serving/10ml	16	0.0	155	0.4	36.9	0.1	0.4
Balsamic, Vinaigrette, Newman's Own*	1 Tbsp/15g	49	5.0	326	0.1	6.4	33.3	0.5
Balsamic, Weight Watchers*	1 Serving/15ml	12	0.3	81	0.1	16.0	1.8	0.5
Balsamic, with Olive Oil, Pizza Express*	1 Serving/10g	42	4.1	421	0.3	10.3	41.2	0.0
Balsamic Vinegar, Light, Kraft*	1 Serving/15ml	15	0.9	100	0.3	9.6	6.3	0.5
Balsamic Vinegar, Morrisons*	1 Serving/15ml	17	0.2	111	0.1	22.9	1.6	0.1
Balsamic Vinegar, Olives & Herb, COU, M&S*	1 Serving/30g	22	0.6	75	0.5	14.3	2.0	0.5
Basil & Pesto, COU, M&S*	1 Serving/50ml	30	1.1	60	0.6	8.3	2.2	0.8
Beetroot, with Balsamic Honey & Orange, Finest, Tesco*	1 Pot/225g	144	3.8	64	1.1	11.1	1.7	2.4
Blue Cheese, 60% Less Fat, BGTY, Sainsbury's*	1 Tbsp/15ml	26	2.3	172	1.9	7.3	15.1	0.2
Blue Cheese, Fresh, Sainsbury's*	1 Dtsp/10ml	42	4.6	423	2.3	0.5	45.7	0.1
Blue Cheese, Hellmann's*	1 Tbsp/15g	69	7.1	459	0.7	6.3	47.2	1.1

DRESSING

INFO/WEIGHT	per Measure KCAL	per Measure FAT	Nutrition Values per 100g / 100ml KCAL	PROT	CARB	FAT	FIBRE
Blue Cheese, Sainsbury's*	1 Serving/20g	64	6.0	321	2.3	10.6	29.9	0.4
Blue Cheese, Salad, Waitrose*	1 Serving/50g	265	25.2	530	2.1	17.3	50.3	4.1
Blue Cheese, True, Briannas*	2 Tbsp/30ml	120	11.0	400	3.3	16.7	36.7	0.0
Caesar, 95% Fat Free, Tesco*	1 Tsp/6g	5	0.2	88	4.1	8.9	3.7	0.3
Caesar, Asiago, Briannas*	1 Tbsp/15ml	70	7.5	467	3.3	3.3	50.0	0.0
Caesar, Chilled, Reduced Fat, Tesco*	1 Tsp/5ml	13	1.2	252	6.5	3.1	23.7	0.1
Caesar, Classic, Sainsbury's*	1 Tsp/5ml	22	2.3	442	2.7	4.6	45.9	0.5
Caesar, Creamy, Get Dressed, Kraft*	1 Serving/67g	68	2.3	102	2.1	15.0	3.5	0.1
Caesar, Fat Free, Average	1 Tsp/5g	4	0.2	84	4.6	11.0	4.1	0.2
Caesar, Finest, Tesco*	1 Tbsp/15ml	72	7.6	477	1.9	2.8	50.9	0.2
Caesar, Fresh, Asda*	1 Dtsp/10ml	45	4.8	454	2.4	3.2	48.0	0.0
Caesar, Fresh, M&S*	1 Tsp/6g	32	3.4	525	2.0	1.8	56.4	0.2
Caesar, Fresh, Sainsbury's*	1 Tbsp/15ml	72	7.5	477	3.7	3.7	49.7	1.9
Caesar, Hellmann's*	1 Tsp/6g	30	3.1	499	2.5	4.5	51.7	0.3
Caesar, LC, Tesco*	1 Serving/15g	9	0.2	60	1.5	9.5	1.5	0.5
Caesar, Less Than 3% Fat, BGTY, Sainsbury's*	1 Serving/20g	10	0.4	48	0.8	7.0	1.9	0.3
Caesar, Light, Kraft*	1 Serving/15g	22	1.6	148	0.5	11.5	11.0	0.2
Caesar, Low Fat, Average	1 Tsp/5g	4	0.1	77	2.3	11.1	2.6	0.4
Caesar, Loyd Grossman*	1 Dtsp/10g	34	3.4	342	2.1	7.0	33.9	0.0
Caesar, Luxury, Hellmann's*	1 Tsp/4g	20	2.1	498	2.5	4.4	51.7	0.3
Caesar, Original, Cardini's*	1 Serving/10g	56	6.0	555	2.3	1.5	60.0	0.2
Caesar, Tesco*	1 Tbsp/15ml	65	6.8	435	0.9	5.4	45.1	0.3
Caesar, Waitrose*	1 Serving/15ml	72	7.6	479	4.5	0.9	50.8	0.2
Caesar Style, GFY, Asda*	1 Sachet/44ml	34	1.0	77	5.0	9.0	2.3	0.0
Citrus Salad, BGTY, Sainsbury's*	1 Tbsp/15ml	14	0.5	90	0.3	14.4	3.1	0.3
Cream Cheese & Chive, Creamy Ranch, Kraft*	1 Serving/15ml	31	2.6	205	1.2	11.0	17.0	0.0
French, BGTY, Organic, Sainsbury's*	1 Tbsp/15ml	11	0.6	71	0.2	8.3	4.1	0.5
French, BGTY, Sainsbury's*	1 Tbsp/15ml	12	0.7	79	1.1	8.8	4.4	0.5
French, Chilled, Tesco*	1 Tbsp/15ml	63	5.9	421	1.1	15.1	39.6	0.0
French, Cider Vinegar & Mustard, Tesco*	1 Tbsp/15ml	45	4.2	300	0.7	9.9	28.1	0.3
French, Classic, Fat Free, Kraft*	1 Tsp/5ml	2	0.0	39	0.1	8.7	0.0	0.5
French, Classic, Sainsbury's*	1 Tbsp/15ml	71	7.4	473	1.0	5.7	49.6	0.5
French, Classics, M&S*	1 Tbsp/15ml	77	8.0	516	0.6	8.2	53.1	0.2
French, COU, M&S*	1/3 Bottle/105g	74	2.7	70	0.7	11.5	2.6	0.7
French, Essential, Waitrose*	1 Serving/15ml	34	2.3	228	0.1	22.9	15.1	0.5
French, Finest, Tesco*	1 Tbsp/15g	56	5.8	370	0.4	5.1	38.7	1.0
French, Fresh, Classic, M&S*	1 Serving/10ml	52	5.3	515	0.6	8.2	53.1	0.2
French, Fresh, Florette*	1 Bottle/175ml	763	73.1	436	0.8	14.1	41.8	0.0
French, Fresh, Morrisons*	1 Tbsp/15ml	75	7.3	499	1.5	13.6	48.7	0.0
French, Fresh, Organic, Sainsbury's*	1 Tbsp/15ml	45	4.6	301	0.4	5.5	31.0	0.4
French, Fresh, Sainsbury's*	1 Tbsp/15ml	64	6.7	429	0.6	6.6	44.6	0.6
French, GFY, Asda*	1 Tbsp/15g	8	0.3	50	0.7	7.0	2.1	0.1
French, Good Intentions, Somerfield*	1 Serving/15ml	12	0.5	83	0.7	12.1	3.5	0.3
French, LC, Tesco*	1 Tbsp/16g	8	0.3	50	0.8	7.6	1.6	1.1
French, Less Than 3% Fat, M&S*	1 Tbsp/15ml	10	0.4	68	0.7	11.5	2.6	0.7
French, Light, Heinz*	1 Sachet/12g	13	0.6	111	0.7	15.4	5.4	0.0
French, Luxury, Hellmann's*	1 Tbsp/15g	45	3.9	297	0.4	14.9	25.9	0.3
French, Organic, M&S*	1 Tbsp/15g	98	10.4	655	0.2	7.5	69.4	0.3
French, Organic, Tesco*	1 Tsp/5ml	23	2.2	451	0.6	11.0	44.9	0.2
French, Reduced Fat, M&S*	1 Tbsp/15g	10	0.4	70	0.7	11.5	2.8	0.7
French, Sainsbury's*	1 Tbsp/15ml	33	2.9	219	0.6	9.8	19.1	0.5
French, Salad, M&S*	1 Serving/25ml	156	16.8	625	0.5	3.8	67.3	0.1
French, Style Calorie-Wise Salad, Kraft*	1 Tbsp/15ml	24	1.6	160	0.0	18.7	10.7	0.0

D

DRESSING

INFO/WEIGHT	Measure	per Measure KCAL	FAT	Nutrition Values per 100g / 100ml KCAL	PROT	CARB	FAT	FIBRE
French, Tesco*	1 Serving/25ml	110	11.2	441	0.7	7.2	44.9	0.2
French, Vinaigrette, TTD, Sainsbury's*	1 Tbsp/15ml	69	6.7	460	0.6	13.9	44.5	0.5
Garlic & Herb, Light, 5% Fat, Get Dressed, Kraft*	1 Serving/25ml	29	1.3	116	1.3	15.5	5.1	0.2
Garlic & Herb, PB, Waitrose*	1 Serving/50ml	68	0.7	135	0.6	29.9	1.4	0.8
Garlic & Herb, Reduced Calorie, Hellmann's*	1 Tbsp/15ml	35	2.9	232	0.6	12.8	19.3	0.4
Garlic & Herb, Tesco*	1 Tbsp/15g	32	3.0	210	0.9	5.8	20.2	0.8
Honey, Orange & Mustard, BGTY, Sainsbury's*	1 Tbsp/15ml	16	0.4	105	1.8	18.6	2.5	1.8
Honey & Mustard, BGTY, Sainsbury's*	1 Tbsp/20g	14	0.1	71	0.4	16.1	0.5	0.2
Honey & Mustard, Finest, Tesco*	1 Serving/25ml	72	5.6	288	1.7	19.6	22.5	0.7
Honey & Mustard, Fresh, M&S*	1 Serving/10ml	43	4.2	430	1.7	9.7	42.4	0.5
Honey & Mustard, GFY, Asda*	1 Tbsp/15g	13	0.5	89	1.5	13.0	3.4	0.8
Honey & Mustard, Hellmann's*	1 Serving/15ml	27	0.2	182	0.7	13.7	1.6	0.3
Honey & Mustard, LC, Tesco*	1 Tbsp/14g	9	0.2	65	1.3	11.6	1.1	0.6
Honey & Mustard, M&S*	1 Tbsp/15ml	64	6.4	427	1.7	9.7	42.4	0.6
Honey & Mustard, Sainsbury's*	1 Serving/10ml	37	3.3	366	1.0	15.4	33.0	0.1
Honey & Mustard, Tesco*	1 Serving/10ml	38	3.6	378	0.8	13.1	35.8	0.6
Honey & Mustard, The English Provender Co.*	1 Tbsp/15ml	17	0.2	111	2.5	21.8	1.5	1.0
Honey Mustard, Dijon, Briannas*	1 Tbsp/15ml	65	6.0	433	0.0	20.0	40.0	0.0
Italian, Classic, Get Dressed, Kraft*	1 Serving/25ml	30	2.6	120	0.1	5.6	10.3	0.5
Italian, Light, Low Fat, Newman's Own*	1 Serving/15g	9	0.4	58	0.1	6.7	2.8	0.5
Italian, Low Fat, Heinz*	1 Pot/30ml	26	1.9	86	0.9	6.3	6.3	2.7
Italian, M&S*	1 Tbsp/15ml	62	6.2	415	0.9	8.9	41.5	1.0
Italian Salad, Hellmann's*	1 Serving/50g	103	8.4	206	0.7	12.8	16.7	0.0
Lemon, Feta & Oregano, M&S*	1 Tbsp/15ml	24	2.0	160	1.3	8.2	13.4	0.6
Lemon & Cracked Black Pepper, GFY, Asda*	1 Tbsp/15g	9	0.0	57	0.2	14.0	0.0	0.3
Lime & Coriander, Sainsbury's*	1 Tbsp/15ml	61	6.1	409	0.4	10.0	40.8	0.5
Lime & Coriander, Thai, The English Provender Co.*	1 Serving/25g	26	0.2	104	1.6	22.3	0.9	1.1
Lime & Coriander, The English Provender Co.*	1 Serving/50g	28	0.2	57	0.3	13.3	0.3	0.0
Mint & Tomato, Mary Berry*	1 Serving/100g	399	37.1	399	0.8	14.8	37.1	0.3
Mustard, Low Fat, Mild, Weight Watchers*	1 Tbsp/10g	6	0.4	63	2.0	5.7	3.6	0.4
Mustard & Dill, PB, Waitrose*	1 Tbsp/15ml	24	0.5	159	1.1	31.5	3.2	1.1
Oil & Lemon	1 Tbsp/15g	97	10.6	647	0.3	2.8	70.6	0.0
Olive Oil, Pizza Express*	1 Tbsp/15g	86	9.4	573	1.4	3.4	63.0	0.0
Olive Oil & Balsamic Vinegar, Sainsbury's*	1 Serving/25ml	104	10.4	415	0.9	9.4	41.8	0.2
Ranch, Creamy, 95% Fat Free, Kraft*	1 Tsp/6ml	7	0.3	111	1.4	14.5	5.0	0.3
Ranch, Texas, Frank Cooper*	1 Pot/28g	128	12.8	457	1.9	9.4	45.8	0.2
Ranch Style, Asda*	1 Serving/44ml	37	1.7	85	3.5	9.0	3.9	0.0
Red Pepper, & Chilli, Less Than 1%, BGTY, Sainsbury's*	1 Serving/20g	9	0.0	45	0.1	10.6	0.2	0.5
Red Pepper, BGTY, Sainsbury's*	1 Bottle/250g	108	0.8	43	0.2	9.8	0.3	0.2
Red Pepper, Fire Roasted, M&S*	1 Serving/30g	14	0.0	45	0.5	10.7	0.1	0.9
Red Pepper, M&S*	1 Tbsp/15ml	58	5.9	385	0.6	7.6	39.2	0.5
Rich Poppy Seed, Briannas*	1 Tbsp/15ml	65	6.5	433	0.0	20.0	43.3	0.0
Salad, Blue Cheese, Heinz*	1 Serving/15g	55	5.5	369	1.2	7.8	36.9	0.2
Salad, Caesar, Light, Fry Light*	1 Spray/0.2ml	1	0.1	321	0.4	9.2	30.7	0.1
Salad, Honey & Mustard, Light, Kraft*	1 Tbsp/15ml	19	0.7	126	1.2	19.0	4.6	1.1
Salad, Italian, Light, Kraft*	1 Tbsp/15ml	5	0.0	31	0.1	6.8	0.0	0.6
Salad, Italian, Newman's Own*	1 Tbsp/15g	82	9.0	545	0.2	1.0	59.8	0.0
Salad, Light, Heinz*	1 Serving/10g	24	2.0	244	1.8	13.5	19.9	0.0
Salad, Low Fat, Weight Watchers*	1 Tbsp/10g	10	0.4	106	1.5	15.4	4.3	0.0
Salad, Mary Berry*	1 Serving/15g	77	6.6	513	0.8	28.5	44.0	0.1
Salad, Oil Free, Caper & Hot Peppercorn, Righteous*	1 Tbsp/15ml	8	0.1	53	1.3	7.3	0.7	0.1
Salad, Pizza Express*	1 Serving/5g	29	3.2	573	1.4	3.4	63.0	0.0
Salad, Raspberry Balsamic, GFY, Asda*	1 Tbsp/15ml	6	0.1	40	0.7	9.3	0.7	1.3

	Measure INFO/WEIGHT	per Measure KCAL	FAT	Nutrition Values per 100g / 100ml KCAL	PROT	CARB	FAT	FIBRE
DRESSING								
Salad, Thousand Island, 95% Fat Free, Asda*	1 Tsp/6g	6	0.3	99	1.6	12.6	4.7	0.5
Salad, Vinaigrette Style, 95% Fat Free, Asda*	1 Tbsp/15ml	6	0.0	42	0.1	10.6	0.0	0.3
Sweet Balsamic & Smoked Garlic, BGTY, Sainsbury's*	1 Serving/20g	10	0.1	51	0.2	11.9	0.3	0.2
Sweet Chilli, COU, M&S*	1 Tbsp/15ml	9	0.1	60	0.5	14.5	0.5	0.4
Sweet Chilli & Mango, Love Life, Waitrose*	1 Serving/16ml	10	0.0	64	1.6	14.0	0.1	0.6
Thousand Island	1 Tsp/6g	19	1.8	323	1.1	12.5	30.2	0.4
Thousand Island, BGTY, Sainsbury's*	1 Serving/20g	19	1.4	95	0.4	7.3	7.2	0.5
Thousand Island, Eat Smart, Morrisons*	1 Tbsp/15ml	38	3.2	253	0.0	0.0	21.3	0.0
Thousand Island, Light, Kraft*	1 Tbsp/15ml	16	0.0	105	0.6	23.0	0.2	3.0
Thousand Island, Reduced Calorie	1 Tsp/6g	12	0.9	195	0.7	14.7	15.2	0.0
Tomato & Red Pepper, BGTY, Sainsbury's*	1 Serving/50ml	42	2.2	83	1.1	10.0	4.3	0.6
Vinegar & Oil Based, Fat Free, Average	1 Tsp/5g	2	0.0	37	0.4	7.9	0.2	0.4
Yoghurt, & Mint, PB, Waitrose*	1 Serving/100ml	130	2.6	130	4.6	22.1	2.6	0.7
Yoghurt, Mint Cucumber, M&S*	1 Tsp/5ml	6	0.4	115	1.0	8.7	8.0	0.0
DRIED FRUIT								
Banana, Bites, Kiddylicious, Babylicious*	1 Serving/15g	43	2.9	285	10.8	43.6	19.3	6.1
Honey Coated Banana Chips, Whitworths*	1 Serving/25g	132	7.8	526	1.0	59.9	31.4	1.7
Mango, Sweetened, Whitworths*	1 Pack/30g	80	0.4	260	0.3	61.3	1.3	0.5
Mixed, Value, Tesco*	1 Serving/25g	71	0.2	285	2.1	67.5	0.7	2.3
Pineapple, Sweetened, Whitworths*	1 Bag/35g	122	0.1	350	0.4	86.3	0.2	0.5
Prunes, Juicy, Whitworths*	1 Pack/500g	740	2.0	148	2.5	34.0	0.4	5.7
Trail Mix, Kick Start, Wholefoods, Asda*	1 Serving/50g	194	10.2	387	10.9	40.0	20.4	10.7
DRIED FRUIT & SEED MIX								
Sainsbury's*	1 Pack/50g	204	10.7	408	11.6	42.0	21.4	5.1
DRIED FRUIT MIX								
Agadoo, Pineapple, Jumbo & Green Raisins, Graze*	1 Pack/40g	110	0.4	275	2.1	69.0	0.9	0.0
Apple Strudel, Graze*	1 Pack/40g	99	0.3	247	2.2	58.7	0.7	5.9
Asda*	1 Serving/50g	152	0.2	305	2.0	74.0	0.5	0.6
Average	1 Tbsp/25g	67	0.1	268	2.3	68.1	0.4	2.2
Beach Bum, Graze*	1 Pack/33g	121	4.1	363	3.3	61.5	12.4	9.7
Berry, Love Life, Waitrose*	1 Serving/30g	89	0.3	296	1.9	70.0	0.9	3.0
Berry, Whole Foods, Tesco*	1 Serving/25g	66	0.2	265	3.3	60.0	0.7	7.5
Dates, Raisins & Apricots, Wholefoods, Tesco*	1 Serving/20g	52	0.1	260	3.1	59.0	0.4	4.0
Dragons Nest, Kids, Graze*	1 Punnet/33g	119	3.3	362	3.0	68.0	10.0	4.0
Exotic Mix, Sundora*	1 Pack/50g	138	1.4	276	2.3	60.6	2.7	3.8
Festival Fruits, Graze*	1 Punnet/32g	84	0.2	261	1.7	67.1	0.6	6.5
Fruit Tumble, Kids, Graze*	1 Punnet/37g	111	0.4	299	2.0	71.0	1.0	3.0
Garden of England, Graze*	1 Punnet/25g	70	0.2	280	1.0	71.2	0.7	5.6
Little Figgy Went to Market, Graze*	1 Punnet/37g	103	0.3	273	1.8	63.9	0.7	7.9
Luxury, Co-Op*	1 Serving/40g	114	0.2	285	2.0	68.0	0.6	4.0
Pear Tatin, Graze*	1 Punnet/35g	143	6.3	408	7.0	57.2	18.1	5.9
Scandinavian Forest, Graze*	1 Punnet/28g	75	0.2	271	1.7	69.0	0.6	6.9
Scrumptious Blueberry Swirl, Graze*	1 Punnet/40g	155	3.2	392	1.2	76.0	8.0	3.0
Sultanas, Currants, Raisins & Citrus Peel, Asda*	1 Serving/100g	283	0.5	283	2.6	67.0	0.5	1.7
Sultanas Raisins & Cranberries, Dunnes*	1 Serving/15g	47	0.1	315	2.0	80.2	0.9	4.7
Tesco*	1 Tbsp/25g	71	0.1	284	2.3	67.9	0.4	2.2
Top Banana, Graze*	1 Serving/40g	115	0.4	287	2.6	70.1	0.9	0.0
Tropical Sundae, Graze*	1 Punnet/29g	86	0.3	299	2.7	72.7	1.0	8.5
Tropical Treasure, Kids, Graze*	1 Punnet/36g	134	2.9	373	3.0	76.0	8.0	5.8
Vine Fruit, Wholesome, Waitrose*	1 Serving/30g	87	0.1	289	2.1	69.3	0.4	5.3
DRIFTER								
Nestle*	1 Finger/20g	99	4.2	482	4.0	69.6	20.5	1.2

	Measure INFO/WEIGHT	per Measure KCAL	FAT	Nutrition Values per 100g / 100ml KCAL	PROT	CARB	FAT	FIBRE
DRINK MIX								
Chocolate, Finest, Tesco*	1 Serving/200ml	242	12.9	121	4.9	10.7	6.4	0.8
Chocolate, Flavia*	1 Serving/18g	64	0.7	368	15.6	67.2	4.0	0.0
Milk Chocolate, Instant Break, Cadbury*	4 Tsp/28g	119	3.9	425	10.9	64.2	14.0	0.0
DRINKING CHOCOLATE								
Cadbury*	1 Tbsp/16g	64	0.4	402	4.4	89.3	2.4	0.0
Dry, M&S*	1 Serving/20g	73	0.9	365	8.4	66.0	4.4	13.0
Dry, Tesco*	3 Tsp/25g	92	1.4	368	6.4	72.6	5.8	4.2
Dry, Waitrose*	3 Tsp/12g	48	0.7	403	7.2	79.9	6.1	2.9
Fairtrade, Truly Irresistible, Co-Op*	1 Serving/20g	73	1.9	365	10.0	60.3	9.4	13.8
LC, Tesco*	1 Cup/11g	38	0.8	345	13.8	54.9	7.7	13.1
Made Up with Semi-Skimmed Milk, Average	1 Mug/227ml	129	4.3	57	3.5	7.0	1.9	0.2
Made Up with Skimmed Milk, Average	1 Mug/227ml	100	1.1	44	3.5	7.0	0.5	0.0
Made Up with Whole Milk, Average	1 Mug/227ml	173	9.5	76	3.4	6.8	4.2	0.2
Powder, Dry, Cocodirect*	1 Serving/18g	67	1.5	372	8.9	65.1	8.4	0.0
Powder, Made Up with Skimmed Milk	1 Mug/227ml	134	1.4	59	3.5	10.8	0.6	0.0
Powder, Made Up with Whole Milk	1 Mug/227ml	204	9.3	90	3.4	10.6	4.1	0.0
DRINKS								
Coca Cola, Diet, Abokado*	1 Serving/330ml	3	0.0	1	0.0	0.0	0.0	0.0
Orange Juice, Abokado*	1 Serving/250ml	78	0.3	31	1.1	8.5	0.1	1.7
Water, Life, Sparkling, Abokado*	1 Serving/500ml	0	0.0	0	0.0	0.0	0.0	0.0
Water, Life, Still, Abokado*	1 Serving/500ml	0	0.0	0	0.0	0.0	0.0	0.0
DRIPPING								
Beef	*1oz/28g*	*249*	*27.7*	*891*	*0.0*	*0.0*	*99.0*	*0.0*
DUCK								
Breast, Meat Only, Cooked, Average	*1oz/28g*	*48*	*2.0*	*172*	*25.3*	*1.8*	*7.0*	*0.0*
Breast, Meat Only, Raw, Average	*1 Serving/160g*	*206*	*6.8*	*128*	*22.6*	*0.0*	*4.2*	*0.2*
Fillets, Gressingham, Mini, TTD, Sainsbury's*	½ Pack/90g	127	2.4	141	29.0	0.0	2.7	0.6
Leg, Meat & Skin, Average	*1oz/28g*	*80*	*5.6*	*286*	*17.2*	*9.5*	*20.0*	*0.4*
Raw, Meat, Fat & Skin	*1oz/28g*	*109*	*10.4*	*388*	*13.1*	*0.0*	*37.3*	*0.0*
Roasted, Meat, Fat & Skin	*1oz/28g*	*118*	*10.7*	*423*	*20.0*	*0.0*	*38.1*	*0.0*
Shredded & Spring Onion Rice Paper Rolls, Waitrose*	1 Pack/95g	101	0.7	104	6.6	17.7	0.8	0.7
DUCK &								
Plum Sauce, Roasted, Sainsbury's*	½ Pack/150g	174	3.8	116	6.9	16.0	2.5	1.8
DUCK A L'ORANGE								
Roast, M&S*	½ Pack/270g	554	42.1	205	12.5	4.1	15.6	0.6
DUCK AROMATIC								
Crispy, Asda*	1/3 Pack/166g	469	24.9	283	19.0	18.0	15.0	0.8
Crispy, Half Duck & Pancakes, M&S*	½ Pack/311g	590	26.7	190	13.9	14.0	8.6	2.1
Crispy, Half with Hoisin Sauce & 12 Pancakes, Tesco*	1/6 Pack/70g	162	7.4	232	18.3	15.9	10.6	1.1
Crispy, Quarter with Hoisin Sauce & Pancakes, Tesco*	1/6 Pack/40g	100	4.2	250	12.3	25.3	10.6	2.0
Crispy, Somerfield*	1 Serving/265g	782	49.0	295	18.1	14.0	18.5	0.7
with Plum Sauce, Finest, Tesco*	1 Serving/250g	400	14.0	160	16.1	11.3	5.6	4.6
with Plum Sauce, Tesco*	½ Pack/250g	350	11.5	140	9.3	15.2	4.6	0.3
DUCK CANTONESE								
Style, Roast, Tesco*	1 Pack/300g	375	6.9	125	8.2	17.9	2.3	0.5
DUCK IN								
Barbecue, Chinese, Wings, Sainsbury's*	1 Serving/175g	430	25.0	246	19.4	9.7	14.3	0.0
Plum & Chilli Sauce, Legs, Aldi*	½ Pack/200g	342	11.6	171	5.7	24.0	5.8	0.6
Plum Sauce, Cantonese Style, Gressingham Foods*	1 Portion/200g	423	18.0	211	14.2	18.5	9.0	0.5
Plum Sauce, Crispy, M&S*	1 Pack/325g	569	31.2	175	10.7	11.2	9.6	0.9
Plum Sauce, Legs, Asda*	1 Leg/200g	452	23.0	226	24.1	6.4	11.5	0.5
DUCK PEKING								
Crispy, Aromatic, Sainsbury's*	½ Pack/300g	1236	110.7	412	19.5	0.6	36.9	0.1

	Measure INFO/WEIGHT	per Measure KCAL	per Measure FAT	Nutrition Values per 100g / 100ml KCAL	PROT	CARB	FAT	FIBRE
DUCK PEKING								
Crispy, Cherry Valley*	1 Serving/270g	702	35.9	260	17.5	17.8	13.3	0.7
DUCK WITH								
Noodles, Fu & Hoisin, Fuller for Longer, M&S*	1 Pack/370g	335	7.4	91	8.2	10.0	2.0	2.0
Noodles, Shanghai Roast, Sainsbury's*	1 Pack/450g	580	17.1	129	5.6	18.0	3.8	1.2
Pancakes, & Hoisin Sauce, M&S*	1 Pack/80g	136	3.2	170	13.0	19.9	4.0	0.9
Pancakes, Shredded, Iceland*	1 Pack/220g	471	5.9	214	20.4	27.0	2.7	1.5
DUMPLING MIX								
Farmhouse, Goldenfry Foods Ltd*	1 Serving/35g	148	5.3	422	9.1	62.0	15.1	1.0
DUMPLINGS								
Average	1oz/28g	58	3.3	208	2.8	24.5	11.7	0.9
Dried Mix, Tesco*	1 Pack/137g	404	16.7	295	5.4	39.9	12.2	2.8
Homestyle, Baked Weight, Frozen, Aunt Bessie's*	1 Dumpling/49g	188	8.6	384	9.7	44.4	17.6	2.8
Pork & Garlic Chive, Waitrose*	1 Pack/115g	215	8.1	187	9.4	20.4	7.0	1.1
Prawn, Cantonese, Crispy, Sainsbury's*	1 Dumpling/11g	27	1.5	241	9.3	20.9	13.4	1.1
Prawn, Siu Mai, Chinese, M&S*	8 Dumplings/170g	170	2.9	100	7.8	13.1	1.7	1.3

EASTER EGG

INFO/WEIGHT	Measure	per Measure KCAL	FAT	Nutrition Values per 100g / 100ml KCAL	PROT	CARB	FAT	FIBRE
Aero Bubbles, Nestle*	1 Egg/235g	1264	72.4	538	6.6	57.6	30.8	2.2
Buttons, Chocolate Egg Shell Only, Cadbury*	1 Egg/162g	859	48.6	530	7.5	56.8	30.0	0.7
Caramel, Chocolate Egg Shell Only, Cadbury*	1 Egg/343g	1801	102.9	525	7.5	56.8	30.0	0.7
Chocolate, Chick, Dairy Milk, Shell Only, Cadbury*	1 Egg/167g	877	50.1	525	7.5	56.8	30.0	0.7
Chocolate Egg Shell Only, Dairy Milk, Cadbury*	1 Egg/178g	943	53.4	530	7.5	56.8	30.0	0.7
Chocolate Orange, Terry's*	1 Egg/120g	636	36.6	530	7.4	57.0	30.5	2.4
Creme Egg, Chocolate Egg Shell Only, Cadbury*	1 Egg/178g	943	53.4	530	7.5	56.8	30.0	0.7
Crunchie, Cadbury*	1 Egg/167g	885	50.1	530	7.5	56.8	30.0	0.7
Dark Chocolate, 70%, Green & Black's*	1 Egg/180g	1026	75.4	570	9.3	33.8	41.9	11.5
Dark Chocolate, Thorncroft's*	1 Egg/360g	1890	134.6	525	6.8	39.4	37.4	9.8
Disney, Nestle*	1 Egg/65g	342	18.9	526	6.3	59.7	29.1	0.6
Flake, Chocolate Egg Shell Only, Cadbury*	1 Shell/153g	811	45.9	530	7.5	56.8	30.0	0.7
Kit Kat, Chunky, Nestle*	1 Egg/235g	1250	67.7	532	5.5	61.7	28.8	1.7
Mars*	1 Serving/63g	281	10.9	449	4.2	69.0	17.4	0.0
Milk Chocolate, Nestle*	½ Egg/42g	205	9.7	489	5.0	65.2	23.1	0.5
Milk Chocolate, Swiss, Hollow, M&S*	1 Egg/18g	100	6.3	555	6.7	53.2	34.8	2.5
Milky Bar, Nestle*	1 Egg/40g	182	6.9	454	4.2	70.8	17.2	0.0
Roses, Chocolate Egg Shell Only, Cadbury*	1 Egg/200g	1060	60.0	530	7.5	56.8	30.0	0.7
Smarties, Nestle*	1 Egg/258g	1367	74.0	530	5.3	62.2	28.7	1.7
Twirl, Chocolate Egg Shell Only, Cadbury*	1 Egg/325g	1722	97.5	530	7.5	56.8	30.0	0.7
White Chocolate, Thorntons*	1 Egg/360g	1958	109.1	544	5.5	62.2	30.3	2.1
Wispa, Chocolate Egg Shell Only, Cadbury*	1 Egg/313g	1643	93.9	525	7.5	56.8	30.0	0.7

ECLAIR

INFO/WEIGHT	Measure	per Measure KCAL	FAT	Nutrition Values per 100g / 100ml KCAL	PROT	CARB	FAT	FIBRE
Belgian Chocolate, Weight Watchers*	1 Eclair/30g	81	3.5	271	3.9	37.6	11.7	6.6
Chocolate, 25% Less Fat, Sainsbury's*	1 Eclair/58g	171	9.3	295	6.8	31.1	16.0	1.2
Chocolate, Asda*	1 Eclair/33g	144	11.0	436	6.7	27.3	33.3	4.8
Chocolate, Cream, Fresh, Tesco*	1 Eclair/66g	285	20.5	430	6.0	31.1	30.9	1.8
Chocolate, Cream filled, VLH Kitchens	1 Serving/66g	286	44.2	434	7.0	36.4	29.2	1.8
Chocolate, Fresh Cream, M&S*	1 Eclair/44g	170	12.2	390	6.3	28.4	27.9	2.0
Chocolate, Fresh Cream, Sainsbury's*	1 Eclair/59g	212	13.9	360	4.2	32.7	23.6	0.5
Chocolate, Frozen, Morrisons*	1 Eclair/31g	116	9.6	374	5.0	18.8	31.0	1.3
Chocolate, Mini, Iceland*	1 Eclair/13g	55	4.6	426	4.9	21.5	35.6	0.4
Chocolate & Fresh Cream, Tempting, Tesco*	1 Eclair/39g	158	11.2	405	6.5	29.1	28.8	1.1
Double Chocolate with Fresh Cream, Tesco*	1 Eclair/69g	275	18.6	400	5.9	33.4	27.0	1.6

EEL

INFO/WEIGHT	Measure	per Measure KCAL	FAT	Nutrition Values per 100g / 100ml KCAL	PROT	CARB	FAT	FIBRE
Cooked or Smoked, Dry Heat, Average	1 Serving/100g	236	15.0	236	23.6	0.0	15.0	0.0
Jellied, Average	1oz/28g	27	2.0	98	8.4	0.0	7.1	0.0
Raw, Average	1oz/28g	47	3.2	168	16.6	0.0	11.3	0.0

EGG

INFO/WEIGHT	Measure	per Measure KCAL	FAT	Nutrition Values per 100g / 100ml KCAL	PROT	CARB	FAT	FIBRE
White, Free Range, Liquid, Two Chicks*	3 Tbsp/45g	23	0.0	50	10.5	1.0	0.0	0.0

EGG SUBSTITUTE

INFO/WEIGHT	Measure	per Measure KCAL	FAT	Nutrition Values per 100g / 100ml KCAL	PROT	CARB	FAT	FIBRE
99% Real Eggs, The Crafty Cook*	¼ Cup/61g	30	0.0	49	10.0	2.0	0.0	0.0

EGGS

INFO/WEIGHT	Measure	per Measure KCAL	FAT	Nutrition Values per 100g / 100ml KCAL	PROT	CARB	FAT	FIBRE
Dried, White, Average	1 Tbsp/14g	41	0.0	295	73.8	0.0	0.0	0.0
Dried, Whole, Average	1oz/28g	159	11.6	568	48.4	0.0	41.6	0.0
Duck, Boiled & Salted, Average, Weight with Shell	1 Egg/75g	169	13.2	225	16.6	0.0	17.6	0.0
Duck, Whole, Raw, Average, Weight with Shell	1 Egg/75g	139	10.0	185	16.2	0.0	13.4	0.0
Free Range, Large, Average, Weight with Shell	1 Egg/68g	109	7.6	161	14.1	0.9	11.2	0.0
Fried in Veg Oil, Average	1 Med/60g	107	8.3	179	13.6	0.0	13.9	0.0
Fried without Fat, Average	1 Med/60g	104	7.6	174	15.0	0.0	12.7	0.0
Goose, Whole, Fresh, Raw, Average, Weight with Shell	1 Egg/144g	267	19.1	185	13.9	1.4	13.3	0.0
Large, Average, Weight with Shell	1oz/28g	37	2.5	131	12.6	0.1	9.0	0.0
Medium, Average, Weight with Shell	1 Egg/58g	76	5.2	131	12.6	0.1	9.0	0.0

	Measure INFO/WEIGHT	per Measure KCAL	FAT	Nutrition Values per 100g / 100ml KCAL	PROT	CARB	FAT	FIBRE
EGGS								
Medium, Boiled, Average, Weight with Shell	1 Egg/50g	83	6.1	165	14.0	0.6	12.1	0.1
Poached, Weight with Shell	1 Med/50g	83	6.1	165	14.0	0.6	12.1	0.6
Quail, Whole, Raw, Weight with Shell	*1 Egg/13g*	*21*	*1.6*	*164*	*14.0*	*0.4*	*12.1*	*0.0*
Scrambled, Average	1 Egg/68g	109	7.9	160	13.8	0.0	11.6	0.0
Scrambled with Milk, Average	1 Egg/60g	154	14.0	257	10.9	0.7	23.4	0.0
Turkey, Whole, Raw, Weight with Shell	*1 Egg/79g*	*154*	*10.9*	*194*	*15.5*	*1.3*	*13.9*	*0.0*
Very Large, Average, Weight with Shell	1 Egg/78g	125	8.7	161	14.1	0.9	11.2	0.0
Whites, Liquid, Myprotein*	1 Serving/32g	16	0.0	50	11.2	0.0	0.0	0.0
Whites Only, Raw, Average	*1 Egg/33g*	*12*	*0.0*	*36*	*9.0*	*0.0*	*0.0*	*0.0*
Yolks, Raw	*1 Yolk/14g*	*47*	*4.3*	*339*	*16.1*	*0.0*	*30.5*	*0.0*
ELDERBERRIES								
Average	*1oz/28g*	*10*	*0.1*	*35*	*0.7*	*7.4*	*0.5*	*0.0*
ELICHE								
Dry Weight, Buitoni*	1 Serving/80g	282	1.5	352	11.2	72.6	1.9	0.0
ELK								
Raw, Meat only	1 Serving/100g	111	1.4	111	23.0	0.0	1.4	0.0
Roasted, Meat only	1 Serving/100g	146	1.9	146	30.2	0.0	1.9	0.0
ENCHILADAS								
3 Bean, Ready Meal, Average	1 Pack/400g	505	16.6	126	4.4	16.9	4.2	3.2
Beef, LC, Tesco*	1 Pack/400g	440	11.2	110	5.4	13.4	2.8	3.1
Chicken, Asda*	1 Serving/500g	690	30.0	138	10.0	17.0	6.0	1.0
Chicken, Average	1 Serving/295g	483	18.8	164	11.6	16.0	6.4	1.7
Chicken, Morrisons*	½ Pack/275g	393	12.6	143	10.0	15.4	4.6	1.8
Chicken, Suiza, Smart Ones, Weight Watchers*	1 Pack/255g	290	5.0	114	4.3	18.0	2.0	1.2
Chicken in a Spicy Salsa & Bean Sauce, Asda*	½ Pack/212g	373	17.0	176	10.0	16.0	8.0	0.0
Spicy, Three Bean, Cooked, CBY, Asda*	1 Pack/400g	466	15.9	117	4.4	13.7	4.0	4.1
ENDIVE								
Raw	*1oz/28g*	*4*	*0.1*	*13*	*1.8*	*1.0*	*0.2*	*2.0*
ENERGY DRINK								
Average	1 Can/250ml	118	0.0	47	0.0	11.4	0.0	0.0
Blue Bolt, Sainsbury's*	1 Can/250ml	124	0.0	49	0.0	11.3	0.0	0.0
Cherry, Lucozade*	1 Bottle/500ml	345	0.0	69	0.0	17.1	0.0	0.0
Isostar Sport, Isostar*	1 Glass/250ml	74	0.0	30	0.0	7.0	0.0	0.0
Juiced Berry, Relentless*	1 Can/500g	230	0.0	46	0.0	10.7	0.0	0.0
Juiced Orange & Tropical Fruit, Relentless*	1 Can/500ml	220	0.0	44	0.0	10.7	0.0	0.0
KX, Sugar Free, Diet, Tesco*	1 Can/250ml	5	0.0	2	0.0	0.0	0.0	0.0
Libertus, Blue, Sugar Free, Relentless*	1 Can/500ml	20	0.0	4	0.0	0.0	0.0	0.0
Monster*	1 Can/500ml	240	0.0	48	0.0	12.0	0.0	0.0
Orange, Active Sport, Tesco*	1 Bottle/500ml	135	0.0	27	0.0	6.5	0.0	0.0
Powerade, Aqua+*	1 Bottle/500ml	80	0.0	16	0.0	3.7	0.0	0.0
Red Thunder, Diet, Low Calorie, Aldi*	1 Can/250ml	5	0.0	2	0.1	0.0	0.0	0.0
Relentless, Original, Relentless*	1 Can/500ml	230	0.0	46	0.0	10.4	0.0	0.0
Relentless, Sugar Free, Coca-Cola*	1 Can/500ml	20	0.0	4	0.0	0.0	0.0	0.0
Revive, Cranberry with Acai, Light Sparkling, Lucozade*	1 Bottle/380ml	50	0.0	13	0.0	2.8	0.0	0.0
Sugar Free, Diet, Mountain Dew, Britvic*	1 Can/440ml	3	0.0	1	0.0	0.0	0.0	0.0
V, Frucor Beverages*	1 Can/250ml	112	0.0	45	0.0	11.2	0.0	0.0

	Measure INFO/WEIGHT	per Measure KCAL	FAT	Nutrition Values per 100g / 100ml KCAL	PROT	CARB	FAT	FIBRE
FAGGOTS								
in Rich Gravy, Iceland*	1 Faggot/81g	116	5.2	143	6.5	15.9	6.4	1.1
Pork, with Streaky Bacon, British, Essential, Waitrose*	2 Faggots/128g	255	14.5	199	16.7	7.5	11.3	0.9
FAJITA								
Beef, GFY, Asda*	½ Pack/208g	354	9.8	170	11.0	21.0	4.7	1.6
Chicken, American Style, Tesco*	1 Pack/275g	388	14.0	141	9.5	14.2	5.1	1.0
Chicken, Asda*	½ Pack/225g	371	10.1	165	11.0	20.0	4.5	3.5
Chicken, Average	1 Serving/275g	409	14.7	149	10.2	15.0	5.4	2.3
Chicken, Co-Op*	1 Serving/230g	391	16.1	170	11.0	15.0	7.0	3.0
Chicken, COU, M&S*	1 Pack/230g	288	5.3	125	10.0	16.5	2.3	1.5
Chicken, M&S*	1 Pack/230g	345	12.2	150	8.6	17.7	5.3	1.0
Chicken, Tesco*	½ Pack/275g	382	14.3	139	9.2	13.9	5.2	1.9
Meal Kit, Tesco*	1 Serving/100g	210	3.4	210	6.1	38.2	3.4	2.1
Vegetable	1 Serving/275g	472	14.9	172	4.9	25.6	5.4	1.9
FALAFEL								
12 Pack, Sainsbury's*	1 Falafel/17g	44	2.5	259	7.3	20.6	14.8	7.2
Asda*	½ Pack/50g	140	9.6	281	8.3	18.9	19.1	8.2
Balls, Meat Free, Meat Free, Tesco*	3 Balls/67g	135	5.3	205	7.1	21.7	8.1	6.3
Fried in Vegetable Oil, Average	1 Falafel/25g	45	2.8	179	6.4	15.6	11.2	3.4
Mini, M&S*	1 Falafel/14g	43	2.5	310	7.9	28.1	18.4	2.6
Mini, Sainsbury's*	1 Serving/168g	499	29.6	297	8.0	26.8	17.6	3.2
Mix, Asda*	1 Pack/120g	313	15.0	261	6.4	30.8	12.5	2.6
Mix, Authentic, Al'fez*	1 Serving/100g	235	13.8	235	7.1	26.3	13.8	8.8
Organic, Cauldron Foods*	1 Falafel/25g	51	2.4	203	8.4	20.3	9.8	7.2
Vegetarian, Organic, Waitrose*	1 Falafel/25g	55	2.6	220	8.0	23.3	10.5	7.6
FANTA								
Fruit Twist, Coca-Cola*	1 Serving/250ml	132	0.0	53	0.0	13.0	0.0	0.0
Icy Lemon, Coca-Cola*	1 Can/330ml	165	0.0	50	0.0	12.2	0.0	0.0
Icy Lemon, Zero, Coca-Cola*	1 Can/330ml	7	0.0	2	0.0	0.2	0.0	0.0
Lemon, Coca-Cola*	1 Can/330ml	165	0.0	50	0.0	12.0	0.0	0.0
Orange, Coca-Cola*	1 Glass/250ml	75	0.0	30	0.0	7.1	0.0	0.0
Orange, Zero, Coca-Cola*	1 Can/330ml	11	0.0	3	0.0	0.5	0.0	0.0
Red Fruits, Coca-Cola*	1 Serving/100ml	37	0.0	37	0.0	9.0	0.0	0.0
Summer Fruits, Z, Coca-Cola*	1 fl oz/30ml	1	0.0	3	0.0	0.6	0.0	0.0
FARFALLE								
Bows, Dry, Average	1 Serving/75g	265	1.4	353	11.4	72.6	1.9	1.9
FENNEL								
Florence, Boiled in Salted Water	1oz/28g	3	0.1	11	0.9	1.5	0.2	2.3
Florence, Raw, Unprepared, Average	1 Bulb/250g	30	0.5	12	0.9	1.8	0.2	2.4
Florence, Steamed	1 Serving/80g	9	0.2	11	9.0	1.5	0.2	2.3
FENUGREEK								
Leaves, Raw, Fresh, Average	1 Serving/80g	28	0.2	35	4.6	4.8	0.2	1.1
FETTUCINI								
Chicken, Cajun, CBY, Asda*	1 Pack/400g	360	5.2	90	6.3	12.6	1.3	1.4
Chicken, Cajun, GFY, Asda*	1 Pack/400g	384	7.6	96	8.9	9.7	1.9	2.4
Chicken, Cajun Spiced, COU, M&S*	1 Pack/400g	400	8.0	100	8.0	12.3	2.0	1.3
Dry Weight, Buitoni*	1 Serving/90g	326	1.5	362	12.2	74.4	1.7	0.0
FIG ROLLS								
Asda*	1 Biscuit/19g	71	1.7	372	4.8	68.0	9.0	0.0
Go Ahead, McVitie's*	1 Biscuit/15g	55	0.7	365	4.2	76.8	4.6	2.9
Jacob's*	1 Biscuit/18g	68	1.5	380	4.0	71.4	8.5	3.3
Sainsbury's*	1 Biscuit/19g	70	1.7	377	4.8	68.3	9.4	2.6
Vitalinea, Jacob's*	1 Biscuit/18g	61	1.0	339	3.7	68.2	5.8	3.8

F

	Measure INFO/WEIGHT	per Measure		Nutrition Values per 100g / 100ml				
		KCAL	FAT	KCAL	PROT	CARB	FAT	FIBRE
FIGS								
Dried, Average	*1 Fig/14g*	*32*	*0.1*	*232*	*3.6*	*53.2*	*1.1*	*8.6*
In Light Syrup, Asda*	1 Serving/100g	75	0.1	75	0.4	18.0	0.1	0.7
Raw, Fresh, Average	*1 Fig/35g*	*16*	*0.1*	*45*	*1.3*	*9.8*	*0.2*	*1.5*
FISH								
Balls, Gefilte, M&S*	1 Pack/200g	280	7.8	140	14.1	11.9	3.9	1.0
Battered, Portion, Ross*	1 Serving/110g	223	11.9	203	10.4	16.1	10.8	0.8
Fillets, Garlic & Herb, Youngs*	1 Fillet/118g	261	14.8	222	11.0	16.2	12.6	1.4
Fillets, Lemon & Pepper, Youngs*	1 Fillet/130g	283	16.7	218	10.3	15.3	12.9	4.3
Fillets, Lime & Chilli, Fish Fusions, Birds Eye*	1 Portion/160g	270	10.1	169	15.0	12.9	6.3	0.5
Fillets, Pollack, Breaded, Cooked, Tesco*	1 Fillet/125g	315	12.2	250	15.0	24.4	9.7	2.0
Fillets, White, Breaded, Tesco*	1 Piece/95g	198	10.4	208	10.6	16.9	10.9	1.0
Fillets, White, Breaded, Value, Tesco*	1 Serving/100g	192	9.7	192	10.6	15.6	9.7	2.2
Fillets, White, Natural, Tesco*	1 Fillet/100g	72	0.6	72	16.6	0.0	0.6	0.0
Goujons, Asda*	1 Serving/125g	240	8.0	192	12.8	20.8	6.4	0.2
Grouper	1 Serving/100g	92	1.0	92	19.4	0.0	1.0	0.0
Medley, SteamFresh, Birds Eye*	1 Bag/170g	170	6.3	100	13.0	2.3	3.7	0.1
Portion, Chip Shop, Youngs*	1 Portion/135g	315	19.7	233	11.0	15.1	14.6	0.6
Pouting, Fillet, Tesco*	1 Serving/100g	85	0.3	85	19.7	0.3	0.3	0.0
River Cobbler, Smoked, Tesco*	1 Fillet/165g	124	3.5	75	13.9	0.0	2.1	1.5
River Cobbler, Value, Tesco*	½ Pack/133g	133	5.3	100	15.1	0.1	4.0	0.1
Salted, Chinese, Steamed	1oz/28g	43	0.6	155	33.9	0.0	2.2	0.0
Steaks, Chip Shop, Youngs*	1 Serving/100g	198	10.4	198	11.0	14.9	10.4	0.9
White, Breaded, Fillets, Ocean Pure*	1 Fillet/113g	276	11.5	245	20.8	16.9	10.2	1.2
White, Smoked, Average	1 Serving/100g	108	0.9	108	23.4	0.0	0.9	0.0
White, Tesco*	1 Fillet/100g	78	0.6	78	16.6	0.0	0.6	0.0
FISH & CHIPS								
Budgens*	1 Pack/284g	625	28.4	220	8.0	24.5	10.0	2.3
Cod, Asda*	1 Serving/280g	450	14.0	161	8.0	21.0	5.0	1.1
Co-Op*	1 Pack/250g	388	15.0	155	6.0	18.0	6.0	2.0
Ross*	1 Serving/250g	415	19.0	166	6.2	18.1	7.6	1.6
Tesco*	1 Serving/300g	489	18.6	163	5.5	21.2	6.2	1.6
with Mushy Peas, Kershaws*	1 Pack/315g	450	18.3	143	6.4	16.4	5.8	1.6
FISH CAKES								
Battered, Bubbly Batter, Youngs*	1 Cake/44g	109	6.7	247	7.1	20.5	15.1	1.4
Breaded, Sainsbury's*	1 Cake/42g	75	3.4	179	10.0	16.2	8.1	0.7
Captain's Coins, Mini, Captain Birds Eye, Birds Eye*	1 Cake/20g	38	1.7	188	9.5	18.7	8.3	1.1
Cod, & Pancetta, Cafe Culture, M&S*	1 Cake/85g	166	13.2	195	9.2	7.2	15.5	2.0
Cod, & Parsley, Waitrose*	1 Cake/85g	147	6.5	173	9.2	16.9	7.6	1.1
Cod, Baked, Tesco*	1 Cake/135g	255	9.9	189	9.1	21.1	7.3	3.2
Cod, Big Time, Birds Eye*	1 Cake/114g	223	11.6	196	8.3	17.8	10.2	1.0
Cod, Birds Eye*	1 Cake/51g	93	4.4	182	10.0	16.0	8.7	1.1
Cod, Cheese & Chive, Finest, Tesco*	1 Cake/100g	212	11.5	212	9.7	18.3	11.5	1.7
Cod, Chunky, Breaded, Chilled, Youngs*	1 Cake/90g	192	11.5	213	9.5	14.9	12.8	1.2
Cod, Fresh, Asda*	1 Cake/75g	164	8.2	219	7.0	23.0	11.0	1.6
Cod, Homemade, Average	1 Cake/50g	120	8.3	241	9.3	14.4	16.6	0.7
Cod, in Crunch Crumb, Birds Eye*	1 Cake/50g	93	4.3	187	11.4	16.0	8.6	1.0
Cod, King Prawn & Pancetta, Extra Special, Asda*	1 Cake/115g	202	7.7	176	11.0	17.8	6.7	15.0
Cod, M&S*	1 Cake/85g	153	7.8	180	8.9	15.4	9.2	1.3
Cod, Mornay, Easy to Cook, Waitrose*	1 Cake/149g	234	9.1	157	10.5	15.0	6.1	1.4
Cod, Tesco*	1 Cake/90g	202	9.4	224	8.9	23.8	10.4	0.2
Crab & Prawn, Thai, Tesco*	1 Cake/115g	269	16.6	234	8.8	17.4	14.4	1.2
Fried in Blended Oil	1 Cake/50g	109	6.7	218	8.6	16.8	13.4	0.0
Frozen, Average	1 Cake/85g	112	3.3	132	8.6	16.7	3.9	0.0

F

FISH CAKES

INFO/WEIGHT	Measure	per Measure		Nutrition Values per 100g / 100ml				
		KCAL	FAT	KCAL	PROT	CARB	FAT	FIBRE
Great Value, Iceland*	1 Cake/42g	74	2.7	175	9.1	20.3	6.4	1.6
Grilled, Average	1 Cake/50g	77	2.2	154	9.9	19.7	4.5	0.0
Haddock, Asda*	1 Cake/88g	181	8.8	206	8.0	21.0	10.0	1.5
Haddock, Breaded, Asda*	1 Cake/90g	187	7.6	208	10.0	22.8	8.5	1.2
Haddock, Fresh Tastes, Asda*	1 Cake/75g	141	5.0	188	9.6	22.2	6.7	1.8
Haddock, in Breadcrumbs, Sainsbury's*	1 Cake/88g	158	6.2	179	10.8	18.2	7.0	1.4
Haddock, Sainsbury's*	1 Cake/135g	253	10.0	188	10.8	18.7	7.4	1.5
Haddock, Smoked, Breaded, Asda*	1 Cake/90g	202	11.7	225	9.0	18.0	13.0	1.6
Haddock, Smoked, Extra Special, Asda*	1 Cake/115g	218	10.9	190	12.8	13.2	9.5	1.3
Haddock, Smoked, Frozen, Waitrose*	1 Cake/85g	186	10.3	219	9.6	17.8	12.1	0.8
Haddock, Smoked, M&S*	1 Cake/85g	153	8.0	180	10.6	13.4	9.4	2.6
Haddock, Smoked, Sainsbury's*	1 Cake/63g	127	6.0	201	11.0	17.8	9.5	2.1
Haddock, Smoked, Tesco*	1 Cake/135g	236	9.3	175	7.7	19.9	6.9	2.8
Haddock, Smoked & Spinach, TTD, Sainsbury's*	½ Pack/107g	213	11.7	199	10.3	14.8	10.9	1.2
Halibut Cod Loin, Finest, Tesco*	1 Cake/115g	213	8.3	185	8.8	21.3	7.2	1.4
Plaice, & Asparagus, Melting Middle, M&S*	1 Cake/145g	239	11.6	165	7.7	15.3	8.0	1.3
Pollock, Cheddar & Sweetcorn, Jamie Oliver, Youngs*	2 Cakes/97g	198	9.1	204	9.8	19.1	9.4	1.6
Pollock, Chive & Cream, Jamie Oliver, Youngs*	1 Cake/84g	160	7.0	190	9.1	18.7	8.3	1.8
Pollock, Parsley Breadcrumbs, Jamie Oliver, Youngs*	2 Cakes/98g	181	7.9	185	8.9	18.0	8.1	2.0
Prawn, Sainsbury's*	1 Cake/90g	184	7.8	204	9.6	21.7	8.7	1.2
Prawn, Thai Style, Finest, Tesco*	1 Cake/145g	305	13.5	210	6.7	24.2	9.3	1.0
Salmon, & Asparagus, Finest, Tesco*	1 Cake/115g	300	17.8	261	10.7	19.6	15.5	0.4
Salmon, & Broccoli, Morrisons*	1 Cake/60g	126	7.1	210	9.8	17.2	11.9	1.3
Salmon, & Dill, Waitrose*	1 Cake/85g	206	11.9	242	11.5	17.5	14.0	1.8
Salmon, & Haddock with Lemon & Dill Sauce, Waitrose*	1 Cake/187g	304	18.1	163	9.2	9.7	9.7	1.5
Salmon, & Leek, Northern Catch, Aldi*	1 Cake/114g	212	9.0	186	9.5	19.3	7.9	0.9
Salmon, & Pollock, Basil Parmesan, Jamie Oliver, Youngs*	1 Cake/85g	157	6.7	184	10.8	16.2	7.8	2.6
Salmon, & Pollock, Lemon Parsley, Jamie Oliver, Youngs*	2 Cakes/96g	190	8.6	198	10.3	18.0	9.0	1.8
Salmon, & Tarragon, Waitrose*	1 Cake/85g	179	10.0	211	11.9	14.3	11.8	2.2
Salmon, Asda*	1 Cake/86g	215	12.0	250	8.0	23.0	14.0	1.4
Salmon, Birds Eye*	1 Cake/50g	84	4.5	168	9.5	12.2	9.0	1.4
Salmon, Chunky, Sainsbury's*	1 Cake/84g	192	10.5	228	13.2	15.8	12.5	2.9
Salmon, Coated in Light & Crispy Breadcrumb, Tesco*	1 Cake/90g	212	10.8	235	9.7	21.0	12.0	1.2
Salmon, Homemade, Average	1 Cake/50g	136	9.8	273	10.4	14.4	19.7	0.7
Salmon, M&S*	1 Cake/86g	180	10.9	210	9.1	15.1	12.7	1.7
Salmon, Melting Middle, Lochmuir, M&S*	1 Pack/290g	551	30.4	190	9.1	14.3	10.5	1.5
Salmon, Sainsbury's*	1 Cake/88g	171	7.6	194	12.6	16.5	8.6	1.6
Salmon, Spinach & Sicilian Lemon, Finest, Tesco*	1 Cake/145g	290	16.2	200	9.9	14.3	11.2	1.4
Salmon, Tesco*	1 Cake/90g	239	13.5	266	11.4	21.3	15.0	0.0
Salmon, VLH Kitchens	1 Serving/56g	156	35.7	278	10.5	14.4	20.0	0.6
Salmon, with Lemon Butter Sauce, Finest, Tesco*	1 Cake/220g	524	40.3	238	7.3	10.9	18.3	1.0
Salmon, with Lemon Butter Sauce, Gastropub, M&S*	1 Cake/107g	188	13.3	175	7.8	8.5	12.4	1.2
Salmon, with Parsley Sauce, Finest, Tesco*	½ Pack/170g	350	23.6	206	8.6	11.7	13.9	1.0
Smart Price, Asda*	1 Cake/42g	78	3.3	188	7.0	22.0	8.0	0.9
Thai, Finest, Tesco*	1 Cake/65g	150	8.6	230	7.5	20.3	13.2	1.6
Thai, Oriental Selection, Waitrose*	1 Cake/11g	18	0.3	161	17.8	15.8	3.0	1.5
Thai, Tesco*	1 Cake/22g	37	1.1	166	17.4	12.8	5.0	1.1
Thai Style, Sainsbury's*	1 Cake/49g	69	2.1	141	12.0	13.8	4.2	1.7
Tuna, Lime & Coriander, BGTY, Sainsbury's*	1 Cake/91g	200	10.7	220	10.7	17.7	11.8	2.6
Tuna, Sainsbury's*	1 Cake/90g	183	7.5	203	13.7	18.4	8.3	2.1
Value, Tesco*	1 Cake/42g	88	4.8	210	8.2	19.5	11.5	1.1

FISH FINGERS

INFO/WEIGHT	Measure	per Measure		Nutrition Values per 100g / 100ml				
Atlantis*	1 Finger/30g	52	2.2	172	12.0	14.0	7.5	0.4

	Measure INFO/WEIGHT	per Measure		Nutrition Values per 100g / 100ml				
		KCAL	FAT	KCAL	PROT	CARB	FAT	FIBRE
FISH FINGERS								
Brilliant, Jamie Oliver, Youngs*	3 Fingers/86g	177	7.9	205	11.7	18.4	9.1	1.2
Chip Shop, Youngs*	1 Finger/30g	75	4.9	251	9.3	16.6	16.4	1.2
Chunky, Cooked, Tesco*	2 Fingers/98g	230	10.0	235	13.2	21.6	10.2	1.3
Cod, 100% Cod Fillet, Tesco*	1 Finger/30g	53	2.2	177	12.4	14.9	7.5	1.4
Cod, Chunky, Tesco*	1 Finger/40g	70	3.0	175	12.3	14.3	7.6	1.6
Cod, Fillet, Asda*	1 Finger/31g	66	3.1	214	13.0	18.0	10.0	0.0
Cod, Fillet, Chunky, M&S*	1 Finger/40g	70	2.4	175	12.0	17.2	6.0	1.0
Cod, Fillet, Chunky, TTD, Sainsbury's*	2 Fingers/120g	274	13.2	228	13.4	18.3	11.0	1.2
Cod, Fillet, Iceland*	1 Finger/30g	62	2.5	205	13.0	19.5	8.3	1.4
Cod, Fillet, Waitrose*	1 Finger/30g	55	2.2	183	11.9	16.9	7.5	0.7
Cod, Fried in Blended Oil, Average	1 Finger/28g	67	3.9	238	13.2	15.5	14.1	0.6
Cod, Frozen, Average	1 Finger/28g	48	2.2	170	11.6	14.2	7.8	0.6
Cod, Grilled, Average	1 Finger/28g	56	2.5	200	14.3	16.6	8.9	0.7
Cod, Morrisons*	1 Finger/30g	54	2.2	180	11.7	16.4	7.5	1.1
Cod, Sainsbury's*	1 Finger/28g	53	2.1	190	12.5	17.7	7.7	1.0
Economy, Sainsbury's*	1 Finger/26g	51	2.2	198	12.6	17.7	8.5	1.3
Farmfoods*	1 Finger/27g	49	2.2	183	12.2	15.6	8.0	1.2
Free From, Sainsbury's*	1 Finger/30g	56	2.3	188	11.4	18.0	7.8	0.7
Haddock, Fillet, Asda*	1 Finger/30g	62	2.7	205	14.0	17.0	9.0	0.0
Haddock, in Crispy Batter, Birds Eye*	1 Finger/30g	56	2.3	188	14.3	15.1	7.8	0.7
Haddock, in Crunchy Crumb, Morrisons*	1 Finger/30g	57	2.4	190	13.1	16.3	8.0	1.1
Omega 3, Grilled, Tesco*	3 Fingers/71g	150	6.8	210	12.4	17.8	9.5	1.3
Sainsbury's*	1 Finger/27g	52	2.3	194	13.4	16.0	8.5	0.7
Salmon, Birds Eye*	1 Finger/28g	63	2.7	225	13.2	21.7	9.5	0.9
Smart Price, Asda*	1 Finger/25g	46	2.0	184	12.0	16.0	8.0	1.1
Value, Tesco*	1 Finger/25g	42	2.0	170	11.5	11.9	8.1	1.7
FISH IN								
Batter, Morrisons*	1 Fish/140g	235	8.1	168	14.0	15.0	5.8	0.2
Batter, Youngs*	1 Serving/100g	315	19.7	315	14.9	20.4	19.7	0.8
Butter Sauce, Steaks, Ross*	1 Serving/150g	126	5.8	84	9.1	3.2	3.9	0.1
Butter Sauce, Steaks, Youngs*	1 Steak/140g	102	2.9	73	9.6	3.7	2.1	0.5
Butter Sauce, Value, Tesco*	1 Portion/150g	128	3.8	85	10.5	5.2	2.5	1.5
Parsley Sauce, Fillets, Light & Easy, Youngs*	1 Pack/224g	139	4.3	62	8.4	2.8	1.9	1.4
Parsley Sauce, Steaks, Ross*	1 Serving/150g	123	5.6	82	9.1	3.1	3.7	0.1
FIVE SPICE								
Powder, Sharwood's*	1 Tsp/2g	3	0.2	172	12.2	11.6	8.6	23.4
FLAKE								
Dipped, Cadbury*	1 Bar/41g	215	12.5	530	7.6	56.1	30.8	0.8
Luxury, Cadbury*	1 Bar/45g	240	13.6	533	7.3	57.8	30.2	0.0
Praline, Cadbury*	1 Bar/38g	201	12.9	535	7.7	49.5	34.3	0.0
Snow, Cadbury*	1 Bar/36g	198	11.1	550	7.2	60.1	30.9	0.0
FLAN								
Pastry with Fruit	1oz/28g	33	1.2	118	1.4	19.3	4.4	0.7
Sponge with Fruit	1oz/28g	31	0.4	112	2.8	23.3	1.5	0.6
FLAN CASE								
Sponge, Average	**1oz/28g**	**90**	**1.5**	**320**	**7.0**	**62.5**	**5.4**	**0.7**
FLAPJACK								
7 Fruits, Graze*	1 Punnet/55g	223	10.5	406	5.1	54.9	19.1	4.3
All Butter, Organic, Sainsbury's*	1 Serving/35g	156	8.0	446	5.3	54.5	23.0	2.7
All Butter, Sainsbury's*	1 Flapjack/35g	156	8.0	446	5.7	54.5	22.8	2.7
All Butter, Squares, M&S*	1 Flapjack/34g	150	7.2	441	6.2	56.2	21.2	4.4
All Butter, Waitrose*	1 Flapjack/34g	126	9.0	376	3.8	52.4	26.8	1.2
Apple & Cinnamon, Graze*	1 Punnet/54g	238	12.3	440	4.6	54.7	22.7	3.7

FLAPJACK

INFO/WEIGHT	Measure	per Measure KCAL	FAT	Nutrition Values per 100g / 100ml KCAL	PROT	CARB	FAT	FIBRE
Apple & Sultana, Blackfriars*	1 Flapjack/110g	507	24.2	461	5.5	61.0	22.0	0.0
Apricot, The Handmade Flapjack Company*	1 Flapjack/90g	321	4.8	357	5.5	71.6	5.4	0.0
Apricot & Raisin, Waitrose*	1 Flapjack/38g	143	4.2	376	4.7	64.3	11.1	5.8
Average	1 Sm/50g	242	13.3	484	4.5	60.4	26.6	2.7
Banana, The Handmade Flapjack Company*	1 Flapjack/90g	379	13.1	421	5.3	67.2	14.6	0.0
Butter, Kate's Cakes Ltd*	1 Serving/100g	425	22.2	425	5.4	51.4	22.2	3.3
Caramel Bake, The Handmade Flapjack Company*	1 Flapjack/90g	375	13.0	417	6.0	65.6	14.5	0.0
Cherry & Coconut, Blackfriars*	1 Flapjack/110g	490	23.1	445	5.0	58.0	21.0	0.0
Cherry Bakewell, Iced, Devondale*	1 Flapjack/95g	432	21.9	455	3.7	54.0	23.1	2.6
Chocolate, Chunky, M&S*	1 Flapjack/80g	348	15.1	435	5.8	59.9	18.9	2.2
Chocolate, McVitie's*	1 Flapjack/85g	422	23.0	496	6.6	56.6	27.1	3.2
Chocolate, The Handmade Flapjack Company*	1 Flapjack/90g	392	17.6	435	6.0	58.6	19.6	0.0
Chocolate Chip, Boots*	1 Flapjack/75g	313	11.2	417	5.6	65.0	15.0	3.5
Chocolate Chip, Devondale*	1 Flapjack/95g	434	24.7	457	4.3	49.0	26.0	3.6
Chocolate Chip, Happy Shopper*	1 Flapjack/35g	163	8.2	467	5.7	58.7	23.3	0.0
Chocolate Chunk, Boots*	1 Slice/75g	351	18.8	468	5.7	55.0	25.0	3.0
Chocolate Dipped, Belgian, Asda*	1 Serving/67g	321	16.8	477	6.0	57.0	25.0	3.2
Chocolate Dipped, M&S*	1 Flapjack/96g	442	21.5	460	6.1	61.3	22.4	3.0
Chocolate Flavour, Blackfriars*	1 Bar/110g	521	26.4	474	5.0	61.0	24.0	0.0
Chocolate Special, The Handmade Flapjack Company*	1 Flapjack/90g	392	17.8	436	5.7	58.7	19.8	0.0
Co-Op*	1 Flapjack/38g	175	9.4	465	5.0	54.0	25.0	4.0
Date & Walnut, The Handmade Flapjack Company*	1 Flapjack/90g	360	13.5	400	6.1	60.2	15.0	0.0
Fingers, Golden, Oaty Fabulous Baking Boys*	1 Finger/28g	130	6.8	464	4.5	60.2	24.3	3.1
Fingers, Golden Oaty, Tesco*	1 Finger/25g	112	5.3	450	5.7	59.6	21.1	3.4
Fruit, Kate's Cakes Ltd*	1 Serving/100g	425	16.7	425	7.3	58.2	16.7	4.7
Fruit, Tesco*	1 Flapjack/33g	136	5.2	412	5.7	62.0	15.7	4.0
Fruit, Weight Watchers*	1 Serving/30g	106	1.9	353	6.0	68.3	6.3	4.7
Fruit with Raisins, Boots*	1 Pack/75g	329	15.8	439	5.4	57.0	21.0	3.5
Fruity, Waitrose*	1 Serving/50g	199	6.8	398	6.1	62.9	13.5	3.9
Fudge, Blackfriars*	1 Serving/110g	528	26.4	480	5.0	60.0	24.0	0.0
Hob Nobs, Milk Chocolate, McVitie's*	1 Flapjack/35g	155	6.0	443	5.8	64.2	17.2	4.2
Jaffa, Kids, Graze*	1 Punnet/54g	244	13.0	451	5.0	54.0	24.0	4.0
M & S*	1 Flapjack/53g	228	10.1	430	6.0	59.1	19.0	3.5
Ma Baker*	1 Serving/90g	381	18.0	423	7.4	56.9	20.0	4.8
Mighty Oat, Fabulous Bakin' Boys*	1 Bar/85g	366	17.0	430	6.0	58.0	20.0	3.0
Millionaire, Anytime, Gu*	1 Flapjack/19g	87	4.8	465	4.9	54.2	25.4	2.2
Mini, Sainsbury's*	1 Slice/15g	65	2.9	431	5.6	59.3	19.0	2.7
Mixed Fruit, Fabulous Bakin' Boys*	1 Serving/90g	350	9.4	389	5.5	71.0	10.5	4.0
Oat, GF, Hale & Hearty*	1 Cake/36g	165	9.1	457	6.8	55.1	25.2	8.9
Oat & Syrup, Oatjacks, McVitie's*	1 Bar/34g	153	7.5	450	5.3	57.6	22.0	5.0
Orange & Ginger, Graze*	1 Punnet/54g	241	12.9	446	5.1	53.0	23.8	4.2
Pecan, Maple Syrup, Wheat Free, Honeyrose Bakery*	1 Flapjack/75g	347	19.5	463	5.4	51.9	26.0	4.2
Plain, The Handmade Flapjack Company*	1 Flapjack/90g	398	19.2	442	5.4	57.1	21.3	0.0
Red Berry, Finger, Fabulous Bakin' Boys*	1 Bar/27g	129	6.2	477	5.5	60.6	22.9	2.9
Snickers, McVitie's*	1 Flapjack/65g	315	18.5	484	7.9	49.0	28.5	6.0
Summer Berry, Graze*	1 Punnet/54g	236	11.4	437	4.6	57.2	21.1	4.2
Toffee, Finest, Tesco*	1 Flapjack/35g	156	6.7	446	4.9	63.6	19.1	1.3
Weight Watchers*	1 Slice/30g	109	1.8	363	6.7	71.0	6.0	4.0
Yoghurt & Apricot, Iced, Devondale*	1 Flapjack/95g	443	25.6	466	4.5	51.0	27.0	3.3
Yoghurt Flavour, Blackfriars*	1 Bar/110g	521	26.4	474	7.0	58.0	24.0	0.0

FLATBREAD

INFO/WEIGHT	Measure	per Measure KCAL	FAT	Nutrition Values per 100g / 100ml KCAL	PROT	CARB	FAT	FIBRE
Cheddar & Garlic, Mature, Finest, Tesco*	¼ Flatbread/66g	188	6.3	285	7.2	41.8	9.6	2.6
Cheese & Tomato, Tesco*	¼ Pack/54g	160	3.5	295	11.6	45.7	6.4	1.9

Product	Measure INFO/WEIGHT	per Measure KCAL	FAT	Nutrition Values per 100g / 100ml KCAL	PROT	CARB	FAT	FIBRE
FLATBREAD								
Chicken, & Mango, Spiced, Love Life, Waitrose*	1 Pack/174g	298	4.7	171	9.7	26.1	2.7	1.9
Chicken, BBQ, Improved, Shapers, Boots*	1 Pack/165g	268	3.8	162	10.0	25.0	2.3	1.2
Chicken, Tikka, Shapers, Boots*	1 Flatbread/164g	269	4.1	164	11.0	24.0	2.5	1.5
Gluten, Wheat & Milk Free, 4 Pack, Free From, Livwell*	1 Flatbread/55g	148	2.9	269	6.4	53.6	5.3	4.6
Greek Style Salad, Waitrose*	1 Pack/172g	280	8.4	163	7.4	22.3	4.9	3.3
FLAXSEED								
Milled, Organic, Linwoods*	2 Dtsp/30g	170	13.9	568	21.9	1.7	46.2	28.9
Organic, Premium Ground, Prewett's*	1 Tbsp/15g	73	6.0	489	24.0	2.0	40.0	23.0
FLOUR								
Arrowroot, Average	*1oz/28g*	*100*	*0.0*	*357*	*0.3*	*88.2*	*0.1*	*3.4*
Bread, Brown, Strong, Average	*1 Serving/100g*	*311*	*1.8*	*311*	*14.0*	*61.0*	*1.8*	*6.4*
Bread, White, Strong, Average	*1oz/28g*	*94*	*0.4*	*336*	*11.8*	*68.4*	*1.5*	*3.4*
Brown, Chapati, Average	*1 Tbsp/20g*	*67*	*0.2*	*333*	*11.5*	*73.7*	*1.2*	*0.0*
Brown, Wheat	*1oz/28g*	*90*	*0.5*	*323*	*12.6*	*68.5*	*1.8*	*6.4*
Chick Pea	*1oz/28g*	*88*	*1.5*	*313*	*19.7*	*49.6*	*5.4*	*10.7*
GF, Alternative, Wellfoods*	1 Serving/100g	351	1.3	351	1.5	83.1	1.3	2.1
Gram, Stoneground, Gluten & Wheat Free, Dove's Farm*	1 Serving/100g	336	5.0	336	12.8	60.0	5.0	9.7
Millet	*1oz/28g*	*99*	*0.5*	*354*	*5.8*	*75.4*	*1.7*	*0.0*
Peanut, Protein Plus*	¼ Cup/30g	110	4.0	367	53.3	26.7	13.3	13.3
Plain, Average	*1oz/28g*	*98*	*0.4*	*349*	*10.3*	*73.8*	*1.5*	*2.2*
Potato	*1oz/28g*	*92*	*0.3*	*328*	*9.1*	*75.6*	*0.9*	*5.7*
Quinoa	1 Serving/100g	349	5.2	349	14.1	61.4	5.2	3.4
Rice	*1 Tsp/5g*	*18*	*0.0*	*366*	*6.4*	*80.1*	*0.8*	*2.0*
Rye, Whole	*1oz/28g*	*94*	*0.6*	*335*	*8.2*	*75.9*	*2.0*	*11.7*
Soya, Full Fat, Average	*1oz/28g*	*118*	*6.1*	*422*	*37.9*	*19.8*	*21.8*	*11.6*
Soya, Low Fat, Average	*1oz/28g*	*99*	*2.0*	*352*	*45.3*	*28.2*	*7.2*	*13.5*
Speciality GF, Dove's Farm*	1 Serving/100g	353	1.8	353	4.7	85.2	1.8	2.7
Spelt, Average	*1 Serving/57g*	*216*	*1.7*	*381*	*14.3*	*74.5*	*3.0*	*6.4*
Strong, Wholemeal, Average	*1 Serving/100g*	*315*	*2.2*	*315*	*13.2*	*60.6*	*2.2*	*9.0*
White, Average	*1oz/28g*	*89*	*0.3*	*319*	*9.8*	*66.8*	*1.0*	*2.9*
White, Chapati, Average	*1 Tbsp/20g*	*67*	*0.1*	*335*	*9.8*	*77.6*	*0.5*	*0.0*
White, Self Raising, Average	*1oz/28g*	*94*	*0.4*	*336*	*9.9*	*71.8*	*1.3*	*2.9*
White, Self Raising, Gluten & Wheat Free, Dove's Farm*	1 Serving/100g	344	1.0	344	5.5	78.1	1.0	1.4
White, Wheat, Average	*1oz/28g*	*95*	*0.4*	*341*	*10.4*	*76.5*	*1.4*	*3.1*
Wholemeal, Average	*1oz/28g*	*87*	*0.6*	*312*	*12.6*	*61.9*	*2.2*	*9.0*
FLYTE								
Mars*	1 Bar/23g	99	3.2	441	3.4	74.8	14.2	0.0
Snacksize, Mars*	1 Bar/23g	98	3.3	436	3.8	72.5	14.5	0.0
FOCACCIA								
Olive, Rosemary & Siciliano Pesto, Graze*	1 Punnet/40g	128	8.2	321	6.3	27.9	20.6	4.2
FOOL								
Blackcurrant, BGTY, Sainsbury's*	1 Pot/113g	89	2.9	79	3.5	10.4	2.6	0.6
Fruit, Average	1 Pot/120g	196	11.2	163	1.0	20.2	9.3	1.2
Gooseberry, Fruit, BGTY, Sainsbury's*	1 Pot/121g	93	3.4	77	2.9	10.0	2.8	0.8
Gooseberry, Fruit, Somerfield*	1 Pot/114g	215	12.5	189	3.0	19.0	11.0	0.0
Gooseberry, PB, Waitrose*	1 Pot/113g	125	2.9	111	3.6	18.3	2.6	0.7
Gooseberry, Sainsbury's*	1 Pot/113g	214	12.9	189	2.6	19.1	11.4	1.1
Gooseberry, Tesco*	1 Pot/112g	225	14.1	200	3.0	17.8	12.5	0.7
Lemon, Fruit, BGTY, Sainsbury's*	1 Pot/113g	94	3.8	83	3.4	9.7	3.4	0.3
Raspberry, Fruit, Tesco*	1 Pot/113g	234	12.8	207	2.6	23.6	11.3	0.3
Rhubarb, Fruit, Waitrose*	1 Pot/114g	182	12.9	160	2.7	11.9	11.3	0.3
Rhubarb, PB, Waitrose*	1 Pot/113g	101	2.9	89	3.5	13.0	2.6	0.3
Rhubarb, Sainsbury's*	1 Pot/113g	180	12.9	159	2.6	11.5	11.4	0.4

	Measure INFO/WEIGHT	per Measure		Nutrition Values per 100g / 100ml				
		KCAL	FAT	KCAL	PROT	CARB	FAT	FIBRE
FRANKFURTERS								
Average	*1 Frankfurter/42g*	*123*	*11.2*	*292*	*12.0*	*1.3*	*26.6*	*0.0*
FRANKFURTERS VEGETARIAN								
Asda*	1 Frankfurter/27g	54	3.4	199	18.0	3.5	12.5	2.5
Tivall*	1 Sausage/30g	73	4.8	244	18.0	7.0	16.0	3.0
FRAZZLES								
Bacon, Smith's, Walkers*	1 Bag/23g	113	5.3	488	7.5	62.0	23.0	1.3
FRENCH FRIES								
Cheese & Onion, Walkers*	1 Pack/22g	95	3.5	430	5.0	66.0	16.0	5.0
Ready Salted, Walkers*	1 Bag/22g	83	3.0	377	4.5	56.4	13.6	4.5
Salt & Vinegar, BGTY, Sainsbury's*	1 Bag/15g	51	0.2	340	6.0	80.1	1.5	4.1
Salt & Vinegar, Walkers*	1 Bag/22g	95	3.5	430	5.0	66.0	16.0	5.0
Worcester Sauce, Walkers*	1 Bag/22g	96	3.5	435	5.0	65.0	16.0	5.0
FRENCH TOAST								
Asda*	1 Toast/8g	30	0.4	381	10.0	74.0	5.0	4.0
Co-Op*	1 Toast/8g	31	0.5	385	10.0	72.0	6.0	5.0
Morrisons*	1 Toast/8g	31	0.5	393	11.0	72.5	6.6	3.0
Sainsbury's*	1 Toast/8g	31	0.5	382	10.0	72.0	6.6	5.0
FRIDGE RAIDERS								
Chicken, Barbeque Flavour, Bites, Mattessons*	1 Bag/60g	134	7.5	223	20.5	6.5	12.5	1.1
Chicken, Hot And Spicy, Bites, Mattessons*	1 Bag/60g	131	7.3	218	21.1	5.4	12.2	1.1
Chicken, Piri Piri, Bites, Mattessons*	1 Bag/60g	122	7.0	203	19.5	4.9	11.6	0.7
Chicken, Southern Fried, Bites, Mattessons*	1 Bag/60g	133	8.5	221	18.8	4.2	14.2	0.8
Chicken, Tikka Flavour, Bites, Mattessons*	1 Bag/60g	110	6.2	184	19.9	2.0	10.4	1.3
FRIES								
9/16" Straight Cut Home, Deep Fried, McCain*	1oz/28g	65	2.8	233	3.2	32.7	9.9	0.0
9/16" Straight Cut Home, Oven Baked, McCain*	1oz/28g	53	1.5	188	3.2	31.5	5.5	0.0
American, 3 Way Cook, Somerfield*	1oz/28g	43	1.4	155	3.0	25.0	5.0	0.0
American Style, Frozen, Thin, Tesco*	1 Serving/125g	208	10.1	166	2.2	21.1	8.1	1.9
American Style, Slim, Iceland*	1 Serving/100g	187	6.1	187	2.4	30.6	6.1	2.4
Crispy French, Weighed Deep Fried, McCain*	1 Serving/100g	193	8.5	193	1.9	27.4	8.5	0.9
Curly, Cajun, Weighed Frozen, McCain*	1 Portion/100g	156	8.7	156	1.6	17.7	8.7	1.8
Curly, Southern Style, Tesco*	1 Serving/50g	124	3.6	248	3.8	41.7	7.3	3.8
Curly, Twisters, Frozen, Conagra Foods*	1 Serving/150g	273	14.0	182	2.5	22.0	9.3	2.2
Extra Chunky, Oven Baked, Homefries, McCain*	1 Serving/200g	306	6.2	153	3.2	28.0	3.1	2.3
Oven, American Style, Frozen, Asda*	1 Serving/180g	407	14.4	226	3.9	34.6	8.0	4.0
Oven, Straight Cut, Morrisons*	1 Serving/100g	149	4.3	149	2.8	24.6	4.3	2.6
Southern, Oven Cook, Baked, Potato Winners, McCain*	1 Serving/100g	232	8.3	232	3.6	35.7	8.3	2.4
Southern, Oven Cook, Frozen, Potato Winners, McCain*	1 Serving/100g	176	6.7	176	2.4	26.5	6.7	1.6
Southern Spicy Spiral, Deep Fried, McCain*	1oz/28g	58	2.9	208	2.7	26.4	10.2	0.0
Southern Spicy Spiral, Oven Baked, McCain*	1oz/28g	46	1.8	165	1.7	24.6	6.6	0.0
FRISPS								
Tangy Salt & Vinegar, KP Snacks*	1 Bag/30g	160	10.0	532	5.0	52.6	33.5	2.9
Tasty Cheese & Onion, KP Snacks*	1 Bag/28g	150	9.4	537	5.5	53.2	33.6	3.2
FRITTATA								
Vegetable, CBY, Asda*	1 Frittata/150g	183	7.8	122	6.2	12.1	5.2	1.0
FROG								
Legs, Raw, Meat Only	*1oz/28g*	*20*	*0.1*	*73*	*16.4*	*0.0*	*0.3*	*0.0*
FROMAGE FRAIS								
0% Fat, Vitalinea, Danone*	1 Tbsp/28g	14	0.0	50	7.4	4.7	0.1	0.0
Apricot, Layered, Weight Watchers*	1 Pot/100g	46	0.1	46	5.4	5.8	0.1	0.2
Blackberry, Layered, Weight Watchers*	1 Pot/100g	49	0.2	49	5.5	5.7	0.2	0.4
Danone*	100g	73	3.1	73	7.2	3.9	3.1	0.0
Fat Free, Average	*1 Pot/60g*	*35*	*0.1*	*58*	*7.7*	*6.8*	*0.2*	*0.0*

F

FROMAGE FRAIS

	INFO/WEIGHT	KCAL	FAT	KCAL	PROT	CARB	FAT	FIBRE
Forest Fruits, Layered, Weight Watchers*	1 Pot/100g	47	0.2	47	5.5	5.7	0.2	0.4
Fruit on the Bottom, BFY, Morrisons*	1 Pot/100g	66	0.2	66	5.6	10.6	0.2	0.0
Kids, Yeo Valley*	1 Serving/90g	111	4.8	123	6.6	12.6	5.3	0.0
Low Fat, Aldi*	1 Pot/100g	52	0.3	52	5.4	7.1	0.3	0.7
Morrisons*	1 Serving/28g	17	0.0	59	9.8	4.8	0.0	0.0
Munch Bunch, Nestle*	1 Pot/42g	44	1.3	105	6.7	12.6	3.0	0.0
Natural, Fat Free, M&S*	1 Serving/100g	60	0.1	60	9.8	4.8	0.1	0.0
Natural, GFY, Asda*	½ Pot/100g	52	0.3	52	7.3	5.0	0.3	0.0
Natural, Plain, Fat Free, Normandy, BGTY, Sainsbury's*	1 Serving/30g	15	0.0	49	8.0	4.2	0.1	0.0
Natural, Virtually Fat Free, French, Waitrose*	1 Tub/500g	260	1.5	52	7.3	5.0	0.3	0.0
Normandy, LC, Tesco*	1 Serving/100g	46	0.2	46	7.8	3.3	0.2	0.0
Normandy, Sainsbury's*	1 Serving/25g	29	2.0	116	7.7	3.4	8.1	0.0
Organic, Vrai*	1 Serving/100g	83	3.6	83	8.1	4.5	3.6	0.0
Peach, Layered, Weight Watchers*	1 Pot/100g	46	0.1	46	5.0	8.0	0.1	0.0
Plain, Average	*1oz/28g*	*32*	*2.0*	*113*	*6.8*	*5.7*	*7.1*	*0.0*
Raspberry, Layered, Weight Watchers*	1 Pot/100g	47	0.2	47	5.5	5.7	0.2	0.4
Raspberry, Low Fat, Sainsbury's*	1 Pot/90g	96	2.3	107	5.8	15.1	2.6	0.1
Raspberry, Value, Tesco*	1 Serving/60g	56	0.8	93	7.2	13.5	1.3	0.0
Strawberry, 0% Fat, Vitalinea, Danone*	1 Serving/150g	82	0.2	55	6.0	7.4	0.2	1.6
Strawberry, 99.9% Fat Free, Onken*	1 Serving/50g	46	0.0	91	6.9	15.3	0.1	0.0
Strawberry, Layered, Weight Watchers*	1 Pot/100g	50	0.1	50	5.4	6.2	0.1	0.0
Strawberry, Petit Filou, Yoplait*	1 Pot/50g	52	1.4	104	6.7	12.6	2.9	0.2
Strawberry, Value, Tesco*	1 Pot/60g	55	0.8	92	7.2	13.0	1.3	0.0
Vanilla, Danone*	1 Serving/200g	274	8.2	137	5.3	19.6	4.1	0.0
Virtually Fat Free, Tesco*	1 Pot/100g	56	0.1	56	5.6	8.2	0.1	0.0
Wildlife, Strawberry, Raspberry Or Peach, Yoplait*	1 Pot/50g	46	0.6	93	7.1	13.2	1.3	0.2
with Fruit, Average	1 Pot/90g	74	2.2	83	6.1	9.0	2.5	0.8
with Real Fruit Puree, Nestle*	1 Serving/50g	65	1.4	130	7.1	18.9	2.7	0.2

FROZEN DESSERT

	INFO/WEIGHT	KCAL	FAT	KCAL	PROT	CARB	FAT	FIBRE
Vanilla, Too Good to Be True, Wall's Ice Cream*	1 Serving/50ml	35	0.2	70	2.0	14.9	0.4	0.1

FROZEN YOGHURT

	INFO/WEIGHT	KCAL	FAT	KCAL	PROT	CARB	FAT	FIBRE
Angelmoo, Yoomoo*	1 Serving/100g	162	2.7	162	3.9	28.7	2.7	3.8
Cherry Garcia, Low Fat, Ben & Jerry's*	1 Serving/100g	143	2.4	143	3.0	26.0	2.4	1.0
Chocmoo, Yoomoo*	1 Serving/100g	142	1.7	142	3.5	26.0	1.7	4.1
Chocolate, Average	1 Portion/100g	120	1.9	120	4.3	22.0	1.9	2.1
Chocolate, Pinkberry*	1 Pot/140g	168	2.1	120	5.0	23.0	1.5	2.0
Chocolate, Snog*	1 Serving/100g	109	1.6	109	4.5	19.9	1.6	1.7
Chocolate Fudge Brownie, Low Fat, Ben & Jerry's*	1 Serving/100g	180	3.0	180	4.0	34.0	3.0	1.5
Coconut, Pinkberry*	1 Pot/140g	196	0.0	140	4.0	30.0	0.0	0.0
Devilmoo, Yoomoo*	1 Serving/100g	167	2.6	167	3.6	30.4	2.6	3.8
Mango, Pinkberry*	1 Cup/140g	140	0.0	100	3.0	22.0	0.0	0.0
Nakedmoo, Yoomoo*	1 Serving/125g	168	2.0	134	3.3	24.5	1.6	4.1
Natural, Average	1 Portion/100g	101	0.8	101	3.8	19.9	0.8	0.9
Natural, Snog*	1 Serving/100g	89	0.2	89	3.3	18.4	0.2	0.5
Original, Pinkberry*	1 Pot/140g	140	0.0	100	3.0	21.0	0.0	0.0
Passionfruit, Pinkberry*	1 Pot/140g	140	0.0	100	3.0	22.0	0.0	0.0
Peanut Butter, Pinkberry*	1 Pot/140g	238	9.8	170	7.0	23.0	7.0	1.0
Phish Food, Lower Fat, Ben & Jerry's*	½ Pot/211g	464	10.6	220	4.0	40.0	5.0	1.5
Pomegranate, Pinkberry*	1 Pot/140g	168	0.0	120	3.0	26.0	0.0	0.0
Raspberry, Handmade Farmhouse, Sainsbury's*	1 Serving/100g	132	3.8	132	2.7	21.8	3.8	2.2
Salted Caramel, Pinkberry*	1 Pot/140g	168	0.0	120	4.0	26.0	0.0	0.0
Strawberry, Average	1 Portion/100g	114	2.2	114	2.6	21.2	2.2	0.5
Strawberry, Tesco*	1 Pot/60g	82	1.3	136	2.6	26.5	2.2	0.8

	Measure INFO/WEIGHT	per Measure		Nutrition Values per 100g / 100ml				
		KCAL	FAT	KCAL	PROT	CARB	FAT	FIBRE
FROZEN YOGHURT								
Strawberry Cheesecake, Low Fat, Ben & Jerry's*	1 Serving/100g	170	3.0	170	4.0	31.0	3.0	1.0
Strawbmoo, Yoomoo*	1 Serving/100g	133	1.5	133	3.2	24.7	1.5	4.1
Tropicoolmoo, Yoomoo*	1 Pot/92g	136	1.2	148	2.8	29.4	1.3	3.6
Vanilla, Less Than 5% Fat, Tesco*	1 Pot/120g	179	2.9	149	8.1	23.8	2.4	0.7
Vanilla Bean & Honey, Yog*	1 Serving/100g	93	1.9	93	3.1	14.3	1.9	0.5
FRUIT								
Apple, Pineapple & Grape, Ready to Eat, Sainsbury's*	1 Pack/180g	94	0.2	52	0.5	8.3	0.1	1.3
Apple & Pear, Snack Pack, Great Stuff, Asda*	1 Pack/80g	42	0.1	52	0.4	11.0	0.1	2.6
Apples & Grape, Snack Pack, Fresh, Tesco*	1 Pack/80g	44	0.1	55	0.3	12.3	0.1	2.6
Baked, Nibbles, Mango Pineapple, We Are Bear*	1 Bag/30g	85	0.0	285	1.4	73.0	0.2	11.0
Bananito, Fresh, Raw, Tesco*	1 Fruit/40g	38	0.1	95	1.2	23.2	0.3	1.1
Berries, Mixed, Frozen, Creative Gourmet*	1 Serving/100g	57	1.0	57	1.1	10.4	1.0	4.1
Berry Medley, Freshly Prepared, M&S*	1 Pack/180g	90	0.4	50	0.7	10.9	0.2	2.9
Black Forest, Frozen, Tesco*	1 Serving/80g	37	0.0	46	0.8	10.5	0.0	1.8
Fabulous Fruity Fingers, Melon & Mango, M&S*	1 Pack/240g	96	0.5	40	0.6	8.2	0.2	1.0
Grapefruit & Orange Segments, Breakfast, Del Monte*	1 Can/411g	193	0.4	47	1.0	10.2	0.1	1.0
Juicy Twist, Tesco*	1 Pack/170g	71	0.3	42	0.4	9.6	0.2	1.2
Melon, Kiwi Fruit & Strawberries, Fresh Tastes, Asda*	1 Pack/240g	96	0.5	40	0.8	7.7	0.2	2.1
Melon, Pineapple & Mango Fingers, Waitrose*	1 Pot/160g	82	0.3	51	0.7	11.6	0.2	1.2
Melon, Wedges, Snack Pack, Tesco*	1 Pack/90g	17	0.1	19	0.4	4.1	0.1	0.6
Melon & Grape, Sainsbury's*	½ Pack/200g	66	0.2	33	0.5	7.1	0.1	0.7
Melon & Grape, Snack Pack, Tesco*	1 Pack/90g	34	0.0	38	0.5	9.0	0.0	0.7
Melon & Grape Munchies, Eat Well, M&S*	½ Pack/200g	70	0.2	35	0.5	8.3	0.1	0.7
Melon & Grape Pot, Co-Op*	1 Pot/125g	44	0.1	35	0.6	7.0	0.1	0.9
Melon & Grapes, Morrisons*	1 Pack/360g	112	0.4	31	0.6	6.4	0.1	0.8
Melon & Pineapple, Fingers, Sainsbury's*	1 Pack/240g	74	0.2	31	0.5	6.5	0.1	0.8
Mixed, Fresh, 5 a Day, Tesco*	1 Pack/400g	136	0.8	34	0.8	7.4	0.2	1.4
Mixed, Fresh, Tesco*	1 Pack/200g	70	0.4	35	0.8	7.4	0.2	1.4
Mixed, Fruitime, Pieces, Tesco*	1 Can/140g	84	0.0	60	0.4	14.0	0.0	1.0
Mixed, Pieces, in Orange Jelly, Fruitini, Del Monte*	1 Can/140g	94	0.1	67	0.3	15.8	0.1	0.0
Mixed, Tropical, Fruit Express, Del Monte*	1 Pot/185g	89	0.2	48	0.2	11.2	0.1	1.2
Outrageously Orange Melon, M&S*	1 Pack/180g	36	0.2	20	0.6	4.2	0.1	0.8
Peach, Slices, Frozen, Sainsbury's*	1 Serving/80g	30	0.0	37	1.0	7.6	0.0	1.5
Peach Pieces in Fruit Juice, Tesco*	1 Pot/125g	60	0.0	48	0.4	11.7	0.0	1.0
Pieces, Mixed in Fruit Juice, Fruitini, Del Monte*	1 Serving/120g	61	0.1	51	0.4	12.0	0.1	0.5
Pineapple, Fingers, Snack Pack, Tesco*	1 Pack/70g	31	0.1	44	0.4	10.1	0.2	2.0
Pineapple, Grape & Kiwi, Fresh Tastes, Asda*	1 Pack/200g	106	0.6	53	0.6	11.0	0.3	1.8
Pineapple, Mango & Nectarine, Fresh Tastes, Asda*	1 Pack/240g	127	0.5	53	0.8	11.0	0.2	2.1
Pineapple & Mango Tango, Eat Well, M&S*	1 Pack/200g	100	0.8	50	1.0	22.2	0.4	2.6
Pineapple Pot, CBY, Asda*	1 Pot/200g	106	0.0	53	0.4	12.5	0.0	0.7
Pink Lady Apple & Grape, Snack Pack, Tesco*	1 Pack/80g	44	0.1	55	0.3	12.3	0.1	2.6
Rolls, Peach, Yo Yo, Bear*	1 Roll/10g	28	0.0	275	1.4	72.0	0.2	10.0
Snack, Sweet Grape, Shapers, Boots*	1 Pack/80g	53	0.1	66	0.4	15.0	0.1	1.0
Snack Pack, Fresh, Sainsbury's*	1 Serving/120g	54	0.1	45	0.1	11.0	0.1	1.3
Strawberries, Apple & Grapes, Fresh Tastes, Asda*	1 Pot/190g	91	0.2	48	0.5	10.6	0.1	0.0
Strawberries, Coconut & Chocolate, Pret a Manger*	1 Serving/125g	194	15.8	155	2.0	8.2	12.6	4.6
Summer Berries, M&S*	1 Pack/160g	80	0.3	50	0.7	10.0	0.2	3.0
Tropical, Tesco*	1 Pack/180g	85	0.4	47	0.6	10.8	0.2	1.9
Tropical in Juice, Dole*	1 Pot/113g	59	0.0	52	0.3	14.2	0.0	1.8
Tropical Sticks, Costa*	1 Pack/210g	86	0.0	41	0.8	8.4	0.0	1.9
Tutti Frutti Collection, Freshly Prepared, Tesco*	1 Pack/200g	86	0.4	43	0.6	9.1	0.2	1.4
FRUIT & NUT MIX								
After Dinner Mint, Graze*	1 Pack/42g	203	12.2	483	10.0	42.0	29.0	7.0

FRUIT & NUT MIX	Measure INFO/WEIGHT	per Measure KCAL	FAT	Nutrition Values per 100g / 100ml KCAL	PROT	CARB	FAT	FIBRE
Almond, Raisin & Berry, Sainsbury's*	1 Bag/50g	188	7.2	377	6.1	57.6	14.3	4.2
Almonds & Raisins, Love Life, Waitrose*	1 Pack/150g	681	42.6	454	11.6	38.1	28.4	4.7
Bakewell Tart, Graze*	1 Pack/37g	154	8.1	416	8.9	48.3	21.8	4.7
Banana Split, Graze*	1 Punnet/35g	160	8.6	458	12.3	50.3	24.7	2.8
Banoffee Pie, Graze*	1 Punnet/33g	154	9.1	468	6.9	48.0	27.6	6.6
Billionaire's Shortbread, Graze*	1 Punnet/38g	177	9.5	465	7.8	53.0	24.9	4.3
Bounty Hunter, Graze*	1 Punnet/31g	145	8.2	473	4.0	54.4	26.8	5.6
Cacao Vine, Graze*	1 Punnet/45g	187	9.4	416	8.5	51.4	20.8	0.0
Cherries, Raisins & Nuts, Love Life, Waitrose*	1 Serving/30g	132	7.5	439	7.7	45.8	25.0	3.4
Date & Banana Loaf, Graze*	1 Punnet/41g	132	1.8	327	3.3	68.3	4.4	6.3
Dried, Selection, Wholesome, Love Life, Waitrose*	1 Serving/30g	144	9.6	479	9.8	38.0	32.0	4.4
Eleanor's Apple Crumble, Graze*	1 Pack/32g	115	4.0	356	6.4	62.0	12.5	8.0
Eton Mess, Graze*	1 Punnet/33g	140	4.6	420	5.4	67.5	13.9	4.5
Exotic, Waitrose*	1 Serving/50g	207	8.8	414	9.0	54.6	17.7	4.6
Flapjack, Fruit & Seed, Graze*	1 Punnet/54g	225	11.0	417	5.2	54.7	20.4	4.3
Fruit Squash, Graze*	1 Pack/41g	183	9.7	451	13.4	47.5	23.8	6.4
Grandma's Apple Crumble, Graze*	1 Punnet/40g	154	7.8	385	0.0	48.9	19.6	4.0
Honeycomb Crunch, Graze*	1 Punnet/40g	181	10.2	452	9.8	48.0	25.4	3.2
Jaffa Cake, Graze*	1 Punnet/44g	210	13.7	476	6.8	43.1	31.0	5.1
Jungle Fever, Graze*	1 Pack/30g	135	8.3	449	7.4	42.3	27.8	6.8
Jungle Trekker, Kids, Graze*	1 Punnet/32g	137	5.8	427	10.0	56.0	18.0	5.0
Limoncello, Graze*	1 Punnet/41g	162	8.4	396	6.3	50.6	20.6	4.3
Luxury, Asda*	1 Serving/50g	226	15.2	451	9.0	33.5	30.5	7.4
M & S*	1 Serving/30g	135	7.6	450	12.4	44.3	25.3	6.0
Marvellous Macaroon, Graze*	1 Pack/28g	158	11.4	566	10.7	37.4	40.9	4.7
Nuts & Raisins, Mixed, Natural, Love Life, Waitrose*	1 Serving/50g	258	16.4	515	16.5	38.4	32.8	7.2
Organic, Waitrose*	1 Pack/100g	489	32.6	489	15.0	33.8	32.6	5.4
Peanuts & Flame Raisins, Wholefoods, Tesco*	1 Serving/30g	142	8.3	475	18.6	34.7	27.8	4.5
Pure Vitality, Graze*	1 Punnet/45g	151	6.4	337	11.2	46.0	14.3	9.5
Seed, Nut & Sultana Sprinkle, Love Life, Waitrose*	1 Serving/30g	177	15.4	591	17.2	15.4	51.2	4.3
Shangri-la, Graze*	1 Punnet/29g	132	8.3	454	15.7	38.2	28.5	8.5
Strawberry Milkshake, Graze*	1 Pack/35g	135	4.0	385	3.6	66.6	11.3	5.2
Sun Dance, Graze*	1 Punnet/38g	136	3.8	358	4.3	67.2	9.9	4.5
The Mix, Whitworths*	1 Pot/90g	341	13.1	379	4.1	63.1	14.6	7.3
Trail Mix, Average	1oz/28g	121	8.0	432	9.1	37.2	28.5	4.3
Trail Mix, Love Life, Waitrose*	1 Portion/30g	126	9.3	506	14.2	28.5	37.2	6.3
Unsalted, Tesco*	1 Serving/25g	112	4.6	449	12.6	58.1	18.5	12.2
Vanilla, Cherry, Frangipane, Graze*	1 Punnet/39g	201	13.2	516	15.0	38.0	34.0	6.0
Walnut & Vanilla Truffle, Graze*	1 Punnet/38g	187	12.1	496	10.0	43.9	32.2	6.0
White Chocolate & Raspberry Cheesecake, Graze*	1 Punnet/39g	204	13.7	524	7.5	44.7	35.1	4.5
Ying & Yang, Graze*	1 Pack/60g	296	19.5	493	6.8	41.2	32.5	0.0
FRUIT COCKTAIL								
Fresh & Ready, Sainsbury's*	1 Pack/300g	117	0.3	39	0.6	9.0	0.1	1.2
in Apple Juice, Asda*	1/3 Can/80g	40	0.1	50	0.3	12.0	0.1	1.6
in Fruit Juice, Sainsbury's*	1 Serving/198g	97	0.2	49	0.3	11.9	0.1	1.3
in Juice, Del Monte*	1 Can/415g	203	0.4	49	0.4	11.2	0.1	0.0
in Light Syrup, Princes*	1 Serving/206g	64	0.0	31	0.4	7.3	0.0	1.0
in Syrup, Del Monte*	1 Can/420g	315	0.4	75	0.4	18.0	0.1	0.0
No Added Sugar, Asda*	1 Serving/134g	67	0.1	50	0.3	12.0	0.1	1.6
FRUIT COMPOTE								
Apple, Strawberry & Blackberry, Organic, Yeo Valley*	½ Pot/112g	73	0.1	65	0.5	15.5	0.1	1.9
Apricot & Prune, Yeo Valley*	1 Pot/225g	207	0.2	92	0.6	22.3	0.1	1.6
Spiced, Tesco*	1 Serving/112g	122	0.6	109	1.7	24.4	0.5	3.1

	Measure INFO/WEIGHT	per Measure KCAL	FAT	Nutrition Values per 100g / 100ml KCAL	PROT	CARB	FAT	FIBRE
FRUIT COMPOTE								
Strawberry & Raspberry, M&S*	1 Serving/80g	72	0.1	90	0.7	23.5	0.1	2.3
Summerfruit, M&S*	¼ Pot/125g	119	0.8	95	0.9	22.7	0.6	0.8
FRUIT DRINK								
Alive Tropical Torrent, Coca-Cola*	1 Glass/200ml	88	0.0	44	0.0	11.0	0.0	0.0
Cherryade, No Added Sugar, Morrisons*	1 Glass/250ml	2	0.0	1	0.0	0.1	0.0	0.0
Pineapple, Sparkling, KA, Barr's*	1 Can/330ml	168	0.0	51	0.0	12.5	0.0	0.0
Sparkling Pink Grapefruit, Shapers, Boots*	1 Serving/200ml	6	0.0	3	0.0	0.3	0.0	0.0
FRUIT FLAKES								
Blackcurrant with Yoghurt Coating, Fruit Bowl*	1 Bag/25g	112	5.1	449	1.7	64.2	20.6	0.0
Raisins with Yoghurt Coating, Fruit Bowl*	1 Pack/30g	133	5.6	440	2.9	66.6	18.4	2.0
Raspberry with Yoghurt Coating, Fruit Bowl*	1 Serving/25g	112	5.2	449	1.7	64.2	20.6	0.0
Strawberry, Fruit Bowl*	1 Pack/20g	66	0.4	330	1.0	78.0	2.0	2.0
Strawberry with Yoghurt Coating, Fruit Bowl*	1 Serving/25g	112	5.2	449	1.7	64.2	20.6	0.0
FRUIT GUMS								
Rowntree's*	1 Tube/49g	170	0.1	344	4.8	81.3	0.2	0.0
FRUIT MEDLEY								
Dried, Tropical, Soft, Love Life, Waitrose*	1 Serving/30g	86	0.0	288	0.2	70.6	0.0	2.5
Exotic, Co-Op*	1 Serving/120g	54	0.2	45	0.6	10.0	0.2	0.0
Fresh, Tesco*	1 Pack/200g	86	0.2	43	0.4	10.0	0.1	1.1
in Fresh Orange Juice, Co-Op*	1 Serving/140g	49	0.0	35	0.5	9.0	0.0	0.0
Mango, Melon, Kiwi & Blueberry, Fresh, M&S*	1 Pack/260g	104	0.8	40	0.7	9.1	0.3	1.6
Melon & Grape, Somerfield*	1 Serving/200g	70	0.2	35	0.5	8.0	0.1	0.7
Nectarine, Mango & Blueberry, Fresh, M&S*	1 Pack/245g	122	0.5	50	1.0	11.1	0.2	2.1
Shapers, Boots*	1 Pack/140g	55	0.3	39	0.7	8.6	0.2	1.0
FRUIT MIX								
Apple Cosmo, Graze*	1 Punnet/34g	100	0.2	292	1.5	69.8	0.7	4.6
Banana, Coconut & Mango, Dried, Graze*	1 Punnet/45g	144	3.7	320	18.7	57.1	8.2	0.0
Banana Coins, Graze*	1 Serving/20g	49	0.1	245	2.4	54.0	0.6	0.0
Berry, Sainsbury's*	1 Serving/20g	64	0.4	319	1.0	78.1	1.9	5.5
Forest Fruit, Dried, Graze*	1 Pack/50g	160	0.4	319	1.8	76.0	0.8	0.0
Frozen, Blueberries & Strawberries, Sainsbury's*	1 Portion/75g	26	0.2	34	0.7	6.5	0.2	1.5
Love Mix, Graze*	1 Pack/40g	99	0.4	245	4.0	58.0	0.9	5.9
Melon, Strawberry & Grape, Sainsbury's*	1 Pack/180g	58	0.4	32	0.5	7.0	0.2	0.4
Nectarine, Raspberry & Blueberry, Seasonal, M&S*	1 Pack/160g	72	0.3	45	1.3	8.3	0.2	2.7
Pineapple, Kiwi, Mango & Blueberry, Waitrose*	1 Pack/330g	208	1.0	63	0.7	14.5	0.3	1.9
Pineapple, Melon, Mango, Tesco*	1 Pack/440g	242	0.9	55	1.1	11.4	0.2	1.3
Scandi Berries, Graze*	1 Punnet/23g	61	0.1	270	1.6	65.3	0.6	6.6
Sour Mango Tangtastic, Graze*	1 Pack/34g	110	0.2	323	1.3	79.8	0.6	2.0
Strawberries, Raspberries & Blackberries, Morrisons*	1 Serving/80g	30	0.2	37	0.9	7.3	0.2	1.6
Summer Fruits, British, Frozen, Waitrose*	1 Pack/380g	99	0.8	26	1.0	5.2	0.2	5.5
Summer Pudding, Graze*	1 Punnet/32g	109	0.4	342	1.6	81.2	1.2	4.2
Super Berry Detox, Graze*	1 Punnet/43g	129	0.3	299	1.7	73.9	0.7	3.4
Tropical, Fresh, Waitrose*	1 Pack/240g	122	0.5	51	0.6	11.6	0.2	1.9
Tutti Frutti, Graze*	1 Punnet/41g	120	0.4	293	1.9	72.3	0.9	4.0
FRUIT PUREE								
Apple & Blueberry, Organic, Clearspring*	1 Tub/100g	76	0.3	76	0.4	17.8	0.3	0.0
Apple & Blueberry, Organix*	1 Pot/100g	54	0.6	54	0.4	11.6	0.6	2.5
Apple & Peach, Organix*	1 Pot/100g	49	0.3	49	0.6	11.0	0.3	2.1
Banana, Apple & Apricot, Organix*	1 Pot/100g	68	0.4	68	0.8	15.4	0.4	2.0
FRUIT SALAD								
Apple, Orange, Pineapple & Grape, Morrisons*	1 Serving/64g	40	0.1	62	0.8	13.1	0.1	2.6
Apple, Pineapple & Grape, Sweet & Tangy, Sainsbury's*	1 Pack/180g	70	0.2	39	0.5	8.3	0.1	1.3
Autumn, Fresh, M&S*	½ Pack/160g	64	0.2	40	0.7	9.4	0.1	2.9

F

FRUIT SALAD

	Measure INFO/WEIGHT	per Measure KCAL	FAT	Nutrition Values per 100g / 100ml KCAL	PROT	CARB	FAT	FIBRE
Berry, Asda*	1 Pack/250g	122	0.2	49	0.6	10.9	0.1	0.0
Berry, Seasonal, Asda*	1 Pack/300g	93	0.3	31	0.6	7.0	0.1	2.1
Chunky in Fruit Juice, Canned, John West*	1 Can/411g	193	0.8	47	0.4	11.0	0.2	0.8
Citrus, Fresh, M&S*	½ Pack/225g	79	0.2	35	0.9	7.7	0.1	1.5
Classic, Co-Op*	1 Box/285g	142	0.3	50	0.6	11.0	0.1	2.3
Classic, Fresh, Prepared, Sainsbury's*	1 Pack/320g	157	0.3	49	0.6	10.3	0.1	2.0
Classic, Shapers, Boots*	1 Pack/200g	75	0.2	38	0.7	8.5	0.1	1.3
Exotic, Fresh, Tesco*	1 Serving/225g	86	0.4	38	0.7	8.4	0.2	1.5
Exotic, Fully Prepared, Sainsbury's*	1 Serving/200g	74	0.4	37	0.6	8.3	0.2	1.3
Exotic, Morrisons*	1 Serving/150g	78	0.3	52	0.6	12.2	0.2	0.0
Exotic, Waitrose*	1 Pack/300g	126	0.6	42	0.6	9.5	0.2	1.1
Exotic with Melon, Mango, Kiwi Fruit & Grapes, Asda*	1 Pot/300g	141	0.9	47	0.6	10.5	0.3	1.4
Fresh, Morrisons*	1 Tub/350g	150	0.4	43	0.7	9.9	0.1	0.0
Fresh, Tesco*	1 Pack/200g	84	0.4	42	0.7	9.3	0.2	1.5
Fresh, Washed, Ready to Eat, Tesco*	1 Pack/200g	92	0.2	46	0.7	10.6	0.1	1.6
Fresh for You, Tesco*	1 Pack/160g	59	0.3	37	0.6	8.2	0.2	1.1
Freshly Prepared, M&S*	1 Pack/350g	140	0.7	40	0.5	9.3	0.2	1.0
Fruit Crunch, Salad Bowl, M&S*	½ Pack/120g	174	4.1	145	3.1	25.5	3.4	0.6
Homemade, Unsweetened, Average	1 Serving/140g	77	0.1	55	0.7	13.8	0.1	1.5
Juicy Melon, Pineapple & Grapes, Asda*	1 Pot/300g	111	0.3	37	0.5	8.4	0.1	0.9
Kiwi, Pineapple & Grape, Fresh Tastes, Asda*	1 Pack/200g	106	0.6	53	0.6	11.0	0.3	1.8
Layered, Tropical Rainbow, Freshly Prepared, M&S*	1 Pack/375g	206	1.1	55	0.7	12.6	0.3	1.7
Luxury, Frozen, Boylans*	1 Serving/100g	54	0.2	54	0.8	12.7	0.2	0.0
Mango, Kiwi, Blueberry & Pomegranate, Fresh, M&S*	1 Pack/350g	210	1.0	60	0.9	13.4	0.3	2.4
Melon, Kiwi, Strawberry, WTF Sainsbury's*	1 Pack/245g	74	0.5	30	0.8	6.3	0.2	1.3
Melon, Pineapple & Grapes, Fresh, Tesco*	1 Pack/300g	120	0.3	40	0.5	9.2	0.1	1.0
Melon & Grapes, Shapers, Boots*	1 Pack/220g	75	0.2	34	0.6	7.7	0.1	0.8
Melon & Mango, Shapers, Boots*	1 Pack/80g	29	0.1	36	0.6	7.8	0.1	1.2
Melon & Red Grape, Freshly Prepared, M&S*	1 Pack/450g	158	0.4	35	0.5	8.4	0.1	0.7
Mixed, Average	1 Bowl/100g	42	0.2	42	0.6	9.4	0.2	1.5
Mixed, Food to Go, M&S*	1 Pack/400g	400	1.2	100	0.9	23.3	0.3	2.8
Mixed, Fresh, Sainsbury's*	1 Pack/200g	84	0.4	42	0.7	9.4	0.2	1.9
Mixed, Tesco*	1 Pack/225g	86	0.4	38	0.7	8.3	0.2	1.3
Oranges, Apple, Pineapple & Grapes, Fresh, Asda*	1 Pack/260g	120	0.3	46	0.6	10.5	0.1	2.1
Papaya, Mango & Lime, Love Life, Waitrose*	½ Pack/100g	60	0.2	60	0.6	13.0	0.2	1.9
Pineapple, Apple & Strawberries, Tesco*	1 Pack/190g	80	0.2	42	0.4	9.8	0.1	1.4
Pineapple, Mango, Apple & Grape, Waitrose*	1 Pack/300g	186	0.6	62	0.5	14.7	0.2	1.7
Pineapple, Mango & Passion Fruit, Prepared, M&S*	1 Pack/400g	200	0.8	50	0.7	10.8	0.2	1.8
Plum, Blackberries, & Fig, Tesco*	1 Pot/260g	109	0.5	42	0.8	8.2	0.2	2.5
Radiant Rainbow, Layered, Eat Well, M&S*	1 Pack/350g	140	0.7	40	0.5	9.1	0.2	0.9
Rainbow, Asda*	1 Pack/350g	140	1.0	40	0.6	8.8	0.3	1.4
Seasonal, Fresh, Asda*	1 Pack/125g	55	0.1	44	0.5	10.4	0.1	1.2
Seasonal Melon & Grapes, Asda*	½ Pack/200g	66	1.0	33	0.5	7.5	0.5	0.4
Shapers, Boots*	1 Pack/140g	55	0.3	39	0.7	8.6	0.2	1.0
Sharing, Fresh Tastes, Asda*	1 Pack/450g	220	0.9	49	0.4	10.4	0.2	0.0
Strawberry & Blueberry, Asda*	1 Pack/240g	86	0.2	36	0.9	7.0	0.1	1.5
Summer, Red, Fresh, M&S*	1 Pack/400g	160	0.8	40	0.0	10.0	0.2	1.2
Sunshine, Fresh, M&S*	1 Serving/200g	70	0.2	35	0.0	8.3	0.1	1.3
Tropical, Fresh, Asda*	1 Pack/400g	164	0.8	41	0.7	9.0	0.2	1.8

FRUIT SHOOT

	Measure INFO/WEIGHT	per Measure KCAL	FAT	Nutrition Values per 100g / 100ml KCAL	PROT	CARB	FAT	FIBRE
Apple, Low Sugar, Robinson's*	1 Bottle/200ml	14	0.0	7	0.0	1.2	0.0	0.0
Apple & Blackcurrant, Robinson's*	1 Bottle/200ml	10	0.0	5	0.1	0.8	0.0	0.0

	Measure INFO/WEIGHT	per Measure KCAL	FAT	Nutrition Values per 100g / 100ml KCAL	PROT	CARB	FAT	FIBRE
FRUIT SPREAD								
Blackcurrant, Weight Watchers*	1 Tsp/6g	6	0.0	106	0.2	26.3	0.0	0.9
Blueberry, High, St Dalfour*	1 Tsp/15g	34	0.0	228	0.5	56.0	0.2	2.2
Cherries & Berries, Organic, Meridian Foods*	1 Tbsp/15g	16	0.0	109	0.5	26.0	0.3	1.1
Cherry & Berry, Meridian Foods*	1 Serving/10g	14	0.1	138	0.7	33.7	0.6	3.2
Orange, Seville, Weight Watchers*	1 Tsp/15g	17	0.0	111	0.2	27.5	0.0	0.3
Raspberry, Weight Watchers*	1 Tsp/6g	7	0.0	111	0.4	27.1	0.1	0.9
Raspberry & Cranberry, No Added Sugar, Superjam*	1 Spread/10g	22	0.0	216	2.1	47.0	0.3	0.0
Strawberry, Weight Watchers*	1 Tbsp/15g	23	0.0	156	0.7	39.8	0.1	1.8
FU YUNG								
Egg, Average	1oz/28g	67	5.8	239	9.9	2.2	20.6	1.3
FUDGE								
All Butter, Finest, Tesco*	1 Sweet/10g	43	1.4	429	1.3	73.4	14.5	0.0
Butter, Milk, Thorntons*	1 Sweet/13g	60	2.5	462	3.7	68.5	19.2	0.0
Butter Tablet, Thorntons*	1oz/28g	116	3.1	414	0.9	77.6	11.1	0.0
Cadbury*	1 Bar/25g	115	4.0	440	2.4	73.7	15.3	0.4
Chocolate, Average	1 Sweet/30g	132	4.1	441	3.3	81.1	13.7	0.0
Chocolate, Double, Bar, M&S*	1 Bar/43g	202	9.0	470	4.2	66.9	21.0	0.7
Chocolate, Thorntons*	1 Bag/100g	459	19.1	459	3.1	69.0	19.1	0.6
Chunks, for Baking	1 Serving/100g	428	12.2	428	1.7	77.2	12.2	0.6
Chunks, Home Cooking, Asda*	1 Portion/10g	45	1.3	446	1.5	79.7	13.2	1.1
Chunks, Mini, Sainsbury's*	1 Pack/100g	409	11.3	409	1.9	74.8	11.3	0.0
Clotted Cream, M&S*	1oz/28g	133	6.2	474	1.7	67.6	22.1	0.0
Clotted Cream, Sainsbury's*	1 Sweet/8g	35	0.9	430	1.9	81.5	10.7	0.7
Dairy, Co-Op*	1 Sweet/9g	39	1.2	430	2.0	76.0	13.0	0.0
Devon, Somerfield*	1 Pack/250g	1060	27.8	424	2.0	78.9	11.1	0.0
Pure Indulgence, Thorntons*	1 Bar/45g	210	9.9	466	1.8	65.9	21.9	0.0
Vanilla, Bar, M&S*	1 Bar/43g	205	10.0	476	3.7	63.0	23.3	0.4
Vanilla, Thorntons*	1 Bag/100g	465	21.9	465	1.8	65.9	21.9	0.0
FUSE								
Cadbury*	1 Bar/49g	238	12.2	485	7.6	58.2	24.8	0.0
FUSILLI								
Chickpea, Dell'ugo*	1 Serving/100g	275	2.4	275	19.2	38.1	2.4	12.1
Cooked, Average	**1 Serving/210g**	**248**	**1.4**	**118**	**4.2**	**23.8**	**0.6**	**1.2**
Dry, Average	**1 Serving/90g**	**316**	**1.4**	**352**	**12.3**	**72.0**	**1.6**	**2.2**
Fresh, Cooked, Average	**1 Serving/200g**	**329**	**3.6**	**164**	**6.4**	**30.6**	**1.8**	**1.8**
Fresh, Dry, Average	**1 Serving/75g**	**208**	**2.0**	**277**	**10.9**	**53.4**	**2.7**	**2.1**
Maize & Rice, Gluten & Wheat Free, Dove's Farm*	1 Serving/75g	260	0.7	347	7.0	76.0	0.9	2.4
Tricolore, Dry, Average	**1 Serving/75g**	**264**	**1.3**	**351**	**12.2**	**71.8**	**1.7**	**2.7**
Whole Wheat, Dry Weight, Average	**1 Serving/90g**	**290**	**2.1**	**322**	**13.1**	**62.3**	**2.3**	**9.0**
FYBOGEL								
Lemon, Reckitt Benckiser*	1 Serving/4g	4	0.0	95	2.4	11.3	1.1	64.8
Orange, Reckitt Benckiser*	1 Serving/4g	5	0.0	106	2.4	12.7	1.1	64.4

F

	Measure INFO/WEIGHT	per Measure KCAL	per Measure FAT	Nutrition Values per 100g / 100ml KCAL	PROT	CARB	FAT	FIBRE
GALANGAL								
Raw, Root, Average	100g	71	0.6	71	1.2	15.3	0.6	2.4
GALAXY								
Bubbles Filled, Chocolate Egg, Galaxy, Mars*	1 Egg/28g	155	9.5	555	6.5	54.7	34.1	1.5
Caramel, Mars*	1 Bar/49g	254	13.0	518	5.8	64.2	26.4	0.0
Caramel Crunch, Promises, Mars*	1 Bar/100g	540	31.8	540	6.1	57.5	31.8	0.0
Cookie Crumble, Mars*	1 Bar/119g	658	40.5	553	6.0	55.0	34.0	2.0
Fruit & Hazelnut, Milk, Mars*	1 Bar/47g	235	13.2	501	7.1	55.2	28.0	0.0
Hazelnut, Mars*	1 Piece/6g	37	2.5	582	7.8	49.4	39.2	0.0
Swirls, Mars*	1 Bag/150g	747	39.8	498	4.9	60.2	26.5	0.0
GAMMON								
Breaded, Average	1oz/28g	34	0.9	120	22.5	1.0	3.0	0.0
Dry Cured, Ready to Roast, M&S*	½ Joint/255g	255	3.8	100	20.5	0.5	1.5	0.5
Honey & Mustard, Average	½ Pack/190g	294	13.5	155	19.1	3.6	7.1	0.1
Joint, Applewood Smoked, Tesco*	1 Serving/100g	152	9.0	152	17.5	0.2	9.0	0.0
Joint, Boiled, Average	*1 Serving/60g*	*122*	*7.4*	*204*	*23.3*	*0.0*	*12.3*	*0.0*
Joint, Dry Cure, Sticky Caramel Glaze, Waitrose*	1/3 Pack/183g	458	28.7	250	14.5	12.6	15.7	1.4
Joint, Raw, Average	*1 Serving/100g*	*138*	*7.5*	*138*	*17.5*	*0.0*	*7.5*	*0.0*
Joint, with Sweet Maple Syrup Glaze, As Sold, Waitrose*	1 Serving/100g	211	12.6	211	14.1	10.2	12.6	0.9
Steaks, Average	*1 Steak/97g*	*157*	*7.1*	*161*	*23.3*	*0.4*	*7.4*	*0.0*
Steaks, Healthy Range, Average	*1 Serving/110g*	*107*	*3.5*	*97*	*18.0*	*0.4*	*3.2*	*0.2*
Steaks, Honey Roast, Average	*1 Steak/100g*	*142*	*5.3*	*142*	*21.5*	*2.3*	*5.3*	*0.0*
Steaks, Pineapple & Mango, Easy to Cook, Waitrose*	1 Steak/163g	239	11.6	146	14.1	6.5	7.1	0.5
Steaks, Smoked, Average	*1 Steak/110g*	*150*	*5.5*	*137*	*22.7*	*0.1*	*5.0*	*0.1*
Steaks, with Egg & Fries	1 Serving/540g	684	26.9	127	10.3	10.1	5.0	0.0
GAMMON &								
Parsley Sauce, Steak, Tesco*	½ Pack/140g	217	7.3	155	23.7	2.9	5.2	0.5
Pineapple, 228, Oakhouse Foods Ltd*	1 Meal/360g	284	4.0	79	7.1	10.9	1.1	1.7
GAMMON WITH								
Cheese Sauce & Crumb, Steaks, Simply Cook, Tesco*	½ Pack/156g	218	12.0	140	14.2	3.1	7.7	1.0
GARAM MASALA								
Dry, Ground, Average	*1 Tbsp/15g*	*57*	*2.3*	*379*	*15.6*	*45.2*	*15.1*	*0.0*
GARLIC								
Crushed, Frozen, Taj*	1 Block/18g	18	0.1	102	7.5	14.0	0.6	4.0
Minced, Nishaan*	1 Tsp/5g	5	0.0	97	6.0	16.2	0.9	0.0
Pickled, Bevellini*	1 Serving/12g	5	0.0	42	2.5	0.8	0.1	0.0
Powder, Average	*1 Tsp/3g*	*7*	*0.0*	*246*	*18.7*	*42.7*	*1.2*	*9.9*
Raw, Average	*1 Clove/3g*	*3*	*0.0*	*98*	*7.9*	*16.3*	*0.6*	*2.1*
Spice Blend, Gourmet Garden*	1 Squeeze/10ml	32	2.4	210	4.5	10.8	16.2	10.3
Very Lazy, The English Provender Co.*	1 Tsp/3g	3	0.0	111	6.0	20.9	0.4	3.0
Wild	1 Clove/3g	1	0.0	23	2.8	1.7	0.6	1.9
GARLIC & GINGER								
Minced, Paste, Nishaan*	1 Tsp/5g	4	0.1	71	2.4	8.5	1.6	0.0
GARLIC PUREE								
Average	*1 Tbsp/18g*	*68*	*6.0*	*380*	*3.5*	*16.9*	*33.6*	*0.0*
in Vegetable Oil, GIA*	1 Tsp/5g	12	0.9	248	3.6	18.8	17.7	0.0
with Tomato, GIA*	10g	7	0.1	70	5.1	0.5	1.2	0.0
GATEAU								
Au Fromage Blanc, Ligne Et Plaisir*	1 Serving/80g	128	2.1	160	8.0	26.0	2.6	0.0
Black Forest, 500g Size, Tesco*	1 Cake/500g	1125	55.0	225	4.0	27.1	11.0	1.8
Black Forest, Mini, Tesco*	1 Serving/55g	136	5.1	247	5.7	35.3	9.2	1.0
Black Forest, Sainsbury's*	1/8 Cake/63g	163	10.8	259	3.9	27.7	17.1	3.5
Black Forest, Sara Lee*	1 Serving/80g	221	9.8	276	3.6	37.9	12.3	1.2
Chocolate, & Vanilla, Ice Cream, Iceland*	1 Serving/130g	252	12.2	194	3.3	24.1	9.4	0.6

	Measure INFO/WEIGHT	per Measure KCAL	per Measure FAT	Nutrition Values per 100g / 100ml KCAL	PROT	CARB	FAT	FIBRE
GATEAU								
Chocolate, Double, Frozen, Tesco*	1/5 Gateau/70g	119	4.7	265	5.0	35.8	10.4	4.0
Chocolate, Layer, M&S*	1 Serving/86g	278	15.7	323	4.2	35.9	18.3	0.9
Chocolate, Swirl, Tesco*	1 Serving/83g	230	13.3	277	3.8	29.3	16.0	0.2
Strawberry, Co-Op*	1 Serving/77g	222	12.9	288	5.1	29.2	16.7	1.0
Strawberry, Double, Sara Lee*	1/8 Cake/199g	533	24.3	268	3.2	36.2	12.2	0.6
Strawberry, Frozen, Tesco*	1/5 Gateau/75g	155	6.3	205	2.8	28.8	8.3	0.9
GELATINE								
Average	*1oz/28g*	*95*	*0.0*	*338*	*84.4*	*0.0*	*0.0*	*0.0*
GHEE								
Butter	*1oz/28g*	*251*	*27.9*	*898*	*0.0*	*0.0*	*99.8*	*0.0*
Palm	*1oz/28g*	*251*	*27.9*	*897*	*0.0*	*0.0*	*99.7*	*0.0*
Vegetable	*1oz/28g*	*251*	*27.8*	*895*	*0.0*	*0.0*	*99.4*	*0.0*
GHERKINS								
Pickled, Average	*1 Gherkin/36g*	*5*	*0.0*	*14*	*0.9*	*2.6*	*0.1*	*1.2*
GIN								
& Diet Tonic, Can, Greenalls*	1 Can/250ml	95	0.0	38	0.0	0.0	0.0	0.0
37.5% Volume	*1 Pub Shot/35ml*	*72*	*0.0*	*207*	*0.0*	*0.0*	*0.0*	*0.0*
40% Volume	*1 Pub Shot/35ml*	*78*	*0.0*	*222*	*0.0*	*0.0*	*0.0*	*0.0*
Gordons & Bitter Lemon, Premixed, Canned, Gordons*	1 Can/250ml	170	0.0	68	0.0	7.1	0.0	0.0
Gordons & Slim Line Tonic, Premixed, Diageo*	1 Can/250ml	90	0.0	36	0.0	0.0	0.0	0.0
Gordons & Tonic, Premixed, Diageo*	1 Can/250ml	152	0.0	61	0.0	6.2	0.0	0.0
London Dry, Bombay Sapphire*	1 Serving/25ml	59	0.0	236	0.0	0.0	0.0	0.0
GINGER								
Chunks, Crystallised, Julian Graves*	1 Serving/10g	28	0.0	283	0.2	70.1	0.2	1.5
Crystallised, Suma*	1 Serving/30g	104	0.0	348	0.2	82.0	0.1	0.3
Ground, Average	*1 Tsp/2g*	*5*	*0.1*	*258*	*7.4*	*60.0*	*3.3*	*0.0*
Root, Raw, Pared, Average	*1 Tsp/2g*	*2*	*0.0*	*86*	*2.0*	*19.1*	*0.8*	*2.2*
Root, Raw, Unprepared, Average	*1 Tsp/2g*	*2*	*0.0*	*80*	*1.8*	*17.8*	*0.8*	*2.0*
Stem in Sugar Syrup, Sainsbury's*	1oz/28g	76	0.0	271	0.2	67.3	0.1	1.4
Stem in Syrup, Waitrose*	1 Jar/350g	1071	7.7	306	0.1	70.4	2.2	0.7
Very Lazy, The English Provender Co.*	1 Tsp/5g	3	0.0	52	0.7	10.9	0.8	0.8
GINGER ALE								
American, Finest, Tesco*	1 Serving/150ml	68	0.0	45	0.0	11.0	0.0	0.0
American, Low Calorie, Tesco*	1 fl oz/30ml	0	0.0	1	0.0	0.0	0.0	0.0
American, Tesco*	1 Glass/250ml	58	0.0	23	0.0	5.5	0.0	0.0
Dry	1 Glass/250ml	38	0.0	15	0.0	3.9	0.0	0.0
Dry, Sainsbury's*	1 Glass/250ml	95	0.2	38	0.1	9.1	0.1	0.1
GINGER BEER								
Alcoholic, Crabbies*	1 Bottle/500ml	254	0.0	51	0.0	7.1	0.0	0.0
Asda*	1 Can/330ml	144	0.0	44	0.0	10.9	0.0	0.0
Classic, Schweppes*	1 Can/330ml	115	0.0	35	0.0	8.4	0.0	0.0
D & G Old Jamaican*	1 Can/330ml	211	0.0	64	0.0	16.0	0.0	0.0
Diet, Crabbies*	1 Bottle/700ml	7	0.0	1	0.0	0.0	0.0	0.0
Fiery, Canned, Waitrose*	1 Can/330ml	178	0.0	54	0.0	13.3	0.0	0.0
Fiery, Low Calorie, Waitrose*	1 Can/330ml	3	0.0	1	0.1	0.0	0.0	0.0
Light, Waitrose*	1 Glass/250ml	2	0.2	1	0.0	0.0	0.1	0.1
No Added Sugar, Aldi*	1 Glass/250ml	5	0.0	2	0.0	0.0	0.0	0.0
Sainsbury's*	1 Can/330ml	69	0.0	21	0.0	5.1	0.0	0.0
Sparkling, Organic, Whole Earth*	1 Can/330ml	116	0.0	35	0.0	8.2	0.0	0.0
Tesco*	1 Serving/200ml	70	0.2	35	0.1	8.2	0.1	0.0
Traditional, Fentiman's*	1 Bottle/275ml	130	0.0	47	0.0	11.3	0.0	0.0
Traditional Style, Tesco*	1 Can/330ml	218	0.0	66	0.0	16.1	0.0	0.0

G

	Measure INFO/WEIGHT	per Measure KCAL	FAT	Nutrition Values per 100g / 100ml KCAL	PROT	CARB	FAT	FIBRE
GINGER WINE								
Green Ginger Wine & Scots Whisky, Crabbies*	1 Glass/125ml	192	0.0	153	14.3	14.3	0.0	0.0
GINGERBREAD								
Average	1oz/28g	106	3.5	379	5.7	64.7	12.6	1.2
Decorate Your Own, CBY, Asda*	1 Serving/100g	414	12.6	414	4.8	70.4	12.6	2.3
Man, Gluten & Wheat Free, Lovemore*	1 Biscuit/37g	179	7.6	485	4.7	70.1	20.5	1.7
Men, Mini, Asda*	1 Biscuit/11g	46	1.4	433	5.0	74.0	13.0	1.8
Men, Mini, M&S*	1 Biscuit/17g	78	3.1	470	6.2	63.9	18.6	1.7
Men, Mini, Sainsbury's*	1 Biscuit/12g	56	1.4	463	5.7	83.4	11.8	1.5
GNOCCHI								
Aldi*	1 Serving/100g	160	0.3	160	3.8	35.6	0.3	0.0
Di Patate, Italfresco*	½ Pack/200g	296	0.4	148	3.3	33.2	0.2	0.0
Fresh, Italian, Chilled, Sainsbury's*	¼ Pack/125g	190	0.4	152	3.8	33.6	0.3	1.4
Potato, Cooked, Average	*1 Serving/150g*	*200*	*0.0*	*133*	*0.0*	*33.2*	*0.0*	*0.0*
GOAT								
Meat, Uncooked	1 Portion/100g	109	2.3	109	20.0	0.0	2.3	0.0
Raw	*1oz/28g*	*31*	*0.6*	*109*	*20.6*	*0.0*	*2.3*	*0.0*
GOJI BERRIES								
Average	*1 Serving/100g*	*287*	*0.7*	*287*	*6.6*	*65.1*	*0.7*	*6.8*
Dried, Love Life, Waitrose*	1 Serving/30g	91	0.5	302	13.6	57.8	1.8	12.2
Whole, Sun-Dried, Linwoods*	1 Serving/30g	80	0.7	268	13.0	48.8	2.3	14.9
GOOSE								
Leg with Skin, Fire Roasted	*1 Leg/174g*	*482*	*29.8*	*277*	*28.8*	*0.0*	*17.1*	*0.0*
Meat, Fat & Skin, Raw	*1oz/28g*	*101*	*9.2*	*361*	*16.5*	*0.0*	*32.8*	*0.0*
Meat, Raw	*1 Portion/185g*	*298*	*13.0*	*161*	*23.0*	*0.0*	*7.0*	*0.0*
Meat, Roasted	*1 Portion/143g*	*340*	*18.6*	*238*	*29.0*	*0.0*	*13.0*	*0.0*
Meat & Skin, Roasted	*½ Goose/774g*	*2361*	*169.5*	*305*	*25.2*	*0.0*	*21.9*	*0.0*
GOOSEBERRIES								
Dessert, Raw, Tops & Tails Removed	*1oz/28g*	*11*	*0.1*	*40*	*0.7*	*9.2*	*0.3*	*2.4*
Stewed with Sugar	*25g*	*14*	*0.1*	*54*	*0.7*	*12.9*	*0.3*	*4.2*
Stewed without Sugar	*25g*	*4*	*0.1*	*16*	*0.9*	*2.5*	*0.3*	*4.4*
GOULASH								
Beef, Average	1 Serving/300g	310	9.5	103	8.1	10.4	3.2	0.9
Beef, Finest, Tesco*	½ Pack/300g	297	9.3	99	11.6	6.2	3.1	0.6
Beef, Weight Watchers*	1 Pack/330g	241	5.6	73	4.8	9.5	1.7	0.6
GRANOLA								
Cranberry & Honey Nut, Graze*	1 Punnet/35g	157	7.1	447	11.0	56.2	20.3	8.0
Nibbles, Tropical Crunch, We Are Bear*	1 Pack/30g	99	1.5	329	13.0	76.0	4.9	15.5
Summer Fruits, Pomegranate Infused, M&S*	1 Serving/50g	200	6.4	400	8.6	63.2	12.7	5.8
GRAPEFRUIT								
Fresh Cut, Graze*	1 Pack/120g	38	0.1	32	1.0	7.0	0.1	2.0
in Juice, Average	*1oz/28g*	*13*	*0.0*	*46*	*0.5*	*10.6*	*0.0*	*0.4*
in Syrup, Average	*1oz/28g*	*19*	*0.0*	*69*	*0.5*	*16.8*	*0.1*	*0.5*
Raw, Flesh Only, Average	*½ Fruit/160g*	*48*	*0.2*	*30*	*0.8*	*6.8*	*0.1*	*1.3*
Raw, Weighed with Skin & Seeds, Average	*1 Fruit/340g*	*109*	*0.3*	*32*	*0.6*	*8.1*	*0.1*	*1.1*
Ruby Red in Juice, Average	*1 Serving/135g*	*54*	*0.1*	*40*	*0.6*	*9.4*	*0.0*	*0.5*
GRAPES								
Green, Average	*1 Grape/5g*	*3*	*0.0*	*62*	*0.4*	*15.2*	*0.1*	*0.7*
Red, Average	*1 Grape/5g*	*3*	*0.0*	*65*	*0.4*	*15.8*	*0.1*	*0.6*
Red & Green Selection, Average	*1 Grape/5g*	*3*	*0.0*	*62*	*0.4*	*15.2*	*0.1*	*0.8*
GRAPPA								
Average	1 Serving/30ml	85	0.0	283	0.0	6.7	0.0	0.0
GRATIN								
Dauphinoise, Budgens*	½ Pack/218g	277	15.7	127	3.0	12.5	7.2	2.5

G

INFO/WEIGHT	Measure	per Measure KCAL	FAT	Nutrition Values per 100g / 100ml KCAL	PROT	CARB	FAT	FIBRE

GRATIN

	Measure INFO/WEIGHT	per Measure KCAL	FAT	KCAL	PROT	CARB	FAT	FIBRE
Potato, Creamy, M&S*	½ Pack/225g	360	25.0	160	2.2	11.9	11.1	0.9
Potato, Sainsbury's*	½ Pack/225g	448	34.0	199	4.4	11.4	15.1	1.0
Potato, Somerfield*	½ Pack/225g	356	27.0	158	2.0	11.0	12.0	0.0
Salmon, Haddock & Prawn, Easy to Cook, Waitrose*	½ Pack/270g	522	35.8	194	9.4	8.8	13.3	0.5
Vegetable, Somerfield*	1 Pack/300g	417	39.0	139	1.0	5.0	13.0	0.0

GRAVLAX

Salmon, Cured with Salt, Sugar & Herbs	1 Serving/100g	119	3.3	119	18.3	3.1	3.3	0.4

GRAVY

Beef, Aunt Bessie's*	1 Serving/100g	73	5.3	73	1.0	5.3	5.3	0.5
Beef, Fresh, Sainsbury's*	1 Serving/83ml	47	2.7	56	2.4	4.5	3.2	0.6
Beef, Fresh, Signature, TTD, Sainsbury's*	¼ Pot/123g	38	1.1	31	1.9	3.7	0.9	0.6
Beef, Fresh, VLH Kitchens	1 Serving/83ml	47	2.7	56	2.4	4.5	3.2	0.6
Beef, Heat & Serve, Morrisons*	1 Serving/150g	27	0.4	18	0.3	3.9	0.3	0.5
Beef, Home Style, Savoury, Heinz*	¼ Cup/60g	30	1.0	50	1.7	6.7	1.7	0.0
Beef, Mix, Classic, Schwartz*	1 Pack/27g	83	0.8	306	11.2	58.8	2.9	3.8
Beef, Pouch, VLH Kitchens	1 Serving/83ml	38	1.1	31	1.9	3.7	0.9	0.6
Beef, Rich, Ready to Heat, Schwartz*	½ Pack/100g	31	1.6	31	0.8	3.4	1.6	0.5
Beef, Roast, Best in Glass Jar, Made Up, Bisto*	1 Serving/70ml	21	0.3	30	0.3	6.1	0.4	0.0
Beef, with Winter Berry & Shallot, Made Up, Oxo*	1 Serving/105ml	24	0.3	23	0.6	4.3	0.3	0.1
Chicken, Fresh, VLH Kitchens	1 Serving/83ml	27	1.2	27	0.8	3.3	1.2	0.5
Chicken, Rich, Ready to Heat, Schwartz*	½ Pack/100g	27	1.2	27	0.8	3.3	1.2	0.5
Chicken, Roast, Mix, Classic, Schwartz*	1 Pack/26g	49	1.5	189	10.3	23.6	5.9	2.5
Fresh, Somerfield*	1 Pack/300g	69	3.0	23	0.0	4.0	1.0	0.0
Granules, Beef, Dry, Tesco*	1 Serving/6g	29	2.1	480	5.5	36.4	34.7	1.5
Granules, Beef, Made Up, Tesco*	1 Serving/140ml	48	3.6	35	0.3	2.6	2.5	0.1
Granules, Chicken, & Hint of Sage & Onion, Oxo*	1 Serving/30g	95	1.8	316	11.1	54.2	6.1	0.7
Granules, Chicken, Dry, Average	1 Tsp/4g	17	0.9	428	4.5	49.4	23.6	1.2
Granules, Chicken, Dry, Oxo*	1oz/28g	83	1.4	296	11.1	54.2	4.9	0.7
Granules, Chicken, Dry Weight, Bisto*	1 Serving/20g	80	3.2	400	1.9	62.5	15.8	0.2
Granules, Chicken, Made Up, Oxo*	1 fl oz/30ml	5	0.1	18	0.7	3.3	0.3	0.0
Granules, Chicken, Made Up, Smart Price, Asda*	1 Serving/100ml	34	2.3	34	0.2	3.0	2.3	0.1
Granules, Chicken, Morrisons*	1 Serving/100ml	34	2.3	34	0.2	3.2	2.3	0.0
Granules, Dry, Bisto*	1 Serving/10g	38	1.6	384	3.1	56.4	16.2	1.5
Granules, Dry, Value, Tesco*	1oz/28g	111	5.2	397	3.2	54.4	18.5	1.0
Granules, Favourite, Made Up, Bisto*	1 Serving/50ml	15	0.6	30	0.2	4.4	1.2	0.0
Granules, Instant, Dry	**1oz/28g**	**129**	**9.1**	**462**	**4.4**	**40.6**	**32.5**	**0.0**
Granules, Instant, Made Up	**1oz/28g**	**10**	**0.7**	**34**	**0.3**	**3.0**	**2.4**	**0.0**
Granules, Lamb, Dry, Average	1 Tsp/4g	14	0.3	344	10.8	56.2	8.4	2.8
Granules, Lamb, Hint of Mint, Made Up, Oxo*	1 Serving/100ml	25	0.5	25	0.7	4.3	0.5	0.0
Granules, Lamb, Twist of Mint, Chef's Specials, Bisto*	½ Pack/13g	42	1.0	326	5.3	58.3	7.8	0.7
Granules, Made Up, Bisto*	1 Serving/50ml	15	0.6	30	0.2	4.4	1.2	0.2
Granules, Made Up, Oxo*	1 Serving/150ml	28	0.4	19	0.6	3.4	0.3	0.0
Granules, Meat, Made Up, Asda*	1 Serving/100ml	38	2.4	38	0.6	4.0	2.4	0.1
Granules, Meat, Made Up, Sainsbury's*	1 Serving/100ml	37	2.4	37	0.4	3.5	2.4	0.1
Granules, Onion, Dry, Morrisons*	1 Serving/25g	124	8.7	495	3.4	44.0	34.7	0.0
Granules, Onion, Dry Weight, Bisto*	4 Tsp/20g	78	2.9	391	2.4	62.3	14.7	2.3
Granules, Onion, Made Up, Bisto*	1 Serving/50ml	14	0.3	28	0.2	5.6	0.6	0.0
Granules, Onion, Made Up, Oxo*	1 fl oz/30ml	6	0.1	20	0.5	3.7	0.3	0.0
Granules, Original, Dry, Oxo*	1oz/28g	88	1.3	313	10.2	57.2	4.8	1.0
Granules, Turkey, Dry Weight, Bisto*	4 Tsp/20g	75	3.1	377	2.4	57.2	15.5	1.0
Granules, Turkey, Made Up, Bisto*	1 Serving/50ml	14	0.6	28	0.2	4.0	1.2	0.2
Granules, Vegetable, Dry, Oxo*	1oz/28g	88	1.4	316	8.4	59.5	4.9	0.9
Granules, Vegetable, Dry, Tesco*	½ Pint/20g	94	6.7	470	3.8	38.5	33.4	3.7

	Measure INFO/WEIGHT	per Measure KCAL	per Measure FAT	Nutrition Values per 100g / 100ml KCAL	PROT	CARB	FAT	FIBRE
GRAVY								
Granules, Vegetable, Dry Weight, Bisto*	1 Tsp/4g	15	0.5	380	2.1	63.0	13.3	4.5
Granules, Vegetable, Made Up, Bisto*	1 Serving/50ml	14	0.2	28	0.2	5.6	0.4	0.2
Granules, Vegetarian, Dry Weight, Bisto*	1 Serving/28g	100	3.7	356	2.7	56.0	13.3	4.5
Granules, Vegetarian, Made Up, Sainsbury's*	1 Serving/50ml	16	1.1	32	0.2	2.8	2.2	0.8
Instant, Dry Weight, BFY, Morrisons*	1 Serving/25g	80	0.1	320	3.5	77.0	0.3	1.2
Instant, Made Up, BGTY, Sainsbury's*	1 fl oz/30ml	10	0.0	32	0.3	7.4	0.1	0.1
Lamb, Roast, Bisto*	1 Serving/20g	60	0.9	302	3.4	62.3	4.3	0.0
Lamb, Roast, Mix, Classic, Schwartz*	1 Pack/26g	87	1.2	336	10.4	63.6	4.5	0.0
Onion, Caramelised, Made Up, Bisto*	1 Serving/70ml	20	0.3	29	0.1	6.1	0.4	0.1
Onion, Fresh, Asda*	1/6 Pot/77g	30	1.6	39	1.7	3.3	2.1	0.4
Onion, Fresh, Somerfield*	1 Pack/300g	195	12.0	65	1.0	7.0	4.0	0.0
Onion, Rich, M&S*	½ Pack/150g	60	1.8	40	2.0	5.9	1.2	0.3
Paste, Beef, Antony Worrall Thompson's*	1 Portion/31g	104	5.7	334	11.8	30.3	18.4	0.6
Pork, & Sage, Roast, Mix, Classic, Schwartz*	1 Pack/25g	88	1.4	354	11.8	63.8	5.8	0.0
Pork, Roast, Best, in Glass Jar, Dry Weight, Bisto*	4 Tsp/20g	63	0.9	314	4.3	64.1	4.5	0.0
Poultry, Fresh, Sainsbury's*	1 Serving/100g	46	1.2	46	3.5	4.9	1.2	0.5
Poultry, TTD, Sainsbury's*	1 Portion/125g	76	5.6	61	1.8	3.5	4.5	0.8
Powder, Made Up, Sainsbury's*	1 Serving/100ml	15	0.1	15	0.4	3.2	0.1	0.1
Powder, Vegetarian, Organic, Marigold*	1 Serving/22g	79	1.7	361	10.6	61.5	7.7	1.3
Turkey, Rich, Ready to Heat, Schwartz*	1 Pack/200g	62	2.4	31	1.9	3.1	1.2	0.5
Turkey, Roast, Mix, As Sold, Schwartz*	1 Pack/25g	91	1.6	365	10.8	64.7	6.5	2.4
GREENGAGES								
Raw, Average	*1 Fruit/23g*	*9*	*0.0*	*38*	*0.8*	*9.4*	*0.1*	*2.0*
GREENS								
Spring, Boiled, Average	*1 Serving/80g*	*16*	*0.6*	*20*	*1.9*	*1.6*	*0.7*	*2.6*
Spring, Raw, Average	*1 Serving/80g*	*26*	*0.8*	*33*	*3.0*	*3.1*	*1.0*	*3.4*
GRILLS								
Bacon & Cheese, Tesco*	1 Grill/78g	222	14.7	284	15.0	13.4	18.9	1.2
Vegetable, Dalepak*	1 Grill/83g	125	4.1	151	4.0	22.5	5.0	1.6
Vegetable, Mediterranean, Cauldron Foods*	1 Grill/88g	145	10.4	166	5.3	15.8	11.9	6.5
Vegetable, Tesco*	1 Grill/72g	129	7.2	179	4.2	18.0	10.0	2.2
GROUSE								
Meat Only, Roasted	*1oz/28g*	*36*	*0.6*	*128*	*27.6*	*0.0*	*2.0*	*0.0*
GUACAMOLE								
Average	1 Tbsp/17g	33	3.3	194	1.6	3.4	19.2	2.4
Avocado, Reduced Fat, The Fresh Dip Company*	1 Serving/113g	128	9.8	113	2.5	6.1	8.7	2.3
Chunky, M&S*	1 Pot/170g	221	19.2	130	1.5	5.1	11.3	1.7
Chunky, Sainsbury's*	½ Pot/65g	120	11.9	185	1.6	3.2	18.4	3.8
Doritos, Walkers*	1 Tbsp/20g	32	3.2	159	1.2	2.6	16.0	0.1
Fresh, VLH Kitchens	1 Serving/17g	26.9	85.9	158	1.5	3.0	14.6	2.5
Fresh, Waitrose*	½ Pack/100g	190	18.4	190	1.9	4.1	18.4	2.5
Mexican Style, Dip Selection, Morrisons*	½ Pack/50g	102	10.2	204	1.5	3.7	20.4	0.9
Reduced Fat Average	1 Serving/100g	129	10.8	129	2.4	5.2	10.8	3.0
GUAVA								
Canned in Syrup	*1oz/28g*	*17*	*0.0*	*60*	*0.4*	*15.7*	*0.0*	*3.0*
Raw, Flesh Only, Average	*1 Fruit/55g*	*37*	*0.6*	*68*	*3.0*	*14.0*	*1.0*	*5.0*
GUINEA FOWL								
Boned & Stuffed, Fresh, Fayrefield Foods*	1 Serving/325g	650	39.3	200	19.1	3.3	12.1	0.5
Fresh, Free Range, Waitrose*	1 Portion/193g	258	11.9	134	19.5	0.0	6.2	0.3
GUMS								
American Hard, Sainsbury's*	1 Sweet/6g	22	0.0	360	0.1	90.0	0.1	0.0
American Hard, Tesco*	1 Serving/200g	646	0.0	323	0.0	80.8	0.0	0.0
Milk Bottles, Bassett's*	1 Pack/25g	88	0.4	353	6.2	78.3	1.6	0.0

G

	Measure INFO/WEIGHT	per Measure KCAL	FAT	Nutrition Values per 100g / 100ml KCAL	PROT	CARB	FAT	FIBRE
GUMS								
Milk Bottles, Milk Flavour, Asda*	1 Pack/100g	369	2.3	369	7.0	80.0	2.3	0.4

G

	Measure INFO/WEIGHT	per Measure		Nutrition Values per 100g / 100ml				
		KCAL	FAT	KCAL	PROT	CARB	FAT	FIBRE
HADDOCK								
Fillet, Smoked, in Mustard & Dill, The Saucy Fish Co.*	2 Fillets/270g	262	9.7	97	15.5	0.1	3.6	0.0
Fillets, Battered, Average	1oz/28g	64	3.4	228	13.4	16.3	12.2	1.1
Fillets, in Breadcrumbs, Average	1 Fillet/125g	253	12.4	203	13.5	14.9	9.9	1.2
Fillets, in Lemon & Chive Butter, Simply, Birds Eye*	1 Portion/148g	190	11.3	128	14.6	0.4	7.6	0.0
Fillets, Lightly Dusted, Seeded, M&S*	1 Fillet/144g	266	12.5	185	14.3	12.2	8.7	1.0
Fillets, Raw, Average	*1 Fillet/140g*	*112*	*1.2*	*80*	*18.0*	*0.2*	*0.8*	*0.0*
Fillets, Smoked, Cooked, Average	*1 Pack/300g*	*337*	*7.7*	*112*	*21.9*	*0.4*	*2.6*	*0.1*
Fillets, Smoked, Raw, Average	*1 Pack/227g*	*194*	*1.0*	*86*	*20.3*	*0.1*	*0.5*	*0.2*
Flour, Fried in Blended Oil	1oz/28g	39	1.1	138	21.1	4.5	4.1	0.2
Goujons, Batter, Crispy, M&S*	1 Serving/100g	250	14.1	250	11.7	18.5	14.1	0.8
Loins, Beer Battered, Chunky, TTD, Sainsbury's*	1 Fillet/93g	177	8.8	191	15.8	10.5	9.5	2.3
Loins, Skinless, Frozen, TTD, Sainsbury's*	1 Serving/100g	116	0.2	116	28.5	0.1	0.2	0.1
with Cheddar & Chive Sauce, The Saucy Fish Co.*	1 Fillet/120g	168	9.0	140	16.6	1.2	7.5	0.0
HADDOCK IN								
Butter Sauce, Steaks, Youngs*	1 Serving/150g	134	5.6	89	9.9	4.0	3.7	0.5
Cheese & Chive Sauce, Fillets, Go Cook, Asda*	1 Pack/360g	400	19.1	111	14.8	1.5	5.3	0.2
Cheese & Leek Sauce, Fillets, SteamFresh, Birds Eye*	1 Serving/190g	165	7.0	87	11.0	2.4	3.7	0.2
Cheese Sauce, Fillets, Fresh Tastes, Asda*	½ Pack/180g	212	9.5	118	16.2	1.3	5.3	0.6
Smoked Leek & Cheese Sauce, Asda*	½ Pack/200g	232	10.0	116	14.0	3.7	5.0	1.5
Tomato Herb Sauce, Fillets, BGTY, Sainsbury's*	½ Pack/165g	150	4.6	91	12.9	3.6	2.8	0.1
HAGGIS								
Neeps & Tatties, M&S*	1 Pack/300g	330	14.4	110	3.8	12.3	4.8	0.8
Traditional, Average	*1 Serving/454g*	*1119*	*66.5*	*246*	*12.4*	*17.2*	*14.6*	*1.0*
Vegetarian, Macsween*	1 Serving/100g	208	11.5	208	5.9	25.9	11.5	2.4
Whole, Hall's*	1 Haggis/454g	1053	64.5	232	9.7	15.1	14.2	2.5
HAKE								
Fillets, Herby Mediterranean Glaze, Sensations, Youngs*	½ Pack/120g	106	2.6	88	16.8	0.4	2.2	0.0
Fillets, in Breadcrumbs, Average	1oz/28g	66	3.7	234	12.9	16.0	13.4	1.0
Fillets, in Tomato & Basil Marinade, Donegal Catch*	1 Fillet/135g	201	8.9	149	15.6	6.7	6.6	1.0
Goujons, Average	1 Serving/150g	345	17.8	230	12.4	18.6	11.9	1.3
Raw, Average	*1oz/28g*	*29*	*0.6*	*102*	*20.4*	*0.0*	*2.2*	*0.0*
HALIBUT								
Cooked, Average	*1oz/28g*	*38*	*1.1*	*135*	*24.6*	*0.4*	*4.0*	*0.0*
Raw	*1oz/28g*	*29*	*0.5*	*103*	*21.5*	*0.0*	*1.9*	*0.0*
with Roasted Pepper Sauce, Fillets, M&S*	1 Serving/145g	218	14.4	150	12.7	2.4	9.9	0.6
HALVA								
Average	*1oz/28g*	*107*	*3.7*	*381*	*1.8*	*68.0*	*13.2*	*0.0*
HAM								
Applewood Smoked, Average	*1 Slice/28g*	*31*	*0.8*	*112*	*21.2*	*0.6*	*2.8*	*0.2*
Baked, Average	*1 Slice/74g*	*98*	*3.7*	*133*	*21.0*	*1.0*	*5.0*	*0.0*
Beechwood Smoked, Morrisons*	1 Slice/20g	32	1.8	160	19.5	0.5	9.0	0.0
Belgian, Sainsbury's*	1 Serving/100g	141	6.1	141	19.4	2.0	6.1	0.0
Boiled, Average	*1 Pack/113g*	*154*	*6.5*	*136*	*20.6*	*0.6*	*5.8*	*0.0*
Breaded, Average	*1 Slice/37g*	*57*	*2.3*	*155*	*23.1*	*1.8*	*6.3*	*1.6*
Breaded, Dry Cured, Average	*1 Slice/33g*	*47*	*1.8*	*142*	*22.2*	*1.4*	*5.4*	*0.0*
Breaded, M&S*	1 Slice/20g	23	0.6	115	22.2	0.7	2.8	0.1
Brunswick, Average	*1 Slice/20g*	*32*	*1.8*	*160*	*19.5*	*0.6*	*8.8*	*0.0*
Cooked, Sliced, Average	*1 Slice/17g*	*18*	*0.5*	*109*	*19.0*	*1.0*	*3.2*	*0.1*
Crumbed, Sliced, Average	*1 Slice/28g*	*33*	*0.9*	*117*	*21.5*	*0.9*	*3.1*	*0.0*
Danish, Average	*1 Slice/11g*	*14*	*0.6*	*125*	*18.4*	*1.0*	*5.4*	*0.0*
Danish, Lean, Average	*1 Slice/15g*	*14*	*0.3*	*92*	*17.8*	*1.0*	*1.8*	*0.0*
Dry Cured, Average	*1 Slice/18g*	*26*	*1.0*	*144*	*22.4*	*1.0*	*5.6*	*0.2*
Extra Lean, Average	*1 Slice/11g*	*10*	*0.2*	*90*	*18.0*	*1.4*	*1.4*	*0.0*

Measure INFO/WEIGHT	per Measure KCAL	FAT	Nutrition Values per 100g / 100ml KCAL	PROT	CARB	FAT	FIBRE

HAM

	Measure INFO/WEIGHT	per Measure KCAL	FAT	KCAL	PROT	CARB	FAT	FIBRE
Gammon, Breaded, Average	1 Serving/25g	31	0.8	122	22.0	1.5	3.1	0.0
Gammon, Dry Cured, Sliced, Average	1 Slice/33g	43	1.4	131	22.9	0.4	4.2	0.0
Gammon, Honey Roast, Average	1 Serving/60g	81	2.8	134	22.4	0.4	4.8	0.0
Gammon, Smoked, Average	1 Slice/43g	59	2.1	137	22.3	0.7	4.9	0.2
German Black Forest, Average	½ Pack/35g	93	6.0	267	27.2	1.3	17.0	0.5
Glazed with Honey & Muscovado Sugar, Waitrose*	1 Slice/21g	25	0.8	119	21.3	0.4	3.6	0.0
Honey & Mustard, Average	1oz/28g	39	1.2	140	20.8	4.6	4.3	0.0
Honey Roast, Average	1 Slice/20g	25	0.8	123	20.3	1.6	3.8	0.1
Honey Roast, Dry Cured, Average	1 Slice/33g	46	1.5	140	22.7	2.3	4.4	0.2
Honey Roast, Lean, Average	1 Serving/25g	28	0.8	111	18.2	2.7	3.1	0.0
Honey Roast, Wafer Thin, Average	1 Slice/10g	11	0.3	113	17.4	3.7	3.2	0.3
Honey Roast, Wafer Thin, Premium, Average	1 Slice/10g	15	0.6	149	22.0	1.6	6.0	0.0
Jamon de Trevelez, Antonio Alvarez Jamones*	1 Slice/10g	19	0.9	192	35.6	0.0	8.6	0.0
Joint, Cured, Roasted, Average	1 Serving/100g	138	5.2	138	21.7	1.0	5.2	0.1
Joint, Easy Carve, Asda*	1oz/28g	41	1.7	146	22.8	1.2	5.9	0.6
Joint, Honey Roast, Asda*	1oz/28g	35	0.8	124	23.9	1.7	2.8	0.7
Joint, Roast, Christmas, Tesco*	1/6 Joint/167g	225	10.8	135	17.9	1.1	6.5	0.0
Lean, Average	1 Slice/18g	19	0.4	104	19.5	1.1	2.4	0.3
Oak Smoked, Average	1 Slice/20g	26	0.9	130	21.0	1.0	4.7	0.3
Parma, Average	1 Slice/10g	21	1.1	213	29.3	0.0	10.6	0.0
Parma, Premium, Average	1 Slice/14g	36	2.3	258	27.9	0.3	16.1	0.0
Peppered, Average	1 Slice/12g	13	0.3	110	18.5	2.0	2.7	0.4
Peppered, Dry Cured, Average	1 Slice/31g	43	1.5	140	23.1	1.3	4.7	0.2
Prosciutto, Average	1 Slice/12g	27	1.5	226	28.7	0.0	12.4	0.4
San Daniele, Finest, Tesco*	1 Slice/10g	24	1.3	242	30.5	0.5	13.1	0.0
Serrano, Average	1 Slice/20g	46	2.4	230	30.5	0.4	11.8	0.0
Smoked, Average	1 Slice/18g	21	0.7	117	19.7	0.9	3.7	0.0
Smoked, Dry Cured, Average	1 Slice/28g	38	1.2	137	23.0	1.4	4.4	0.2
Smoked, Wafer Thin, Average	1 Serving/40g	41	1.2	102	17.7	1.2	2.9	0.2
Suffolk Black, TTD, Sainsbury's*	1 Slice/42g	58	1.7	139	22.3	3.5	4.0	0.0
Thick Cut, Average	1 Slice/74g	94	2.9	127	22.4	0.6	3.9	0.1
Tinned, Average	½ Can/100g	136	8.8	136	12.2	2.0	8.8	0.0
Tinned, Lean, Average	½ Can/100g	94	2.3	94	18.1	0.2	2.3	0.4
Wafer Thin, Applewood Smoked, British, Finest, Tesco*	1 Slice/14g	19	0.5	135	22.8	2.2	3.8	0.5
Wafer Thin, Average	1 Slice/10g	10	0.3	101	17.9	1.4	2.6	0.1
Wafer Thin, Weight Watchers*	1 Serving/60g	58	1.1	97	18.2	1.8	1.8	0.1
Wiltshire, Average	1oz/28g	41	1.7	148	23.1	0.0	6.0	0.0
Wiltshire, Breaded, Average	1oz/28g	41	1.4	145	23.9	1.0	5.0	0.0
Wiltshire, Orange Marmalade Roasted, Finest, Tesco*	1 Slice/40g	67	2.4	167	26.0	2.0	6.1	0.3

HARE

	Measure INFO/WEIGHT	per Measure KCAL	FAT	KCAL	PROT	CARB	FAT	FIBRE
Raw, Lean Only, Average	1oz/28g	35	1.0	125	23.5	0.2	3.5	0.0
Stewed, Lean Only, Average	1oz/28g	48	1.5	170	29.5	0.2	5.5	0.0

HARIBO*

	Measure INFO/WEIGHT	per Measure KCAL	FAT	KCAL	PROT	CARB	FAT	FIBRE
American Hard Gums, Haribo*	1 Pack/175g	630	3.3	360	0.3	85.5	1.9	0.2
Build a Burger, Haribo*	1oz/28g	96	0.1	344	6.6	79.0	0.2	0.3
Chamallows, Haribo*	1oz/28g	92	0.0	330	2.0	80.0	0.0	0.0
Cola Bottles, Fizzy, Haribo*	1 Pack/175g	595	0.4	340	6.3	78.3	0.2	0.3
Cola Bottles, Haribo*	1 Pack/16g	56	0.0	348	7.7	78.9	0.2	0.3
Dinosaurs, Haribo*	1oz/28g	95	0.1	340	6.3	78.3	0.2	0.5
Dolly Mixtures, Haribo*	1 Pack/175g	719	8.4	411	1.8	90.2	4.8	0.2
Fantasy Mix, Haribo*	1 Pack/100g	344	0.2	344	6.6	79.0	0.2	0.3
Fried Eggs/eggstras, Haribo*	1oz/28g	96	0.1	344	6.6	79.0	0.2	0.0
Gold Bears, Haribo*	1 Pack/100g	348	0.2	348	7.7	78.9	0.2	0.3

	Measure INFO/WEIGHT	per Measure KCAL	FAT	Nutrition Values per 100g / 100ml KCAL	PROT	CARB	FAT	FIBRE
HARIBO*								
Happy Cherries, Haribo*	1 Serving/40g	139	0.1	348	7.7	78.9	0.2	0.3
Horror Mix, Haribo*	1 Pack/100g	344	0.2	344	6.6	79.0	0.2	0.3
Jelly Babies, Haribo*	1oz/28g	97	0.1	348	4.5	82.1	0.2	0.5
Jelly Beans, Haribo*	1 Pack/100g	379	0.2	379	0.6	93.8	0.2	0.1
Kiddies Super Mix, Haribo*	1 Pack/100g	344	0.2	344	6.6	79.0	0.2	0.3
Liquorice Cream Rock, Haribo*	1oz/28g	107	1.5	382	2.3	81.2	5.3	0.3
Liquorice Favourite, Haribo*	1oz/28g	100	0.8	357	2.8	78.8	3.0	2.3
Liquorice with Stevia, Stevi-Lakritz, Haribo*	¼ Bag/25g	46	0.0	185	8.1	16.0	0.1	48.6
Magic Mix, Haribo*	1oz/28g	102	0.5	366	5.4	82.0	1.9	0.3
Maoam Stripes, Haribo*	1 Chew/7g	27	0.4	384	1.2	81.7	6.1	0.3
Mega Roulette, Haribo*	1oz/28g	97	0.1	348	7.7	78.9	0.2	0.3
Mega Roulette Sour, Haribo*	1oz/28g	95	0.1	340	6.3	78.3	0.2	0.5
Micro Mix, Haribo*	1oz/28g	106	0.7	379	4.7	84.5	2.5	0.4
Milky Mix, Haribo*	1 Pack/175g	607	0.4	347	7.1	79.6	0.2	0.4
Mint Imperials, Haribo*	1 Pack/175g	695	0.9	397	0.4	98.8	0.5	0.1
Peaches, Haribo*	1oz/28g	98	0.4	350	4.3	82.1	0.0	0.0
Pontefract Cakes, Haribo*	1 Serving/40g	118	0.1	296	5.3	68.2	0.2	0.5
Shrimps, Haribo*	1oz/28g	99	0.1	352	6.1	81.5	0.2	0.1
Snakes, Haribo*	1 Snake/8g	28	0.0	348	7.7	78.9	0.2	0.3
Starmix, Haribo*	1 Pack/100g	344	0.2	344	6.6	79.0	0.2	0.3
Tangfastics, Haribo*	1 Pack/100g	359	2.3	359	6.3	78.3	2.3	0.5
Tropifruit, Haribo*	1oz/28g	97	0.1	348	4.5	82.1	0.2	0.5
HARISSA PASTE								
Average	1 Tsp/5g	6	0.3	123	2.9	12.9	6.7	2.8
Barts*	1 Tbsp/15g	11	0.3	76	4.0	10.7	1.9	0.0
Easy, M&S*	1 Tbsp/15g	16	0.8	105	2.5	11.2	5.5	4.4
Moroccan Style, Al'fez*	1 Tsp/10g	19	1.1	190	4.0	18.2	11.2	3.4
Sainsbury's*	¼ Jar/19g	43	3.8	226	2.1	6.6	20.1	5.1
HASH								
Corned Beef, M&S*	½ Pack/321g	385	20.2	120	8.1	7.4	6.3	1.3
Corned Beef, Tesco*	1 Serving/400g	416	10.4	104	5.3	14.8	2.6	1.7
HASH BROWNS								
Oven Baked, Weighed Cooked, McCain*	1 Piece/38g	80	4.3	214	2.1	25.7	11.4	2.2
Oven Baked, Weighed Frozen, McCain*	1 Hash Brown/40g	75	4.1	187	1.7	21.8	10.3	2.1
Uncooked, Average	1 Hash Brown/45g	78	3.7	173	2.0	22.5	8.3	1.9
HAZELNUTS								
Blanched, Average	1 Serving/25g	164	15.9	656	15.4	5.8	63.5	6.5
Chopped, Average	*1 Serving/10g*	*67*	*6.4*	*666*	*16.8*	*5.6*	*64.0*	*6.6*
Whole, Average	*10 Whole/10g*	*66*	*6.4*	*655*	*15.4*	*5.8*	*63.5*	*6.5*
HEART								
Lambs, Average	*1 Heart/75g*	*92*	*4.5*	*122*	*16.0*	*1.0*	*6.0*	*0.0*
Ox, Raw	*1oz/28g*	*29*	*1.0*	*104*	*18.2*	*0.0*	*3.5*	*0.0*
Ox, Stewed	*1oz/28g*	*44*	*1.4*	*157*	*27.8*	*0.0*	*5.1*	*0.0*
Pig, Raw	*1oz/28g*	*27*	*0.9*	*97*	*17.1*	*0.0*	*3.2*	*0.0*
Pig, Stewed	*1oz/28g*	*45*	*1.9*	*162*	*25.1*	*0.0*	*6.8*	*0.0*
HERMESETAS								
The Classic Sweetener, Hermes*	1 Tablet/0.5g	0	0.0	294	14.2	59.3	0.0	0.0
HEROES								
Cadbury*	1 Chocolate/11g	60	3.9	545	9.1	48.2	35.2	0.0
HERRING								
Canned in Tomato Sauce, Average	1oz/28g	57	4.3	204	11.9	4.1	15.5	0.1
Dried, Salted, Average	*1oz/28g*	*47*	*2.1*	*168*	*25.3*	*0.0*	*7.4*	*0.0*
Fillets, Raw, Average	*1 Herring/100g*	*185*	*12.6*	*185*	*18.4*	*0.0*	*12.6*	*0.0*

H

	Measure INFO/WEIGHT	per Measure KCAL	per Measure FAT	Nutrition Values per 100g / 100ml KCAL	PROT	CARB	FAT	FIBRE
HERRING								
Fillets in Mustard & Dill Sauce, John West*	1 Can/190g	332	26.6	175	9.4	2.9	14.0	0.1
Fillets in Olive Oil, Succulent, Princes*	1 Serving/50g	108	7.5	215	20.0	0.0	15.0	0.0
Grilled, Average	*1oz/28g*	*51*	*3.1*	*181*	*20.1*	*0.0*	*11.2*	*0.0*
Pickled, Average	1oz/28g	73	5.0	262	14.2	9.6	18.0	0.0
Pickled in Mustard Sauce, Abba*	1 Serving/58g	150	10.9	260	7.0	16.0	19.0	0.0
Rollmop with Onion, Asda*	1 Rollmop/65g	89	3.1	137	13.2	10.3	4.8	0.8
Rollmops, Tesco*	1 Rollmop/65g	110	5.5	170	12.0	10.4	8.4	0.4
Smoked, Pepper in Oil, Glyngøre*	1 Can/130g	338	24.7	260	21.0	0.0	19.0	0.0
Whole, Raw, Average	*1 Serving/100g*	*190*	*13.2*	*190*	*17.8*	*0.0*	*13.2*	*0.0*
HIGHLIGHTS								
Caffe Latte, Made Up, Cadbury*	1 Serving/200g	40	1.4	20	1.0	2.5	0.7	0.0
Choc Mint, Made Up, Cadbury*	1 Serving/200ml	40	1.4	20	1.0	2.5	0.7	0.3
Chocolate, Dairy Fudge, Dry Weight, Cadbury*	1 Serving/11g	40	1.1	363	17.0	50.0	10.0	0.0
Chocolate Delights, Cadbury*	1 Bar/13g	60	2.6	480	6.4	67.0	20.5	1.2
Chocolate Orange, Made Up, Cadbury*	1 Serving/200ml	40	1.4	20	1.0	2.3	0.7	0.3
Dairy Fudge, Hot Chocolate, Made Up, Cadbury*	1 Serving/200ml	40	1.0	20	1.0	2.7	0.5	0.2
Dark, Hot Chocolate, Bournville, Made Up, Cadbury*	1 Serving/200ml	35	0.9	18	1.2	2.0	0.4	0.0
Dark Chocolate, Cadbury*	1 Sachet/11g	35	0.9	315	23.1	37.3	8.1	0.0
Espresso, Made Up, Cadbury*	1 Serving/200ml	35	0.9	18	1.2	2.0	0.4	0.0
Hot Chocolate Drink, Instant, Dry Weight, Cadbury*	1 Sachet/11g	42	1.4	380	16.8	46.9	13.1	3.4
Hot Chocolate Drink, Instant, Made Up, Cadbury*	1 Cup/200ml	40	1.4	20	1.0	2.5	0.7	0.3
Instant Hot Chocolate, Cadbury*	1 Sachet/22g	80	2.8	364	17.3	44.6	12.7	0.0
Mint, Cadbury*	1 Serving/200ml	40	1.4	20	1.0	2.5	0.7	0.0
Toffee Flavour, Made Up, Cadbury*	1 Serving/200ml	40	1.4	20	1.0	2.6	0.7	0.0
HOKI								
Grilled	*1oz/28g*	*34*	*0.8*	*121*	*24.1*	*0.0*	*2.7*	*0.0*
in Breadcrumbs, Average	1 Piece/156g	298	13.8	191	14.5	13.9	8.9	1.2
Raw	*1oz/28g*	*24*	*0.5*	*85*	*16.9*	*0.0*	*1.9*	*0.0*
HONEY								
Acacia, Tesco*	1 Tsp/4g	12	0.0	307	0.4	76.4	0.0	0.0
Acacia Blossom, Sainsbury's*	1 Serving/24g	81	0.0	339	0.1	84.7	0.1	0.3
Australian Eucalyptus, Finest, Tesco*	1 Tsp/4g	12	0.0	307	0.4	76.4	0.0	0.0
Bio Active, New Zealand Honey Co*	1 Serving/10g	32	0.0	325	1.0	80.0	0.0	0.0
Clear, Basics, Sainsbury's*	1 Tsp/15g	46	0.0	307	0.4	76.4	0.1	0.0
Clear, Runny, Sainsbury's*	1 Serving/15g	51	0.0	339	0.1	84.7	0.1	0.3
Clear, Value, Tesco*	1 Serving/27g	86	0.0	320	1.0	78.0	0.0	0.0
Clover, Canadian, TTD, Sainsbury's*	1 Tbsp/15g	50	0.0	336	0.2	83.6	0.1	0.1
Florida Orange, Extra Special, Asda*	1 Tbsp/15g	50	0.0	334	0.5	83.0	0.0	0.0
Greek, Waitrose*	1 Tsp/6g	18	0.0	307	0.4	76.4	0.0	0.0
Pure, Clear, Average	*1 Tbsp/20g*	*63*	*0.0*	*315*	*0.5*	*78.5*	*0.0*	*0.0*
Pure, Clear, Squeezy, Oak Lane*	1 Tsp/5ml	16	0.0	330	0.5	81.0	0.0	0.0
Pure, Set, Average	*1 Tbsp/20g*	*62*	*0.0*	*312*	*0.4*	*77.6*	*0.0*	*0.0*
Scottish Heather, Waitrose*	1 Serving/20g	61	0.0	307	0.4	76.4	0.0	0.0
Spanish Orange Blossom, Sainsbury's*	1 Tbsp/15g	51	0.0	339	0.1	84.7	0.0	0.3
HONEYCOMB								
Natural, Epicure*	1 Serving/100g	290	4.6	290	0.4	74.4	4.6	0.0
HOOCH*								
Vodka, Calculated Estimate, Hooch*	1 Bottle/330ml	244	0.0	74	0.3	5.1	0.0	0.0
HORLICKS								
Malted Drink, Chocolate, Extra Light, Dry, Horlicks*	1 Serving/32g	95	2.5	296	9.2	47.0	7.8	17.3
Malted Drink, Extra Light, Instant, Dry, Horlicks*	1 Serving/11g	35	0.7	319	8.4	57.4	6.2	10.5
Malted Drink, Light, Dry, Horlicks*	1 Serving/32g	116	1.2	364	14.8	72.2	3.8	1.9
Malted Drink, Light, Made Up, Horlicks*	1 Mug/200ml	116	1.2	58	2.4	11.6	0.6	0.3

	Measure INFO/WEIGHT	per Measure KCAL	FAT	Nutrition Values per 100g / 100ml KCAL	PROT	CARB	FAT	FIBRE
HORLICKS								
Powder, Made Up with Semi-Skimmed Milk	1 Mug/227ml	184	4.3	81	4.3	12.9	1.9	0.0
Powder, Made Up with Skimmed Milk	1 Mug/227ml	159	1.1	70	4.3	12.9	0.5	0.0
Powder, Made Up with Whole Milk	1 Mug/227ml	225	8.9	99	4.2	12.7	3.9	0.0
HORSE								
Meat, Raw, Average	*1 Serving/110g*	*146*	*5.1*	*133*	*21.4*	*0.0*	*4.6*	*0.0*
HORSERADISH								
Prepared, Average	*1 Tsp/5g*	*3*	*0.0*	*62*	*4.5*	*11.0*	*0.3*	*6.2*
HOT CHOCOLATE								
Balanced Lifestyle, Camelot*	1 Sachet/11g	40	1.6	363	18.5	40.6	14.1	0.5
Cadbury*	1 Serving/12g	44	0.7	370	6.3	73.3	5.9	0.0
Caramel, Whittards of Chelsea*	1 Serving/20g	71	1.5	355	7.5	64.5	7.5	13.0
Chococino, Dulce Gusto, Nescafe*	1 Serving/34g	149	5.5	437	14.6	58.6	16.1	4.6
Chocolate Break, Dry, Tesco*	1 Serving/21g	110	6.0	524	7.9	58.9	28.5	1.7
Cocoa, Lidl*	1 Serving/20g	77	1.2	386	6.1	74.1	6.2	0.0
Dreamtime, Whittards of Chelsea*	5 Tsp/20g	72	1.0	361	6.6	72.4	5.1	8.7
Drink, Organic, Green & Black's*	1 Tsp/4g	13	0.3	374	9.1	63.5	9.3	0.1
Drink, Twinings*	3 Tbsp/21g	81	0.7	387	5.0	82.0	3.3	6.0
Dry Weight, Tassimo, Suchard*	1 Serving/27g	88	2.4	325	3.2	58.0	8.9	2.6
Fairtrade, Whittards of Chelsea*	4 Tsp/20g	68	0.8	342	7.8	69.0	3.9	10.9
From Coffee Shop, Waitrose*	1 Serving/298ml	217	5.9	73	3.6	10.9	2.0	0.0
Galaxy, Mars*	1 Sachet/25g	97	1.9	386	4.8	71.9	7.7	4.7
Horlicks*	1 Serving/32g	128	2.6	400	8.8	72.5	8.1	3.8
Impress*	1 Serving/25g	90	0.9	360	5.6	76.0	3.6	6.0
Instant, BGTY, Made Up, Sainsbury's*	1 Sachet/28g	16	0.2	56	2.1	10.6	0.6	0.3
Instant, GFY, Asda*	1 Tsp/10g	32	1.3	321	13.2	37.0	13.4	7.7
Instant, Low Fat, Solo Slim, Rosemary Conley*	1 Sachet/18g	66	0.5	368	17.0	66.7	2.8	3.8
Instant, Skinny Cow*	1 Sachet/10g	37	1.5	370	19.7	39.3	14.6	0.0
Instant, Tesco*	1 Serving/32g	155	10.3	485	10.5	38.1	32.3	5.0
Instant Break, Cadbury*	1 Sachet/28g	119	3.9	425	10.9	64.2	14.0	0.0
Light, Caramel Flavour, Kruger*	1 Sachet/10g	37	1.4	370	13.0	41.4	14.2	6.8
Luxury, Skinny, Whittards of Chelsea*	1 Serving/28g	92	0.8	328	12.9	67.1	2.8	13.5
Made Up, Tassimo, Suchard*	1 Serving/280ml	88	2.4	31	0.3	5.5	0.9	0.2
Maltesers, Malt Drink, Instant, Made Up, Mars*	1 Serving/220ml	104	3.0	47	0.9	7.7	1.4	0.0
Milk Drink, Low Calorie, You Count, Love Life, Waitrose*	1 Serving/11g	37	0.3	339	21.2	57.1	2.9	5.5
Velvet, Cadbury*	1 Serving/28g	136	6.9	487	8.6	57.8	24.6	2.0
Wispa, Hot Frothy, Cadbury*	1 Sachet/27g	107	1.4	395	11.0	74.0	5.3	2.9
HOT DOG								
American Style, Hunters*	1 Sausage/23g	50	3.4	220	12.5	8.7	15.0	0.1
Feasters, Eat Well, M&S*	1 Sausage/140g	326	11.3	233	11.0	29.1	8.1	1.6
Sausage, American Style, Average	1 Sausage/75g	180	14.3	241	11.6	6.2	19.0	0.0
Sausage, Average	1 Sausage/23g	40	3.0	175	10.8	4.3	12.8	0.3
HOT DOG VEGETARIAN								
Meat Free, Sainsbury's*	1 Sausage/30g	71	4.5	237	18.0	7.6	15.0	1.0
Tesco*	1 Sausage/30g	66	4.5	220	18.0	2.7	15.0	2.0
HOT POT								
Beef, & Vegetable, Minced, COU, M&S*	1 Pack/400g	380	6.8	95	10.3	9.0	1.7	2.4
Beef, Classic, 800g, Asda*	1 Serving/400g	400	20.8	100	5.7	7.1	5.2	1.2
Beef, Minced, Bisto*	1 Pack/375g	364	13.5	97	4.1	11.3	3.6	1.4
Beef, Minced, Frozen, Tesco*	1 Pack/450g	338	11.2	75	4.0	9.1	2.5	1.4
Beef, Minced, Sainsbury's*	1 Pack/450g	464	22.0	103	5.3	9.5	4.9	2.2
Beef, Ross*	1 Pack/310g	255	11.2	82	2.2	9.4	3.6	1.5
Beef, Weight Watchers*	1 Pack/320g	231	7.7	72	3.6	8.4	2.4	1.6
Chicken, & Cider, Ready Meals, Waitrose*	1 Pack/400g	500	20.4	125	6.8	12.9	5.1	1.1

H

INFO/WEIGHT	Measure	per Measure KCAL	FAT	Nutrition Values per 100g / 100ml KCAL	PROT	CARB	FAT	FIBRE

HOT POT

	Measure INFO/WEIGHT	per Measure KCAL	FAT	Per 100g KCAL	PROT	CARB	FAT	FIBRE
Chicken, Chunky, Weight Watchers*	1 Pack/320g	275	9.0	86	4.7	10.4	2.8	0.6
Chicken, Co-Op*	1 Pack/340g	289	10.2	85	6.0	9.0	3.0	0.7
Chicken, Frozen, Asda*	1 Pack/400g	300	6.0	75	5.5	9.9	1.5	0.8
Chicken, GFY, Asda*	1 Serving/400g	256	5.2	64	4.8	8.2	1.3	1.4
Chicken, LC, Tesco*	1 Pack/361g	250	4.6	70	5.1	9.1	1.3	1.5
Chicken, Sainsbury's*	1 Pack/400g	340	11.0	85	5.2	9.8	2.8	1.3
Chicken, Weight Watchers*	1 Pack/320g	226	4.5	71	6.4	7.3	1.4	1.8
Lamb, & Vegetable, Asda*	1 Hotpot/500g	240	2.0	48	4.0	7.0	0.4	0.0
Lamb, & Vegetable, Minced, COU, M&S*	1 Pack/400g	340	10.8	85	5.7	12.5	2.7	1.8
Lamb, Cumbrian, Look What We Found*	1 Pack/300g	276	5.4	92	8.9	10.1	1.8	3.0
Lamb, Diet Chef Ltd*	1 Pack/300g	276	5.4	92	8.9	10.1	1.8	3.0
Lamb, Low Fat, Solo Slim, Rosemary Conley*	1 Pack/300g	276	5.4	92	8.9	10.1	1.8	3.0
Lamb, Shank, Extra Special, Asda*	1 Pack/450g	508	20.2	113	10.2	7.8	4.5	1.3
Lancashire, M&S*	1 Pack/454g	431	15.0	95	10.1	6.7	3.3	1.0
Lancashire, Sainsbury's*	½ Pack/225g	220	8.8	98	6.1	9.5	3.9	1.0
Lancashire, Tesco*	½ Pack/225g	205	7.0	91	6.0	9.7	3.1	0.5
Lancashire, Weight-Away*	1 Pack/250g	214	5.3	85	8.8	7.2	2.1	1.5
Liver & Bacon, Tesco*	1 Pack/550g	693	31.4	126	6.4	12.3	5.7	1.5
Sausage, Aunt Bessie's*	¼ Pack/200g	212	9.2	106	3.6	12.6	4.6	1.9
Sausage, Smart Price, Asda*	1 Pack/300g	239	7.0	80	3.7	11.0	2.3	0.4
Vegetable, & Tomato, Chunky, Big Eat, Heinz*	1 Pot/355g	213	1.4	60	2.5	11.7	0.4	4.1
Vegetable, Ready Meal, Average	1 Serving/400g	261	7.4	65	1.9	10.7	1.9	1.9
Vegetable, Weight Watchers*	1 Pack/335g	228	6.4	68	2.6	9.9	1.9	1.5
Vegetarian Sausage & Vegetable, Linda McCartney*	1 Pot/400g	516	20.4	129	6.4	15.7	5.1	2.3

HOUMOUS

	Measure INFO/WEIGHT	per Measure KCAL	FAT	Per 100g KCAL	PROT	CARB	FAT	FIBRE
40% Less fat, Eat Smart, Morrisons*	½ Pack/85g	209	15.0	246	7.9	13.8	17.7	2.7
Avocado, Fresh, San Amvrosia*	1 Serving/50g	172	16.0	344	5.4	8.5	32.1	2.5
Balsamic Caramelised Red Onion, Extra Special, Asda*	½ Pack/50g	146	10.7	293	6.8	18.2	21.4	1.0
Broad Bean, Asparagus & Mint, Tesco*	¼ Pot/42g	120	9.7	285	7.1	9.7	23.0	3.7
Caramelised Onion, Tesco*	¼ Pack/50g	125	9.7	250	5.5	13.0	19.4	4.2
Carrot with Lemon & Coriander, Shapers, Boots*	1 Pack/75g	64	1.9	85	3.0	11.0	2.5	3.4
Chargrilled Red Pepper & Chilli, 30% Less Fat, Asda*	1 Serving/50g	116	8.2	233	7.5	11.5	16.4	4.9
Chilli & Red Pepper, Topped, Tesco*	½ Pack/100g	281	25.1	281	7.1	6.6	25.1	8.1
Fresh, Sainsbury's*	1 Serving/50g	156	13.8	312	7.3	8.9	27.5	2.2
Fresh, Waitrose*	1 Serving/75g	219	19.8	292	7.2	6.3	26.4	7.6
Garlic & Pesto, Asda*	1 Serving/34g	107	8.8	314	8.0	12.0	26.0	0.0
GFY, Asda*	1 Serving/50g	136	10.0	272	9.0	14.0	20.0	3.8
Greek, Somerfield*	1 Serving/50g	152	13.4	304	7.6	8.2	26.8	5.5
Jalapeno, Asda*	1 Serving/50g	166	14.5	331	7.0	10.6	29.0	4.5
Jalapeno, Sainsbury's*	¼ Pot/50g	148	13.4	296	6.4	7.2	26.8	5.7
Jalapeno, Tesco*	½ Pot/100g	360	31.1	360	7.5	11.4	31.1	3.9
Lemon & Coriander, BGTY, Sainsbury's*	½ Tub/100g	145	9.0	145	6.3	9.7	9.0	5.9
Lemon & Coriander, GFY, Asda*	1 Serving/50g	130	9.9	259	8.3	12.0	19.8	5.1
Lemon & Coriander, Reduced Fat, Tesco*	1 Pot/60g	135	9.2	225	7.4	13.8	15.3	4.7
Lemon & Coriander, Sainsbury's*	¼ Tub/50g	146	12.6	291	7.0	9.1	25.1	6.0
Lemon & Coriander, Tesco*	1 Serving/50g	170	14.5	340	7.0	12.7	29.0	2.1
Light, Morrisons*	½ Pack/85g	200	15.3	235	7.4	10.9	18.0	0.0
Mediterranean Deli, M&S*	¼ Pack/70g	203	17.7	290	7.8	8.0	25.3	6.5
Mixed Olive, Sainsbury's*	¼ Pot/50g	134	11.6	268	6.7	8.4	23.1	7.7
Moroccan, Tesco*	¼ Pot/50g	144	12.8	289	6.8	8.1	25.5	7.3
Moroccan Style, Sainsbury's*	¼ Pot/50g	114	9.8	227	5.5	7.3	19.5	6.6
Moroccan Style Topped, M&S*	1 Serving/100g	220	15.3	220	6.5	13.2	15.3	9.2
Moroccan with Coriander & Spices, Tesco*	¼ Pot/50g	131	9.9	262	9.4	11.6	19.8	5.2

H

	Measure INFO/WEIGHT	per Measure KCAL	FAT	Nutrition Values per 100g / 100ml KCAL	PROT	CARB	FAT	FIBRE

HOUMOUS

	Measure INFO/WEIGHT	KCAL	FAT	KCAL	PROT	CARB	FAT	FIBRE
Organic, M&S*	¼ Pack/25g	82	7.4	330	6.9	9.1	29.7	3.3
Organic, Sainsbury's*	¼ Pot/43g	139	12.1	326	6.8	10.7	28.4	3.5
Organic, Tesco*	¼ Tub/42g	134	11.4	320	6.5	12.3	27.2	2.4
Red Pepper, Reduced Fat, Tesco*	¼ Pot/57g	120	7.4	205	7.7	12.5	12.6	5.3
Red Pepper Pesto, Tesco*	¼ Pot/50g	138	11.3	275	7.4	9.7	22.6	5.7
Reduced Fat, Average	1 Tbsp/30g	72	5.0	241	9.2	13.3	16.8	3.6
Reduced Fat, BGTY, Sainsbury's*	1 Serving/50g	84	5.0	167	7.1	12.3	10.0	6.0
Reduced Fat, Budgens*	1 Serving/50g	130	9.6	261	9.1	12.6	19.3	3.3
Reduced Fat, Co-Op*	¼ Pack/50g	72	4.3	145	6.5	10.7	8.6	7.3
Reduced Fat, Mediterranean Deli, M&S*	1 Mini Pot/60g	126	9.7	210	7.5	8.3	16.2	9.3
Reduced Fat, Moroccan Style, Topped, M&S*	1 Tub/170g	374	26.0	220	6.6	13.2	15.3	9.2
Reduced Fat, Snack Pots, Mini, BGTY, Sainsbury's*	1 Mini Pot/60g	100	7.3	167	7.0	13.8	12.1	5.5
Roasted Red Pepper, 50% Less Fat, Tesco*	½ Pot/85g	156	10.5	184	7.3	10.9	12.4	9.5
Roasted Red Pepper, BGTY, Sainsbury's*	¼ Tub/50g	64	3.4	129	4.9	11.9	6.9	5.3
Roasted Red Pepper, Sainsbury's*	½ Pot/100g	317	27.2	317	6.2	9.0	27.2	5.7
Roasted Red Pepper, Somerfield*	½ Pot/85g	244	21.3	287	7.1	8.1	25.1	5.2
Roasted Red Pepper, Tesco*	1 Serving/75g	255	22.3	340	7.1	11.1	29.7	2.4
Roasted Red Pepper VLH Kitchens	1 Serving/17g	31	49.4	183	6.5	15.6	8.4	6.2
Roasted Vegetable, Fresh, Sainsbury's*	¼ Pot/50g	144	13.6	287	5.9	4.9	27.1	7.8
So Organic, Sainsbury's*	¼ Pack/50g	157	13.5	314	6.7	8.5	27.0	5.0
Somerfield*	1 Pot/170g	517	45.6	304	7.6	6.2	26.8	5.5
Spicy Red Pepper with Crudite Dippers, M&S*	1 Pack/130g	124	7.9	95	3.3	7.1	6.1	3.4
Sun Dried Tomato, Chunky, Tesco*	½ Pot/95g	322	27.0	339	6.7	14.0	28.4	3.3
Sweet Chilli, Tesco*	¼ Pot/50g	120	8.4	240	6.9	15.2	16.7	5.4
Tesco*	¼ Pot/51g	160	13.6	315	7.4	9.8	26.8	3.4
with Extra Virgin Olive Oil, Tesco*	1 Pack/190g	564	46.2	297	7.9	11.7	24.3	5.1
Zorba Delicacies Ltd*	1 Serving/50g	156	13.3	313	7.6	10.7	26.6	3.0

HULA HOOPS

	Measure INFO/WEIGHT	KCAL	FAT	KCAL	PROT	CARB	FAT	FIBRE
Bacon & Ketchup Flavour, KP Snacks*	1 Bag/27g	140	8.3	517	3.4	56.3	30.9	2.0
BBQ Beef, 55% Less Saturated Fat, KP Snacks*	1 Pack/34g	174	9.7	511	3.6	60.3	28.4	1.8
Cheese & Onion 55% Less Saturated Fat, KP Snacks*	1 Bag/34g	175	9.7	515	3.6	61.0	28.5	1.9
Chilli Salsa, Tortilla, KP Snacks*	1 Bag/25g	124	6.8	494	4.9	57.2	27.3	5.3
Minis, Original, KP Snacks*	1 Tub/140g	752	48.7	537	3.0	52.9	34.8	1.7
Multigrain, KP Snacks*	1 Pack/23g	113	5.9	491	5.6	60.0	25.6	4.4
Original, 55% Less Saturated Fat, KP Snacks*	1 Bag/34g	175	9.7	515	3.2	61.6	28.4	1.8
Roast Chicken, 50% Less Saturated Fat, KP Snacks*	1 Bag/34g	175	9.7	514	3.4	61.0	28.5	1.7
Salt & Vinegar, 50% Less Saturated Fat, KP Snacks*	1 Pack/25g	128	7.0	510	3.1	60.9	28.2	1.8
Sizzling Bacon, KP Snacks*	1 Bag/34g	175	9.7	514	3.4	60.9	28.5	1.7

ICE CREAM

INFO/WEIGHT	Measure	per Measure		Nutrition Values per 100g / 100ml				
		KCAL	FAT	KCAL	PROT	CARB	FAT	FIBRE
After Dinner, Mint, Dairy, Asda*	1 Serving/100g	182	8.0	182	3.4	24.0	8.0	0.4
After Dinner Bites, Vanilla, Magnum, Wall's Ice Cream*	1 Serving/29g	100	6.7	344	3.4	31.0	23.0	1.4
After Eight, Nestle*	1 Serving/55g	114	5.2	207	3.6	27.1	9.4	0.3
Almond Indulgence, Sainsbury's*	1 Serving/120g	286	18.8	238	2.8	21.4	15.7	0.6
Baked Alaska, Ben & Jerry's*	1 Serving/100g	260	15.0	260	4.0	29.0	15.0	0.1
Banana, Thorntons*	1oz/28g	63	3.5	225	4.0	23.8	12.6	0.0
Bananas Foster, Haagen-Dazs*	1 Serving/125ml	260	15.0	208	3.2	22.4	12.0	0.0
Banoffee, Haagen-Dazs*	1 Serving/120ml	274	15.6	228	4.0	23.0	13.0	0.0
Bar, Belgian Chocolate & Vanilla, Giant, M&S*	1 Bar/120g	384	26.3	320	3.5	27.7	21.9	0.1
Billionaire Shortcake, Chokablok*	1 Scoop/100ml	225	11.4	225	2.8	27.0	11.4	0.7
Bounty, Mini Bar, Mars*	1 Bar/25ml	72	4.8	288	4.5	24.8	19.0	1.0
Bournville, Cadbury*	1 Bar/120g	258	13.9	215	3.5	26.0	11.6	0.0
Brandy, Luxurious, M&S*	1 Serving/100g	228	13.3	228	3.8	19.1	13.3	0.2
Caramel, Carte d'Or*	2 Boules/50g	106	4.4	212	2.6	30.8	8.7	0.0
Caramel & Cinnamon Waffle, Carte d'Or*	2 Scoops/55g	121	6.0	220	3.0	27.0	11.0	0.0
Caramel Chew Chew, Ben & Jerry's*	1 Tub/113g	305	18.1	270	3.0	29.0	16.0	0.0
Caramel Craze, Organic, Tesco*	1 Serving/100g	253	15.3	253	3.3	25.5	15.3	0.0
Caramella, Sundae, Tesco*	1 Sundae/80g	165	5.5	205	2.2	32.9	6.8	1.9
Caramella, Tesco*	1 Serving/51g	120	5.5	235	2.6	32.0	10.7	1.1
Cheesecake Brownie, Ben & Jerry's*	1 Serving/100g	260	16.0	260	4.0	26.0	16.0	0.0
Cherry Bomb Brownie, Chokablok*	1 Scoop/87g	191	8.3	220	3.3	29.9	9.5	1.4
Cherry Garcia, Ben & Jerry's*	1 Serving/100g	250	15.0	250	3.0	26.0	15.0	0.0
Choc Chip, Cookie Dough, Haagen-Dazs*	1oz/28g	74	4.7	266	3.8	24.9	16.9	0.0
Choc Chip, Haagen-Dazs*	1oz/28g	80	5.2	286	4.7	24.8	18.7	0.0
Chocolate, Belgian, Haagen-Dazs*	1 Tub/78g	249	16.2	318	4.6	28.4	20.7	0.0
Chocolate, Chunky, Giant, M&S*	1 Lolly/90g	300	20.6	335	4.0	28.0	23.0	2.3
Chocolate, Double, Nestle*	1 Serving/78g	248	14.3	320	4.8	33.7	18.4	0.0
Chocolate, Easy Serve, Co-Op*	1oz/28g	46	2.0	165	3.0	22.0	7.0	0.3
Chocolate, Flavour, Average	1 Serving/70g	149	7.9	212	4.1	23.7	11.3	0.6
Chocolate, Flavour, Healthy Option, Average	1 Serving/70g	89	1.2	127	3.5	25.9	1.7	0.3
Chocolate, Flavour, Soft Scoop, Sainsbury's*	1 Serving/70g	122	5.2	174	3.1	23.6	7.5	0.3
Chocolate, Haagen-Dazs*	1 Serving/120ml	269	18.0	224	4.0	19.0	15.0	0.0
Chocolate, Milk, Belgian, Tesco*	1 Lolly/85g	255	15.5	300	3.9	29.8	18.2	0.7
Chocolate, Milk, Mini Sticks, Weight Watchers*	1 Stick/45ml	96	5.0	213	2.7	25.8	11.1	0.7
Chocolate, Organic, Green & Black's*	1 Serving/125g	310	17.6	248	5.0	25.3	14.1	1.1
Chocolate, Organic, M&S*	1oz/28g	71	4.5	255	5.0	24.0	16.0	1.5
Chocolate, Really Creamy, Asda*	1 Serving/100g	227	11.0	227	4.1	28.0	11.0	0.4
Chocolate, Soft Scoop, Asda*	1 Scoop/47g	84	3.8	179	3.7	23.0	8.0	0.0
Chocolate, Soft Scoop, Morrisons*	1 Serving/50g	100	5.3	199	3.3	22.3	10.6	1.1
Chocolate, Soft Scoop, Tesco*	1 Serving/50g	93	4.0	186	3.2	25.1	8.1	0.3
Chocolate, Stick, Chocolate Covered, Green & Black's*	1 Stick/100g	214	13.6	214	3.7	19.3	13.6	2.1
Chocolate, Thorntons*	1oz/28g	67	3.6	238	4.6	25.1	12.9	0.0
Chocolate, Triple, Carte d'Or*	1 Serving/58g	122	5.7	210	3.7	27.0	9.8	0.0
Chocolate, Triple, Dairy, Sainsbury's*	1/8 Litre/67g	123	4.4	184	3.5	27.6	6.6	1.0
Chocolate, Weight Watchers*	1 Serving/100ml	140	1.2	140	4.3	28.7	1.2	0.0
Chocolate & Orange, Organic, Green & Black's*	1 Serving/100g	248	14.1	248	5.0	25.3	14.1	0.1
Chocolate Brownie with Walnuts, Haagen-Dazs*	1 Cup/101g	223	16.4	221	4.4	21.0	16.2	0.0
Chocolate Chip, Baskin Robbins*	1 Serving/75g	170	10.0	227	4.0	24.0	13.3	0.0
Chocolate Fudge Brownie, Ben & Jerry's*	1 Tub/114g	285	14.8	250	4.0	32.0	13.0	1.5
Chocolate Fudge Swirl, Haagen-Dazs*	1oz/28g	77	4.8	276	4.6	25.6	17.2	0.0
Chocolate Honeycomb, Co-Op*	¼ Pot/81g	186	10.5	230	4.0	26.0	13.0	0.3
Chocolate Honeycomb, COU, M&S*	1 Serving/100ml	150	2.6	150	3.5	31.5	2.6	0.7
Chocolate Macadamia, Ben & Jerry's*	1 Serving/100g	260	18.0	260	4.0	22.0	18.0	0.8

ICE CREAM

INFO/WEIGHT	Measure per Measure		Nutrition Values per 100g / 100ml				
	KCAL	FAT	KCAL	PROT	CARB	FAT	FIBRE
Chocolate Midnight Cookies, Haagen-Dazs* — 1oz/28g	81	4.8	289	4.9	28.7	17.2	0.0
Chocolate Stick, Milk Chocolate, Mini, Weight Watchers* — 1 Stick/32g	95	5.1	296	3.7	33.8	15.9	1.6
Chocolate Trio, Thorntons* — 1 Bar/100g	310	20.6	310	3.3	28.0	20.6	1.8
Chocolate with Chocolate Chips, Milfina* — 1oz/28g	66	3.5	235	3.8	26.7	12.5	0.8
Chocolatino, Sundae, Tesco* — 1 Tub/80g	160	5.9	200	4.4	29.0	7.4	2.4
Chocolatino, Tesco* — 1 Serving/56g	115	3.8	205	3.4	31.4	6.8	1.8
Chunky Monkey, Fairtrade, Ben & Jerry's* — 1 Serving/100g	290	17.0	290	4.0	27.0	17.0	1.0
Clotted Cream, Cornish, Kelly's Of Cornwall* — 1 Serving/125g	282	18.6	226	2.9	20.1	14.9	0.1
Coconut, Carte d'Or* — 1 Serving/100ml	125	7.1	125	1.8	14.0	7.1	0.5
Coffee, Finest, Tesco* — ¼ Pot/93g	236	14.9	254	4.9	22.5	16.0	0.0
Coffee, Haagen-Dazs* — 1 Serving/120ml	271	18.4	226	4.1	17.9	15.3	0.0
Coffee, Waitrose* — ¼ Tub/125ml	292	16.4	234	3.6	25.4	13.1	0.0
Cookie Dough, Ben & Jerry's* — 1 Serving/100g	270	14.0	270	4.0	31.0	14.0	0.0
Cookies & Cream, Haagen-Dazs* — 1 Tub/100ml	226	14.7	226	4.0	19.5	14.7	0.0
Cornetto Soft, Chocolate Chip, Wall's Ice Cream* — 1 Serving/80g	256	13.6	320	3.5	37.0	17.0	1.5
Cornetto Soft, Mint Chocolate Chip, Wall's Ice Cream* — 1 Serving/80g	240	13.6	300	4.0	33.0	17.0	1.0
Cornetto Soft, Strawberry, Wall's Ice Cream* — 1 Serving/80g	208	8.0	260	3.5	38.0	10.0	1.0
Cornetto Soft, Vanilla, Wall's Ice Cream* — 1 Serving/80g	264	16.0	330	4.5	33.0	20.0	0.0
Cornish, Asda* — 1 Serving/100ml	100	5.0	100	1.8	12.0	5.0	0.0
Cornish Clotted, M&S* — 1 Pot/90g	207	13.0	230	2.8	21.8	14.5	0.1
Cornish Dairy, Waitrose* — 1 Serving/125ml	121	6.6	97	1.7	10.7	5.3	0.1
Cornish Style, Co-Op* — 1oz/28g	53	2.5	190	4.0	23.0	9.0	0.1
Crema Di Mascarpone, Carte d'Or* — 1 Serving/100g	207	8.9	207	2.8	29.0	8.9	0.0
Crunchie, Blast, Cadbury* — 1 Lolly/100ml	230	13.9	230	2.8	23.1	13.9	0.1
Dairy, Flavoured — 1oz/28g	50	2.2	179	3.5	24.7	8.0	0.0
Dairy Cornish, Tesco* — 1 Serving/49g	112	6.0	228	3.2	24.7	12.3	0.1
Date & Almond Cream, Haagen-Dazs* — 1 Serving/120ml	254	15.6	212	5.0	19.0	13.0	0.0
Dream, Cadbury* — 1 Bar/120ml	264	14.3	220	3.6	26.0	11.9	0.0
Dulce De Leche, Bar, Haagen-Dazs* — 1 Bar/105g	370	24.0	352	3.8	32.3	22.9	0.0
Farmhouse Toffee, TTD, Sainsbury's* — ¼ Pot/100g	293	18.6	293	3.2	28.3	18.6	0.6
Fig & Orange Blossom Honey, Waitrose* — 1 Serving/100g	219	11.8	219	3.9	24.3	11.8	0.4
Forest Fruits & Mascarpone Forest Fruits, Aldi* — 1 Pot/73g	159	7.4	217	1.8	29.6	10.1	0.6
Fruit & Fresh Tropical, Carte d'Or* — 1 Serving/83g	154	7.1	185	2.5	24.5	8.5	0.0
Galaxy, Mars* — 1 Bar/60ml	203	13.4	339	4.7	29.7	22.4	0.0
Gelato, Vanilla — 1 Serving/100g	162	7.2	162	2.4	22.6	7.2	0.3
Get Fruit, Tropical, Solero* — 1 Serving/125ml	162	5.5	130	1.6	20.6	4.4	0.4
Gold Digger Dynamite, Chokablok* — ¼ Tub/125ml	288	14.0	230	3.2	28.2	11.2	0.9
Half Baked, Ben & Jerry's* — 1 Serving/100g	270	13.0	270	5.0	32.0	13.0	1.0
Honeycomb Harvest, Mackies* — 1 Serving/100g	209	10.0	209	4.0	25.0	10.0	0.0
Knickerbocker Glory — 1oz/28g	31	1.4	112	1.5	16.4	5.0	0.2
Lactose Free, Hacendado* — 1 Serving/100g	141	4.9	141	4.0	27.6	4.9	6.6
Lavazza, Carte d'Or* — 1 Serving/55g	120	5.4	218	3.5	29.0	9.9	0.0
Lemon Cream, Dairy, Sainsbury's* — 1 Serving/100g	199	9.3	199	3.0	25.9	9.3	0.1
Lemon Curd Swirl, Duchy Originals* — ¼ Pot/101g	247	14.2	245	3.7	25.8	14.1	0.0
Lemon Meringue, Really Creamy, Asda* — 1 Serving/100ml	100	5.0	100	1.8	12.0	5.0	0.1
Lemon Meringue, Zesty, COU, M&S* — ¼ Pot/73g	120	1.8	165	2.6	33.0	2.5	0.5
Lychee Cream & Ginger, Haagen-Dazs* — 1 Serving/120ml	258	12.7	215	3.6	26.1	10.6	0.0
Magic Stars, Milky Way* — 1 Ice Cream/53ml	67	3.3	127	2.1	15.5	6.2	0.0
Magnum Moments, Wall's Ice Cream* — 1 Serving/18ml	58	3.7	323	4.0	30.0	20.8	0.0
Mango, 98% Fat Free, Bulla* — 1 Serving/70g	94	1.1	134	4.2	25.4	1.6	0.0
Maple, Magic, M&S* — 1 Ice Cream/93g	259	11.4	278	2.9	39.0	12.3	0.6
Maple & Walnut, American, Sainsbury's* — 1/8 Pot/68g	121	4.9	179	3.1	25.6	7.2	0.2
Mince Pie, Finest, Tesco* — ¼ Pack/188g	476	22.1	254	3.9	33.0	11.8	1.1

ICE CREAM

INFO/WEIGHT	Measure Measure	per KCAL	FAT	KCAL	PROT	CARB	FAT	FIBRE
Mint, Majestic Luxury, Iceland*	1 Serving/80g	269	14.6	337	3.8	39.3	18.3	1.3
Mint & Chocolate, Sainsbury's*	1 Serving/71g	137	6.7	192	3.4	23.5	9.4	0.4
Mint & Chocolate Flavour, Average	1 Serving/70g	129	6.3	184	3.0	22.6	9.0	1.2
Mint & Chocolate Flavour, Healthy Option, Average	1 Serving/70g	101	1.8	144	4.1	29.9	2.6	4.1
Mint Choc Chip, Luscious, Morrisons*	1 Serving/50g	99	5.2	198	2.9	23.1	10.5	0.7
Mint Choc Chip Soft Scoop, Asda*	1 Serving/46g	86	4.1	189	2.9	24.0	9.0	0.3
Mint Chocolate Chip, Baskin Robbins*	1 Scoop/113g	270	16.0	239	4.4	24.8	14.2	0.9
Mocha Coffee Indulgence, Sainsbury's*	¼ Pot/82g	178	10.6	217	3.2	22.1	12.9	0.1
My Carte D'or, Caramel, Carte d'Or*	1 Tub/200ml	210	8.0	105	1.5	16.0	4.0	0.4
My Carte D'or, Chocolate, Carte d'Or*	1 Tub/200ml	220	11.0	110	1.8	12.5	5.5	0.4
Neapolitan, Average	1 Serving/70g	111	4.6	158	3.1	21.9	6.5	0.6
Neapolitan, Brick, Tesco*	1 Serving/50g	82	3.4	163	3.3	21.9	6.9	0.4
Neapolitan, Iceland*	1oz/28g	46	2.1	164	3.0	21.3	7.4	0.0
Neapolitan, Lidl*	1 Serving/48g	108	4.8	226	4.3	29.5	10.0	0.0
Neapolitan, Soft Scoop, Asda*	1 Scoop/47g	82	3.8	175	2.8	23.0	8.0	0.2
Neapolitan, Soft Scoop, Sainsbury's*	1 Serving/75g	124	5.2	165	2.8	22.8	6.9	0.2
Neapolitan, Soft Scoop, Value, Tesco*	1 Serving/100g	125	5.1	125	2.7	16.2	5.1	1.4
Neapolitan Easy Serve, Co-Op*	1oz/28g	42	2.0	150	3.0	20.0	7.0	0.2
Neapolitan Sandwich, Gelatelli*	1 Sandwich/106g	233	9.5	220	4.9	29.0	9.0	1.9
Neopolitian, Soft Scoop, Tesco*	1 Serving/43g	70	3.0	163	3.3	21.9	6.9	0.4
Non-Dairy, Reduced Calorie	1oz/28g	33	1.7	119	3.4	13.7	6.0	0.0
Nuts About Caramel, Cadbury*	1 Serving/100ml	290	17.1	290	4.3	28.1	17.1	2.6
Panna Cotta, Haagen-Dazs*	1 Serving/120ml	248	16.0	207	3.4	18.4	13.3	0.0
Peach Melba, Soft Scoop, M&S*	1oz/28g	46	2.1	165	2.8	21.4	7.6	0.3
Pistachio, Haagen-Dazs*	1 Serving/120ml	276	18.8	230	4.4	17.7	15.7	0.0
Praline, Green & Black's*	1 Pot/100g	191	10.8	191	3.5	20.0	10.8	0.9
Praline & Chocolate, Thorntons*	1oz/28g	87	6.4	309	4.6	21.3	22.9	0.6
Pralines & Cream, Baskin Robbins*	1 Serving/100g	252	13.6	252	4.5	27.7	13.6	0.3
Pralines & Cream, Haagen-Dazs*	1 Tub/78g	213	12.9	272	3.9	27.2	16.5	0.0
Raspberries, Clotted Cream, Waitrose*	1 Tub/500ml	790	39.5	158	2.9	18.9	7.9	0.1
Raspberry Ripple, Average	1 Serving/70g	93	3.3	134	1.9	20.8	4.7	0.1
Raspberry Ripple, Co-Op*	1oz/28g	45	2.0	160	3.0	23.0	7.0	0.2
Raspberry Ripple, Dairy, Waitrose*	1 Serving/186ml	195	10.0	105	1.9	12.3	5.4	0.0
Raspberry Ripple, Soft Scoop, Asda*	1 Scoop/46g	78	3.2	170	2.5	24.0	7.0	0.3
Raspberry Ripple, Soft Scoop, Sainsbury's*	1 Serving/75g	128	5.2	170	2.6	24.2	7.0	0.3
Raspberry Ripple, Soft Scoop, Tesco*	1 Scoop/25g	39	1.5	157	2.5	23.0	6.1	0.2
Rocky Road, Sainsbury's*	1/8 Pot/67g	137	4.9	205	3.8	30.9	7.3	1.0
Rolo, Nestle*	½ Tub/500ml	1180	52.5	236	3.4	31.9	10.5	0.2
Rum & Raisin, Carte d'Or*	2 Scoops/50g	100	4.0	200	2.5	24.0	8.0	1.0
Rum & Raisin, Haagen-Dazs*	1 Serving/120ml	264	17.6	220	3.4	18.6	14.7	0.0
Rum & Raisin, TTD, Sainsbury's*	¼ Pot/100g	220	10.4	220	3.8	27.7	10.4	1.0
Screwball, Asda*	1 Screwball/60g	122	6.0	203	3.3	25.0	10.0	1.5
Screwball, Morrisons*	1 Screwball/100ml	133	6.3	133	2.0	17.0	6.3	0.0
Screwball, Raspberry Ripple, Asda*	1 Screwball/100ml	100	3.7	100	1.3	15.4	3.7	0.1
Screwball, Tesco*	1 Screwball/61g	116	5.2	190	2.9	25.2	8.6	0.3
Smarties, Nestle*	1 Serving/50g	125	6.0	250	3.6	32.3	11.9	0.2
Stem Ginger with Belgian Chocolate, Waitrose*	1 Lolly/110g	255	14.4	232	2.9	25.5	13.1	1.7
Strawberry, Haagen-Dazs*	1oz/28g	67	4.3	241	4.0	21.5	15.5	0.0
Strawberry, Soft Scoop, Tesco*	1 Serving/46g	78	3.4	170	2.8	23.1	7.4	0.1
Strawberry, Thorntons*	1oz/28g	52	2.6	185	3.2	22.5	9.3	0.1
Strawberry, Weight Watchers*	1 Pot/57g	81	2.2	142	2.5	23.4	3.9	0.2
Strawberry & Cream, Mivvi, Nestle*	1 Serving/60g	118	4.6	196	2.6	29.4	7.6	0.2
Strawberry & Cream, Organic, Sainsbury's*	1 Serving/100g	193	9.8	193	3.6	22.6	9.8	0.4

ICE CREAM

	Measure INFO/WEIGHT	per Measure		Nutrition Values per 100g / 100ml				
		KCAL	FAT	KCAL	PROT	CARB	FAT	FIBRE
Strawberry & Yoghurt Delice, Carte d'Or*	1 Portion/54g	95	2.0	175	1.5	34.0	3.6	0.0
Strawberry Cheesecake, Ben & Jerry's*	1 Serving/100g	240	14.0	240	3.0	27.0	14.0	0.0
Strawberry Cheesecake, Co-Op*	1/6 Pot/86g	163	6.0	190	3.0	29.0	7.0	0.2
Strawberry Cheesecake, Haagen-Dazs*	¼ Tub/125ml	295	17.0	236	3.3	25.1	13.6	0.3
Tantilising Toffee, COU, M&S*	¼ Pot/125ml	125	3.5	100	0.6	18.0	2.8	0.0
Terry's Chocolate Orange, Carte d'Or*	1 Serving/100g	182	7.1	182	2.8	27.0	7.1	0.0
Tiramisu, Haagen-Dazs*	1 Serving/120ml	303	19.6	253	3.8	22.7	16.3	0.0
Toblerone, Carte d'Or*	1 Serving/100g	211	9.1	211	3.7	29.0	9.1	0.0
Toffee, Deliciously Dairy, Co-Op*	1oz/28g	45	2.0	160	3.0	21.0	7.0	0.2
Toffee, Really Creamy, Asda*	1 Serving/120ml	146	6.0	122	1.8	17.5	5.0	0.1
Toffee, Thorntons*	1oz/28g	61	3.2	218	4.1	24.5	11.6	0.0
Toffee & Biscuit, Weight Watchers*	1 Pot/100ml	93	2.7	93	1.5	14.9	2.7	0.1
Toffee & Honeycomb Sundaes, Weight Watchers*	1 Pot/150g	183	2.7	122	1.7	18.1	1.8	5.9
Toffee & Vanilla, Sainsbury's*	1 Serving/71g	146	6.8	205	3.1	26.7	9.5	0.1
Toffee Fudge, Soft Scoop, Asda*	1 Serving/50g	92	3.5	185	2.6	28.0	7.0	0.0
Toffee Ripple, Tesco*	1 Serving/100g	173	7.2	173	2.7	24.4	7.2	0.1
Vanilla, & Cinnamon, Finest, Tesco*	1 Serving/50g	114	7.4	229	3.9	20.2	14.7	0.4
Vanilla, & Cinnamon, Spar*	1 Serving/120g	247	10.3	206	3.8	28.0	8.6	0.0
Vanilla, Bean, Light, Deluxe*	1 Serving/64g	110	2.5	172	4.7	26.6	3.9	0.0
Vanilla, Bean, Purbeck*	1 Serving/100g	198	11.5	198	4.8	18.7	11.5	0.0
Vanilla, Ben & Jerry's*	1 Tub/112g	258	16.8	230	4.0	20.0	15.0	0.1
Vanilla, Budgens*	1oz/28g	45	1.9	159	3.0	21.7	6.7	0.1
Vanilla, Caramel Brownie, Haagen-Dazs*	1 Serving/150g	410	24.8	273	4.5	26.8	16.5	0.0
Vanilla, Carte d'Or*	1 Serving/50g	105	4.8	210	3.0	26.0	9.5	0.0
Vanilla, Choc Fudge, Haagen-Dazs*	1oz/28g	75	4.8	267	4.3	23.5	17.2	0.0
Vanilla, Chocolate, Taste Sensation, Frosty's, Aldi*	1 Pot/73g	164	7.0	224	2.1	32.4	9.6	0.7
Vanilla, Cornish, Organic, Iceland*	1oz/28g	60	3.5	214	4.1	21.4	12.4	0.0
Vanilla, Cornish, Soft Scoop, M&S*	1oz/28g	56	3.0	199	3.9	21.8	10.7	0.2
Vanilla, COU, M&S*	¼ Pot/79g	111	2.2	140	1.7	25.9	2.8	0.8
Vanilla, Criminally Creamy, Co-Op*	1oz/28g	60	4.2	215	3.0	18.0	15.0	0.1
Vanilla, Dairy, Average	1 Scoop/40g	80	4.4	201	3.5	23.6	11.0	0.7
Vanilla, Dairy, Finest, Tesco*	1 Serving/92g	227	16.0	247	4.5	18.0	17.4	0.3
Vanilla, Dairy, Organic, Yeo Valley*	1 Serving/100g	206	11.2	206	4.9	21.3	11.2	0.0
Vanilla, Dairy Milk, Cadbury*	1 Serving/120g	259	13.9	216	3.5	26.0	11.6	0.1
Vanilla, Easy Serve, Co-Op*	1oz/28g	39	2.0	140	3.0	18.0	7.0	0.0
Vanilla, Everyday, Co-Op*	1oz/28g	41	2.0	145	3.0	18.0	7.0	0.2
Vanilla, Haagen-Dazs*	1oz/28g	70	4.8	250	4.5	19.7	17.1	0.0
Vanilla, Heavenly, Cadbury*	1 Serving/250ml	355	23.2	142	2.5	12.8	9.3	0.0
Vanilla, Light, Carte d'Or*	1 Serving/100g	136	4.4	136	2.4	22.0	4.4	4.0
Vanilla, Light Soft Scoop, 25% Less Fat, Morrisons*	1 Scoop/50g	75	2.5	150	2.9	23.2	5.0	0.2
Vanilla, Low Fat, Average	1 Scoop/50g	59	1.7	118	2.3	19.4	3.4	0.6
Vanilla, Low Fat, Weight Watchers*	1 Scoop/125ml	75	2.1	60	1.1	9.7	1.7	0.1
Vanilla, Mackies*	1 Serving/100g	193	11.0	193	4.0	18.0	11.0	0.0
Vanilla, Madagascan, Organic, Yeo Valley*	1 Serving/40ml	45	2.5	112	2.4	11.4	6.3	0.1
Vanilla, Non-Dairy, Average	1 Serving/60g	107	5.2	178	3.2	23.1	8.7	0.0
Vanilla, Organic, Waitrose*	1 Serving/125g	178	11.2	142	2.7	12.4	9.0	0.0
Vanilla, Pecan, Haagen-Dazs*	1 Serving/120ml	316	23.5	263	4.3	17.1	19.6	0.0
Vanilla, Pizza Express*	1 Serving/100g	119	6.8	119	0.9	13.8	6.8	0.0
Vanilla, Really Creamy, Asda*	1 Serving/50g	98	5.0	196	3.5	23.0	10.0	0.1
Vanilla, Sandwich, Skinny Cow*	1 Portion/36g	100	3.0	277	5.4	45.1	8.2	2.1
Vanilla, Smart Price, Asda*	1 Scoop/40g	55	2.4	137	2.8	19.0	6.0	0.2
Vanilla, Soft, Non Milk Fat, Waitrose*	1 Serving/125ml	78	3.4	62	1.3	8.0	2.7	0.1
Vanilla, Soft Scoop, 25% Less Fat, Asda*	1oz/28g	42	1.4	149	2.9	23.0	5.0	0.0

ICE CREAM	Measure INFO/WEIGHT	per Measure KCAL	FAT	KCAL	PROT	CARB	FAT	FIBRE
Vanilla, Soft Scoop, BGTY, Sainsbury's*	1 Serving/75g	88	1.3	117	3.1	22.2	1.7	0.2
Vanilla, Soft Scoop, Light, Wall's*, Wall's Ice Cream*	1 Scoop/50ml	31	1.3	62	1.3	7.0	2.6	0.9
Vanilla, Soft Scoop, Light, Weighed in Grams, Wall's*	1 Serving/100g	140	6.0	140	3.0	19.0	6.0	2.0
Vanilla, Soft Scoop, Sainsbury's*	1 Serving/71g	96	3.9	136	2.9	18.8	5.5	0.2
Vanilla, Soft Scoop, Tesco*	1oz/28g	46	2.0	164	3.1	21.8	7.1	0.1
Vanilla, Soft Scoop, Value, Tesco*	1 Scoop/42g	57	2.4	137	2.8	18.7	5.7	0.2
Vanilla, Soft Scoop, Wall's*	1 Scoop/45ml	38	1.8	84	1.3	10.0	4.1	0.1
Vanilla, Soft Slice, Wall's Ice Cream*	1 Serving/100ml	90	4.4	90	1.4	11.2	4.4	0.1
Vanilla, Thorntons*	1oz/28g	63	3.8	225	4.9	20.5	13.6	0.0
Vanilla, Toffee Crunch, Ben & Jerry's*	1 Tub/407g	1099	65.1	270	4.0	29.0	16.0	0.5
Vanilla, Too Good to Be True, Wall's Ice Cream*	1 Serving/50ml	35	0.2	70	2.0	14.9	0.4	0.1
Vanilla, TTD, Sainsbury's*	¼ Pot/100g	246	16.9	246	5.2	18.2	16.9	0.0
Vanilla, Waitrose*	1 Serving/100ml	156	10.8	156	2.6	12.0	10.8	0.0
Vanilla, with Strawberry Swirl, Weight Watchers*	1 Mini Tub/57g	81	2.2	142	2.5	23.4	3.9	0.2
Vanilla, with Vanilla Pods, Sainsbury's*	1 Serving/100g	195	10.1	195	3.5	22.5	10.1	0.1
Vanilla Flavour, Soft VLH Kitchens	1 Serving/100g	235	15.0	235	4.0	22.1	15.0	0.2
Vanilletta, Tesco*	1 Serving/47g	82	3.8	175	4.0	21.6	8.1	0.0
Viennetta, Biscuit Caramel, Wall's Ice Cream*	1/6 Serving/58g	183	12.1	315	3.3	27.8	20.9	0.0
Viennetta, Chocolate, Wall's Ice Cream*	¼ Pot/80g	200	12.2	250	4.1	24.0	15.2	0.0
Viennetta, Mint, Wall's Ice Cream*	1 Serving/80g	204	13.3	255	3.4	23.0	16.6	0.0
Viennetta, Selection Brownie, Wall's Ice Cream*	1 Serving/70g	194	11.3	277	4.2	28.5	16.2	0.0
Viennetta, Strawberry, Wall's Ice Cream*	1 Serving/80g	204	13.4	255	3.4	22.1	16.8	0.0
Viennetta, Vanilla, Wall's Ice Cream*	¼ Bar/80g	204	13.4	255	3.3	23.0	16.7	0.0
Walnut & Maple, Waitrose*	1 Serving/60g	68	2.3	114	1.8	18.2	3.8	0.0
with Raspberry Sauce, Movenpick*	1 Serving/50g	130	7.0	260	4.0	27.0	14.0	0.2

ICE CREAM BAR

	Measure INFO/WEIGHT	per Measure KCAL	FAT	KCAL	PROT	CARB	FAT	FIBRE
Bailey's, Haagen-Dazs*	1oz/28g	86	5.9	307	4.1	24.8	21.2	0.0
Bounty, 100 Ml Bar, Mars*	1 Bar/100ml	278	18.5	278	3.4	24.7	18.5	0.7
Choc Chip, Haagen-Dazs*	1oz/28g	90	6.0	320	4.3	27.4	21.5	0.0
Chocolate, Chunky, Co-Op*	1 Bar/60g	204	12.0	340	5.0	35.0	20.0	1.0
Chocolate Covered	1 Bar/40g	128	9.3	320	5.0	24.0	23.3	0.0
Dairy Milk, Caramel, Cadbury*	1 Bar/60ml	175	10.3	290	3.6	30.2	17.1	0.0
Dairy Milk, Fudge, Cadbury*	1 Bar/60g	165	10.3	275	3.0	27.6	17.2	0.0
Dairy Milk, Lolly, Cadbury*	1 Lolly/100g	235	15.0	235	3.0	25.1	15.0	0.0
Galaxy, Mars*	1 Bar/54g	184	12.2	341	3.8	30.7	22.5	0.6
Lion, Nestle*	1 Bar/45g	166	9.9	370	4.2	39.1	21.9	1.0
Maltesers, Mars*	1 Bar/45ml	113	7.0	252	2.9	25.0	15.6	0.7
Mars, Mars*	1 Bar/65g	182	10.5	280	3.4	29.7	16.2	0.8
Peanut, Farmfoods*	1 Bar/60ml	216	12.8	360	5.3	36.6	21.4	1.2
Racer, Aldi*	1 Bar/59g	194	11.0	328	6.0	34.2	18.6	0.0
Red Fruits, Solero*	1 Bar/80g	99	2.2	124	1.6	25.0	2.7	0.0
Snickers, Mars*	1 Bar/67g	250	15.0	373	6.0	37.3	22.4	0.0
Toffee Cream, Haagen-Dazs*	1oz/28g	97	6.2	345	4.0	31.0	22.0	0.0
Toffee Crunch, English, Weight Watchers*	1 Bar/40g	110	6.0	275	2.5	32.5	15.0	5.0
Twix, Mars*	1 Serving/43ml	130	7.8	306	4.0	30.8	18.3	1.2

ICE CREAM CONE

	Measure INFO/WEIGHT	per Measure KCAL	FAT	KCAL	PROT	CARB	FAT	FIBRE
Average	1 Cone/75g	140	6.4	186	3.5	25.5	8.5	0.0
Carousel Wafer Company*	1 Cone/5g	19	0.2	392	9.8	78.6	4.2	0.0
Choc 'n' Nut, Farmfoods*	1 Cone/120ml	334	16.8	278	5.0	33.0	14.0	1.0
Chocolate, Mini, Cornetto, Wall's Ice Cream*	1 Cone/36g	110	5.9	300	3.5	34.0	16.0	2.0
Chocolate, Vanilla & Hazelnut, Sainsbury's*	1 Cone/62g	190	10.5	306	4.5	33.9	16.9	0.6
Chocolate & Caramel, Skinny Cow*	1 Cone/110ml	121	2.8	110	2.5	19.3	2.5	2.7
Chocolate & Nut, Co-Op*	1 Cone/110g	307	17.0	279	3.9	31.0	15.5	0.6

	Measure INFO/WEIGHT	per Measure		Nutrition Values per 100g / 100ml				
		KCAL	FAT	KCAL	PROT	CARB	FAT	FIBRE
ICE CREAM CONE								
Chocolate & Vanilla, Good Choice, Iceland*	1 Cone/110ml	161	7.2	146	2.7	22.9	6.5	0.8
Chocolate & Vanilla, M&S*	1oz/28g	83	4.8	295	4.2	31.8	17.0	0.7
Classico, Mini, Cornetto, Wall's Ice Cream*	1 Cone/36g	120	6.8	320	3.5	35.0	18.0	1.0
Cornet, Wafer Cone, Askeys*	1 Cone/4g	13	0.1	376	10.7	77.6	2.5	0.0
Cornetto, Classico, Wall's Ice Cream*	1 Cone/98g	200	12.6	205	2.7	19.7	12.9	0.0
Cornetto, Flirt, Choc Chip & Hazelnut, Wall's Ice Cream*	1 Cone/70g	223	11.2	320	4.0	40.0	16.0	0.0
Cornetto, GFY, Asda*	1 Cone/67g	162	6.0	241	3.0	37.0	9.0	0.1
Cornetto, Mint, Wall's Ice Cream*	1 Cone/75g	190	9.9	250	4.0	31.0	13.0	0.8
Cornetto, Wall's Ice Cream*	1 Cone/75g	195	9.7	260	3.7	34.5	12.9	0.0
Creme Egg, Cadbury*	1 Cone/115ml	270	13.3	235	2.9	29.3	11.6	0.0
Cup Cornet, Wafer Cone, Askeys*	1 Cone/4g	13	0.1	376	10.7	77.6	2.5	0.0
Dairy Milk, Mint, Cadbury*	1 Cone/115ml	190	8.9	165	2.4	21.5	7.7	0.0
Extreme Raspberry, Cornetto, Nestle*	1 Cone/88g	220	8.8	250	2.5	36.0	10.0	0.2
Flake 99, Cadbury*	1 Cone/125ml	244	12.5	195	2.6	23.2	10.0	0.0
Mini, Tesco*	1 Cone/48g	152	9.3	316	4.1	31.5	19.3	0.8
Mint Choc Chip, Iceland*	1 Cone/72g	210	9.4	292	3.3	40.4	13.0	1.0
Smarties, Nestle*	1 Cone/100g	177	8.1	177	2.4	23.6	8.1	0.7
Sticky Toffee, Farmfoods*	1 Cone/120ml	326	15.4	272	3.2	36.0	12.8	2.0
Strawberry, Co-Op*	1 Cone/110g	283	13.3	257	3.5	33.6	12.1	0.5
Strawberry & Vanilla, Asda*	1 Cone/115ml	193	9.0	168	1.8	22.6	7.8	0.1
Strawberry & Vanilla, Iceland*	1 Serving/70g	182	7.6	260	3.3	37.5	10.8	0.7
Strawberry & Vanilla, M&S*	1oz/28g	81	4.6	290	4.2	30.9	16.5	0.7
Strawberry & Vanilla, Sainsbury's*	1 Cone/70g	171	6.8	243	3.4	35.6	9.7	1.0
Strawberry & Vanilla, Tesco*	1 Cone/70g	194	9.4	277	3.0	35.9	13.5	0.3
Tropical, GFY, Asda*	1 Cone/100g	135	5.0	135	2.6	20.0	5.0	0.3
Vanilla & Chocolate, Everyday Value, Tesco*	1 Cone/58g	170	7.4	285	3.8	38.9	12.4	1.3
ICE CREAM ROLL								
Arctic, Average	1 Serving/70g	140	4.6	200	4.1	33.3	6.6	0.0
Mini, Cadbury*	1 Roll/45ml	99	5.9	220	3.4	24.3	13.1	0.0
Tesco*	¼ Roll/57g	131	4.9	230	3.7	34.5	8.6	0.4
ICE CREAM SANDWICH								
Vanilla, Chocolate Coated, Lidl*	1 Serving/51g	145	9.5	284	1.8	21.6	18.6	0.0
Wich, Ben & Jerry's*	1 Pack/117g	398	19.9	340	4.0	44.0	17.0	1.0
ICE CREAM STICK								
Berry Blast, Smoothie, Skinny Cow*	1 Stick/110ml	71	0.1	65	0.9	15.1	0.1	1.9
Chocolate Cookies, Haagen-Dazs*	1 Stick/43g	162	10.9	376	4.9	31.8	25.4	0.0
Cookies 'n' Cream, Skinny Cow*	1 Stick/67g	89	1.0	133	4.8	23.5	1.5	3.6
Mint Double Chocolate, Skinny Cow*	1 Stick/110ml	94	1.8	85	2.7	15.1	1.6	2.4
Toffee, Skinny Cow*	1 Stick/72g	87	0.4	121	3.9	25.2	0.5	4.2
Triple Chocolate, Skinny Cow*	1 Stick/68g	87	1.5	128	4.3	22.8	2.2	2.8
Tropical Moment, Asda*	1 Lolly/75g	112	3.1	150	1.7	26.1	4.2	0.4
ICE LOLLY								
Assorted, De Roma*	1 Lolly/55ml	48	0.2	87	0.2	20.9	0.4	0.2
Assorted, Farmfoods*	1 Lolly/56ml	35	0.0	62	0.0	15.6	0.0	0.0
Assorted, Iceland*	1 Lolly/51g	33	0.0	65	0.0	16.2	0.0	0.0
Baby, Tesco*	1 Lolly/32g	26	0.0	80	0.1	20.0	0.0	0.1
Berry Burst, Sainsbury's*	1 Serving/90ml	93	1.6	103	1.1	20.8	1.8	0.7
Blackcurrant, Dairy Split, Sainsbury's*	1 Lolly/73ml	88	2.6	121	1.8	20.4	3.6	0.1
Blackcurrant, Ribena*	1 Lolly/35ml	25	0.0	68	0.0	16.4	0.0	0.0
Blackcurrant Split, Iceland*	1 Lolly/75g	61	2.4	81	1.1	12.0	3.2	0.1
Calippo, Lemon Lime, Mini, Wall's Ice Cream*	1 Lolly/80g	68	0.0	85	0.0	21.0	0.0	0.2
Calippo, Orange, Mini, Wall's Ice Cream*	1 Lolly/78g	70	0.0	90	0.0	21.9	0.0	0.2
Calippo, Strawberry Tropical, Wall's Ice Cream*	1 Lolly/105g	89	0.1	85	0.1	21.0	0.1	0.0

ICE LOLLY

INFO/WEIGHT	per Measure KCAL	FAT	Nutrition Values per 100g / 100ml KCAL	PROT	CARB	FAT	FIBRE
Choc Lime Split, Morrisons*	1 Lolly/73ml	120	6.1	164	1.6	20.4	8.4	0.1
Chocolate, Mini Milk, Milk Time, Wall's Ice Cream*	1 Lolly/23g	31	0.7	135	4.3	22.0	3.1	1.0
Chocolate, Plain, Mini, Tesco*	1 Lolly/31g	94	6.6	304	3.1	24.8	21.4	1.2
Chocolate & Vanilla, Sainsbury's*	1 Lolly/40g	143	10.1	357	3.7	28.7	25.3	2.2
Chocolate Wonderpops, Sainsbury's*	1 Lolly/43g	118	8.3	276	2.6	21.8	19.4	0.7
Cider Refresher, Treats*	1 Lolly/70ml	54	0.0	77	0.0	19.2	0.0	0.0
Cola Lickers, Farmfoods*	1 Lolly/56ml	38	0.0	68	0.0	17.0	0.0	0.0
Exotic Split, Bars, M&S*	1oz/28g	36	0.5	127	2.5	25.0	1.9	0.4
Fab, Nestle*	1 Lolly/64g	90	3.2	141	0.5	23.4	5.0	0.4
Fab, Orange, Nestle*	1 Lolly/58g	81	2.7	140	0.6	24.0	4.7	0.0
Feast, Chocolate, Mini, Wall's Ice Cream*	1 Lolly/52g	165	11.9	318	3.3	24.0	23.0	0.0
Feast, Ice Cream, Original, Wall's Ice Cream*	1 Lolly/90ml	252	18.0	280	2.5	20.0	20.0	0.0
Feast, Toffee, Mini, Wall's Ice Cream*	1 Lolly/52g	163	12.0	313	3.0	24.0	23.0	0.0
Fruit, Assorted, Waitrose*	1 Lolly/73g	59	0.0	81	0.0	20.0	0.0	0.1
Fruit, Blackcurrant, Jubbly, Calypso*	1 Serving/200ml	66	0.0	33	0.0	7.7	0.0	0.0
Fruit, Red, Tesco*	1 Lolly/32g	40	0.6	128	1.8	25.6	2.0	0.6
Fruit Flavour, Assorted, Basics, Sainsbury's*	1 Lolly/50g	33	0.0	66	0.0	16.5	0.0	0.0
Fruit Ices, Made with Orange Juice, Del Monte*	1 Lolly/75ml	79	0.0	105	0.5	25.7	0.0	0.0
Fruit Pastilles, Rowntree's*	1 Lolly/65ml	61	0.0	94	0.2	23.2	0.0	0.0
Fruit Split, Asda*	1 Lolly/74g	85	2.7	115	1.7	19.0	3.6	0.0
Fruit Split, Assorted, Co-Op*	1 Lolly/73g	80	2.2	110	1.0	20.0	3.0	0.1
Fruit Split, Waitrose*	1 Lolly/73g	91	2.6	124	2.5	21.7	3.6	0.4
Fruit Splits, Assorted, Somerfield*	1 Lolly/73ml	74	2.2	102	0.0	18.0	3.0	0.0
Fruit Splits, Treats*	1 Lolly/75ml	77	3.1	103	1.4	17.6	4.1	0.0
Funny Foot, Wall's Ice Cream*	1 Lolly/81ml	83	4.9	102	2.0	12.5	6.0	0.0
Lemonade & Cola, Morrisons*	1 Lolly/55ml	36	0.0	65	0.0	16.2	0.0	0.0
Lemonade Flavour, R White*	1 Ice Lolly/75ml	56	1.1	75	0.5	15.1	1.5	0.1
Mango & Passion Fruit Smoothie, Waitrose*	1 Lolly/73g	60	0.3	82	0.7	18.9	0.4	0.7
Milk, Blue Parrot Cafe, Sainsbury's*	1 Lolly/30ml	34	1.0	113	2.7	18.0	3.3	0.3
Milk Flavour, Farmfoods*	1 Lolly/50ml	91	5.0	182	2.8	20.1	10.1	0.1
Mint Chocolate, Tesco*	1 Lolly/70g	234	13.9	334	3.6	35.4	19.8	1.2
Morrisons*	1 Lolly/100g	30	0.0	30	0.0	7.4	0.0	0.0
Nobbly Bobbly, Nestle*	1 Lolly/70ml	219	11.6	312	2.9	38.1	16.5	0.6
Orange, Average	1 Lolly/72g	66	0.0	92	0.4	22.4	0.0	0.1
Orange, Real Fruit Juice, Sainsbury's*	1 Lolly/73ml	49	0.1	67	0.2	16.5	0.1	0.1
Orange, Real Juice, Tesco*	1 Lolly/32g	25	0.0	78	0.6	18.7	0.0	0.3
Orange, Tesco*	1 Lolly/77g	53	0.0	68	0.2	16.8	0.0	0.3
Orange Juice, Asda*	1 Lolly/70g	58	0.0	83	0.7	20.0	0.0	0.0
Orange Juice, Bar, M&S*	1 Lolly/75g	64	0.0	86	0.5	21.0	0.0	0.1
Orange Juice, Co-Op*	1 Lolly/73g	51	0.1	70	0.4	17.0	0.1	0.1
Orange Juice, Freshly Squeezed, Finest, Tesco*	1 Lolly/80ml	89	0.0	111	0.7	27.0	0.00	0.0
Orange Juice, Freshly Squeezed, Waitrose*	1 Lolly/73g	88	0.1	120	0.6	29.7	0.1	0.0
Orange Maid, Nestle*	1 Lolly/73ml	66	0.0	91	0.5	21.6	0.0	0.0
Pineapple, Dairy Split, Sainsbury's*	1 Lolly/72ml	84	2.6	116	1.8	19.0	3.6	0.1
Pineapple, Real Fruit Juice, Sainsbury's*	1 Lolly/73ml	55	0.1	76	0.1	19.0	0.1	0.1
Pop Up, CBY, Asda*	1 Ice Lolly/80ml	65	0.0	81	0.0	20.1	0.0	0.3
Raspberry, Real Fruit Juice, Sainsbury's*	1 Lolly/72g	62	0.1	86	0.3	21.0	0.1	0.1
Raspberry, Smoothie, Iced, Del Monte*	1 Lolly/90ml	84	0.0	94	0.3	22.8	0.0	0.8
Raspberry & Apple, Sainsbury's*	1 Lolly/57ml	39	0.1	68	0.1	17.1	0.1	0.1
Real Fruit, Dairy Split, Sainsbury's*	1 Lolly/73ml	100	3.1	137	2.1	22.8	4.2	0.1
Real Orange, Kids, Tesco*	1 Lolly/32g	25	0.0	78	0.6	18.7	0.0	0.3
Refresher, Fruit Flavour, Bassett's*	1 Lolly/45g	56	0.7	125	1.6	26.0	1.6	0.3
Rocket, Co-Op*	1 Lolly/60g	42	0.0	70	0.0	17.0	0.0	0.0

	Measure INFO/WEIGHT	per Measure KCAL	per Measure FAT	Nutrition Values per 100g / 100ml KCAL	PROT	CARB	FAT	FIBRE
ICE LOLLY								
Rocket, Sainsbury's*	1 Lolly/58g	42	0.1	72	0.1	17.8	0.1	0.1
Rolo, Nestle*	1 Lolly/75ml	243	14.1	324	3.8	36.5	18.8	0.0
Scooby-Doo, Freezepops, Calypso*	1 Lolly/50ml	14	0.0	28	0.0	7.0	0.0	0.0
Seriously Fruity, Mango Sorbet, Waitrose*	1 Lolly/100ml	79	0.3	79	0.8	18.4	0.3	0.5
Solero, Exotic, Wall's Ice Cream*	1 Lolly/82g	99	2.3	121	1.6	22.0	2.8	0.5
Solero, Orange Fresh, Wall's Ice Cream*	1 Lolly/96g	78	0.0	81	0.2	20.0	0.0	0.0
Solero, Red Fruits, Wall's Ice Cream*	1 Lolly/95g	99	2.1	104	1.3	21.0	2.2	0.0
Sprinkle Tops, Sainsbury's*	1 Lolly/40g	51	1.2	126	0.2	24.8	2.9	0.1
Strawberries & Cream, Cadbury*	1 Lolly/100ml	225	11.7	225	2.9	27.0	11.7	0.0
Strawberry, Dairy Split, Sainsbury's*	1 Lolly/73ml	86	2.6	118	1.7	19.8	3.6	0.1
Strawberry, Fruit Split, Iceland*	1 Lolly/73g	77	2.4	105	0.9	17.8	3.3	0.5
Strawberry, Mini Milk, Milk Time, Wall's Ice Cream*	1 Lolly/23g	30	0.7	131	4.0	22.0	2.9	0.5
Strawberry, Orange & Pineapple, Rocket, Iceland*	1 Lolly/47g	38	0.0	81	0.0	20.2	0.0	0.1
Strawberry Fruit, Double, Del Monte*	1 Lolly/76g	84	2.0	111	1.8	20.1	2.6	0.0
Strawberry Split, Average	1 Lolly/72g	78	2.3	108	1.5	18.5	3.2	0.2
Strawberry Split, Co-Op*	1 Lolly/71ml	75	2.1	105	1.0	17.0	3.0	0.1
Tip Top, Calypso*	1 Lolly/20ml	6	0.0	30	0.1	7.1	0.1	0.0
Tropical Fruit Sorbet, Waitrose*	1 Lolly/110g	90	2.2	82	1.5	14.5	2.0	0.2
Twister, Choc, Mini, Wall's Ice Cream*	1 Lolly/27g	40	1.6	150	3.5	22.0	6.0	0.9
Twister, Wall's Ice Cream*	1 Lolly/80ml	76	1.5	95	0.6	18.4	1.9	0.0
Vanilla, Mini Milk, Milk Time, Wall's Ice Cream*	1 Lolly/23g	29	0.7	127	3.8	21.0	2.9	0.3
ICED DESSERT								
Cafe Latte, BGTY, Sainsbury's*	1 Serving/75g	104	2.7	139	2.9	23.7	3.6	3.3
Chocolate, Honeycomb Pieces, Weight Watchers*	1 Pot/58g	92	2.5	159	3.1	26.2	4.3	0.8
Chocolate Mint Crisp, COU, M&S*	¼ Pot/85g	115	2.5	135	5.4	21.9	2.9	1.0
Raspberry Swirl, Weight Watchers*	1 Scoop/60g	74	1.5	124	1.7	23.4	2.5	0.3
Vanilla, 3% Fat, M&S*	1oz/28g	40	0.8	143	3.5	25.9	2.8	0.7
Vanilla, Dairy, BGTY, Sainsbury's*	1 Serving/65g	78	1.0	120	3.0	23.6	1.5	0.6
Vanilla, Non Dairy, Soft, Swedish Glace*	1 Serving/100g	200	10.0	200	2.5	25.0	10.0	1.0
INDIAN MEAL								
Banquet for One, COU, M&S*	1 Pack/500g	400	6.0	80	6.7	10.2	1.2	3.1
for One, Asda*	1 Pack/550g	834	25.3	152	6.7	20.9	4.6	1.4
for One, Vegetarian, Asda*	1 Pack/499g	789	44.9	158	3.2	16.0	9.0	1.4
for Two, Hot, Takeaway, Tesco*	1 Pack/825g	1215	60.6	147	6.6	13.6	7.4	1.9
for Two, Menu, Tesco*	1 Serving/537g	811	34.4	151	6.3	17.0	6.4	0.8
for Two, Peshwari Naan, Finest, Tesco*	½ Pack/200g	612	17.8	306	8.3	48.3	8.9	5.2
INSTANT WHIP								
Chocolate Flavour, Dry, Bird's*	1oz/28g	109	1.7	390	3.8	80.5	5.9	0.7
Strawberry Flavour, Dry, Bird's*	1oz/28g	112	1.5	400	2.5	85.0	5.4	0.4
IRN BRU								
Diet, Barr's*	1 Can/330ml	2	0.0	1	0.1	0.1	0.0	0.0
Original, Barr's*	1 Bottle/500ml	214	0.0	43	0.0	10.5	0.0	0.0

INFO/WEIGHT	Measure	per Measure KCAL	FAT	Nutrition Values per 100g / 100ml KCAL	PROT	CARB	FAT	FIBRE
JACKFRUIT								
Raw, Average, Flesh Only	*1 Portion/162g*	*155*	*0.5*	*95*	*1.5*	*24.4*	*0.3*	*1.6*
JALFREZI								
Chicken, & Coriander Rice, TTD, Sainsbury's*	1 Pack/473g	501	15.1	106	6.2	13.2	3.2	3.1
Chicken, & Pilau Rice, Sainsbury's*	1 Pack/500g	600	20.5	120	6.9	13.9	4.1	1.5
Chicken, & Pilau Rice, Takeaway, Asda*	1 Pack/558g	792	23.4	142	7.0	19.0	4.2	1.3
Chicken, Asda*	1 Pack/340g	415	20.4	122	10.0	7.0	6.0	1.6
Chicken, Finest, Tesco*	1 Pack/350g	402	16.4	115	10.4	6.9	4.7	1.2
Chicken, Hot & Spicy, Sainsbury's*	½ Pack/200g	228	11.4	114	12.8	2.9	5.7	1.0
Chicken, Indian Takeaway, Tesco*	1 Serving/350g	245	8.7	70	7.4	4.3	2.5	1.8
Chicken, with Pilau Rice, CBY, Asda*	1 Pack/450g	682	15.4	151	8.1	21.5	3.4	1.2
Chicken, with Rice, Ready Meal, Average	1 Serving/450g	557	18.9	124	6.9	14.5	4.2	1.5
Chicken. Canned, Tesco*	½ Can/200g	190	6.8	95	10.8	4.1	3.4	1.4
Chicken. with Lemon Pilau Rice, Finest, Tesco*	1 Pack/493g	665	21.7	135	6.9	16.4	4.4	1.8
Chicken. with Pilau Rice, Tesco*	1 Pack/460g	506	17.5	110	5.3	13.6	3.8	0.9
Chicken. with Rice, Morrisons*	1 Pack/400g	564	20.8	141	7.7	15.9	5.2	1.4
Chicken. with Rice, Tesco*	1 Pack/550g	732	26.4	133	5.5	17.0	4.8	1.0
Meal for One, M&S*	1 Serving/500g	700	35.0	140	6.1	13.4	7.0	3.0
Vegetable, Eastern Indian, Sainsbury's*	1 Pack/400g	208	13.6	52	3.4	2.0	3.4	1.7
Vegetable, Indian, Sainsbury's*	½ Pack/200g	156	9.0	78	2.0	5.3	4.5	4.2
JAM								
Apricot, Average	*1 Tbsp/15g*	*37*	*0.0*	*248*	*0.2*	*61.6*	*0.0*	*1.5*
Apricot, Reduced Sugar, Average	*1 Serving/20g*	*37*	*0.1*	*186*	*0.4*	*46.0*	*0.3*	*0.4*
Black Cherry, Average	*1 Tsp/5g*	*12*	*0.0*	*247*	*0.4*	*61.2*	*0.3*	*0.4*
Blackberry, Extra Special, Asda*	1 Tbsp/15g	29	0.1	190	0.9	45.0	0.7	0.0
Blackcurrant, Average	*1 Tbsp/15g*	*38*	*0.0*	*250*	*0.2*	*62.3*	*0.0*	*1.0*
Blackcurrant, Reduced Sugar, Average	*1 Tsp/6g*	*10*	*0.0*	*178*	*0.4*	*44.4*	*0.2*	*1.0*
Blueberry, Best, Hartley's*	1 Tsp/20g	49	0.0	244	0.3	60.6	0.1	0.0
Blueberry, St Dalfour*	1 Serving/20g	46	0.0	228	0.5	56.0	0.2	2.2
Blueberry. & Blackberry, Baxters*	1 Tsp/15g	38	0.0	252	0.0	63.0	0.0	1.2
Blueberry. & Blackcurrant, 100% Pure Fruit, Super Jam*	1 Tsp/5g	11	0.0	222	0.3	55.0	0.1	0.0
Country Berries, Luxury, Baxters*	1 Tsp/15g	37	0.0	247	0.5	60.0	0.1	2.0
Damson, Extra Fruit, Best, Hartley's*	1 Tsp/5g	12	0.0	244	0.2	60.8	0.0	0.0
Fig	1 Tsp/15g	36	0.0	242	0.5	60.0	0.0	0.0
Grape, Jelly, Concorde, Organic, Smucker's*	1 Tbsp/20g	50	0.0	250	0.0	65.0	0.0	0.0
Kiwi & Gooseberry, 66% Fruit, Asda*	1 Serving/30g	56	0.2	187	0.5	45.0	0.5	0.0
Mixed Fruit, Average	*1 Tbsp/15g*	*38*	*0.0*	*252*	*0.3*	*63.5*	*0.0*	*0.5*
Peach, Golden, Rhapsodie De Fruit, St Dalfour*	1 Tsp/10g	23	0.0	227	0.5	56.0	0.1	1.3
Plum, Tesco*	1 Serving/50g	130	0.0	261	0.2	64.4	0.0	0.6
Raspberry, Average	*1 Tbsp/15g*	*36*	*0.0*	*239*	*0.6*	*58.6*	*0.1*	*0.9*
Raspberry, Reduced Sugar, Average	*1 Tsp/6g*	*10*	*0.0*	*160*	*0.5*	*39.3*	*0.2*	*0.6*
Raspberry, Seedless, Average	*1 Tsp/10g*	*26*	*0.0*	*257*	*0.4*	*63.6*	*0.0*	*0.3*
Rhubarb & Ginger, Baxters*	1 Tsp/15g	40	0.0	264	0.4	65.0	0.1	0.8
Strawberry, & Redcurrant, Reduced Sugar, Streamline*	1 Tbsp/15g	29	0.0	192	0.4	46.8	0.3	0.0
Strawberry, & Vanilla, Best, Hartley's*	1 Tsp/5g	12	0.0	244	0.4	60.6	0.0	0.0
Strawberry, Average	*1 Tsp/10g*	*24*	*0.0*	*243*	*0.3*	*60.2*	*0.1*	*0.7*
Strawberry, Reduced Sugar, Average	*1 Tbsp/15g*	*28*	*0.0*	*187*	*0.4*	*45.8*	*0.3*	*0.2*
Wild Blackberry Jelly, Baxters*	1 Tsp/15g	32	0.0	210	0.0	53.0	0.0	1.2
JAMBALAYA								
American Style, Tesco*	1 Serving/275g	432	19.2	157	7.7	16.0	7.0	0.5
Cajun Chicken, Cooked, BGTY, Sainsbury's*	1 Pack/400g	392	6.5	103	6.6	14.6	1.7	1.6
Chicken, & Prawn, Love Life, Waitrose*	1 Pack/390g	417	10.9	107	5.2	14.3	2.8	1.9
Chicken, & Prawn, with Brown Rice, Waitrose*	1 Pack/390g	390	14.0	100	4.7	12.1	3.6	1.8
COU, M&S*	1 Pack/400g	340	8.0	85	6.5	10.8	2.0	0.9

J

	Measure INFO/WEIGHT	per Measure KCAL	FAT	Nutrition Values per 100g / 100ml KCAL	PROT	CARB	FAT	FIBRE
JAMBALAYA								
M & S*	1 Pack/480g	552	16.8	115	5.8	14.6	3.5	1.2
Ready Meal, Average	1 Pack/450g	569	18.2	126	6.4	15.7	4.0	1.3
JELLY								
Apple & Watermelon, Low Calorie, Hartley's*	1 Serving/175g	5	0.0	3	0.0	0.3	0.0	0.3
Blackberry, Unprepared, Morrisons*	1 Serving/20g	52	0.0	261	0.3	65.0	0.0	0.0
Blackcurrant, Made Up, Rowntree's*	¼ Jelly/140ml	100	0.1	71	1.4	16.4	0.1	0.0
Blackcurrant, Made Up, Sainsbury's*	¼ Jelly/150g	98	0.0	65	1.2	15.1	0.0	0.0
Blackcurrant, Sugar Free, Unprepared, Rowntree's*	1 Pack/24g	73	0.0	305	50.0	25.0	0.0	25.0
Blackcurrant, Tesco*	1 Serving/100g	84	0.1	84	0.2	20.5	0.1	0.4
Bramble, Tesco*	1 Serving/100g	257	0.1	257	0.3	63.7	0.1	1.3
Crystals, Orange, Sugar Free, Bird's*	1 Sachet/12g	39	0.1	335	62.5	6.4	0.9	0.0
Crystals, Strawberry, Made Up, Tesco*	1 Serving/145g	9	0.0	6	1.3	0.3	0.0	0.0
Crystals Apple & Blackcurrant, Weight Watchers*	1 Pack/204g	14	0.2	7	0.1	1.4	0.1	0.1
Exotic Fruit, M&S*	1 Pot/175g	140	0.4	80	0.1	18.9	0.2	0.9
Fresh Fruit, M&S*	1 Pot/175g	131	0.2	75	0.2	18.4	0.1	0.3
Fruit Cocktail, M&S*	1oz/28g	31	1.3	110	0.4	16.4	4.7	0.3
Fruitini, Del Monte*	1 Serving/120g	78	0.1	65	0.3	15.3	0.1	0.5
Lemon & Lime, Sugar Free, Unprepared, Rowntree's*	1oz/28g	85	0.0	305	4.5	60.7	0.0	0.0
Lime, Made Up, Rowntree's*	¼ Jelly/140ml	100	0.1	71	1.4	16.4	0.1	0.0
Lime Flavour, Cubes, Hartley's*	1 Cube/12g	36	0.0	296	5.1	68.9	0.0	0.0
Made Up with Water, Average	*1oz/28g*	*17*	*0.0*	*61*	*1.2*	*15.1*	*0.0*	*0.0*
Mandarin & Pineapple, Sainsbury's*	1 Pot/125g	95	0.1	76	0.2	18.9	0.1	1.2
Orange, Sugar Free, Crystals, Dry Weight, Hartley's*	1 Pack/26g	66	0.0	254	57.4	6.1	0.0	0.0
Orange, Sugar Free, Made Up, Hartley's*	1 Serving/140ml	9	0.0	6	1.3	0.3	0.0	0.0
Orange, Sugar Free, Rowntree's*	1 Serving/140ml	8	0.0	6	1.4	0.1	0.0	0.0
Orange, Unprepared, Rowntree's*	1 Square/11g	33	0.0	296	4.4	69.6	0.0	0.0
Peach Melba, Eat Well, M&S*	1 Pot/175g	114	0.4	65	0.2	15.9	0.2	0.2
Pineapple with Pineapple Pieces, Tesco*	1 Serving/120g	96	0.1	80	1.2	18.6	0.1	0.7
Raspberry, Crystals, Vegetarian, Just Wholefoods*	1 Pack/85g	293	0.0	345	0.5	85.7	0.0	0.0
Raspberry & Rose, Aroma, M&S*	1oz/28g	14	0.1	50	0.2	11.9	0.2	0.4
Raspberry Flavour, Sugar Free, Made Up, Rowntree's*	1 Serving/140ml	9	0.0	6	1.4	0.1	0.0	0.0
Raspberry Flavour, Tesco*	1 Serving/34g	22	0.0	64	1.0	15.0	0.0	0.1
Redcurrant, Average	*1oz/28g*	*70*	*0.0*	*250*	*0.2*	*64.4*	*0.0*	*0.0*
Strawberry, No Added Sugar, Hartley's*	1 Pot/115g	4	0.0	4	0.0	0.4	0.0	0.3
Strawberry, Sugar Free, Crystals, Dry Weight, Hartley's*	1 Sachet/26g	73	0.0	280	56.8	13.1	0.0	0.0
Strawberry, Sugar Free, Made Up, Rowntree's*	1 Serving/140ml	10	0.0	7	1.5	0.1	0.0	0.0
Strawberry, Sugar Free, Unprepared, Rowntree's*	1oz/28g	84	0.0	300	64.9	3.0	0.0	0.0
Strawberry & Raspberry, Sainsbury's*	½ Pot/280g	230	0.0	82	0.2	20.2	0.0	1.2
Sugar Free, Dry, Tesco*	1 Pack/13g	36	0.0	285	55.4	15.6	0.0	0.2
JELLY BABIES								
Bassett's*	1 Baby/6g	20	0.0	335	4.0	79.5	0.0	0.0
M & S*	1 Pack/125g	418	0.0	334	5.2	78.0	0.0	0.0
Mini, Rowntree's*	1 Bag/35g	128	0.0	366	4.6	86.9	0.0	0.0
Mini, Waitrose*	1 Bag/125g	370	0.5	296	4.3	68.7	0.4	0.0
Sainsbury's*	1 Serving/70g	247	0.5	353	4.1	82.5	0.7	0.3
Somerfield*	1 Sweet/6g	21	0.0	343	4.7	80.7	0.0	0.0
JELLY BEANS								
Asda*	1 Bag/100g	364	0.4	364	0.1	90.0	0.4	0.2
Average	1 Serving/100g	365	0.1	365	0.1	91.2	0.1	0.1
Jelly Belly*	35 Beans/40g	140	0.0	350	0.0	90.0	0.0	0.0
M & S*	1 Bag/113g	407	0.0	360	0.1	89.6	0.0	0.0
No Added Sugar, Jelly Belly*	1 Serving/40g	80	0.0	200	0.0	50.0	0.0	20.0
Rowntree's*	1 Pack/35g	128	0.0	367	0.0	91.8	0.0	0.0

J

	Measure INFO/WEIGHT	per Measure KCAL	FAT	Nutrition Values per 100g / 100ml KCAL	PROT	CARB	FAT	FIBRE
JELLY BEARS								
Co-Op*	1 Sweet/3g	10	0.0	325	6.0	76.0	0.1	0.0
JELLY TOTS								
Rowntree's*	1 Pack/42g	145	0.0	346	0.1	86.5	0.0	0.0
JERKY								
Beef, Peppered, Jack Link's*	1 Serving/28g	80	0.5	286	53.6	14.3	1.8	0.0
Beef, with Tomato Relish, Graze*	1 Pack/36g	91	1.0	253	22.2	30.6	2.8	2.5
JUICE								
& Water, Orange & Pear, Planet Lunch*	1 Serving/150ml	60	0.0	40	0.0	0.0	0.0	0.0
100% Vegetable, V8*	1 Bottle/354ml	71	1.1	20	0.8	3.2	0.3	0.5
Apple, Cloudy, Pressed, Copella*	1 Glass/100ml	46	0.0	46	0.2	10.7	0.0	0.7
Apple, Concentrate, Average	*1 Tbsp/15ml*	*45*	*0.0*	*302*	*0.0*	*73.6*	*0.2*	*0.0*
Apple, English with Cherry, Cawston Vale*	1 Can/250ml	118	0.2	47	0.4	11.6	0.1	0.0
Apple, Juice & Water, Tropicana Kids, Tropicana*	1 Bottle/200ml	70	0.0	35	0.0	8.7	0.0	0.0
Apple, Peach & Pear, Innocent*	1 Serving/100ml	45	0.1	45	0.4	10.0	0.1	1.4
Apple, Pressed, Not from Concentrate, Co-Op*	1 Glass/100ml	45	0.1	45	0.1	10.4	0.1	0.0
Apple, Pure, Average	1 Glass/100ml	47	0.0	47	0.1	11.2	0.0	0.0
Apple, Pure, Organic, Average	*1 Serving/200ml*	*92*	*0.1*	*46*	*0.0*	*11.2*	*0.0*	*0.0*
Apple, Pure, Value, Tesco*	1 Glass/200ml	94	0.0	47	0.1	11.4	0.0	0.0
Apple, Vitafit, Lidl*	1 Carton/250ml	110	0.2	44	0.1	10.0	0.1	0.1
Apple & Cherry, Sainsbury's*	1 Serving/200ml	96	0.0	48	0.3	10.8	0.0	0.8
Apple & Cranberry, Average	*1 Glass/250ml*	*114*	*0.0*	*46*	*0.1*	*10.2*	*0.0*	*0.0*
Apple & Elderflower, Copella*	1 Glass/250ml	108	0.2	43	0.4	10.2	0.1	0.0
Apple & Mango, Average	*1 Glass/200ml*	*108*	*0.1*	*54*	*0.3*	*12.6*	*0.0*	*0.1*
Apple & Mango, Pressed, Waitrose*	1 Glass/100ml	54	0.0	54	0.3	12.6	0.0	0.0
Apple & Orange, Fresh Up*	1 Serving/250ml	105	0.0	42	0.0	10.3	0.0	0.0
Apple & Raspberry, Average	*1 Serving/200ml*	*89*	*0.1*	*44*	*0.4*	*10.2*	*0.0*	*0.2*
Apple & Rhubarb, Caxton Vale*	1 Glass/250ml	115	1.0	46	0.2	9.7	0.4	0.0
Apple & Rhubarb, Pressed, Cawston Press*	1 Serving/200ml	92	0.8	46	0.2	9.7	0.4	0.0
Apple & Rhubarb, Pressed, Cawston Vale*	1 Glass/200ml	92	0.8	46	0.2	9.7	0.4	0.0
Apple with Ginger, Waitrose*	1 Glass/150ml	72	0.0	48	0.3	11.0	0.0	0.5
Beetroot, Organic, James White*	1 Glass/250ml	105	0.2	42	0.9	9.3	0.1	0.0
Berry Tasty, Smoothie, Nak'd*	1 Bottle/450ml	243	0.0	54	0.4	12.1	0.0	0.0
Breakfast, Ruby, Tropicana*	1 Glass/200ml	90	0.0	45	0.8	9.7	0.0	0.7
Breakfast, Sainsbury's*	1 Serving/200ml	94	0.2	47	0.7	11.3	0.1	0.3
Carrot, Average	*1 Glass/200ml*	*48*	*0.2*	*24*	*0.5*	*5.7*	*0.1*	*0.0*
Clementine, Morrisons*	1 Serving/100ml	48	0.1	48	0.5	10.9	0.1	0.1
Cranberry, Average	*1 Bottle/250ml*	*139*	*0.2*	*56*	*0.1*	*13.4*	*0.1*	*0.3*
Cranberry, No Added Sugar, Average	*1 Glass/200ml*	*11*	*0.1*	*6*	*0.1*	*0.8*	*0.0*	*0.0*
Fruit, Tropical, Pure Premium, Tropicana*	1 Glass/200ml	98	0.0	49	0.5	11.0	0.0	0.8
Fruit, Tropical in Sparkling Spring Water, Light, Rio*	1 Can/330ml	17	0.0	5	0.1	1.1	0.0	0.0
Grape, Purple, Light, Welch's*	1 Serving/100ml	27	0.3	27	0.2	6.1	0.3	0.3
Grape, Purple, Welch's*	1 Serving/200ml	136	0.0	68	0.1	16.5	0.0	0.0
Grape, Red, Average	*1 Serving/100ml*	*62*	*0.0*	*62*	*0.2*	*15.2*	*0.0*	*0.0*
Grape, White, Average	*1 Can/160ml*	*95*	*0.1*	*60*	*0.2*	*14.3*	*0.1*	*0.1*
Grape & Peach, Don Simon*	1 Serving/200ml	94	0.0	47	0.4	11.3	0.0	0.0
Grapefruit, Pink, Average	*1 Glass/200ml*	*81*	*0.1*	*40*	*0.6*	*9.0*	*0.0*	*0.2*
Grapefruit, Pure, Average	*1 Glass/200ml*	*77*	*0.2*	*38*	*0.5*	*8.5*	*0.1*	*0.1*
Lemon, Fresh, Average	*1 Lemon/36ml*	*2*	*0.0*	*7*	*0.3*	*1.6*	*0.0*	*0.1*
Lime, Fresh, Average	*1 Tsp/5ml*	*0*	*0.0*	*9*	*0.4*	*1.6*	*0.1*	*0.1*
Lime from Concentrate, Asda*	1 Tbsp/17g	1	0.0	6	0.3	0.8	0.1	0.2
Mandarin Orange, Tropicana*	1 Serving/200ml	94	0.0	47	0.6	10.0	0.0	0.8
Mango, Peach, Papaya, Pure, Premium, Tropicana*	1 Glass/200ml	88	0.0	44	0.5	9.8	0.0	0.1
Mango, Pure, Canned	*1 Glass/250ml*	*98*	*0.5*	*39*	*0.1*	*9.8*	*0.2*	*0.1*

J

JUICE

	Measure INFO/WEIGHT	per Measure KCAL	FAT	Nutrition Values per 100g / 100ml KCAL	PROT	CARB	FAT	FIBRE
Mango Veggie, Naked Juice Co*	1 Serving/240ml	150	1.0	62	1.2	15.8	0.4	2.1
Orange, 100% from Concentrate, Farmfoods*	1 Serving/200ml	84	0.2	42	0.6	9.1	0.1	0.1
Orange, 100% Pure Squeezed, Smooth, Tesco*	1 Glass/250ml	115	0.0	46	0.4	10.6	0.0	0.0
Orange, C, No Added Sugar, Libby's*	1 Serving/250ml	32	0.0	13	0.1	2.7	0.0	0.0
Orange, Freshly Squeezed, Average	1 Serving/200ml	66	0.0	33	0.6	8.1	0.0	1.0
Orange, No Bits, Innocent*	1 Glass/250ml	120	0.0	48	0.8	10.9	0.0	0.2
Orange, Pure, Smooth, Average	*1 Glass/200ml*	*88*	*0.1*	*44*	*0.7*	*9.8*	*0.0*	*0.2*
Orange, Pure, Smooth, From Concentrate, Sainsbury's*	1 Serving/200ml	84	0.2	42	0.5	9.1	0.1	0.1
Orange, Pure, Tesco*	1 Glass/200ml	94	0.0	47	0.5	10.5	0.0	0.0
Orange, Pure from Concentrate, Carton, Value, Tesco*	1 Serving/250ml	115	0.0	46	0.5	10.4	0.0	0.0
Orange, Pure Premium, Smooth, No Bits, Tropicana*	1 Glass/200ml	96	0.0	48	0.8	10.0	0.0	0.4
Orange, Pure with Bits, Average	*1 Glass/200ml*	*90*	*0.1*	*45*	*0.6*	*10.2*	*0.1*	*0.1*
Orange, Smooth, Freshly Squeezed, TTD, Sainsbury's*	1 Serving/249g	132	0.0	53	0.7	11.4	0.0	0.2
Orange, Smooth, Happy Shopper*	1 Serving/150ml	63	0.2	42	0.5	9.1	0.1	0.2
Orange, with Bits, Freshly Squeezed, TTD, Sainsbury's*	1 Serving/249g	132	0.0	53	0.7	11.4	0.0	0.2
Orange, with Bits, Innocent*	1 Glass/250ml	120	0.0	48	0.8	10.9	0.0	0.3
Orange, with Bits, Not From Concentrate, Tesco*	1 Glass/250ml	110	0.0	44	0.4	10.6	0.0	0.0
Orange & Carrot, Love Life, Waitrose*	1 Serving/150ml	57	0.3	38	0.6	8.5	0.2	1.2
Orange & Grapefruit, Average	*1 Glass/200ml*	*84*	*0.2*	*42*	*0.8*	*9.2*	*0.1*	*0.4*
Orange & Lime, Tropicana*	1 Serving/250ml	115	0.0	46	1.1	9.4	0.0	0.6
Orange & Mango, Average	*1 Bottle/375ml*	*176*	*0.4*	*47*	*0.5*	*10.7*	*0.1*	*0.2*
Orange & Passionfruit, Tropicana*	1 Serving/200ml	94	0.0	47	0.8	10.0	0.0	0.7
Orange & Pineapple, Average	*1 Glass/120ml*	*56*	*0.6*	*46*	*0.4*	*10.5*	*0.5*	*0.5*
Orange & Raspberry, Average	*1 fl oz/30ml*	*15*	*0.0*	*50*	*0.6*	*11.4*	*0.1*	*0.2*
Orange & Raspberry, Tropicana*	1 Glass/200ml	92	0.0	46	1.2	9.0	0.0	0.9
Orange & Strawberry, Average	*1 Serving/125ml*	*64*	*0.5*	*51*	*0.6*	*10.9*	*0.4*	*0.8*
Passion Fruit, Average	*1 Glass/200ml*	*94*	*0.2*	*47*	*0.8*	*10.7*	*0.1*	*0.0*
Peach, Mango & Passion Fruit, Sainsbury's*	1 Glass/200ml	92	0.2	46	0.3	10.3	0.1	0.5
Pear, with a Hint of Ginger, Pressed, M&S*	1 Glass/250ml	125	0.2	50	0.3	11.7	0.1	0.0
Pineapple, Average	*1 Glass/200ml*	*100*	*0.1*	*50*	*0.3*	*11.7*	*0.1*	*0.2*
Pineapple, Pure, From Concentrate, Sainsbury's*	1 Serving/200ml	95	0.2	48	0.3	10.8	0.1	0.0
Pineapple & Coconut, Tesco*	1 Serving/250ml	138	1.0	55	0.4	11.3	0.4	0.0
Pineapple & Coconut, Waitrose*	1 Serving/250ml	125	0.8	50	0.2	11.5	0.3	0.2
Pineapple Mango Crush, Just Juice*	1 Glass/250ml	108	0.0	43	0.0	10.6	0.0	0.0
Pomegranate, & Blueberry, Sainsbury's*	1oz/28g	14	0.0	49	0.0	11.7	0.0	0.1
Pomegranate, Grape & Apple, Tropicana*	1 Bottle/330ml	211	0.0	64	0.2	15.5	0.0	0.6
Pomegranate, Pomegreat*	1 Glass/200ml	88	0.0	44	0.1	11.1	0.0	0.0
Pomegranate, with Cherry, Pomegreat*	1 Serving/200ml	75	0.0	38	0.1	8.8	0.0	0.1
Prune, Average	*1 Serving/200ml*	*123*	*0.1*	*61*	*0.6*	*15.3*	*0.1*	*1.8*
Prune, Pure Squeezed, Sunraysia*	1 Glass/250ml	182	0.2	73	0.6	18.4	0.1	0.6
Tomato, Average	*1 Glass/200ml*	*40*	*0.1*	*20*	*0.8*	*4.0*	*0.0*	*0.4*
Tomato, from Concentrate, Sainsbury's*	1 Glass/250ml	40	0.2	16	0.7	2.7	0.1	0.7
Tomato, Princes*	1 Serving/100g	16	0.0	16	0.8	3.1	0.0	0.6
Tropical, Fruit, Plenty*	1 Glass/200ml	120	0.2	60	0.5	13.7	0.1	0.0
Tropical, Fruit & Vegetable, V8*	1 Serving/150ml	0	0.0	35	0.4	8.1	0.1	1.1
Tropical, Pure, Sainsbury's*	1 Glass/200ml	104	0.2	52	0.5	12.0	0.1	0.1
Vegetable, Organic, James White*	1 Serving/100g	22	0.2	22	0.6	4.4	0.2	0.0
White Apple & Ginger, James White*	1 Glass/250ml	122	0.0	49	0.1	11.8	0.0	0.0

JUICE DRINK

	Measure INFO/WEIGHT	per Measure KCAL	FAT	Nutrition Values per 100g / 100ml KCAL	PROT	CARB	FAT	FIBRE
Apple, Cranberry, & Blueberry, Waitrose*	1 Serving/150ml	75	0.0	50	0.1	11.9	0.0	0.1
Apple, Juiceburst, Purity*	1 Bottle/500ml	220	0.0	44	0.0	11.0	0.0	0.0
Apple, Libby's*	1 Serving/100ml	43	0.0	43	0.0	10.3	0.0	0.0
Apple, No Added Sugar, Asda*	1 Glass/200ml	10	0.0	5	0.0	1.0	0.0	0.0

J

JUICE DRINK

INFO/WEIGHT	Measure	per Measure KCAL	FAT	Nutrition Values per 100g / 100ml KCAL	PROT	CARB	FAT	FIBRE
Apple, No Added Sugar, LC, Tesco*	1 Glass/250ml	12	0.0	5	0.0	0.9	0.0	0.0
Apple, Plum & Pear, Pure Pressed, CBY, Asda*	1 Glass/200ml	92	0.0	46	0.4	10.5	0.0	0.2
Apple, Sparkling, Zing*	1 Can/250ml	92	0.0	37	0.1	8.5	0.0	0.0
Apple & Blueberry, The Feel Good Drinks Co*	1 Serving/375ml	163	0.4	44	0.1	10.6	0.1	0.0
Apple & Elderflower, Tesco*	1 Serving/200ml	76	0.0	38	0.0	9.4	0.0	0.0
Apple & Mango, CBY, Asda*	1 Carton/250ml	115	0.0	46	0.0	11.0	0.0	0.0
Apple & Raspberry, Sainsbury's*	1 Serving/200ml	112	0.2	56	0.1	13.8	0.1	0.1
Apple & Raspberry, Tesco*	1 Serving/300ml	138	0.0	46	0.0	11.2	0.0	0.0
Berry Blast, 5 Alive*	1 Glass/200ml	50	0.0	25	0.0	6.1	0.0	0.0
Blackcurrant, Extra Light, Ribena*	1 Serving/200ml	8	0.0	4	0.0	0.5	0.0	0.0
Blackcurrant & Apple, Oasis*	1 Serving/500ml	90	0.0	18	0.0	4.1	0.0	0.0
Cranberry, Classic, Ocean Spray*	1 Bottle/500ml	245	0.5	49	0.1	11.7	0.1	0.1
Cranberry, Grape & Apple, Ocean Spray*	1 Glass/200ml	108	0.0	54	0.1	12.9	0.0	0.0
Cranberry, Light, Classic, Ocean Spray*	1 Glass/200ml	16	0.0	8	0.0	1.4	0.0	0.0
Cranberry, M&S*	1 Serving/100ml	60	0.0	60	0.1	14.3	0.0	0.0
Cranberry, Morrisons*	1 Glass/200ml	92	0.0	46	0.0	11.6	0.0	0.0
Cranberry, No Added Sugar, BGTY, Sainsbury's*	1 Glass/200ml	4	0.0	2	0.0	0.3	0.0	0.0
Cranberry, Organic, Sainsbury's*	1 Serving/200ml	100	0.0	50	0.0	11.9	0.0	0.0
Cranberry, Original, Concentrated, Ocean Spray*	1 Serving/15ml	27	0.0	183	0.2	44.1	0.0	0.0
Cranberry, Tesco*	1 Serving/330ml	152	0.0	46	0.0	11.1	0.0	0.0
Cranberry, Waitrose*	1 Serving/250ml	145	0.0	58	0.1	13.9	0.0	0.1
Cranberry & Apple, Ocean Spray*	1 Glass/200ml	92	0.0	46	0.0	11.1	0.0	0.0
Cranberry & Blackberry, Ocean Spray*	1 Glass/250ml	120	0.2	48	0.1	11.3	0.1	0.2
Cranberry & Blueberry, Ocean Spray*	1 Serving/100ml	48	0.0	48	0.0	11.6	0.0	0.0
Cranberry & Lime, Sparkling, The Feel Good Drinks Co.*	1 Bottle/375ml	142	0.0	38	0.1	9.0	0.0	0.1
Cranberry & Orange, No Added Sugar, Sainsbury's*	1 Glass/250ml	15	0.2	6	0.1	1.2	0.1	0.1
Cranberry & Pomegranate, Ocean Spray*	1 Glass/250ml	120	0.0	48	0.0	11.5	0.0	0.0
Cranberry & Raspberry, No Add Sugar, LC, Tesco*	1 Serving/250ml	12	0.0	5	0.0	0.8	0.0	0.0
Cranberry & Raspberry, Ocean Spray*	1 Glass/200ml	104	0.0	52	0.0	12.6	0.0	0.0
Cranberry & Raspberry, Sainsbury's*	1 Serving/250ml	105	0.0	42	0.1	9.9	0.0	0.0
Cranberry & Raspberry, Tesco*	1 Serving/200ml	96	0.0	48	0.0	11.6	0.0	0.0
Cranberry Blend, Ocean Spray*	1 Glass/250ml	148	0.0	59	0.1	13.9	0.0	0.0
Exotic, Tesco*	1 Serving/250ml	128	0.0	51	0.1	12.3	0.0	0.0
Forest Fruits, Asda*	1 Serving/200ml	88	0.0	44	0.3	10.9	0.0	0.3
Fruit Cocktail, Sainsbury's*	1 Glass/200ml	90	0.0	45	0.2	10.6	0.0	0.1
Grape, & Elderflower, White, Sparkling, Shloer*	1 Glass/200ml	74	0.0	37	0.0	9.2	0.0	0.0
Grape, Apple & Raspberry, Asda*	1 Glass/200ml	90	0.0	45	0.2	11.0	0.0	0.0
Grape, Apple & Raspberry, Co-Op*	1 Serving/150ml	75	0.0	50	0.4	12.0	0.0	0.1
Grape, Red, Sparkling, Shloer*	1 Glass/200ml	84	0.0	42	0.0	10.4	0.0	0.0
Grape, White, Sparkling, Shloer*	1 Serving/120ml	59	0.0	49	0.0	11.6	0.0	0.0
Guava Exotic, Rubicon*	1 Carton/288ml	150	0.3	52	0.2	12.9	0.1	0.0
J20, Apple & Mango, Britvic*	1 Bottle/275ml	83	0.0	30	0.1	6.8	0.0	0.2
J20, Apple & Raspberry, Britvic*	1 Bottle/275ml	88	0.0	32	0.1	7.3	0.0	0.3
J20, Glitterberry, Britvic*	1 Bottle/275ml	110	0.0	40	0.2	9.4	0.0	0.2
J20, Orange & Passion Fruit, Britvic*	1 Bottle/275ml	88	0.0	32	0.3	7.2	0.0	0.2
Lemon, The Feel Good Drinks Co*	1 Bottle/171ml	78	0.2	46	0.1	10.8	0.1	0.0
Lemonade, Asda*	1 Glass/200ml	88	0.0	44	0.1	11.0	0.0	0.0
Lychee, Sparkling, Rubicon*	1 Can/330g	182	0.0	55	0.0	13.6	0.0	0.0
Mango, Rubicon*	1 Serving/100ml	54	0.1	54	0.1	13.1	0.1	0.0
Mango, Sparkling, Rubicon*	1 Can/330ml	172	0.0	52	0.0	12.8	0.0	0.0
Mixed Berry Crush, Sparkling, CBY, Asda*	1 Glass/250ml	8	0.0	3	0.0	0.5	0.0	0.0
Orange, Caprisun*	1 Pouch/200ml	89	0.0	45	0.0	10.8	0.0	0.0
Orange, Carrot & Lemon, Pago*	1 Serving/200g	90	0.2	45	0.2	10.5	0.1	0.0

J

	Measure INFO/WEIGHT	per Measure KCAL	FAT	Nutrition Values per 100g / 100ml KCAL	PROT	CARB	FAT	FIBRE
JUICE DRINK								
Orange, Diluted, Mi Wadi*	1 Serving/250ml	26	0.0	10	0.0	2.3	0.0	0.0
Orange, Juice Burst, Purity*	1 Bottle/500ml	220	0.0	44	1.0	10.2	0.0	0.0
Orange, Morrisons*	1 Serving/250ml	12	0.2	5	0.1	0.9	0.1	0.1
Orange, No Added Sugar, Tesco*	1 fl oz/30ml	1	0.0	4	0.0	0.7	0.0	0.0
Orange, Sainsbury's*	1 Serving/250ml	18	0.2	7	0.1	1.4	0.1	0.1
Orange, Value, Tesco*	1 Glass/250ml	32	0.0	13	0.0	3.3	0.0	0.0
Passion Fruit, Exotic, Rubicon*	1 Serving/200ml	110	0.0	55	0.1	13.6	0.0	0.0
Pomegranate, Rubicon*	1 Can/330ml	108	0.0	54	0.0	13.5	0.0	0.0
Raspberry, Ribena*	1 Bottle/500ml	215	0.0	43	0.0	10.4	0.0	0.0
Raspberry & Apple, No Added Sugar, Ribena*	1 Serving/200ml	8	0.0	4	0.0	0.5	0.0	0.0
Summer Fruits, Fresh, Tesco*	1 Glass/250ml	112	0.2	45	0.1	10.8	0.1	0.3
Summer Fruits, Oasis*	1 Bottle/500ml	90	0.0	18	0.0	4.2	0.0	0.0
Tropical, No Added Sugar, Tesco*	1 Carton/250ml	12	0.0	5	0.0	1.1	0.0	0.0
Tropical Fruit, Tesco*	1 Glass/250ml	118	0.0	47	0.0	11.4	0.0	0.0
Tropical Fruit, Waitrose*	1 Glass/250ml	118	0.0	47	0.2	11.2	0.0	0.0
White Grape, Raspberry & Cranberry, Sparkling, Shloer*	1 Serving/250ml	117	0.0	47	0.0	11.0	0.0	0.0
White Grape & Peach, Sainsbury's*	1 Glass/250ml	95	0.2	38	0.2	9.0	0.1	0.1
JUNIPER								
Berries, Dried, Average	1 Tsp/2g	6	0.3	292	4.0	33.0	16.0	0.0

J

Measure INFO/WEIGHT	per Measure KCAL	FAT	Nutrition Values per 100g / 100ml KCAL	PROT	CARB	FAT	FIBRE

KALE

	Measure INFO/WEIGHT	per Measure KCAL	FAT	KCAL	PROT	CARB	FAT	FIBRE
Curly, Boiled in Salted Water, Average	*1 Serving/60g*	*14*	*0.7*	*24*	*2.4*	*1.0*	*1.1*	*2.8*
Curly, Raw, Average	*1 Serving/90g*	*30*	*1.4*	*33*	*3.4*	*1.4*	*1.6*	*3.1*

KANGAROO

	Measure INFO/WEIGHT	per Measure KCAL	FAT	KCAL	PROT	CARB	FAT	FIBRE
Raw, Average	*1 Serving/200g*	*196*	*2.0*	*98*	*22.0*	*1.0*	*1.0*	*0.0*
Steak, Grilled, Average*	*1 Fillet/150g*	*198*	*1.8*	*132*	*30.0*	*0.0*	*1.2*	*0.0*

KEBAB

	Measure INFO/WEIGHT	per Measure KCAL	FAT	KCAL	PROT	CARB	FAT	FIBRE
Beef, Kofta, PepperWaitrose*	1 Kebab/138g	223	13.9	162	14.8	2.9	10.1	0.6
Beef, Kofta, Uncooked, Tesco*	1 Kebab/73g	163	12.5	225	14.0	3.2	17.3	1.2
Beef, with Sweet Chilli Seasoning, Sainsbury's*	1 Kebab/61g	151	8.0	248	24.1	8.5	13.1	0.8
Chicken, & Pineapple, Aldi*	1 Kebab/85g	89	2.6	105	13.9	5.3	3.1	0.0
Chicken, Barbecue, Sainsbury's*	1 Pack/200g	238	3.4	119	24.4	1.5	1.7	1.8
Chicken, Breast, Mediterranean, Sainsbury's*	1 Kebab/65g	73	2.1	113	16.5	4.6	3.2	0.6
Chicken, Breast, Salsa, Sainsbury's*	1 Kebab/80g	94	0.9	118	20.1	6.5	1.1	0.6
Chicken, Chilli & Lime, Breast Fillet, Sainsbury's*	1 Kebab/77g	120	0.7	156	29.9	6.2	0.9	0.3
Chicken, Fillet, Mini with a Tikka Marinade, Sainsbury's*	1 Kebab/25g	41	0.8	164	33.4	0.6	3.1	0.1
Chicken, Green Thai, Waitrose*	1 Serving/180g	223	7.2	124	20.5	1.4	4.0	1.4
Chicken, Mango & Lime, PB, Waitrose*	1 Kebab/83g	103	1.3	125	26.0	1.2	1.6	1.1
Chicken, Mini Fillet, M&S*	1 Serving/150g	210	8.7	140	20.2	2.0	5.8	0.3
Chicken, Shish, Meat Only, Average	1 Kebab/250g	312	5.2	125	25.7	0.9	2.1	0.1
Chicken, Shish in Pitta Bread with Salad	1 Kebab/250g	388	10.2	155	13.5	17.2	4.1	1.0
Chicken, Sweet Chilli, PB, Waitrose*	1 Kebab/83g	111	0.9	135	28.6	1.7	1.1	0.5
Chicken, Thigh, Sticky Barbecue, M&S*	1 Kebab/100g	160	7.5	160	15.6	7.4	7.5	0.8
Chicken, Tikka, Citrus, Breast, Sainsbury's*	1 Kebab/61g	79	0.3	129	25.6	5.4	0.5	0.9
Chicken, with Sweet Chilli Sauce, Finest, Tesco*	½ Pack/175g	242	1.4	138	17.9	14.7	0.8	1.2
Halloumi & Vegetable, Waitrose*	1 Kebab/127g	235	21.6	185	5.6	2.2	17.0	2.4
King Prawn, Spicy Tomato Creole, M&S*	1 Pack/240g	240	7.9	100	14.3	2.9	3.3	0.7
Lamb, Greek Style, Sainsbury's*	1 Serving/70g	196	15.3	282	16.1	4.9	22.0	1.8
Lamb, Kofta, Citrus Tikka, Sainsbury's*	1 Kebab/84g	199	11.6	235	18.1	9.8	13.7	2.6
Lamb, Kofta, Indian Style, Waitrose*	1 Kebab/125g	266	19.8	213	12.3	5.5	15.8	1.6
Lamb, Shami with a Mint Raita Dip, M&S*	½ Pack/90g	189	12.1	210	12.8	9.7	13.4	3.5
Lamb, Shish, Sainsbury's*	1 Kebab/85g	178	11.3	210	19.7	2.8	13.3	0.7
Lamb, Shish, Waitrose*	1 Kebab/56g	114	7.1	203	15.3	6.8	12.7	1.1
Lamb, Shoulder, M&S*	½ Pack/250g	312	10.8	125	20.4	0.9	4.3	1.7
Lamb, with Mint, Tesco*	1 Serving/80g	192	13.4	240	16.0	5.5	16.7	0.4
Pork, & Pepper, BBQ, Sainsbury's*	1 Kebab/41g	65	2.2	158	24.1	3.1	5.4	1.9
Pork, & Pepper, Co-Op*	1 Kebab/74g	78	3.0	105	17.0	1.0	4.0	0.5
Pork, BBQ, Sainsbury's*	1 Serving/90g	65	2.2	72	11.0	1.4	2.4	0.9
Salmon, Cajun, Tesco*	1 Kebab/75g	100	3.2	133	19.8	3.9	4.2	1.3

KEDGEREE

	Measure INFO/WEIGHT	per Measure KCAL	FAT	KCAL	PROT	CARB	FAT	FIBRE
Average	1oz/28g	48	2.4	171	15.9	7.8	8.7	0.1
COU, M&S*	1 Pack/370g	388	8.1	105	7.6	13.7	2.2	2.1
Smoked Haddock, Big Dish, M&S*	1 Pack/450g	585	22.5	130	8.5	13.0	5.0	1.9

KETCHUP

	Measure INFO/WEIGHT	per Measure KCAL	FAT	KCAL	PROT	CARB	FAT	FIBRE
Barbeque, Asda*	1 Tbsp/15g	20	0.0	136	0.9	33.0	0.0	0.0
BBQ, Heinz*	1 Serving/10g	14	0.0	137	1.3	31.3	0.3	0.3
Mild Chilli, Twisted, Heinz*	1 Tbsp/15g	16	0.0	108	1.0	24.9	0.2	0.7
Tomato, Average	*1 Tsp/5g*	*6*	*0.0*	*120*	*1.5*	*28.1*	*0.2*	*0.8*
Tomato, Reduced Sugar, Average	*1 Tbsp/10g*	*9*	*0.1*	*87*	*2.0*	*16.9*	*1.2*	*0.9*
Tomato,with Balsamic Vinegar, Basil & Oregano, Heinz*	1 Serving/15g	16	0.0	110	1.4	25.3	0.1	1.3
Tomato with Indian Spices, Heinz*	1 Tbsp/15g	17	0.1	114	1.1	24.8	0.4	0.8
Tomato with Roasted Garlic, Thyme & Honey, Heinz*	1 Serving/15g	17	0.0	114	1.4	26.0	0.2	1.3

KIDNEY

	Measure INFO/WEIGHT	per Measure KCAL	FAT	KCAL	PROT	CARB	FAT	FIBRE
Lamb, Raw, Average	*1oz/28g*	*44*	*2.2*	*156*	*21.5*	*0.0*	*7.7*	*0.0*

K

	Measure INFO/WEIGHT	per Measure KCAL	FAT	Nutrition Values per 100g / 100ml KCAL	PROT	CARB	FAT	FIBRE
KIDNEY								
Ox, Raw	**1oz/28g**	**25**	**0.6**	**88**	**17.2**	**0.0**	**2.1**	**0.0**
Ox, Stewed	**1oz/28g**	**39**	**1.2**	**138**	**24.5**	**0.0**	**4.4**	**0.0**
Pig, Fried	**1oz/28g**	**57**	**2.7**	**202**	**29.2**	**0.0**	**9.5**	**0.0**
Pig, Raw	**1oz/28g**	**24**	**0.8**	**86**	**15.5**	**0.0**	**2.7**	**0.0**
Pig, Stewed	**1oz/28g**	**43**	**1.7**	**153**	**24.4**	**0.0**	**6.1**	**0.0**
Veal, Raw, Average	1 Serving/100g	99	3.1	99	15.8	0.8	3.1	0.0
KIEV								
Cheese & Herb, Mini, Bernard Matthews*	1 Kiev/23g	46	2.3	199	15.7	12.1	9.8	0.0
Cheese & Mushroom Chicken, Somerfield*	½ Pack/142g	294	15.6	207	14.0	15.0	11.0	0.0
Chicken, BFY, Morrisons*	1 Kiev/134g	304	17.4	227	16.1	11.5	13.0	1.0
Chicken, Breast, Hand Filled, Birds Eye*	1 Kiev/172g	330	17.2	192	15.5	9.9	10.0	2.0
Chicken, Cooked, M Kitchen, Fresh Ideas, Morrisons*	1 Kiev/145g	359	20.8	248	17.5	12.0	14.4	0.9
Chicken, Creamy Garlic, Chilled, Tesco*	½ Pack/143g	285	17.1	200	12.9	9.7	12.0	1.3
Chicken, Creamy Peppercorn, Tesco*	1 Kiev/132g	290	17.3	220	13.1	12.1	13.1	0.6
Chicken, Fillets, Whole, Frozen, Cooked, Birds Eye*	1 Portion/150g	300	16.0	200	14.7	11.3	10.7	1.4
Chicken, Finest, Tesco*	1 Kiev/237g	504	26.6	212	19.5	8.2	11.2	2.6
Chicken, Garlic, 25% Less Fat, GFY, Asda*	1 Kiev/134g	296	15.7	221	17.0	11.9	11.7	0.5
Chicken, Garlic, Breast, Frozen, Tesco*	1 Kiev/141g	430	34.7	305	13.0	6.9	24.6	1.3
Chicken, Garlic, M&S*	1 Kiev/150g	370	24.8	247	15.6	8.2	16.5	2.9
Chicken, Garlic, Morrisons*	1 Kiev/122g	289	19.2	237	14.3	9.8	15.7	0.0
Chicken, Garlic, Whole Breast, Asda*	1 Pack/290g	638	38.0	220	15.2	10.4	13.1	0.0
Chicken, Garlic & Herb, Sainsbury's*	1 Kiev/134g	319	19.6	239	15.0	11.7	14.7	1.3
Chicken, Garlic & Parsley, BGTY, Sainsbury's*	1 Kiev/126g	289	15.3	229	14.0	15.9	12.1	1.1
Chicken, Garlic & Parsley, Sainsbury's*	1 Kiev/120g	365	25.6	304	11.1	17.1	21.3	0.8
Chicken, Garlic Butter, Breast, Sun Valley*	1 Kiev/141g	436	32.7	309	13.2	11.8	23.2	0.9
Chicken, Garlic Butter, Somerfield*	1 Kiev/142g	425	33.9	299	12.6	8.5	23.9	1.2
Chicken, Ham & Cheese, BGTY, Sainsbury's*	1 Kiev/132g	264	10.2	200	13.2	19.5	7.7	0.8
Chicken, Ham & Cheese, Tesco*	1 Serving/143g	307	18.6	215	14.4	9.3	13.0	1.3
Chicken, in Crispy Breadcrumbs, Sainsbury's*	1 Kiev/117g	310	22.4	266	12.8	10.6	19.2	1.1
Chicken, Maitre Jean-Pierre*	1 Kiev/140g	385	26.7	275	13.3	12.7	19.1	0.8
Chicken, Tomato & Mozzarella, Tesco*	1 Kiev/143g	285	17.4	200	13.4	9.0	12.2	1.4
Turkey, Mini, Baked, Bernard Matthews*	1 Kiev/23g	50	2.7	221	17.5	11.2	11.8	1.1
KIEV VEGETARIAN								
Aduki Bean, Cauldron Foods*	1 Kiev/110g	223	5.4	203	6.2	30.0	4.9	7.0
Cheesy Garlic, Meat Free, Sainsbury's*	1 Kiev/123g	274	15.1	223	13.8	14.3	12.3	3.5
Garlic, Meat Free, Asda*	1 Kiev/125g	239	11.2	191	15.0	12.5	9.0	2.6
Garlic, Meat Free, Tesco*	1 Kiev/125g	244	11.2	195	15.0	12.5	9.0	2.6
Sweet Potato, Spinach & Quinoa, Linda McCartney*	1 Kiev/145g	319	13.5	220	3.8	28.7	9.3	3.4
Vegetable, M&S*	1 Kiev/155g	279	16.6	180	4.2	17.2	10.7	3.7
KIPPER								
Baked, Average	**1oz/28g**	**57**	**3.2**	**205**	**25.5**	**0.0**	**11.4**	**0.0**
Fillets, Raw, Average	**1 Serving/200g**	**451**	**34.3**	**226**	**17.0**	**0.0**	**17.1**	**0.0**
Fillets, Smoked with Butter, Scottish, Boil in Bag, Tesco*	1 Serving/100g	225	17.2	225	17.0	0.0	17.2	0.0
Fillets in Brine, John West*	1 Can/140g	269	16.8	192	21.0	0.0	12.0	0.0
Fillets in Sunflower Oil, John West*	1 Can/140g	321	23.8	229	19.0	0.0	17.0	0.0
Grilled, Average	**1oz/28g**	**71**	**5.4**	**255**	**20.1**	**0.0**	**19.4**	**0.0**
Smoked, Average	**1 Serving/150g**	**322**	**23.0**	**214**	**18.9**	**0.0**	**15.4**	**0.0**
KIT KAT								
2 Finger, Nestle*	2 Fingers/21g	107	5.4	510	6.4	62.8	25.6	2.3
4 Finger, Nestle*	4 Fingers/46g	233	11.8	512	6.3	62.6	25.9	1.1
Caramac, 4 Finger, Nestle*	4 Fingers/49g	259	14.1	532	5.9	61.9	29.0	0.6
Chunky, Caramel, Nestle*	1 Bar/48g	259	15.3	539	5.2	58.6	31.8	0.0
Chunky, Nestle*	1 Bar/48g	248	12.6	516	5.9	62.5	26.3	2.1

K

	Measure INFO/WEIGHT	per Measure		Nutrition Values per 100g / 100ml				
		KCAL	FAT	KCAL	PROT	CARB	FAT	FIBRE
KIT KAT								
Chunky, Orange, Nestle*	1 Bar/48g	247	12.5	515	5.8	62.0	26.1	0.0
Chunky, Peanut, Nestle*	1 Bar/50g	268	15.8	537	8.4	54.9	31.5	0.0
Chunky, Snack Size, Nestle*	1 Bar/26g	133	7.1	513	6.6	60.4	27.2	1.1
Cookies & Cream, Nestle*	2 Fingers/21g	107	5.2	510	6.3	64.0	25.0	1.4
Kubes, Nestle*	1 Pack/50g	258	13.8	515	5.9	60.9	27.5	1.0
Mini, Nestle*	1 Bar/15g	75	3.9	502	7.5	59.4	26.0	0.0
Mint, 4 Finger, Nestle*	4 Fingers/48g	244	12.7	508	6.0	61.5	26.4	1.1
Orange, 2 Finger, Nestle*	2 Fingers/21g	107	5.6	507	5.5	61.7	26.5	0.0
Senses, Nestle*	1 Bar/31g	165	9.5	531	7.5	56.3	30.7	0.0
White, Chunky, Nestle*	1 Bar/53g	276	14.6	521	8.3	60.3	27.5	0.7
KIWI FRUIT								
Fresh, Raw, Flesh & Seeds, Average	*1 Kiwi/60g*	*29*	*0.3*	*49*	*1.1*	*10.6*	*0.5*	*1.9*
Weighed with Skin, Average	*1 Kiwi/60g*	*29*	*0.3*	*49*	*1.1*	*10.6*	*0.5*	*1.9*
KOHLRABI								
Boiled in Salted Water	*1oz/28g*	*5*	*0.1*	*18*	*1.2*	*3.1*	*0.2*	*1.9*
Raw	*1oz/28g*	*6*	*0.1*	*23*	*1.6*	*3.7*	*0.2*	*2.2*
KORMA								
Chicken, & Basmati Rice, Tesco*	1 Pot/350g	588	32.6	168	4.3	16.9	9.3	2.3
Chicken, & Pilau Rice, Asda*	1 Serving/350g	735	49.0	210	12.0	9.0	14.0	2.0
Chicken, & Pilau Rice, BGTY, Sainsbury's*	1 Pack/400g	404	5.2	101	8.0	14.3	1.3	0.6
Chicken, & Pilau Rice, Indian, Asda*	1 Pack/456g	643	22.8	141	8.0	16.0	5.0	2.4
Chicken, & Pilau Rice, PB, Waitrose*	1 Pack/400g	452	6.8	113	8.9	15.4	1.7	1.3
Chicken, & Pilau Rice, Sharwood's*	1 Pack/375g	489	16.2	130	5.2	17.1	4.3	1.2
Chicken, & Pilau Rice, Tesco*	1 Serving/460g	722	45.1	157	5.6	11.5	9.8	1.3
Chicken, & Rice, Everyday, Value, Tesco*	1 Pack/400g	625	28.9	160	7.3	13.8	7.4	2.6
Chicken, & Rice, Indian Meal for Two, Sainsbury's*	1 Pack/500g	785	40.5	157	6.8	14.3	8.1	3.1
Chicken, & Rice, LC, Tesco*	1 Pack/450g	495	9.0	110	7.2	16.0	2.0	0.8
Chicken, Breast, Chunks, Sainsbury's*	1 Serving/227g	354	9.3	156	28.0	1.7	4.1	0.8
Chicken, Diet Chef Ltd*	1 Pack/300g	324	15.0	108	11.1	4.6	5.0	0.6
Chicken, Fresh, Chilled, Tesco*	1 Pack/350g	819	60.9	234	13.1	6.3	17.4	2.3
Chicken, Indian, Take Away, Tesco*	½ Pack/175g	222	13.5	127	9.0	5.5	7.7	1.8
Chicken, Indian Meal for 2, Finest, Tesco*	½ Pack/200g	348	24.0	174	10.3	6.2	12.0	2.5
Chicken, Indian Takeaway for One, Sainsbury's*	1 Serving/300g	498	30.9	166	13.0	5.3	10.3	1.6
Chicken, Morrisons*	1 Pack/350g	707	46.6	202	13.6	7.0	13.3	0.7
Chicken, Solo Slim, Rosemary Conley*	1 Pack/300g	315	12.9	105	8.7	7.9	4.3	0.8
Chicken, Tesco*	1 Pack/350g	620	41.3	177	10.8	6.8	11.8	0.6
Chicken, Waitrose*	1 Pack/400g	680	46.8	170	13.7	2.4	11.7	1.9
Chicken, with Rice, Ready Meal, Average	1 Pack/350g	648	30.4	185	8.4	18.1	8.7	1.7
Chicken, with Rice, Ready Meal, Healthy Range	1 Serving/400g	450	8.2	112	7.3	16.1	2.1	1.2
Vegetable, Sainsbury's*	1 Serving/200g	302	25.2	151	2.7	6.6	12.6	2.2
KRISPROLLS								
Cracked Wheat, Original, Pagen*	1 Krisproll/13g	48	0.9	380	12.0	67.0	7.0	9.0
Golden, Swedish Toasts, Pagen*	1 Krisproll/12g	48	1.0	400	11.0	69.0	8.5	5.0
Organic, Bio, Pagen*	1 Krisproll/12g	46	0.8	380	12.0	67.0	7.0	8.0
Swedish Toasts, Wholegrain, Pagen*	1 Toast/13g	51	0.8	390	11.0	67.0	6.5	8.5
KULFI								
Average	*1oz/28g*	*119*	*11.2*	*424*	*5.4*	*11.8*	*39.9*	*0.6*
KUMQUATS								
Raw	*1oz/28g*	*12*	*0.1*	*43*	*0.9*	*9.3*	*0.5*	*3.8*

	Measure INFO/WEIGHT	per Measure KCAL	FAT	Nutrition Values per 100g / 100ml KCAL	PROT	CARB	FAT	FIBRE
LACES								
Apple Flavour, Tesco*	5 Laces/15g	52	0.5	347	3.6	74.8	3.2	2.1
Strawberry, Fizzy, Somerfield*	1 Pack/100g	380	2.0	380	3.0	86.0	2.0	0.0
Strawberry, Sainsbury's*	1 Serving/25g	94	1.2	377	3.3	76.3	4.6	0.1
Strawberry, Tesco*	1 Serving/75g	260	2.4	347	3.6	74.8	3.2	2.1
LAGER								
Alcohol Free, Becks*	1 Serving/275ml	55	0.0	20	0.7	5.0	0.0	0.0
Amstel, Heineken*	1 Pint/568ml	227	0.0	40	0.5	3.0	0.0	0.0
Average	1 Pint/568ml	233	0.0	41	0.3	3.1	0.0	0.0
Becks*	1 Can/275ml	113	0.0	41	0.0	3.0	0.0	0.0
Blanc, Kronenbourg*	½ Pint/284ml	119	0.0	42	0.0	3.3	0.0	0.0
Boston, Samuel Adams*	1 Bottle/355ml	160	0.0	45	0.0	0.0	0.0	0.0
Bottled, Brahma*	1 Bottle/330ml	125	0.0	38	0.0	0.0	0.0	0.0
Budweiser, 66, Anheuser-Busch*	1 Bottle/330ml	102	0.0	31	0.0	0.0	0.0	0.0
C2, Carling*	½ Pint/284ml	80	0.0	28	0.0	3.5	0.0	0.0
Can, Carlsberg*	1 Can/440ml	141	0.0	32	0.0	2.0	0.0	0.0
Draught, Carling*	1 Pint/568ml	189	0.0	33	0.0	1.4	0.0	0.0
Export, Carlsberg*	1 Can/440ml	185	0.0	42	0.4	2.8	0.0	0.4
Export, Foster's*	1 Pint/568ml	210	0.0	37	0.0	2.2	0.0	0.0
Foster's*	1 Pint/568ml	193	0.0	34	0.0	3.1	0.0	0.0
Gold, Foster's, Heineken*	1 Can/440ml	145	0.0	33	0.3	1.2	0.0	0.0
Grolsch*	1 Can/330ml	145	0.0	44	0.0	2.2	0.0	0.0
Heineken v 5, Heineken*	1 Pint/568ml	256	0.0	45	0.5	3.0	0.0	0.0
Heineken*, 5%, Heineken*	1 Bottle/250ml	110	0.0	44	0.4	3.4	0.0	0.0
Kaliber, Guinness*	1 Can/440ml	110	0.0	25	0.2	6.0	0.0	0.0
Light, Coors*	1 Serving/500ml	150	0.0	30	0.3	1.5	0.0	0.0
Light, Corona*	1 Bottle/330ml	105	0.0	32	1.5	0.0	0.0	0.0
Light, Michelob*	1 Serving/340ml	113	0.0	33	0.3	2.0	0.0	0.0
Lite, Carlsberg*	1 Bottle/330ml	89	0.0	27	0.1	0.5	0.0	0.0
Low Alcohol	1 Can/440ml	44	0.0	10	0.2	1.5	0.0	0.0
Pils, Holsten*	1 Can/440ml	167	0.0	38	0.3	2.4	0.0	0.0
Pilsner, Efes*	1 Can/500ml	226	0.0	45	0.0	7.6	0.0	0.0
Premier, Kronenbourg*	½ Pint/284ml	136	0.0	48	0.0	0.0	0.0	0.0
Premium	1 Can/440ml	260	0.0	59	0.3	2.4	0.0	0.0
Premium, Co-Op*	1 Can/440ml	132	0.4	30	0.4	0.9	0.1	0.0
Premium, French, Biere Speciale, Tesco*	1 Serving/250ml	105	0.0	42	0.3	3.3	0.0	0.0
Premium, Light, Amstel*	1 Can/355ml	95	0.0	27	0.0	1.4	0.0	0.0
Premium, Tesco*	1 Can/440ml	145	0.0	33	0.3	4.0	0.0	0.0
Shandy, Traditional Style, Asda*	1 Serving/200ml	44	0.0	22	0.0	4.6	0.0	0.0
Tuborg Green, Carlsberg*	1 Serving/200ml	78	0.0	39	0.5	2.5	0.0	0.0
Ultra Low Carb, Michelob*	1 Bottle/275ml	88	0.0	32	0.2	0.9	0.0	0.0
Vier, Becks*	1 Bottle/275ml	110	0.0	40	0.0	3.0	0.0	0.0
LAKSA								
Thai Noodle with Chicken, M&S*	1 Pack/400g	460	21.6	115	7.0	9.8	5.4	1.1
LAMB								
Breast, Lean, Roasted, Average	1 Serving/100g	273	18.5	273	26.7	0.0	18.5	0.0
Chops, Average	*1 Chop/82g*	*190*	*13.4*	*231*	*20.6*	*0.4*	*16.4*	*0.0*
Chops, Minted, Average	*1 Chop/100g*	*260*	*15.1*	*260*	*25.9*	*5.1*	*15.1*	*0.3*
Cutlets, Neck, Raw, Lean & Fat, Weighed with Bone	*1 Pack/210g*	*485*	*42.8*	*231*	*11.9*	*0.0*	*20.4*	*0.0*
Diced, From Supermarket, Healthy Range, Average	*½ Pack/200g*	*277*	*8.9*	*138*	*24.6*	*0.1*	*4.5*	*0.0*
Escalope, Asda*	1 Serving/100g	173	5.0	173	32.0	0.0	5.0	0.0
Fillet, Indian, Somerfield*	1 Pack/300g	570	36.0	190	17.0	4.0	12.0	0.0
Grill Steak, Average	*1oz/28g*	*70*	*4.7*	*250*	*20.2*	*4.4*	*16.9*	*0.4*
Grill Steak, Prime, Average	*1 Steak/63g*	*197*	*16.1*	*312*	*18.5*	*2.0*	*25.5*	*0.1*

L

Measure INFO/WEIGHT		per Measure		Nutrition Values per 100g / 100ml				
		KCAL	FAT	KCAL	PROT	CARB	FAT	FIBRE
LAMB								
Grill Steak, Rosemary & Mint, Tesco*	1 Steak/62g	172	10.9	277	24.4	5.6	17.6	1.8
Leg, Joint, Raw, Average	*1 Joint/510g*	*858*	*45.5*	*168*	*20.9*	*1.4*	*8.9*	*0.2*
Leg, Roasted, Lean, Average	*1oz/28g*	*58*	*2.7*	*206*	*29.9*	*0.0*	*9.6*	*0.0*
Leg, Roasted, Lean & Fat, Average	*1oz/28g*	*66*	*3.8*	*237*	*28.6*	*0.0*	*13.6*	*0.0*
Loin, Chops, Grilled, Lean & Fat, Weighed with Bone	1 Serving/100g	247	17.9	247	21.5	0.0	17.9	0.0
Loin, Chops, Raw, Lean & Fat, Weighed with Bone	1 Serving/100g	216	17.9	216	13.7	0.0	17.9	0.0
Mince, Average	*1oz/28g*	*58*	*4.2*	*207*	*17.6*	*0.5*	*14.8*	*0.0*
Mince, Extra Lean, Sainsbury's*	1 Serving/225g	324	11.9	144	24.1	0.0	5.3	0.1
Mince, Lean, Raw, Tesco*	1 Pack/400g	860	63.6	215	17.6	0.0	15.9	0.0
Neck Fillet, Lean, Raw	1 Serving/100g	232	17.6	232	18.4	0.0	17.6	0.0
Rack, Raw, Lean & Fat	*1oz/28g*	*79*	*6.7*	*283*	*17.3*	*0.0*	*23.8*	*0.0*
Rack, Raw, Lean Only, Weighed with Bone	*1oz/28g*	*48*	*2.6*	*169*	*20.0*	*0.0*	*9.2*	*0.0*
Rack, Roasted, Lean	*1oz/28g*	*63*	*3.6*	*225*	*27.1*	*0.0*	*13.0*	*0.0*
Rack, Roasted, Lean & Fat	*1oz/28g*	*102*	*8.4*	*363*	*23.0*	*0.0*	*30.1*	*0.0*
Rump, Mint & Balsamic Crust, Easy to Cook, Waitrose*	½ Pack/167g	261	11.9	156	18.1	5.0	7.1	0.1
Rump, Parsnip, Rosemary & Breadcrumb, COOK!, M&S*	½ Pack/190g	360	19.6	189	16.3	7.5	10.3	0.5
Shoulder, Cooked, Lean & Fat	*1oz/28g*	*84*	*6.3*	*301*	*24.4*	*0.0*	*22.5*	*0.0*
Shoulder, Fillet, Average	*1oz/28g*	*66*	*5.1*	*235*	*17.6*	*0.0*	*18.3*	*0.0*
Shoulder, Raw, Average	*1oz/28g*	*70*	*5.7*	*248*	*16.8*	*0.0*	*20.2*	*0.0*
Shoulder, Roasted, Whole, Lean	*1oz/28g*	*61*	*3.4*	*218*	*27.2*	*0.0*	*12.1*	*0.0*
Steak, Leg, Raw, Average	*1 Steak/150g*	*169*	*5.5*	*112*	*20.0*	*0.0*	*3.6*	*0.0*
Steak, Minted, Average	*1 Steak/125g*	*212*	*9.0*	*170*	*22.7*	*3.4*	*7.2*	*0.9*
Steak, Raw, Average	*1 Steak/140g*	*190*	*7.6*	*136*	*21.7*	*0.2*	*5.4*	*0.0*
Stewing, Raw, Lean & Fat	*1oz/28g*	*57*	*3.5*	*203*	*22.5*	*0.0*	*12.6*	*0.0*
Stewing, Stewed, Lean	*1oz/28g*	*67*	*4.1*	*240*	*26.6*	*0.0*	*14.8*	*0.0*
Stewing, Stewed, Lean & Fat	*1oz/28g*	*78*	*5.6*	*279*	*24.4*	*0.0*	*20.1*	*0.0*
Trimmed Fat, Raw, Average	1 Serving/100g	518	51.6	518	13.3	0.0	51.6	0.0
LAMB BRAISED								
Shanks, with Chunky Vegetables, M&S*	½ Pack/425g	808	38.2	190	24.7	2.0	9.0	0.7
LAMB DINNER								
Roast, Birds Eye*	1 Dinner/340g	370	14.0	109	5.9	12.1	4.1	1.5
LAMB IN								
Garlic & Rosemary Gravy, Shank, Asda*	1 Shank/280g	451	23.2	161	19.8	1.7	8.3	0.5
Gravy, Minted, Rich, Shank, Morrisons*	1 Pack/400g	612	26.4	153	18.8	5.2	6.6	0.0
Gravy, Minted, Roast, M&S*	1 Pack/200g	140	3.0	70	6.8	6.6	1.5	0.9
Gravy, Minted, Shank, Iceland*	1 Shank/350g	651	45.2	186	15.0	2.4	12.9	0.5
LAMB RAGU								
with Tagliatelle, Slow Cooked, Finest, Tesco*	1 Pack/400g	560	19.2	140	8.5	14.9	4.8	1.1
LAMB TAGINE								
Moroccan Style with Couscous, COU, M&S*	1 Pack/400g	340	5.6	85	8.9	8.3	1.4	1.6
LAMB WITH								
Cous Cous, Moroccan Style, Tesco*	1 Pack/550g	710	14.9	129	6.6	19.6	2.7	1.3
Gravy, Joint, Tesco*	1 Serving/225g	277	13.0	123	14.9	2.8	5.8	0.0
Gravy, Mint, Joint, Tesco*	1 Serving/100g	88	1.7	88	16.6	1.8	1.7	0.1
Gravy, Mint, Leg Chops, Tesco*	1 Serving/175g	214	9.8	122	15.0	3.2	5.6	1.7
Gravy, Mint, Shanks, Frozen, Tesco*	1 Shank/200g	420	26.4	210	20.1	1.6	13.2	0.7
Honey Roast Vegetables, Extra Special, Asda*	1 Pack/400g	400	14.8	100	9.9	6.7	3.7	2.5
Mango & Mint, Shoulder Chops, Waitrose*	1 Chop/250g	555	40.5	222	16.7	2.3	16.2	0.5
Mint, Butter, Leg Steaks, Waitrose*	1 Serving/155g	270	16.3	174	19.6	0.4	10.5	0.0
Mint, Glaze & Redcurrant Sauce, Steaks, Leg, Asda*	½ Pack/145g	247	8.7	170	18.0	11.0	6.0	0.5
Mint, Leg Chops, Morrisons*	2 Chops/350g	858	45.2	245	29.4	2.4	12.9	0.9
Redcurrant & Rosemary Sauce, Chops, Leg, Tesco*	1 Pack/325g	604	36.1	186	17.6	4.0	11.1	0.5
Roasted Vegetables, Shank, M&S*	½ Pack/420g	660	30.6	157	14.9	8.3	7.3	0.7

L

	Measure INFO/WEIGHT	per Measure KCAL	FAT	Nutrition Values per 100g / 100ml KCAL	PROT	CARB	FAT	FIBRE
LAMB WITH								
Rosemary, Joint, Tesco*	1 Serving/125g	250	17.6	200	17.5	0.8	14.1	0.5
Rosemary Gravy, Shank, Sainsbury's*	1 Serving/200g	204	8.2	102	13.2	3.1	4.1	0.3
Sweet Mint Dressing, Joint, Tesco*	1 Serving/50g	96	5.9	193	19.9	1.8	11.8	0.6
LARD								
Average	*1oz/28g*	*249*	*27.7*	*891*	*0.0*	*0.0*	*99.0*	*0.0*
LASAGNE								
Al Forno, Beef, with a Chianti Classico Ragu, M&S*	1 Pack/400g	640	38.0	160	8.2	10.7	9.5	2.8
Al Forno, Finest, Tesco*	1 Pack/400g	700	38.4	175	8.4	13.3	9.6	1.0
Al Forno, TTD, Sainsbury's*	1 Pack/383g	571	30.3	149	8.6	10.9	7.9	2.1
Alla Bolognese, Weight Watchers*	1 Pack/350g	416	8.8	119	8.0	16.0	2.5	0.0
Asda*	1 Pack/398g	502	23.9	126	7.3	10.6	6.0	1.1
Basics, Sainsbury's*	1 Pack/300g	330	12.9	110	4.8	13.1	4.3	1.2
Beef, BGTY, Sainsbury's*	1 Pack/390g	376	8.5	102	6.2	13.2	2.3	1.7
Beef, Frozen, Co-Op*	1 Pack/340g	388	15.6	114	7.5	10.7	4.6	1.4
Beef, Frozen, Eat Smart, Morrisons*	1 Pack/380g	331	10.3	87	6.1	9.5	2.7	1.3
Beef, Frozen, Morrisons*	1 Serving/250g	417	23.2	167	6.5	14.3	9.3	0.9
Beef, Frozen, Tesco*	1 Pack/450g	608	25.2	135	7.5	12.6	5.6	0.8
Beef, Frozen, Weight Watchers*	1 Pack/300g	257	7.8	86	6.1	9.3	2.6	0.4
Beef, Italian, Sainsbury's*	½ Pack/350g	494	27.0	141	7.5	10.3	7.7	2.0
Beef, Less Than 3% Fat, Frozen, GFY, Asda*	1 Pack/400g	369	10.0	92	7.3	8.9	2.5	2.5
Beef, Less Than 5% Fat, Asda*	1 Pack/400g	460	17.2	115	5.0	14.0	4.3	0.6
Beef, Ready Meal, Average	1 Serving/400g	553	24.0	138	8.2	12.7	6.0	1.4
Beef, Ready Meals, Waitrose*	1 Pack/400g	444	20.5	111	5.8	10.4	5.1	0.8
Beef, with Fresh Pasta, Birds Eye*	1 Pack/400g	396	9.2	99	7.3	12.2	2.3	0.5
BFY, Morrisons*	1 Pack/350g	340	14.0	97	7.1	8.6	4.0	0.2
Bolognese, & Vegetable, Weight Watchers*	1 Pack/300g	279	7.8	93	5.0	12.4	2.6	0.0
Bolognese, Co-Op*	1 Pack/500g	758	35.5	152	8.1	13.8	7.1	0.0
Bolognese, Lidl*	1 Serving/200g	336	18.0	168	8.0	13.7	9.0	0.0
Bolognese, Trattorie Alfredo*	1 Serving/125g	204	11.2	163	9.0	13.0	9.0	0.0
Chicken, Italian, Sainsbury's*	1 Pack/450g	549	18.9	122	8.4	12.6	4.2	0.5
Chicken, Italiano, Tesco*	1 Serving/450g	490	13.5	109	8.6	12.0	3.0	0.6
Chicken, LC, Tesco*	1 Pack/400g	344	6.8	86	7.1	10.5	1.7	1.8
Classic, Deep Filled, M&S*	1 Pack/400g	760	47.6	190	10.0	11.2	11.9	0.6
Extra Special, Asda*	½ Pack/291g	416	20.4	143	7.0	13.0	7.0	0.3
Family, Big Value Pack, Iceland*	¼ Pack/237g	322	14.0	136	5.0	15.9	5.9	1.4
Family, M&S*	¼ Pack/225g	281	14.0	125	10.3	6.9	6.2	1.1
Frozen, You Count, Love Life, Waitrose*	1 Pack/380g	359	10.3	94	5.0	12.2	2.7	0.6
GFY, Asda*	1 Pack/410g	344	8.2	84	5.5	11.0	2.0	0.3
Iceland*	1 Pack/400g	548	22.0	137	7.5	14.3	5.5	0.9
Italian, Family, Asda*	¼ Pack/185g	306	18.5	166	8.0	11.0	10.0	1.7
Italian, Fresh, Chilled, Sainsbury's*	1 Pack/400g	480	22.0	120	10.1	7.5	5.5	1.4
Italian, Tesco*	1 Pack/400g	540	28.8	135	6.3	11.1	7.2	1.5
Layered, Asda*	1 Pack/300g	444	24.0	148	5.0	14.0	8.0	0.3
LC, Tesco*	1 Pack/430g	396	11.2	92	5.8	11.3	2.6	1.6
Low Fat, Co-Op*	1 Pack/300g	255	9.0	85	6.0	10.0	3.0	1.0
Low Saturated Fat, Waitrose*	1 Pack/400g	312	6.0	78	4.7	11.4	1.5	0.4
M & S*	1/3 Pack/333g	466	24.6	140	8.5	10.4	7.4	0.9
Mushroom & Spinach, Waitrose*	1 Pack/400g	373	14.0	93	3.1	12.3	3.5	1.3
Primana, Aldi*	1 Serving/250g	422	22.5	169	8.0	14.0	9.0	0.0
Reduced Calorie, CBY, Asda*	1 Pack/400g	332	10.0	83	6.0	8.4	2.5	1.3
Salmon, King Prawn & Spinach, Finest, Tesco*	1 Pack/400g	600	29.6	150	10.6	9.6	7.4	0.8
Sheets, Boiled, Average	**1 Sheet/20g**	**20**	**0.1**	**100**	**3.0**	**22.0**	**0.6**	**0.9**
Sheets, Dry, Average	**1 Sheet/20g**	**70**	**0.3**	**349**	**11.9**	**72.1**	**1.5**	**2.9**

L

INFO/WEIGHT	Measure	per Measure		Nutrition Values per 100g / 100ml				
		KCAL	FAT	KCAL	PROT	CARB	FAT	FIBRE
LASAGNE								
Sheets, Fresh, Dry, Average	**1 Sheet/21g**	**56**	**0.4**	**271**	**10.9**	**52.7**	**2.1**	**1.9**
Spinach & Ricotta, Asda*	1 Pack/400g	488	24.0	122	4.9	12.0	6.0	1.5
Spinach & Ricotta, Finest, Tesco*	1 Pack/350g	584	37.1	167	6.1	11.7	10.6	1.2
Value, Tesco*	1 Pack/300g	330	15.0	110	3.3	12.9	5.0	0.8
Vegetable, BGTY, Sainsbury's*	1 Pack/385g	339	7.7	88	3.5	13.9	2.0	2.3
Vegetable, Healthy Range, Average	1 Serving/400g	318	8.2	80	3.5	11.8	2.1	1.5
Vegetable, Italian Roasted, Asda*	1 Serving/200g	234	14.0	117	2.6	11.0	7.0	0.7
Vegetable, Italian Three Layer, Sainsbury's*	1 Pack/450g	554	23.4	123	4.8	14.3	5.2	0.5
Vegetable, Low Saturated Fat, Waitrose*	1 Pack/400g	340	11.6	85	2.9	11.9	2.9	0.9
Vegetable, Morrisons*	1 Pack/400g	464	22.8	116	3.8	12.3	5.7	0.7
Vegetable, Ready Meal, Average	1 Serving/400g	408	17.6	102	4.1	12.4	4.4	1.0
Vegetable, Roasted, GFY, Asda*	1 Pack/425g	306	7.2	72	3.3	10.9	1.7	1.6
Vegetable, Roasted, M&S*	1 Pack/400g	440	20.4	110	3.4	12.8	5.1	1.7
Vegetable, Waitrose*	1 Pack/400g	440	23.2	110	3.2	11.3	5.8	1.2
Vegetable, Weight Watchers*	1 Pack/330g	251	5.6	76	3.6	11.8	1.7	0.7
Vegetable, You Count, Love Life, Waitrose*	1 Pack/400g	319	28.3	80	3.2	11.9	7.1	1.5
You Count, Love Life, Waitrose*	1 Pack/400g	306	6.4	76	6.7	8.1	1.6	1.2
LASAGNE VEGETARIAN								
Linda McCartney*	1 Pack/360g	451	20.2	125	6.3	12.4	5.6	1.4
Tesco*	1 Pack/450g	630	34.6	140	6.0	11.6	7.7	1.6
LAVERBREAD								
Average	**1oz/28g**	**15**	**1.0**	**52**	**3.2**	**1.6**	**3.7**	**0.0**
LEEKS								
Boiled, Average	**1oz/28g**	**6**	**0.2**	**21**	**1.2**	**2.6**	**0.7**	**1.7**
Creamed, Frozen, Waitrose*	1 Serving/225g	115	5.4	51	1.8	5.5	2.4	0.0
Raw, Unprepared, Average	**1 Leek/166g**	**64**	**1.5**	**39**	**2.8**	**5.1**	**0.9**	**3.9**
LEMON								
Extract	¼ Tsp/1ml	5	0.0	400	0.0	0.0	0.0	0.0
Fresh, Raw, Average	1 Slice/5g	1	0.0	20	1.0	3.2	0.3	2.4
Fresh, Raw, Unwaxed, Sainsbury's*	½ Lemon/60g	12	0.2	20	1.0	3.2	0.3	0.0
Peel, Raw, Average	**1 Tbsp/6g**	**3**	**0.0**	**47**	**1.5**	**16.0**	**0.3**	**10.6**
LEMON CURD								
Average	**1 Tbsp/15g**	**44**	**0.7**	**294**	**0.7**	**62.9**	**4.7**	**0.1**
Luxury, Average	**1 Tsp/7g**	**23**	**0.6**	**326**	**2.8**	**59.7**	**8.4**	**0.1**
Sainsbury's*	1 Portion/20g	51	1.0	254	0.7	51.3	4.8	1.3
Value, Tesco*	1 Serving/15g	44	0.7	290	0.7	61.1	4.8	0.4
LEMON GRASS								
Stalks, Tesco*	1 Stalk/13g	12	0.1	99	1.8	25.3	0.5	0.0
LEMON SOLE								
Fillets, Raw, Average	**1 Serving/220g**	**180**	**2.8**	**82**	**17.3**	**0.2**	**1.3**	**0.3**
Goujons, Average	1 Serving/150g	359	18.3	239	13.9	18.5	12.2	1.0
Grilled, Average	**1oz/28g**	**27**	**0.5**	**97**	**20.2**	**0.0**	**1.7**	**0.0**
in Breadcrumbs, Average	1 Fillet/142g	322	17.4	228	13.7	15.7	12.3	1.0
in White Wine & Herb Butter, Fillets, M&S*	1 Pack/220g	385	27.7	175	15.1	0.1	12.6	0.0
Steamed, Average	**1oz/28g**	**25**	**0.3**	**91**	**20.6**	**0.0**	**0.9**	**0.0**
with Lemon Mayonnaise, Goujons, Finest, Tesco*	1 Pack/230g	713	52.4	310	10.6	15.6	22.8	1.0
LEMONADE								
7 Up, Zero, Britvic*	1 Can/330ml	6	0.0	2	0.1	0.1	0.0	0.0
7-Up, Light, Britvic*	1 Can/330ml	4	0.0	1	0.1	0.2	0.0	0.0
Asda*	1 Glass/250ml	82	0.0	33	0.0	8.0	0.0	0.0
Average	1 Glass/250ml	52	0.2	21	0.1	5.0	0.1	0.1
Cloudy, Diet, Sainsbury's*	1 Can/330ml	7	0.3	2	0.1	0.2	0.1	0.3
Cloudy, Diet, Tesco*	1 Serving/200ml	6	0.0	3	0.0	0.8	0.0	0.0

	Measure INFO/WEIGHT	per Measure KCAL	FAT	Nutrition Values per 100g / 100ml KCAL	PROT	CARB	FAT	FIBRE
LEMONADE								
Cloudy, Gastropub, M&S*	1 Bottle/500ml	25	0.0	5	0.0	0.0	0.0	0.0
Cloudy, Sainsbury's*	1 Glass/250ml	118	0.2	47	0.1	12.0	0.1	0.1
Cloudy, Shapers, Boots*	1 Bottle/500ml	15	0.0	3	0.0	0.3	0.0	0.0
Cloudy, Waitrose*	1 Glass/250ml	125	0.0	50	0.0	12.2	0.0	0.0
Diet, Average	1 Glass/250ml	4	0.1	2	0.1	0.2	0.0	0.0
Diet, Premium, Tesco*	1 Glass/250ml	8	0.0	3	0.0	0.4	0.0	0.0
Low Calorie, Smart Price, Asda*	1 Glass/250ml	1	0.0	0	0.0	0.1	0.0	0.0
Pink, Pret a Manger*	1 Serving/250ml	75	0.0	30	0.1	7.1	0.0	0.0
R White*	1 Glass/250ml	65	0.0	26	0.1	6.2	0.0	0.0
Sainsbury's*	1 Glass/250ml	52	0.2	21	0.1	4.9	0.1	0.1
Schweppes*	1 Glass/250ml	45	0.0	18	0.0	4.2	0.0	0.0
Sicilian, Sainsbury's*	1 Glass/200ml	98	0.2	49	0.1	11.5	0.1	0.1
Sparkling, Co-Op*	1 Can/330ml	25	0.0	8	0.0	1.5	0.0	0.0
Sparkling, Morrisons*	1 Glass/250ml	63	0.0	25	0.0	6.1	0.0	0.0
Still, Freshly Squeezed, M&S*	½ Bottle/250ml	100	0.5	40	0.1	9.0	0.2	0.5
Sugar Free, Everyday Value, Tesco*	1 Glass/250ml	1	0.0	0	0.0	0.0	0.0	0.0
Tesco*	1 Glass/200ml	30	0.0	15	0.0	3.6	0.0	0.0
Traditional Style, Tesco*	1 Glass/200ml	100	0.0	50	0.0	12.3	0.0	0.0
TTD, Sainsbury's*	1 Serving/248g	159	0.0	64	0.1	14.8	0.0	0.2
Victorian, Fentiman's*	1 Bottle/275ml	130	0.0	47	0.0	11.3	0.0	0.0
LEMSIP								
Beechams*	1 Sachet/3g	11	0.0	387	0.0	100.0	0.0	0.0
LENTILS								
Black Beluga, Ready to Eat, Merchant Gourmet*	1 Serving/63g	92	0.8	147	10.9	20.5	1.2	5.2
Green, Organic, Dry, Love Life, Waitrose*	1 Serving/40g	125	0.8	313	24.3	48.8	1.9	8.9
Green & Brown, Dried, Boiled in Salted Water, Average	*1 Tbsp/30g*	*32*	*0.2*	*105*	*8.8*	*16.9*	*0.7*	*3.8*
Green or Brown, Dried, Average	*1 Serving/50g*	*150*	*0.8*	*301*	*22.8*	*49.8*	*1.5*	*9.6*
Green or Brown in Water, Tinned, Average	*½ Can/132g*	*131*	*0.8*	*99*	*8.1*	*15.4*	*0.6*	*3.8*
Puy, Green, Dry, Average	1 Serving/100g	306	1.4	306	24.7	49.5	1.4	10.3
Red, Boiled in Unsalted Water, Average	*1oz/28g*	*28*	*0.1*	*102*	*7.6*	*17.5*	*0.4*	*2.6*
Red, Dried, Average	*1oz/28g*	*88*	*0.4*	*315*	*23.8*	*53.8*	*1.3*	*4.9*
Red, Split, Great Scot*	1 Serving/50g	152	0.5	304	23.8	53.2	1.0	0.0
Red, Split, Wholefoods, Tesco*	1 Serving/100g	335	1.3	335	23.8	56.3	1.3	4.9
Red, Split, Wholesome, Love Life, Waitrose*	1 Serving/80g	270	1.0	337	23.8	56.3	1.3	4.9
LETTUCE								
Average, Raw	1 Serving/28g	4	0.1	14	1.1	1.8	0.3	1.2
Cos, Sweet, Baby, Somerfield*	1 Pack/600g	90	3.0	15	0.8	1.7	0.5	0.9
Crest, Sainsbury's*	1 Serving/80g	11	0.4	14	0.8	1.7	0.5	0.0
Curly Leaf, Sainsbury's*	1 Serving/80g	11	0.4	14	0.8	1.7	0.5	0.0
Iceberg, Average	*1 Serving/80g*	*11*	*0.3*	*13*	*0.8*	*1.8*	*0.3*	*0.5*
Lamb's, Average	*1 Serving/80g*	*12*	*0.2*	*14*	*1.4*	*1.6*	*0.2*	*1.0*
Leafy, Tesco*	1 Serving/80g	11	0.3	14	1.2	1.5	0.4	1.9
Radicchio, Red, Raw, Average	*1 Head/220g*	*29*	*0.2*	*13*	*1.4*	*1.6*	*0.1*	*3.0*
Romaine, Average	*1 Serving/80g*	*12*	*0.4*	*15*	*0.9*	*1.7*	*0.5*	*0.7*
Romaine, Hearts, Average	*1 Serving/80g*	*12*	*0.4*	*16*	*0.9*	*1.7*	*0.6*	*1.0*
Romaine, Sweet, Average	*1 Serving/80g*	*12*	*0.4*	*16*	*0.9*	*1.6*	*0.6*	*0.8*
Round, Average	1 Serving/80g	10	0.2	13	1.4	2.2	0.2	1.1
Sweet Gem, TTD, Sainsbury's*	1 Serving/100g	15	0.5	15	0.8	1.7	0.5	0.9
LILT								
Fruit Crush, Coca-Cola*	1 Can/330ml	66	0.0	20	0.0	4.6	0.0	0.0
Fruit Crush, Zero, Coca-Cola*	1 Can/330ml	12	0.0	4	0.0	0.3	0.0	0.0
Z, Coca-Cola*	1 Can/330ml	10	0.0	3	0.0	0.4	0.0	0.0

L

INFO/WEIGHT	Measure	per Measure		Nutrition Values per 100g / 100ml				
		KCAL	FAT	KCAL	PROT	CARB	FAT	FIBRE

LIME
Peel, Raw	1 Tbsp/6g	3	0.0	47	1.5	16.0	0.3	10.6
Raw, Flesh Only, Average	1 Lime/71g	18	0.1	25	0.6	8.8	0.2	2.4
Raw, Weighed with Peel & Seeds, Average	1 Lime/85g	26	0.2	30	0.7	10.5	0.2	2.8

LINGUINE
Cooked	1 Serving/100g	133	0.7	133	5.1	26.3	0.7	1.1
Crab, Rocket & Chilli, Italian, Finest, Tesco*	1 Pack/350g	718	36.4	205	6.5	20.7	10.4	1.7
Crab & Chilli, Waitrose*	1 Pack/350g	770	45.0	220	7.7	18.0	12.9	1.8
Dry, Average	1 Serving/100g	352	2.2	352	13.1	70.0	2.2	2.8
Fresh, Dry, Average	1 Pack/250g	681	6.5	272	12.3	51.7	2.6	4.0
King Prawn, & Calamari, Olive Oil & Lemon, M&S*	1 Pack/245g	320	13.5	131	0.0	1.0	5.5	0.0
King Prawn, & Roasted Garlic, LC, Tesco*	1 Pack/400g	340	5.2	85	5.6	11.9	1.3	1.5
King Prawn, Asda*	1 Pack/400g	380	10.4	95	6.4	11.5	2.6	1.5
King Prawn, FreshTastes, Asda*	1 Serving/356g	338	9.3	95	6.4	11.5	2.6	1.5
King Prawn, Meal For One, CBY, Asda*	1 Pack/380g	338	9.1	89	5.1	10.5	2.4	2.3
King Prawn, Meal for One, M&S*	1 Pack/400g	380	6.8	95	6.6	13.1	1.7	2.2
King Prawn, Tomato & Chilli, City Kitchen, Tesco*	1 Pack/385g	424	16.2	110	4.0	13.5	4.2	1.4
Pomodoro, M&S*	1 Pack/300g	360	10.5	120	4.1	17.6	3.5	1.2
Prawn & Scallops, BGTY, Sainsbury's*	1 Pack/400g	320	2.0	80	6.2	12.7	0.5	0.8
Salmon, Smoked, Sainsbury's*	1 Serving/400g	586	28.8	146	6.2	14.2	7.2	1.2
Salmon & Prawn, Iceland*	1 Meal/450g	540	19.8	120	4.5	15.8	4.4	1.5
with Mushrooms, Vegelicious, Tesco*	1 Bowl/380g	399	12.5	105	4.3	13.7	3.3	2.0

LINSEEDS
Average	1 Tsp/5g	23	1.7	464	21.7	18.5	33.5	26.3
Brown, Wholefoods, Tesco*	1 Portion/10g	52	4.2	515	18.3	1.6	42.2	27.3

LION BAR
Mini, Nestle*	1 Bar/16g	80	3.6	486	4.6	67.7	21.7	0.0
Nestle*	1 Bar/52g	248	11.2	478	6.5	64.6	21.6	0.0
Peanut, Nestle*	1 Bar/49g	256	14.5	522	7.1	56.9	29.6	0.0

LIQUEURS
Amaretto, Average	1 Pub Shot/25ml	97	0.0	388	0.0	60.0	0.0	0.0
Cointreau, Specialite De France	1 Serving/37ml	80	0.0	215	0.0	0.0	0.0	0.0
Cream, Average	1 Shot/25ml	81	4.0	325	0.0	22.8	16.1	0.0
*Grand Marnier**	1 Pub Shot/35ml	94	0.0	268	0.0	22.9	0.0	0.0
High Strength, Average	1 Shot/25ml	78	0.0	314	0.0	24.4	0.0	0.0
Kirsch, Average	1 Shot/25ml	67	0.0	267	0.0	20.0	0.0	0.0
Marula Fruit & Cream Cocktail, Amarula*	1 fl oz/30ml	103	0.0	343	0.0	36.7	0.0	0.0
Raspberry, Vanilla, Honey, Herbs & Brandy, Chambord*	1 Serving/35ml	79	0.0	225	0.0	29.3	0.0	0.0

LIQUORICE
Allsorts, Average	1 Bag/56g	195	2.9	349	3.7	76.7	5.2	2.0
Allsorts, Bassett's*	1 Pack/225g	855	11.0	380	5.6	77.8	4.9	1.6
Allsorts, Fruit, Bassett's*	1 Serving/50g	160	0.2	320	1.8	76.9	0.4	0.0
Allsorts, Julian Graves*	1 Serving/30g	113	2.2	376	3.4	78.7	7.2	1.2
Assorted, Filled, Panda*	1 Sweet/4g	15	0.4	385	3.7	68.0	11.0	0.0
Bars, Panda*	1 Bar/32g	99	0.1	308	3.7	72.0	0.4	0.9
Catherine Wheels, Barratt*	1 Wheel/22g	65	0.1	290	3.8	67.2	0.3	0.7
Catherine Wheels, Sainsbury's*	1 Wheel/17g	49	0.1	286	3.8	67.2	0.3	0.7
Comfits, M&S*	1oz/28g	100	0.1	357	2.4	86.2	0.3	0.7
Log, Raspberry, Choc, RJ's Licorice Ltd*	1 Log/45g	178	4.5	395	3.9	74.0	10.0	0.9
Organic, Laidback Liquorice*	1 Bar/28g	90	0.3	320	4.7	75.0	1.0	3.0
Panda*	1 Bar/32g	109	0.2	340	3.8	78.0	0.5	0.0
Red, Fresh, 98% Fat Free, RJ's Licorice Ltd*	1oz/28g	96	0.5	342	3.0	75.0	1.7	0.0
Shapes, Average	1oz/28g	78	0.4	278	5.5	65.0	1.4	1.9
Soft Eating, Australia, Darrell Lea*	1 Piece/20g	68	0.4	338	2.8	76.1	1.9	0.0

	Measure INFO/WEIGHT	per Measure KCAL	FAT	Nutrition Values per 100g / 100ml KCAL	PROT	CARB	FAT	FIBRE
LIQUORICE								
Sweets, Blackcurrant, Tesco*	1 Sweet/8g	32	0.3	410	0.0	92.3	3.8	0.0
Torpedos, Panda*	1 Serving/25g	92	0.0	366	1.9	88.0	0.2	1.4
Twists, Tesco*	1 Serving/63g	186	0.2	297	2.7	71.0	0.3	0.7
LIVER								
Calves, Fried	*1oz/28g*	*49*	*2.7*	*176*	*22.3*	*0.0*	*9.6*	*0.0*
Calves, Raw	*1oz/28g*	*29*	*1.0*	*104*	*18.3*	*0.0*	*3.4*	*0.0*
Calves with Fresh Sage Butter, M&S*	1 Serving/117g	210	12.5	180	12.8	10.1	10.7	1.5
Chicken, Cooked, Simmered, Average	*1 Serving/100g*	*167*	*6.5*	*167*	*24.5*	*0.9*	*6.5*	*0.0*
Chicken, Fried, Average	*1oz/28g*	*47*	*2.5*	*169*	*22.1*	*0.0*	*8.9*	*0.0*
Chicken, Raw, Average	*1oz/28g*	*26*	*0.6*	*92*	*17.7*	*0.0*	*2.3*	*0.0*
Lamb's, Braised, Average	*1 Serving/100g*	*220*	*8.8*	*220*	*30.6*	*2.5*	*8.8*	*0.0*
Lamb's, Fried, Average	*1oz/28g*	*66*	*3.6*	*237*	*30.1*	*0.0*	*12.9*	*0.0*
Lamb's, Raw, Average	*1 Serving/125g*	*171*	*7.8*	*137*	*20.3*	*0.0*	*6.2*	*0.0*
Ox, Raw	*1oz/28g*	*43*	*2.2*	*155*	*21.1*	*0.0*	*7.8*	*0.0*
Ox, Stewed	*1oz/28g*	*55*	*2.7*	*198*	*24.8*	*3.6*	*9.5*	*0.0*
Pig's, Raw	*1oz/28g*	*32*	*0.9*	*113*	*21.3*	*0.0*	*3.1*	*0.0*
Pig's, Stewed	*1 Serving/70g*	*132*	*5.7*	*189*	*25.6*	*3.6*	*8.1*	*0.0*
LIVER & BACON								
Meal for One, M&S*	1 Pack/452g	430	16.7	95	7.0	8.0	3.7	1.2
with Creamy Mash, GFY, Asda*	1 Pack/386g	282	5.4	73	5.5	9.6	1.4	2.2
with Fresh Mashed Potato, Waitrose*	1 Pack/400g	416	17.2	104	7.3	9.0	4.3	1.3
with Mash, Cooked, British Classics, Tesco*	1 Pack/450g	562	20.2	125	11.9	7.6	4.5	1.0
with Mash, M Kitchen, Morrisons*	1 Pack/450g	463	16.6	103	7.4	9.3	3.7	1.4
LIVER & ONIONS								
British Classics, Tesco*	1 Pack/250g	265	12.0	106	9.7	5.9	4.8	0.5
M & S*	1 Serving/200g	250	12.0	125	7.6	10.5	6.0	0.9
LIVER SAUSAGE								
Average	*1 Slice/10g*	*22*	*1.5*	*216*	*15.3*	*4.4*	*15.2*	*0.2*
LOBSTER								
Boiled, Average	*1oz/28g*	*29*	*0.4*	*103*	*22.1*	*0.0*	*1.6*	*0.0*
Crepes, Finest, Tesco*	1 Serving/160g	250	10.2	156	10.7	14.0	6.4	1.2
Dressed, John West*	1 Can/43g	45	2.2	105	13.0	2.0	5.0	0.0
Dressed, M&S*	1oz/28g	76	6.6	273	14.3	0.8	23.6	0.1
Half, M&S*	1oz/28g	66	5.5	235	12.1	2.4	19.6	0.2
Raw, Average	1 Serving/100g	92	1.4	92	18.7	0.3	1.4	0.0
Squat, Tails, Youngs*	½ Pack/125g	246	10.8	197	9.8	20.1	8.6	1.1
Thermidor, Finest, Tesco*	½ Pack/140g	381	25.2	272	15.3	12.1	18.0	1.0
Thermidor, M&S*	1 Serving/140g	287	19.2	205	10.7	9.7	13.7	0.0
LOGANBERRIES								
Raw	*1oz/28g*	*5*	*0.0*	*17*	*1.1*	*3.4*	*0.0*	*2.5*
LOLLIPOPS								
Assorted, Co-Op*	1 Lolly/10g	40	0.0	400	0.0	97.0	0.0	0.0
Assorted Flavours, Asda*	1 Lolly/7g	27	0.0	380	0.0	95.0	0.0	0.0
Blackcurrant, Sugar Free, Rowntree's*	1 Lolly/15g	35	0.0	233	0.1	89.4	0.0	0.0
Chocolate Lolly, M&S*	1 Lolly/45g	248	15.8	550	6.8	54.0	35.1	2.7
Chupa Chups*	1 Lolly/18g	44	0.2	247	0.0	96.5	1.3	0.0
Orange, Sugar Free, Rowntree's*	1 Lolly/15g	35	0.0	235	0.1	89.5	0.0	0.6
Refreshers, Bassett's*	1 Lolly/6g	25	0.0	417	0.0	108.3	0.0	0.0
LOQUATS								
Raw	*1oz/28g*	*8*	*0.1*	*28*	*0.7*	*6.3*	*0.2*	*0.0*
LOZENGES								
Original, Victory V*	1 Lozenge/3g	9	0.0	350	0.0	91.0	0.0	0.0
Original Extra Strong Lozenge, Fisherman's Friend*	1 Lozenge/1g	4	0.0	382	0.3	94.9	0.0	0.5

Measure INFO/WEIGHT	per Measure KCAL	FAT	Nutrition Values per 100g / 100ml KCAL	PROT	CARB	FAT	FIBRE
LUCOZADE							
Apple, Energy Drink, GlaxoSmithKline UK Limited*	1 Bottle/380ml	262	0.0	69	0.0	17.1	0.0	0.0
Caribbean Crush, Energy, Lucozade*	1 Bottle/380ml	217	0.0	57	0.0	13.9	0.0	0.0
Cherry, Sport, Lite, GlaxoSmithKline UK Limited*	1 Bottle/500ml	50	0.0	10	0.0	2.0	0.0	0.0
Citrus Fruits, Hydro Active, Sport, Lucozade*	1 Bottle/500ml	50	0.0	10	0.0	2.0	0.0	0.0
Energy, Original, GlaxoSmithKline UK Limited*	1 Bottle/380ml	266	0.0	70	0.0	17.2	0.0	0.0
Orange, Sport Lite, GlaxoSmithKline UK Limited*	1 Serving/500g	50	0.0	10	0.0	2.0	0.0	0.0
Orange Energy Drink, GlaxoSmithKline UK Limited*	1 Bottle/500ml	350	0.0	70	0.0	17.2	0.0	0.0
LUNCHEON MEAT							
Pork, Average	*1oz/28g*	*81*	*6.8*	*288*	*13.3*	*4.0*	*24.3*	*0.0*
LYCHEES							
Fresh, Raw, Flesh Only	*1oz/28g*	*16*	*0.0*	*58*	*0.9*	*14.3*	*0.1*	*0.7*
in Juice, Amoy*	1oz/28g	13	0.0	46	0.4	10.9	0.0	0.0
in Syrup, Average	*1oz/28g*	*19*	*0.0*	*69*	*0.4*	*17.7*	*0.0*	*0.4*
Raw, Weighed with Skin & Stone	*1oz/28g*	*10*	*0.0*	*36*	*0.5*	*8.9*	*0.1*	*0.4*

L

	Measure INFO/WEIGHT	per Measure KCAL	FAT	Nutrition Values per 100g / 100ml KCAL	PROT	CARB	FAT	FIBRE
M&M'S								
Crispy, Mars*	1 Serving/36g	177	8.8	492	4.1	63.9	24.4	2.7
Mars*	1 Pack/45g	218	9.7	485	5.0	68.0	21.5	0.0
Mini, Mars*	1 Pack/36g	176	8.4	489	6.3	63.6	23.2	0.0
Peanut, Mars*	1 Pack/45g	228	11.4	506	9.4	60.1	25.4	2.7
Peanut Butter, Mars*	1 Pack/42g	230	12.0	548	9.5	57.1	28.6	4.8
MACADAMIA NUTS								
Plain, Average	**1 Pack/100g**	**750**	**77.6**	**750**	**7.9**	**4.8**	**77.6**	**5.3**
Roasted, Salted, Average	**6 Nuts/10g**	**75**	**7.8**	**748**	**7.9**	**4.8**	**77.6**	**5.3**
MACARONI								
Dry, Average	**1oz/28g**	**99**	**0.5**	**354**	**11.9**	**73.5**	**1.7**	**2.6**
MACARONI CHEESE								
& Spinach, TTD, Sainsbury's*	1 Pack/500g	1025	57.5	205	6.5	18.9	11.5	1.3
Birds Eye*	1 Pack/300g	470	15.0	157	5.7	22.3	5.0	0.8
Canned	1oz/28g	39	1.8	138	4.5	16.4	6.5	0.4
COU, M&S*	1 Pack/360g	360	8.6	100	5.8	13.9	2.4	1.2
Creamy Cheddar Cheese Sauce, McIntosh of Dyce*	1 Pack/250g	370	21.2	148	6.5	11.4	8.5	1.7
Finest, Tesco*	1 Serving/450g	735	30.3	165	7.6	17.8	6.8	1.8
Four Cheese, Extra Special, Asda*	1 Pack/400g	664	30.8	166	7.7	16.4	7.7	1.1
Italian, Sainsbury's*	½ Pack/225g	360	15.8	160	6.9	17.3	7.0	1.5
Italian, Tesco*	1 Pack/420g	830	40.7	198	9.2	18.2	9.7	1.2
M & S*	1 Pack/400g	700	28.4	175	7.0	20.9	7.1	0.9
Made with Fresh Pasta, Findus*	1 Pack/360g	360	7.2	100	5.0	16.0	2.0	0.5
Morrisons, Canned, Morrisons*	1 Can/410g	279	5.7	68	5.1	8.8	1.4	1.0
Ready Meal, Average	1 Serving/300g	435	19.1	145	6.0	15.8	6.4	1.0
Value, Tesco*	1 Pack/300g	375	14.7	125	4.4	15.0	4.9	1.2
Waitrose*	1 Pack/350g	466	32.9	133	6.8	5.2	9.4	0.0
You Count, Love Life, Waitrose*	1 Pack/370g	424	8.5	115	5.6	17.4	2.3	0.8
MACAROONS								
Butterscotch, Picard*	1 Macaroon/20g	85	3.6	424	9.7	55.1	18.2	0.0
Coconut, Sainsbury's*	1 Macaroon/33g	146	6.1	441	4.7	63.7	18.6	0.8
Coconut, Tesco*	1 Macaroon/33g	140	6.1	425	4.4	59.0	18.6	5.7
French, Average	1 Serving/60g	225	11.0	375	6.7	46.7	18.3	3.3
MACKEREL								
Atlantic, Raw, Average	**1 Fillet/75g**	**154**	**10.4**	**205**	**18.6**	**0.0**	**13.9**	**0.0**
Fillets, Honey Roast, Smoked, Sainsbury's*	1 Serving/100g	349	27.3	349	21.5	4.5	27.3	12.4
Fillets, Hot Smoked, Peppered, Asda*	1 Fillet/100g	341	28.0	341	19.0	3.3	28.0	0.6
Fillets, in a Hot Chilli Dressing, Princes*	1 Pack/125g	370	33.8	296	13.3	0.0	27.0	0.0
Fillets, in Brine, Average	**1 Can/88g**	**206**	**15.3**	**234**	**19.4**	**0.0**	**17.4**	**0.0**
Fillets, in Curry Sauce, John West*	1 Can/125g	275	20.8	220	14.2	3.5	16.6	0.2
Fillets, in Mustard Sauce, Average	1 Can/125g	274	19.4	219	14.1	5.4	15.5	0.0
Fillets, in Olive Oil, Average	1 Serving/50g	149	12.2	298	18.5	1.0	24.4	0.0
Fillets, in Spicy Tomato Sauce, Average	1oz/28g	56	3.9	199	14.3	3.8	14.0	0.0
Fillets, in Sunflower Oil, Average	1 Can/94g	262	20.6	279	20.2	0.2	21.9	0.2
Fillets, in Teriyaki Sauce, Boneless & Skinless, Tesco*	1 Can/125g	320	20.3	255	12.6	13.4	16.2	2.0
Fillets, in Tomato Sauce, Average	1 Can/125g	251	18.3	200	14.3	2.7	14.7	0.0
Fillets, Smoked, Average	**1 Fillet/75g**	**251**	**21.2**	**335**	**19.8**	**0.5**	**28.2**	**0.3**
Fillets, with Red Pepper & Onion, Smoked, Asda*	1 Serving/90g	319	27.9	354	18.0	0.8	31.0	1.2
Fried, in Blended Oil	**1oz/28g**	**76**	**5.5**	**272**	**24.0**	**0.0**	**19.5**	**0.0**
Grilled	**1oz/28g**	**67**	**4.8**	**239**	**20.8**	**0.0**	**17.3**	**0.0**
Raw, with Skin, Weighed with Bone, Average	**1oz/28g**	**67**	**4.9**	**238**	**19.9**	**0.0**	**17.6**	**0.0**
Roasted, with Piri-piri, Tesco*	1 Fillet/80g	240	19.0	300	20.7	0.0	23.8	1.0
Smoked, Lemon & Parsley, Morrisons*	½ Pack/100g	282	20.0	282	20.9	4.6	20.0	1.0
Smoked, Peppered, Average	**1oz/28g**	**87**	**7.0**	**310**	**20.4**	**0.3**	**25.2**	**0.2**

	Measure INFO/WEIGHT	per Measure KCAL	FAT	Nutrition Values per 100g / 100ml KCAL	PROT	CARB	FAT	FIBRE
MACKEREL								
Whole, Raw, Average	1 Serving/100g	220	16.1	220	18.7	0.0	16.1	0.0
MADRAS								
Beef, Indian, Takeaway, CBY, Asda*	½ Pack/200g	246	14.2	123	8.9	4.7	7.1	2.5
Beef, Tesco*	1 Pack/460g	616	37.7	134	10.6	4.5	8.2	1.2
Chicken, & Pilau Rice, Asda*	1 Pack/400g	588	28.0	147	8.0	13.0	7.0	1.7
Chicken, & Rice, Hot & Spicy, Sainsbury's*	1 Pack/500g	670	25.5	134	7.1	14.9	5.1	2.2
Chicken, Asda*	1 Serving/350g	430	31.5	123	7.0	3.6	9.0	2.3
Chicken, Iceland*	1 Pack/400g	376	19.2	94	7.7	4.9	4.8	1.1
Chicken, Indian, Tesco*	1 Pack/350g	518	31.2	148	11.3	5.6	8.9	1.9
Chicken, Indian Take Away, Tesco*	1 Serving/175g	254	17.7	145	8.2	4.8	10.1	1.7
Chicken, Morrisons*	1 Pack/350g	448	30.4	128	9.6	2.8	8.7	2.4
Chicken, Sainsbury's*	1 Pack/400g	468	27.2	117	11.7	2.2	6.8	2.8
Chicken, Tesco*	1 Pack/350g	326	14.3	93	10.6	3.6	4.1	0.6
Chicken, Waitrose*	1 Pack/400g	672	42.0	168	14.6	3.7	10.5	1.8
MAGNUM								
Almond, Wall's Ice Cream*	1 Bar/82g	270	17.2	330	5.0	30.0	21.0	1.5
Caramel & Almond, Temptation, Wall's Ice Cream*	1 Lolly/68g	239	15.0	351	5.4	34.0	22.0	0.0
Caramel & Nuts Bar, Wall's Ice Cream*	1 Bar/60g	132	9.0	220	4.0	19.0	15.0	0.0
Classic, Mini, Wall's Ice Cream*	1 Lolly/50g	170	11.0	340	4.0	30.0	22.0	0.0
Classic, Wall's Ice Cream*	1 Lolly/86g	239	15.0	278	3.5	26.7	17.4	1.2
Double Chocolate, Wall's Ice Cream*	1 Bar/92g	346	22.0	378	4.5	36.0	24.0	0.0
Gluttony, Wall's Ice Cream*	1 Lolly/110ml	425	29.0	386	4.6	32.7	26.4	0.0
Greed, Wall's Ice Cream*	1 Bar/110ml	307	18.0	279	3.6	29.1	16.4	0.0
White, Wall's Ice Cream*	1 Lolly/87g	256	14.7	296	3.8	32.0	17.0	0.0
MAKHANI								
Chicken, Sainsbury's*	½ Pack/199g	313	21.3	157	12.2	2.9	10.7	2.5
Chicken Tikka, Waitrose*	1 Pack/400g	560	30.4	140	14.0	3.8	7.6	2.1
King Prawns, Finest, Tesco*	1 Pack/350g	514	38.8	147	6.0	6.0	11.1	1.3
Paneer, Ashoka*	½ Pouch/150g	283	23.0	189	4.7	8.0	15.3	1.0
MALTESERS								
MaltEaster, Chocolate Bunny, Mars*	1 Bunny/29g	157	9.2	541	6.9	57.0	31.7	0.0
Mars*	1 Bag/37g	187	9.2	505	8.0	61.8	25.0	0.9
Mini Bunnies, Mars*	1 Bunny/12g	64	3.6	534	8.0	53.5	30.2	0.0
White Chocolate, Mars*	1 Pack/37g	186	9.4	504	7.9	61.0	25.4	0.0
MANDARIN ORANGES								
in Juice, Average	1oz/28g	11	0.0	39	0.7	9.0	0.0	0.5
in Light Syrup, Average	1 Can/298g	201	0.1	68	0.6	16.0	0.0	0.1
Weighed with Peel, Average	1 Sm/50g	18	0.0	36	0.9	8.4	0.1	1.2
MANGE TOUT								
& Sugar Snap Peas, Tesco*	1 Pack/150g	102	0.6	68	7.0	9.2	0.4	3.8
Boiled in Salted Water	1oz/28g	7	0.0	26	3.2	3.3	0.1	2.2
Raw, Average	1 Serving/80g	26	0.2	32	3.6	4.2	0.2	1.2
Stir-Fried in Blended Oil	1oz/28g	20	1.3	71	3.8	3.5	4.8	2.4
MANGO								
Dried, Average	1 Serving/50g	174	0.5	347	1.4	83.1	1.0	4.9
in Syrup, Average	1oz/28g	22	0.0	80	0.3	20.5	0.0	0.9
Ripe, Raw, Weighed with Skin & Stone, Average	1 Mango/225g	88	0.2	39	0.5	9.6	0.1	1.8
Ripe, Raw, without Peel & Stone, Flesh Only, Average	1 Mango/207g	81	1.0	39	0.5	9.6	0.5	1.8
MANGOSTEEN								
Raw, Fresh, Average	1 Serving/80g	50	0.5	63	0.6	15.6	0.6	5.1
MARGARINE								
Average	1 Thin Spread/7g	51	5.7	726	0.1	0.5	81.0	0.0
Butter Style, Average	1 Thin Spread/7g	44	4.8	627	0.7	1.1	68.9	0.0

	Measure INFO/WEIGHT	per Measure KCAL	per Measure FAT	Nutrition Values per 100g / 100ml KCAL	PROT	CARB	FAT	FIBRE

MARGARINE

	Measure INFO/WEIGHT	KCAL	FAT	KCAL	PROT	CARB	FAT	FIBRE
Buttery, Pro Activ, Flora*	1 Serving/10g	55	6.0	550	0.0	0.0	60.0	0.0
for Baking, Average	*1 Thin Spread/7g*	*42*	*4.7*	*607*	*0.2*	*0.4*	*67.2*	*0.0*
No Salt, Flora*	1 Thin Spread/7g	37	4.1	531	0.0	0.0	59.0	0.0
Omega 3 Plus, Flora*	1 Thin Spread/7g	24	2.7	350	0.1	3.0	38.0	0.0
Pro Activ, Extra Light, Flora*	1 Thin Spread/7g	15	1.6	218	0.1	2.9	23.0	0.2
Pro Activ, Light, Flora*	1 Thin Spread/7g	23	2.4	331	0.1	4.0	35.0	0.0
Pro Activ, with Olive Oil, Flora*	1 Thin Spread/7g	23	2.4	331	0.1	4.0	35.0	0.0
Pro Active, Becel*	1 Serving/7g	22	1.8	320	0.0	0.0	25.0	0.0
Reduced Fat, Average	*1 Thin Spread/7g*	*25*	*2.7*	*356*	*0.6*	*3.0*	*38.0*	*0.0*
Soya, Granose*	1 Thin Spread/7g	52	5.7	745	0.1	0.1	82.0	0.0
Utterly Butterly*	1 Thin Spread/7g	32	3.4	452	0.3	2.5	49.0	0.0
White, Flora*	1 Thin Spread/7g	60	6.6	855	0.0	0.0	95.0	0.0

MARGARITA

	Measure INFO/WEIGHT	KCAL	FAT	KCAL	PROT	CARB	FAT	FIBRE
Sainsbury's*	1 Serving/100ml	53	0.1	53	0.1	12.8	0.1	0.1

MARINADE

	Measure INFO/WEIGHT	KCAL	FAT	KCAL	PROT	CARB	FAT	FIBRE
Barbeque, Sticky, Sainsbury's*	¼ Jar/77g	112	2.8	145	0.8	26.7	3.6	1.0
BBQ, Sticky, Newman's Own*	1/3 Jar/83ml	139	0.7	167	0.9	39.0	0.8	2.5
Cajun Spice, The English Provender Co.*	1 Serving/50g	94	6.7	187	1.3	15.3	13.4	1.6
Lime & Coriander with Peri Peri, Nando's*	1 Tsp/5g	9	0.8	182	0.0	13.1	16.6	0.0
Peri Peri, Hot, Nando's*	1 Serving/40g	46	2.2	115	1.4	15.2	5.4	0.9
Peri Peri, Portuguese Bbq, Nando's*	1 Serving/40g	36	0.6	90	1.1	17.7	1.6	1.0
Tomato & Basil, Sun Dried, with Peri-Peri, Nando's*	1 Bottle/270g	319	25.6	118	0.1	15.3	9.5	0.8

MARJORAM

	Measure INFO/WEIGHT	KCAL	FAT	KCAL	PROT	CARB	FAT	FIBRE
Dried	*1 Tsp/1g*	*2*	*0.0*	*271*	*12.7*	*42.5*	*7.0*	*0.0*

MARLIN

	Measure INFO/WEIGHT	KCAL	FAT	KCAL	PROT	CARB	FAT	FIBRE
Steaks, Raw, Sainsbury's*	1 Steak/110g	109	0.2	99	24.3	0.0	0.2	0.0

MARMALADE

	Measure INFO/WEIGHT	KCAL	FAT	KCAL	PROT	CARB	FAT	FIBRE
3 Fruit, Thick Cut, Waitrose*	1 Tsp/15g	39	0.0	262	0.4	64.8	0.1	0.7
Blood Orange, Grandessa*	1 Serving/15g	36	0.0	240	0.4	59.0	0.1	0.7
Blood Orange, TTD, Sainsbury's*	1 Tbsp/15g	40	0.0	264	0.3	65.7	0.0	0.8
Citrus Shred, Robertson*	1 Tsp/5g	13	0.0	253	0.2	63.0	0.0	0.0
Five Fruit, Tesco*	1 Serving/10g	28	0.0	278	0.2	68.2	0.1	0.9
Grapefruit, Fine Cut, Duerr's*	1 Tsp/15g	39	0.0	261	0.2	65.0	0.0	0.0
Lemon, Fine Cut, Tesco*	1 Serving/15g	39	0.0	257	0.2	64.0	0.0	0.5
Lemon, Jelly, No Peel, Tesco*	1 Tsp/15g	39	0.0	263	0.1	65.0	0.0	0.4
Lemon, with Shred, Average	*1 Serving/20g*	*50*	*0.0*	*248*	*0.2*	*61.6*	*0.0*	*0.6*
Lemon & Lime, Average	*1 Tbsp/20g*	*53*	*0.0*	*267*	*0.2*	*66.4*	*0.1*	*0.4*
Lime, with Shred, Average	*1 Tbsp/15g*	*39*	*0.0*	*261*	*0.2*	*65.0*	*0.1*	*0.4*
Onion, Organic, Antony Worrall Thompson's*	1 Serving/11g	20	0.1	191	1.1	44.9	0.8	1.8
Onion, Organic, Duchy Originals*	1 Serving/40g	103	1.0	257	1.0	57.8	2.4	2.6
Orange, & Ginger, Average	*1 Tbsp/15g*	*40*	*0.0*	*264*	*0.2*	*65.7*	*0.1*	*0.3*
Orange, & Tangerine, Tiptree, Wilkin & Sons*	1 Tsp/15g	40	0.0	268	0.0	67.0	0.0	0.0
Orange, Lemon & Grapefruit, Baxters*	1 Tsp/15g	38	0.0	252	0.0	63.0	0.0	0.1
Orange, Reduced Sugar, Average	*1 Tbsp/15g*	*26*	*0.0*	*170*	*0.4*	*42.0*	*0.1*	*0.6*
Orange, Reduced Sugar, Thin Cut, Streamline*	1 Serving/10g	18	0.0	178	0.5	43.0	0.3	0.0
Orange, Seville, Thick Cut, Organic, Fair Trade, Tesco*	1 Tbsp/15g	37	0.0	245	0.3	60.3	0.1	0.7
Orange, Shred, Medium Cut, Tesco*	1 Serving/15g	39	0.0	260	0.3	64.7	0.0	0.5
Orange, Shredless, Average	*1 Tsp/10g*	*26*	*0.0*	*261*	*0.2*	*65.0*	*0.0*	*0.1*
Orange, with Shred, Average	*1 Tsp/5g*	*13*	*0.0*	*263*	*0.2*	*65.2*	*0.0*	*0.3*
Orange & Whisky, Christmas, M&S*	1oz/28g	67	0.1	240	0.3	59.5	0.2	1.9
Pink Grapefruit, Thin Cut, Waitrose*	1 Serving/10g	26	0.0	261	0.2	65.0	0.0	0.4
Three Fruit, Fresh Fruit, Sainsbury's*	1 Tsp/15g	38	0.0	250	0.0	61.3	0.0	0.0
Three Fruits, Fresh Fruit, TTD, Sainsbury's*	1 Tbsp/15g	40	0.0	268	0.3	66.7	0.0	0.8

	Measure INFO/WEIGHT	per Measure KCAL	FAT	Nutrition Values per 100g / 100ml KCAL	PROT	CARB	FAT	FIBRE
MARMITE*								
Xo, Marmite*	1 Serving/4g	10	0.0	250	37.5	25.0	0.2	0.2
Yeast Extract, Marmite*	1 Tsp/9g	22	0.0	250	39.0	24.0	0.1	3.5
Yeast Extract, with Gold Coloured Flecks, Marmite*	1 Serving/4g	10	0.0	250	39.0	24.0	0.1	3.5
MARROW								
Boiled, Average	***1oz/28g***	***3***	***0.1***	***9***	***0.4***	***1.6***	***0.2***	***0.6***
Raw	***1oz/28g***	***3***	***0.1***	***12***	***0.5***	***2.2***	***0.2***	***0.5***
MARS								
Bar, 5 Little Ones, Mars*	1 Piece/8g	38	1.5	477	4.5	73.6	18.3	0.0
Bar, Duo, Mars*	1 Bar/42g	191	7.6	450	4.4	67.5	18.0	1.2
Bar, Funsize, Mars*	1 Bar/18g	80	3.0	446	3.5	70.1	16.8	1.1
Bar, Mars*	1 Bar/58g	260	10.2	448	4.1	68.1	17.6	1.1
Bar, Medium, 58g, Mars*	1 Bar/58g	263	10.5	453	4.6	67.9	18.1	0.0
Bar, Minis, Mars*	1 Bar/18g	80	11.6	444	3.3	0.0	64.4	1.1
Delight, Mars*	1 Bar/20g	110	6.7	552	4.5	57.8	33.6	1.3
MARSHMALLOWS								
Average	1 Mallow/5g	16	0.0	327	3.9	83.1	0.0	0.0
Chocolate, Mallows, Cadbury*	1 Mallow/13g	56	2.2	435	4.7	64.7	17.4	0.8
Fat Free, Tesco*	1 Mallow/7g	24	0.0	339	3.4	80.8	0.2	0.5
Haribo*	1 Mallow/5g	16	0.0	330	3.0	80.0	0.0	0.0
No Added Sugar, Sainsbury's*	1 Mallow/2g	5	0.0	206	3.3	77.0	0.1	0.0
Pascall*	1 Mallow/5g	15	0.0	335	2.6	80.0	0.0	0.0
Pink & White, Co-Op*	1 Mallow/7g	24	0.0	340	3.0	82.0	0.0	0.0
Princess*	1 Mallow/5g	16	0.0	314	3.4	80.0	0.0	0.0
Sainsbury's*	1 Mallow/7g	23	0.0	330	4.1	78.5	0.0	0.5
MARZIPAN								
Chocolate, Bar, Plain, Thorntons*	1 Bar/46g	206	8.0	448	5.2	69.1	17.4	2.0
Dark Chocolate, Thorntons*	1 Serving/46g	207	8.0	451	5.2	69.4	17.4	2.1
Plain, Average	***1oz/28g***	***115***	***4.0***	***412***	***5.8***	***67.5***	***14.2***	***1.7***
MASALA								
Dal, with Channa & Toor Lentils, Waitrose*	½ Pack/150g	166	6.2	111	6.6	12.0	4.1	5.0
Prawn, King, Waitrose*	1 Pack/350g	385	25.9	110	7.1	3.8	7.4	1.8
Prawn, Mango, Waitrose*	½ Pack/175g	175	11.2	100	5.8	4.3	6.4	1.3
Vegetable, Waitrose*	1 Serving/400g	288	19.2	72	2.2	4.9	4.8	2.5
MASH								
Carrot, Parsnip & Turnip, Mash Direct*	1 Serving/100g	63	2.0	63	1.0	10.2	2.0	2.8
Carrot, Swede, & Potato, Butter & Seasoning, Sainsbury's*	½ Pack/200g	110	3.4	55	0.9	8.1	1.7	1.8
Parsnip, & Parmesan, Finest, Tesco*	½ Pack/250g	245	12.2	98	1.6	11.9	4.9	2.4
Potato, Carrot, Swede, Parsnip, Cream & Butter, Asda*	½ Pack/200g	94	3.0	47	1.0	7.2	1.5	3.3
Potato, Carrot & Swede, Buttery, Waitrose*	½ Pack/225g	116	3.1	52	1.0	7.1	1.4	3.3
Root, Asda*	½ Pack/200g	142	8.0	71	0.7	8.0	4.0	3.1
Root, Vegetable, Finest, Tesco*	½ Pack/250g	225	12.5	90	1.1	9.1	5.0	3.4
Vegetables, Mousline, Maggi*	1 Bag/39g	127	1.2	328	8.2	67.0	3.0	10.4
MAYONNAISE								
50% Less Fat, GFY, Asda*	1 Tbsp/10g	32	3.1	322	0.8	10.0	31.0	0.0
60% Less Fat, BGTY, Sainsbury's*	1 Tbsp/15ml	42	4.1	277	0.4	7.3	27.3	0.0
Aioli, Finest, Tesco*	1 Tsp/5g	20	2.1	408	0.8	8.5	41.2	0.0
Average	***1 Tsp/5g***	***35***	***3.8***	***690***	***0.9***	***1.6***	***75.5***	***0.0***
Caramelised Onion, Deli, Heinz*	1 Serving/20g	110	11.5	548	1.4	5.9	57.5	0.1
Dijon, Light, Benedicta*	1 Tbsp/15g	44	4.4	292	0.7	6.7	29.2	0.0
Dijon, Mustard, Hellmann's*	1 Tbsp/15ml	32	3.0	210	2.9	5.1	19.7	0.0
Egg & Dairy Free, Life Free From*	1 Serving/15g	76	8.0	508	0.9	5.6	53.3	0.2
Extra Light, Asda*	1 Tbsp/10ml	12	0.7	119	0.7	13.1	7.1	0.2
Extra Light, Average	***1 Tbsp/33g***	***34***	***2.0***	***102***	***0.7***	***10.5***	***6.2***	***0.8***

MAYONNAISE

	Measure INFO/WEIGHT	per Measure		Nutrition Values per 100g / 100ml				
		KCAL	FAT	KCAL	PROT	CARB	FAT	FIBRE
Extra Light, Bramwells, Specially Selected, Aldi*	1 Tbsp/33g	40	3.2	121	1.1	7.2	9.7	2.4
Extra Light, Heinz*	1 Tbsp/12ml	9	0.4	75	0.6	11.4	3.0	0.6
Extra Light, Now Only 3% Fat, Hellmann's*	1 Serving/16g	12	0.5	73	0.6	11.0	3.0	0.6
Extra Light, Sainsbury's*	1 Tbsp/15ml	17	1.0	115	0.7	11.9	7.0	0.0
Extra Light, Squeezy, Oak Lane, Tesco*	1 Tbsp/15g	20	1.4	130	0.6	9.4	9.6	0.0
Extra Light, Tesco*	1 Serving/45ml	40	2.1	90	0.6	10.2	4.7	0.0
Extra Light, Top Down, Tesco*	1 Tbsp/15g	14	0.8	95	0.6	10.4	5.5	0.0
Extra Light, Weight Watchers*	1 Serving/15g	15	0.9	97	1.1	9.6	5.9	3.2
Finest, Tesco*	1 Dtsp/22g	155	16.9	703	1.1	1.5	77.0	0.0
Free Range, M&S*	1 Tbsp/15g	108	11.8	720	1.1	1.2	78.5	0.0
French, Light, Sainsbury's*	1 Tbsp/15ml	46	4.7	307	0.4	6.1	31.1	0.2
French, Style, BGTY, Sainsbury's*	1 Tbsp/15ml	55	5.5	366	0.6	7.5	36.9	0.0
Garlic, Frank Cooper*	1 Tsp/6g	28	2.8	460	2.2	8.8	46.2	0.1
Garlic, Morrisons*	1 Tbsp/15ml	55	5.4	365	0.7	8.8	36.0	0.0
Garlic, Retail, Average	1 Tsp/11g	44	4.4	403	1.2	8.6	40.3	0.0
Garlic, Roasted, Beolive, Vandemooetele*	1 Tbsp/15ml	46	4.2	305	1.3	11.3	28.2	0.0
Garlic, Roasted, Deli, Heinz*	1 Tbsp/15g	81	8.5	537	1.1	5.5	56.6	0.0
Garlic, Waitrose*	1 Tsp/6g	21	2.1	346	0.6	8.6	34.3	0.0
Garlic & Herb, M&S*	1 Tsp/6g	43	4.6	712	3.4	2.4	76.9	0.9
Garlic & Herb, Reduced Calorie, Hellmann's*	1 Serving/25ml	58	4.8	233	0.7	13.1	19.3	0.4
Heinz*	1 Tbsp/15g	99	10.8	663	0.9	3.0	71.8	0.0
Lemon, & Roast Garlic, Twist of, Branston*	1 Tbsp/15ml	64	6.2	428	0.9	13.8	41.0	0.3
Lemon, Waitrose*	1 Tsp/8ml	56	6.1	694	1.2	1.3	76.0	5.4
Light, & Squeezy, Co-Op*	1 Tbsp/15ml	45	4.2	315	1.0	11.4	29.6	0.0
Light, Asda*	2 Tsp/10g	36	3.3	364	1.0	16.1	32.8	0.0
Light, BGTY, Sainsbury's*	1 Tsp/11g	33	3.2	296	0.5	7.2	29.3	0.0
Light, Hellmann's*	1 Serving/10g	30	3.0	298	0.7	6.5	29.8	0.1
Light, Kraft*	1 Serving/25g	61	5.0	245	0.6	15.0	20.0	0.0
Light, Morrisons*	1 Tsp/11g	32	3.0	287	1.4	8.5	27.5	0.0
Light, Reduced Calorie, Hellmann's*	1 Tsp/10g	30	3.0	297	0.7	6.5	29.8	0.0
Light, Reduced Fat, Heinz*	1 Tbsp/15g	42	4.0	279	1.1	7.7	26.8	0.5
Light, Squeezable, Hellmann's*	1 Tbsp/15g	44	4.4	293	0.7	6.4	29.4	0.0
Light, Squeezy, Oak Lane*	1 Tbsp/15ml	46	4.4	305	0.5	9.1	29.4	0.0
Light, Tesco*	1 Tbsp/15ml	41	4.0	275	0.8	7.1	26.7	0.0
Lighter than Light, Bramwells, Aldi*	1 Tbsp/15ml	10	0.4	67	0.4	10.4	2.6	0.0
Low Fat, Belolive*	1 Tbsp/15ml	45	4.4	298	0.8	11.1	29.0	0.0
Organic, Evernat*	1 Tsp/11g	83	8.9	752	1.3	2.8	81.0	0.0
Organic, Whole Foods*	1 Tbsp/14g	100	11.0	714	0.0	7.1	78.6	0.0
Original, Egg, Dairy & Gluten Free, Tiger Tiger*	1 Tbsp/15g	66	6.8	440	1.4	5.8	45.6	0.3
Pesto, Twist of, Branston*	1 Tbsp/30ml	124	11.6	412	1.2	14.1	38.6	0.2
Real, Asda*	1 Serving/10g	72	7.9	721	1.3	1.2	79.0	0.1
Real, Hellmann's*	1 Tsp/13g	94	10.3	720	1.1	1.5	79.1	0.0
Real, The Big Squeeze, Hellmann's*	1 Tbsp/15ml	101	11.1	676	1.0	1.2	74.0	0.0
Reduced Calorie, Average	*2 Tsp/11g*	*33*	*3.2*	*301*	*0.7*	*8.9*	*29.0*	*0.1*
Reduced Calorie, Tesco*	1 Tbsp/15g	49	4.7	326	0.8	9.8	31.5	0.0
Reduced Calorie, Waitrose*	1 Tsp/11g	32	3.0	287	1.4	8.5	27.5	0.0
Reduced Fat, Tesco*	1 Tbsp/15ml	44	4.3	292	0.8	7.9	28.6	0.0
Sainsbury's*	1 Tsp/11g	75	8.3	686	0.4	1.2	75.4	0.0
Sundried Tomato, Deli, Heinz*	1 Tbsp/15g	88	9.4	589	1.3	4.9	62.5	0.0
Sweet Chilli, Twist of, Branston*	1 Tbsp/15g	64	5.6	430	0.9	21.4	37.5	0.2
Value, Tesco*	1 Tbsp/15g	73	7.7	488	0.8	5.4	51.4	0.0
Vegetarian, Tesco*	1 Tsp/12g	89	9.7	738	1.5	0.8	81.0	0.0
Waitrose*	1 Tbsp/15ml	106	11.7	709	1.3	0.8	77.8	0.0

INFO/WEIGHT	Measure	per Measure		Nutrition Values per 100g / 100ml				
		KCAL	FAT	KCAL	PROT	CARB	FAT	FIBRE
MAYONNAISE								
with a Spark of Chilli, Hellmann's*	1 Tbsp/15ml	41	4.0	276	0.8	7.5	27.0	0.3
with Coarse Ground Mustard, French, Sainsbury's*	1 Tbsp/15ml	93	10.1	618	0.8	1.7	67.3	0.3
MEAT LOAF								
Beef, Wrapped In Prosciutto Crudo, Waitrose*	1/3 Pack/196g	378	27.4	193	14.2	2.6	14.0	0.7
Beef & Pork, Co-Op*	¼ Loaf/114g	314	25.1	275	13.0	7.0	22.0	1.0
in Onion Gravy, M&S*	¼ Pack/140g	203	11.9	145	11.3	6.3	8.5	1.2
Somerfield*	1 Pack/454g	867	59.0	191	10.0	8.0	13.0	0.0
MEATBALLS								
& Mashed Potato, Tesco*	1 Pack/450g	526	29.7	117	4.0	10.4	6.6	1.0
& Pasta, in Tomato Sauce, Wayfayrer*	1 Pack/300g	375	17.4	125	9.0	9.2	5.8	1.0
& Pasta, Sainsbury's*	1 Serving/300g	333	9.3	111	5.3	15.5	3.1	1.9
Beef, Aberdeen Angus, 12 Pack, Waitrose*	1 Meatball/36g	93	7.1	259	18.0	2.3	19.8	0.1
Beef, Aberdeen Angus, Fresh, Chilled, Waitrose*	1 Meatball/36g	92	7.1	256	18.0	1.5	19.8	0.0
Beef, in Sauce, Aberdeen Angus, PB, Waitrose*	½ Pack/240g	228	7.2	95	10.5	6.5	3.0	1.1
Beef, in Tomato Sauce, Diet Chef Ltd*	1 Pack/300g	408	18.6	136	11.3	8.7	6.2	2.7
Beef, Morrisons*	3 Meatballs/85g	213	13.8	251	23.1	3.1	16.2	0.9
Beef, Sainsbury's*	1 Meatball/29g	75	5.1	257	21.7	3.4	17.4	0.8
Beef, Tesco*	3 Meatballs/53g	140	11.4	265	15.0	2.9	21.5	0.9
Beef, TTD, Sainsbury's*	1 Meatball/35g	73	5.2	208	16.7	1.5	15.0	0.1
Beef, with Italian Herbs, Finest, Tesco*	1oz/28g	63	4.7	225	15.4	2.1	16.8	1.7
Chicken, in Tomato Sauce, Average	1 Can/392g	580	32.9	148	7.7	10.4	8.4	0.0
Chicken, Lemon, with Rice, BGTY, Sainsbury's*	1 Pack/400g	388	8.4	97	6.8	12.8	2.1	1.4
Greek, M&S*	1 Serving/350g	402	18.9	115	7.7	9.1	5.4	1.5
in Bolognese Sauce, Fray Bentos*	½ Can/204g	188	5.9	92	4.8	11.6	2.9	0.7
in Bolognese Sauce, Somerfield*	1 Pack/454g	704	49.9	155	7.0	7.0	11.0	0.0
in Gravy, Campbell's*	½ Can/205g	164	5.3	80	5.6	8.6	2.6	0.0
in Gravy, Fray Bentos*	1 Meatball/21g	17	0.6	79	4.6	8.7	2.9	0.6
in Sherry Sauce, Tapas, Waitrose*	1 Serving/185g	272	7.4	147	18.8	5.9	4.0	1.2
in Spicy Tomato & Bacon Sauce, M Kitchen, Morrisons*	½ Pack/90g	123	8.1	136	6.5	5.5	9.0	3.6
in Tomato & Basil Sauce, Go Cook, Asda*	½ Pack/270g	526	38.3	195	12.4	4.4	14.2	2.4
in Tomato Sauce, Canned, Average	1 Can/410g	387	15.1	94	5.6	9.8	3.7	0.0
in Tomato Sauce, Tapas, Waitrose*	1 Pack/185g	285	16.8	154	10.8	7.2	9.1	1.3
Lamb, Asda*	1 Pack/340g	928	71.4	273	16.0	5.1	21.0	0.6
M & S*	1oz/28g	58	3.8	208	10.9	10.7	13.5	2.4
Pork, & Beef, Swedish Style, Tesco*	1 Meatball/14g	34	2.5	245	14.3	6.5	17.7	2.0
Pork, & Chorizo with Paprika Potatoes, Finest, Tesco*	½ Pack/425g	527	25.9	124	7.5	9.8	6.1	2.8
Pork, British, Simply, M&S*	½ Pack/180g	396	27.2	220	17.0	4.3	15.1	0.5
Pork, Italian, Al Forno, Sainsbury's*	1 Pack/450g	644	23.8	143	6.1	17.6	5.3	1.4
Spaghetti, Tesco*	1 Pack/385g	377	16.0	98	5.4	9.8	4.2	1.2
Swedish, Average	¼ Pack/88g	198	13.8	224	14.0	7.4	15.7	1.3
Turkey, GFY, Asda*	½ Pack/330g	333	12.2	101	10.0	7.0	3.7	0.0
with Spicy Tomato Sauce, Just Cook, Sainsbury's*	½ Pack/170g	246	11.9	145	14.8	5.7	7.0	0.9
MEATBALLS VEGETARIAN								
Swedish Style, Sainsbury's*	1 Ball/27g	53	2.6	194	21.5	5.5	9.5	4.0
MEDLAR								
Raw, Flesh Only	*1 Fruit/28g*	*11*	*0.1*	*40*	*0.5*	*10.6*	*0.4*	*10.0*
MELBA TOAST								
Asda*	1 Slice/3g	13	0.2	395	12.0	76.0	4.8	4.6
Average	1 Serving/3g	13	0.2	396	12.0	76.0	4.9	4.6
Buitoni*	1 Serving/33g	130	1.6	395	12.1	75.5	4.9	4.6
Dutch, LC, Tesco*	1 Pack/20g	75	0.5	375	13.1	75.0	2.4	4.6
Organic Spelt, Amisa*	2 Slices/24g	95	1.9	395	12.4	68.5	7.9	0.0

	Measure INFO/WEIGHT	per Measure KCAL	FAT	Nutrition Values per 100g / 100ml KCAL	PROT	CARB	FAT	FIBRE
MELBA TOAST								
Original, Van Der Meulen*	1 Slice/3g	12	0.1	399	12.8	80.5	2.9	3.9
Thinly Sliced Toasted Wheat Bread, Sainsbury's*	1 Slice/3g	12	0.1	374	13.1	75.1	2.4	4.6
Tomato & Basil, Morrisons*	1 Pack/20g	77	0.6	383	13.6	75.7	2.9	2.4
Van Der Meulen*	3 Slices/39g	151	0.9	388	13.1	75.1	2.4	0.0
Wholegrain, Morrisons*	6 Toasts/20g	73	1.0	367	16.8	63.8	4.9	8.9
with Sesame, Tesco*	1 Slice/3g	11	0.2	370	12.8	61.7	8.0	3.8
MELON								
Cantaloupe, Flesh Only, Average	½ Melon/255g	87	0.5	34	0.8	8.2	0.2	0.9
Cantaloupe, Weighed with Rind, Average	1 Wedge/100g	35	0.3	35	0.8	8.3	0.3	0.8
Galia, Average	1 Serving/240g	60	0.1	25	0.8	5.8	0.0	0.2
Honeydew, Raw, Flesh Only, Average	1oz/28g	8	0.0	30	0.7	7.0	0.1	0.5
Medley, Pre Packed, Average	1 Pack/240g	66	0.3	27	0.6	6.0	0.1	0.5
Pineapple & Strawberry, Fully Prepared, Sainsbury's*	1 Serving/245g	86	0.2	35	0.6	7.8	0.1	0.9
MENTOS								
Cola, Mentos*	1 Pack/38g	146	0.8	390	0.0	93.0	2.0	0.0
MERINGUE								
Average	1 Meringue/8g	30	0.0	379	5.3	95.4	0.0	0.0
Bombe, Raspberry & Vanilla, M&S*	1 Bombe/100g	155	1.8	155	3.4	33.3	1.8	2.6
Chocolate, Belgian, Mini, Extra Special, Asda*	1 Meringue/6g	28	0.9	459	6.0	75.0	15.0	0.7
Chocolate, Waitrose*	1 Meringue/77g	341	11.3	444	2.6	75.3	14.7	0.5
Cream, Fresh, Sainsbury's*	1 Meringue/35g	142	5.1	407	3.5	65.4	14.6	0.5
Cream, M&S*	1 Meringue/34g	145	7.6	425	4.1	52.6	22.2	1.4
Layered, Tesco*	1/5 Meringue/52g	146	0.8	280	3.5	63.2	1.5	1.4
Lemon, Morrisons*	1 Serving/120g	295	14.4	246	2.5	32.0	12.0	0.5
Mini, Extra Special, Asda*	1 Meringue/4g	14	0.0	394	5.0	93.0	0.2	0.5
Mini, M&S*	1 Meringue/4g	15	0.0	395	6.1	91.6	0.0	0.2
Nests, Asda*	1 Nest/15g	59	0.0	394	5.0	93.0	0.2	0.5
Nests, Average	1 Nest/16g	63	0.0	397	4.8	93.3	0.1	0.1
Nests, M&S*	1 Nest/12g	47	0.0	390	6.1	91.6	0.0	0.0
Nests, Mini, Tesco*	1 Nest/5g	19	0.0	386	4.8	91.2	0.2	0.0
Nests, Morrisons*	1 Nest/15g	62	0.0	414	4.5	94.7	0.0	0.0
Nests, Sainsbury's*	1 Nest/13g	52	0.0	392	4.2	93.6	0.1	0.1
Raspberry, M&S*	1 Serving/105g	215	13.8	205	1.8	20.6	13.1	3.1
Shells, Sainsbury's*	2 Shells/24g	93	0.0	387	3.9	92.8	0.0	0.0
Summer Fruits, 90% Fat Free, Sara Lee*	1 Meringue/135g	308	11.5	228	2.5	35.7	8.5	2.2
Toffee, M&S*	1 Meringue/30g	124	6.3	415	4.1	52.2	20.9	0.8
Toffee, Mini, COU, M&S*	1 Meringue/5g	20	0.1	395	5.0	95.3	1.7	0.7
MIDGET GEMS								
M & S*	1 Bag/113g	367	0.1	325	6.3	75.1	0.1	0.0
Smart Price, Asda*	1 Pack/178g	586	0.2	329	6.0	76.0	0.1	0.0
MILK								
1% Fat, Fresh, Arla*	1 Glass/202ml	83	2.0	41	3.3	4.8	1.0	0.0
2% Low Fat, Dunkley's*	1 Cup/240ml	120	5.0	50	2.9	4.2	2.1	0.0
Alternative, Original, Good Hemp*	1 Glass/250ml	90	6.0	36	1.3	2.2	2.4	0.2
Condensed, Caramel, Carnation, Nestle*	1 Serving/50g	148	3.0	296	5.5	55.1	6.0	0.0
Condensed, Semi Skimmed, Sweetened	1oz/28g	75	0.1	267	10.0	60.0	0.2	0.0
Condensed, Skimmed, Unsweetened, Average	1oz/28g	30	1.1	108	7.5	10.5	4.0	0.0
Condensed, Whole, Sweetened, Average	1oz/28g	93	2.8	333	8.5	55.5	10.1	0.0
Dried, Skimmed, Average	1oz/28g	99	0.3	355	35.4	52.3	0.9	0.0
Dried, Skimmed, Powder, Value, Tesco*	1 Serving/50g	180	0.3	361	36.1	52.9	0.6	0.0
Dried, Whole, Average	1oz/28g	137	7.4	490	26.3	39.4	26.3	0.0
Evaporated, Average	1 Serving/85g	136	7.6	160	8.2	11.6	9.0	0.0
Evaporated, Reduced Fat, Average	1oz/28g	33	1.5	118	7.4	10.5	5.2	0.0

	Measure INFO/WEIGHT	per Measure KCAL	per Measure FAT	Nutrition Values per 100g / 100ml KCAL	PROT	CARB	FAT	FIBRE
MILK								
Goats, Pasteurised	*1 fl oz/30ml*	*18*	*1.0*	*60*	*3.1*	*4.4*	*3.5*	*0.0*
Goats, Semi Skimmed, St Helen's Farm*	1 Serving/250ml	109	4.0	44	3.0	4.3	1.6	0.0
Goats, Semi Skimmed, Waitrose*	1 Serving/250ml	98	4.0	39	3.0	4.5	1.6	0.0
Goats, Skimmed, St Helen's Farm*	1 Serving/125ml	38	0.1	30	3.0	4.3	0.1	0.0
Low Fat, Calcia Extra Calcium, Unigate*	1 fl oz/30ml	14	0.2	45	4.3	6.3	0.5	0.0
Semi Skimmed, Average	*1 fl oz/30ml*	*15*	*0.5*	*49*	*3.4*	*5.0*	*1.7*	*0.0*
Semi Skimmed, Long Life, Average	*1 fl oz/30ml*	*15*	*0.5*	*49*	*3.4*	*5.0*	*1.7*	*0.0*
Semi Skimmed, Low Lactose, Lactofree, Arla*	1 Glass/125ml	50	1.9	40	3.6	3.0	1.5	0.0
Semi Skimmed, Low Lactose, UHT, Lactofree, Arla*	1 Serving/100ml	38	1.7	38	3.2	2.6	1.7	0.0
Skimmed, Average	*1 Pint/568ml*	*194*	*0.5*	*34*	*3.3*	*5.0*	*0.1*	*0.0*
Skimmed, Lactofree, Arla*	1 Serving/200ml	78	0.8	39	3.8	3.6	0.4	0.0
Skimmed, Uht, Average	*1 fl oz/30ml*	*10*	*0.0*	*34*	*3.4*	*5.0*	*0.1*	*0.0*
Skimmed 1% Fat, Waitrose*	1 Serving/200ml	70	0.2	35	3.4	5.0	0.1	0.0
Soya, Vitasoy*	1 Serving/250ml	130	3.8	52	3.0	5.5	1.5	2.0
Whole, Average	*1 Serving/200ml*	*134*	*7.8*	*67*	*3.3*	*4.7*	*3.9*	*0.0*
Whole, Buffalo, Laverstoke Park Farm*	1 Serving/200ml	220	16.0	110	4.5	4.9	8.0	0.0
Whole, Lactose Free, Lactofree, Arla*	1 Serving/200ml	116	7.0	58	3.9	2.7	3.5	0.0
MILK DRINK								
Chocolate Coconut, Free From, Tesco*	1 Serving/250ml	125	5.4	49	0.4	6.8	2.1	0.7
Chocolate Flavoured, Goodness for Kids, Tesco*	1 Bottlel/330ml	248	5.9	75	3.8	10.3	1.8	0.7
Hazelnut, Free From, Tesco*	1 Serving/250ml	85	2.5	34	0.2	5.2	1.0	1.5
Original, Mars*	1 Serving/330g	284	6.9	86	3.1	13.7	2.1	0.0
Refuel, Mars*	1 Bottle/388ml	299	5.8	77	3.1	13.5	1.5	0.0
Semi Skimmed, Cholesterol Lowering, Pro Activ, Flora*	1 Serving/250ml	125	4.5	50	3.6	4.8	1.8	0.0
Strawberry Flavoured, Goodness for Kids, Tesco*	1 Bottle/330ml	248	5.6	75	4.0	9.9	1.7	0.4
MILK SHAKE								
Banana, Yazoo, Campina*	1 Bottle/200ml	120	2.4	60	3.1	9.6	1.2	0.0
Banana Flavour, Frijj*	1 Bottle/500ml	325	4.5	65	3.7	10.5	0.9	0.0
Cafe Latte, Diet Chef Ltd*	1 Carton/330ml	218	3.3	66	4.2	8.9	1.0	2.0
Chocolate, Asda*	1 Serving/250ml	198	9.2	79	4.4	7.0	3.7	0.4
Chocolate, Extreme, Frijj*	1 Bottle/500g	425	10.5	85	3.9	12.7	2.1	0.0
Chocolate Flavour, Diet Chef Ltd*	1 Drink/330ml	210	2.3	64	4.1	8.5	0.7	1.9
Chocolate Flavoured, Fresh, Thick, Frijj*	1 Bottle/500ml	350	5.0	70	3.5	11.7	1.0	0.0
Honeycomb Choc Swirl Flavour, The Incredible, Frijj*	1 Bottle/500ml	450	12.5	90	4.0	13.0	2.5	0.2
Measure Up, Asda*	1 Glass/250ml	200	2.4	80	6.0	12.0	1.0	2.4
Powder, Made Up with Semi-Skimmed Milk	1 Serving/250ml	172	4.0	69	3.2	11.3	1.6	0.0
Powder, Made Up with Whole Milk	1 Serving/250ml	218	9.2	87	3.1	11.1	3.7	0.0
Sticky Toffee Pudding Flavour, The Incredible, Frijj*	1 Bottle/500ml	445	10.0	89	4.0	13.7	2.0	0.1
Strawberry, Yazoo, Campina*	1 Bottle/475ml	300	6.0	60	3.1	9.5	1.2	0.0
Strawberry Flavour, Thick, Low Fat, Frijj*	1 Bottle/250ml	155	2.0	62	3.4	10.1	0.8	0.0
Vanilla, Diet Chef Ltd*	1 Pack/330ml	225	3.0	68	4.2	10.5	0.9	1.5
Vanilla, Frijj*	1 Bottle/500ml	320	4.0	64	3.4	10.7	0.8	0.0
Vanilla Flavour, BGTY, Sainsbury's*	1 Bottle/500ml	230	0.5	46	5.3	5.9	0.1	0.4
MILKY BAR								
Buttons, Nestle*	1 Pack/30g	164	9.5	547	7.3	58.4	31.7	0.0
Choo, Nestle*	1 Bar/25g	116	4.3	464	4.2	73.1	17.2	0.0
Chunky, Nestle*	¼ Bar/38g	207	12.0	547	7.3	58.4	31.7	0.0
Eggs, Mini, Nestle*	1 Pack/100g	500	23.3	500	4.2	68.4	23.3	0.0
Funsize, Mars*	1 Bar/17g	75	2.7	449	3.8	71.8	16.3	0.6
Munchies, Nestle*	1 Serving/70g	392	24.3	560	7.0	54.9	34.7	0.1
Nestle*	1 Bar/13g	68	4.0	547	7.3	58.4	31.7	0.0
MILKY WAY								
Funsize, Mars*	1 Bar/16g	70	2.5	450	3.9	71.6	16.3	0.6

	Measure INFO/WEIGHT	per Measure KCAL	FAT	Nutrition Values per 100g / 100ml KCAL	PROT	CARB	FAT	FIBRE
MILKY WAY								
Magic Stars, Mars*	1 Bag/33g	183	11.5	555	6.2	54.1	34.9	1.8
Mars*	1 Bar/22g	98	3.5	448	3.7	72.4	15.9	0.6
MINCEMEAT								
Asda*	1 Serving/100g	285	3.5	285	0.8	62.8	3.5	2.1
Average	*1oz/28g*	*77*	*1.2*	*274*	*0.6*	*62.1*	*4.3*	*1.3*
Finest, Tesco*	1 Tbsp/15g	44	0.4	290	1.2	61.1	2.7	2.9
Organic, Waitrose*	1oz/28g	81	0.7	290	0.9	65.8	2.6	2.0
Tesco*	1 Serving/20g	58	0.7	292	0.8	64.2	3.5	1.6
Traditional, Robertson*	1 Tbsp/17g	49	0.6	286	0.6	62.5	3.4	2.5
Traditional, Sainsbury's*	1 Tbsp/23g	65	0.7	282	0.9	62.4	3.2	1.4
MINI BITES								
Blueberry & Yoghurt Clusters, M&S*	1 Bite/13g	60	2.7	465	5.0	64.4	20.7	4.7
Chocolate Caramel, M&S*	1 Bite/21g	95	5.1	460	5.6	53.5	24.6	1.6
Chocolate Cornflake, M&S*	1 Bite/12g	55	2.4	470	6.2	66.3	20.1	3.6
Chocolate Orange, M&S*	1 Bite/22g	95	4.8	430	5.5	54.6	21.6	1.8
Extremely Chocolatey, M&S*	1 Bite/20g	90	4.9	450	5.7	52.4	24.6	1.6
Extremely Chocolatey Caramel Crispy, M&S*	1 Bite/11g	50	2.0	455	4.7	68.2	17.9	2.8
Flapjack, M&S*	1 Bite/14g	70	3.5	500	6.4	62.1	25.0	3.6
Rocky Road, M&S*	1 Bite/12g	50	1.6	410	5.2	66.9	13.3	2.5
MINIS								
Cream Cheese & Chives, Ryvita*	1 Pack/30g	114	2.3	380	8.7	75.7	7.7	13.0
Salt & Vinegar, Ryvita*	1 Pack/24g	90	1.9	376	8.2	74.0	7.8	11.4
Sweet Chilli, Ryvita*	1 Pack/24g	90	1.8	376	8.5	75.9	7.4	10.3
MINSTRELS								
Galaxy, Mars*	1 Serving/100g	503	22.3	503	5.2	70.3	22.3	1.1
MINT								
Dried, Average	*1 Tsp/5g*	*14*	*0.2*	*279*	*24.8*	*34.6*	*4.6*	*0.0*
Fresh, Average	*2 Tbsp/3g*	*1*	*0.0*	*43*	*3.8*	*5.3*	*0.7*	*0.0*
MINTS								
After Dinner, Dark, Elizabeth Shaw*	1 Sweet/9g	42	2.1	469	2.8	62.5	23.1	0.0
After Dinner, Sainsbury's*	1 Mint/7g	32	1.5	456	4.1	62.1	21.2	4.1
Butter Mintoes, M&S*	1 Sweet/9g	35	0.6	391	0.0	84.0	6.8	0.0
Butter Mintoes, Tesco*	1 Sweet/7g	24	0.5	349	0.0	71.3	7.1	0.0
Clear, Co-Op*	1 Sweet/6g	24	0.0	395	0.0	98.0	0.0	0.0
Cream, Luxury, Thorntons*	1 Sweet/13g	62	3.1	477	4.2	62.3	23.8	2.3
Creams, Bassett's*	1 Sweet/11g	40	0.0	365	0.0	91.8	0.0	0.0
Curiously Strong, M&S*	1 Sweet/1g	4	0.0	390	0.4	97.5	0.0	0.0
Everton, Co-Op*	1 Sweet/6g	25	0.2	410	0.6	92.0	4.0	0.0
Extra, Wrigleys*	1 Sweet/1g	3	0.0	240	0.0	64.0	1.0	0.0
Extra Strong, Peppermint, Trebor*	1 Roll/46g	180	0.1	395	0.4	98.1	0.2	0.0
Extra Strong, Spearmint, Trebor*	1 Pack/44g	174	0.0	395	0.4	98.7	0.0	0.0
Glacier, Fox's*	1 Sweet/5g	19	0.0	386	0.0	96.4	0.0	0.0
Humbugs, Co-Op*	1 Sweet/8g	34	0.6	425	0.6	89.9	7.0	0.0
Humbugs, M&S*	1 Sweet/9g	37	0.4	407	0.6	91.1	4.4	0.0
Humbugs, Thorntons*	1 Sweet/9g	31	0.4	340	1.0	87.8	4.4	0.0
Imperials, Co-Op*	1 Sweet/3g	12	0.0	395	0.3	98.0	0.2	0.0
Imperials, M&S*	1 Sweet/3g	12	0.0	391	0.0	97.8	0.0	0.0
Imperials, Sainsbury's*	1 Sweet/3g	10	0.0	374	0.0	92.1	0.0	0.0
Imperials, Tesco*	1 Sweet/3g	12	0.0	397	0.6	98.7	0.0	0.0
Mento, Sugar Free, Mentos*	1 Sweet/2g	5	0.1	260	1.0	87.0	5.5	0.0
Mint Assortment, M&S*	1 Sweet/7g	26	0.5	375	0.4	78.2	6.9	0.0
Mint Favourites, Bassett's*	1 Sweet/6g	22	0.4	367	0.9	77.4	5.9	0.0
Peppermints, Strong, Altoids*	1 Sweet/1g	3	0.0	385	0.5	96.0	0.0	0.0

M

	Measure INFO/WEIGHT	per Measure KCAL	FAT	Nutrition Values per 100g / 100ml KCAL	PROT	CARB	FAT	FIBRE
MINTS								
Soft, Trebor*	1 Pack/48g	182	0.0	380	0.0	94.9	0.0	0.0
Softmints, Peppermint, Trebor*	1 Pack/48g	170	0.0	355	0.0	88.9	0.0	0.0
Softmints, Spearmint, Trebor*	1 Pack/45g	170	0.0	375	0.0	94.3	0.0	0.0
Thins, Chocolate, Waitrose*	1 Thin/5g	27	1.3	509	4.2	69.6	23.8	0.2
MIRIN								
Rice Wine, Sweetened, Average	*1 Tbsp/15ml*	*35*	*0.0*	*231*	*0.2*	*41.6*	*0.0*	*0.0*
MISO								
Average	*1oz/28g*	*57*	*1.7*	*203*	*13.3*	*23.5*	*6.2*	*0.0*
MIXED HERBS								
Average	*1 Tsp/5g*	*13*	*0.4*	*260*	*13.0*	*37.5*	*8.5*	*6.7*
MIXED VEGETABLES								
Baby, Corn, Mange Tout & Baby Carrots, Tesco*	1 Pack/220g	64	0.9	29	2.3	4.3	0.4	2.2
Baby, Iceland*	1 Serving/100g	20	0.0	20	1.2	3.9	0.0	2.7
Baby, Steam, Fresh, Tesco*	1 Pack/160g	72	1.3	45	2.7	6.7	0.8	3.8
Bag, M&S*	1 Serving/200g	70	0.4	35	2.9	5.6	0.2	0.0
Broccoli & Cauliflower Florets, Baby Carrots, Asda*	1 Serving/113g	28	0.7	25	2.2	2.6	0.6	2.4
Canned, Drained, Co-Op*	½ Can/100g	45	0.1	45	2.0	9.0	0.1	2.0
Canned, Drained, Sainsbury's*	1 Can/200g	114	0.6	57	3.0	10.6	0.3	2.3
Canned, Re-Heated, Drained	1oz/28g	11	0.2	38	1.9	6.1	0.8	1.7
Carrot, Cauliflower & Broccoli, Prepared, Co-Op*	1 Pack/250g	100	1.5	40	2.4	5.0	0.6	2.7
Carrot, Cauliflower & Fine Beans, Steam Veg, Tesco*	1 Bag/160g	37	0.5	23	1.4	3.6	0.3	2.9
Carrot, Swede, Leek & Onion for Casserole, M&S*	1 Serving/100g	35	0.4	35	0.8	5.6	0.4	2.6
Carrot Batons, Cauliflower & Broccoli, Steamed, Asda*	1 Bag/120g	28	0.7	23	1.8	2.6	0.6	3.1
Carrots, Broccoli & Sweetcorn, EasySteam, Sainsbury's*	1 Pack/120g	67	1.4	56	2.6	8.7	1.2	2.0
Carrots, Broccoli & Sweetcorn, Steam Veg, Tesco*	1 Sachet/160g	80	1.8	50	2.5	7.5	1.1	3.0
Carrots, Cauliflower & Broccoli, Waitrose*	1 Serving/100g	35	0.6	35	2.4	4.9	0.6	2.9
Carrots, Peas, Green Beans & Sweetcorn, Tesco*	1 Serving/80g	38	0.6	48	3.1	7.3	0.7	3.9
Casserole, Frozen, Tesco*	1 Serving/100g	26	0.4	26	0.8	4.8	0.4	2.0
Casserole, Tesco*	1 Pack/440g	176	1.3	40	1.2	8.0	0.3	2.3
Cauliflower, Carrots, Green Beans, SteamFresh, Birds Eye*	1 Bag/120g	40	0.6	33	2.0	5.0	0.5	2.2
Chef's Style, Ready Prepared, M&S*	1 Pack/240g	72	1.2	30	2.6	4.5	0.5	2.9
Chinese, Stir Fry, Amoy*	1 Serving/110g	27	0.3	25	1.8	3.7	0.3	0.0
Chunky, Frozen, Sainsbury's*	1 Serving/85g	31	0.6	37	2.9	4.7	0.7	3.1
Corn Baby, Fine Beans & Baby Carrots, Tesco*	1 Pack/250g	68	1.2	27	1.7	4.0	0.5	2.2
Crunchy, Tesco*	1 Pack/210g	63	0.8	30	1.7	5.0	0.4	2.4
Farmhouse, Frozen, Waitrose*	1 Serving/90g	22	0.5	25	1.9	3.1	0.6	2.4
Fine Beans & Baby Carrots, Sweet, Tender, Waitrose*	½ Pack/125g	42	0.6	34	1.3	4.6	0.5	2.8
Freshly Frozen, Asda*	1 Serving/80g	42	0.6	52	3.2	8.0	0.8	3.0
Freshly Frozen, Iceland*	1 Serving/100g	54	0.8	54	3.3	8.3	0.8	3.7
Frozen, Aldi*	1 Serving/100g	34	0.7	34	2.8	4.3	0.7	0.0
Frozen, Boiled in Salted Water	1oz/28g	12	0.1	42	3.3	6.6	0.5	0.0
Frozen, Waitrose*	1 Serving/80g	43	0.6	54	3.1	8.7	0.8	3.5
Green, Microwave, Aldi*	1 Serving/300g	189	9.0	63	3.5	5.6	3.0	4.1
Layered, Classics, M&S*	½ Pack/160g	112	6.2	70	1.2	7.3	3.9	1.2
Peas, Carrots, & Baby Leeks, Prepared, Tesco*	½ Pack/130g	57	1.2	44	3.1	5.8	0.9	3.5
Peas & Carrots Crinkle Cut, D'Aucy*	1 Serving/265g	138	1.3	52	3.2	6.5	0.5	4.3
Potatoes, Broad Beans & Peas, M&S*	1 Pack/245g	147	3.2	60	2.9	12.9	1.3	3.4
Ready to Roast, Asda*	½ Pack/362g	315	11.6	87	1.6	13.0	3.2	2.4
Red Peppers & Courgette, Tesco*	1 Pack/250g	68	1.2	27	1.7	3.8	0.5	2.0
Roast, Four Seasons*	1 Serving/187g	79	0.4	42	1.2	8.8	0.2	0.0
Sainsbury's*	1 Serving/230g	55	1.4	24	2.1	2.5	0.6	0.0
Seasonal Selection, Tesco*	1 Serving/100g	37	0.4	37	1.1	7.2	0.4	2.2
Special, Freshly Frozen, Morrisons*	1 Serving/100g	48	0.8	48	3.2	7.2	0.8	0.0

	Measure INFO/WEIGHT	per Measure		Nutrition Values per 100g / 100ml				
		KCAL	FAT	KCAL	PROT	CARB	FAT	FIBRE
MIXED VEGETABLES								
Special, Sainsbury's*	1 Serving/120g	68	1.2	57	3.2	8.9	1.0	2.9
Tenderstem Broccoli, Carrots & Mange Tout, M&S*	½ Pack/100g	35	0.2	35	2.9	5.6	0.2	2.1
Thai Style in a Herb Marinade, Straight to Wok, Amoy*	1 Pouch/400g	74	0.8	19	0.7	3.5	0.2	0.0
MOLASSES								
Average	*1 Tsp/5g*	*13*	*0.0*	*266*	*0.0*	*68.8*	*0.1*	*0.0*
MONKEY NUTS								
without Shell, Average	*1oz/28g*	*158*	*13.4*	*565*	*25.6*	*8.2*	*48.0*	*6.3*
MONKFISH								
Grilled	*1oz/28g*	*27*	*0.2*	*96*	*22.7*	*0.0*	*0.6*	*0.0*
Raw	*1oz/28g*	*18*	*0.1*	*66*	*15.7*	*0.0*	*0.4*	*0.0*
MONSTER MUNCH								
Flamin' Hot, Walkers*	1 Bag/22g	108	5.5	490	7.0	59.0	25.0	1.5
Pickled Onion, Walkers*	1 Bag/22g	108	5.5	490	6.0	60.0	25.0	1.7
Roast Beef, Walkers*	1 Bag/22g	108	5.5	490	7.0	59.0	25.0	1.7
Spicy, Walkers*	1 Bag/25g	125	7.2	500	5.0	55.0	29.0	1.3
MORNAY								
Cod, Gratin, Cooked, Just Cook, Sainsbury's*	1 Pack/320g	518	32.2	185	13.3	6.9	11.5	0.5
Cod, Mash, Peas & Runner Beans, Fuller Longer, M&S*	1 Pack/390g	312	10.1	80	6.2	6.8	2.6	2.2
Cod, Nutritionally Balanced, M&S*	1 Pack/400g	320	10.4	80	6.8	7.2	2.6	1.6
Haddock, COU, M&S*	½ Pack/194g	165	3.9	85	14.5	2.6	2.0	0.6
Haddock, in Cheese Sauce with Chives, Morrisons*	½ Pack/170g	192	7.5	113	15.5	2.6	4.4	0.4
Salmon, with Broccoli, Weight Watchers*	1 Pack/320g	231	9.6	72	4.5	6.5	3.0	0.5
Spinach, Waitrose*	½ Pack/125g	112	8.6	90	3.3	3.6	6.9	1.6
MOUSSAKA								
Aubergine, Veg Pot, Innocent*	1 Pot/380g	258	4.6	68	2.4	10.4	1.2	3.0
Aubergine & Lentil, Asda*	1 Pack/451g	370	17.1	82	3.9	8.1	3.8	2.9
Beef, BGTY, Sainsbury's*	1 Pack/400g	300	10.4	75	6.1	6.8	2.6	1.2
COU, M&S*	1 Pack/340g	272	9.9	80	5.3	8.5	2.9	1.4
Lamb, Sainsbury's*	1 Pack/329g	497	32.3	151	8.4	7.2	9.8	1.0
TTD, Sainsbury's*	1 Pack/399g	546	35.9	137	8.1	5.8	9.0	0.6
Vegetable, COU, M&S*	1 Pack/400g	280	10.8	70	2.7	9.1	2.7	2.4
MOUSSE								
Banoffee, COU, M&S*	1 Pot/70g	102	1.5	145	2.9	28.8	2.1	1.5
Cappuccino & Chocolate, Aero Twist, Nestle*	1 Pot/75g	135	8.1	180	4.2	16.8	10.8	0.2
Chocolate	1 Pot/60g	83	3.2	139	4.0	19.9	5.4	0.0
Chocolate, Aero, Nestle*	1 Pot/58g	101	3.0	174	4.8	27.3	5.1	1.1
Chocolate, Asda*	1 Pot/61g	134	6.1	219	3.7	26.0	10.0	1.0
Chocolate, Basics, Sainsbury's*	1 Pot/63g	94	3.8	150	5.1	18.9	6.0	0.0
Chocolate, Belgian, Finest, Tesco*	1 Pot/120g	360	22.7	300	5.1	26.6	18.9	1.1
Chocolate, BGTY, Sainsbury's*	1 Pot/63g	83	1.8	133	4.9	21.8	2.9	0.5
Chocolate, Cadbury*	1 Pot/55g	107	4.5	195	6.1	24.6	8.2	0.0
Chocolate, COU, M&S*	1 Pot/70g	84	1.9	120	5.2	20.3	2.7	1.0
Chocolate, Finest, Tesco*	1 Pot/82g	321	26.4	391	3.7	21.7	32.2	0.0
Chocolate, GFY, Asda*	1 Pot/60g	70	1.7	117	4.8	17.9	2.9	3.5
Chocolate, Iceland*	1 Pot/62g	113	4.3	183	4.0	26.3	6.9	0.0
Chocolate, Italian Style, Tesco*	1 Pot/90g	243	11.9	270	5.0	32.8	13.2	2.4
Chocolate, LC, Light Choices, Tesco*	1 Pot/63g	80	1.3	125	5.0	20.8	2.1	1.5
Chocolate, Light, Cadbury*	1 Pot/55g	60	1.9	110	4.6	14.2	3.4	0.0
Chocolate, Light, Cadbury's, St Ivel*	1 Pot/64g	79	2.0	123	6.2	17.3	3.2	0.0
Chocolate, Low Fat, Danette, Danone*	1 Pot/60g	73	1.1	121	5.1	20.8	1.9	1.5
Chocolate, Milk, M&S*	1 Pot/90g	180	7.8	200	5.3	24.8	8.7	1.5
Chocolate, Mint, Cadbury*	1 Pot/45g	90	3.6	200	6.0	25.6	8.1	0.0
Chocolate, Minty, Bubbly, Dessert, Aero, Nestle*	1 Pot/58g	108	5.9	186	4.6	18.9	10.2	0.3

	Measure INFO/WEIGHT	per Measure		Nutrition Values per 100g / 100ml				
		KCAL	FAT	KCAL	PROT	CARB	FAT	FIBRE
MOUSSE								
Chocolate, Plain, Low Fat, Nestle*	1 Pot/120g	71	0.9	59	2.4	10.4	0.8	0.0
Chocolate, Sainsbury's*	1 Pot/63g	119	5.3	190	4.7	23.8	8.5	1.0
Chocolate, Shapers, Boots*	1 Pot/70g	97	1.9	138	5.3	23.0	2.7	1.7
Chocolate, Tesco*	1 Pot/60g	120	5.0	200	3.6	27.6	8.4	0.9
Chocolate, Value, Tesco*	1 Pot/63g	101	3.3	161	4.9	23.3	5.2	1.3
Chocolate, White, Bubbly, Dessert, Aero, Nestle*	1 Pot/58g	99	4.4	170	4.3	21.0	7.5	0.2
Chocolate, White, Finest, Tesco*	1 Pot/92g	436	34.5	474	3.9	30.2	37.5	0.0
Chocolate & Hazelnut, Creamy, Dr Oetker*	1 Pot/115g	158	6.9	137	3.3	17.6	6.0	0.6
Chocolate & Mint, COU, M&S*	1 Pot/70g	84	1.8	120	6.2	18.7	2.5	1.0
Chocolate & Orange, COU, M&S*	1 Pot/70g	77	1.8	110	5.9	16.0	2.6	0.9
Chocolate & Vanilla, Belgian, Weight Watchers*	1 Pot/80g	106	2.2	132	4.4	22.2	2.8	0.9
Lemon, COU, M&S*	1 Pot/70g	91	1.8	130	3.1	23.7	2.5	0.6
Lemon, Dessert, Sainsbury's*	1 Pot/63g	114	5.9	182	3.6	20.7	9.4	0.6
Lemon, Low Fat, Morrisons*	1 Pot/63g	99	5.8	158	3.7	15.4	9.3	0.3
Lemon, Tesco*	1 Pot/60g	67	1.6	111	3.4	18.2	2.7	0.0
Lemon with Meringue Style Sauce, Ski, Nestle*	1 Pot/60g	81	2.8	137	3.1	19.8	4.8	0.0
Pineapple, COU, M&S*	1 Pot/70g	84	1.7	120	3.3	20.7	2.4	3.5
Raspberry & Cranberry, Luxury, Weight Watchers*	1 Pot/80g	62	1.0	78	3.8	13.0	1.2	1.0
Strawberry, Light, Muller*	1 Pot/150g	147	0.6	98	4.3	19.4	0.4	0.0
Strawberry, Shape, Danone*	1 Pot/100g	44	1.8	44	3.0	4.0	1.8	0.0
Strawberry, Tesco*	1 Pot/63g	106	5.8	169	3.5	17.9	9.3	0.2
Strawberry, with Strawberry Sauce, Ski, Nestle*	1 Pot/60g	79	3.1	131	3.1	18.1	5.2	0.0
Strawberry & Vanilla, Weight Watchers*	1 Pot/80g	87	1.9	109	3.8	18.1	2.4	0.4
Summer Fruits, Light, Muller*	1 Pot/149g	143	0.6	96	4.3	18.7	0.4	0.0
Vanilla, Finesse, Aero, Rowntree's*	1 Pot/57g	127	8.3	223	3.7	18.8	14.6	0.0
MUFFIN								
All Butter, M&S*	1 Muffin/65g	175	4.7	270	10.3	40.8	7.3	2.1
Apple, Sultana & Cinnamon, GFY, Asda*	1 Muffin/50g	134	1.8	268	6.0	53.0	3.5	3.9
Banana & Walnut, The Handmade Flapjack Company*	1 Muffin/135g	520	30.6	385	5.3	40.5	22.7	0.0
Banana Pecan, Organic, Honeyrose Bakery*	1 Muffin/110g	300	12.6	273	4.1	38.3	11.5	4.3
Berry Burst, Asda*	1 Muffin/60g	139	1.4	232	6.2	46.7	2.3	1.7
Blueberry, American Style, Sainsbury's*	1 Muffin/72g	256	13.1	355	5.1	42.7	18.2	1.9
Blueberry, Asda*	1 Muffin/77g	273	13.1	353	5.0	45.0	17.0	1.3
Blueberry, Kate's Cakes Ltd*	1 Serving/100g	315	14.5	315	5.3	40.9	14.5	1.6
Blueberry, M&S*	1 Muffin/75g	255	12.6	340	4.9	41.9	16.8	1.3
Blueberry, Mini, Sainsbury's*	1 Muffin/28g	82	2.3	293	6.3	48.9	8.1	1.9
Blueberry, Mini, Tesco*	1 Muffin/28g	104	5.4	370	5.6	43.5	19.3	1.2
Blueberry, Tesco*	1 Muffin/73g	248	12.5	340	4.7	41.0	17.1	1.9
Blueberry, The Handmade Flapjack Company*	1 Muffin/135g	479	26.6	355	4.7	39.9	19.7	0.0
Blueberry, Waitrose*	1 Muffin/65g	239	9.2	367	4.7	55.2	14.2	1.7
Blueberry, Weight Watchers*	1 Muffin/63g	156	2.0	247	4.8	46.4	3.1	7.0
Blueberry Buster, McVitie's*	1 Muffin/95g	408	22.4	429	4.3	49.9	23.6	1.1
Bran, Average	1 Muffin/57g	155	4.4	272	7.8	45.6	7.7	7.7
Bran & Sultana, Weight Watchers*	1 Muffin/60g	144	1.3	240	4.5	50.7	2.1	2.3
Carrot, Asda*	1 Muffin/59g	138	1.4	233	6.0	47.0	2.3	1.6
Carrot Cake, Entenmann's*	1 Muffin/105g	344	15.9	328	5.1	45.8	15.1	3.0
Cheese, Tesco*	1 Muffin/67g	150	1.9	224	13.0	36.4	2.9	3.0
Chocolate Chip, American Style, Sainsbury's*	1 Muffin/72g	284	14.4	395	5.0	48.8	20.0	2.1
Chocolate Chip, BGTY, Sainsbury's*	1 Muffin/75g	282	12.3	376	5.2	51.8	16.4	1.6
Chocolate Chip, Double, Weight Watchers*	1 Muffin/65g	189	5.4	291	6.8	47.2	8.3	3.6
Chocolate Chip, Mini, Asda*	1 Muffin/22g	77	2.9	349	7.0	51.0	13.0	2.1
Chocolate Chip, Mini, BGTY, Sainsbury's*	1 Muffin/28g	91	2.4	324	6.5	55.1	8.7	1.6
Chocolate Chip, Mini, CBY, Asda*	1 Serving/100g	425	22.5	425	5.0	50.0	22.5	0.0

MUFFIN

	Measure INFO/WEIGHT	per Measure KCAL	FAT	Nutrition Values per 100g / 100ml KCAL	PROT	CARB	FAT	FIBRE
Chocolate Chip, Mini, Essential, Waitrose*	1 Muffin/27g	108	5.1	399	5.9	49.8	19.0	2.5
Chocolate Chip, Plain, Tesco*	1 Muffin/72g	270	12.7	375	5.0	48.1	17.6	1.4
Cinnamon & Sultana, Morrisons*	1 Muffin/75g	183	1.0	244	8.3	48.2	1.4	2.9
Cranberry & White Chocolate, Sainsbury's*	1 Muffin/72g	253	13.3	352	5.7	40.7	18.5	1.5
Double Chocolate, CBY, Asda*	1 Serving/100g	398	19.8	398	6.0	47.9	19.8	0.0
Double Chocolate, Chocolate Chip, Mini, Tesco*	1 Muffin/28g	116	6.4	414	6.3	45.7	23.0	1.4
Double Chocolate, Free From, Tesco*	1 Muffin/70g	281	12.7	402	4.7	54.8	18.2	1.7
Double Chocolate, Mini, CBY, Asda*	1 Serving/100g	400	18.7	400	5.6	51.0	18.7	0.0
Double Chocolate, Mini, M&S*	1 Muffin/32g	133	6.9	416	5.4	49.8	21.7	1.1
Double Chocolate Chip, American Style, Sainsbury's*	1 Muffin/72g	276	14.6	384	5.2	45.0	20.3	2.9
Double Chocolate Chip, Co-Op*	1 Muffin/70g	308	16.8	440	6.6	49.4	24.0	2.5
Double Chocolate Chip, Mini, Asda*	1 Muffin/19g	76	3.7	400	7.4	48.5	19.6	2.7
Double Chocolate Chip, Mini, Weight Watchers*	1 Muffin/15g	45	1.3	300	7.0	48.5	8.7	3.5
Double Chocolate Chip, Tesco*	1 Muffin/100g	360	17.9	360	6.1	44.9	17.9	5.4
English	1 Muffin/57g	120	1.0	211	7.0	43.9	1.8	1.8
English, Butter, Tesco*	1 Muffin/67g	170	3.6	253	11.2	39.8	5.4	2.0
English, Gluten, Wheat & Milk Free, Free From, Livwell*	1 Muffin/50g	160	4.9	320	4.6	52.8	9.8	3.2
English, Kingsmill*	1 Muffin/75g	167	1.4	222	9.7	40.4	1.8	2.6
English, M&S*	1 Muffin/60g	135	1.1	225	11.2	43.7	1.9	2.9
English, Tesco*	1 Muffin/72g	171	2.3	238	11.2	41.7	3.2	2.8
Family, Irwin's Bakery*	1 Muffin/40g	116	2.5	291	8.9	50.0	6.2	0.0
Fruit, Spiced, TTD, Sainsbury's*	1 Muffin/70g	181	3.6	259	10.1	43.1	5.1	2.1
Lemon & Poppy Seed, M&S*	1 Muffin/72g	281	14.3	390	6.3	46.1	19.8	1.5
Mini, Tesco*	1 Muffin/28g	120	6.3	428	6.4	50.0	22.6	1.2
Orange, Apricot & Almond, Organic, Honeyrose Bakery*	1 Muffin/110g	312	11.4	284	3.5	44.2	10.4	1.9
Organic Wholemeal, Love Life, Waitrose*	1 Serving/100g	245	3.6	245	11.7	40.8	3.6	6.3
Oven Bottom, Aldi*	1 Muffin/68g	173	1.0	255	10.0	50.4	1.5	2.2
Oven Bottom, Asda*	1 Muffin/68g	173	1.0	255	10.0	50.4	1.5	2.2
Oven Bottom, Mini, Morrisons*	1 Muffin/42g	107	0.6	255	10.0	50.4	1.5	2.2
Oven Bottom, Tesco*	1 Muffin/68g	173	1.0	255	10.0	50.4	1.5	2.2
Oven Bottom, Warburton's*	1 Muffin/69g	175	2.0	253	10.9	45.8	2.9	0.0
Plain, Co-Op*	1 Muffin/60g	135	1.1	225	11.2	41.3	1.9	2.4
Plain, Morrisons*	1 Muffin/70g	140	0.8	200	8.0	41.4	1.1	0.0
Plain, Prepared From Recipe, Average	1 Muffin/57g	169	6.5	296	6.9	41.4	11.4	2.7
Raspberry, PB, Waitrose*	1 Muffin/101g	220	2.1	219	4.7	45.4	2.1	3.7
Raspberry Cream, Sainsbury's*	1 Muffin/90g	314	19.8	349	3.9	33.8	22.0	1.3
Strawberry Cakelet, The Handmade Flapjack Company*	1 Muffin/135g	526	29.6	390	4.5	43.6	21.9	0.0
Toasting, Warburton's*	1 Muffin/64g	138	1.0	216	8.9	41.4	1.6	2.9
Triple Chocolate, Triumph, Fabulous Bakin' Boys*	1 Muffin/40g	160	9.6	400	4.5	42.0	24.0	0.0
Vanilla & Choc Chip, GFY, Asda*	1 Muffin/59g	152	1.3	260	7.0	53.0	2.2	1.6
White, All Butter, Sainsbury's*	1 Muffin/67g	173	4.2	258	10.6	39.6	6.3	3.6
White, Asda*	1 Muffin/67g	148	1.3	222	11.0	40.0	2.0	2.5
White, Finest, Tesco*	1 Muffin/70g	159	0.8	227	8.4	45.7	1.2	2.1
White, M&S*	1 Muffin/60g	135	1.1	225	11.2	43.7	1.9	2.9
White, Tesco*	1 Muffin/72g	173	2.3	240	11.3	41.6	3.2	2.8
White Chocolate & Strawberry Filled, Tesco*	1 Muffin/103g	415	20.3	405	5.2	51.3	19.8	1.3
White Chocolate Chunk Lemon, Mini, M&S*	1 Muffin/28g	130	6.7	464	6.4	55.4	23.9	2.1
Wholemeal, Tesco*	1 Muffin/65g	130	1.3	200	12.6	32.9	2.0	5.7

MULBERRIES

	Measure INFO/WEIGHT	per Measure KCAL	FAT	Nutrition Values per 100g / 100ml KCAL	PROT	CARB	FAT	FIBRE
Raw	1oz/28g	10	0.0	36	1.3	8.1	0.0	0.0

MULLET

	Measure INFO/WEIGHT	per Measure KCAL	FAT	Nutrition Values per 100g / 100ml KCAL	PROT	CARB	FAT	FIBRE
Grey, Grilled	1oz/28g	42	1.5	150	25.7	0.0	5.2	0.0
Grey, Raw	1oz/28g	32	1.1	115	19.8	0.0	4.0	0.0

	Measure INFO/WEIGHT	per Measure KCAL	FAT	KCAL	PROT	CARB	FAT	FIBRE
MULLET								
Red, Grilled	1oz/28g	34	1.2	121	20.4	0.0	4.4	0.0
Red, Raw, Weighed Whole, Flesh Only	1 Serving/100g	109	3.8	109	18.7	0.0	3.8	0.0
MUNCHIES								
Mint, Nestle*	1 Pack/62g	267	10.1	432	3.8	67.5	16.4	0.0
Original, Tube, Nestle*	1 Pack/55g	266	12.3	487	5.4	64.6	22.5	1.4
MUSHROOMS								
Breaded, Average	**3 Mushrooms/51g**	77	2.9	152	4.3	20.8	5.7	0.6
Breaded, Garlic, Average	3 Mushrooms/50g	92	4.9	183	5.2	18.7	9.7	1.7
Buna Shimeji, Livesey Brothers*	½ Pack/75g	29	0.3	39	2.7	5.9	0.4	1.2
Button, Average	1 Serving/50g	7	0.2	15	2.3	0.5	0.4	1.2
Cheesey, Stuffed, Asda*	1 Serving/290g	322	17.4	111	4.3	10.0	6.0	0.0
Chestnut, Average	**1 Med/5g**	1	0.0	13	1.8	0.4	0.5	0.6
Chinese, Dried, Raw	1oz/28g	80	0.5	284	10.0	59.9	1.8	0.0
Closed Cup, Average	1oz/28g	4	0.1	14	1.8	0.4	0.5	1.1
Common, Boiled in Salted Water, Average	1oz/28g	3	0.1	11	1.8	0.4	0.3	1.1
Common, Fried, Average	1oz/28g	44	4.5	157	2.4	0.3	16.2	1.5
Common, Raw, Average	1 Serving/80g	10	0.4	13	1.9	0.3	0.5	1.1
Creamed, Average	1oz/28g	23	1.5	82	1.3	6.8	5.5	0.5
Crispy, M&S*	1 Serving/130g	390	33.4	300	4.2	12.5	25.7	1.8
Dried	1oz/28g	45	1.7	159	21.8	4.8	6.0	13.3
Enoki, Average	**1 Serving/80g**	34	0.0	42	3.0	7.0	0.0	3.0
Flat, Large, Average	**1 Mushroom/52g**	10	0.3	20	3.3	0.5	0.5	0.7
Frozen, Cooks' Ingredients, Waitrose*	1 Portion/75g	14	0.2	18	2.1	1.8	0.3	2.5
Garlic, Average	½ Pack/150g	159	14.0	106	2.1	3.7	9.3	1.7
Garlic, Fresh Tastes, Asda*	½ Pack/125g	101	8.7	81	3.1	3.9	7.0	2.6
Giant with Tomatoes & Mozzarella, M&S*	1 Serving/145g	218	15.8	150	6.3	7.1	10.9	5.5
Oyster, Average	**1 Serving/80g**	12	0.2	15	1.6	1.6	0.2	1.3
Porcini, Dried, Asda*	1 Bag/25g	65	1.2	260	30.4	24.1	4.7	17.5
Porcini, Wild, Dried, Merchant Gourmet*	1 Pack/25g	66	0.8	265	27.9	30.6	3.4	18.7
Shiitake, Cooked	1oz/28g	15	0.1	55	1.6	12.3	0.2	0.0
Shiitake, Dried, Raw	1oz/28g	83	0.3	296	9.6	63.9	1.0	0.0
Sliced, Average	1oz/28g	3	0.1	12	1.8	0.4	0.3	1.1
Sliced, in Water, Canned, Drained, Value, Tesco*	½ Can/78g	8	0.2	10	1.6	0.2	0.3	2.2
Straw, Canned, Drained	1oz/28g	4	0.1	15	2.1	1.2	0.2	0.0
Stuffed, Ready to Roast, Waitrose*	1 Serving/125g	94	4.6	75	3.9	6.5	3.7	1.5
Stuffed with Cheese, Parsley & Butter, Sainsbury's*	½ Pack/110g	246	24.2	224	4.1	2.3	22.0	2.6
Whole Button, Canned, Drained, Morrisons*	1 Can/142g	18	0.4	13	1.8	0.4	0.3	1.1
MUSSELS								
Boiled, Flesh Only, Average	1 Mussel/2g	2	0.1	104	16.7	3.5	2.7	0.0
Boiled, Weighed in Shell, Average	1 Mussel/7g	7	0.2	104	16.7	3.5	2.7	0.0
Pickled, Drained, Average	1oz/28g	32	0.6	112	20.0	1.5	2.2	0.0
Raw, Weighed in Shell, Average	1oz/28g	24	0.7	87	12.7	3.6	2.5	0.2
MUSSELS IN								
Garlic Butter Sauce, Cooked, Scottish, Sainsbury's*	1 Pack/155g	141	6.8	91	8.4	4.2	4.4	0.6
Garlic Butter Sauce, with Shells, Aldi*	1 Serving/113g	93	3.9	82	7.8	4.7	3.4	0.5
Thai Sauce, Scottish, Waitrose*	1 Serving/250g	135	6.2	54	5.4	2.6	2.5	0.6
Tomato & Garlic, Fresh, M&S*	1 Serving/650g	455	10.4	70	7.9	6.5	1.6	0.1
White Wine, Cream, Shallot & Garlic Sauce, COOK!, M&S*	1 Pack/450g	360	12.6	80	11.7	1.6	2.8	2.1
White Wine Sauce, Sainsbury's*	½ Pack/250g	221	9.2	88	8.0	5.8	3.7	0.0
White Wine Sauce, Scottish, Cooked, Norprawn, Lidl*	¼ Pack/45g	37	1.6	83	8.3	4.0	3.6	0.8
White Wine Sauce, Seasoned, Bantry Bay*	1 Serving/450g	270	9.0	60	6.3	4.1	2.0	0.1
MUSTARD								
American, Average	**1 Tsp/5g**	5	0.2	102	4.4	10.5	5.0	2.5

	Measure INFO/WEIGHT	per Measure KCAL	FAT	Nutrition Values per 100g / 100ml KCAL	PROT	CARB	FAT	FIBRE
MUSTARD								
Cajun, Colman's*	1 Tsp/6g	11	0.4	187	7.0	23.0	6.5	2.7
Coarse Grain, Average	*1 Tsp/5g*	*7*	*0.4*	*141*	*7.7*	*8.4*	*8.3*	*5.9*
Dijon, Average	*1 Tsp/5g*	*8*	*0.6*	*163*	*7.4*	*7.7*	*11.3*	*1.1*
English, Average	*1 Tsp/5g*	*9*	*0.4*	*173*	*6.8*	*19.2*	*7.6*	*1.2*
French, Average	*1 Tsp/5g*	*5*	*0.3*	*106*	*5.4*	*8.1*	*5.6*	*1.8*
German Style, Sainsbury's*	1 Serving/10g	9	0.6	92	5.5	2.8	6.5	0.0
Honey, Colman's*	1 Tsp/6g	12	0.5	208	7.4	24.0	8.2	0.0
Powder, Average	*1 Tsp/3g*	*15*	*0.9*	*452*	*28.9*	*20.7*	*28.7*	*0.0*
Powder, Made Up, Average	*1oz/28g*	*63*	*4.0*	*226*	*14.5*	*10.4*	*14.4*	*0.0*
Smooth, Average	*1 Tsp/8g*	*11*	*0.7*	*139*	*7.1*	*9.7*	*8.2*	*0.0*
Whole Grain, Average	*1 Tsp/8g*	*11*	*0.8*	*140*	*8.2*	*4.2*	*10.2*	*4.9*
Yellow, Prepared	*1 Tbsp/15ml*	*11*	*0.6*	*73*	*4.0*	*6.0*	*4.0*	*0.0*
MUSTARD CRESS								
Raw	*1oz/28g*	*4*	*0.2*	*13*	*1.6*	*0.4*	*0.6*	*1.1*
MUTTON								
Lean, Raw, Average	1 Serving/100g	236	13.4	236	17.9	0.1	13.4	0.0

INFO/WEIGHT	Measure	per Measure		Nutrition Values per 100g / 100ml				
		KCAL	FAT	KCAL	PROT	CARB	FAT	FIBRE

NACHOS
American Chilli Beef, Asda*	1 Serving/200g	208	10.0	104	10.0	4.7	5.0	0.8
Cheesy with Salsa & Soured Cream, Sainsbury's*	½ Pack/170g	449	26.9	264	8.8	21.5	15.8	1.4
Chilli, Sainsbury's*	½ Pack/250g	695	32.2	278	10.9	29.5	12.9	1.3
Kit, Old El Paso*	½ Pack/260g	598	26.0	230	4.0	31.0	10.0	0.0

NASI GORENG
Indonesian, Asda*	1 Pack/360g	778	22.7	216	7.4	32.3	6.3	1.3

NECTARINES
Fresh, Raw, Weighed with Stone, Average	*1 Med/140g*	*53*	*0.1*	*38*	*1.3*	*8.5*	*0.1*	*1.2*
White Flesh, Love Life, Waitrose*	1 Fruit/130g	60	0.1	46	1.4	9.0	0.1	1.6

NESQUIK
Chocolate Flavour, Powder, Dry Weight, Nestle*	1 Serving/15g	56	0.5	372	3.0	82.9	3.1	6.5
Strawberry Flavour, Powder, Dry Weight, Nestle*	1 Serving/15g	59	0.0	393	0.0	98.1	0.0	0.0
Strawberry Milk, Fresh, Nestle*	1 Glass/250ml	175	4.0	70	3.3	10.4	1.6	0.3

NIK NAKS
Cream 'n' Cheesy, KP Snacks*	1 Bag/34g	196	13.0	575	5.2	52.7	38.1	0.2
Nice 'n' Spicy, KP Snacks*	1 Bag/30g	171	11.5	571	4.6	51.6	38.4	1.6
Rib 'n' Saucy, Golden Wonder*	1 Bag/25g	143	9.4	571	4.5	53.7	37.6	0.5
Scampi 'n' Lemon, KP Snacks*	1 Bag/25g	143	9.4	573	4.9	53.1	37.5	0.1

NOODLES
Beef, BBQ, Instant, Asda*	1 Pack/333g	420	16.0	126	2.6	18.0	4.8	0.0
Beef, Chilli, Ramen, M&S*	1 Pack/484g	532	17.4	110	8.1	11.9	3.6	0.8
Beef, Chilli, Finest, Tesco*	1 Pack/450g	486	8.6	108	7.7	15.2	1.9	0.9
Beef, Shanghai, COU, M&S*	1 Pack/400g	380	6.4	95	6.8	13.1	1.6	1.5
Cellophane, Glass, Dry Weight	1 Serving/100g	351	0.1	351	0.1	86.1	0.1	0.5
Chicken, & Coconut & Lime, Fuller Longer, M&S*	1 Pack/390g	448	17.6	115	8.7	10.0	4.5	1.6
Chicken, Chinese, Asda*	1 Pot/302g	305	4.2	101	6.0	16.0	1.4	0.8
Chicken, Curry Flavour, Instant, Sainsbury's*	1 Pack/85g	167	6.2	196	4.6	27.9	7.3	0.8
Chicken, Flavour, Dry, Eldorado*	1 Pack/85g	360	12.8	423	14.0	61.0	15.0	0.0
Chicken, Flavour, Instant, Cooked, Smart Price, Asda*	1 Serving/246g	293	11.1	111	2.8	14.9	4.2	1.0
Chicken, Flavour, Instant, Made Up, Kohlico Group*	1 Serving/265g	236	11.4	89	1.7	10.8	4.3	5.5
Chicken, Flavour, Instant, Made Up, Tesco*	½ Pack/168g	285	10.6	170	4.1	23.7	6.3	1.5
Chicken, Flavour, Instant, Sainsbury's*	1 Pack/335g	549	21.4	164	4.4	22.3	6.4	1.3
Chicken, Flavour, Made Up, Mug Shot, Symingtons*	1 Mug/243g	246	1.5	101	2.7	21.0	0.6	1.0
Chicken, Instant, Basics, Sainsbury's*	½ Pack/132g	209	7.0	158	4.0	23.5	5.3	0.6
Chicken, Instant, Weight Watchers*	1 Pack/385g	270	0.4	70	2.3	14.9	0.1	0.6
Chicken, Singapore, Meal for One, CBY, Asda*	1 Pack/400g	348	10.0	87	7.0	8.4	2.5	1.6
Chow Mein, Sainsbury's*	1 Pack/125g	136	2.2	109	3.9	19.2	1.8	0.8
Chow Mein, Stir Fry, Tesco*	1 Serving/200g	116	2.4	58	2.1	9.7	1.2	1.0
Crispy, Dry, Blue Dragon*	1 Box/125g	438	0.6	350	2.4	84.0	0.5	0.0
Curry, Flavour, Instant, Dry, Asda*	1 Serving/65g	415	11.0	638	20.0	101.5	16.9	0.9
Curry, Flavour, Instant, Sainsbury's*	1 Pack/335g	412	15.4	123	2.6	17.8	4.6	0.1
Curry, Flavour, Instant, Value, Made Up, Tesco*	1 Pack/65g	83	2.4	127	3.1	20.3	3.7	0.8
Curry, Instant, Dry, Heinz*	1 Serving/85g	261	0.3	307	9.5	66.4	0.4	2.7
Curry, Spicy, Flavour, Dry, Princes*	1 Pack/85g	395	16.0	465	9.6	64.1	18.8	0.0
Egg, Asda*	1 Pack/184g	213	12.9	116	2.3	11.0	7.0	0.6
Egg, Boiled	*1oz/28g*	*17*	*0.1*	*62*	*2.2*	*13.0*	*0.5*	*0.6*
Egg, Cooked, Somerfield*	½ Pack/150g	189	8.2	126	3.2	16.0	5.5	0.6
Egg, Dry, Average	*1 Block/63g*	*218*	*1.2*	*348*	*12.1*	*70.1*	*1.9*	*2.6*
Egg, Fine, Blue Dragon*	1 Serving/100g	356	1.7	356	13.8	70.0	1.7	3.4
Egg, Fine, Dry Weight, Sharwood's*	1 Block/63g	216	1.3	346	12.0	70.0	2.1	2.5
Egg, Fine, Fresh, M&S*	1 Pack/275g	330	6.0	120	4.4	20.7	2.2	1.5
Egg, Fine, Waitrose*	¼ Pack/63g	221	1.6	353	15.0	67.3	2.6	3.8
Egg, Fine Thread, Dry, M&S*	1 Serving/63g	220	0.6	350	14.3	71.6	0.9	5.1

NOODLES

	Measure INFO/WEIGHT	per Measure KCAL	FAT	Nutrition Values per 100g / 100ml KCAL	PROT	CARB	FAT	FIBRE
Egg, Free Range, Asda*	1 Serving/125g	205	4.9	164	5.1	27.0	3.9	1.8
Egg, Free Range, Fresh, Sainsbury's*	½ Pack/205g	340	7.0	166	5.0	28.0	3.4	1.8
Egg, Free Range, Morrisons*	1 Pack/300g	372	8.7	124	4.9	19.7	2.9	1.3
Egg, Fresh, Just Stir Fry, Sainsbury's*	½ Pack/192g	314	6.5	163	5.0	28.1	3.4	1.8
Egg, Fresh, Tesco*	½ Pack/205g	287	3.9	140	4.9	25.3	1.9	2.0
Egg, M&S*	½ Pack/110g	165	1.9	150	4.9	28.3	1.7	2.8
Egg, Medium, Asda*	1 Serving/83g	125	0.7	150	4.8	31.0	0.8	1.3
Egg, Medium, Dry, Blue Dragon*	1 Serving/50g	158	1.2	317	10.1	62.3	2.4	3.1
Egg, Medium, Dry, Sharwood's*	1 Serving/63g	216	1.3	346	12.0	70.0	2.1	2.5
Egg, Medium, Dry Nests, Cooks' Ingredients, Waitrose*	1 Nest/54g	189	0.9	350	13.2	70.4	1.7	2.4
Egg, Medium, Sainsbury's*	1 Serving/122g	168	1.0	138	5.7	26.9	0.8	1.0
Egg, Ramen, Fresh, The Original Noodle Company*	1 Serving/63g	186	1.7	298	11.3	57.0	2.7	0.0
Egg, Raw, Medium, Waitrose*	¼ Pack/63g	221	1.6	353	15.0	67.3	2.6	3.8
Egg, Thick, Dry Weight, Sharwood's*	1 Serving/63g	214	1.1	342	10.8	71.0	1.7	2.5
Egg, Thread, Cooked Weight, Sharwood's*	1oz/28g	30	0.2	107	3.6	21.8	0.6	1.1
Egg, Tossed in Sesame Oil, Asda*	½ Pack/150g	174	10.5	116	2.3	11.0	7.0	0.6
Fried, Average	*1oz/28g*	*43*	*3.2*	*153*	*1.9*	*11.3*	*11.5*	*0.5*
Garlic, Chilli & Ginger, Tesco*	1 Serving/350g	508	11.2	145	4.8	24.1	3.2	2.6
Instant, Dry, Sainsbury's*	1 Pack/100g	392	14.0	392	9.4	57.0	14.0	0.2
Instant, Value, Tesco*	1 Pack/265g	334	9.0	126	3.2	20.7	3.4	0.9
Japanese Udon, Sainsbury's*	1 Serving/150g	210	2.7	140	3.9	27.1	1.8	1.2
King Prawn, in Sweet Chilli Sauce, COU, M&S*	1 Pack/400g	260	1.6	65	4.8	10.3	0.4	1.5
Medium, Traditional, Straight to Wok, Amoy*	1 Serving/150g	243	2.2	162	4.3	34.3	1.5	1.3
Nest, Medium, Cooked, Waitrose*	1 Nest/63g	88	0.3	139	5.0	28.6	0.5	0.6
Pad Thai, Ribbon, Ready to Wok, Sharwood's*	1 Serving/150g	206	1.6	137	5.0	26.3	1.1	1.0
Pasta, 100% Hard Durum Wheat, Dry, Goody*	1 Serving/100g	362	1.7	362	12.5	73.0	1.7	0.0
Plain, Boiled	*1oz/28g*	*17*	*0.1*	*62*	*2.4*	*13.0*	*0.4*	*0.7*
Plain, Dry	*1oz/28g*	*109*	*1.7*	*388*	*11.7*	*76.1*	*6.2*	*2.9*
Rice, Brown, 100%, Organic, King Soba*	1 Pack/83g	252	2.0	303	6.0	64.4	2.4	0.0
Rice, Cooked	1 Cup/176g	192	0.4	109	0.9	24.9	0.2	1.0
Rice, Cooked, Sharwood's*	1 Serving/200g	239	0.6	120	2.0	27.2	0.3	0.8
Rice, Dry, Amoy*	1oz/28g	101	0.3	361	6.5	86.6	1.0	0.0
Rice, Dry, Blue Dragon*	1 Serving/30g	113	0.0	376	7.0	84.0	0.0	0.0
Rice, Medium, Blue Dragon*	1 Serving/63g	235	0.0	376	7.0	84.0	0.0	0.0
Rice, Oriental, Thai, Stir Fry, Dry Weight, Sharwood's*	1 Serving/63g	226	0.6	361	6.5	86.8	1.0	2.4
Rice, Stir Fry, Tesco*	½ Pack/190g	304	10.8	160	2.0	24.8	5.7	1.0
Rice, Thai, Wheat & GF, King Soba*	1 Serving/55g	193	0.8	351	8.9	75.6	1.4	0.0
Rice, Thick, Thai, Dry, M&S*	1 Serving/100g	355	0.7	355	6.5	80.6	0.7	1.4
Rice, with Spring Onions, Fresh Tastes, Asda*	½ Pack/188g	248	4.1	132	2.2	25.9	2.2	1.4
Rice Stick, Aroy-d*	1 Serving/75g	273	0.8	364	7.0	82.0	1.0	0.0
Singapore, LC, Tesco*	1 Pack/450g	338	7.6	75	4.8	9.8	1.7	1.2
Singapore, Morrisons*	1 Serving/400g	480	26.8	120	4.8	11.6	6.7	1.6
Singapore, Sainsbury's*	1 Pack/400g	368	6.8	92	7.5	11.6	1.7	0.9
Singapore, Style, Asda*	1 Pack/400g	688	32.0	172	7.0	18.0	8.0	1.0
Singapore, Waitrose*	1 Pack/400g	476	17.6	119	7.3	12.6	4.4	2.1
Singapore, You Count, Love Life, Waitrose*	1 Pot/260g	243	5.0	97	5.4	13.3	2.0	2.2
Special, Chinese Takeaway, Iceland*	1 Pack/340g	422	10.9	124	6.5	17.2	3.2	0.6
Stir Fry, Tesco*	1 Serving/150g	202	3.6	135	5.3	23.0	2.4	1.5
Straight to Wok, Medium, Amoy*	1 Pack/150g	240	2.2	160	5.8	31.7	1.5	0.0
Straight to Wok, Rice, Amoy*	1 Pack/150g	174	0.2	116	1.6	27.4	0.1	0.0
Straight to Wok, Singapore, Amoy*	1 Serving/150g	232	4.2	155	4.8	28.4	2.8	0.0
Straight to Wok, Thread, Fine, Amoy*	1 Pack/150g	237	3.9	158	5.0	28.7	2.6	0.0
Straight to Wok, Udon, Amoy*	1 Pack/150g	212	2.0	141	4.4	28.8	1.3	0.0

Measure INFO/WEIGHT		per Measure		Nutrition Values per 100g / 100ml				
		KCAL	FAT	KCAL	PROT	CARB	FAT	FIBRE

NOODLES

	Measure INFO/WEIGHT	KCAL	FAT	KCAL	PROT	CARB	FAT	FIBRE
Super, Bacon Flavour, Dry Weight, Batchelors*	1 Pack/100g	526	23.6	526	9.4	69.2	23.6	1.6
Super, Barbecue Beef, Made Up, Batchelors*	1 Serving/100g	156	6.7	156	3.2	20.9	6.7	1.1
Super, BBQ Beef, to Go, 98% Fat Free, Batchelors*	1 Pack/380g	308	0.6	81	2.4	17.6	0.2	0.6
Super, Chicken & Ham, Dry Weight, Batchelors*	1 Pack/100g	472	20.2	472	9.4	63.2	20.2	1.5
Super, Chicken & Herb, Low Fat, Dry, Batchelors*	½ Pack/43g	161	0.8	379	12.2	78.4	1.9	2.4
Super, Chicken & Herb, Low Fat, Made Up, Batchelors*	1 Pack/170g	322	1.6	189	6.1	39.2	0.9	1.2
Super, Chicken Flavour, Dry Weight, Batchelors*	1 Serving/100g	449	19.2	449	8.7	60.3	19.2	2.5
Super, Chicken Flavour, Made Up, Batchelors*	1 Serving/100g	170	7.3	170	3.3	22.9	7.3	0.9
Super, Chow Mein Flavour, Made Up, Batchelors*	½ Pack/150g	262	11.8	175	3.0	23.0	7.9	0.4
Super, Mild Curry, Dry Weight, Batchelors*	½ Pack/50g	260	11.7	520	9.4	67.8	23.4	1.4
Super, Mild Curry Flavour, Made Up, Batchelors*	1 Serving/100g	157	6.7	157	3.2	20.9	6.7	1.0
Super, Roast Chicken, to Go, 98% Fat Free, Batchelors*	1 Serving/380g	308	0.8	81	2.6	17.2	0.2	0.5
Super, Sweet Thai Chilli, 98% Fat Free, Batchelors*	1 Pack/270g	292	1.1	108	3.3	22.8	0.4	0.9
Sweet Chilli, Sainsbury's*	½ Pack/110g	172	6.0	156	4.0	24.6	5.5	1.0
Thai, Waitrose*	1 Pack/300g	357	6.3	119	6.8	18.4	2.1	1.7
Thai Chicken, Takeaway, Somerfield*	1 Pack/300g	426	16.8	142	7.8	16.0	5.6	0.8
Thai Glass, Vermicelli, Wai Wai*	1oz/28g	112	0.3	400	7.3	89.1	0.9	1.8
Tiger Prawn, Stir Fry, Tesco*	1 Pack/400g	596	14.8	149	6.0	23.0	3.7	2.7
Udon Japanese & Dashi Soup Stock, Yutaka*	1 Pack/230g	290	1.2	126	3.0	26.8	0.5	0.0
Udon Style, Thick, Ready to Wok, Sharwood's*	1 Pack/150g	233	0.6	155	5.4	32.5	0.4	2.1
Vermicelli Rice, Mama*	1 Serving/45g	166	0.4	370	7.0	81.0	1.0	0.0
Whole Wheat, Dry, Blue Dragon*	1 Serving/65g	208	1.3	320	12.5	63.0	2.0	8.0
Yaki Udan, Chicken & Prawn, M&S*	1 Pack/395g	434	14.2	110	8.1	11.9	3.6	0.8
Zero, Glow Nutrition Ltd*	1 Serving/100g	5	0.0	5	0.0	4.0	0.0	4.0

NOUGAT

	Measure INFO/WEIGHT	KCAL	FAT	KCAL	PROT	CARB	FAT	FIBRE
Almond & Cherry, M&S*	1 Sweet/7g	28	0.6	405	4.5	76.0	9.1	1.1
Average	1 Bar/28g	108	2.4	384	4.4	77.3	8.5	0.9
Bassetts & Beyond, Cadbury*	1oz/28g	105	1.1	375	4.0	82.0	4.0	0.0
Soft, Bar, Bassett's*	1 Bar/25g	94	1.0	375	4.0	82.0	4.0	0.0

NUT ROAST

	Measure INFO/WEIGHT	KCAL	FAT	KCAL	PROT	CARB	FAT	FIBRE
Asda*	1 Roast/230g	389	16.3	169	8.7	23.2	7.1	5.6
Average	1 Serving/200g	704	51.4	352	13.3	18.3	25.7	4.2
Courgette & Spiced Tomato, Cauldron Foods*	1 Serving/100g	208	12.3	208	11.7	12.5	12.3	4.9
Leek, Cheese & Mushroom, Organic, Cauldron Foods*	½ Pack/143g	343	21.3	240	13.2	13.2	14.9	4.1
Lentil, Average	1oz/28g	62	3.4	222	10.6	18.8	12.1	3.8
Tomato & Courgette, Vegetarian, Organic, Waitrose*	½ Pack/142g	295	17.5	208	11.7	12.5	12.3	4.9

NUTMEG

	Measure INFO/WEIGHT	KCAL	FAT	KCAL	PROT	CARB	FAT	FIBRE
Ground, Average	1 Tsp/3g	16	1.1	525	5.8	45.3	36.3	0.0

NUTS

	Measure INFO/WEIGHT	KCAL	FAT	KCAL	PROT	CARB	FAT	FIBRE
Almond, Sweet Pecan & Peanut, Clusters, Red Sky*	1 Serving/30g	182	13.9	607	17.9	32.1	46.4	7.1
Assortment, Eat Well, M&S*	1 Pack/70g	441	41.2	630	16.7	8.5	58.9	5.3
Bento Box, Mix, Graze*	1 Portion/30g	141	6.6	469	17.9	50.1	22.1	3.7
Honey Roasted, M&S*	1oz/28g	175	14.6	625	18.1	20.5	52.2	5.1
Luxury, Organic, M&S*	1oz/28g	179	15.8	640	21.1	11.6	56.6	6.1
Mixed	1 Pack/40g	243	21.6	607	22.9	7.9	54.1	6.0
Mixed, Almonds, Brazil, Hazel & Walnuts, M&S*	1 Serving/25g	168	16.0	670	16.0	4.8	64.0	5.4
Mixed, Americas, Graze*	1 Punnet/40g	263	25.6	658	15.5	5.2	64.0	5.6
Mixed, Ancient Forest, Graze*	1 Pack/36g	229	21.9	636	17.4	8.3	60.7	7.0
Mixed, Chocolate Orange Granola, Graze*	1 Punnet/41g	195	11.3	475	12.0	43.7	27.5	7.7
Mixed, Chopped, Julian Graves*	1 Pack/300g	1773	152.7	591	23.2	10.0	50.9	0.0
Mixed, Chopped, Sainsbury's*	1 Serving/100g	605	50.9	605	27.1	9.6	50.9	6.0
Mixed, Chopped, Tesco*	1 Serving/25g	149	12.6	595	23.5	10.5	50.6	6.0
Mixed, Cookies & Cream, Graze*	1 Punnet/38g	214	16.0	562	12.0	36.0	42.0	5.0

NUTS

Measure INFO/WEIGHT	per Measure KCAL	per Measure FAT	Nutrition Values per 100g / 100ml KCAL	PROT	CARB	FAT	FIBRE

	Measure INFO/WEIGHT	KCAL	FAT	KCAL	PROT	CARB	FAT	FIBRE
Mixed, Copacabana, Brazil, with Choc Buttons, Graze*	1 Pack/40g	249	21.3	621	10.4	24.4	53.1	4.5
Mixed, Delicious, Boots*	1 Pack/50g	332	29.0	663	16.0	16.0	58.0	8.1
Mixed, Hickory Almonds, Cashews & Seeds, Graze*	1 Punnet/35g	209	17.0	598	20.6	16.4	48.6	6.7
Mixed, Honey Roasted, Waitrose*	1 Serving/50g	292	22.5	583	17.1	27.5	45.0	5.3
Mixed, Natural, Asda*	1 Snack/30g	197	18.8	656	18.0	4.3	62.7	7.4
Mixed, Natural, Luxury, Tesco*	1oz/28g	179	16.2	639	22.6	6.9	57.9	5.6
Mixed, Nature's Harvest*	1 Serving/25g	145	13.4	581	17.5	7.7	53.4	6.3
Mixed, Organic, Waitrose*	1oz/28g	179	16.5	640	19.3	7.7	59.1	8.4
Mixed, Roast, Salted, Somerfield*	1oz/28g	175	15.1	625	24.0	11.0	54.0	0.0
Mixed, Roasted, Salted, Waitrose*	1 Pack/200g	1252	116.8	626	13.7	11.3	58.4	4.4
Mixed, Roasted, Waitrose*	1 Serving/25g	166	16.0	662	15.2	6.2	64.0	8.2
Mixed, Unsalted, Sainsbury's*	1 Serving/50g	311	28.8	622	18.5	7.2	57.7	8.7
Mixed, Wholesome, Love Life, Waitrose*	1 Serving/30g	206	19.6	685	14.6	5.0	65.2	5.4
Natural, Mixed, Love Life, Waitrose*	1 Serving/50g	314	25.8	628	17.4	24.9	51.6	12.1
Natural Assortment, Tesco*	1 Serving/50g	338	32.3	676	17.5	6.1	64.6	5.0
Natural Roasted Peanuts, Love Life, Waitrose*	1 Pack/250g	1595	131.5	638	27.1	15.6	52.6	5.1
Omega Booster Seeds, Graze*	1 Punnet/34g	189	16.5	553	22.1	16.4	48.3	11.1
Peanuts, Roasted, Salted, Value, Tesco*	1/8 Pack/25g	151	12.4	604	25.5	13.8	49.6	6.8
Peanuts & Cashews, Honey Roast, Tesco*	1 Serving/25g	145	10.7	579	21.6	26.6	42.9	4.2
Pecan, Wholesome, Love Life, Waitrose*	1 Serving/30g	207	21.0	691	9.2	5.8	70.1	9.6
Pine, Tesco*	1 Pack/100g	699	68.6	699	16.5	4.0	68.6	1.9
Pine, Wholefoods, Tesco*	1 Serving/10g	69	6.9	690	14.0	4.0	68.6	1.9
Roast Salted, Luxury, KP Snacks*	1oz/28g	181	16.1	646	21.9	10.1	57.6	5.9
Roasted, Salted, Assortment, Luxury, Tesco*	1 Serving/25g	161	14.5	643	21.1	9.4	57.9	8.1
Soya, Dry Roasted, The Food Doctor*	1 Serving/50g	203	10.7	406	37.5	15.9	21.4	16.1
Soya, Roast, Wholefoods, Tesco*	1/5 Pack/20g	80	3.8	400	38.0	19.1	19.0	13.4
Unsalted, Selection, Sainsbury's*	1 Serving/75g	491	48.0	655	14.7	5.0	64.0	6.7
Walnut Pieces, Morrisons*	7 Peices/6g	41	4.1	689	14.7	3.3	68.5	3.5

NUTS & RAISINS

	Measure INFO/WEIGHT	KCAL	FAT	KCAL	PROT	CARB	FAT	FIBRE
Mixed, Average	1 Serving/30g	144	10.2	481	14.1	31.5	34.1	4.5
Mixed, KP Snacks*	1 Serving/50g	273	20.2	546	21.4	24.4	40.3	5.2
Mixed, Tesco*	1 Serving/25g	115	6.9	450	18.6	32.6	26.8	12.5
Peanuts, Mixed, Average	1 Pack/40g	174	10.4	435	15.3	37.5	26.0	4.4
Yoghurt Coated, Waitrose*	1 Serving/50g	264	18.4	527	10.9	38.2	36.7	3.0

	Measure INFO/WEIGHT	per Measure KCAL	FAT	Nutrition Values per 100g / 100ml KCAL	PROT	CARB	FAT	FIBRE
OAT BAKES								
Cheese, Nairn's*	1 Bag/30g	130	4.7	432	15.0	57.4	15.8	1.3
Sweet Chilli, Nairn's*	1 Bag/30g	128	4.0	426	8.1	68.4	13.3	7.2
OAT CAKES								
Bran, Paterson's*	1 Cake/13g	52	2.0	416	10.0	58.5	15.8	9.5
Cheese, Nairn's*	1 Cake/9g	42	2.4	471	13.2	43.3	27.2	6.8
Fine Milled, Nairn's*	1 Cake/8g	35	1.7	449	10.5	52.6	21.8	8.6
Herb & Pumpkin Seed, Nairn's*	1 Cake/10g	43	2.1	426	12.2	46.8	21.1	13.0
Highland, Organic, Sainsbury's*	1 Cake/13g	57	2.4	456	10.2	59.8	19.5	5.5
Highland, Walkers*	1 Cake/12g	54	2.5	451	10.3	56.0	20.6	6.7
Oatmeal, Rough, Nairn's*	1 Cake/11g	45	2.0	421	10.6	52.8	18.6	10.5
Oatmeal, Rough, Organic, Nairn's*	1 Cake/10g	43	1.7	418	10.2	57.7	16.3	7.5
Organic, The Village Bakery*	1 Cake/13g	56	2.7	452	10.9	54.5	21.3	5.6
Orkney, Stockan's*	1 Oatcake/14g	63	3.2	453	11.1	50.3	23.0	6.0
Retail, Average	1 Cake/13g	57	2.4	441	10.0	63.0	18.3	0.0
Rough, Sainsbury's*	1 Cake/11g	45	1.8	426	11.7	65.2	16.9	8.6
Rough, Scottish, Tesco*	1 Cake/10g	45	1.9	435	11.4	55.3	18.4	8.0
Rough Scottish, Sainsbury's*	1 Cake/11g	51	2.1	462	12.3	59.9	19.3	6.5
Rough with Bran, Walkers*	1 Cake/13g	55	2.2	424	11.0	57.1	16.8	8.1
Rough with Olive Oil, Paterson's*	1 Cake/13g	54	2.2	431	10.6	58.4	17.2	8.1
Scottish, Organic, Waitrose*	1 Cake/13g	58	2.5	447	11.2	57.0	19.4	6.6
Scottish, Rough, Waitrose*	1 Cake/13g	55	2.3	438	10.4	57.4	18.5	8.0
Traditional, M&S*	1 Cake/11g	49	2.0	445	11.0	59.3	18.3	6.6
with Cracked Black Pepper, Walkers*	1 Cake/10g	41	1.8	433	10.4	55.0	19.0	8.5
OAT DRINK								
Healthy Oat, Enriched, Oatly*	1 Serving/250ml	112	3.8	45	1.0	6.5	1.5	0.8
Healthy Oat Milk, Organic, Oatly*	1 Serving/250ml	88	1.8	35	1.0	6.5	0.7	0.8
OATBRAN								
Original Pure, Mornflake*	1 Serving/30g	104	2.9	345	14.8	49.7	9.7	15.2
OATMEAL								
Raw	*1oz/28g*	*112*	*2.4*	*401*	*12.4*	*72.8*	*8.7*	*6.8*
OCTOPUS								
Chunks in Olive Oil, Palacio De Oriente*	1 Tin/111g	148	4.0	133	21.6	4.5	3.6	0.0
Raw	*1oz/28g*	*23*	*0.4*	*83*	*17.9*	*0.0*	*1.3*	*0.0*
OIL								
Again & Again, No Cholesterol, Anglia*	1 Tbsp/15ml	124	13.8	828	0.0	0.0	92.0	0.0
Avocado, Olivado*	1 Tsp/5ml	40	4.4	802	0.0	0.0	88.0	0.0
Black Truffle, Grapeseed, Cuisine Perel*	1 Tsp/5ml	43	5.0	857	0.0	7.1	100.0	0.0
Chilli, Average	*1 Tsp/5ml*	*41*	*4.6*	*824*	*0.0*	*0.0*	*91.5*	*0.0*
Chinese Stir Fry, Asda*	1 Tbsp/15ml	123	13.7	823	0.0	0.0	91.4	0.0
Coconut, Average	*1 Tsp/5ml*	*45*	*5.0*	*899*	*0.0*	*0.0*	*99.9*	*0.0*
Cod Liver, Average	*1 Capsule/1g*	*9*	*1.0*	*900*	*0.0*	*0.0*	*100.0*	*0.0*
Corn, Average	*1 Tsp/5ml*	*43*	*4.8*	*864*	*0.0*	*0.0*	*96.0*	*0.0*
Cuisine, Flora*	1 Tsp/5ml	32	3.5	630	0.1	1.0	70.3	0.0
Dipping with Balsamic Vinegar, Finest, Tesco*	1 Tsp/5ml	33	3.6	668	0.0	4.4	71.7	0.0
Evening Primrose, Average	*1 Serving/1g*	*9*	*1.0*	*900*	*0.0*	*0.0*	*100.0*	*0.0*
Fish, Average	*1 Serving/1g*	*9*	*1.0*	*900*	*0.0*	*0.0*	*100.0*	*0.0*
Fish, Omega 3, Capsule, Holland & Barrett*	1 Capsule/1g	10	1.0	1000	0.1	0.1	100.0	0.1
Flax Seed, Average	*1 Tbsp/15ml*	*124*	*13.9*	*829*	*0.0*	*0.0*	*92.6*	*0.0*
Fry Light, Bodyline*	1 Spray/0.25ml	1	0.1	522	0.0	0.0	55.2	0.0
Grapeseed, Average	*1 Tsp/5ml*	*43*	*4.8*	*866*	*0.0*	*0.0*	*96.2*	*0.0*
Groundnut, Average	*1 Tsp/5ml*	*41*	*4.6*	*824*	*0.0*	*0.0*	*91.8*	*0.0*
Hazelnut, Average	*1 Tsp/5ml*	*45*	*5.0*	*899*	*0.0*	*0.0*	*99.9*	*0.0*
Linseed, Organic, Biona*	1 Serving/10ml	84	9.3	837	0.0	0.0	93.0	0.0

	Measure INFO/WEIGHT	per Measure KCAL	FAT	Nutrition Values per 100g / 100ml KCAL	PROT	CARB	FAT	FIBRE
OIL								
Macadamia Nut, Oz Tukka*	1 Tsp/5ml	40	4.6	805	0.0	0.0	91.0	0.0
Olive, Average	*1 Tsp/5ml*	*43*	*4.7*	*855*	*0.0*	*0.0*	*94.9*	*0.0*
Olive, Basil Infused, Tesco*	1 Serving/20ml	180	20.0	900	0.0	0.0	100.0	0.0
Olive, Evo Filtered, Italian, Parioli, Cucina*	1 Serving/100ml	825	91.6	825	0.0	0.0	91.6	0.0
Olive, Extra Virgin, Average	*1 Tsp/5ml*	*42*	*4.7*	*848*	*0.0*	*0.0*	*94.5*	*0.0*
Olive, Extra Virgin, Mist Spray, Belolive*	1 Serving/5ml	25	2.8	500	0.0	0.0	55.0	0.0
Olive, Extra Virgin, Only 1 Cal, Spray, Fry Light*	1 Spray/0.2ml	1	0.1	498	0.0	0.0	55.2	0.0
Olive, Garlic, Average	*1 Tbsp/15ml*	*127*	*14.1*	*848*	*0.0*	*0.0*	*94.3*	*0.0*
Olive, Lemon Flavoured, Sainsbury's*	1 Tbsp/15ml	123	13.7	823	0.1	0.0	91.4	0.1
Olive, Mild, Average	*1 Tbsp/15ml*	*129*	*14.4*	*862*	*0.0*	*0.0*	*95.7*	*0.0*
Olive, Spray, Fry Light*	5 Sprays/1ml	5	0.5	521	0.0	0.0	54.2	0.0
Omega, Organic, Clearspring*	1 Tbsp/15ml	124	13.8	828	0.0	0.0	92.0	0.0
Palm, Average	*1 Tsp/5ml*	*45*	*5.0*	*899*	*0.0*	*0.0*	*99.9*	*0.0*
Peanut, Average	*1 Tsp/5ml*	*45*	*5.0*	*899*	*0.0*	*0.0*	*99.9*	*0.0*
Rapeseed, Average	*1 Tbsp/15ml*	*130*	*14.4*	*864*	*0.0*	*0.0*	*96.0*	*0.0*
Red Palm & Canola, Carotino*	1 Tsp/5ml	41	4.6	812	0.0	0.0	92.0	0.0
Rice Bran, Average	1 Tbsp/14g	120	13.6	884	0.0	0.0	100.0	0.0
Safflower, Average	*1 Tsp/5ml*	*45*	*5.0*	*899*	*0.0*	*0.0*	*99.9*	*0.0*
Sesame, Average	*1 Tsp/5ml*	*45*	*5.0*	*892*	*0.1*	*0.0*	*99.9*	*0.0*
Soya, Average	*1 Tsp/5ml*	*45*	*5.0*	*899*	*0.0*	*0.0*	*99.9*	*0.0*
Stir Fry, Sharwood's*	1 fl oz/30ml	269	29.9	897	0.0	0.0	99.7	0.0
Sunflower, Average	*1 Tsp/5ml*	*43*	*4.8*	*869*	*0.0*	*0.0*	*96.6*	*0.0*
Sunflower, Cooking Spray, LC Spray*	1 Spray/10ml	21	2.2	210	0.0	0.0	22.0	0.0
Sunflower, Spray, Fry Light*	1 Spray/0.2ml	1	0.1	522	0.0	0.0	55.2	0.0
Ultimate Blend, Udo's Choice*	1 Capsule/1ml	9	1.0	900	1.3	0.0	96.8	0.0
Vegetable, Average	*1 Tbsp/15ml*	*129*	*14.3*	*858*	*0.0*	*0.0*	*95.3*	*0.0*
Walnut, Average	*1 Tsp/5ml*	*45*	*5.0*	*899*	*0.0*	*0.0*	*99.9*	*0.0*
Wheatgerm, Average	*1 Tsp/5ml*	*45*	*5.0*	*899*	*0.0*	*0.0*	*99.9*	*0.0*
OKRA								
Boiled in Unsalted Water, Average	*1 Serving/80g*	*22*	*0.7*	*28*	*2.5*	*2.7*	*0.9*	*3.6*
Canned, Drained, Average	*1 Serving/80g*	*17*	*0.6*	*21*	*1.4*	*2.5*	*0.7*	*2.6*
Raw, Average	*1 Serving/80g*	*25*	*0.8*	*31*	*2.8*	*3.0*	*1.0*	*4.0*
Stir-Fried in Corn Oil, Average	*1 Serving/80g*	*215*	*20.9*	*269*	*4.3*	*4.4*	*26.1*	*6.3*
OLIVES								
Black, & Green with Greek Feta Cheese, Tesco*	1 Pot/100g	200	20.1	200	3.4	0.3	20.1	4.6
Black, Pitted, Average	*½ Jar/82g*	*135*	*13.3*	*164*	*1.0*	*3.5*	*16.2*	*3.1*
Green, & Harissa, Graze*	1 Punnet/44g	109	11.6	248	1.0	2.0	26.3	2.9
Green, Lightly Flavoured with Lemon & Garlic, Attis*	1 Serving/50g	82	8.2	164	1.7	2.2	16.5	0.0
Green, Pimiento Stuffed, Somerfield*	1 Olive/3g	4	0.4	126	1.0	4.0	12.0	0.0
Green, Pitted, Average	*1 Olive/3g*	*4*	*0.4*	*130*	*1.1*	*0.9*	*13.3*	*2.5*
Green, Pitted, Stuffed with Anchovies, Sainsbury's*	1 Serving/50g	78	8.0	155	1.8	0.6	16.1	3.2
Green, Stuffed with Almonds, Pitted, Waitrose*	1 Serving/50g	90	8.4	180	3.8	3.2	16.9	2.5
Green, Stuffed with Anchovy, Waitrose*	½ Can/40g	38	3.1	94	1.5	4.7	7.7	2.3
Green, Stuffed with Minced Pimiento, Sainsbury's*	1 Olive/5g	8	0.8	147	1.2	3.9	14.1	2.0
Green, with Chilli & Garlic, Delicious, Boots*	1 Pack/60g	97	9.0	161	1.3	4.4	15.0	2.0
Green, with Chilli & Garlic, Graze*	1 Punnet/44g	133	13.6	301	0.6	1.4	30.9	2.9
Kalamata, & Halkidiki with Chilli & Garlic, Graze*	1 Punnet/51g	144	14.8	281	0.7	1.5	28.8	3.0
*Kalamata, Kalamata**	*1 Olive/3g*	*9*	*0.9*	*300*	*1.0*	*6.7*	*30.0*	*0.0*
Kalamata, with Herbs, Graze*	1 Punnet/52g	144	15.3	277	0.6	1.7	29.4	3.1
Marinated, Mixed, M&S*	1 Serving/20g	33	3.0	165	1.6	6.5	14.9	3.0
Marinated, Selection, M&S*	4 Olives/20g	44	4.4	225	1.4	3.9	22.6	2.1
Mixed, Chilli & Garlic, Asda*	1 Serving/30g	43	4.7	144	0.9	0.0	15.6	6.1
Mixed, Marinated, Anti Pasti, Asda*	1 Serving/100g	215	22.0	215	1.8	0.7	22.0	3.1

O

	Measure INFO/WEIGHT	per Measure		Nutrition Values per 100g / 100ml				
		KCAL	FAT	KCAL	PROT	CARB	FAT	FIBRE
OLIVES								
Mixed, Marinated with Feta & Red Peppers, Asda*	1 Pot/120g	233	21.6	194	5.8	2.2	18.0	1.7
Pimento Stuffed, in Brine, Tesco*	1 Serving/25g	38	4.1	153	0.8	0.1	16.4	2.1
OMELETTE								
Cheese, 2 Egg, Average	1 Omelette/180g	479	40.7	266	15.9	0.0	22.6	0.0
Cheese, Asda*	1 Omelette/119g	268	22.6	225	12.0	1.5	19.0	0.0
Cheese, Findus*	1 Serving/200g	400	26.0	200	9.5	14.0	13.0	0.0
Cheese & Mushroom, Apetito*	1 Serving/320g	486	25.0	152	6.2	14.4	7.8	1.9
Cheese & Mushroom, Tesco*	1 Omelette/120g	248	21.5	207	9.8	1.6	17.9	0.2
Ham & Mushroom, Farmfoods*	1 Omelette/120g	200	16.7	167	8.7	1.8	13.9	0.1
Plain, 2 Egg	1 Omelette/120g	229	19.7	191	10.9	0.0	16.4	0.0
Spanish	1oz/28g	34	2.3	120	5.7	6.2	8.3	1.4
Spanish, Potato, Rapido, Unearthed*	1 Pack/175g	273	13.6	156	4.6	15.8	7.8	2.2
ONION RINGS								
Battered, Asda*	1 Serving/100g	343	22.7	343	3.8	31.0	22.7	1.7
Battered, Oven Baked, Tesco*	1 Serving/50g	110	5.0	219	3.9	28.4	10.0	3.5
Battered, Oven Crisp, Tesco*	1 Ring/17g	40	2.3	236	4.2	24.8	13.3	2.5
Battered, Sainsbury's*	1 Ring/12g	26	1.2	219	3.9	28.4	10.0	3.5
Breadcrumbs, Tesco*	1 Serving/100g	294	15.6	294	4.3	34.1	15.6	2.3
Breaded, Asda*	1 Serving/10g	29	1.5	289	4.4	34.0	15.0	2.7
Breaded, Iceland*	1 Ring/11g	33	1.7	293	4.4	34.2	15.4	2.7
Breaded, Sainsbury's*	1 Serving/100g	280	12.4	280	4.6	37.6	12.4	4.1
Value, Tesco*	1 Bag/14g	73	3.8	520	7.0	61.4	27.0	1.2
ONIONS								
Baked	**1oz/28g**	**29**	**0.2**	**103**	**3.5**	**22.3**	**0.6**	**3.9**
Boiled in Unsalted Water	**1oz/28g**	**5**	**0.0**	**17**	**0.6**	**3.7**	**0.1**	**0.7**
Borettane, Char-Grilled, Sacla*	1 Serving/100g	90	5.6	90	0.9	8.9	5.6	2.5
Dried, Raw, Average	**1oz/28g**	**88**	**0.5**	**313**	**10.2**	**68.6**	**1.7**	**12.1**
Fried, Average	**1oz/28g**	**46**	**3.1**	**164**	**2.3**	**14.1**	**11.2**	**3.1**
Pickled, Average	**1 Onion/15g**	**3**	**0.0**	**23**	**0.8**	**4.9**	**0.1**	**0.7**
Powder	1 Tsp/2g	7	0.0	341	10.4	79.1	1.0	15.2
Raw, Average	**1 Med/180g**	**69**	**0.4**	**38**	**1.2**	**7.9**	**0.2**	**1.3**
Red, Raw, Average	**1 Med/180g**	**66**	**0.4**	**37**	**1.2**	**7.9**	**0.2**	**1.5**
Sliced, Frozen, Farmfoods*	1 Serving/80g	29	0.2	36	1.2	7.9	0.2	1.4
Spring, Raw, Average	**1 Med/15g**	**4**	**0.1**	**25**	**2.0**	**3.0**	**0.5**	**1.5**
Sweet, TTD, Sainsbury's*	1 Serving/100g	39	0.2	39	1.3	7.9	0.2	1.4
OPTIONS								
Choca Mocha Drink, Ovaltine*	1 Sachet/11g	39	1.3	359	14.1	50.1	11.4	7.0
Chocolate Au Lait, Ovaltine*	1 Sachet/10g	36	1.0	355	11.8	54.5	10.0	7.3
Dreamy Caramel, Hot Chocolate, Ovaltine*	1 Sachet/11g	39	0.9	354	12.3	48.5	7.8	0.0
Mint Madness, Belgian, Ovaltine*	1 Serving/11g	38	0.8	348	12.3	49.2	6.9	20.0
Outrageous Orange, Hot Chocolate, Ovaltine*	1 Serving/11g	38	0.8	348	12.3	49.3	6.9	20.0
Tempting Toffee, Ovaltine*	1 Sachet/11g	43	1.0	391	13.6	66.4	9.1	0.0
Wicked White, Hot Chocolate, Ovaltine*	1 Sachet/11g	44	1.1	398	10.5	64.6	10.0	3.7
ORANGES								
Blood, Average	**1 Orange/140g**	**82**	**0.0**	**58**	**0.8**	**13.3**	**0.0**	**2.5**
Fresh, Weighed with Peel, Average	**1 Med/185g**	**115**	**0.5**	**62**	**1.0**	**15.6**	**0.3**	**3.2**
Fresh, without Peel, Average	**1 Med/145g**	**54**	**0.1**	**37**	**1.1**	**8.5**	**0.1**	**1.7**
Peel Only, Raw, Average	**1 Tbsp/6g**	**6**	**0.0**	**97**	**1.5**	**25.0**	**0.2**	**10.6**
Ruby Red, Tesco*	1 Med/130g	51	0.1	39	1.1	8.5	0.1	1.7
OREGANO								
Dried,	**1 Tsp/1g**	**3**	**0.1**	**306**	**11.0**	**49.5**	**10.3**	**0.0**
Fresh	**1 Tsp/1g**	**1**	**0.0**	**66**	**2.2**	**9.7**	**2.0**	**0.0**

	Measure INFO/WEIGHT	per Measure		Nutrition Values per 100g / 100ml				
		KCAL	FAT	KCAL	PROT	CARB	FAT	FIBRE
ORO BLANCO								
Fruit, Citrus	½ Fruit/150g	98	0.0	65	1.0	14.0	0.0	3.0
OVALTINE*								
Chocolate, Light, Ovaltine*	4 Tsp/20g	76	1.2	380	8.5	70.5	6.0	4.5
Chocolate, Light, Sachet, Ovaltine*	1 Sachet/25g	96	1.5	384	7.4	73.0	5.9	4.7
Hi Malt, Light, Instant Drink, Ovaltine*	1 Sachet/20g	72	1.2	358	9.1	67.1	5.9	2.8
Powder, Made Up with Semi-Skimmed Milk, Ovaltine*	1 Mug/227ml	179	3.9	79	3.9	13.0	1.7	0.0
Powder, Made Up with Whole Milk, Ovaltine*	1 Mug/227ml	220	8.6	97	3.8	12.9	3.8	0.0
OXTAIL								
Raw	*1oz/28g*	*48*	*2.8*	*171*	*20.0*	*0.0*	*10.1*	*0.0*
Stewed, Bone Removed	*1oz/28g*	*68*	*3.8*	*243*	*30.5*	*0.0*	*13.4*	*0.0*
OYSTERS								
in Vegetable Oil, Smoked, John West*	1oz/28g	64	3.9	230	16.0	10.0	14.0	0.0
Raw, Shelled, Shucked	*1 Oyster/14g*	*9*	*0.2*	*65*	*10.8*	*2.7*	*1.3*	*0.0*

	Measure INFO/WEIGHT	per Measure		Nutrition Values per 100g / 100ml				
		KCAL	FAT	KCAL	PROT	CARB	FAT	FIBRE
PAELLA								
Bistro, Waitrose*	1 Serving/300g	534	19.8	178	7.4	22.2	6.6	0.7
Chicken & Chorizo, Asda*	1 Pack/390g	484	8.6	124	10.0	16.0	2.2	2.6
Chicken & Chorizo, Big Dish, M&S*	1 Pack/450g	630	17.6	140	7.9	18.4	3.9	1.6
Chicken & Chorizo, M Kitchen, Morrisons*	1 Pack/402g	482	14.1	120	4.4	18.3	3.5	1.3
Chicken & Chorizo, with King Prawns, City Kitchen, Tesco*	1 Pack/400g	540	20.0	135	4.7	17.0	5.0	1.4
Chicken & Chorizo, with King Prawns, Finest, Tesco*	½ Pack/400g	520	19.6	130	7.0	14.2	4.9	1.2
Chicken & Chorizo, with King Prawns, Fuller Longer, M&S*	1 Pack/390g	410	11.3	105	9.8	10.1	2.9	1.6
Chicken & King Prawn, BGTY, Sainsbury's*	1 Pack/400g	336	5.2	84	5.4	11.8	1.3	1.9
Diet Chef Ltd*	1 Pack/250g	355	3.0	142	11.2	21.7	1.2	0.4
Seafood, Espana, M&S*	1 Bowl/380g	565	12.1	150	5.5	25.2	3.2	0.5
Seafood, Finest, Tesco*	1 Pack/400g	756	23.6	189	6.8	27.2	5.9	1.0
Seafood, M&S*	1 Pack/450g	518	17.1	115	6.4	13.7	3.8	3.2
Seafood, Sainsbury's*	1 Pack/400g	504	5.2	126	8.3	20.3	1.3	0.6
Spanish Style, with Spices, Dinner Kit, Ainsley Harriott*	½ Pack/136g	473	1.9	348	10.0	73.7	1.4	2.7
TTD, Sainsbury's*	½ Pack/374g	475	20.9	127	9.4	9.9	5.6	4.8
Vegetable, Espana, M&S*	1 Pack/375g	505	13.5	135	2.8	22.4	3.6	1.3
Vegetable, Waitrose*	1 Serving/174g	202	3.1	116	2.2	22.7	1.8	1.5
PAIN AU CHOCOLAT								
All Butter, Tesco*	1 Serving/59g	242	11.6	410	8.2	49.4	19.7	2.3
Average	1 Serving/60g	253	13.7	422	8.0	45.8	22.8	3.1
Chocolate Filled, CBY, Asda*	1 Pain/45g	198	11.3	441	7.1	44.9	25.2	2.9
Mini, Asda*	1 Pastry/23g	96	5.5	420	8.0	43.0	24.0	3.3
Mini, Cafe Simple*	1 Pastry/27g	122	7.2	452	10.2	42.8	26.7	2.5
Small, Asda*	1 Serving/23g	106	6.0	462	8.0	49.0	26.0	0.0
Waitrose*	1 Pastry/53g	230	12.6	435	8.8	45.5	23.9	3.7
PAIN AU RAISIN								
Takeaway, Average	1 Pastry/100g	313	13.2	313	5.2	43.0	13.2	1.3
PAK CHOI								
Raw, Average	**1 Leaf/14g**	**2**	**0.0**	*13*	*1.5*	*2.2*	*0.2*	*1.0*
PAKORA								
Bhaji, Onion, Fried in Vegetable Oil	1oz/28g	76	4.1	271	9.8	26.2	14.7	5.5
Bhajia, Potato Carrot & Pea, Fried in Vegetable Oil	1oz/28g	100	6.3	357	10.9	28.8	22.6	6.1
Bhajia, Vegetable, Retail	1oz/28g	66	4.1	235	6.4	21.4	14.7	3.6
Chicken, Tikka, Asda*	1 Pack/350g	696	38.5	199	16.0	9.0	11.0	1.1
Potato & Spinach, Waitrose*	1 Pakora/50g	120	8.2	240	5.5	17.3	16.5	4.7
Prawn, Indian Appetisers, Waitrose*	1 Pakora/21g	35	1.7	165	16.8	5.9	8.2	1.5
Sainsbury's*	1 Pakora/55g	166	10.1	302	7.3	26.8	18.3	1.1
Spinach, Mini, Indian Selection, Somerfield*	1 Serving/22g	61	3.5	277	6.2	26.9	16.1	4.9
Spinach, Sainsbury's*	1 Pakora/18g	35	1.9	195	5.1	19.4	10.8	3.8
Vegetable, Indian Selection, Party, Co-Op*	1 Pakora/23g	47	1.6	205	6.0	28.0	7.0	4.0
Vegetable, Indian Starter Selection, M&S*	1 Pakora/23g	61	4.2	265	6.3	19.6	18.1	2.9
Vegetable, Mini, Indian Snack Collection, Tesco*	1 Pakora/21g	36	1.9	173	6.0	16.8	9.1	4.9
Vegetable, Somerfield*	1 Pakora/15g	46	3.4	305	7.0	19.0	23.0	0.0
PANCAKE								
Apple, Bramley, Sainsbury's*	1 Pancake/85g	114	2.1	134	4.2	23.6	2.5	1.0
Apple, GFY, Asda*	1 Pancake/74g	100	1.8	135	4.2	24.0	2.5	1.0
Asda*	1 Pancake/23g	59	1.6	254	4.8	43.0	7.0	4.0
Big, Crafty, Genesis*	1 Pancake/71g	171	3.7	241	6.2	42.3	5.2	2.1
Chinese Roll, Farmfoods*	1 Pancake/88g	125	3.8	142	4.3	21.6	4.3	1.0
Chocolate, M&S*	1 Pancake/80g	125	4.9	156	3.1	22.1	6.1	0.2
for Duck, Sainsbury's*	1 Pancake/10g	33	0.9	333	10.9	51.7	9.3	2.4
Golden Syrup, Value, Tesco*	1 Pancake/24g	61	1.5	255	5.1	44.1	6.3	1.9
Golden Syrup, Warburton's*	1 Pancake/26g	65	1.6	250	6.3	40.7	6.3	2.4

PANCAKE	Measure INFO/WEIGHT	per Measure KCAL	FAT	Nutrition Values per 100g / 100ml KCAL	PROT	CARB	FAT	FIBRE
Irish, Rankin Selection, Irwin's Bakery*	1 Pancake/40g	101	1.3	252	6.2	49.2	3.2	2.5
Lemon, M&S*	1 Pancake/38g	90	2.8	235	4.5	38.5	7.2	2.8
Low Calorie, Eurodiet*	1 Serving/30g	112	2.9	373	57.5	9.2	9.8	8.4
M & S*	1 Pancake/62g	170	7.7	275	5.7	33.9	12.5	1.5
Maple & Raisin, M&S*	1 Pancake/35g	102	2.4	290	5.6	50.4	6.9	2.2
Mini, for Kids, Tesco*	1 Pancake/16g	45	0.9	283	6.6	51.7	5.5	1.3
Mini, Scotch, Tesco*	1 Pancake/16g	44	0.9	277	6.7	50.0	5.6	1.4
Morrisons*	1 Pancake/60g	133	3.0	221	8.4	37.3	5.0	1.5
North Staffordshire Oatcakes Ltd*	1 Pancake/71g	166	4.3	234	5.0	40.9	6.1	1.0
Perfect, Kingsmill*	1 Pancake/27g	71	1.2	264	6.2	49.7	4.5	1.2
Plain, Sainsbury's*	1 Pancake/46g	102	2.4	221	6.9	36.1	5.3	1.2
Raisin & Lemon, Asda*	1 Serving/30g	92	2.4	304	6.0	52.0	8.0	1.4
Raisin & Lemon, Morrisons*	1 Pancake/36g	55	0.4	153	5.3	30.4	1.2	0.9
Raisin & Lemon, Sainsbury's*	1 Pancake/35g	95	1.5	272	6.3	51.8	4.4	2.2
Savoury, Made with Skimmed Milk, Average	6" Pancake/77g	192	11.3	249	6.4	24.1	14.7	0.8
Savoury, Made with Whole Milk, Average	6" Pancake/77g	210	13.5	273	6.3	24.0	17.5	0.8
Scotch	1 Pancake/50g	146	5.8	292	5.8	43.6	11.7	1.4
Scotch, BGTY, Sainsbury's*	1 Pancake/30g	76	1.2	252	5.3	48.5	4.1	1.3
Scotch, Essential, Waitrose*	1 Pancake/31g	82	2.6	265	6.4	40.9	8.4	2.4
Scotch, Low Fat, Asda*	1 Pancake/32g	87	0.7	272	6.0	57.0	2.2	1.3
Sultana & Syrup, Asda*	1 Pancake/34g	89	2.4	263	5.9	43.7	7.2	1.5
Sultana & Syrup, Scotch, Sainsbury's*	1 Pancake/35g	113	2.9	322	6.7	55.2	8.3	1.7
Sweet, Made with Skimmed Milk	1oz/28g	78	3.9	280	6.0	35.1	13.8	0.8
Sweet, Made with Whole Milk	1oz/28g	84	4.5	301	5.9	35.0	16.2	0.8
Syrup, American Style, Large, Tesco*	1 Pancake/38g	102	1.3	268	5.1	54.2	3.4	0.9
Syrup, Tesco*	1 Pancake/30g	80	2.5	265	4.7	42.1	8.2	1.5
Traditional, Aunt Bessie's*	1 Pancake/60g	90	1.9	150	6.1	24.6	3.1	1.1
Traditional, Tesco*	1 Pancake/62g	137	3.1	221	8.4	35.6	5.0	1.5
Vegetable Roll	1 Roll/85g	185	10.6	218	6.6	21.0	12.5	0.0
PANCAKE MIX								
4 Grain, Wheat & GF, Organic, Hale & Hearty*	½ Pack/180g	562	2.9	312	7.8	66.6	1.6	5.7
Batter, Shake to Make, Made Up, Betty Crocker*	1 Serving/74g	114	4.0	154	3.5	22.7	5.4	1.0
Fresh, M&S*	1 Pancake/38g	90	5.0	235	7.5	22.4	13.1	0.5
Traditional, Asda*	1 Pack/256g	545	23.0	213	6.0	27.0	9.0	1.8
PANCETTA								
Average	*½ Pack/65g*	*212*	*18.7*	*326*	*17.0*	*0.1*	*28.7*	*0.0*
PANINI								
Bacon, British Midland*	1 Serving/150g	273	9.9	182	9.1	21.6	6.6	0.0
Cheese, Tesco*	1 Panini/100g	249	9.1	249	10.5	31.3	9.1	3.1
Chicken, Mozzarella, & Pesto, Chargrilled, Udo's Choice*	1 Panini/170g	389	14.6	229	16.4	21.6	8.6	2.0
Ham & Cheese, Ginsters*	1 Panini/200g	567	25.6	283	13.3	28.7	12.8	1.6
Mozzarella & Tomato, M&S*	1 Serving/176g	484	28.5	275	11.3	21.3	16.2	2.1
Tuna & Sweetcorn, Tesco*	1 Serving/250g	559	16.4	224	12.0	29.3	6.6	1.4
PANNA COTTA								
Caramel, Sainsbury's*	1 Pot/120g	335	15.7	279	2.5	34.6	13.1	3.3
Sainsbury's*	1 Pot/100g	304	15.7	304	3.0	41.5	15.7	4.0
Strawberry, COU, M&S*	1 Pot/145g	145	3.8	100	2.6	15.7	2.6	0.8
PAPAYA								
Dried, Pieces, Nature's Harvest*	1 Serving/50g	178	0.0	355	0.2	85.4	0.0	2.6
Dried, Strips, Tropical Wholefoods*	1 Strip/10g	31	0.1	310	3.9	71.4	0.9	1.5
Dried, Sweetened, Tesco*	4 Pieces/25g	59	0.2	235	0.4	56.3	0.9	2.9
Raw, Flesh Only, Average	*1 Serving/140g*	*37*	*0.1*	*26*	*0.4*	*6.6*	*0.1*	*1.2*
Raw, Unripe, Flesh Only	1 Serving/100g	27	0.1	27	0.9	5.5	0.1	1.0

INFO/WEIGHT	Measure	per Measure		Nutrition Values per 100g / 100ml				
		KCAL	FAT	KCAL	PROT	CARB	FAT	FIBRE
PAPAYA								
Raw, Unripe, Weighed with Seeds & Skin	*1oz/28g*	*8*	*0.0*	*27*	*0.9*	*5.5*	*0.1*	*1.5*
Raw, Weighed with Seeds & Skin	*1 Serving/140g*	*55*	*0.2*	*39*	*0.6*	*9.8*	*0.1*	*1.8*
PAPPARDELLE								
Egg, Dry, Average	*1 Serving/100g*	*364*	*3.7*	*364*	*14.1*	*68.5*	*3.7*	*2.1*
Egg, Fresh, Waitrose*	¼ Pack/125g	350	3.4	280	12.9	51.0	2.7	1.9
Portobello & Chestnut Mushroom, M&S*	1 Serving/368g	405	16.9	110	4.8	12.3	4.6	2.0
with Salmon, COU, M&S*	1 Pack/358g	340	6.8	95	6.3	13.0	1.9	0.8
PAPRIKA								
Average	*1 Tsp/2g*	*6*	*0.3*	*289*	*14.8*	*34.9*	*13.0*	*0.0*
PARATHA								
Average	*1 Paratha/80g*	*258*	*11.4*	*322*	*8.0*	*43.2*	*14.3*	*4.0*
Roti, Plain, Crown Farms*	1 Slice/80g	250	10.0	312	5.0	46.2	12.5	1.2
PARCELS								
Brie & Cranberry, Filo, Finest, Tesco*	1 Parcel/22g	73	3.7	330	9.8	33.2	17.0	1.4
Cheese & Ham, Sainsbury's*	1 Pack/250g	445	19.0	178	7.4	19.9	7.6	1.5
Mushroom, Leek, & Gruyere, Filo, Finest, Tesco*	1 Serving/160g	440	33.6	275	6.9	20.5	21.0	1.5
Salmon, in Lemon Sauce, M&S*	1 Serving/185g	350	27.9	189	12.1	1.4	15.1	0.5
Salmon, Smoked, Sainsbury's*	1 Pack/115g	269	20.2	234	15.8	3.5	17.6	0.2
Salmon, with Soft Cheese & Herb, Smoked, Waitrose*	1 Pack/100g	246	20.2	246	14.6	1.2	20.2	0.0
Turkey, with Cheddar Cheese & Chive, Breast, Asda*	1 Parcel/140g	242	9.8	173	23.0	4.6	7.0	0.9
PARSLEY								
Dried	*1 Tsp/1g*	*2*	*0.1*	*181*	*15.8*	*14.5*	*7.0*	*26.9*
Fresh, Average	*1 Tbsp/4g*	*1*	*0.0*	*34*	*3.0*	*2.7*	*1.3*	*5.0*
PARSNIP								
Boiled, Average	*1 Serving/80g*	*53*	*1.0*	*66*	*1.6*	*12.9*	*1.2*	*4.7*
Fragrant, Tesco*	1 Serving/50g	34	0.6	67	1.8	12.5	1.1	4.6
Honey Glazed, Roasting, Cooked, Betty Smith's*	1 Serving/80g	177	11.9	221	1.4	18.7	14.9	3.4
Honey Roasted, Tesco*	½ Pack/125g	165	6.6	130	1.3	16.7	5.2	5.2
Raw, Unprepared, Average	*1oz/28g*	*19*	*0.3*	*66*	*1.8*	*12.5*	*1.1*	*4.6*
Roast, Honey Glazed, Baked, Aunt Bessie's*	1 Serving/80g	177	11.9	221	1.4	18.7	14.9	3.4
Roasting, Freshly Frozen, CBY, Asda*	1 Serving/110g	221	8.5	201	2.5	30.4	7.7	7.8
PARTRIDGE								
Breast, Fillets, Raw, Skinned, Abel & Cole*	1 Serving/100g	145	4.7	145	25.8	0.0	4.7	0.0
Meat Only, Roasted	*1oz/28g*	*59*	*2.0*	*212*	*36.7*	*0.0*	*7.2*	*0.0*
PASANDA								
Chicken, M&S*	½ Pack/150g	240	16.4	160	11.3	3.8	10.9	1.3
Chicken, Waitrose*	1oz/28g	52	3.4	185	14.8	3.8	12.3	1.1
PASSATA								
Napolina*	1 Bottle/690g	172	0.7	25	1.4	4.5	0.1	0.0
Onion & Garlic, Italian, Classic, Sainsbury's*	1oz/28g	10	0.0	37	1.4	7.7	0.1	1.3
Smart Price, Asda*	1 Serving/100g	25	0.1	25	1.4	4.5	0.1	0.2
So Organic, Sainsbury's*	¼ Jar/175g	38	0.7	22	0.9	3.8	0.4	0.9
Tomato, Sieved, Valfrutta*	1 Pack/500g	110	0.5	22	1.2	4.0	0.1	0.0
with Fresh Leaf Basil, Waitrose*	¼ Jar/170g	44	0.2	26	1.0	5.2	0.1	0.8
with Garlic & Italian Herbs, Tesco*	1 Serving/165g	53	0.3	32	1.2	6.4	0.2	1.1
PASSION FRUIT								
Raw, Fresh, Average	*1 Fruit/30g*	*11*	*0.1*	*36*	*2.6*	*5.8*	*0.4*	*3.3*
Weighed with Skin, Average	*1 Fruit/30g*	*11*	*0.1*	*36*	*2.6*	*5.8*	*0.4*	*3.3*
PASTA								
Angel Hair, Konjac, Slim Pasta*	1 Serving/100g	8	0.0	8	0.6	0.6	0.0	5.6
Arrabbiata Nodini, Asda*	1 Serving/150g	302	8.7	201	7.8	29.3	5.8	2.7
Boccoletti, Dried, Sainsbury's*	1 Serving/90g	321	1.5	357	12.3	73.1	1.7	2.5
Bolognese, Diet Chef Ltd*	1 Serving/300g	288	10.2	96	7.9	5.8	3.4	4.4

PASTA

	Measure INFO/WEIGHT	per Measure KCAL	per Measure FAT	Nutrition Values per 100g / 100ml KCAL	PROT	CARB	FAT	FIBRE
Bolognese, Fusilli, Pastavita, Dolmio*	1 Serving/300g	333	5.1	111	5.3	17.9	1.7	0.0
Brown Rice, Fusilli, GF, Dove's Farm*	1 Serving/30g	101	0.4	338	7.9	70.3	1.5	4.1
Brown Rice & Maize, Ditalini, Organic, Dove's Farm*	1 Serving/100g	347	0.9	347	7.0	76.0	0.9	2.4
Cappalletti, Meat, Sainsbury's*	1 Pack/420g	816	23.9	195	10.0	25.8	5.7	2.3
Carbonara, with Cheese & Bacon, Slim Fast*	1 Serving/70g	240	4.4	343	22.7	48.9	6.3	5.7
Cheese, & Tortellini in Tomato Sauce, Heinz*	1 Pack/250g	229	7.6	92	2.2	13.7	3.0	0.2
Cheese, Tomato & Pesto, Boots*	1 Pack/250g	355	11.0	142	5.9	20.0	4.4	2.0
Cheese,& Broccoli, LC, Tesco*	1 Pack/348g	435	8.0	125	4.4	21.2	2.3	2.4
Chicken, & Bacon, Chargrilled, Tesco*	1 Pack/200g	420	23.6	210	6.7	18.8	11.8	1.3
Chicken, & Chorizo, Average	1 Pack/400g	174	5.7	174	10.1	20.3	5.7	1.5
Chicken, & Mushroom Panzerotti, CBY, Asda*	½ Pack/209g	310	6.7	148	5.7	22.7	3.2	2.6
Chicken, Sicilian, City Kitchen, Tesco*	1 Pack/385g	500	13.5	130	9.1	14.6	3.5	0.6
Chicken, Tomato & Basil, GFY, Asda*	1 Pack/400g	404	9.2	101	6.4	13.6	2.3	1.4
Elicoidali, Waitrose*	1 Serving/200g	682	2.6	341	11.5	70.7	1.3	3.7
Fiorelli, Goats Cheese & Red Onion, Waitrose*	½ Pack/155g	226	8.8	146	6.3	17.3	5.7	2.2
Garlic Mushroom Filled, Extra Special, Asda*	1 Serving/125g	224	8.8	179	8.0	21.0	7.0	2.5
Girasole, Filled with Red Pepper & Goats Cheese, Asda*	½ Pack/150g	261	9.9	174	7.2	21.4	6.6	1.8
High Fibre, Uncooked, Fiber Gourmet*	1 Serving/56g	130	1.0	232	12.5	75.0	1.8	32.1
Lumache, Tesco*	1 Serving/100g	345	2.0	345	13.2	68.5	2.0	2.9
Margherite, Basil & Pinenut, TTD, Sainsbury's*	½ Pack/150g	309	10.5	206	12.6	23.2	7.0	2.7
Mushroom, Creamy, LC, Tesco*	1 Pack/350g	455	4.9	130	4.3	25.0	1.4	1.3
Mushroom, Creamy, Sainsbury's*	1 Serving/63g	148	9.1	237	4.5	21.7	14.6	1.2
Organic, GF, Dove's Farm*	1 Serving/100g	338	1.5	338	7.9	70.3	1.5	4.1
Orzo, Dry, Average	1 Serving/100g	348	1.5	348	12.4	71.9	1.5	3.0
Orzo, with Chicken, Tomato & Basil, Eat Well, M&S*	1 Pack/300g	390	11.1	130	7.9	16.5	3.7	1.9
Paccheri, Finest, Tesco*	1 Serving/100g	360	1.5	360	13.5	72.5	1.5	1.6
Pomodoro, Pasta King*	1 Serving/100g	109	1.8	109	3.6	19.6	1.8	1.8
Quadrotti, Pumpkin & Sage, TTD, Sainsbury's*	½ Pack/159g	287	8.1	180	7.6	25.8	5.1	3.0
Raviolini, Gorgonzola & Walnut, M&S*	½ Pack/125g	381	16.5	305	12.6	33.6	13.2	2.0
Riccioli, Dry Weight, Buitoni*	1 Serving/75g	264	1.4	352	11.2	72.6	1.9	0.0
Salmon, Hot Smoked, Tesco*	1 Pack/275g	426	17.0	155	7.1	16.6	6.2	4.1
Sausage & Tomato, Italiano, Tesco*	1 Serving/450g	680	26.6	151	5.7	18.8	5.9	1.6
Seafood, Retail	1oz/28g	31	1.3	110	8.9	7.6	4.8	0.4
Shapes, Dried, Tesco*	1 Serving/100g	345	2.0	345	13.2	68.5	2.0	2.9
Spirals, Co-Op*	1 Serving/100g	350	1.0	350	12.0	73.0	1.0	3.0
Stuffed Mushroom & Emmental, Sainsbury's*	1 Pack/250g	650	23.0	260	11.3	33.5	9.2	3.7
Sweet Pepper, Pastavita, Dolmio*	1 Pot/300g	327	5.7	109	4.4	17.9	1.9	1.4
Tomato, & Vegetable, Diet Chef Ltd*	1 Pack/300g	216	6.0	72	2.6	10.9	2.0	1.8
Tomato & Basil, Pastavita, Dolmio*	1 Pot/300g	327	5.1	109	4.5	18.2	1.7	1.5
Tomato & Chilli, Pastavita, Dolmio*	1 Pot/300g	330	5.4	110	4.4	18.4	1.8	1.5
Tomato & Herb, Snackpot, Made Up, CBY, Asda*	1 Pot/225g	259	1.6	115	3.8	23.4	0.7	2.0
Tomato & Mozzarella, Filled, Caramella, Jamie Oliver*	½ Pack/165g	294	9.2	178	8.9	24.9	5.6	2.0
Tortelloni, Spinach & Ricotta, Emma Giordani*	1 Pack/250g	685	15.0	274	10.0	45.0	6.0	0.0
Tortelloni, Spinach & Ricotta, Giovanni Rana*	½ Pack/125g	248	8.1	198	7.8	27.0	6.5	3.1
Tuna Rigatoni, Diet Chef Ltd*	1 Pack/300g	336	13.2	112	5.9	12.2	4.4	1.0
Twists, Dry, Average	1oz/28g	99	0.4	354	12.2	71.8	1.5	2.2
Twists, Quick Cook, Morrisons*	1 Serving/75g	265	1.5	353	12.0	72.0	2.0	3.1
Twists, with Tuna, Italian, Weight Watchers*	1 Can/385g	239	5.4	62	4.3	8.2	1.4	0.6
Vegetable, Mediterranean, Sainsbury's*	1 Pack/400g	504	11.6	126	4.0	20.9	2.9	1.8
Vegetable Rice, Dry Weight, Orgran*	1 Serving/66g	233	1.3	353	6.8	80.0	2.0	4.8
Wheat Free, Delverde*	1 Serving/63g	229	1.2	366	0.5	86.9	1.9	1.2
Wholewheat, Cooked, Tesco*	1 Serving/200g	284	1.8	142	5.7	27.9	0.9	4.5

	Measure INFO/WEIGHT	per Measure KCAL	FAT	Nutrition Values per 100g / 100ml KCAL	PROT	CARB	FAT	FIBRE
PASTA BAKE								
Bacon, & Leek, Average	1 Serving/400g	633	32.3	158	6.7	14.8	8.1	1.3
Bolognese, Baked, CBY, Asda*	½ Pack/200g	315	12.0	157	7.5	17.6	6.0	1.5
Bolognese, Finest, Tesco*	1 Serving/250g	375	15.8	150	7.3	16.1	6.3	1.1
Bolognese, Italiano, Tesco*	1/3 Pack/284g	409	14.5	144	8.7	15.7	5.1	2.3
Bolognese, Weight Watchers*	1 Pack/400g	324	8.0	81	6.1	9.6	2.0	1.3
Cheese & Bacon, Asda*	1 Serving/120g	168	14.4	140	3.0	5.2	12.0	0.3
Cheese & Bacon, Fresh Italian, Asda*	1 Serving/250g	265	20.0	106	6.0	2.6	8.0	0.5
Cheese & Tomato, Italiano, Tesco*	1 Bake/300g	354	12.6	118	3.9	16.1	4.2	1.0
Cheese & Tomato, LC, Tesco*	1 Pack/350g	385	4.6	110	3.2	20.9	1.3	1.5
Cheese & Tomato, Tesco*	1 Pack/400g	388	5.6	97	3.4	17.8	1.4	1.2
Chicken, Bacon, & Mushroom, Average	1 Serving/400g	632	29.2	158	7.8	15.1	7.3	2.3
Chicken, Bacon, & Mushroom, Sainsbury's*	1 Serving/400g	548	20.0	137	7.0	15.3	5.0	1.3
Chicken, Tomato, & Mascarpone, Tesco*	1 Serving/400g	448	8.4	112	8.0	15.2	2.1	1.7
Chicken, Weight Watchers*	1 Pack/300g	249	2.7	83	6.0	12.1	0.9	1.1
Chicken & Bacon, Asda*	1 Pack/400g	592	25.2	148	8.6	14.2	6.3	3.0
Chicken & Bacon, Average	1 Serving/400g	627	28.7	157	9.0	13.7	7.2	1.6
Chicken & Broccoli, Morrisons*	1 Pack/400g	452	16.0	113	6.1	13.3	4.0	0.6
Chicken & Broccoli, Weight Watchers*	1 Bake/305g	290	4.6	95	6.0	14.2	1.5	0.9
Chicken & Mushroom, Waitrose*	1 Pack/400g	532	30.8	133	6.7	9.1	7.7	0.8
Meatball, Aberdeen Angus, Waitrose*	½ Pack/350g	501	28.0	143	5.2	12.5	8.0	0.9
Mozzarella, & Tomato, Asda*	1 Pack/400g	532	19.2	133	4.4	18.1	4.8	1.8
Mozzarella, Penne, Tesco*	1 Pack/340g	408	8.5	120	4.7	19.7	2.5	0.6
Mozzarella & Tomato, Average	1 Serving/400g	500	12.4	125	5.3	17.3	3.1	1.5
Mozzarella & Tomato, Italiano, Tesco*	1 Pack/340g	398	8.5	117	4.8	18.9	2.5	1.7
Mozzarella & Tomato, LC, Tesco*	1 Pack/400g	380	4.4	95	3.4	17.2	1.1	1.2
Mozzarella & Tomato, Sainsbury's*	1 Pack/400g	480	12.8	120	5.0	17.9	3.2	2.1
Pepperoni, & Tomato, Spicy, Asda*	1 Pack/440g	431	26.4	98	1.1	10.0	6.0	1.2
Sausage, Average	1 Serving/400g	591	24.0	148	5.5	17.7	6.0	1.9
Tomato & Herb, Asda*	1 Jar/436g	715	56.7	164	1.8	10.0	13.0	1.2
Tuna & Sweetcorn, Asda*	1 Serving/250g	332	22.5	133	5.0	8.0	9.0	0.9
Tuna & Sweetcorn, Average	1 Pack/400g	423	22.4	106	5.0	8.6	5.6	1.9
Tuna & Tomato, BGTY, Sainsbury's*	1 Pack/450g	554	18.9	123	8.7	12.6	4.2	0.4
Tuna Conchiglie, M&S*	1 Pack/400g	520	17.2	130	8.6	14.3	4.3	1.1
Vegetable, Asda*	1 Serving/300g	231	10.5	77	2.4	9.0	3.5	0.8
Vegetable, M&S*	½ Pack/175g	201	8.8	115	4.1	12.6	5.0	2.2
Vegetable, Mediterranean, Roasted, Dolmio*	1 Portion/125g	66	2.1	53	1.3	8.1	1.7	1.2
Vegetable, Mediterranean, Tesco*	1 Serving/450g	495	20.7	110	4.3	12.9	4.6	1.3
Vegetable, Tesco*	1 Pack/380g	467	21.3	123	5.6	12.6	5.6	1.6
PASTA 'N' SAUCE								
Carbonara, Dry, Batchelors*	1 Pack/120g	463	6.0	386	14.3	71.0	5.0	3.1
Cheese, Leek & Ham, Batchelors*	1 Pack/120g	454	6.1	378	16.1	67.0	5.1	2.0
Cheese & Broccoli Sauce Mix, Made Up, Sainsbury's*	1 Pack/120g	164	6.8	137	4.2	17.2	5.7	1.1
Chicken & Mushroom, Batchelors*	½ Pack/63g	227	1.1	361	14.1	72.3	1.7	2.8
Chicken & Mushroom, Made Up, Morrisons*	1 Pack/110g	166	6.2	151	5.0	20.3	5.6	2.1
Macaroni Cheese, Dry, Batchelors*	1 Pack/108g	402	5.1	372	17.2	65.2	4.7	2.7
Mild Cheese & Broccoli, Batchelors*	½ Pack/61g	221	2.4	363	15.0	67.0	3.9	4.0
Mushroom & Wine, Batchelors*	½ Pack/50g	242	2.8	483	18.5	89.9	5.5	4.4
Tomato, Onion & Herb, Made Up, Morrisons*	1 Serving/110g	141	5.0	128	3.2	18.7	4.5	2.3
Tomato, Onion & Herbs, Dry, Batchelors*	1 Pack/135g	455	1.8	337	12.8	68.5	1.3	5.8
Tomato & Mascarpone, BGTY, Sainsbury's*	1 Pack/380g	555	7.2	146	6.6	25.6	1.9	1.3
PASTA QUILLS								
Dry, Average	**1 Serving/75g**	**256**	**0.9**	**342**	**12.0**	**72.3**	**1.2**	**2.0**
GF, Salute*	1 Serving/75g	269	1.4	359	7.5	78.0	1.9	0.0

PASTA SALAD

INFO/WEIGHT	Measure	per Measure KCAL	per Measure FAT	KCAL	PROT	CARB	FAT	FIBRE
Basil & Parmesan, Tesco*	1 Serving/50g	65	1.8	130	4.3	20.2	3.6	0.6
Basil Pesto Dressing, Mixed Leaf, Tesco*	1 Pack/220g	528	37.6	240	4.7	16.9	17.1	0.7
Bean, Mixed, Diet Chef Ltd*	1 Pack/300g	300	3.6	100	4.7	17.5	1.2	2.8
Caesar, & Santa Tomatoes, M&S*	1 Serving/220g	495	33.7	225	5.2	15.9	15.3	0.8
Caesar, Chicken, Asda*	1 Pack/297g	683	41.3	230	9.6	16.6	13.9	2.5
Caesar, Chicken, Shapers, Boots*	1 Pack/218g	288	8.3	132	6.7	18.0	3.8	1.8
Cheese, Average	1 Serving/370g	782	56.8	211	5.5	12.8	15.4	1.2
Cheese, Cheddar, Tesco*	1 Pot/215g	546	43.9	254	5.7	12.0	20.4	0.8
Cheese, Morrisons*	½ Pot/125g	341	26.6	273	5.7	14.7	21.3	1.0
Cheese, with Mayonnaise & Vinaigrette, Sainsbury's*	¼ Pot/50g	124	8.6	249	6.1	17.0	17.3	1.7
Chicken, & Pesto, Chargrilled, Sainsbury's*	1 Pack/240g	454	22.1	189	7.2	19.4	9.2	0.0
Chicken, & Red Pepper, Chargrilled, Tesco*	1 Pack/270g	554	24.0	205	9.8	20.3	8.9	3.1
Chicken, Chargrilled, M&S*	1 Serving/190g	285	5.5	150	9.6	23.6	2.9	1.6
Chicken, Honey & Mustard, M&S*	1 Serving/190g	304	4.8	160	8.7	26.7	2.5	1.5
Chicken, Honey & Mustard, Sainsbury's*	1 Pack/190g	344	16.9	181	7.1	18.0	8.9	0.0
Chicken, Honey & Mustard, Shapers, Boots*	1 Serving/252g	350	5.5	139	8.4	22.0	2.2	2.8
Chicken, Italian Style, Chargrilled, Fresh, Asda*	1 Pack/200g	318	14.0	159	7.0	17.0	7.0	0.4
Chicken & Bacon, Layered, Fresh Tastes, Asda*	1 Pack/197g	290	16.9	147	6.5	10.3	8.6	0.0
Chicken & Bacon, Smoked, M&S*	1 Pack/380g	817	46.7	215	7.5	19.0	12.3	1.9
Chicken & Bacon, Tesco*	½ Pack/200g	450	29.0	225	6.3	16.8	14.5	3.2
Chicken & Sweetcorn, Morrisons*	1 Serving/220g	255	3.5	116	6.7	18.7	1.6	1.0
Goats Cheese, & Mixed Pepper, Sainsbury's*	1 Pack/200g	366	18.8	183	6.4	18.2	9.4	1.5
Ham, Sainsbury's*	1 Pot/250g	610	48.2	244	4.1	13.4	19.3	0.8
Italian, Bowl, Sainsbury's*	1 Serving/210g	309	15.5	147	3.1	16.9	7.4	1.9
Italian, Tesco*	½ Pack/225g	315	8.3	140	3.5	22.6	3.7	2.3
Italian Style, Iceland*	1 Serving/75g	97	4.5	129	2.6	16.2	6.0	1.6
Mozzarella, & Plum Tomatoes, COU, M&S*	1 Bowl/255g	204	4.1	80	4.6	11.5	1.6	1.7
Pepper, & Tomato, Fire Roasted, Finest, Tesco*	1 Pack/200g	260	8.2	130	3.7	19.4	4.1	2.5
Pesto, with Pine Nuts & Spinach, Salad Bar, Waitrose*	1 Serving/100g	178	7.7	178	0.0	0.0	7.7	0.0
Prawn, King & Juicy Fresh Tomatoes, COU, M&S*	1 Serving/270g	256	4.0	95	5.1	16.4	1.5	0.9
Prawn, Layered, Asda*	½ Pack/220g	279	11.4	127	5.2	14.2	5.2	2.0
Prawn, Shapers, Boots*	1 Pot/250g	250	7.8	100	4.1	14.0	3.1	0.4
Prawn, Tesco*	½ Pack/250g	488	27.8	195	4.9	18.9	11.1	2.0
Prawn Cocktail, Shapers, Boots*	1 Pack/248g	255	6.7	103	5.0	15.0	2.7	1.6
Red Pepper & Sunblush Tomato, Finest, Tesco*	1 Serving/100g	165	4.3	165	4.9	26.0	4.3	3.3
Salmon, & Beans, Poached, Fuller Longer, M&S*	1 Pack/330g	380	12.2	115	10.0	10.0	3.7	6.3
Salmon, Hot Smoked, No Mayonnaise, Tesco*	1 Pack/275g	426	17.0	155	7.1	16.6	6.2	4.1
Tomato, Diet Chef Ltd*	1 Pack/300g	264	5.4	88	2.3	15.6	1.8	1.2
Tomato, Morrisons*	1 Serving/50g	46	0.6	92	3.0	17.3	1.2	2.4
Tomato & Basil, Chicken, Waitrose*	1 Pack/205g	434	24.6	212	8.3	17.7	12.0	1.1
Tomato & Basil, M&S*	1 Pot/225g	484	35.8	215	2.9	15.0	15.9	1.2
Tomato & Basil, Sainsbury's*	1 Serving/62g	87	4.3	141	3.2	16.4	6.9	3.8
Tomato & Basil Chicken, M&S*	1 Serving/279g	446	22.0	160	7.0	14.8	7.9	1.8
Tomato & Basil with Red & Green Pepper, Sainsbury's*	¼ Pot/63g	89	4.3	141	3.2	16.4	6.9	3.8
Tomato & Mozzarella, Sainsbury's*	1 Pack/200g	440	22.6	220	7.5	22.2	11.3	1.3
Tuna, Mediterranean, Shapers, Boots*	1 Serving/239g	232	3.1	97	6.2	15.0	1.3	0.9
Tuna & Sweetcorn, COU, M&S*	1 Pack/200g	210	1.8	105	7.1	18.3	0.9	1.2
Tuna & Sweetcorn, Morrisons*	1 Serving/100g	227	15.1	227	5.0	16.1	15.1	2.2
Tuna & Sweetcorn, Sainsbury's*	1 Serving/100g	111	1.2	111	7.1	18.3	1.2	1.2
Tuna Nicoise, Waitrose*	1 Pot/190g	306	17.1	161	5.1	14.9	9.0	1.1
Vegetable, & Bean, Mediterranean, BGTY, Sainsbury's*	1 Serving/66g	53	1.3	80	3.2	12.5	1.9	2.8
Vegetable, & Tomato, Chargrilled, Shapers, Boots*	1 Pack/175g	187	5.4	107	2.8	17.0	3.1	1.5
Vegetable, Chargrilled, Sainsbury's*	1 Serving/178g	192	4.8	108	2.7	15.9	2.7	4.7

	Measure INFO/WEIGHT	per Measure KCAL	FAT	Nutrition Values per 100g / 100ml KCAL	PROT	CARB	FAT	FIBRE
PASTA SALAD								
Vegetable, Healthy Selection, Somerfield*	1 Pot/200g	180	0.0	90	2.8	19.6	0.0	0.7
Vegetable, Roasted, Waitrose*	1 Pack/190g	270	8.7	142	6.8	18.2	4.6	1.1
PASTA SAUCE								
Amatriciana, Italian, Sainsbury's*	½ Pot/175g	136	3.0	78	2.6	5.7	1.7	0.5
Amatriciana, Italiano, Tesco*	½ Pot/175g	124	6.6	71	4.1	5.3	3.8	0.9
Amatriciana, M&S*	1 Jar/340g	425	32.3	125	3.4	6.3	9.5	2.9
Amatriciana, Tesco*	1 Serving/175g	108	7.2	62	2.3	4.0	4.1	0.7
Arrabbiata, Barilla*	1 Serving/100g	47	3.0	47	1.5	3.5	3.0	0.0
Arrabbiata, Fresh, Co-Op*	½ Pot/150g	82	4.5	55	1.0	5.0	3.0	1.0
Arrabbiata, Fresh, Morrisons*	1 Pot/350g	139	5.2	40	1.9	5.4	1.5	0.0
Arrabbiata, GFY, Asda*	1 Serving/350g	133	3.9	38	1.1	6.0	1.1	0.0
Arrabbiata, Italian, Waitrose*	1 Jar/320g	115	3.2	36	1.5	6.7	1.0	1.4
Arrabbiata, M&S*	1 Jar/320g	240	17.0	75	1.2	6.2	5.3	0.8
Arrabbiata, Red Pepper, Sainsbury's*	½ Pot/175g	79	5.1	45	1.4	3.3	2.9	1.6
Arrabbiata, Romano*	1 Serving/100g	69	3.4	69	2.5	7.0	3.4	0.6
Bacon, Smoky, Loyd Grossman*	½ Jar/175g	142	8.4	81	3.0	6.1	4.8	0.8
Basil & Oregano, Ragu, Knorr*	1 Jar/500g	215	0.0	43	1.3	9.4	0.0	1.1
Bolognese, CBY, Asda*	¼ Jar/125g	55	0.8	44	1.3	7.6	0.6	1.5
Bolognese, Extra Mushrooms, Dolmio*	1 Jar/500g	240	6.5	48	1.6	7.6	1.3	1.1
Bolognese, Extra Onion & Garlic, Dolmio*	1 Serving/125g	51	0.8	41	1.4	6.6	0.6	1.0
Bolognese, Extra Spicy, Dolmio*	1 Jar/500g	260	5.5	52	1.7	8.8	1.1	0.8
Bolognese, Finest, Tesco*	1 Serving/175g	170	10.7	97	7.0	3.8	6.1	0.5
Bolognese, Fresh, Sainsbury's*	½ Pot/150g	120	6.2	80	6.0	4.7	4.1	1.2
Bolognese, Italiano, Tesco*	1 Serving/175g	194	13.1	111	5.9	4.8	7.5	0.8
Bolognese, Light, Original, Ragu, Knorr*	1 Jar/515g	196	0.5	38	1.4	8.2	0.1	1.2
Bolognese, Mediterranean Vegetable, Chunky, Dolmio*	½ Jar/250g	138	4.0	55	1.3	8.8	1.6	1.1
Bolognese, Organic, Seeds of Change*	1 Jar/500g	290	6.0	58	1.3	10.4	1.2	0.8
Bolognese, Original, Asda*	1 Serving/158g	73	2.2	46	1.4	7.0	1.4	0.8
Bolognese, Original, Light, Low Fat, Dolmio*	1 Serving/125g	44	0.4	35	1.5	6.7	0.3	0.9
Bolognese, Seasonal, Dolmio*	1 Jar/500g	205	1.0	41	1.5	7.4	0.2	1.4
Bolognese, Smart Price, Asda*	½ Jar/226g	88	1.8	39	0.9	7.0	0.8	0.6
Bolognese, Spicy, Ragu, Knorr*	1 Jar/500g	260	1.0	52	1.9	9.7	0.2	1.4
Bolognese, Tesco*	¼ Jar/125g	51	1.8	41	1.0	6.1	1.4	2.3
Bolognese, Tomato, Beef & Red Wine, Fresh, Waitrose*	1 Pot/350g	301	17.2	86	5.4	5.3	4.9	2.0
Bolognese, Traditional, Ragu, Knorr*	1 Jar/320g	157	5.4	49	1.3	7.1	1.7	1.2
Bolognese, VLH Kitchens	1 Serving/380g	316	1.1	83	6.0	4.7	4.1	1.2
Bolognese, with Beef, Tesco*	½ Can/213g	179	10.0	84	4.9	5.5	4.7	0.0
Bolognese, with Red Wine, Weight Watchers*	1 Jar/350g	98	0.4	28	1.4	5.3	0.1	1.3
Cacciatore, Fresh, Sainsbury's*	½ Pot/150g	152	8.8	101	5.4	8.1	5.9	1.5
Carbonara, Asda*	½ Pot/175g	359	29.8	205	7.0	6.0	17.0	0.1
Carbonara, Bottled, Tesco*	1 Jar/315g	504	41.6	160	3.2	6.8	13.2	0.1
Carbonara, CBY, Asda*	1 Serving/100g	162	12.6	162	7.3	4.5	12.6	0.5
Carbonara, Co-Op*	½ Pot/150g	270	25.5	180	3.0	4.0	17.0	0.1
Carbonara, Creamy, Dolmio Express, Dolmio*	1 Pack/150g	166	13.2	111	3.3	4.7	8.8	0.1
Carbonara, Creamy, Stir in Sauce, Dolmio*	1 Serving/75g	98	8.0	130	3.3	5.2	10.6	0.2
Carbonara, Fresh, Chilled, Finest, Tesco*	½ Tub/175g	298	24.8	170	5.5	4.2	14.2	0.0
Carbonara, Italian, Fresh, Sainsbury's*	½ Pot/176g	209	16.3	119	5.4	3.4	9.3	0.9
Carbonara, Reduced Fat, BFY, Morrisons*	½ Pot/175g	135	5.8	77	6.6	5.1	3.3	0.5
Carbonara, with Pancetta, Loyd Grossman*	½ Pack/170g	209	15.5	123	2.8	7.5	9.1	0.1
Cheese, Five, Italiano, Tesco*	½ Tub/175g	271	20.1	155	6.8	6.0	11.5	0.0
Cheese, Fresh, PB, Waitrose*	½ Pot/175g	144	5.1	82	6.1	7.9	2.9	0.5
Cheese, Italian, Finest, Tesco*	½ Pot/175g	172	8.9	98	4.8	8.4	5.1	0.0
Cherry Tomato, & Basil, Sacla*	1 Serving/96g	90	7.1	94	1.2	5.3	7.4	0.0

PASTA SAUCE

	Measure INFO/WEIGHT	per Measure KCAL	FAT	Nutrition Values per 100g / 100ml KCAL	PROT	CARB	FAT	FIBRE
Cherry Tomato, & Roasted Pepper, Asda*	1 Jar/172g	91	5.2	53	1.5	5.0	3.0	2.4
Four Cheese, BGTY, Sainsbury's*	1 Serving/150g	104	6.0	69	2.9	5.5	4.0	0.1
Four Cheese, Fresh, Asda*	½ Pot/162g	309	28.8	191	5.4	2.2	17.8	0.5
Four Cheese, GFY, Asda*	½ Pot/175g	144	8.0	82	4.0	6.3	4.6	0.5
Garlic & Chilli, Slow Roasted, Seeds of Change*	½ Jar/175g	158	9.3	90	1.7	8.7	5.3	2.0
Garlic & Herbs, Low Fat, LC, Tesco*	1 Jar/500g	200	1.5	40	1.6	6.8	0.3	1.9
Garlic & Onion, Roasted, Weight Watchers*	1 Jar/175g	65	0.7	37	1.3	6.4	0.4	1.2
Ham & Mushroom, Pasta Bake, Creamy, Homepride*	1 Pack/425g	489	45.5	115	1.8	2.8	10.7	0.0
Hot & Spicy, Morrisons*	1 Serving/130g	81	3.1	62	1.4	8.5	2.4	1.1
Lasagne, Tomato, Red, Ragu, Knorr*	1 Jar/500g	215	0.0	43	1.1	9.7	0.0	1.1
Mushroom, Co-Op*	¼ Jar/125g	75	2.5	60	2.0	9.0	2.0	1.0
Mushroom, Fresh, Waitrose*	1 Serving/175g	142	10.0	81	1.6	5.7	5.7	0.5
Mushroom, Italian, Sainsbury's*	1 Serving/85g	56	1.8	66	2.0	9.8	2.1	1.7
Napoletana, Buitoni*	½ Jar/200g	146	8.2	73	1.6	7.3	4.1	2.2
Napoletana, Fresh, Waitrose*	1 Serving/175g	82	3.0	47	1.3	6.6	1.7	1.0
Napoletana, Morrisons*	1 Serving/175g	82	2.6	47	2.6	6.7	1.5	0.0
Onion & Roasted Garlic, Knorr*	1 Jar/500g	210	0.0	42	1.3	9.2	0.0	1.1
Original, Tesco*	1 Jar/300g	123	4.2	41	1.0	6.1	1.4	2.3
Original, with Tomato & Onions, Morrisons*	1 Serving/125g	51	1.4	41	1.4	6.3	1.1	1.2
Parmesan & Pesto, Weight Watchers*	½ Jar/175g	86	2.8	49	1.8	6.7	1.6	1.0
Pomodoro, Cirio*	1 Serving/200g	116	4.6	58	1.4	8.4	2.3	0.0
Primavera, Loyd Grossman*	1 Jar/350g	343	25.9	98	1.4	6.3	7.4	0.9
Puttanesca, Italian, Waitrose*	1 Jar/350g	195	9.8	56	1.5	6.1	2.8	1.3
Puttanesca, Loyd Grossman*	1 Jar/350g	315	21.7	90	1.7	6.8	6.2	0.9
Puttanesca, M&S*	1 Jar/320g	256	17.6	80	1.5	6.2	5.5	1.9
Red Pepper & Italian Cheese, Stir Through, Asda*	½ Jar/95g	86	4.7	90	2.9	8.5	4.9	0.9
Red Pepper & Tomato, Roasted, Finest, Tesco*	1 Serving/145g	117	7.8	81	1.2	6.8	5.4	2.2
Siciliana, Sainsbury's*	1/3 Jar/113g	168	14.7	149	1.8	6.2	13.0	0.0
Spinach & Ricotta, Asda*	½ Pot/175g	175	12.2	100	3.2	6.0	7.0	0.5
Sweet Pepper, Dolmio*	1 Serving/150g	238	20.1	159	1.6	8.8	13.4	0.0
Sweet Red Pepper, Loyd Grossman*	1 Jar/350g	304	19.6	87	1.7	7.3	5.6	1.2
Three Cheese, Co-Op*	1 Pack/300g	405	27.0	135	6.0	6.0	9.0	0.1
Tomato, Black Olive, Caper, Finest, Tesco*	1 Serving/145g	146	11.2	101	1.5	6.4	7.7	3.3
Tomato, Creamy, Pasta Bake, Dolmio*	1 Serving/125g	141	9.0	113	2.3	8.4	7.2	0.0
Tomato, Garlic & Basil, Sun Dried, Finest, Tesco*	1 Jar/340g	493	39.1	145	1.8	7.7	11.5	2.3
Tomato, Low Price, Sainsbury's*	1 Jar/440g	220	3.1	50	0.6	10.1	0.7	0.4
Tomato, Mushroom & Pancetta, Italian, Sainsbury's*	½ Jar/75g	125	11.2	167	2.2	6.1	14.9	1.3
Tomato, Sun Dried, Stir In, Light, Dolmio*	1 Serving/75g	62	3.5	83	1.7	9.8	4.7	0.0
Tomato & Bacon, Creamy, Pasta Bake, Homepride*	1 Serving/110g	99	6.9	90	1.9	6.5	6.3	0.0
Tomato & Bacon, Smoky, Dolmio*	1 Pot/150g	240	19.6	160	5.5	5.8	13.1	0.0
Tomato & Bacon, Stir & Serve, Homepride*	1 Serving/96g	81	4.3	84	2.7	8.1	4.5	0.0
Tomato & Basil, Bertolli*	1 Jar/500g	215	5.0	43	1.2	7.3	1.0	0.4
Tomato & Basil, Classic, Sacla*	1 Serving/100g	137	11.1	137	2.0	7.2	11.1	2.8
Tomato & Basil, Creamy, BGTY, Sainsbury's*	½ Jar/250g	172	9.0	69	1.7	7.6	3.6	1.0
Tomato & Basil, Dolmio*	1 Serving/170g	95	3.6	56	1.4	7.9	2.1	0.0
Tomato & Basil, Loyd Grossman*	½ Jar/175g	107	6.0	61	1.5	5.8	3.4	0.8
Tomato & Basil, M&S*	1 Jar/340g	119	7.1	35	2.0	2.1	2.1	0.9
Tomato & Basil, Organic, Pasta Reale*	1 Pack/300g	216	15.9	72	1.0	5.1	5.3	0.4
Tomato & Basil, Organic, Simply Organic*	1 Pot/300g	183	12.9	61	1.5	4.2	4.3	0.6
Tomato & Basil, Pesto, Rich, Express, Dolmio*	1 Pack/170g	146	10.0	86	2.0	6.2	5.9	0.0
Tomato & Basil, Sun Dried, Free From, Sainsbury's*	½ Jar/172g	124	4.8	72	2.9	8.7	2.8	1.5
Tomato & Basil, Sun Dried, Organic, Seeds of Change*	½ Jar/100g	155	13.1	155	1.6	7.7	13.1	0.0
Tomato & Basil, Sun Ripened, Dolmio*	1 Serving/150g	117	6.9	78	1.3	7.9	4.6	0.0

PASTA SAUCE	Measure INFO/WEIGHT	per Measure KCAL	FAT	Nutrition Values per 100g / 100ml KCAL	PROT	CARB	FAT	FIBRE
Tomato & Basil, Sun Ripened, Express, Dolmio*	1 Pouch/170g	88	2.7	52	1.5	7.9	1.6	0.0
Tomato & Basil, Sun Ripened, Microwaveable, Dolmio*	½ Pack/190g	106	4.0	56	1.4	7.9	2.1	0.0
Tomato & Cheese, Pasta Bake, Dolmio*	¼ Jar/125g	70	1.5	56	2.1	9.1	1.2	1.2
Tomato & Chilli, Pour Over, M&S*	1 Jar/330g	231	12.5	70	1.3	7.6	3.8	1.8
Tomato & Chilli, Whole Cherry Tomatoes, Sacla*	½ Jar/175g	238	19.2	136	2.0	7.2	11.0	3.1
Tomato & Garlic, & Pecorino Romano Cheese, Bertolli*	1 Serving/125g	76	3.5	61	2.3	6.5	2.8	0.9
Tomato & Garlic, CBY, Asda*	½ Jar/160g	74	0.8	46	1.6	7.9	0.5	1.7
Tomato & Garlic, Roasted, Loyd Grossman*	½ Jar/175g	107	5.4	61	1.5	6.3	3.1	0.8
Tomato & Garlic, Sun Dried, Sacla*	1 Serving/95g	177	14.0	186	3.0	10.3	14.7	0.0
Tomato & Herb, Creamy, Pasta Bake, Homepride*	1 Serving/125g	128	8.8	102	1.5	8.3	7.0	0.9
Tomato & Herb, M&S*	1 Jar/500g	400	15.5	80	2.6	10.1	3.1	1.7
Tomato & Herb, Organic, M&S*	1 Jar/550g	302	19.8	55	1.4	4.2	3.6	2.6
Tomato & Herb, with Extra Garlic, Sainsbury's*	½ Pot/150g	62	1.6	41	1.4	6.3	1.1	1.6
Tomato & Mascarpone, Finest, Tesco*	1 Serving/175g	135	8.8	77	2.7	5.4	5.0	0.8
Tomato & Mascarpone, Fresh, Sainsbury's*	1 Serving/150g	177	15.4	118	2.2	4.2	10.3	1.1
Tomato & Mascarpone, Morrisons*	½ Pot/175g	217	16.8	124	2.9	6.5	9.6	1.1
Tomato & Mascarpone, Sacla*	½ Jar/95g	161	14.2	169	2.2	6.2	15.0	0.0
Tomato & Mascarpone, Sainsbury's*	½ Pot/150g	137	9.9	91	2.1	5.9	6.6	1.2
Tomato & Mascarpone, Waitrose*	½ Pot/175g	184	14.7	105	1.9	5.5	8.4	1.1
Tomato & Mushroom, & Roasted Garlic, Bertolli*	1 Jar/500g	235	9.5	47	1.9	5.3	1.9	0.0
Tomato & Mushroom, CBY, Asda*	½ Jar/160g	70	1.0	44	2.1	7.0	0.6	1.1
Tomato & Mushroom, Cucina, Aldi*	1 Jar/500g	165	1.0	33	1.1	5.7	0.2	1.9
Tomato & Mushroom, Organic, Sainsbury's*	1 Serving/150g	87	3.9	58	1.6	7.1	2.6	1.5
Tomato & Mushroom, Wild, Loyd Grossman*	½ Jar/175g	154	9.8	88	2.1	7.4	5.6	1.5
Tomato & Olive, Sacla*	1 Serving/95g	87	7.6	92	1.3	3.6	8.0	0.0
Tomato & Parmesan, Seeds of Change*	1 Serving/150g	100	4.4	67	2.5	7.8	2.9	1.1
Tomato & Pepper, M&S*	1 Jar/320g	224	13.4	70	1.6	6.1	4.2	0.9
Tomato & Ricotta, Italian, Sainsbury's*	1 Pack/390g	238	11.7	61	2.5	6.1	3.0	1.2
Tomato & Roasted Pepper, Whole Cherry Tomatoes, Sacla*	½ Jar/145g	93	5.9	64	1.5	5.2	4.1	0.0
Tomato & Sausage, Spicy, M&S*	1 Jar/330g	214	9.9	65	4.0	5.5	3.0	0.8
Tomato & Tuna, Loyd Grossman*	½ Jar/175g	154	7.7	88	4.4	7.5	4.4	0.8
Tomato & Vegetable, Chargrilled, Loyd Grossman*	1 Serving/150g	134	8.4	89	1.8	7.9	5.6	0.9
Tuna, Pasta Bake, Homepride*	½ Jar/250g	208	13.0	83	1.4	7.6	5.2	0.9
Tuna, Pasta Bake, Mix, Dry, Colman's*	1 Sachet/45g	145	2.3	323	9.2	60.0	5.2	4.7
Vegetable, Chargrilled, with Extra Virgin Olive Oil, Bertolli*	½ Jar/250g	150	4.8	60	2.1	8.7	1.9	2.4
Vegetable, Chunky, Tesco*	1 Jar/500g	235	5.0	47	1.8	6.8	1.0	1.8
Vegetable, Mediterranean, Organic, Seeds of Change*	1 Jar/350g	245	12.2	70	1.5	8.3	3.5	1.1
Vegetable, Roasted, Sainsbury's*	½ Pot/151g	103	5.9	68	1.6	6.7	3.9	0.4
Vegetable, Roasted, Tesco*	1 Pack/175g	114	5.2	65	1.5	8.0	3.0	0.8
PASTA SHAPES								
Alphabetti, in Tomato Sauce, Heinz*	1 Can/200g	118	1.0	59	1.8	11.7	0.5	1.5
Bob The Builder, in Tomato Sauce, Heinz*	1 Can/205g	111	0.6	54	1.7	11.3	0.3	1.5
Cooked, Tesco*	1 Serving/260g	356	2.1	137	5.1	26.3	0.8	1.1
Disney Princess in Tomato Sauce, Heinz*	1 Can/200g	114	0.6	57	1.8	11.9	0.3	1.5
Durum Wheat, Dry, Basics, Sainsbury's*	1 Serving/75g	260	1.5	346	12.0	70.0	2.0	4.0
Postman Pat, HP*	1 Can/410g	279	1.6	68	1.8	14.3	0.4	0.7
Scooby Doo, HP*	1 Can/410g	279	1.6	68	1.8	14.3	0.4	0.7
Shrek, in Tomato Sauce, Multigrain, Omega 3, Heinz*	1 Can/200g	120	1.0	60	1.9	12.0	0.5	1.5
Thomas Tank Engine, in Tomato Sauce, Heinz*	1 Can/205g	109	0.4	53	1.7	11.0	0.2	0.5
Tweenies, in Tomato Sauce, Heinz*	1 Can/205g	121	1.0	59	1.8	11.7	0.5	1.5
PASTA SHELLS								
Dry, Average	1 Serving/75g	265	1.5	353	11.1	71.8	2.0	2.0
Egg, Fresh, Average	1 Serving/125g	344	3.6	275	11.5	49.8	2.8	3.4

	Measure INFO/WEIGHT	per Measure		Nutrition Values per 100g / 100ml				
		KCAL	FAT	KCAL	PROT	CARB	FAT	FIBRE

PASTA SHELLS

	Measure INFO/WEIGHT	KCAL	FAT	KCAL	PROT	CARB	FAT	FIBRE
Fresh, Dry, Average	**1 Serving/125g**	**216**	**2.1**	**173**	**7.4**	**32.0**	**1.6**	**1.6**
Wholewheat, Healthy Living, Co-Op*	1 Serving/75g	232	0.8	310	11.0	64.0	1.0	12.0

PASTA SNACK

Cheese, Creamy, Mug Shot, Made Up, Symingtons*	1 Serving/271g	301	6.0	111	3.7	19.1	2.2	1.0
Cheese & Ham, Pot, Tesco*	1 Serving/208g	254	8.5	122	3.4	17.9	4.1	1.5
Chicken, Roast, Mug Shot, Made Up, Symingtons*	1 Serving/258g	204	2.6	79	1.4	16.2	1.0	0.8
Sweet & Sour, Mug Shot, Made Up, Symingtons*	1 Serving/275g	239	1.9	87	2.2	19.5	0.7	1.2
Tomato & Herb in a Pot, Dry, Tesco*	1 Pot/59g	207	1.4	352	11.8	70.7	2.4	2.6
Tomato 'n' Herb, Made Up, Mug Shot*	1 Serving/257g	265	2.1	103	2.3	21.6	0.8	1.2

PASTA TWIRLS

Dry, Asda*	1 Serving/50g	173	0.8	346	12.0	71.0	1.5	3.0
Tri-Colour, Sainsbury's*	1 Serving/75g	268	1.3	357	12.3	73.1	1.7	2.5

PASTA TWISTS

Wheat & GF, Glutafin*	1 Serving/75g	262	1.5	350	8.0	75.0	2.0	0.1

PASTA WITH

Cheese & Tomato, Al Forno, Sainsbury's*	½ Pack/499g	749	29.0	150	5.5	18.9	5.8	1.8
Chicken, Spicy, Sainsbury's*	1 Pot/300g	489	18.3	163	7.1	20.1	6.1	2.3
Chicken, Tomato & Basil, BGTY, Sainsbury's*	1 Pack/189g	250	2.1	132	9.2	21.2	1.1	2.7
Feta Cheese & Slow Roasted Tomatoes, M&S*	1 Pack/190g	332	13.3	175	6.0	22.3	7.0	2.4
Pesto, Spinach & Pine Nuts, Tesco*	1 Pack/300g	480	22.2	160	5.2	17.1	7.4	1.5
Salmon & Broccoli, Lemon Dressed, Sainsbury's*	1 Serving/300g	486	17.7	162	6.9	20.4	5.9	2.1
Tuna & Roasted Peppers, M&S*	1 Serving/220g	308	8.6	140	9.1	17.7	3.9	0.9
Vegetables, Mediterranean, Pasta King*	1 Serving/100g	121	3.2	121	3.7	19.3	3.2	2.1
Vegetables & Tomatoes, Chargrilled, BGTY, Sainsbury's*	1 Serving/100g	96	1.6	96	2.9	17.4	1.6	0.0

PASTE

Beef, Asda*	1 Serving/37g	72	5.2	194	17.0	0.1	14.0	0.0
Beef, Princes*	1 Serving/18g	40	2.8	220	14.4	5.2	15.8	0.0
Beef, Sainsbury's*	1 Jar/75g	142	9.9	189	16.0	1.5	13.2	1.4
Chicken, Princes*	1 Thin Spread/9g	22	1.7	240	12.6	5.6	18.5	0.0
Chicken, Tesco*	1 Serving/12g	30	2.4	248	14.8	2.3	20.0	0.1
Chicken, Value, Tesco*	1 Thin Spread/9g	18	1.3	196	15.1	1.8	14.3	0.1
Chicken & Ham, Asda*	½ Jar/38g	82	6.5	217	14.0	2.1	17.0	0.0
Chicken & Ham, Princes*	1 Jar/100g	233	18.6	233	13.6	2.8	18.6	0.0
Chicken & Ham, Sainsbury's*	1 Thin Spread/9g	14	0.9	158	16.0	1.1	10.0	1.1
Crab, Princes*	1 Pot/35g	36	1.2	104	13.4	4.8	3.5	0.0
Crab, Sainsbury's*	1 Thick Spread/5g	6	0.2	115	16.5	1.7	4.7	0.5
Crab, Tesco*	1 Jar/75g	116	6.3	155	14.4	4.6	8.4	0.1
Fruit, Golden Quince, Lowry Peaks*	1 Tsp/5g	16	0.0	321	0.8	83.6	0.2	0.0
Salmon, Asda*	1 Serving/53g	76	3.7	143	15.0	5.0	7.0	0.0
Salmon, Princes*	1 Serving/30g	58	3.8	195	13.5	6.5	12.8	0.0
Salmon, Value, Tesco*	1 Serving/10g	16	1.0	165	14.0	4.6	10.1	0.8
Salmon & Shrimp, Tesco*	1 Jar/75g	83	2.6	111	15.1	5.0	3.4	0.1
Sardine & Tomato, Asda*	1 Thin Spread/9g	11	0.5	123	14.0	3.3	6.0	0.0
Sardine & Tomato, Princes*	1 Jar/75g	130	8.1	173	13.9	3.4	10.8	3.2
Sardine & Tomato, Sainsbury's*	1 Mini Pot/35g	60	3.8	170	16.9	1.2	10.8	1.3
Sardine & Tomato, Tesco*	1 Jar/75g	98	4.4	130	14.6	4.8	5.8	0.1
Tagine, Lemon, Spicy, Al'fez*	1 Tsp/6g	13	0.9	216	3.1	17.6	14.8	4.6
Tuna & Mayonnaise, Princes*	1 Pot/75g	86	12.3	115	16.8	3.8	16.4	0.0
Tuna & Mayonnaise, Sainsbury's*	1 Tbsp/17g	41	3.1	242	19.2	0.6	18.1	1.6
Tuna & Mayonnaise, Tesco*	1 Serving/15g	31	2.4	209	14.9	2.1	15.7	0.1

PASTILLES

Blackcurrant, Rowntree's*	1 Tube/53g	188	0.0	353	4.4	84.0	0.0	0.0
Fruit, Average	1 Tube/33g	108	0.0	327	2.8	84.2	0.0	0.0

INFO/WEIGHT	Measure	per Measure		Nutrition Values per 100g / 100ml				
		KCAL	FAT	KCAL	PROT	CARB	FAT	FIBRE
PASTILLES								
Fruit, Co-Op*	1 Sweet/6g	20	0.0	337	2.8	81.5	0.0	0.0
Fruit, Rowntree's*	1 Tube/53g	186	0.0	351	4.4	83.7	0.0	0.0
Fruit, Sainsbury's*	1 Sweet/7g	23	0.0	332	3.4	78.7	0.1	0.1
Wine, Maynards*	1 Sweet/5g	15	0.0	325	6.1	75.0	0.0	0.0
PASTRAMI								
Beef, Average	**1 Serving/40g**	**51**	**1.4**	**128**	**23.1**	**1.1**	**3.6**	**0.2**
Coriander, Paprika & Black Pepper, TTD, Sainsbury's*	1 Slice/10g	12	0.3	121	21.6	1.0	3.4	0.0
Turkey, Average	**½ Pack/35g**	**38**	**0.5**	**107**	**21.8**	**1.7**	**1.5**	**0.5**
PASTRY								
Case, From Supermarket, Average	**1 Case/230g**	**1081**	**58.9**	**470**	**5.8**	**55.9**	**25.6**	**1.2**
Choux, Cooked, Average	**1oz/28g**	**91**	**5.5**	**325**	**8.5**	**29.8**	**19.8**	**1.2**
Choux, Raw, Average	**1oz/28g**	**59**	**3.6**	**211**	**5.5**	**19.4**	**12.9**	**0.8**
Filo, Average	**1 Sheet/45g**	**137**	**1.2**	**304**	**9.0**	**61.4**	**2.7**	**0.9**
Flaky, Chinese, Average	**1oz/28g**	**110**	**4.6**	**392**	**5.4**	**59.3**	**16.4**	**0.0**
Flaky, Cooked, Average	**1oz/28g**	**157**	**11.4**	**560**	**5.6**	**45.9**	**40.6**	**1.8**
Flaky, Raw, Average	**1oz/28g**	**119**	**8.6**	**424**	**4.2**	**34.8**	**30.7**	**1.4**
Flan Case, Average	**1 Case/113g**	**615**	**38.0**	**544**	**7.1**	**56.7**	**33.6**	**1.8**
Greek, Average	**1oz/28g**	**90**	**4.8**	**322**	**4.7**	**40.0**	**17.0**	**0.0**
Puff, Frozen, Average	**1 Serving/47g**	**188**	**12.0**	**400**	**5.0**	**29.2**	**25.6**	**0.0**
Shortcrust, Cooked, Average	**1oz/28g**	**146**	**9.0**	**521**	**6.6**	**54.2**	**32.3**	**2.2**
Shortcrust, Raw, Average	**1oz/28g**	**127**	**8.1**	**453**	**5.6**	**44.0**	**29.1**	**1.3**
Spring Roll, Wrapper, TYJ Food Manufacturing*	1 Sheet/18g	54	0.0	300	0.0	73.0	0.0	0.0
Wholemeal, Cooked, Average	**1oz/28g**	**140**	**9.2**	**499**	**8.9**	**44.6**	**32.9**	**6.3**
Wholemeal, Raw, Average	**1oz/28g**	**121**	**8.0**	**431**	**7.7**	**38.5**	**28.4**	**5.4**
PASTY								
Beef, Port Royal*	1 Pattie/130g	299	13.3	230	10.2	24.4	10.2	0.0
Cheese & Onion, Average	1 Pasty/150g	435	27.6	290	7.3	24.5	18.4	1.4
Cheese & Onion, Farmfoods*	1 Pasty/191g	485	26.7	254	6.6	25.5	14.0	2.0
Cheese & Onion, Geo Adams*	1 Pasty/150g	420	23.4	280	6.9	27.9	15.6	1.1
Cheese & Onion, Sainsbury's*	1 Serving/150g	486	32.7	324	7.4	24.5	21.8	1.3
Cheese & Onion, Tesco*	1 Pasty/150g	416	26.4	277	5.9	23.7	17.6	2.2
Cheese & Onion, Three Cheese, Ginsters*	1 Pasty/180g	531	36.9	295	8.0	19.7	20.5	3.1
Chese & Onion, Cheddar, Hand Crimped, Waitrose*	1 Pasty/200g	546	42.2	273	8.8	22.5	21.1	2.2
Chicken, & Bacon, Ginsters*	1 Pasty/180g	457	29.0	254	8.0	19.3	16.1	2.8
Chicken, & Vegetable, Proper Cornish Ltd*	1 Pasty/255g	671	34.7	263	7.4	30.2	13.6	2.4
Chicken, Port Royal*	1 Pattie/130g	289	10.9	222	5.5	31.2	8.4	0.0
Cornish, Asda*	1 Pasty/100g	287	19.0	287	7.0	22.0	19.0	1.2
Cornish, Average	1 Pasty/160g	450	27.7	281	7.0	24.2	17.3	1.6
Cornish, BGTY, Sainsbury's*	1 Pasty/135g	308	12.7	228	7.7	28.2	9.4	1.6
Cornish, Cheese & Onion, Ginsters*	1 Pasty/130g	511	33.0	393	10.4	30.7	25.4	2.3
Cornish, Co-Op*	1 Pasty/75g	200	12.3	267	6.4	23.4	16.4	1.6
Cornish, Crimped, TTD, Sainsbury's*	1 Pasty/200g	515	28.7	258	8.3	23.7	14.4	1.2
Cornish, Frozen, Oven Baked, Iceland*	1 Pasty/167g	501	29.2	300	7.5	22.0	17.5	0.0
Cornish, Mini, Iceland*	1 Pasty/70g	215	14.8	306	7.0	22.1	21.1	1.2
Cornish, Mini, M&S*	1 Pasty/75g	244	17.6	325	7.3	21.9	23.4	1.8
Cornish, Mini, Sainsbury's*	1 Pasty/70g	280	20.1	400	7.3	28.1	28.7	1.5
Cornish, Mini, Tesco*	1 Pasty/24g	66	4.2	274	5.6	23.2	17.7	0.5
Cornish, Morrisons*	1 Pasty/200g	626	37.0	313	7.5	29.1	18.5	0.0
Cornish, Original, Ginsters*	1 Pasty/227g	549	32.2	242	5.3	23.2	14.2	3.1
Cornish, Roaster, Ginsters*	1 Pasty/130g	417	24.2	321	8.5	29.9	18.6	1.3
Cornish, Sainsbury's*	1 Pasty/150g	489	32.1	326	6.7	26.6	21.4	2.0
Cornish, Smart Price, Asda*	1 Pasty/94g	286	15.0	304	8.0	32.0	16.0	1.7
Cornish, Snack Pack, Six, Ginsters*	1 Pasty/40g	116	8.0	289	7.2	20.3	19.9	2.8

	Measure INFO/WEIGHT	per Measure		Nutrition Values per 100g / 100ml				
		KCAL	FAT	KCAL	PROT	CARB	FAT	FIBRE
PASTY								
Cornish, Tesco*	1 Pasty/150g	466	32.7	311	6.8	21.9	21.8	1.6
Cornish, Traditional Style, Geo Adams*	1 Pasty/165g	488	30.4	296	7.1	25.4	18.4	1.3
Cornish, Value, Tesco*	1 Pasty/150g	425	26.6	283	6.7	24.2	17.7	2.2
Lamb, Port Royal*	1 Pattie/130g	352	17.4	271	7.2	30.5	13.4	0.0
Olive & Cheese, Tapas, Waitrose*	1 Pack/130g	455	25.2	350	8.1	35.8	19.4	1.3
Salt Fish, Port Royal*	1 Pattie/130g	300	13.4	231	6.8	27.8	10.3	0.0
Vegetable	1oz/28g	77	4.2	274	4.1	33.3	14.9	1.9
Vegetable, Hand Crimped, Waitrose*	1 Pasty/200g	454	22.6	227	4.5	26.8	11.3	2.2
Vegetarian, Country Slice, Linda McCartney*	1 Pasty/150g	373	20.2	249	5.6	26.5	13.5	2.9
Vegetarian, Port Royal*	1 Pattie/130g	315	13.8	242	12.5	24.1	10.6	0.0
PATE								
Apricot, Asda*	1 Serving/50g	156	14.0	312	12.0	3.0	28.0	0.0
Ardennes, Asda*	1 Serving/50g	143	12.0	286	13.9	3.6	24.0	1.3
Ardennes, BGTY, Sainsbury's*	¼ Pack/50g	90	5.7	180	16.6	2.9	11.4	0.0
Ardennes, Iceland*	1 Serving/70g	223	20.0	318	12.0	3.4	28.5	0.5
Ardennes, Reduced Fat, Waitrose*	¼ Pack/42g	94	7.1	224	15.4	2.6	16.9	0.5
Ardennes, Tesco*	1 Tbsp/15g	53	5.0	354	13.3	0.5	33.2	1.2
Ardennes, with Bacon, Tesco*	½ Pack/85g	241	20.6	284	11.4	5.1	24.2	1.1
Aubergine, Spiced, Waitrose*	¼ Pack/38g	71	5.2	186	4.9	10.9	13.6	2.4
Breton, Country with Apricots, Coarse, Sainsbury's*	1 Serving/21g	60	4.7	285	13.5	7.0	22.5	0.5
Brussels, & Garlic, Reduced Fat, Tesco*	1 Serving/65g	135	8.0	208	16.2	8.1	12.3	0.6
Brussels, & Garlic, Tesco*	1 Serving/40g	145	13.5	363	8.7	6.0	33.8	0.0
Brussels, & Mushroom, Mini, GFY, Asda*	1 Pack/40g	67	4.4	167	14.7	2.3	11.0	3.9
Brussels, 25% Less Fat, Morrisons*	¼ Pack/43g	106	8.8	249	14.2	0.7	20.6	0.0
Brussels, BGTY, 50% Less Fat, Sainsbury's*	1 Serving/100g	223	16.0	223	14.6	5.1	16.0	0.1
Brussels, Co-Op*	1 Serving/15g	51	4.6	340	11.0	4.0	31.0	2.0
Brussels, Fat Reduced, Somerfield*	1 Serving/50g	96	7.0	192	14.0	2.0	14.0	0.0
Brussels, Finest, Tesco*	½ Pack/85g	306	28.7	360	8.6	5.2	33.8	0.8
Brussels, M&S*	1 Pot/170g	518	45.2	305	13.3	2.8	26.6	1.0
Brussels, Reduced Fat, Tesco*	1 Pack/175g	420	33.2	240	11.1	5.8	19.0	1.4
Brussels, Sainsbury's*	1 Pack/170g	663	64.9	390	10.6	1.1	38.2	0.1
Brussels, Smooth, 50% Less Fat, Tesco*	1 Pack/175g	350	26.8	200	14.1	1.2	15.3	1.8
Brussels, Smooth, Reduced, Tesco*	1 Serving/40g	82	6.4	205	10.7	4.5	16.0	0.6
Brussels, Smooth, Reduced Fat, Tesco*	1 Serving/15g	30	2.3	200	14.1	1.2	15.3	1.8
Brussels, Smooth, Spreadable, Sainsbury's*	1 Serving/30g	97	8.7	323	10.7	4.7	29.0	0.0
Brussels, Style, Organic, The Redwood Co*	¼ Pack/30g	82	6.1	273	15.2	8.0	20.4	1.3
Brussels, Tesco*	1 Serving/28g	92	8.5	330	11.0	3.0	30.5	1.1
Brussels, with Forest Mushroom, Co-Op*	1 Serving/57g	180	16.5	315	12.0	2.0	29.0	1.0
Brussels, with Garlic, Asda*	1 Serving/50g	170	15.6	340	10.7	4.0	31.3	2.5
Brussels, with Herbs, Tesco*	1 Serving/25g	87	8.2	347	8.4	6.4	32.6	1.5
Celery, Stilton & Walnut, Waitrose*	1 Pot/115g	294	26.4	256	9.0	3.2	23.0	2.2
Chick Pea & Black Olive, Cauldron Foods*	1 Pot/113g	193	11.9	171	7.6	11.4	10.5	6.6
Chicken & Brandy, Morrisons*	1 Serving/44g	133	11.8	303	10.8	4.3	26.9	0.8
Chicken Liver, Asda*	1 Serving/65g	131	10.4	202	13.0	4.0	16.0	0.8
Chicken Liver, BGTY, Sainsbury's*	1 Serving/30g	64	4.8	214	11.5	6.0	16.0	0.5
Chicken Liver, M&S*	1oz/28g	79	6.7	281	14.0	1.9	24.1	0.1
Chicken Liver, Organic, Waitrose*	½ Tub/88g	204	16.1	233	12.6	1.8	18.4	1.4
Chicken Liver & Brandy, Asda*	1 Serving/50g	176	16.4	353	9.0	5.5	32.8	3.2
Chicken Liver & Garlic, Smooth, Asda*	1 Serving/31g	119	11.1	388	9.0	7.0	36.0	3.2
Chicken Liver with Brandy, Tesco*	1oz/28g	82	7.2	293	11.8	3.5	25.8	1.4
Chicken Liver with Madeira, Sainsbury's*	1 Serving/30g	84	7.3	279	13.1	1.9	24.3	0.0
Chickpea, Moroccan, Organic, Cauldron Foods*	½ Pot/58g	119	7.9	207	6.8	16.3	13.7	4.9
Crab, M&S*	1oz/28g	63	4.8	225	12.1	5.9	17.3	0.0

F

PATE

PATE	Measure INFO/WEIGHT	per Measure KCAL	FAT	Nutrition Values per 100g / 100ml KCAL	PROT	CARB	FAT	FIBRE
Crab, Terrine, Orkney, Luxury, Castle MacLellan*	1 Tub/113g	250	21.4	221	7.3	5.5	18.9	0.9
Crab, Waitrose*	1 Pot/113g	218	16.7	193	12.4	2.5	14.8	0.9
De Campagne, Sainsbury's*	1 Serving/55g	129	10.0	235	16.3	1.4	18.2	0.0
Duck, & Champagne, Luxury, M&S*	1oz/28g	106	9.9	380	8.3	8.3	35.2	7.8
Duck, & Orange, Asda*	1 Serving/40g	94	7.2	235	16.0	2.2	18.0	0.0
Duck, & Orange, Smooth, Tesco*	1 Serving/50g	188	17.7	377	10.5	4.0	35.4	0.5
Duck, & Truffle, Medallions, M&S*	1 Serving/25g	91	8.8	365	9.0	4.8	35.0	1.4
Farmhouse, Coarse, Organic, Sainsbury's*	1 Serving/56g	138	11.0	246	13.3	3.7	19.7	0.8
Farmhouse, Mushroom, Asda*	1 Serving/50g	126	10.0	252	13.0	5.0	20.0	0.7
Farmhouse, Style, Finest, Tesco*	1 Serving/28g	83	7.3	295	11.9	3.6	25.9	1.0
Farmhouse, Style, M&S*	¼ Pack/42g	90	7.1	215	14.4	1.9	16.9	1.2
Farmhouse, with Christmas Ale, Sainsbury's*	1oz/28g	67	5.3	239	15.4	1.6	19.1	0.0
Farmhouse, with Herbes De Provence, Tesco*	1 Serving/50g	136	10.8	273	13.9	5.4	21.6	1.0
Farmhouse, with Mushrooms & Garlic, Tesco*	1 Serving/90g	256	22.8	285	13.8	0.6	25.3	1.3
Forestiere, M&S*	1 Serving/20g	61	5.3	305	11.5	4.2	26.6	1.4
Kipper, Waitrose*	¼ Tub/28g	105	9.2	370	16.8	2.0	32.7	0.6
Liver, Value, Tesco*	1 Serving/50g	151	13.0	302	13.0	4.1	26.0	0.5
Liver & Bacon, Spreading, Value, Tesco*	1 Roll/150g	423	37.2	282	12.7	2.1	24.8	1.4
Mackerel, Smoked	1oz/28g	103	9.6	368	13.4	1.3	34.4	0.0
Mackerel, Smoked, M&S*	1oz/28g	104	9.7	370	13.4	0.7	34.7	0.3
Mackerel, Smoked, Sainsbury's*	½ Pot/57g	215	20.1	378	14.2	0.8	35.3	0.0
Mackerel, Smoked, Scottish, M&S*	½ Pot/58g	158	13.3	275	15.9	0.6	23.2	0.1
Mackerel, Tesco*	1 Serving/29g	102	9.5	353	14.3	0.5	32.6	0.0
Mushroom, & Tarragon, Waitrose*	1 Serving/30g	46	4.0	155	2.8	5.5	13.5	1.4
Mushroom, BGTY, Sainsbury's*	½ Pot/58g	29	0.3	50	4.6	6.7	0.5	3.0
Mushroom, M&S*	1 Pot/115g	224	20.1	195	4.2	4.8	17.5	1.5
Mushroom, Roast, Tesco*	1 Serving/25g	36	3.2	145	3.6	3.6	12.9	4.5
Mushroom, Sainsbury's*	½ Pot/58g	89	7.0	153	3.3	7.8	12.1	2.1
Mushroom, Tesco*	1oz/28g	39	2.7	138	3.3	9.8	9.5	1.0
Parsnip, & Carrot, Roasted, Organic, Cauldron Foods*	1 Pot/115g	132	7.7	115	3.5	10.2	6.7	4.9
Pork, & Garlic, Somerfield*	1oz/28g	83	7.0	295	14.0	3.0	25.0	0.0
Pork, & Mushroom, Somerfield*	1oz/28g	95	8.7	339	11.0	3.0	31.0	0.0
Pork, with Apple & Cider, Sainsbury's*	1 Serving/50g	152	12.6	303	12.5	6.3	25.3	1.1
Pork, with Peppercorns, Tesco*	1 Serving/28g	84	7.5	300	12.9	1.4	26.8	0.7
Pork Liver, with Garlic, Coarse, Asda*	1 Pack/40g	130	12.0	326	13.0	1.0	30.0	0.0
Red Pepper & Houmous, Roasted, Princes*	¼ Jar/27g	32	1.6	120	4.6	12.4	5.8	0.0
Salmon, Dill, Princes*	1 Serving/70g	124	7.8	177	15.4	4.0	11.1	0.5
Salmon, Organic, M&S*	1oz/28g	76	6.3	270	16.9	0.0	22.5	0.0
Salmon, Scottish, Smoked, M&S*	1 Serving/30g	81	6.7	270	17.0	0.2	22.3	0.0
Salmon, Smoked, Isle of Skye, TTD, Sainsbury's*	½ Pot/58g	133	9.8	231	17.5	1.8	17.1	0.2
Salmon, Smoked, Luxury, Morrisons*	½ Pot/57g	150	12.4	266	16.0	0.9	22.0	0.5
Salmon, Smoked, M&S*	1oz/28g	74	6.2	265	16.9	0.0	22.0	0.0
Salmon, Smoked, Organic, Waitrose*	1oz/28g	83	7.2	296	13.9	2.4	25.6	0.0
Salmon, Smoked, Scottish, Castle MacLellan*	¼ Tub/28g	62	4.5	220	13.5	5.6	16.0	0.0
Salmon, Smoked, Tesco*	1 Pack/115g	282	22.0	245	15.0	3.0	19.1	1.0
Salmon, Smoked, Waitrose*	½ Pot/57g	120	8.9	212	17.1	0.5	15.7	0.6
Tofu, Spicy Mexican, Organic, GranoVita*	1 Serving/50g	108	10.0	216	6.0	3.0	20.0	0.0
Tomato, Lentil & Basil, Cauldron Foods*	1 Pot/115g	161	7.8	140	6.8	14.0	6.8	3.2
Trout, Smoked, Waitrose*	½ Pot/56g	130	10.3	232	15.8	0.9	18.4	0.0
Tuna, M&S*	1oz/28g	106	9.5	380	17.0	0.8	33.8	0.7
Tuna, Tesco*	1 Pack/115g	332	26.7	289	19.8	0.3	23.2	0.2
Tuna, with Butter & Lemon Juice, Sainsbury's*	½ Pot/58g	209	18.3	360	19.0	0.1	31.6	0.3
Vegetable	1oz/28g	48	3.8	173	7.5	5.9	13.4	0.0

	Measure INFO/WEIGHT	per Measure KCAL	FAT	Nutrition Values per 100g / 100ml KCAL	PROT	CARB	FAT	FIBRE
PATE								
Vegetable, Mediterranean, Roast, Tesco*	1 Serving/28g	31	2.6	112	2.4	4.3	9.4	1.2
Vegetarian, with Mushrooms, Organic, Tartex*	¼ Tube/50g	102	8.0	203	7.7	7.0	16.0	0.0
Yeast, Garlic & Herb, Tartex*	1 Serving/30g	69	5.4	230	7.0	10.0	18.0	0.0
Yeast, Pateole, GranoVita*	1 Portion/30g	66	5.3	219	10.2	4.5	17.8	0.0
Yeast, Wild Mushroom, GranoVita*	1oz/28g	60	4.8	213	10.0	5.0	17.0	0.0
PAVLOVA								
Raspberry, & Lemon, Asda*	1 Serving/43g	102	1.9	235	2.8	46.0	4.4	0.5
Raspberry, Co-Op*	1/6 Pavlova/49g	147	5.9	300	3.2	44.8	12.0	1.1
Raspberry, Individual, M&S*	1 Pavlova/65g	133	1.6	205	4.0	41.8	2.4	0.2
Raspberry, M&S*	1 Serving/84g	193	8.1	230	2.3	33.3	9.6	0.3
Raspberry, Sara Lee*	1/6 Pavlova/55g	168	8.5	303	2.7	38.5	15.3	1.1
Raspberry, Tesco*	1 Serving/65g	191	8.4	294	2.7	41.8	12.9	1.1
Sticky Toffee, Sainsbury's*	1/6 Pavlova/60g	249	9.8	415	3.7	63.1	16.4	0.9
Strawberry, Co-Op*	1 Serving/52g	177	7.3	340	3.0	50.0	14.0	0.4
Strawberry, COU, M&S*	1 Pot/95g	147	2.3	155	2.4	30.5	2.4	0.8
Strawberry, Farmfoods*	1/6 Pavlova/52g	152	7.8	292	2.3	36.9	15.0	2.2
Toffee, Co-Op*	1/6 Pavlova/53g	193	8.5	365	3.0	52.0	16.0	0.6
PAW-PAW								
Raw, Fresh	*1oz/28g*	*10*	*0.0*	*36*	*0.5*	*8.8*	*0.1*	*2.2*
Raw, Weighed with Skin & Pips	*1oz/28g*	*8*	*0.0*	*27*	*0.4*	*6.6*	*0.1*	*1.7*
PEACH								
Dried, Average	*1 Pack/250g*	*472*	*1.6*	*189*	*2.6*	*45.0*	*0.6*	*6.9*
in Fruit Juice, Average	*1oz/28g*	*13*	*0.0*	*47*	*0.5*	*11.2*	*0.0*	*0.7*
in Light Syrup, Average	*1 Serving/100g*	*66*	*0.0*	*66*	*0.4*	*15.9*	*0.0*	*1.0*
in Strawberry Jelly, Pieces, Fruitini, Del Monte*	1 Can/140g	91	0.1	65	0.3	15.3	0.1	0.0
in Syrup, Average	*1oz/28g*	*19*	*0.0*	*67*	*0.4*	*16.3*	*0.1*	*0.4*
Raw, Stoned, Average	1oz/28g	9	0.0	33	1.0	7.6	0.1	1.5
Raw, Weighed with Stone, Average	*1 Peach/125g*	*41*	*0.1*	*33*	*1.0*	*7.6*	*0.1*	*1.4*
Slices, in Fruit Juice, Average	1 Serving/100g	49	0.0	49	0.6	11.6	0.0	0.5
PEANUT BRITTLE								
Thorntons*	2 Pieces/32g	163	8.6	509	12.4	54.3	26.9	2.6
PEANUT BUTTER								
25% Less Fat, Tesco*	1 Tbsp/16g	85	5.6	529	22.6	30.7	35.1	6.7
Crunchy, Basics, Sainsbury's*	1 Serving/10g	61	5.3	610	22.2	12.0	52.6	5.6
Crunchy, Bettabuy, Morrisons*	1 Serving/10g	61	5.2	606	22.5	17.3	52.2	5.7
Crunchy, CBY, Asda*	1 Serving/10g	60	4.9	603	24.5	15.5	49.2	6.6
Crunchy, Extra, Skippy*	2 Tbsps/40g	252	20.0	630	22.7	22.9	50.0	7.7
Crunchy, Extra, Sun Pat*	1 Serving/20g	119	10.2	597	21.9	12.6	51.0	7.3
Crunchy, Harvest Spread*	1 Serving/25g	148	12.4	592	23.6	12.5	49.7	6.9
Crunchy, No Added Sugar, Organic, Whole Earth*	1 Serving/25g	148	12.6	592	24.9	10.1	50.2	7.3
Crunchy, Organic, Evernat*	1 Tsp/10g	64	5.3	641	29.0	13.0	53.0	7.0
Crunchy, Organic, No Added Sugar, Waitrose*	1 Serving/12g	71	6.0	592	24.9	10.1	50.2	7.3
Crunchy, Organic, Tesco*	1 Serving/25g	149	12.4	595	23.6	12.5	49.7	6.9
Crunchy, Original Style, No Added Sugar, Whole Earth*	1 Serving/20g	127	10.2	637	25.7	16.8	51.1	8.7
Crunchy, Sainsbury's*	1 Serving/10g	62	5.0	620	28.6	12.6	49.6	4.3
Crunchy, Smart Price, Asda*	1 Thin Spread/12g	73	6.0	610	23.2	16.0	50.4	6.2
Crunchy, Somerfield*	1 Tsp/10g	59	4.9	586	24.4	11.8	49.0	7.1
Crunchy, Sun Pat*	1 Serving/50g	308	24.4	615	25.3	15.1	48.9	6.8
Crunchy, Tesco*	1 Serving/20g	123	10.2	615	23.8	14.6	50.8	6.4
Crunchy, Value, Tesco*	1 Serving/10g	62	5.4	615	21.5	11.7	53.6	5.4
Crunchy, Whole Nut, Organic, Meridian Foods*	1 Serving/28g	171	13.6	612	31.2	12.2	48.7	6.5
GFY, Asda*	1 Serving/15g	80	5.2	531	28.0	31.0	35.0	0.0
Powdered, PB2, Bell Plantation*	2 Tbsp/12g	45	1.5	375	41.7	41.7	12.5	16.7

INFO/WEIGHT	Measure		per Measure		Nutrition Values per 100g / 100ml				
			KCAL	FAT	KCAL	PROT	CARB	FAT	FIBRE
PEANUT BUTTER									
Smart Price, Asda*	1 Serving/15g		87	7.5	582	23.0	10.0	50.0	6.0
Smooth, 30% Reduced Fat, Duerr's*	1 Serving/20g		107	7.0	533	22.6	31.7	35.1	6.7
Smooth, 33% Less Fat, BGTY, Sainsbury's*	1 Serving/10g		53	3.5	533	22.6	31.7	35.1	6.7
Smooth, Average	1 Serving/20g		125	10.7	623	22.6	13.1	53.7	5.4
Smooth, CBY, Asda*	1 Serving/15g		91	7.4	604	24.1	15.7	49.4	6.0
Smooth, Creamy, Sun Pat*	1 Serving/15g		93	7.5	620	24.0	17.5	50.2	6.1
Smooth, Kernel King, Duerr's*	1 Serving/15g		89	7.5	596	23.3	12.4	50.3	6.8
Smooth, Kraft*	1 Serving/20g		127	10.7	636	23.1	17.6	53.5	0.0
Smooth, Light, Kraft*	1 Serving/20g		114	7.7	571	16.3	40.1	38.6	0.0
Smooth, Morrisons*	1 Serving/15g		92	7.8	616	23.1	14.5	51.8	6.2
Smooth, No Added Sugar, Organic, Whole Earth*	1 Serving/20g		119	10.2	595	24.5	9.9	50.8	7.1
Smooth, Organic, Meridian Foods*	1 Serving/10g		61	4.9	612	31.2	12.2	48.7	6.5
Smooth, Organic, Tesco*	1 Serving/15g		90	7.5	600	23.3	12.4	50.3	6.5
Smooth, Organic, Waitrose*	1 Serving/12g		71	6.1	595	24.6	9.9	50.8	7.1
Smooth, Original, No Added Sugar, Whole Earth*	1 Serving/10g		60	5.1	595	24.6	9.9	50.8	7.1
Smooth, Sun Pat*	1 Serving/20g		123	9.8	614	25.0	15.2	48.9	6.7
Smooth, Tesco*	1 Serving/20g		123	10.1	614	27.8	12.0	50.5	6.5
Wholenut, Crunchy, Average	1 Tsp/10g		61	5.3	606	24.9	7.7	53.1	6.0
Wholenut, Sainsbury's*	1 Serving/15g		90	7.7	598	24.2	9.8	51.3	7.0
Wholenut, Tesco*	1 Tbsp/15g		90	7.6	590	24.9	10.1	50.0	6.3
Wholenut, Waitrose*	1 Serving/12g		70	6.0	587	24.9	9.3	50.0	6.3
PEANUTS									
Chilli, Average	½ Pack/50g		303	25.3	605	28.2	9.3	50.6	6.8
Dry Roasted, Average	1 Serving/20g		117	9.8	587	25.7	11.5	48.8	6.5
Honey Roasted, Average	1oz/28g		169	13.2	605	26.8	23.6	47.0	5.5
Plain, Average	*10 Whole/10g*		*59*	*5.0*	*592*	*24.7*	*11.0*	*50.0*	*6.3*
Roast, Salted, Average	10 Whole/12g		74	6.3	614	27.8	7.9	52.4	4.9
Salted, Average	10 Whole/6g		37	3.1	609	27.0	8.3	54.4	5.4
Sweet Chilli, Nobby's*	1 Bag/40g		214	13.6	535	15.0	42.0	34.0	3.0
Yoghurt Coated, Graze*	1 Pack/35g		189	12.3	540	9.9	48.1	35.1	0.0
PEARL BARLEY									
Boiled	*1oz/28g*		*34*	*0.1*	*123*	*2.3*	*28.2*	*0.4*	*3.8*
Raw, Average	*1oz/28g*		*99*	*0.3*	*352*	*9.9*	*77.7*	*1.2*	*15.6*
PEARS									
Abate Fetel, Average	*1 Med/133g*		*48*	*0.1*	*36*	*0.4*	*8.3*	*0.1*	*2.2*
Asian, Nashi, Raw, Average	*1 Pear/209g*		*88*	*0.5*	*42*	*0.5*	*10.6*	*0.2*	*3.6*
Blush, Morrisons*	1 Sm/148g		86	0.2	58	0.4	15.5	0.1	3.1
Cape, Quartered, Tesco*	1 Serving/100g		35	0.0	35	0.3	8.5	0.0	1.4
Comice, Raw, Weighed with Core	*1 Med/170g*		*56*	*0.0*	*33*	*0.3*	*8.5*	*0.0*	*2.0*
Conference, Average	*1 Pear/209g*		*88*	*0.2*	*42*	*0.3*	*10.1*	*0.1*	*2.0*
Dessert, Green, Sainsbury's*	1 Sm/135g		53	0.1	39	0.3	9.2	0.1	2.0
Dried, Average	*½ Pear/16g*		*33*	*0.1*	*204*	*1.9*	*48.4*	*0.5*	*9.7*
in Fruit Juice, Average	*1 Serving/225g*		*102*	*0.1*	*45*	*0.3*	*10.9*	*0.0*	*1.2*
in Syrup, Average	*1oz/28g*		*16*	*0.0*	*58*	*0.2*	*14.4*	*0.1*	*1.4*
Prickly, Raw, Fresh	*1oz/28g*		*14*	*0.1*	*49*	*0.7*	*11.5*	*0.3*	*0.0*
Raw, Weighed with Core, Average	*1 Med/166g*		*62*	*0.2*	*38*	*0.3*	*9.1*	*0.1*	*1.4*
Red, Tesco*	1 Med/180g		65	0.2	36	0.4	8.3	0.1	2.2
William, Raw, Average	*1 Med/170g*		*58*	*0.2*	*34*	*0.4*	*8.3*	*0.1*	*2.2*
PEAS									
& Sweetcorn, Supersweet, Frozen, Birds Eye*	1 Serving/120g		92	0.8	77	4.0	11.3	0.7	4.6
Dried, Boiled in Unsalted Water, Average	*1oz/28g*		*31*	*0.2*	*109*	*6.9*	*19.9*	*0.8*	*5.5*
Dried, Raw, Average	*1oz/28g*		*85*	*0.7*	*303*	*21.6*	*52.0*	*2.4*	*13.0*
Edible Podded, Raw	*1 Cup/63g*		*26*	*0.1*	*42*	*2.8*	*7.6*	*0.2*	*2.6*

	Measure INFO/WEIGHT	per Measure KCAL	FAT	Nutrition Values per 100g / 100ml KCAL	PROT	CARB	FAT	FIBRE
PEAS								
Frozen, Average	1 Serving/85g	62	0.8	73	6.0	9.7	1.0	4.5
Frozen, Boiled, Average	1 Serving/75g	51	0.7	68	6.0	9.4	0.9	5.1
Garden, Canned, No Sugar Or Salt, Average	1 Can/80g	36	0.3	45	4.4	6.0	0.4	2.8
Garden, Canned with Sugar & Salt, Average	1 Serving/90g	59	0.6	66	5.3	9.3	0.7	5.1
Garden, Frozen, Average	1 Serving/90g	66	1.0	74	6.3	9.8	1.1	3.3
Garden, Minted, Average	1 Serving/80g	59	0.9	74	6.3	9.7	1.1	5.9
Gungo, Canned, Drained, Dunn's River*	½ Can/115g	137	3.3	119	7.2	16.1	2.9	4.1
Marrowfat, Canned, Average	1 Can/160g	140	0.9	88	6.4	14.3	0.6	3.9
Mushy, Canned, Average	1 Can/200g	173	1.0	86	6.2	14.4	0.5	2.2
Mushy, Frozen, Cooked, Asda*	1 Serving/80g	75	0.6	94	6.3	11.8	0.8	7.2
Processed, Canned, Average	1 Can/220g	176	1.8	80	6.1	12.3	0.8	3.6
Snow	1 Serving/80g	24	0.2	29	3.3	3.9	0.2	2.1
Sugar Snap, Average	1 Serving/80g	27	0.2	34	3.3	4.9	0.2	1.4
Wasabi, Average	1 Serving/28g	114	3.8	406	15.2	54.0	13.7	8.6
PEASE PUDDING								
Canned, Re-Heated, Drained	1oz/28g	26	0.2	93	6.8	16.1	0.6	1.8
PECAN NUTS								
Average	3 Nuts/6g	42	4.2	692	10.0	5.6	70.1	4.7
Honey, Golden, Graze*	1 Pack/26g	168	15.4	647	7.6	23.4	59.4	0.0
PENNE								
Arrabbiata, BGTY, Sainsbury's*	1 Pack/450g	414	7.2	92	2.9	16.5	1.6	1.9
Brown Rice, GF, Organic, Dove's Farm*	1 Serving/100g	338	1.5	338	7.9	70.3	1.5	4.1
Chilli, Asda*	1 Serving/100g	148	0.7	148	5.1	30.2	0.7	2.4
Cooked, Average	1 Serving/185g	244	1.3	132	4.7	26.7	0.7	1.1
Dry, Average	1 Serving/100g	352	1.9	352	12.4	71.3	1.9	2.7
Dry, Organic, Average	1 Serving/100g	352	1.8	352	12.4	71.6	1.8	1.9
Egg, Fresh, Average	1 Serving/125g	352	4.0	282	11.1	52.2	3.2	2.0
Free From, Tesco*	1 Serving/100g	340	2.0	340	8.0	72.5	2.0	2.5
Fresh, Dry, Average	1 Serving/125g	222	2.4	178	7.3	32.2	1.9	1.6
in Mushroom & Red Pepper Sauce, Creamy, Heinz*	1 Pack/250g	230	6.7	92	3.2	13.4	2.7	0.4
in Tomato & Basil Sauce, Sainsbury's*	½ Pack/110g	118	0.7	107	3.6	21.8	0.6	1.1
Rigate, Dry Weight, Average	1 Serving/90g	318	1.6	353	12.3	72.1	1.8	1.8
Tomato & Basil Sauce, Asda*	½ Pack/314g	185	11.0	59	0.8	6.0	3.5	2.0
Whole Wheat, Asda*	1 Serving/100g	333	2.1	333	12.1	66.3	2.1	6.9
Wholewheat, Authentic, Cooked, Italiano, Tesco*	1 Portion/75g	244	1.9	325	12.5	62.5	2.5	9.0
PEPERAMI*								
Firestick, Peperami*	1 Stick/25g	127	11.0	508	24.5	3.5	44.0	1.2
Hot, Peperami*	1 Stick/25g	126	11.0	504	24.5	2.5	44.0	1.2
Lunchbox Minis, 30% Less Fat, Peperami*	1 Stick/10g	38	3.0	379	25.0	1.5	30.0	3.0
Original, Peperami*	1 Stick/25g	126	11.0	504	24.0	2.5	44.0	0.1
Wideboy, Peperami*	1 Stick/40g	202	17.6	504	24.0	2.5	44.0	0.1
PEPPER								
Black, Freshly Ground, Average	1 Tsp/2g	5	0.1	255	11.0	64.8	3.3	26.5
Black, Whole Peppercorns, Schwartz*	1 Tsp/2g	11	0.4	529	13.0	68.7	22.5	27.0
Cayenne, Ground	1 Tsp/2g	6	0.3	318	12.0	31.7	17.3	0.0
White	½ Tsp/1g	3	0.0	296	10.4	68.6	2.1	26.2
PEPPERS								
Chilli, Crushed, Schwartz*	1 Tsp/0.5g	2	0.1	321	12.0	29.0	17.0	27.0
Chilli, Dried, Flakes, Average	1 Tsp/3g	13	0.4	425	16.0	56.0	15.0	44.0
Chilli, Dried, Whole, Red, Schwartz*	1 Tsp/0.5g	2	0.1	425	15.9	56.4	15.1	0.0
Chilli, Green, Raw, Unprepared, Average	1 Med/13g	5	0.0	40	2.0	9.5	0.2	1.5
Chilli, Green, Very Lazy, The English Provender Co.*	1 Serving/10g	11	0.4	114	4.2	15.3	4.0	0.5
Chilli, Red, Raw, Unprepared, Average	1 Pepper/13g	5	0.0	40	2.0	9.5	0.2	1.5

	Measure INFO/WEIGHT	per Measure		Nutrition Values per 100g / 100ml				
		KCAL	FAT	KCAL	PROT	CARB	FAT	FIBRE
PEPPERS								
Chilli, Red, Very Lazy, The English Provender Co.*	1 Serving/15g	17	0.6	114	4.2	15.3	4.0	0.5
Flame Seared with Greek Feta, M&S*	½ Tub/85g	106	8.2	125	3.6	5.4	9.7	1.8
Greek, Roasted Red in Brine, Kunapi*	1/3 Jar/120g	31	0.2	26	1.9	3.5	0.2	1.3
Green, Boiled in Salted Water	*1oz/28g*	*5*	*0.1*	*18*	*1.0*	*2.6*	*0.5*	*1.8*
Green, Filled, Tesco*	1 Pepper/150g	117	5.2	78	2.6	9.0	3.5	0.7
Green, Raw, Unprepared, Average	*1 Med/160g*	*24*	*0.5*	*15*	*0.8*	*2.6*	*0.3*	*1.6*
Italian Style, Sainsbury's*	1 Serving/150g	160	7.5	107	3.5	14.1	5.0	2.1
Jalapeno, Crushed, Schwartz*	1 Tsp/0.5g	1	0.1	136	15.9	56.4	15.1	0.0
Jalapeno, Raw	*1 Cup/90g*	*27*	*0.6*	*30*	*1.4*	*5.9*	*0.6*	*2.8*
Mixed, Sliced, Morrisons*	1 Pack/120g	34	0.4	28	1.0	4.5	0.3	1.6
Mixed Bag, From Supermarket, Average	*1oz/28g*	*7*	*0.1*	*25*	*1.0*	*4.4*	*0.4*	*1.7*
Orange, Sweet, Raw, Average	*1oz/28g*	*8*	*0.1*	*30*	*1.8*	*5.0*	*0.3*	*1.5*
Pickled, Hot, Turkish, Melis, Melis*	1 Serving/25g	9	0.0	35	1.0	7.9	0.0	1.0
Ramiro, Red, Sainsbury's*	1 Serving/100g	30	0.3	30	1.6	5.1	0.3	2.2
Red, Boiled in Salted Water	*1oz/28g*	*10*	*0.1*	*34*	*1.1*	*7.0*	*0.4*	*1.7*
Red, Filled, Halves, Vegetarian, M&S*	1 Pack/295g	280	10.3	95	2.9	12.3	3.5	1.1
Red, Filled with Feta, COU, M&S*	1 Pepper/154g	200	11.1	130	4.1	12.4	7.2	0.6
Red, Raw, Unprepared, Average	1oz/28g	9	0.1	32	1.0	6.4	0.4	1.6
Red, Roasted, in Brine, Cooks & Co*	1 Serving/100g	23	0.3	23	1.6	4.5	0.3	0.0
Red, Roasted, Melis*	1 Serving/100g	90	1.0	90	1.1	18.8	1.0	0.2
Red, Sweet, Pointed, Organic, Tesco*	1 Serving/100g	33	0.4	33	1.0	6.4	0.4	1.6
Red, Sweet, Pointed, TTD, Sainsbury's*	1 Serving/100g	32	0.4	32	1.0	6.4	0.4	0.0
Stuffed, Fresh, Asda*	1 Pepper/150g	144	7.5	96	3.8	9.0	5.0	1.2
Stuffed, PB, Waitrose*	1 Pack/300g	243	7.2	81	3.0	11.8	2.4	1.3
Stuffed, Sainsbury's*	1 Serving/137g	169	9.5	123	3.3	11.8	6.9	1.0
Stuffed, with Rice Based Filling, Average	1oz/28g	24	0.7	85	1.5	15.4	2.4	1.3
Stuffed, with Vegetables, Cheese Topping, Average	1oz/28g	31	1.9	111	3.4	9.8	6.7	1.5
Stuffed, Yellow, Italian, Ready to Roast, Sainsbury's*	1 Pack/136g	144	6.8	106	5.3	9.9	5.0	1.3
Sweet, Pointed, Extra Special, Asda*	1 Serving/100g	36	0.4	36	1.0	6.4	0.4	1.6
Sweet, Raw, Average	*1 Serving/100g*	*16*	*0.3*	*16*	*0.8*	*2.6*	*0.3*	*1.6*
Sweet, Tinned, Sainsbury's*	½ Can/125g	45	0.5	36	1.1	7.0	0.4	1.7
Yellow, Raw, Unprepared, Average	*1 Med/160g*	*42*	*0.3*	*26*	*1.2*	*5.3*	*0.2*	*1.7*
PERCH								
Raw, Atlantic	*1oz/28g*	*26*	*0.5*	*94*	*18.6*	*0.0*	*1.6*	*0.0*
PERNOD*								
*19% Volume, Pernod***	*1 Pub Shot/35ml*	*46*	*0.0*	*130*	*0.0*	*0.0*	*0.0*	*0.0*
PESTO								
Sauce, & Balsamic Vinegar, Extra Special, Asda*	1 Tbsp/15g	33	3.0	213	0.3	8.6	19.7	0.0
Sauce, Basil, M&S*	1 Serving/65g	348	30.5	535	7.5	20.7	46.9	1.4
Sauce, Dressing, Finest, Tesco*	1 Serving/30ml	108	11.1	360	3.5	2.9	37.1	0.9
Sauce, Fiery Chilli, Sacla*	½ Jar/95g	342	29.3	360	4.8	16.0	30.8	3.4
Sauce, Green, Alla Genovese, Finest, Tesco*	1 Serving/65g	188	25.7	290	5.7	1.5	39.6	2.8
Sauce, Green, Alla Genovese, TTD, Sainsbury's*	1 Serving/30g	192	19.8	640	6.2	5.4	65.9	3.1
Sauce, Green, Asda*	2 Dtsp/25g	92	7.4	368	7.6	16.6	29.7	2.0
Sauce, Green, Average	¼ Jar/48g	246	22.6	517	20.4	2.0	47.5	0.0
Sauce, Green, Classic, Sacla*	1 Serving/40g	185	18.6	462	5.2	7.6	46.5	0.0
Sauce, Green, Fresh, Sainsbury's*	1 Serving/60g	328	31.7	546	9.4	8.3	52.8	0.1
Sauce, Green, Fresh, Tesco*	1oz/28g	141	13.4	505	6.5	12.2	48.0	0.1
Sauce, Green, Italiano, Tesco*	1 Serving/50g	251	24.5	502	9.6	5.6	49.0	1.2
Sauce, Green, Less Than 60% Fat, BGTY, Sainsbury's*	¼ Jar/48g	61	5.3	128	4.2	2.6	11.2	0.0
Sauce, Green, Morrisons*	1 Serving/50g	255	24.9	510	10.7	4.7	49.8	0.0
Sauce, Green, Sainsbury's*	1 Tsp/5g	23	2.2	451	5.9	10.1	43.0	2.0
Sauce, Green, Tesco*	¼ Jar/48g	192	20.0	405	5.6	0.6	42.2	4.4

	Measure INFO/WEIGHT	per Measure KCAL	FAT	Nutrition Values per 100g / 100ml KCAL	PROT	CARB	FAT	FIBRE
PESTO								
Sauce, Green, Verde, Bertolli*	¼ Jar/46g	266	27.5	575	5.7	4.3	59.5	0.0
Sauce, M&S*	1oz/28g	115	12.1	411	3.2	3.5	43.3	3.9
Sauce, Red, Garlic & Chilli, Jamie Oliver*	1 Jar/190g	494	48.8	260	1.1	5.6	25.7	1.1
Sauce, Red, Italian, Tesco*	1 Serving/38g	128	11.5	340	8.2	8.2	30.6	1.2
Sauce, Red, M&S*	1oz/28g	93	9.3	331	3.6	6.9	33.2	3.5
Sauce, Red, Morrisons*	1 Tbsp/15g	47	4.4	311	5.7	6.6	29.0	5.9
Sauce, Red, Rosso, Bertolli*	1 Jar/185g	703	64.8	380	6.8	9.5	35.0	2.0
Sauce, Red, Smart Price, Asda*	1 Tsp/10g	15	0.9	147	3.8	12.1	9.3	2.4
Sauce, Red, Tesco*	¼ Jar/50g	162	15.2	325	5.6	6.3	30.3	6.0
Sauce, Ricotta & Red Pepper, CBY, Asda*	1 Jar/190g	486	37.2	256	4.2	14.4	19.6	2.4
Sauce, Spinach & Parmesan, Sainsbury's*	¼ Jar/46g	162	16.0	349	4.6	5.3	34.4	2.5
Sauce, Sun Dried Tomato, Sacla*	1 Serving/30g	87	8.4	289	4.2	5.2	27.9	0.0
PETIT POIS								
& Baby Carrots, Canned, Drained, Average	½ Can/122g	58	0.8	47	2.9	7.0	0.7	3.2
& Baby Carrots, in a Jar, Drained, Tesco*	½ Jar/110g	47	0.5	43	3.0	4.4	0.5	4.2
Canned, Drained, Average	1 Can/200g	125	1.0	63	4.8	8.9	0.5	2.6
Fresh, Frozen, Average	1 Serving/80g	51	0.8	63	5.4	7.1	1.0	4.8
PHEASANT								
Breast, Fillets, Skinless, Cooked, Gressingham Foods*	1 Serving/100g	127	2.4	127	32.7	0.0	2.4	0.0
Meat Only, Roasted	**1oz/28g**	**62**	**3.4**	**220**	**27.9**	**0.0**	**12.0**	**0.0**
Meat Only, Roasted, Weighed with Bone	**1oz/28g**	**61**	**3.3**	**219**	**27.9**	**0.0**	**11.9**	**0.0**
Stuffed, Easy Carve, Finest, Tesco*	1 Serving/200g	540	37.4	270	23.2	2.2	18.7	0.9
Whole, with Bacon, Cooked, Gressingham Foods*	1 Serving/100g	220	14.5	220	21.9	0.0	14.5	0.0
PHYSALIS								
Raw, without Husk, Average	**5 Fruits/30g**	**16**	**0.2**	**53**	**1.9**	**11.2**	**0.7**	**0.4**
PICCALILLI								
Haywards*	1 Serving/28g	18	0.1	66	1.4	13.9	0.5	0.0
Heinz*	1 Serving/10g	10	0.1	99	1.0	20.5	0.6	0.6
Morrisons*	1 Serving/50g	38	0.4	75	1.6	15.0	0.7	0.6
Sainsbury's*	1 Dtsp/15g	9	0.1	60	1.8	11.9	0.6	0.7
Sandwich, Tesco*	1 Serving/20g	16	0.0	80	0.4	18.5	0.0	1.6
Spicy, Sainsbury's*	1 Serving/15g	12	0.1	80	0.7	15.3	0.5	1.0
Sweet, Asda*	1 Tbsp/15g	17	0.0	112	0.5	27.0	0.2	0.6
Tesco*	1 Serving/50g	51	1.8	102	0.5	17.8	3.6	2.0
Three Mustard, Finest, Tesco*	1 Serving/30g	40	0.2	134	1.3	30.7	0.7	1.0
TTD, Sainsbury's*	1 Serving/19g	13	0.2	67	0.7	13.9	0.9	1.8
PICKLE								
Branston, Beetroot, Crosse & Blackwell*	1 Tsp/20g	25	0.1	123	1.2	28.2	0.3	1.6
Branston, Red Onion & Cranberry, Crosse & Blackwell*	1 Tbsp/14g	13	0.1	92	0.6	21.4	0.4	0.8
Branston, Red Pepper & Tomato, Crosse & Blackwell*	1 Tbsp/14g	12	0.0	84	1.2	17.7	0.3	1.1
Branston, Small Chunk, Squeezy, Crosse & Blackwell*	1 Serving/15g	19	0.0	127	0.9	29.8	0.2	1.1
Branston, Smooth, Squeezy, Crosse & Blackwell*	1 Serving/15g	19	0.0	127	0.9	29.8	0.2	1.1
Branston, Sweet, Original, Crosse & Blackwell*	1 Serving/15g	17	0.0	112	0.8	26.1	0.2	1.1
Branston, Sweet, Small Chunk, Crosse & Blackwell*	1 Serving/20g	22	0.0	109	0.8	26.1	0.2	1.1
Brinjal, Patak's*	1 Tsp/16g	59	3.9	367	2.2	34.6	24.4	0.9
Chilli, Patak's*	1 Tsp/16g	52	5.4	325	4.3	1.3	33.7	0.0
Chilli Tomato, Patak's*	1oz/28g	27	0.9	95	2.5	16.0	3.2	1.5
Cornichons, in Sweet & Sour Vinegar, Waitrose*	1 Serving/10g	3	0.0	28	0.6	6.1	0.1	0.6
Garlic, Patak's*	1 Tsp/16g	42	3.0	261	3.6	20.0	18.5	1.6
Green Chilli, Priya*	1 Tsp/10g	19	1.7	190	3.3	6.7	16.7	4.8
Hot Chilli Jam, What A Pickle*	1 Tsp/8g	14	0.0	178	0.6	44.0	0.1	1.2
Lime, Hot, Asda*	1 Dtsp/10g	12	1.0	123	2.2	6.0	10.0	1.0
Lime, Hot, Patak's*	1 Tsp/16g	31	3.0	194	2.2	4.0	18.7	0.4

	Measure INFO/WEIGHT	per Measure KCAL	FAT	Nutrition Values per 100g / 100ml KCAL	PROT	CARB	FAT	FIBRE
PICKLE								
Lime, M&S*	1 Tsp/16g	34	0.8	215	0.8	42.5	4.8	2.4
Lime, Oily	*2 Tbsp/39g*	*70*	*6.1*	*178*	*1.9*	*8.3*	*15.5*	*0.0*
Lime, Sharwood's*	1 Tbsp/20g	28	2.0	142	1.7	11.5	9.9	1.3
Mango, Hot, Patak's*	1 Tsp/16g	43	4.1	270	2.3	7.4	25.7	1.9
Mild Mustard, Heinz*	1 Tbsp/10g	13	0.1	129	2.2	25.7	1.3	0.9
Mixed, Drained	1 Serving/100g	14	0.2	14	1.0	1.9	0.2	1.0
Mixed, Drained, Haywards*	½ Jar/120g	22	0.4	18	1.4	2.4	0.3	0.0
Mixed, Patak's*	1 Serving/30g	78	7.7	259	2.3	4.7	25.7	0.8
Mixed, Salad Bar, Asda*	1oz/28g	11	0.0	40	0.5	9.2	0.1	0.0
Red Cabbage, Asda*	1 Serving/50g	16	0.0	32	1.6	6.0	0.1	0.0
Sandwich, Somerfield*	1 Tsp/10g	15	0.0	150	1.0	36.0	0.0	0.0
Sandwich, Tesco*	1 Serving/5g	7	0.0	138	1.0	33.1	0.2	1.0
Sweet	*1 Tsp/10g*	*14*	*0.0*	*141*	*0.6*	*36.0*	*0.1*	*1.2*
Sweet, Country, Morrisons*	1 Tbsp/15g	20	0.0	130	0.9	31.1	0.2	0.0
Sweet, Low Price, Sainsbury's*	1 Serving/23g	23	0.1	98	0.7	23.2	0.3	0.7
Sweet, Value, Tesco*	1 Serving/10g	10	0.0	96	0.6	23.0	0.2	0.7
Sweet Harvest, Asda*	1 Serving/25g	38	0.1	154	0.8	37.0	0.3	0.8
Tangy, Sandwich, Heinz*	1 Tsp/10g	13	0.0	134	0.7	31.4	0.2	0.9
Tomato, Tangy, Heinz*	1 Tsp/10g	10	0.0	102	2.0	22.0	0.3	1.5
PICNIC								
Cadbury*	1 Bar/48g	230	10.9	475	7.3	60.9	22.6	2.1
PIE								
Admiral's, Light & Easy, Youngs*	1 Pack/360g	342	14.0	95	4.1	10.9	3.9	0.8
Admiral's, Ross*	1 Pie/340g	357	15.6	105	4.8	10.9	4.6	0.7
Apple, & Custard, Bramley, Lattice Topped, Mr Kipling*	1 Pie/64g	236	9.9	369	3.8	53.7	15.4	1.1
Apple, American, Iceland*	1 Serving/92g	258	10.7	280	4.8	39.2	11.6	2.2
Apple, Asda*	¼ Pack/107g	287	11.7	269	3.6	39.0	11.0	1.7
Apple, Bramley, Aunt Bessie's*	¼ Pie/138g	351	15.1	255	2.8	36.2	11.0	1.2
Apple, Bramley, Deep Filled, Sainsbury's*	1/6 Pie/120g	329	14.3	274	3.7	38.0	11.9	1.9
Apple, Bramley, Individual, Mr Kipling*	1 Pie/66g	228	8.6	346	3.4	53.8	13.0	1.4
Apple, Bramley, Individual, Sainsbury's*	1 Pie/54g	165	5.0	307	3.6	52.2	9.3	1.3
Apple, Bramley, Individual, Tesco*	1 Pie/61g	210	7.9	344	3.4	53.1	13.0	1.5
Apple, Bramley, Large, Tesco*	1/8 Pie/87g	311	13.0	358	3.9	51.9	15.0	1.9
Apple, Bramley, M&S*	1 Pie/55g	184	6.4	335	2.9	57.6	11.7	1.6
Apple, Bramley, Somerfield*	1/6 Pie/70g	193	9.0	275	3.5	34.0	12.8	2.4
Apple, Bramley, Tesco*	1 Serving/106g	284	11.6	268	3.6	38.8	10.9	1.7
Apple, Deep Filled, Sainsbury's*	¼ Pie/137g	374	17.5	273	3.8	35.6	12.8	1.6
Apple, Family, Asda*	1/6 Pie/119g	314	13.0	265	3.6	38.0	11.0	2.9
Apple, Family, Morrisons*	1/6 Pie/116g	326	14.0	281	3.1	39.9	12.1	3.1
Apple, Lattice, Tesco*	1 Serving/145g	325	13.3	224	2.2	33.2	9.2	1.4
Apple, Low Price, Sainsbury's*	¼ Pie/103g	291	15.0	283	4.4	33.5	14.6	1.3
Apple, Pastry Top & Bottom	1oz/28g	74	3.7	266	2.9	35.8	13.3	1.7
Apple, Puff Pastry, M&S*	1 Pie/135g	338	17.1	250	2.4	31.3	12.7	1.0
Apple, Sainsbury's*	1/6 Pie/118g	314	13.6	266	3.4	37.1	11.5	0.6
Apple, Sultana & Cinnamon, Finest, Tesco*	1 Slice/83g	193	7.3	233	2.8	35.6	8.8	5.0
Apple, Tesco*	1 Pie/47g	191	8.1	406	3.3	59.4	17.2	1.5
Apple, Value, Tesco*	1 Pie/47g	127	4.7	270	2.8	41.5	9.9	1.7
Apple, VLH Kitchens	1 Serving/50g	136	22.4	272	3.7	40.0	11.2	1.7
Apple, with Custard	1 Serving/217g	353	18.8	163	2.4	25.2	8.7	1.1
Apple & Blackberry, Bramley, Aunt Bessie's*	¼ Pie/138g	344	12.5	250	2.1	40.1	9.1	2.6
Apple & Blackberry, Bramley, M&S*	¼ Pie/146g	380	14.5	260	3.4	39.8	9.9	1.3
Apple & Blackberry, Co-Op*	1 Serving/138g	338	15.2	245	3.0	33.0	11.0	2.0
Apple & Blackberry, Fruit, Finest, Tesco*	1 Pie/95g	265	11.3	279	13.7	29.3	11.9	2.8

PIE

Measure INFO/WEIGHT		per Measure		Nutrition Values per 100g / 100ml				
		KCAL	FAT	KCAL	PROT	CARB	FAT	FIBRE
Apple & Blackberry, Shortcrust, M&S*	1 Serving/142g	469	17.8	330	4.3	50.2	12.5	1.1
Apple & Blackberry, Somerfield*	¼ Pie/106g	280	12.7	264	4.0	36.0	12.0	0.0
Apple & Blackberry, Tesco*	1 Serving/106g	287	11.9	271	4.2	38.4	11.2	1.7
Apple & Blackcurrant, Mr Kipling*	1 Pie/66g	211	8.4	320	3.3	47.9	12.8	1.2
Apple & Damson, Bramley, M&S*	¼ Pie/142g	370	13.9	260	3.3	39.7	9.8	2.1
Banoffee, Cream, American Dream, McVitie's*	1 Serving/70g	277	17.8	396	4.3	36.7	25.5	0.8
Banoffee, Individual, Sainsbury's*	1 Pie/104g	365	21.0	351	3.2	39.2	20.2	2.2
Banoffee, Mini, Waitrose*	1 Pie/26g	115	5.8	444	3.3	57.0	22.5	1.2
Banoffee, Tesco*	1/6 Pie/94g	365	19.7	390	3.9	45.8	21.1	1.5
Beef, & Vegetable, Macdougalls, McDougalls*	¼ Pie/114g	292	19.3	256	5.3	20.6	16.9	0.3
Beef, Lean, BGTY, Sainsbury's*	1 Serving/212g	280	12.7	132	7.3	12.2	6.0	1.5
Beef, Minced, Aberdeen Angus, Shortcrust, M&S*	1 Pie/171g	435	26.6	255	9.3	19.3	15.6	3.0
Beef, Minced, with Mash, & Herb Liquor, Kershaws*	1 Meal/346g	595	28.3	172	5.2	19.3	8.2	4.3
Beef, Sainsbury's*	1 Pie/210g	535	30.0	255	10.3	21.2	14.3	2.0
Beef, Shamrock, Pieminister*	1 Pie/270g	648	30.8	240	8.8	24.5	11.4	1.8
Beef, Steak, Aberdeen Angus, Top Crust, Waitrose*	½ Pie/280g	476	24.1	170	10.0	13.4	8.6	4.1
Beef & Onion, Minced, Frozen, Baked, Greggs, Iceland*	½ Pie/125g	390	25.8	310	0.0	25.0	20.5	0.0
Beef & Onion, Minced, Tesco*	1 Pie/150g	454	28.5	303	5.7	27.4	19.0	1.7
Beef & Onion, Pukka Pies Ltd*	1 Serving/231g	529	32.6	229	7.6	17.9	14.1	3.0
Beef & Potato, Minced, Weight Watchers*	1 Pie/200g	328	12.4	164	6.7	20.2	6.2	3.6
Blackcurrant, Shortcrust, M&S*	1 Pie/142g	412	14.3	290	3.9	45.6	10.1	1.3
Butternut Squash, Skinny, & Red Pepper, Little, Higgidy*	1 Pie/180g	367	23.6	204	4.2	17.2	13.1	1.6
Cheese & Onion, Hollands*	1 Pie/200g	516	24.4	258	6.3	30.9	12.2	0.0
Cheese & Onion, Oven Baked, Average	1 Serving/200g	654	40.0	327	8.2	30.4	20.0	1.2
Cheese & Potato	1oz/28g	39	2.3	139	4.8	12.6	8.1	0.7
Cheese & Potato, Aunt Bessie's*	¼ Serving/200g	288	18.8	144	4.6	11.7	9.4	1.5
Cherry, Asda*	1/6 Pie/117g	337	14.5	289	3.1	41.2	12.4	1.8
Cherry, Sainsbury's*	1 Serving/117g	325	13.6	278	3.9	39.6	11.6	1.7
Cherry, Tesco*	1 Serving/106g	294	12.7	277	4.0	38.3	12.0	1.8
Chicken, Cottage, Frozen, Tesco*	1 Pack/450g	292	2.2	65	2.8	11.7	0.5	1.0
Chicken, Deep Filled, Puff Pastry, Sainsbury's*	1 Pie/210g	538	31.9	256	10.0	19.9	15.2	3.1
Chicken, Finest, Tesco*	1 Pie/250g	615	32.2	246	10.7	21.9	12.9	1.2
Chicken, Individual, Made with 100% Breast, Birds Eye*	1 Pie/154g	455	28.1	296	7.9	25.0	18.3	1.0
Chicken, Individual, Shortcrust, Asda*	1 Pie/175g	534	29.8	305	10.0	28.0	17.0	1.0
Chicken, Puff Pastry, Tesco*	¼ Pie/114g	250	12.7	220	8.6	21.3	11.2	1.4
Chicken, Roast, In Gravy, Deep Fill, Tesco*	1 Pie/700g	1540	68.6	220	11.2	20.2	9.8	2.0
Chicken, Roast, M&S*	1/3 Pie/182g	465	24.1	255	7.8	26.4	13.2	2.2
Chicken, Roast, Puff Pastry, Deep Fill, Asda*	½ Pie/259g	739	44.1	285	10.0	23.0	17.0	0.8
Chicken, Short Crust, M&S*	1 Pie/170g	510	29.6	300	9.7	26.2	17.4	1.7
Chicken & Asparagus, Lattice, Waitrose*	1 Serving/100g	295	19.6	295	7.4	22.3	19.6	1.8
Chicken & Asparagus, McDougalls*	1 Serving/170g	394	21.9	232	7.4	21.6	12.9	1.5
Chicken & Asparagus, Tesco*	1 Serving/170g	468	28.7	275	8.3	22.4	16.9	0.8
Chicken & Bacon, Filo Pastry, Finest, Tesco*	1 Serving/160g	362	18.7	226	11.3	18.9	11.7	1.7
Chicken & Bacon, Puff Pastry, Deep Fill, Sainsbury's*	1/3 Pie/200g	532	34.0	266	9.1	19.1	17.0	1.3
Chicken & Broccoli, COU, M&S*	1 Serving/320g	272	6.1	85	8.1	8.8	1.9	1.3
Chicken & Broccoli, Lattice, Tesco*	½ Pie/200g	496	30.8	248	8.5	18.9	15.4	2.1
Chicken & Broccoli, LC, Tesco*	1 Pack/450g	382	7.2	85	7.0	10.3	1.6	0.8
Chicken & Broccoli Potato, Top, Asda*	1 Pack/400g	319	7.0	80	5.2	10.8	1.8	0.6
Chicken & Gravy, Deep Fill, Asda*	1 Serving/130g	370	22.1	285	10.0	23.0	17.0	0.8
Chicken & Gravy, Just Chicken, Fray Bentos*	½ Pie/212g	324	17.4	153	5.4	14.3	8.2	0.6
Chicken & Gravy, Shortcrust Pastry, Large, Tesco*	1 Pie/600g	1578	91.2	263	8.2	23.4	15.2	1.0
Chicken & Gravy, Shortcrust Pastry, Sainsbury's*	1 Serving/250g	638	35.2	255	8.0	24.1	14.1	1.0
Chicken & Gravy, Shortcrust Pastry, Tesco*	1 Pie/250g	618	34.5	247	6.8	23.9	13.8	1.0

PIE

Measure INFO/WEIGHT	per Measure KCAL	FAT	Nutrition Values per 100g / 100ml KCAL	PROT	CARB	FAT	FIBRE
Chicken & Ham, Deep Filled, Sainsbury's*	1 Pie/210g	594	37.2	283	8.0	23.0	17.7	1.0
Chicken & Ham, Deep Filled, Somerfield*	¼ Pie/138g	348	19.3	252	11.0	21.0	14.0	0.0
Chicken & Ham, Morrisons*	¼ Pie/115g	267	13.7	232	8.7	22.5	11.9	0.8
Chicken & Ham, Sainsbury's*	1 Pie/128g	461	28.7	360	11.0	28.5	22.4	2.0
Chicken & Ham, Tesco*	1 Serving/113g	293	17.6	259	9.4	20.2	15.6	1.2
Chicken & Ham, Wiltshire, Finest, Tesco*	1 Pie/250g	688	37.2	275	11.6	22.7	14.9	1.1
Chicken & Leek, Deep Filled, Puff Pastry, Sainsbury's*	1/3 Pie/451g	1109	65.4	246	10.1	18.7	14.5	1.5
Chicken & Leek, LC, Tesco*	1 Pie/350g	298	5.6	85	6.6	10.3	1.6	1.3
Chicken & Leek, Shortcrust, TTD, Sainsbury's*	½ Pie/300g	824	48.8	275	12.2	19.8	16.3	1.1
Chicken & Leek, with Bacon, Filo, Finest, Tesco*	½ Pie/225g	574	33.1	255	11.1	18.5	14.7	1.4
Chicken & Leek, with Cheese, Lattice, Sun Valley*	1 Lattice/125g	315	21.9	252	15.2	8.6	17.5	1.0
Chicken & Leek, with Ham, Morrisons*	1 Serving/113g	305	16.6	270	8.8	25.7	14.7	1.1
Chicken & Leek, with Ham, Pot, Higgidy*	1 Pie/250g	710	33.5	284	13.1	19.1	13.4	1.1
Chicken & Mushroom, Asda*	1 Pie/150g	384	24.0	256	9.0	19.0	16.0	1.0
Chicken & Mushroom, Average	1 Serving/200g	540	31.7	270	8.0	23.8	15.9	1.0
Chicken & Mushroom, Chilled, Weight Watchers*	1 Pack/400g	304	4.8	76	5.7	9.8	1.2	1.5
Chicken & Mushroom, Co-Op*	1 Pie/150g	442	27.0	295	8.0	27.0	18.0	0.8
Chicken & Mushroom, Dietary Specials*	1 Pie/140g	300	14.0	214	6.3	24.7	10.0	0.9
Chicken & Mushroom, Farmfoods*	1 Pie/110g	271	16.4	246	5.6	22.4	14.9	0.9
Chicken & Mushroom, Finest, Tesco*	1 Pie/250g	742	46.8	297	9.3	21.1	18.7	0.9
Chicken & Mushroom, Fray Bentos*	1 Pie/425g	684	40.4	161	6.7	11.5	9.5	0.0
Chicken & Mushroom, Individual, Co-Op*	1 Pie/149g	465	29.7	312	8.6	24.5	19.9	1.2
Chicken & Mushroom, Individual, Frozen, Tesco*	1 Pie/142g	347	17.9	245	8.9	23.5	12.6	1.2
Chicken & Mushroom, Luxury, M&S*	½ Pie/275g	880	61.9	320	9.9	20.0	22.5	1.0
Chicken & Mushroom, Puff Pastry, Birds Eye*	1 Pie/152g	415	21.3	273	11.9	24.9	14.0	1.6
Chicken & Mushroom, Puff Pastry, Sainsbury's*	1 Pie/150g	450	25.0	300	7.8	29.6	16.7	0.9
Chicken & Mushroom, Pukka Pies Ltd*	1 Pie/226g	475	29.2	210	7.6	15.7	12.9	3.5
Chicken & Mushroom, Weight Watchers*	1 Pie/136g	317	15.1	233	8.0	25.1	11.1	1.5
Chicken & Vegetable, Individual, Somerfield*	1 Pie/142g	382	22.0	269	7.6	24.8	15.5	1.3
Chicken & Vegetable, PB, Waitrose*	1 Serving/375g	285	5.2	76	5.1	10.8	1.4	1.3
Chicken & Vegetable, Value, Tesco*	1 Pie/121g	321	16.9	265	6.6	26.9	14.0	1.1
Chicken Curry, Iceland*	1 Pie/156g	440	23.7	282	10.2	26.2	15.2	2.0
Cod & Smoked Haddock, COU, M&S*	1 Pack/400g	320	9.6	80	6.1	9.0	2.4	1.2
Cottage, Aberdeen Angus, Bistro, M Kitchen, Morrisons*	1 Pack/700g	791	30.8	113	7.0	10.4	4.4	1.7
Cottage, Aberdeen Angus, Large, Finest, Tesco*	½ Pack/400g	420	17.2	105	7.1	8.7	4.3	1.8
Cottage, Aberdeen Angus, Waitrose*	1 Pie/350g	340	12.2	97	5.3	11.0	3.5	0.9
Cottage, Aldi*	1 Pack/440g	484	27.3	110	4.1	9.5	6.2	0.2
Cottage, Asda*	1 Pack/400g	360	9.6	90	6.5	10.6	2.4	1.0
Cottage, Aunt Bessie's*	1 Pack/350g	413	18.2	118	4.8	12.1	5.2	1.0
Cottage, Basics, Sainsbury's*	1 Pack/300g	228	9.0	76	4.4	7.9	3.0	1.5
Cottage, British Pies, Chilled, Tesco*	1 Pack/500g	450	14.0	90	4.6	10.3	2.8	1.5
Cottage, Chicken, Tesco*	1 Pack/400g	340	2.8	85	6.0	12.8	0.7	1.7
Cottage, Classic British, Sainsbury's*	1 Pack/450g	436	16.2	97	5.3	9.9	3.6	1.7
Cottage, Classics, Asda*	½ Pack/450g	531	27.0	118	7.0	9.0	6.0	1.0
Cottage, COU, M&S*	1 Pack/400g	340	8.0	85	6.0	11.0	2.0	1.5
Cottage, Diet Chef Ltd*	1 Pack/270g	235	9.7	87	3.7	9.8	3.6	1.7
Cottage, Family, Iceland*	¼ Pack/259g	262	10.6	101	4.2	11.8	4.1	0.8
Cottage, Fresh, M&S*	1 Pie/400g	460	22.4	115	6.8	9.9	5.6	0.6
Cottage, Frozen, CBY, Asda*	1 Pack/400g	368	9.6	92	6.5	10.6	2.4	1.0
Cottage, Healthy Living, Co-Op*	1 Pack/400g	320	6.4	80	5.0	11.0	1.6	2.0
Cottage, Iceland*	1 Pack/400g	468	18.8	117	5.1	13.6	4.7	0.7
Cottage, Individual, Smart Price, Asda*	1 Pie/159g	149	5.9	94	3.1	12.0	3.7	0.7
Cottage, LC, Tesco*	1 Pack/500g	400	8.5	80	4.5	11.4	1.7	1.7

PIE

	Measure INFO/WEIGHT	per Measure KCAL	per Measure FAT	Nutrition Values per 100g / 100ml KCAL	PROT	CARB	FAT	FIBRE
Cottage, Lentil & Vegetable, Linda McCartney*	1 Pot/398g	374	10.3	94	2.8	13.5	2.6	2.5
Cottage, Luxury, M&S*	½ Pack/310g	403	21.7	130	7.9	8.3	7.0	1.8
Cottage, Meal for One, M&S*	1 Pack/445g	356	16.0	80	5.4	6.2	3.6	1.7
Cottage, Morrisons*	1 Pack/450g	450	18.4	100	5.2	10.7	4.1	1.2
Cottage, Ready Meals, Tesco*	1 Pack/400g	380	12.0	95	6.1	10.8	3.0	1.6
Cottage, Retail, Average	1 Pack/400g	399	15.7	100	5.5	10.5	3.9	1.3
Cottage, Sainsbury's*	1 Pack/300g	297	10.2	99	6.4	10.7	3.4	1.1
Cottage, Waitrose*	1 Pack/400g	424	19.6	106	3.4	12.1	4.9	1.2
Cottage, Weight Watchers*	1 Pack/300g	186	3.9	62	3.6	9.0	1.3	0.3
Cottage, with Cheddar Mash, TTD, Sainsbury's*	1 Pack/400g	582	27.7	145	9.2	11.6	6.9	2.4
Cottage, You Count, Love Life, Waitrose*	1 Pack/402g	338	9.1	84	4.0	11.5	2.2	1.1
Cumberland, M&S*	1 Pie/195g	312	20.3	160	6.9	10.1	10.4	1.1
Cumberland, Mashed Potato Topped, M&S*	1/3 Pie/300g	360	17.7	120	5.8	9.6	5.9	1.0
Farmhouse, Vegetable, Linda McCartney*	1 Pie/146g	380	23.2	260	5.8	23.4	15.9	1.6
Fish	1 Serving/250g	262	7.5	105	8.0	12.3	3.0	0.7
Fish, & Prawn, PB, Waitrose*	1 Serving/375g	379	13.5	101	6.8	10.4	3.6	0.7
Fish, BFY, Morrisons*	1 Pack/350g	301	10.2	86	5.0	10.0	2.9	0.9
Fish, Co-Op*	1 Pack/400g	380	16.0	95	4.0	12.0	4.0	0.9
Fish, Creamy, Classics, Large, Finest, Tesco*	½ Pack/350g	402	19.6	115	6.4	8.6	5.6	0.9
Fish, Cumberland, BGTY, Sainsbury's*	1 Serving/450g	342	8.6	76	7.3	7.3	1.9	1.8
Fish, Extra Special, Asda*	1 Pack/400g	540	30.8	135	9.8	6.5	7.7	1.1
Fish, Frozen, GFY, Asda*	1 Pack/360g	342	8.6	95	5.8	12.5	2.4	0.9
Fish, Large (700g), Extra Special, Asda*	1 Serving/350g	525	30.8	150	9.9	7.8	8.8	0.6
Fish, Luxury, M&S*	1 Pack/300g	330	16.8	110	7.3	7.6	5.6	1.5
Fish, Mariner's, Frozen, Youngs*	1 Pack/360g	382	16.2	106	5.3	11.0	4.5	1.0
Fish, Pollock, Yummy, Jamie Oliver, Youngs*	1 Pie/217g	204	7.2	94	6.8	8.6	3.3	1.5
Fish, Seasonal, Mix, Sainsbury's*	1 Pack/320g	480	28.2	150	17.7	0.0	8.8	0.0
Fish, The Best, Morrisons*	½ Pack/225g	250	11.9	111	6.6	9.3	5.3	0.8
Fish, TTD, Sainsbury's*	½ Pack/390g	386	12.9	99	7.1	10.3	3.3	1.6
Fish, with Cheddar, Grated, Asda*	¼ Pie/250g	262	12.5	105	7.0	8.0	5.0	1.0
Fish, with Cheddar & Parsley Sauce, Go Cook, Asda*	½ Pack/450g	428	16.2	95	7.8	7.9	3.6	0.8
Fish, with Cheese, Ross*	1 Pack/300g	321	13.5	107	4.7	12.0	4.5	0.8
Fisherman's, Chilled, Co-Op*	1 Pie/300g	345	18.0	115	4.0	11.0	6.0	0.7
Fisherman's, Famous, Chilled, Youngs*	1 Pack/400g	448	22.8	112	7.6	7.6	5.7	0.9
Fisherman's, M&S*	1 Pie/248g	335	15.9	135	9.3	9.8	6.4	0.3
Fisherman's, PB, Waitrose*	1 Pack/376g	380	13.5	101	6.8	10.4	3.6	0.7
Fisherman's, Smart Price, Asda*	1 Pack/300g	213	3.6	71	3.1	12.0	1.2	1.9
Fisherman's, Value, Tesco*	1 Pie/300g	195	3.0	65	3.3	9.1	1.0	1.6
Fruit, Pastry Top & Bottom	1oz/28g	73	3.7	260	3.0	34.0	13.3	1.8
Fruit, Selection, Mr Kipling*	1 Pie/66g	232	9.0	350	3.5	53.5	13.6	1.3
Gala, Tesco*	1 Serving/70g	241	17.6	344	10.6	24.5	25.2	0.0
Key Lime, Sainsbury's*	¼ Pie/80g	280	11.2	350	4.2	51.8	14.0	0.7
Lamb, & Mint, Shortcrust Pasty, Tesco*	¼ Pack/150g	412	26.1	275	5.9	23.6	17.4	1.6
Lemon Meringue	1 Portion/120g	383	17.3	319	4.5	45.9	14.4	0.7
Lemon Meringue, Frozen, Baked, Aunt Bessie's*	½ Pie/117g	370	12.6	315	3.6	49.6	10.7	3.1
Lemon Meringue, Lyons*	1 Serving/100g	310	14.4	310	0.0	45.9	14.4	0.0
Lemon Meringue, Mini, Asda*	1 Pie/26g	101	3.3	396	3.7	66.0	13.0	1.8
Lemon Meringue, Sainsbury's*	¼ Pie/110g	351	9.9	319	2.3	57.3	9.0	0.5
Lemon Meringue, Tesco*	1 Pie/385g	989	28.1	257	4.0	43.7	7.3	0.5
Macaroni Cheese, Countryside*	1 Serving/144g	282	10.1	196	4.9	28.3	7.0	1.2
Mariner's, Light & Easy, Youngs*	1 Pack/350g	368	14.3	105	5.0	12.0	4.1	1.1
Meat, Freshbake*	1 Pie/49g	152	10.5	313	6.6	23.2	21.6	1.0
Meat & Potato, Farmfoods*	1 Pie/158g	416	26.9	263	5.4	22.0	17.0	1.0

PIE

	Measure INFO/WEIGHT	per Measure KCAL	FAT	Nutrition Values per 100g / 100ml KCAL	PROT	CARB	FAT	FIBRE
Meat & Potato, Hollands*	1 Pie/175g	410	19.2	234	6.1	27.5	11.0	0.0
Meat & Potato, Shortcrust, Co-Op*	¼ Pie/137g	403	26.2	294	7.3	23.3	19.1	1.4
Meat & Potato, Tesco*	1 Serving/150g	414	26.8	276	5.1	23.6	17.9	1.6
Meat & Potato, Value, Tesco*	1 Pie/95g	274	17.5	288	6.9	23.8	18.4	3.5
Mince, Asda*	1 Pie/53g	204	8.0	382	3.8	58.0	15.0	1.5
Mince, Christmas, Finest, Tesco*	1 Pie/64g	255	9.4	395	4.6	60.3	14.5	1.4
Mince, Christmas, Sainsbury's*	1 Pie/37g	147	6.0	397	4.5	58.0	16.3	2.6
Mince, Deep, Morrisons*	1 Pie/65g	243	9.1	371	3.7	57.8	13.9	1.5
Mince, Deep Filled, Christmas, Tesco*	1 Pie/65g	255	9.3	395	4.0	60.0	14.4	2.8
Mince, Deep Filled, Morrisons*	1 Pie/66g	257	9.7	386	3.7	57.9	14.6	4.2
Mince, Deep Filled, Sainsbury's*	1 Pie/61g	251	9.0	406	4.1	63.6	14.5	2.5
Mince, Dusted, Mini, Finest, Tesco*	1 Pie/20g	76	2.4	379	7.3	62.9	12.2	5.0
Mince, Extra Special, Asda*	1 Pie/60g	225	8.3	378	3.9	59.0	14.0	2.2
Mince, Iced Top, Asda*	1 Pie/57g	221	6.7	391	2.7	67.3	11.9	1.9
Mince, Iced Top, Tesco*	1 Pie/56g	220	6.0	390	3.2	69.1	10.7	1.2
Mince, Iceland*	1 Pie/39g	156	6.4	405	4.4	59.6	16.6	3.8
Mince, Individual, Average	1 Pie/48g	203	9.8	423	4.3	59.0	20.4	2.1
Mince, Individual, Mr Kipling*	1 Pie/66g	253	9.2	381	3.7	59.5	13.8	1.3
Mince, Lattice, Classics, M&S*	1 Pie/53g	210	8.0	400	4.0	61.7	15.2	2.4
Mince, Luxury, Deep Filled, M&S*	1 Pie/65g	234	9.0	360	4.3	55.0	13.8	3.8
Mince, Mini, M&S*	1 Pie/28g	105	4.0	380	4.3	57.8	14.6	4.0
Mince, Mini, Waitrose*	1 Pie/30g	150	9.1	501	5.7	51.3	30.3	1.7
Mince, Organic, Sainsbury's*	1 Pie/46g	177	7.5	384	5.0	54.5	16.2	5.6
Mince, Puff, Tesco*	1 Pie/25g	105	4.4	420	3.3	62.0	17.6	2.0
Mince, Rowan Hill Bakery*	1 Pie/55g	202	8.2	370	3.8	54.8	15.1	0.0
Mince, Shortcrust, Waitrose*	1 Pie/55g	210	8.0	385	3.6	60.0	14.6	20.9
Mince, Smart Price, Asda*	1 Pie/44g	178	7.6	409	4.6	55.6	17.4	3.2
Mince, Star Motif, Mini, Finest, Tesco*	1 Pie/17g	62	2.1	365	3.8	59.9	12.1	3.8
Mince, Tesco*	1 Pie/47g	180	7.8	383	3.9	54.7	16.5	1.5
Mince, Value, Tesco*	1 Pie/41g	168	7.0	410	4.4	58.8	17.0	1.6
Mississippi Mud, Tesco*	1 Serving/104g	399	26.6	384	5.3	33.1	25.6	1.8
Mushroom, & Leaf Spinach, Little, Higgidy*	1 Pie/180g	441	25.9	245	6.6	22.3	14.4	0.7
Ocean, Original, Frozen, Youngs*	1 Pack/375g	420	21.4	112	7.6	7.6	5.7	0.9
Ocean, The Original, Light & Easy, Youngs*	1 Pack/415g	432	18.7	104	6.4	9.5	4.5	1.0
Ocean, Weight Watchers*	1 Pack/300g	196	3.3	65	4.2	9.2	1.1	0.8
Pork, & Egg, M&S*	¼ Pie/108g	379	28.0	351	9.7	19.8	25.9	0.8
Pork, & Pickle, Bowyers*	1 Pie/150g	576	41.0	384	10.0	26.3	27.3	0.0
Pork, Buffet, Bowyers*	1 Pie/60g	217	14.7	362	10.4	24.9	24.5	0.0
Pork, Buffet, Farmfoods*	1 Pie/65g	252	17.4	388	8.8	28.2	26.7	1.0
Pork, Buffet, Mini, Somerfield*	1 Pie/70g	292	19.9	418	10.8	29.5	28.5	0.2
Pork, Cheddar & Pickle, Mini, Finest, Tesco*	1 Pie/50g	185	10.8	365	10.0	31.3	21.4	1.9
Pork, Cheese & Pickle, Mini, Tesco*	1 Pie/49g	191	12.8	389	9.2	29.3	26.1	1.2
Pork, Crusty Bake, Mini, Sainsbury's*	1 Pie/43g	165	11.2	384	11.5	26.0	26.0	1.5
Pork, Crusty Bake, Sainsbury's*	1 Pie/75g	292	20.0	390	10.5	27.0	26.7	1.0
Pork, Geo Adams*	1 Pie/125g	488	34.8	390	11.8	23.1	27.8	0.9
Pork, Individual	1 Pie/75g	272	19.3	363	10.8	23.7	25.7	0.9
Pork, Melton Mowbray, Cured, M&S*	1 Pie/290g	1044	71.0	360	10.1	25.9	24.5	1.0
Pork, Melton Mowbray, Cured, Mini, M&S*	1 Pie/50g	192	12.2	385	9.8	32.6	24.4	1.0
Pork, Melton Mowbray, Individual, Sainsbury's*	1 Pie/75g	296	20.8	395	10.2	26.1	27.7	2.4
Pork, Melton Mowbray, Large, Co-Op*	¼ Pie/110g	418	35.2	380	11.0	12.0	32.0	5.0
Pork, Melton Mowbray, Lattice, Sainsbury's*	1 Serving/100g	342	23.6	342	10.8	21.7	23.6	1.2
Pork, Melton Mowbray, Mini, Co-Op*	1 Pie/49g	189	13.2	385	11.0	24.0	27.0	2.0
Pork, Melton Mowbray, Mini, Finest, Tesco*	1 Pie/50g	180	11.4	359	12.1	26.6	22.7	0.9

PIE

INFO/WEIGHT	Measure	per Measure KCAL	per Measure FAT	Nutrition Values per 100g / 100ml KCAL	PROT	CARB	FAT	FIBRE
Pork, Melton Mowbray, Mini, Morrisons*	1 Pie/50g	197	12.5	393	10.9	31.3	24.9	0.9
Pork, Melton Mowbray, Mini, Tesco*	1 Pie/50g	196	14.4	392	12.6	20.8	28.7	2.9
Pork, Melton Mowbray, Snack, Tesco*	1 Pie/75g	289	19.4	385	10.1	27.0	25.9	2.7
Pork, Melton Mowbray, Tesco*	1 Pie/148g·	679	49.9	459	10.0	29.0	33.7	1.3
Pork, Mini	1 Pie/50g	196	13.9	391	10.6	26.3	27.8	1.0
Pork, Mini, Tesco*	1 Pie/45g	162	10.7	359	10.2	25.9	23.8	1.0
Pork, Mini, Value, Tesco*	1 Pie/70g	266	17.8	380	9.0	28.5	25.5	3.5
Pork, Ploughmans, Mini, Ginsters*	1 Pie/50g	190	12.6	380	8.9	29.2	25.3	2.0
Pork, Sliced	1 Slice/100g	380	29.9	380	10.2	18.7	29.9	0.0
Pork, VLH Kitchens	1 Serving/36g	168	100.0	466	11.0	26.0	36.0	2.5
Pork, with Cheese & Pickle, Waitrose*	1 Pack/150g	568	36.9	379	10.3	29.1	24.6	2.7
Rhubarb, Sara Lee*	1 Serving/90g	224	12.4	250	2.9	28.7	13.8	1.3
Salmon, & Broccoli, LC, Tesco*	1 Pack/400g	350	7.2	88	7.0	10.2	1.8	1.7
Salmon, Crumble, Light & Easy, Youngs*	1 Pack/320g	282	6.4	88	5.7	11.8	2.0	1.0
Sausage, & Onion, Lattice, Puff Pastry, Tesco*	1/3 Pie/133g	480	22.5	361	9.1	20.6	16.9	4.6
Scotch, Co-Op*	1 Pie/132g	408	24.9	309	7.3	27.3	18.9	1.5
Scotch, Farmfoods*	1 Pie/151g	430	24.6	285	7.8	26.8	16.3	1.2
Shepherd's, Average	1oz/28g	31	1.7	112	6.0	9.3	5.9	0.7
Shepherd's, British Classic, Serves 1, Sainsbury's*	1 Pack/450g	454	22.0	101	6.2	7.9	4.9	1.7
Shepherd's, British Classics, Chilled, Tesco*	1 Pack/500g	500	20.5	100	4.8	10.6	4.1	1.2
Shepherd's, Chilled, Finest, Tesco*	½ Pack/400g	460	16.4	115	6.9	8.0	4.1	1.9
Shepherd's, Chilled, Value, Tesco*	1 Pack/300g	210	4.5	70	3.0	11.0	1.5	1.0
Shepherd's, Classics, Asda*	1 Pack/455g	459	22.7	101	5.0	9.0	5.0	1.1
Shepherd's, Cooked, BGTY, Sainsbury's*	1 Pack/450g	359	8.0	85	4.2	11.8	1.9	1.3
Shepherd's, COU, M&S*	1 Pack/300g	210	3.9	70	5.2	8.6	1.3	1.6
Shepherd's, Diet Chef Ltd*	1 Serving/270g	235	10.5	87	3.2	9.8	3.9	1.9
Shepherd's, Frozen, Tesco*	1 Pack/400g	270	9.1	68	4.1	7.6	2.3	1.2
Shepherd's, Sweet Potato & Carrot, Fuller Longer, M&S*	1 Pack/420g	357	11.3	85	6.6	8.7	2.7	4.5
Shepherd's, TTD, Sainsbury's*	1 Pack/397g	524	27.8	132	7.6	9.7	7.0	1.7
Shepherd's, Vegetarian, Average	1 Serving/400g	371	14.6	93	4.0	10.4	3.6	2.5
Shepherd's, Weight Watchers*	1 Pack/320g	211	5.8	66	3.2	8.8	1.8	1.1
Shepherd's, Welsh Hill Lamb, Gastropub, M&S*	½ Pack/330g	314	11.6	95	5.4	10.2	3.5	1.5
Steak, All Steak, Pukka Pies Ltd*	1 Pie/233g	534	29.8	229	8.8	18.2	12.8	3.1
Steak, Deep Fill, Tesco*	¼ Pie/195g	468	25.5	240	9.7	20.0	13.1	1.5
Steak, in Rich Gravy, Shortcrust Pastry, Sainsbury's*	1/3 Pie/200g	528	30.4	264	12.0	19.6	15.2	3.6
Steak, Individual, British Classics, Tesco*	1 Pie/150g	450	27.6	300	9.1	23.3	18.4	2.5
Steak, Mini, Asda*	1 Serving/67g	117	5.3	176	9.0	17.0	8.0	0.9
Steak, Puff Pastry, Deep Filled, Sainsbury's*	1 Pie/210g	536	30.0	255	10.3	21.2	14.3	2.0
Steak, Scotch, Bell's Bakery*	1 Serving/150g	378	20.2	252	13.6	18.6	13.5	0.7
Steak, Short Crust, Sainsbury's*	½ Pie/118g	314	24.1	267	10.9	22.2	20.5	1.7
Steak, Shortcrust Pastry, Finest, Tesco*	1 Pie/250g	660	37.8	264	10.9	21.2	15.1	0.8
Steak, Tesco*	1 Serving/205g	556	33.8	271	7.2	23.3	16.5	1.4
Steak, Top Crust, TTD, Sainsbury's*	½ Pie/299g	530	23.1	177	15.4	11.4	7.7	0.5
Steak, TTD, Sainsbury's*	½ Pie/300g	713	35.4	238	12.6	20.3	11.8	1.0
Steak & Ale, Average	1 Pie/200g	507	28.7	253	9.8	21.1	14.4	1.3
Steak & Ale, Budgens*	1 Pack/225g	583	38.0	259	7.2	19.5	16.9	0.9
Steak & Ale, Deep Fill, Puff Pastry, Tesco*	¼ Pie/150g	324	19.6	216	8.0	16.6	13.1	2.3
Steak & Ale, Deep Filled, Somerfield*	1 Pie/200g	550	32.0	275	12.0	22.0	16.0	0.0
Steak & Ale, Dorset, Mini, Finest, Tesco*	1 Pie/30g	92	4.9	305	7.9	31.4	16.4	1.9
Steak & Ale, Fray Bentos*	1 Pie/425g	697	38.7	164	7.6	13.0	9.1	0.0
Steak & Ale, Pub Style, Co-Op*	1 Pie/250g	538	30.0	215	9.0	17.0	12.0	2.0
Steak & Ale, Puff Pastry, Asda*	1/3 Pie/200g	520	30.2	260	10.6	20.4	15.1	1.6
Steak & Ale, Sainsbury's*	1 Serving/190g	445	23.4	234	8.3	22.6	12.3	0.9

	Measure INFO/WEIGHT	per Measure KCAL	FAT	Nutrition Values per 100g / 100ml KCAL	PROT	CARB	FAT	FIBRE
PIE								
Steak & Ale, TTD, Sainsbury's*	1 Pie/250g	681	35.6	272	11.6	24.4	14.2	1.4
Steak & Ale, with Chips & Gravy	1 Serving/400g	825	42.2	206	7.2	20.5	10.6	0.5
Steak & Ale, with Mushroom, Topcrust, Waitrose*	1 Pie/250g	500	29.5	200	11.1	12.2	11.8	1.1
Steak & Gravy, Rich, Aunt Bessie's*	¼ Pie/200g	440	20.6	220	9.6	22.0	10.3	1.5
Steak & Guinness, Sainsbury's*	¼ Pie/137g	399	25.5	291	8.7	22.2	18.6	1.0
Steak & Kidney, Individual	1 Pie/200g	646	42.4	323	9.1	25.6	21.2	0.9
Steak & Kidney, Premium, Tesco*	1 Serving/170g	428	26.4	252	9.9	18.3	15.5	1.2
Steak & Kidney, Princes*	½ Pack/212g	379	19.9	179	8.8	14.8	9.4	0.0
Steak & Kidney, Puff Pastry, Sainsbury's*	1 Pie/150g	423	23.6	282	8.2	26.9	15.7	0.9
Steak & Kidney, Pukka Pies Ltd*	1 Pie/238g	488	25.9	205	9.1	17.7	10.9	3.6
Steak & Kidney, Tinned, Fray Bentos*	½ Pie/212g	346	18.7	163	8.2	12.9	8.8	0.0
Steak & Mushroom, Deep Fill, Puff Pastry, Tesco*	1 Slice/150g	339	20.7	226	9.1	16.3	13.8	1.9
Steak & Mushroom, Luxury Mash, Fuller Longer, M&S*	1 Pack/430g	408	9.0	95	9.3	10.0	2.1	1.3
Steak & Onion, Farmfoods*	1 Pie/127g	382	24.3	301	6.0	26.4	19.1	1.0
Steak & Onion, Minced, Puff, Individual, Sainsbury's*	1 Pie/150g	484	29.6	323	7.4	29.0	19.7	1.5
Steak & Potato, Asda*	1/3 Pie/173g	442	26.0	255	6.9	23.1	15.0	0.9
Steak & Red Wine, Puff Pastry, Pub, Sainsbury's*	1 Pie/240g	497	29.5	207	7.2	16.8	12.3	2.1
Summer Fruits, Orchard Tree*	1/8 Pie/75g	242	10.4	323	3.0	46.6	13.8	1.2
Turkey & Ham, Farmfoods*	1 Pie/147g	404	21.9	275	8.6	26.5	14.9	1.4
Turkey & Ham, Shortcrust, M&S*	1/3 Pie/183g	494	29.1	270	11.9	19.5	15.9	1.0
Vegetable	1oz/28g	42	2.1	151	3.0	18.9	7.6	1.5
Vegetable, & Cheddar Cheese, Waitrose*	1 Pie/210g	475	31.5	226	4.9	17.8	15.0	1.2
Vegetable, Moroccan, & Feta, Little, Higgidy*	1 Pie/180g	418	22.5	232	5.1	24.7	12.5	0.6
Vegetable, Retail, Average	1 Serving/200g	348	19.0	174	3.7	18.6	9.5	1.1
Vegetarian, Deep Country, Linda McCartney*	1 Pie/166g	413	23.6	249	5.2	24.9	14.2	2.6
Vegetarian, Mushroom & Ale, Linda McCartney*	1 Pie/200g	439	23.5	219	4.1	25.0	11.7	1.2
Vegetarian, Shepherd's, Linda McCartney*	1 Pack/340g	286	7.5	84	3.7	12.3	2.2	2.3
PIE FILLING								
Apple, Sainsbury's*	1 Serving/75g	67	0.1	89	0.1	22.1	0.1	1.0
Black Cherry, Fruit, Sainsbury's*	1 Serving/100g	73	0.1	73	0.3	17.7	0.1	0.3
Cherry	1oz/28g	23	0.0	82	0.4	21.5	0.0	0.4
Fruit	1oz/28g	22	0.0	77	0.4	20.1	0.0	1.0
PIGEON								
Meat Only, Roasted, Average	**1 Pigeon/115g**	**215**	**9.1**	**187**	**29.0**	**0.0**	**7.9**	**0.0**
Meat Only, Roasted, Weighed with Bone, Average	**1oz/28g**	**25**	**1.0**	**88**	**13.6**	**0.0**	**3.7**	**0.0**
PIKELETS								
Classics, M&S*	1 Pikelet/35g	70	0.5	200	7.3	39.1	1.3	1.6
Tesco*	1 Pikelet/35g	68	0.2	193	5.8	40.9	0.7	1.7
PILAF								
Bulgar Wheat, Sainsbury's*	1 Pack/381g	347	11.1	91	3.9	12.3	2.9	6.3
Forest Mushroom & Pine Nut, Bistro, Waitrose*	1 Serving/225g	338	14.6	150	7.0	15.8	6.5	1.5
with Tomato, Average	1oz/28g	40	0.9	144	2.5	28.0	3.3	0.4
PILCHARDS								
Fillets, in Tomato Sauce, Average	1 Can/120g	158	7.8	132	16.2	2.2	6.5	0.1
Fillets, in Virgin Olive Oil, Glenryck*	1 Serving/92g	223	14.4	242	23.3	2.0	15.7	0.0
in Brine, Average	**½ Can/77g**	**114**	**5.6**	**148**	**20.8**	**0.0**	**7.3**	**0.0**
PIMMS*								
& Lemonade, Premixed, Canned, Pimms*	1 Can/250ml	160	0.0	64	0.0	8.4	0.0	0.0
*25% Volume, Pimms**	**1 Serving/50ml**	**80**	**0.0**	**160**	**0.0**	**5.0**	**0.0**	**0.0**
PINE NUTS								
Average	**1oz/28g**	**195**	**19.2**	**695**	**15.7**	**3.9**	**68.6**	**1.9**
PINEAPPLE								
& Papaya, Dried, Garden Gang, Asda*	1 Pack/50g	142	0.8	283	2.8	64.0	1.7	8.0

	Measure INFO/WEIGHT	per Measure KCAL	FAT	Nutrition Values per 100g / 100ml KCAL	PROT	CARB	FAT	FIBRE
PINEAPPLE								
Dried, Sweetened, Ready to Eat, Tesco*	1/5 Pack/50g	118	1.0	235	0.4	52.9	1.9	1.7
Dried, Tropical Wholefoods*	1 Slice/10g	30	0.0	305	2.9	73.9	0.2	5.2
Dried, Unsweetened, Sainsbury's*	1 Bag/75g	255	1.5	340	1.7	84.7	2.0	6.0
in Juice, Average	*1 Can/106g*	*57*	*0.0*	*53*	*0.3*	*12.9*	*0.0*	*0.6*
in Syrup, Average	*1 Can/240g*	*158*	*0.0*	*66*	*0.3*	*16.1*	*0.0*	*0.8*
Pieces, Yoghurt Coated, Holland & Barrett*	1 Pack/100g	344	19.3	344	2.1	46.8	19.3	0.6
Raw, Diced, Medley, Lozzas	1 Fruit/400g	200	0.9	42	0.4	10.0	0.2	1.0
Raw, Flesh Only, Average	*1 Pineapple/472g*	*200*	*0.9*	*42*	*0.4*	*10.0*	*0.2*	*1.0*
Tidbits, Dried, Graze*	1 Pack/30g	79	0.2	263	0.6	72.0	0.6	1.0
PISTACHIO NUTS								
Black Pepper, Graze*	1 Punnet/31g	104	9.7	331	10.0	5.0	31.0	3.0
Lightly Toasted, Graze*	1 Punnet/31g	104	9.7	331	10.0	5.0	31.0	3.0
Raw, Average, without Shells	1 Serving/20g	111	8.9	557	20.6	28.0	44.4	10.3
Roasted & Salted, without Shells, Average	*1 Serving/25g*	*152*	*13.6*	*608*	*19.6*	*9.9*	*54.5*	*6.1*
Salted, Roasted, without Shells	*1 Serving/100g*	*601*	*55.4*	*601*	*17.9*	*8.2*	*55.4*	*6.1*
Shelled, Kernels, Wholesome, Love Life, Waitrose*	1 Serving/30g	181	16.6	603	17.9	8.2	55.4	10.3
PIZZA								
American Hot, 12 Inch, Supermarket, Pizza Express*	½ Pizza/264g	562	19.8	213	10.5	25.9	7.5	2.6
American Hot, 8 Inch, Supermarket, Pizza Express*	1 Pizza/295g	652	22.4	221	11.0	27.3	7.6	3.5
American Hot, Chicago Town*	1 Pizza/170g	445	20.1	262	8.2	30.8	11.8	0.9
Bacon & Mushroom, & Tomato, Deep Pan, Loaded, Tesco*	½ Pizza/219g	464	12.7	212	9.3	30.6	5.8	1.5
Bacon & Mushroom, & Tomato, Stonebaked, Tesco*	1 Serving/173g	351	12.8	203	9.9	24.1	7.4	2.0
Bacon & Mushroom, Pizzeria, Sainsbury's*	1 Pizza/355g	880	24.8	248	11.7	34.5	7.0	3.7
Bacon & Mushroom, Stone Bake, M&S*	1 Pizza/375g	750	24.0	200	9.9	27.2	6.4	1.6
Bacon & Mushroom, Stonebaked, Tesco*	1 Serving/157g	352	14.8	224	10.5	24.3	9.4	3.3
Bacon & Mushroom, Thin & Crispy, Sainsbury's*	½ Pizza/150g	396	15.9	264	12.9	29.2	10.6	1.7
Bacon & Mushroom, Thin & Crispy, Somerfield*	¼ Pizza/81g	189	8.1	233	11.0	24.0	10.0	0.0
Bacon & Mushroom, with Capers, Lozzas	1 Slice/157g	352	14.8	224	10.5	24.3	9.4	3.3
BBQ Chicken, M&S*	½ Pizza/210g	430	11.8	205	11.6	27.5	5.6	1.8
BBQ Chicken, Stonebaked, Tesco*	½ Pizza/158g	285	9.5	180	10.5	20.9	6.0	3.9
BBQ Chicken, Stuffed Crust, Asda*	½ Pizza/245g	612	24.5	250	13.0	27.0	10.0	2.7
BBQ Chicken, Thin & Crispy, Sainsbury's*	½ Pizza/167g	399	12.4	238	11.4	30.4	7.4	2.2
BBQ Chicken, Thin & Crispy, Tesco*	1 Serving/165g	355	7.4	215	11.9	31.6	4.5	1.2
Calzone, Speciale, Ristorante, Dr Oetker*	½ Pizza/145g	378	23.2	261	11.5	22.1	16.0	0.0
Capricciosa, Pizza Express*	1 Serving/300g	753	29.3	251	13.6	29.0	9.8	0.0
Caprina, Pizza Express*	1 Pizza/300g	635	22.0	212	8.0	31.0	7.3	0.0
Caramelised Onion, Feta & Rosemary, Bistro, Waitrose*	½ Pizza/230g	607	32.0	264	8.6	26.1	13.9	2.4
Cheese, Double, Chicago Town*	1 Pizza/405g	932	27.1	230	11.7	30.6	6.7	0.0
Cheese, Thin & Crispy, Goodfella's*	1 Serving/275g	729	27.8	265	15.7	27.6	10.1	1.8
Cheese, Three, Slice, Microwaveable, Tesco*	1 Slice/160g	486	18.7	304	13.3	36.7	11.7	1.6
Cheese & Onion, Tesco*	1 Serving/22g	56	2.0	255	10.5	32.7	9.1	2.7
Cheese & Tomato, 12 inch, Fresh, Tesco*	1/3 Pizza/160g	413	13.8	258	9.6	36.3	8.6	1.4
Cheese & Tomato, Average	1 Serving/300g	711	35.4	237	9.1	25.2	11.8	1.4
Cheese & Tomato, Baguette, Tesco*	1 Baguette/125g	275	8.5	220	11.0	28.0	6.8	2.8
Cheese & Tomato, Basics, Somerfield*	1 Serving/80g	194	5.6	242	9.7	35.1	7.0	1.9
Cheese & Tomato, Bistro, Waitrose*	½ Pizza/205g	488	19.9	238	10.0	27.6	9.7	1.2
Cheese & Tomato, Deep Pan, Goodfella's*	¼ Pizza/102g	259	10.8	253	11.5	29.6	10.5	3.7
Cheese & Tomato, Deep Pan, Sainsbury's*	1 Pizza/182g	470	15.8	258	11.7	33.1	8.7	1.9
Cheese & Tomato, Economy, Sainsbury's*	1 Pizza/60g	142	3.7	237	11.2	34.1	6.2	1.8
Cheese & Tomato, Everyday Value, Tesco*	1 Pizza/150g	423	9.2	282	9.6	46.0	6.1	2.2
Cheese & Tomato, French Bread, Co-Op*	1 Pizza/135g	270	8.1	200	9.0	27.0	6.0	2.0
Cheese & Tomato, French Bread, Findus*	1 Serving/143g	322	11.6	225	9.4	29.0	8.1	0.0
Cheese & Tomato, Frozen, Sainsbury's*	1 Serving/122g	300	10.7	246	13.7	28.0	8.8	3.0

PIZZA

INFO/WEIGHT	Measure	per Measure		Nutrition Values per 100g / 100ml				
		KCAL	FAT	KCAL	PROT	CARB	FAT	FIBRE
Cheese & Tomato, Italiano, Tesco*	1 Pizza/380g	969	35.0	255	11.4	31.7	9.2	3.3
Cheese & Tomato, Kids, Tesco*	1 Pizza/95g	219	5.2	231	11.5	33.9	5.5	1.9
Cheese & Tomato, Mini, Bruschetta, Iceland*	1 Pizza/34g	63	2.3	188	8.0	23.0	7.0	2.1
Cheese & Tomato, Mini, M&S*	1 Pizza/95g	233	5.5	245	10.0	38.7	5.8	1.6
Cheese & Tomato, Retail, Frozen	1oz/28g	70	3.0	250	7.5	32.9	10.7	1.4
Cheese & Tomato, Sainsbury's*	1 Pizza/247g	706	24.5	286	13.7	35.4	9.9	2.4
Cheese & Tomato, Slice, Ross*	1 Slice/77g	148	6.6	192	6.5	22.2	8.6	2.0
Cheese & Tomato, Slices, CBY, Asda*	1 Slice/14g	62	2.5	453	8.2	63.2	18.1	2.3
Cheese & Tomato, Smart Price, Asda*	1 Pizza/151g	393	7.6	260	4.7	27.0	5.0	1.6
Cheese & Tomato, Stone Bake, M&S*	1 Pizza/340g	782	28.6	230	10.8	30.1	8.4	1.6
Cheese & Tomato, Stonebaked, Co-Op*	1 Pizza/325g	699	26.0	215	10.0	26.0	8.0	3.0
Cheese & Tomato, Stonebaked, Thin & Crispy, Tesco*	½ Pizza/161g	388	13.8	241	11.6	29.4	8.6	2.1
Cheese & Tomato, Thin & Crispy, Asda*	1 Pizza/366g	827	36.6	226	11.0	23.0	10.0	2.0
Cheese & Tomato, Thin & Crispy, Morrisons*	1 Pizza/335g	734	23.8	219	11.2	27.7	7.1	3.1
Cheese & Tomato, Thin & Crispy, Sainsbury's*	1 Serving/135g	344	10.0	255	14.9	32.2	7.4	5.0
Cheese & Tomato, Thin & Crispy, Stonebaked, Tesco*	1/3 Pizza/212g	509	19.5	240	10.1	29.2	9.2	1.4
Cheese & Tomato, Thin & Crispy, Stonebaked, Tesco*	1 Pizza/155g	355	12.1	229	11.6	28.1	7.8	1.3
Cheese & Tomato, Thin & Crispy, Waitrose*	1 Pizza/280g	658	28.3	235	12.3	23.6	10.1	2.3
Cheese Feast, Deep Pan, Asda*	½ Pizza/210g	422	18.9	201	13.0	17.0	9.0	2.3
Cheese Feast, Thin Crust, Chilled, Tesco*	½ Pizza/175g	467	22.4	267	14.7	23.4	12.8	2.5
Chicken, Cajun, Sainsbury's*	½ Pizza/146g	285	2.6	195	12.9	31.8	1.8	2.6
Chicken, Chargrilled, Thin & Crispy, Asda*	1 Pizza/373g	780	18.6	209	9.0	32.0	5.0	1.6
Chicken, Fajita, COU, M&S*	1 Pizza/255g	434	6.1	170	9.9	25.5	2.4	1.2
Chicken, Fajita, Takeaway, Goodfella's*	¼ Pizza/150g	339	12.0	226	10.8	27.5	8.0	1.7
Chicken, Garlic, Thin & Crispy, Stonebake, Sainsbury's*	½ Pizza/160g	386	17.3	241	10.7	25.2	10.8	3.5
Chicken, Hot & Spicy, Deep Pan, Morrisons*	½ Pizza/233g	521	13.0	224	10.5	32.9	5.6	1.0
Chicken & Bacon, Loaded, Tesco*	1 Serving/258g	622	25.3	241	12.8	25.4	9.8	1.9
Chicken & Bacon, Pizzeria, Italian, Sainsbury's*	½ Pizza/170g	508	24.1	300	13.6	29.4	14.2	2.7
Chicken & Chorizo, 12", TTD, Sainsbury's*	½ Pizza/290g	702	20.9	242	12.2	32.1	7.2	2.6
Chicken & Vegetable, Stone Baked, GFY, Asda*	½ Pizza/161g	349	3.7	217	13.0	36.0	2.3	1.7
Chicken Provencal, Goodfella's*	½ Pizza/143g	388	18.0	272	13.7	25.9	12.6	2.1
Chorizo, Red Pepper & Chilli, Spicy, Classico, Tesco*	1 Serving/218g	474	17.4	218	10.3	26.4	8.0	2.5
Diavolo, Pizza Express*	½ Pizza/164g	322	11.0	197	9.4	24.6	6.7	2.1
Five Cheese, & Pepperoni, Deep & Crispy, Waitrose*	1/3 Pizza/200g	560	23.2	280	11.7	32.3	11.6	1.3
Four Cheese, Finest, Tesco*	½ Pizza/230g	575	21.2	250	12.1	29.8	9.2	1.3
Four Cheese, Stuffed Crust, Takeaway, Chicago Town*	¼ Pizza/158g	433	17.0	275	10.8	33.0	10.8	1.9
Four Cheese, Thin & Crispy, Sainsbury's*	1 Pizza/265g	729	32.6	275	11.8	29.3	12.3	3.5
Four Cheese, Thin Crust, Tesco*	½ Pizza/142g	386	13.6	272	14.5	31.8	9.6	1.8
Four Seasons, Stonebaked, Truly Irresistible, Co-Op*	½ Pizza/245g	502	16.2	205	9.5	26.6	6.6	2.6
Four Seasons, Waitrose*	1/3 Pizza/174g	382	14.6	220	9.9	26.2	8.4	2.6
Frutti Di Mare, Express, Pizza Express*	1 Pizza/373g	500	9.5	134	9.1	20.1	2.6	0.0
Funghi, Ristorante, Dr Oetker*	1 Pizza/365g	865	43.4	237	7.9	22.5	11.9	0.0
Garlic Bread, Stonebaked, Italiono, Tesco*	1 Serving/117g	403	18.2	346	7.8	43.6	15.6	1.5
Giardiniera, from Supermarket, Pizza Express*	½ Pizza/144g	291	10.5	202	8.6	25.5	7.3	2.1
Ham & Cheese, Chunky, Asda*	1 Serving/90g	211	3.0	234	12.0	39.0	3.3	4.7
Ham & Mushroom, & Mascarpone, Italian Style, M&S*	1 Pizza/224g	515	21.7	230	10.0	25.5	9.7	2.9
Ham & Mushroom, Average	1 Serving/250g	533	16.0	213	10.5	28.4	6.4	2.1
Ham & Mushroom, Calzone, Waitrose*	½ Pizza/145g	362	13.5	250	10.0	31.6	9.3	1.6
Ham & Mushroom, COU, M&S*	1 Pizza/245g	355	4.4	145	8.8	24.0	1.8	2.2
Ham & Mushroom, Deep Pan, Asda*	½ Pizza/223g	444	15.6	199	9.0	25.0	7.0	1.2
Ham & Mushroom, Deep Pan, Waitrose*	½ Pizza/220g	453	13.6	206	10.9	26.6	6.2	1.0
Ham & Mushroom, Finest, Tesco*	½ Pizza/240g	576	26.4	240	9.5	25.9	11.0	2.2
Ham & Mushroom, Slices, Farmfoods*	1 Slice/89g	170	2.3	191	8.0	34.0	2.6	0.9

PIZZA

	Measure INFO/WEIGHT	per Measure KCAL	per Measure FAT	Nutrition Values per 100g / 100ml KCAL	PROT	CARB	FAT	FIBRE
Ham & Mushroom, Smoked, Thin & Crispy, Co-Op*	1 Pizza/400g	792	18.0	198	9.0	30.3	4.5	1.7
Ham & Mushroom, Thin & Crispy, Asda*	1 Pizza/360g	760	25.2	211	11.0	26.0	7.0	2.4
Ham & Mushroom, Thin & Crispy, Tesco*	½ Pizza/185g	380	11.1	205	11.2	25.6	6.0	2.3
Ham & Pepperoni, Milano, M&S*	1 Pizza/290g	696	28.4	240	14.0	23.3	9.8	1.1
Ham & Pineapple, American Deep Pan, Sainsbury's*	1 Pizza/412g	1001	32.1	243	10.5	32.6	7.8	1.7
Ham & Pineapple, Average	1 Serving/250g	555	16.8	222	11.0	29.2	6.7	2.1
Ham & Pineapple, Deep, Asda*	1 Pizza/486g	1055	22.4	217	11.3	32.5	4.6	3.0
Ham & Pineapple, Deep Dish, Individual, Chicago Town*	1 Pizza/170g	410	15.1	241	9.9	30.4	8.9	1.6
Ham & Pineapple, Deep Pan, Tesco*	1 Pizza/237g	437	6.9	184	9.8	29.8	2.9	1.9
Ham & Pineapple, Hand Made, Thin & Crispy, Waitrose*	¼ Pizza/113g	250	7.9	221	11.0	27.3	7.0	2.5
Ham & Pineapple, Pizzerai, Simply Italian, Sainsbury's*	½ Pizza/178g	434	15.1	244	11.5	30.4	8.5	2.4
Ham & Pineapple, Stonebaked, Tesco*	1 Pizza/161g	293	9.2	182	9.2	23.5	5.7	3.5
Ham & Pineapple, Tesco*	1/6 Pizza/56g	134	4.6	240	10.4	30.9	8.3	2.1
Ham & Pineapple, Thin & Crispy, Good Choice, Iceland*	1 Pizza/600g	1338	29.4	223	11.7	33.1	4.9	1.7
Ham & Pineapple, Thin & Crispy, Sainsbury's*	1 Pizza/330g	719	21.1	218	10.8	29.4	6.4	2.4
Ham & Pineapple, Thin & Crispy, Waitrose*	1 Pizza/220g	616	21.1	280	12.8	33.3	9.6	2.2
Ham & Pineapple, Thin & Crispy Italian, Morrisons*	1 Pizza/375g	746	22.9	199	10.2	24.9	6.1	0.0
Ham & Pineapple, Thin Crust, Tesco*	½ Pizza/175g	385	10.0	220	12.3	29.6	5.7	2.5
Hawaiian, Thin Crust, Tesco*	½ Pizza/192g	365	9.4	190	10.3	25.6	4.9	1.8
Hot & Spicy, Pizzeria Style, Sainsbury's*	1 Pizza/376g	986	46.3	262	12.5	25.5	12.3	2.4
Hot & Spicy, Thin & Crispy, Morrisons*	½ Pizza/170g	393	15.8	231	10.5	26.5	9.3	3.2
Le Reine, 8 Inch, Supermarket, Pizza Express*	1 Pizza/283g	546	16.4	193	10.2	25.0	5.8	2.7
Margherita, 12 Inch, Supermarket, Pizza Express*	½ Pizza/230g	494	13.8	215	10.1	28.3	6.0	3.6
Margherita, 12", Finest, Tesco*	½ Pizza/255g	433	9.2	170	8.1	26.4	3.6	2.7
Margherita, Average	1 Slice/108g	239	8.6	239	11.0	30.5	8.6	1.2
Margherita, Classico, Italiano, Tesco*	½ Pizza/191g	414	11.8	217	11.2	29.1	6.2	2.5
Margherita, Finest, Tesco*	1 Serving/207g	441	10.8	213	11.0	30.5	5.2	1.2
Margherita, Italian Stonebaked, Asda*	¼ Pizza/135g	323	10.8	240	11.0	31.0	8.0	1.8
Margherita, LC, Tesco*	1 Pizza/200g	410	5.0	205	11.0	33.8	2.5	1.7
Margherita, Morrisons*	½ Pizza/163g	416	18.0	256	12.9	26.1	11.1	2.3
Margherita, Pizzeria, Italian, Sainsbury's*	½ Pizza/169g	426	17.4	253	12.2	27.9	10.3	2.5
Margherita, Stone Baked, GFY, Asda*	¼ Pizza/73g	158	1.4	217	11.0	39.0	1.9	1.8
Margherita, Stone Baked, Goodfella's*	1 Slice/36g	95	4.1	263	10.9	31.9	11.4	7.6
Margherita, Stonebaked, Co-Op*	1 Pizza/350g	840	29.1	240	13.2	27.6	8.3	3.0
Margherita, Stonebaked Ciabatta, Goodfella's*	½ Pizza/150g	404	17.2	270	11.3	32.8	11.5	2.6
Margherita, Thin & Crispy, Iceland*	½ Pizza/170g	391	14.4	230	12.7	25.9	8.5	2.8
Margherita, Thin Crust, Tesco*	1 Serving/170g	354	13.4	208	10.1	24.1	7.9	3.6
Margherita, Truly Irresistible, Co-Op*	1 Pizza/465g	1023	36.7	220	8.1	27.4	7.9	3.3
Meat, Italian, Finest, Tesco*	½ Pizza/217g	449	8.5	207	13.6	29.4	3.9	1.3
Meat Feast, American Style, Sainsbury's*	½ Pizza/263g	642	26.0	244	12.6	26.2	9.9	2.9
Meat Feast, Deep & Loaded, Sainsbury's*	½ Pizza/298g	818	30.0	275	13.2	32.7	10.1	2.6
Meat Feast, Hot & Spicy, Thin & Crispy, Sainsbury's*	½ Pizza/170g	462	21.6	272	13.0	26.5	12.7	3.2
Meat Feast, Italian, Thin & Crispy, Waitrose*	1 Pizza/182g	477	22.9	262	10.7	26.5	12.6	1.8
Meat Feast, Loaded, Deep Pan, Large, Tesco*	½ Pizza/282g	776	38.4	275	12.0	26.1	13.6	1.9
Meat Feast, Stuffed Crust, Asda*	½ Pizza/238g	597	24.0	251	14.6	25.5	10.1	3.1
Meat Feast, Thin & Crispy, Asda*	½ Pizza/183g	410	14.6	224	11.0	27.0	8.0	1.4
Meat Feast, Thin Crust, Tesco*	½ Pizza/178g	430	20.2	242	13.6	21.3	11.4	2.3
Mini, Party, Tesco*	1 Pizza/11g	26	1.1	248	11.4	28.6	10.5	1.9
Mozzarella, & Sunblush Tomato, 12", TTD, Sainsbury's*	½ Pizza/251g	638	17.8	254	12.4	35.0	7.1	2.6
Mozzarella, Buffalo, & Rustic Tomato, Finest, Tesco*	½ Pizza/172g	354	11.4	206	6.8	29.8	6.6	1.9
Mozzarella, Ristorante, Dr Oetker*	1 Pizza/335g	890	13.6	266	10.5	24.2	4.1	0.5
Mushroom, & Mascarpone, 12", TTD, Sainsbury's*	½ Pizza/255g	638	18.6	250	12.1	34.0	7.3	2.4
Mushroom, Garlic, Ciabatta Style, Stonebake, Goodfella's*	½ Pizza/187g	474	23.0	254	10.0	27.9	12.3	2.2

	Measure INFO/WEIGHT	per Measure KCAL	FAT	Nutrition Values per 100g / 100ml KCAL	PROT	CARB	FAT	FIBRE

PIZZA

	Measure INFO/WEIGHT	KCAL	FAT	KCAL	PROT	CARB	FAT	FIBRE
Pepper, Grilled, Weight Watchers*	1 Pizza/220g	392	5.1	178	10.0	29.3	2.3	1.8
Pepperoni, & Cheese, Asda*	½ Pizza/150g	386	13.5	257	10.0	34.0	9.0	2.7
Pepperoni, & Jalapeno Chill, Asda*	1 Pizza/277g	742	22.2	268	10.0	39.0	8.0	1.8
Pepperoni, Aldi*	1 Serving/55g	123	4.3	224	8.7	29.5	7.9	1.4
Pepperoni, Asda*	½ Pizza/150g	386	13.5	257	10.0	34.0	9.0	2.7
Pepperoni, Average	1 Serving/250g	671	28.4	269	11.8	29.6	11.4	2.1
Pepperoni, Chicago Town*	1 Pizza/170g	471	21.9	277	11.5	28.8	12.9	0.0
Pepperoni, Deep Filled, Chicago Town*	1 Serving/202g	621	33.6	307	11.5	28.0	16.6	1.3
Pepperoni, Deep Pan, Frozen, Tesco*	½ Pizza/215g	527	17.4	245	11.9	31.1	8.1	2.6
Pepperoni, Deep Pan, Goodfella's*	¼ Pizza/109g	294	12.6	270	12.7	28.9	11.6	1.6
Pepperoni, Double, Italian, Chilled, Tesco*	½ Pizza/160g	455	23.3	285	12.4	25.6	14.6	2.4
Pepperoni, Etruscan, TTD, Sainsbury's*	½ Pizza/252g	676	20.9	268	13.2	35.1	8.3	2.4
Pepperoni, Goodfella's*	1 Pizza/337g	900	43.5	267	13.2	26.3	12.9	1.7
Pepperoni, Hot & Spicy, Stuffed Crust, Asda*	1 Pizza/245g	666	30.0	272	13.9	26.5	12.2	2.4
Pepperoni, Hot & Spicy, Thin Crust, Chilled, Tesco*	½ Pizza/174g	486	25.5	280	12.4	24.0	14.7	2.2
Pepperoni, Italian, Tesco*	½ Pizza/186g	484	20.6	260	11.4	28.0	11.1	1.1
Pepperoni, Italian Stonebaked, Asda*	¼ Pizza/132g	329	13.2	250	12.0	28.0	10.0	2.8
Pepperoni, Pizzeria, Sainsbury's*	½ Pizza/197g	559	25.8	284	13.4	28.3	13.1	2.4
Pepperoni, Pizzeria Style, Sainsbury's*	½ Pizza/183g	515	23.3	281	13.5	28.0	12.7	2.2
Pepperoni, Sauce Stuffed Crust, Chicago Town*	¼ Pizza/151g	427	18.4	283	12.4	31.0	12.2	2.1
Pepperoni, Stonebake, 10", Asda*	½ Pizza/170g	435	19.0	256	12.9	25.9	11.2	2.5
Pepperoni, Stonebaked, American Hot, Sainsbury's*	½ Pizza/276g	674	30.9	244	11.6	24.1	11.2	2.9
Pepperoni, Stonebaked Ciabatta, Goodfella's*	½ Pizza/181g	503	26.1	278	11.9	27.4	14.4	2.4
Pepperoni, Thin & Crispy, Co-Op*	1 Pizza/270g	688	29.7	255	11.0	26.0	11.0	1.0
Pepperoni, Thin & Crispy, Essential, Waitrose*	½ Pizza/133g	380	18.0	286	12.3	28.8	13.5	1.0
Pepperoni, Thin & Crispy, Goodfella's*	1 Pizza/593g	1595	70.0	269	13.8	26.9	11.8	2.3
Pepperoni, Thin & Crispy, Sainsbury's*	½ Pizza/132g	405	18.9	307	13.9	30.7	14.3	2.6
Pepperoni, Thin Crust, Chilled, Tesco*	½ Pizza/163g	479	24.4	295	13.5	25.4	15.0	1.8
Pepperoni, Weight Watchers*	1 Pizza/300g	501	9.3	167	8.0	25.4	3.1	2.8
Pollo, Ad Astra, Pizza Express*	1 Pizza/317g	602	14.9	190	11.6	25.2	4.7	2.7
Pollo, Pesto, Supermarket, Pizza Express*	1 Pizza/265g	500	10.1	189	9.2	25.0	3.8	2.0
Pollo, Ristorante, Dr Oetker*	½ Pizza/178g	383	16.9	216	8.9	23.4	9.5	0.0
Prosciutto, Ristorante, Dr Oetker*	1 Pizza/330g	752	32.3	228	10.3	24.6	9.8	0.0
Quattro Formaggi, 8 Inch, Supermarket, Pizza Express*	1 Pizza/266g	646	26.1	243	12.1	26.5	9.8	2.3
Quattro Formaggi, Ristorante, Dr Oetker*	½ Pizza/175g	472	25.0	270	11.4	23.9	14.3	0.0
Quattro Formaggi Pizzeria, Sainsbury's*	½ Pizza/175g	490	21.2	280	12.8	30.8	12.1	2.5
Quattro Formaggio, Tesco*	½ Pizza/219g	583	27.4	266	13.3	25.1	12.5	1.8
Salame, Ristorante, Dr Oetker*	½ Pizza/160g	455	24.5	285	10.4	26.3	15.3	0.0
Salami, Con Mozarella, Lidl*	½ Pizza/200g	534	22.4	267	9.9	31.5	11.2	0.0
Salami, Lidl*	1 Pizza/350g	854	32.2	244	8.1	29.4	9.2	0.0
Salami & Pepperoni, Bistro, Waitrose*	½ Pizza/190g	492	19.4	259	12.9	28.8	10.2	1.5
Sausage, & Roasted Peppers, Italian, Finest, Tesco*	1 Pizza/325g	650	13.6	200	7.8	31.7	4.2	1.9
Slice, Selection, M&S*	1 Serving/52g	120	4.1	230	9.4	30.3	7.8	1.9
Spinach & Ricotta, BGTY, Sainsbury's*	1 Pizza/265g	535	6.6	202	10.4	34.4	2.5	2.6
Spinach & Ricotta, Extra Special, Asda*	1 Pizza/400g	940	28.0	235	9.0	34.0	7.0	1.9
Spinach & Ricotta, Italian, Chilled, Sainsbury's*	1 Pizza/361g	859	34.7	238	9.3	28.7	9.6	2.3
Spinach & Ricotta, Pizzaria, Waitrose*	½ Pizza/238g	501	21.1	211	10.7	21.9	8.9	2.6
Spinach & Ricotta, Thin Crust, Italian, Tesco*	½ Pizza/190g	365	16.7	192	9.6	18.7	8.8	1.9
Spinach & Rocotta, Classic Italian, Stonebaked, Tesco*	½ Pizza/190g	460	16.3	240	10.3	29.0	8.5	1.2
Supreme, Deep Dish, Individual, Chicago Town*	1 Pizza/170g	456	20.4	268	9.2	30.8	12.0	1.0
Three Cheese, & Tomato, Stonebaked, Co-Op*	1 Pizza/415g	888	33.6	214	10.0	25.2	8.1	1.5
Three Cheese, Calzone, Waitrose*	1 Pizza/265g	747	31.8	282	10.4	33.0	12.0	1.4
Tomato	1oz/28g	54	3.0	193	3.3	22.6	10.6	1.4

	Measure INFO/WEIGHT	per Measure		Nutrition Values per 100g / 100ml				
		KCAL	FAT	KCAL	PROT	CARB	FAT	FIBRE
PIZZA								
Tomato, Aubergine & Spinach, Pizzeria, Waitrose*	½ Pizza/193g	403	7.7	209	7.8	35.4	4.0	3.6
Tomato, Basil & Buffalo Mozzarella, Campanina, Waitrose*	¼ Pack/126g	316	13.8	251	9.0	29.0	11.0	3.4
Tomato, Basil & Garlic, Weight Watchers*	1 Serving/85g	169	2.9	199	12.3	29.8	3.4	1.6
Triple Cheese, Deep Dish, Chicago Town*	1 Serving/170g	418	18.2	246	9.9	27.6	10.7	0.0
Triple Cheese, Deep Pan, Morrisons*	1/6 Pizza/75g	198	9.2	265	10.4	28.2	12.3	1.9
Tuna, & Caramelised Red Onion, COU, M&S*	1 Pizza/245g	429	5.6	175	9.6	26.7	2.3	1.2
Vegetable & Mozzarella, Roast, Balsamic, Sainsbury's*	½ Pizza/200g	444	15.6	222	8.5	29.4	7.8	2.4
Vegetable, Average	1 Serving/250g	475	13.1	190	8.2	27.5	5.2	2.4
Vegetable, Chargrilled, Frozen, BGTY, Sainsbury's*	1 Pizza/290g	548	13.3	189	10.2	26.7	4.6	3.0
Vegetable, Chargrilled, Thin & Crispy, GFY, Asda*	1 Serving/188g	290	3.8	154	6.0	28.0	2.0	3.1
Vegetable, Deep Pan, Co-Op*	1 Pizza/425g	829	29.8	195	8.0	25.0	7.0	2.0
Vegetable, Feast, Thin & Crispy, Iceland*	1 Slice/63g	148	6.9	237	7.8	26.5	11.1	1.8
Vegetable, GFY, Asda*	¼ Pizza/94g	141	2.7	150	7.0	24.0	2.9	3.7
Vegetable, Mediterranean, Pizzeria, Sainsbury's*	1 Serving/211g	397	13.5	188	8.0	24.7	6.4	3.2
Vegetable, Mediterranean, Stonebaked, Sainsbury's*	½ Pizza/260g	622	16.4	239	9.8	35.7	6.3	3.1
Vegetable, Stone Bake, M&S*	1 Serving/465g	837	26.0	180	7.8	25.0	5.6	1.5
Vegetable, Stonebaked, Thin & Crispy, Sainsbury's*	½ Pizza/160g	362	14.2	225	7.4	29.0	8.8	2.8
Vegetable, Thin & Crispy, Iceland*	½ Pizza/200g	442	21.2	221	8.3	23.2	10.6	1.7
Vegetable & Peppers, Fire Roasted, Waitrose*	½ Pizza/235g	442	16.7	188	9.8	21.3	7.1	2.7
Vegetale, Ristorante, Dr Oetker*	½ Pizza/185g	386	16.6	209	8.1	23.9	9.0	0.0
Vitabella, with Peppers & Asparagus, Pizza Express*	1 Pizza/290g	430	6.6	148	7.0	27.0	2.3	2.3
PIZZA BASE								
Deep Pan, Napolina*	1 Base/260g	757	7.8	291	7.9	58.0	3.0	0.2
Everyday Value, Tesco*	½ Base/125g	401	2.8	320	9.6	65.2	2.2	0.7
Garlic Bread, Sainsbury's*	¼ Base/59g	109	4.2	186	5.1	25.4	7.1	1.8
GF, Wellfoods*	½ Pizza/150g	482	16.2	321	1.9	53.9	10.8	1.4
Gluten, Wheat & Dairy Free, Free From, Livwell*	1 Base/100g	237	2.6	237	5.2	48.3	2.6	4.7
Italian, Classic, Sainsbury's*	1 Base/150g	452	7.2	301	7.6	57.0	4.8	1.5
Italian, The Pizza Company*	1 Base/260g	624	6.8	240	7.6	46.5	2.6	0.0
Light & Crispy, Napolina*	1 Base/150g	436	4.5	291	7.9	58.0	3.0	0.2
Mini, Napolina*	1 Base/75g	218	2.2	291	7.9	58.0	3.0	0.2
Thin & Crispy, Sainsbury's*	1 Base/150g	504	7.8	336	9.9	62.3	5.2	4.3
Thin & Crispy, Tesco*	1 Serving/110g	348	8.2	316	9.2	52.9	7.5	1.5
PIZZA BASE MIX								
Made Up as per Instructions, Tesco*	½ Base/126g	360	4.7	285	13.7	48.6	3.7	3.0
Morrisons*	1 Serving/77g	313	3.8	407	12.7	77.9	5.0	3.6
Sainsbury's*	1 Pack/145g	486	5.5	335	12.8	62.3	3.8	2.9
PLAICE								
Fillets, in Breadcrumbs, Average	1 Serving/150g	331	17.9	221	12.8	15.5	11.9	0.8
Fillets, Lightly Dusted, Average	1 Fillet/113g	188	9.2	166	12.9	10.4	8.2	0.6
Fillets, Raw, Average	*1oz/28g*	*24*	*0.4*	*87*	*18.2*	*0.0*	*1.5*	*0.0*
Goujons, Baked	1oz/28g	85	5.1	304	8.8	27.7	18.3	0.0
Goujons, Fried in Blended Oil	1oz/28g	119	9.0	426	8.5	27.0	32.3	0.0
Grilled	*1oz/28g*	*27*	*0.5*	*96*	*20.1*	*0.0*	*1.7*	*0.0*
in Batter, Fried in Blended Oil	1oz/28g	72	4.7	257	15.2	12.0	16.8	0.5
Steamed	*1oz/28g*	*26*	*0.5*	*93*	*18.9*	*0.0*	*1.9*	*0.0*
PLAICE WITH								
Prawns, & Garlic, Filled, Somerfield*	1 Serving/171g	366	20.3	214	12.0	14.8	11.9	0.7
Prawns, in Breadcrumbs, Aldi*	1 Serving/100g	212	8.4	212	8.6	25.4	8.4	0.0
Spinach & Ricotta Cheese, Whole, Sainsbury's*	1 Serving/159g	334	16.7	210	11.6	17.2	10.5	0.8
PLANTAIN								
Boiled in Unsalted Water	*1oz/28g*	*31*	*0.1*	*112*	*0.8*	*28.5*	*0.2*	*1.2*
Raw, Average	*1 Med/179g*	*218*	*0.7*	*122*	*1.3*	*31.9*	*0.4*	*2.3*

	Measure INFO/WEIGHT	per Measure KCAL	FAT	Nutrition Values per 100g / 100ml KCAL	PROT	CARB	FAT	FIBRE
PLANTAIN								
Ripe, Fried in Vegetable Oil	*1oz/28g*	*75*	*2.6*	*267*	*1.5*	*47.5*	*9.2*	*2.3*
PLUMS								
Average, Stewed without Sugar	*1oz/28g*	*8*	*0.0*	*30*	*0.5*	*7.3*	*0.1*	*1.3*
Fresh, Raw, Weighed without Stone, Average	1 Plum/66g	24	0.1	36	0.6	8.6	0.1	1.9
Weighed with Stone, Average	*1 Plum/90g*	*33*	*0.1*	*36*	*0.6*	*8.6*	*0.1*	*1.9*
Whole, Dried, Graze*	1 Pack/60g	143	0.3	239	2.6	56.0	0.5	0.0
Yellow, Waitrose*	1 Plum/50g	20	0.0	39	0.6	8.8	0.1	1.5
POLENTA								
Dry, Merchant Gourmet*	1 Serving/65g	232	0.9	357	7.4	78.8	1.4	1.3
POLLOCK								
Breaded, Asda*	1 Serving/97g	200	9.7	206	12.0	17.0	10.0	1.0
Fillet, Florentine Crusted, Gastro, Youngs*	1 Fillet/170g	203	29.8	119	35.9	10.2	17.5	1.5
POLO								
Citrus Sharp, Nestle*	1 Tube/34g	134	0.3	393	0.0	96.6	1.0	0.0
Fruits, Nestle*	1 Tube/37g	142	0.0	383	0.0	96.0	0.0	0.0
Mints, Clear Ice, Nestle*	1 Sweet/4g	16	0.0	390	0.0	97.5	0.0	0.0
Mints, Original, Nestle*	1 Sweet/2g	8	0.0	402	0.0	98.2	1.0	0.0
Spearmint, Nestle*	1 Tube/35g	141	0.4	402	0.0	98.2	1.1	0.0
POMEGRANATE								
Raw, Fresh, Flesh Only, Average	*1 Fruit/86g*	*59*	*0.3*	*68*	*1.0*	*17.2*	*0.3*	*0.6*
Raw, Weighed with Rind & Skin, Average	*1 Fruit/154g*	*105*	*0.5*	*68*	*1.0*	*17.2*	*0.3*	*0.1*
POMELO								
Fresh, Raw, Weighed with Skin & Seeds	*100 Grams/100g*	*18*	*0.1*	*18*	*0.4*	*4.1*	*0.1*	*0.0*
Raw, Flesh Only, Average	1 Fruit/340g	129	0.1	38	0.8	9.6	0.0	1.0
POP TARTS								
Chocolate, Kellogg's*	1 Pastry/50g	198	8.5	396	5.0	136.0	17.0	2.0
Chocolate Chip, Kellogg's*	1 Pastry/52g	210	6.0	404	5.8	69.2	11.5	1.9
Chocolate Chip Cookie Dough, Kellogg's*	1 Pastry/50g	190	5.0	380	4.0	70.0	10.0	2.0
Cinnamon Roll, Kelloggs*	1 Pastry/50g	210	7.0	420	4.0	68.0	14.0	2.0
Cookies 'n' Creme, Kellogg's*	1 Pastry/50g	190	5.0	380	4.0	70.0	10.0	2.0
Frosted Blueberry, Kellogg's*	1 Pastry/52g	200	5.0	385	3.8	73.1	9.6	1.9
Frosted Confetti Cupcake, Kellogg's*	1 Pastry/50g	190	4.0	380	4.0	72.0	8.0	2.0
Frosted S'mores, Kellogg's*	1 Pastry/52g	200	5.0	385	5.8	69.2	9.6	1.9
Frosted Strawberry, Oatmeal Delights, Kellogg's*	1 Pastry/50g	200	5.0	400	4.0	72.0	10.0	6.0
Strawberry Sensation, Kellogg's*	1 Tart/50g	198	5.5	395	4.0	70.0	11.0	2.0
POPCORN								
94% Fat Free, Orville Redenbacher's*	1 Bag/76g	220	0.0	289	13.2	65.8	0.0	0.0
Air Popped, Plain, Average	1oz/28g	110	1.3	387	12.9	77.9	4.5	14.5
Butter, Microwave, 94% Fat Free, Act II*	½ Bag/41g	130	2.5	317	9.8	68.3	6.1	12.2
Butter, Microwave, Act II*	1 Bag/90g	425	16.2	472	9.0	69.0	18.0	9.0
Butter, Microwave, Butterkist*	1 Bag/100g	395	18.5	395	8.3	49.5	18.5	8.5
Butter, Microwave, Popz*	1 Serving/100g	480	27.5	480	7.5	51.1	27.5	9.2
Butter Toffee, Asda*	1 Serving/100g	364	8.0	364	2.1	71.0	8.0	4.1
Butter Toffee, Belgian Milk Chocolate Coated, M&S*	1 Pack/100g	505	25.0	505	6.5	60.4	25.0	4.1
Butter Toffee, Snack-A-Jacks, Quaker Oats*	1 Bag/35g	149	3.2	425	3.5	86.0	9.0	4.5
Butter Toffee, Tesco*	1 Pack/350g	1418	27.0	405	2.2	81.7	7.7	4.3
Choc Full Of, Cadbury*	¼ Bag/32g	160	7.6	495	4.5	64.5	23.5	2.9
Chocolate, & Pecan, M&S*	1 Pack/27g	130	5.2	480	3.3	72.9	19.3	3.6
Chocolate, & Pecan Clusters, Extra Special, Asda*	1/3 Bag/50g	232	10.0	463	3.7	67.0	20.0	6.2
Chocolate, Toffee, Snack-A-Jacks, Quaker Oats*	1 Bag/35g	126	3.4	359	2.2	65.0	9.8	3.0
Chocolate, Trickle, Skinny, Topcorn, Metcalfe's Food Co*	1 Pack/55g	221	8.4	401	5.2	59.6	15.2	7.1
Maize, Unpopped, Love Life, Waitrose*	1 Serving/33g	200	14.1	605	6.2	48.7	42.8	12.7
Maple, Shapers, Boots*	1 Bag/20g	94	3.6	469	12.0	59.0	18.0	10.0

POPCORN

	Measure INFO/WEIGHT	per Measure KCAL	FAT	Nutrition Values per 100g / 100ml KCAL	PROT	CARB	FAT	FIBRE
Plain, Oil Popped, Average	1 Bag/74g	439	31.7	593	6.2	48.7	42.8	0.0
Salt & Sweet, Pure*	1 Serving/25g	119	5.5	476	6.0	61.1	22.1	7.8
Salt & Vinegar, Diet Chef Ltd*	1 Serving/23g	106	3.6	461	10.4	69.8	15.8	13.0
Salt & Vinegar, Snack-A-Jacks, Quaker Oats*	1 Pack/13g	47	1.3	360	12.0	55.0	9.9	14.0
Salted, Blockbuster*	1 Bowl/25g	99	2.9	397	10.6	62.2	11.7	8.6
Salted, Bop, Microwave, Zanuy*	1 Serving/25g	119	5.8	477	10.7	56.9	23.0	0.0
Salted, Diet Chef Ltd*	1 Pack/23g	107	3.8	465	10.5	68.6	16.6	14.0
Salted, Light, Microwave, Act II*	1 Pack/85g	336	6.5	395	10.6	71.0	7.6	15.8
Salted, Lightly, Snack-A-Jack, Quaker Oats*	1 Bag/13g	48	1.3	370	12.1	58.0	9.9	14.6
Salted, M&S*	1 Pack/25g	132	7.8	530	9.4	50.4	31.1	6.4
Salted, Manhatten Peanuts Limited*	1 Bag/30g	135	4.3	450	10.0	70.0	14.3	13.7
Salted, Microwave, 93% Fat Free, Act II*	1 Pack/85g	345	6.0	406	10.0	76.0	7.0	13.0
Salted, Microwave, Popz*	1 Serving/20g	101	6.0	504	7.0	51.5	30.0	9.2
Salted, Microwave, Sunsnacks*	1 Pack/100g	498	22.9	498	10.7	51.3	22.9	10.8
Salted, Sea Salt, Skinny, Topcorn, Metcalfe's Food Co*	1 Pack/23g	108	5.6	471	6.6	63.7	24.4	15.2
Salted, Sea Salt & Vinegar, Sainsbury's*	1 Bag/11g	52	2.7	474	4.8	53.6	24.6	9.7
Salted, Sold At Cinema, Playtime Popcorn*	1 Sm/74g	384	24.9	519	8.3	45.9	33.6	0.0
Super, Perri*	1 Pack/30g	139	7.0	464	8.4	55.5	23.2	8.5
Sweet, Butterkist, Butterkist*	1 Pack/120g	612	29.8	510	2.8	68.5	24.8	5.6
Sweet, Cinema Style, Basics, Sainsbury's*	1 Handful/20g	90	4.4	450	5.9	57.5	21.8	11.1
Sweet, Cinema Style, Butterkist*	1 Bag/120g	612	29.8	510	2.8	68.5	24.8	5.6
Sweet, Microwave, Butterkist*	½ Pack/50g	235	10.0	470	9.8	60.5	20.1	4.4
Sweet, Microwave, Cinema, Popz*	1 Bag/85g	420	21.7	494	6.0	60.0	25.5	8.2
Sweet & Salty, Shapers, Boots*	1 Bag/20g	89	3.2	443	5.8	65.0	16.0	10.0
Sweet Maple, Diet Chef Ltd*	1 Pack/23g	111	3.6	483	9.7	75.2	15.7	13.0
Sweet 'n' Salt, Skinny, Topcorn, Metcalfe's Food Co*	1 Bag/25g	115	4.8	459	6.4	71.0	19.2	11.7
Toffee, Best-In*	1 Bag/90g	356	3.2	396	5.0	85.9	3.6	0.0
Toffee, Butterkist*	1 Bag/30g	124	3.0	415	2.3	79.3	10.0	4.4
Toffee, Chicago Joes*	1 Serving/10g	31	0.5	314	3.1	84.6	4.8	0.0
Toffee, Milk Chocolate Coated, Morrisons*	1 Serving/25g	119	5.0	479	4.1	68.9	20.0	3.3
Toffee, Milk Chocolate Coated, Sainsbury's*	¼ Bag/25g	130	6.6	520	6.5	64.1	26.4	1.3
Toffee, Sainsbury's*	1 Serving/50g	208	6.4	415	1.8	73.8	12.7	3.3
Toffee, Snack Pack, Butterkist*	1 Bag/25g	105	2.2	420	2.1	81.3	9.0	3.5
Vanilla, Cinema Sweet Microwave, Act II*	½ Pack/50g	234	8.0	468	9.0	71.0	16.0	12.0
Wasabi, Flavour, Skinny, Topcorn, Metcalfe's Food Co*	1 Bag/25g	121	6.6	484	8.4	54.1	26.2	9.7
Wasabi, Pret a Manger*	1 Pack/29g	137	6.4	472	7.2	55.2	22.1	10.7
White Cheddar Cheese, Manhatten Peanuts Limited*	1 Bag/30g	132	4.1	440	10.0	70.0	13.7	13.0

POPPADOMS

	Measure INFO/WEIGHT	per Measure KCAL	FAT	Nutrition Values per 100g / 100ml KCAL	PROT	CARB	FAT	FIBRE
Fried in Vegetable Oil, Takeaway, Average	1 Poppadom/13g	65	5.0	501	11.5	28.3	38.8	5.8
Garlic & Coriander, Ready to Eat, Sharwood's*	1 Poppadom/9g	39	1.9	438	18.4	43.0	21.4	6.5
Indian, Asda*	1 Pack/45g	232	15.7	516	14.5	36.2	34.8	7.8
Mini, Sainsbury's*	½ Pack/50g	249	16.2	498	14.9	36.9	32.3	7.6
Plain, Asda*	1 Poppadom/9g	44	2.5	484	18.0	40.0	28.0	0.0
Plain, Cook to Eat, Sharwood's*	1 Poppadom/12g	32	0.1	273	21.9	45.7	1.0	10.1
Plain, Indian to Go, Sainsbury's*	1 Poppadom/8g	34	1.5	405	18.4	43.4	17.5	9.0
Plain, Mini, Cook to Eat, Sharwood's*	1 Poppadom/4g	11	0.0	273	21.9	45.7	0.3	10.1
Plain, Ready to Eat, Sharwood's*	1 Poppadom/8g	37	1.8	461	19.4	46.3	22.0	5.6
Plain, Tesco*	1 Serving/9g	41	2.0	439	17.8	44.4	21.1	4.6
Plain, Waitrose*	1 Serving/9g	37	1.7	408	21.0	39.3	18.6	9.1
Spicy, Cook to Eat, Sharwood's*	1 Poppadom/12g	30	0.1	257	20.2	43.0	0.5	13.0
Tesco*	1 Poppadum/9g	39	1.9	440	17.8	44.4	21.1	4.6

POPPETS*

	Measure INFO/WEIGHT	per Measure KCAL	FAT	Nutrition Values per 100g / 100ml KCAL	PROT	CARB	FAT	FIBRE
Chocolate Raisins, Poppets*	1 Pack/35g	140	4.7	401	4.9	65.4	13.3	0.0

	Measure INFO/WEIGHT	per Measure KCAL	FAT	Nutrition Values per 100g / 100ml KCAL	PROT	CARB	FAT	FIBRE
POPPETS*								
Mint Cream, Poppets*	1oz/28g	119	3.6	424	2.0	75.0	13.0	0.0
Peanut, Poppets*	1 Box/100g	544	37.0	544	16.4	37.0	37.0	0.0
Toffee, Milk Chocolate, Poppets*	1 Box/100g	491	23.0	491	5.3	68.0	23.0	0.0
POPPING CORN								
Average	1 Serving/30g	112	1.3	375	10.9	73.1	4.3	12.7
Lightly Salted, Graze*	1 Punnet/23g	95	4.0	412	9.1	48.6	17.6	13.3
Slightly Sweet, Graze*	1 Punnet/23g	95	3.6	415	8.1	55.9	15.5	13.3
Twist of Black Pepper, Graze*	1 Punnet/28g	125	6.9	452	8.0	44.0	25.0	13.0
PORK								
Belly, Fresh, Raw, Weighed with Skin, Average	1 Serving/100g	518	53.0	518	9.3	0.0	53.0	0.0
Belly, Roasted, Lean & Fat	1oz/28g	82	6.0	293	25.1	0.0	21.4	0.0
Belly, Slow Cooked, Waitrose*	1 Serving/225g	590	45.9	262	17.3	2.2	20.4	0.0
Chop, Lean & Fat, Boneless, Raw, Average	*1oz/28g*	*67*	*3.8*	*240*	*29.2*	*0.0*	*13.7*	*0.0*
Cooked with Herbs, Italian, Finest, Tesco*	2 Slices/50g	117	8.8	234	18.0	1.0	17.5	0.0
Diced, Lean, Average	*1oz/28g*	*31*	*0.5*	*109*	*22.0*	*0.0*	*1.8*	*0.0*
Ham, Hock, Raw, Weighed with Bone, Fat & Skin	100g	139	5.6	139	20.6	0.0	5.6	0.0
Haslet, Somerfield*	1oz/28g	57	3.4	205	15.0	10.0	12.0	0.0
Joint, Ready to Roast, Average	*½ Joint/254g*	*375*	*18.0*	*148*	*19.2*	*2.3*	*7.1*	*0.2*
Joint, with Crackling, Ready to Roast, Average	*1 Joint/567g*	*1283*	*80.1*	*226*	*24.2*	*0.8*	*14.1*	*0.0*
Leg, Joint, Healthy Range, Average	*1 Serving/200g*	*206*	*4.4*	*103*	*20.0*	*0.6*	*2.2*	*0.0*
Loin, Applewood Smoked, Asda*	1 Slice/15g	18	0.5	122	21.8	0.5	3.6	0.0
Loin, Chops, Boneless, Grilled, Average	*1oz/28g*	*90*	*4.4*	*320*	*29.0*	*0.0*	*15.7*	*0.0*
Loin, Chops, Grilled, Lean	*1oz/28g*	*52*	*1.8*	*184*	*31.6*	*0.0*	*6.4*	*0.0*
Loin, Chops, Raw, Lean & Fat, Weighed with Bone	1 Chop/130g	295	23.7	227	15.7	0.0	18.2	0.0
Loin, Joint, Roast, Lean	*1oz/28g*	*51*	*1.9*	*182*	*30.1*	*0.0*	*6.8*	*0.0*
Loin, Joint, Roasted, Lean & Fat	*1oz/28g*	*71*	*4.3*	*253*	*26.3*	*0.0*	*15.3*	*0.0*
Loin, Roasted with Rosemary, Arista, Sainsbury's*	1 Slice/17g	24	1.2	144	20.8	0.1	6.8	0.7
Loin, Slices, Sweet Cure, Tesco*	1 Slice/13g	19	0.8	146	20.9	2.5	5.8	0.6
Loin, Steak, Fried, Lean	*1oz/28g*	*53*	*2.0*	*191*	*31.5*	*0.0*	*7.2*	*0.0*
Loin, Steak, Fried, Lean & Fat	*1oz/28g*	*77*	*5.2*	*276*	*27.5*	*0.0*	*18.4*	*0.0*
Loin, Steak, Lean, Raw, Average	*1 Serving/175g*	*345*	*19.6*	*197*	*22.7*	*1.8*	*11.2*	*0.4*
Loin, Steak, with Bramley Apple & Cider Sauce, Tesco*	½ Pack/154g	190	11.7	123	12.8	0.6	7.6	0.2
Loin, Stuffed, Roast, M&S*	1 Slice/12g	22	0.9	180	24.4	2.4	7.9	0.0
Medallions, Average	*1 Pack/220g*	*359*	*5.5*	*163*	*35.1*	*0.0*	*2.5*	*0.4*
Mince, & Beef, Frozen, Basics, Sainsbury's*	1 Serving/100g	320	25.2	320	21.2	1.8	25.2	0.5
Mince, Lean, Healthy Range, Average	*1 Pack/400g*	*504*	*20.2*	*126*	*19.8*	*0.4*	*5.0*	*0.3*
Mince, Raw	*1oz/28g*	*46*	*2.7*	*164*	*19.2*	*0.0*	*9.7*	*0.0*
Mince, Stewed	*1oz/28g*	*53*	*2.9*	*191*	*24.4*	*0.0*	*10.4*	*0.0*
Rashers, Streaky, British, Sainsbury's*	1 Serving/100g	320	23.4	320	27.4	0.0	23.4	0.0
Raw, Lean, Average	*1oz/28g*	*42*	*1.2*	*151*	*28.6*	*0.0*	*4.1*	*0.0*
Rib, Chops, Raw, Lean & Fat, Weighed with Bone	1 Chop/130g	287	19.2	221	22.0	0.0	14.8	0.0
Roast, Lean Only, Average	*1oz/28g*	*34*	*0.9*	*121*	*22.7*	*0.3*	*3.3*	*0.0*
Roast, Slices, Average	*1 Slice/30g*	*40*	*1.4*	*134*	*22.7*	*0.4*	*4.5*	*0.0*
Shoulder, Joint, Roasted, Trimmed of Fat, Value, Tesco*	1 Serving/100g	260	16.5	260	27.5	0.0	16.5	0.0
Shoulder, Slices, Cured	*1oz/28g*	*29*	*1.0*	*103*	*16.9*	*0.9*	*3.6*	*0.0*
Shoulder, Steak, Boneless, Grilled, Tesco*	1 Steak/125g	156	4.9	125	0.0	0.0	3.9	0.0
Shoulder, Whole, Lean & Fat, Raw, Average	*100g*	*236*	*18.0*	*236*	*17.2*	*0.0*	*18.0*	*0.0*
Shoulder, Whole, Lean Only, Roasted	1 Serving/150g	345	20.3	230	25.3	0.0	13.5	0.0
Shoulder, with Honey Garlic & Rosemary, Waitrose*	1 Pack/500g	820	48.5	164	18.6	0.6	9.7	0.5
Steak, Lean, Stewed	*1oz/28g*	*49*	*1.3*	*176*	*33.6*	*0.0*	*4.6*	*0.0*
Steak, Lean & Fat, Average	*1oz/28g*	*61*	*3.8*	*219*	*23.8*	*0.0*	*13.7*	*0.1*
Stir Fry Strips, Lean, Healthy Range, Average	*¼ Pack/113g*	*118*	*2.3*	*104*	*21.3*	*0.0*	*2.0*	*0.0*
Tenderloin, Lean, Boneless, Raw, Average	1 Serving/100g	109	2.2	109	21.0	0.0	2.2	0.0

	Measure INFO/WEIGHT	per Measure KCAL	FAT	Nutrition Values per 100g / 100ml KCAL	PROT	CARB	FAT	FIBRE
PORK								
Tenderloin, Roulade, Waitrose*	1 Pack/171g	282	12.8	165	18.4	5.9	7.5	1.8
Tenderloin, Separable Lean & Fat, Raw, Average	1 Loin/265g	318	9.4	120	20.6	0.0	3.5	0.0
PORK CHAR SUI								
Chinese, Tesco*	1 Pack/400g	520	17.2	130	7.2	15.7	4.3	0.6
Oriental, Finest, Tesco*	1 Pack/350g	245	5.2	70	6.8	6.2	1.5	2.1
with Chicken & Egg Fried Rice, Tesco*	1 Serving/450g	602	16.2	134	7.1	18.3	3.6	0.9
PORK CHINESE								
Sliced, M&S*	1 Serving/140g	224	4.3	160	26.4	6.1	3.1	0.0
PORK DINNER								
Roast, Birds Eye*	1 Pack/340g	410	12.0	121	7.6	14.7	3.5	1.6
with Roast Potatoes & Yorkshire Pudding, for One, M&S*	1 Pack/361g	470	17.7	130	8.4	12.1	4.9	1.3
PORK ESCALOPE								
Average	*1 Escalope/75g*	*108*	*1.7*	*144*	*31.0*	*0.0*	*2.2*	*0.0*
Lean, Healthy Range, Average	*1 Escalope/75g*	*80*	*1.5*	*106*	*22.0*	*0.0*	*2.0*	*0.0*
with Gruyere & Mustard Crust, Easy to Cook, Waitrose*	1 Escalope/122g	239	10.7	196	19.8	9.3	8.8	0.8
PORK IN								
Light Mustard Sauce, Fillet, COU, M&S*	1 Pack/390g	312	9.4	80	10.9	3.5	2.4	0.7
Mustard & Cream, Chops	1oz/28g	73	6.0	261	14.5	2.4	21.6	0.3
PORK SCRATCHINGS								
Crunch, Mr Porky*	1 Pack/30g	159	9.6	531	60.4	0.5	31.9	4.6
KP Snacks*	1 Pack/20g	125	9.6	624	47.3	0.5	48.1	0.5
Tavern Snacks*	1 Pack/30g	187	14.4	624	47.3	0.5	48.1	0.5
PORK WITH								
Honey & Mustard Sauce, Steaks, Tesco*	½ Pack/160g	258	11.8	161	16.3	8.7	7.4	1.4
Leek & Bacon Stuffing, Roast, Shoulder, Sainsbury's*	1 Serving/150g	237	12.4	158	18.8	2.4	8.3	0.5
Maple & BBQ Sauce, Loin Steaks, Somerfield*	½ Pack/160g	336	16.0	210	20.4	9.2	10.0	0.0
Medallions with Bramley Apple, M&S*	1 Serving/380g	418	12.9	110	17.7	2.5	3.4	0.5
Peppers, Marinated, Tapas, Waitrose*	1 Serving/105g	181	6.7	172	26.3	2.2	6.4	0.3
Sage, Onion & Lemon Stuffing, Joint, Sainsbury's*	1 Serving/260g	699	43.4	269	27.4	2.2	16.7	1.4
Sage & Onion Stuffing, Joint, Tesco*	1 Serving/200g	208	5.6	104	17.1	2.7	2.8	0.0
Spiced Apple Stuffing, Steaks, Easy Cook, Waitrose*	1 Serving/190g	237	7.8	124	19.3	2.4	4.1	0.5
Stuffing, Belly, Norfolk Outdoor Reared, Finest, Tesco*	1 Serving/180g	524	44.8	291	14.9	1.7	24.9	0.0
with Cannellini Beans & Migas, Braised Belly, M&S*	1 Pack/350g	700	45.8	200	11.2	7.7	13.1	3.4
PORT								
Average	*1 Serving/50ml*	*78*	*0.0*	*157*	*0.1*	*12.0*	*0.0*	*0.0*
POT NOODLE*								
Beef & Tomato, Made Up, Pot Noodle*	1 Pot/300g	378	14.1	126	3.1	18.1	4.7	1.1
Beef & Tomato, Pot Noodle*	1 Pot/319g	424	14.7	133	3.4	19.4	4.6	1.3
Bombay Bad Boy, Made Up, Pot Noodle*	1 Pot/305g	384	14.0	126	3.1	17.9	4.6	1.1
Chicken & Mushroom, King, Pot Noodle*	1 Pack/401g	513	19.2	128	3.2	18.1	4.8	1.1
Chicken & Mushroom, Made Up, Pot Noodle*	1 Pot/300g	384	14.1	128	3.2	18.0	4.7	1.1
Chicken & Mushroom, Mini, Made Up, Pot Noodle*	1 Pot/190g	243	8.5	128	3.8	18.2	4.5	1.4
Chicken Curry, Hot, Made Up, Pot Noodle*	1 Pot/300g	384	14.1	128	2.8	18.7	4.7	1.1
Chow Mein Flavour, Made Up, Pot Noodle*	1 Pot/320g	416	14.7	130	3.2	19.0	4.6	1.3
Spicy Chilli, Posh, Made Up, Pot Noodle*	1 Pot/301g	328	17.8	109	2.5	11.7	5.9	1.0
Spicy Curry, Made Up, Pot Noodle*	1 Pot/300g	393	14.4	131	2.9	19.1	4.8	1.1
Sweet & Sour, Dry, Pot Noodle*	1 Pot/86g	376	13.8	437	12.1	60.9	16.1	3.1
POTATO BOMBAY								
Aloo, M&S*	½ Pack/114g	108	5.2	95	1.8	10.3	4.6	2.3
Average	½ Pack/150g	176	10.2	117	2.0	13.7	6.8	1.2
Indian Meal for Two, Sainsbury's*	½ Pack/151g	154	8.5	102	1.6	11.4	5.6	3.1
Indian Takeaway for 1, Sainsbury's*	1 Serving/200g	202	10.4	101	1.8	11.8	5.2	1.7
Morrisons*	1 Serving/175g	180	8.8	103	1.5	13.0	5.0	1.7

	Measure INFO/WEIGHT	per Measure KCAL	per Measure FAT	Nutrition Values per 100g / 100ml KCAL	PROT	CARB	FAT	FIBRE
POTATO BOMBAY								
Sainsbury's*	1 Pack/300g	285	14.7	95	1.8	10.8	4.9	2.5
Tesco*	1 Pack/300g	240	12.6	80	1.3	9.3	4.2	2.1
Waitrose*	1 Pack/300g	246	12.9	82	1.6	9.3	4.3	2.2
POTATO CAKES								
Average	1 Cake/70g	127	1.2	180	3.8	37.5	1.7	2.4
Fried, Average	1oz/28g	66	2.5	237	4.9	35.0	9.0	0.8
POTATO FRITTERS								
Crispy, Oven Baked, Birds Eye*	1 Fritter/20g	29	1.6	145	2.0	16.3	8.0	1.2
with Sweetcorn, M&S*	1 Pack/135g	304	17.0	225	4.4	24.1	12.6	2.3
POTATO SKINS								
¼ Cut, Deep Fried, McCain*	1oz/28g	52	1.7	186	3.0	30.1	6.0	0.0
¼ Cut, Oven Baked, McCain*	1oz/28g	53	1.3	190	3.6	33.1	4.8	0.0
American Style, Loaded, Asda*	1 Serving/78g	294	18.0	375	15.0	27.0	23.0	2.4
American Style, Loaded, Tesco*	1 Serving/340g	388	8.2	114	6.8	16.3	2.4	3.3
Cheese & Bacon, Loaded, Asda*	½ Pack/125g	275	15.0	220	13.0	15.0	12.0	3.3
Cheese & Bacon, Loaded, Tesco*	1 Skin/59g	150	9.1	255	9.2	19.5	15.5	3.0
Cheese & Bacon, Sainsbury's*	1 Serving/140g	349	21.6	249	10.3	17.3	15.4	2.5
Cheese & Ham, Iceland*	2 Skins/108g	155	4.9	143	6.3	19.3	4.5	2.0
Cheese & Onion, Loaded, Tesco*	1 Skin/60g	114	6.5	190	5.8	17.6	10.8	1.4
Cheese & Onion, Sour Cream & Chive, Loaded, Tesco*	1 Skin/60g	114	6.5	190	5.8	17.6	10.8	1.4
Soured Cream, Loaded, M&S*	½ Pack/150g	308	17.8	205	9.1	15.8	11.9	0.9
with Sour Cream	1 Serving/275g	541	34.6	197	7.2	13.8	12.6	2.2
POTATO SMILES								
Weighed Baked, McCain*	1 Serving/100g	237	10.1	237	3.4	33.4	10.1	3.1
Weighed Frozen, McCain*	1 Serving/100g	191	8.0	191	2.6	27.0	8.0	2.7
POTATO WAFFLES								
Frozen, Cooked	1oz/28g	56	2.3	200	3.2	30.3	8.2	2.3
Frozen, Grilled, Asda*	1 Waffle/57g	104	5.8	183	2.0	21.0	10.1	1.7
Mini, Farmfoods*	1oz/28g	41	1.6	145	1.9	21.6	5.7	1.7
Mini, Sainsbury's*	1 Waffle/11g	27	1.8	242	2.8	20.1	16.7	1.0
Oven Baked, Mini, McCain*	1oz/28g	62	2.4	221	3.9	32.0	8.6	0.0
Uncooked, Average	1 Waffle/62g	113	5.1	182	2.4	24.4	8.3	1.8
POTATO WEDGES								
Aldi*	1 Serving/100g	150	6.8	150	2.1	20.2	6.8	0.0
Asda*	1 Wedge/40g	57	2.0	142	3.4	21.0	4.9	1.7
Baked, GFY, Asda*	1 Pack/450g	616	11.7	137	3.4	25.0	2.6	3.4
BBQ Flavour, Asda*	1 Serving/100g	185	9.0	185	2.9	23.0	9.0	1.7
BGTY, Sainsbury's*	½ Pack/190g	179	3.4	94	3.0	16.4	1.8	3.4
Co-Op*	1oz/28g	38	1.7	135	2.0	20.0	6.0	2.0
Crispy, M&S*	1 Serving/200g	340	14.2	170	1.3	25.3	7.1	1.7
Four Cheese & Red Onion, Chicago Town*	1 Serving/150g	210	8.0	140	2.1	21.0	5.3	2.4
Frozen, Average	1 Serving/120g	145	4.1	121	2.0	20.5	3.4	2.2
Garlic & Herb, COU, M&S*	1 Pack/300g	300	7.8	100	2.3	16.4	2.6	3.2
Garlic & Herb, Kitchen Range Foods*	1oz/28g	42	2.2	151	1.6	18.5	7.8	0.0
Garlic & Herb Crusted, Chicago Town*	1 Serving/150g	216	6.4	144	1.9	24.4	4.3	2.2
Jacket, Spicy, American Style, Frozen, Sainsbury's*	1 Serving/125g	156	5.0	125	1.9	20.3	4.0	1.1
Jumbo, Finest, Tesco*	1 Serving/126g	145	2.6	115	1.4	22.7	2.1	1.7
Jumbo, TTD, Sainsbury's*	1 Serving/165g	279	6.8	169	2.4	30.7	4.1	3.1
Mexican, Inspire, Asda*	1 Pack/500g	525	17.0	105	2.2	16.5	3.4	1.8
Onion & Garlic, Spicy, Cooked, Champion, Aldi*	1 Serving/100g	135	4.7	135	2.5	19.4	4.7	2.7
Only 5% Fat, Weighed Baked, McCain*	1 Serving/100g	173	4.3	173	3.3	30.2	4.3	2.8
Only 5% Fat, Weighed Frozen, McCain*	1 Serving/100g	123	3.0	123	2.2	21.8	3.0	1.9
Oven Baked, Waitrose*	1oz/28g	46	1.2	165	2.4	29.2	4.3	2.1

	Measure INFO/WEIGHT	per Measure KCAL	per Measure FAT	Nutrition Values per 100g / 100ml KCAL	PROT	CARB	FAT	FIBRE
POTATO WEDGES								
PB, Waitrose*	1 Serving/275g	278	4.7	101	2.5	19.0	1.7	3.5
Savoury, Waitrose*	1/3 Bag/250g	350	10.8	140	2.3	22.9	4.3	1.9
Slightly Spiced, Baked, Potato Winners, McCain*	1 Serving/100g	187	5.2	187	2.7	26.9	5.2	1.8
Slightly Spiced, Frozen, Potato Winners, McCain*	1 Serving/100g	144	5.9	144	2.0	20.8	5.9	1.7
Southern Fried, Asda*	1 Serving/100g	157	4.5	157	3.0	26.0	4.5	3.5
Southern Fried, Champion*	1oz/28g	41	1.7	147	2.1	20.8	6.2	2.8
Southern Fried, Style, Tesco*	1 Serving/155g	232	14.1	150	3.0	14.1	9.1	2.0
Spicy, Asda*	1 Serving/100g	145	5.7	145	1.8	21.8	5.7	2.1
Spicy, Deep Fried, McCain*	1oz/28g	52	2.3	187	3.6	27.3	8.1	0.0
Spicy, M&S*	½ Pack/225g	349	14.6	155	2.4	21.8	6.5	1.3
Spicy, Occasions, Sainsbury's*	1 Serving/100g	144	4.3	144	2.5	23.7	4.3	0.4
Spicy, Simple Solutions, Tesco*	1 Serving/150g	141	4.5	94	4.6	12.2	3.0	1.4
with a Parsley & Oil Dressing, Tesco*	½ Pack/280g	168	2.8	60	1.0	11.5	1.0	1.8
POTATOES								
Alphabites, Captain Birds Eye, Birds Eye*	9 Bites/56g	75	3.0	134	2.0	19.5	5.3	1.4
Anya, Raw, TTD, Sainsbury's*	1 Serving/100g	75	0.3	75	1.5	17.8	0.3	1.1
Baby, Dressed with Garlic & Rosemary, M&S*	1 Serving/185g	130	5.2	70	2.0	9.0	2.8	2.4
Baby, Garlic & Sea Salt Roasted, Finest, Tesco*	1 Serving/200g	192	6.6	96	3.1	13.5	3.3	1.0
Baby, New with Butter, Mint & Parsley, Organic, Asda*	1 Pack/360g	414	10.4	115	1.7	20.4	2.9	2.5
Baby, Oven Bake, Aunt Bessie's*	1 Serving/120g	103	1.7	86	2.2	16.3	1.4	3.0
Baby, with Butter & Herbs, Sainsbury's*	¼ Pack/148g	103	0.9	70	1.9	14.2	0.6	2.0
Baby, with Garlic & Rosemary, Ready to Roast, Waitrose*	½ Pack/200g	271	15.3	136	2.3	14.3	7.7	3.1
Baby, with Herbs & Butter, Morrisons*	1 Serving/100g	94	2.3	94	1.9	14.6	2.3	1.9
Baby, with Paprika & Chilli Dressing, Morrisons*	1 Serving/120g	124	5.3	103	1.7	13.6	4.4	1.3
Baked, Flesh & Skin, Average	**1 Med/200g**	**218**	**0.2**	**109**	**2.3**	**25.2**	**0.1**	**2.4**
Baked, Flesh & Skin, Microwaved, Average	**1oz/28g**	**29**	**0.0**	**105**	**2.4**	**24.1**	**0.1**	**2.3**
Baked, Flesh Only, Microwaved, Average	**1oz/28g**	**28**	**0.0**	**100**	**2.1**	**23.3**	**0.1**	**1.6**
Baked, Flesh Only, Weighed with Skin, Average	**1oz/28g**	**26**	**0.0**	**93**	**2.0**	**21.6**	**0.1**	**1.5**
Baked, Jacket, Beef Chilli Filled, GFY, Asda*	1 Serving/300g	261	1.5	87	4.6	16.0	0.5	3.2
Baked, Jacket, Cheddar Cheese, COU, M&S*	1 Potato/164g	164	3.1	100	2.9	17.3	1.9	2.0
Baked, Jacket, Cheese, M&S*	1oz/28g	24	0.7	85	4.5	11.1	2.5	1.6
Baked, Jacket, Cheese & Beans, Somerfield*	1 Pack/340g	306	6.8	90	4.1	13.8	2.0	2.2
Baked, Jacket, Cheesy, GFY, Asda*	1 Serving/155g	129	1.6	83	2.6	16.0	1.0	2.1
Baked, Jacket, Chicken Tikka, Spar*	1 Serving/300g	309	3.1	103	5.5	19.2	1.0	5.0
Baked, Jacket, Chilli, BGTY, Sainsbury's*	1 Pack/350g	318	4.9	91	5.3	14.3	1.4	1.2
Baked, Jacket, Chilli Con Carne, COU, M&S*	1 Pack/300g	270	6.3	90	6.0	11.1	2.1	1.2
Baked, Jacket, Chilli Con Carne, Pro Cuisine*	1 Pack/340g	347	3.4	102	4.6	18.7	1.0	0.0
Baked, Jacket, Chilli Con Carne, Somerfield*	1 Pack/340g	319	11.6	94	5.5	10.3	3.4	1.2
Baked, Jacket, Creamy Mushroom, Asda*	1 Serving/100g	124	2.4	124	3.5	22.0	2.4	1.7
Baked, Jacket, Garlic, Mini, Asda*	1 Serving/65g	59	2.1	91	2.2	13.0	3.3	0.0
Baked, Jacket, Halves, M&S*	1 Serving/250g	188	2.8	75	2.0	14.2	1.1	1.7
Baked, Jacket, Mature Cheddar Cheese, Finest, Tesco*	1 Potato/245g	360	18.4	147	5.4	14.6	7.5	2.3
Baked, Jacket, Mature Cheddar Cheese, M&S*	½ Pack/206g	225	6.6	109	3.6	16.9	3.2	1.0
Baked, Jacket, Stuffed, Garlic & Herb Butter, Tesco*	1 Pack/435g	570	32.6	131	1.3	14.6	7.5	1.0
Baked, Jacket, Stuffed, Mini, Tesco*	1 Serving/108g	130	6.3	120	2.3	14.6	5.8	2.3
Baked, Jacket, Tuna & Sweetcorn, Average	1 Serving/300g	273	6.8	91	5.0	12.6	2.2	0.9
Baked, Jacket, Tuna & Sweetcorn, BGTY, Sainsbury's*	1 Pack/350g	360	9.5	103	6.5	13.2	2.7	1.3
Baked, Jacket, Tuna & Sweetcorn, COU, M&S*	1 Pack/300g	270	5.4	90	5.1	12.8	1.8	1.4
Baked, Jacket, Tuna & Sweetcorn, Somerfield*	1 Pack/340g	333	13.3	98	3.2	12.5	3.9	1.0
Baked, Jacket with Beef Chilli, Asda*	1 Pack/300g	381	7.8	127	5.0	21.0	2.6	2.0
Baked, Jacket with Beef Chilli, M&S*	1 Pack/360g	288	7.2	80	5.9	9.6	2.0	0.9
Baked, Jacket with Cheese, Freshly Prepared, Tesco*	½ Pack/215g	150	3.0	70	3.9	9.7	1.4	2.8
Baked, Jacket with Cheese & Bacon, Finest, Tesco*	1 Potato/245g	360	19.6	147	6.0	12.6	8.0	2.5

POTATOES

INFO/WEIGHT	Measure	per Measure KCAL	FAT	Nutrition Values per 100g / 100ml KCAL	PROT	CARB	FAT	FIBRE
Baked, Jacket with Cheese & Butter, Tesco*	1 Potato/225g	263	11.2	117	3.1	14.9	5.0	2.3
Baked, Jacket with Cheese Mash, GFY, Asda*	1 Potato/200g	192	5.6	96	4.8	13.0	2.8	2.2
Baked, Jacket with Chicken Tikka, LC, Tesco*	1 Potato/247g	185	2.2	75	3.4	12.6	0.9	1.3
Baked, M&S*	1 Potato/205g	215	5.1	105	3.6	16.9	2.5	1.0
Baked, Skin Only, Average	*1oz/28g*	*55*	*0.0*	*198*	*4.3*	*46.1*	*0.1*	*7.9*
Baked, Skin Only, Microwaved, Average	*1oz/28g*	*37*	*0.0*	*132*	*4.4*	*29.6*	*0.1*	*5.5*
Baked, with Cheddar Cheese, Farmfoods*	1 Potato/143g	196	5.4	137	4.7	21.0	3.8	1.9
Baked, with Cheese & Chive, LC, Tesco*	1 Potato/263g	250	3.7	95	3.2	16.7	1.4	1.6
Baking, Raw, Average	*1 Med/250g*	*198*	*0.2*	*79*	*2.1*	*18.0*	*0.1*	*1.6*
Boiled, Average	*1 Serving/120g*	*86*	*0.1*	*72*	*1.8*	*17.0*	*0.1*	*1.2*
Boiled with Skin	*1 Potato/125g*	*98*	*0.1*	*78*	*2.9*	*17.2*	*0.1*	*3.3*
Bombay, TTD, Sainsbury's*	½ Pack/113g	79	3.2	70	1.9	9.3	2.8	3.9
Boulangere, M&S*	½ Pack/225g	180	2.0	80	2.8	15.9	0.9	0.9
Charlotte, Average	*1 Serving/184g*	*139*	*0.5*	*76*	*1.6*	*17.4*	*0.2*	*3.3*
Crispy Slices, M&S*	1/3 Pack/159g	231	8.3	145	2.9	22.2	5.2	1.9
Crispy Slices, Weighed Baked, McCain*	1 Serving/100g	240	11.0	240	3.2	32.1	11.0	2.1
Dauphinoise, Average	*1 Serving/200g*	*335*	*23.9*	*168*	*2.2*	*12.8*	*12.0*	*1.5*
Dauphinoise, Cook*	1 Pack/225g	320	18.7	142	5.3	11.0	8.3	1.8
Dauphinoise, TTD, Sainsbury's*	½ Pack/174g	240	16.2	138	2.9	10.8	9.3	2.7
Desiree, Average	*1 Serving/200g*	*152*	*0.4*	*76*	*2.2*	*16.4*	*0.2*	*0.6*
Exquisa, Finest, Tesco*	¼ Pack/247g	185	0.7	75	1.7	16.1	0.3	1.0
Frites, Fries, Golden, Crunchy, M&S*	½ Pack/100g	158	6.2	158	2.2	23.4	6.2	1.0
Garlic, Tapas Selection, Sainsbury's*	1 Serving/22g	49	4.2	224	2.6	10.4	19.1	0.7
Hasselback, Average	*1 Serving/175g*	*182*	*1.6*	*104*	*1.9*	*22.0*	*0.9*	*2.9*
Jacket, Filled with Cheese & Chives, GFY, Asda*	1 Pack/340g	289	4.4	85	4.1	14.2	1.3	2.4
Jacket, Ready Baked, Frozen, McCain*	1 Potato/200g	190	1.0	95	1.7	20.9	0.5	1.4
Jersey Royal, Canned, Average	*1 Can/186g*	*116*	*0.2*	*62*	*1.4*	*14.0*	*0.1*	*1.2*
Jersey Royal, New, Raw, Average	*1oz/28g*	*21*	*0.1*	*75*	*1.6*	*17.2*	*0.2*	*1.5*
Jersey Royal, with Mint Butter, Extra Special, Asda*	½ Pack/172g	148	5.3	86	1.6	13.0	3.1	1.5
King Edward, Tesco*	1 Serving/100g	77	0.2	77	2.1	16.8	0.2	1.3
Lemon & Rosemary, Finest, Tesco*	½ Pack/200g	200	7.4	100	2.1	14.7	3.7	2.0
Maris Piper, Raw, Average	*1 Serving/200g*	*151*	*0.4*	*75*	*2.0*	*16.5*	*0.2*	*1.4*
Mashed, Buttery, Sainsbury's*	1 Pack/450g	454	25.6	101	1.3	11.1	5.7	3.0
Mashed, CBY, Asda*	½ Pack/250g	177	5.5	71	1.0	10.3	2.2	2.8
Mashed, Colcannon, Co-Op*	1 Pack/500g	325	10.0	65	2.0	10.0	2.0	2.0
Mashed, Colcannon, Sainsbury's*	½ Pack/300g	192	12.0	64	0.4	6.7	4.0	1.4
Mashed, Colcannon, Tesco*	1 Serving/250g	225	13.5	90	1.6	8.4	5.4	1.8
Mashed, Colcannon, Waitrose*	½ Pack/225g	207	8.6	92	1.7	12.8	3.8	1.4
Mashed, Fresh, LC, Tesco*	1 Pack/400g	280	8.8	70	2.0	9.3	2.2	1.6
Mashed, From Supermarket, Average	½ Pack/200g	197	8.1	98	1.8	13.3	4.1	1.5
Mashed, From Supermarket, Healthy Range, Average	1 Serving/200g	160	3.1	80	1.8	14.6	1.6	1.3
Mashed, From Supermarket, Premium, Average	1 Serving/225g	305	17.8	136	1.7	14.4	7.9	1.1
Mashed, Home Prepared with Whole Milk	1 Cup/210g	162	1.2	77	1.9	17.6	0.6	2.0
Mashed, Maris Piper, Tesco*	½ Pack/213g	180	4.0	85	1.9	14.7	1.9	1.6
Mashed, Maris Piper with Cream & Butter, M&S*	½ Pack/200g	180	7.2	90	1.1	12.9	3.6	0.4
Mashed, Mash Direct*	½ Pack/200g	190	3.8	95	1.7	17.7	1.9	1.3
Mashed, Ready to Eat, Sainsbury's*	½ Pack/200g	142	3.8	71	1.4	12.1	1.9	2.0
Mashed, Vintage Cheddar Cheese, M&S*	½ Pack/225g	248	11.9	110	4.6	12.6	5.3	1.0
Mashed, with Cabbage & Spring Onion, COU, M&S*	½ Pack/225g	158	4.0	70	1.7	11.4	1.8	2.1
Mashed, with Carrot & Swede, COU, M&S*	1oz/28g	20	0.6	70	1.1	12.1	2.1	2.9
Mashed, with Carrot & Swede, M&S*	1 Serving/225g	214	14.4	95	1.6	8.3	6.4	1.4
Mashed, with Carrot & Swede, Morrisons*	1 Serving/100g	71	1.6	71	1.5	12.6	1.6	2.2
Mashed, with Carrot & Swede, Sainsbury's*	½ Pack/226g	125	3.9	55	0.9	8.1	1.7	1.8

POTATOES

INFO/WEIGHT	Measure	per Measure KCAL	per Measure FAT	KCAL	PROT	CARB	FAT	FIBRE
Mashed, with Creme Fraiche & Seasoning, Waitrose*	½ Pack/225g	189	6.3	84	2.0	12.7	2.8	1.4
Mashed, with Leeks, Creamy, Birds Eye*	1 Pack/300g	300	21.0	100	2.0	7.3	7.0	0.8
Mashed, with Spring Onion, Weight Watchers*	1 Serving/100g	77	2.2	77	1.9	10.9	2.2	1.4
New, Average	*1 Serving/100g*	*75*	*0.3*	*75*	*1.5*	*17.8*	*0.3*	*1.1*
New, Baby, Average	*1 Serving/180g*	*135*	*0.5*	*75*	*1.7*	*17.1*	*0.3*	*1.6*
New, Baby, Canned, Average	*1 Can/120g*	*70*	*0.2*	*59*	*1.4*	*13.2*	*0.2*	*1.4*
New, Baby, with Herb Dressing & Seasoned Butter, Tesco*	½ Pack/160g	112	4.2	70	1.5	10.2	2.6	2.6
New, Easy Steam with Herbs & Butter, Tesco*	1 Serving/125g	94	3.5	75	1.8	9.6	2.8	1.7
New, Garlic, Herb & Parsley Butter, Co-Op*	1 Serving/100g	115	5.0	115	1.0	15.0	5.0	2.0
New, in a Herb Marinade, Tesco*	¼ Pack/150g	152	7.4	101	1.3	13.0	4.9	1.5
New, with Butter, Chives & Mint, M&S*	¼ Pack/145g	116	2.0	80	1.1	16.2	1.4	2.3
New, with English Churned Butter, M&S*	1 Pack/180g	261	4.0	145	1.3	29.5	2.2	2.1
New, with Herbs & Butter, Asda*	½ Pack/170g	146	2.9	86	1.7	16.0	1.7	1.5
New, with Herbs & Butter, Waitrose*	1 Serving/385g	443	22.7	115	1.7	13.8	5.9	1.2
Organics, Boiled, Asda*	1 Serving/200g	152	0.2	76	1.8	16.0	0.1	1.2
Pan Fried, Aldi*	1 Serving/250g	182	2.0	73	2.7	13.7	0.8	0.0
Patatas Bravas, Bistro, M Kitchen, Morrisons*	½ Pack/126g	113	4.0	90	1.1	13.6	3.2	1.3
Raw, Peeled, Flesh Only	*1 Serving/100g*	*75*	*0.2*	*75*	*2.0*	*17.3*	*0.2*	*1.4*
Red, Flesh Only, Average	*1 Serving/300g*	*218*	*0.4*	*72*	*2.0*	*16.4*	*0.2*	*1.2*
Roast, Basted in Beef Dripping, Waitrose*	1 Serving/165g	213	8.9	129	2.2	18.0	5.4	1.9
Roast, Dry, No Oil, No fat	1 Serving/100g	79	0.1	79	2.7	18.0	0.1	1.6
Roast, Extra Crispy, Oven Baked, Aunt Bessie's*	1 Serving/100g	223	11.8	223	2.9	26.1	11.8	3.6
Roast, Frozen, Average	1 Potato/70g	105	3.5	149	2.6	23.5	5.0	1.4
Roast, Frozen, Healthy Range, Average	1 Potato/70g	70	1.7	100	2.6	18.2	2.4	2.1
Roast, Garlic, Sainsbury's*	½ Pack/225g	358	21.8	159	3.2	14.6	9.7	1.4
Roast, in Lard, Average	*1oz/28g*	*42*	*1.3*	*149*	*2.9*	*25.9*	*4.5*	*1.8*
Roast, in Oil, Average	*1oz/28g*	*42*	*1.3*	*149*	*2.9*	*25.9*	*4.5*	*1.8*
Roast, New, Rosemary, Ainsley Harriott*	1 Serving/150g	133	4.0	89	2.0	16.0	2.7	1.3
Roast, Oven Baked, Aunt Bessie's*	1 Serving/165g	305	15.3	185	2.3	22.9	9.3	1.8
Roast, Seasoned, Butter Basted, Tesco*	½ Pack/225g	338	12.8	150	2.3	21.9	5.7	2.4
Roast, with Caramelised Onions, Finest, Tesco*	½ Pack/200g	500	16.4	250	5.5	38.6	8.2	2.9
Roast, with Goose Fat, TTD, Sainsbury's*	½ Pack/185g	216	4.4	117	2.7	21.1	2.4	3.0
Roasting, Average	*1 Serving/150g*	*202*	*5.2*	*135*	*2.5*	*23.4*	*3.5*	*1.6*
Rooster, Boiled, Albert Bartlett & Sons Ltd*	1 Potato/175g	126	0.2	72	1.8	17.0	0.1	1.2
Salad, Value, Tesco*	1 Serving/150g	111	0.4	74	1.7	16.1	0.3	1.0
Saute, Deep Fried, McCain*	1oz/28g	47	2.0	167	2.6	23.3	7.0	0.0
Saute, Oven Baked, McCain*	1oz/28g	56	1.1	199	4.4	36.9	3.8	0.0
Saute, with Onion & Bacon, Country Supper, Waitrose*	¼ Pack/100g	112	4.3	112	1.9	16.4	4.3	1.3
Slices, Garlic & Herb, Heinz*	1oz/28g	23	1.1	82	1.7	10.2	3.9	0.7
Slices, in Batter, Crispy, Ready To Bake, Waitrose*	1 Pack/475g	860	45.1	181	2.5	21.4	9.5	3.1
Vivaldi, Boiled in Unsalted Water, Sainsbury's*	1 Serving/200g	144	0.2	72	1.8	17.0	0.1	1.2
White, Raw, Flesh & Skin	1 Large/369g	284	0.3	77	2.0	17.5	0.1	2.2
White, Raw, Weighed with Skin, Flesh Only, Average	*1 Med/213g*	*160*	*0.3*	*75*	*2.0*	*16.8*	*0.2*	*1.3*
White, Vivaldi, TTD, Sainsbury's*	1 Serving/100g	76	0.1	76	1.8	17.0	0.1	1.2
with Chorizo, Spicy, Tapas, Waitrose*	1 Serving/260g	512	35.6	197	6.7	11.8	13.7	1.1
with Garlic & Parsley Butter, Herb Oil Dressed, Co-Op*	1 Serving/178g	205	8.9	115	1.0	15.0	5.0	2.0
with Seafood & Seasoned Butter, Tapas, Waitrose*	1 Pack/170g	330	19.4	194	6.2	16.7	11.4	2.1

POTATOES INSTANT

INFO/WEIGHT	Measure	per Measure KCAL	per Measure FAT	KCAL	PROT	CARB	FAT	FIBRE
Mashed, Butter Flavour, Premier Foods*	1 Serving/180g	288	4.1	160	1.4	9.1	2.3	0.8
Mashed, Dry, Tesco*	1 Serving/70g	225	0.1	321	7.7	72.0	0.2	7.1
Mashed, Made Up with Water, Average	1 Serving/180g	118	0.3	66	1.7	14.5	0.2	1.3
Mashed, Original, Dry Weight, Smash*	1 Serving/30g	107	1.4	358	10.7	68.1	4.8	3.4
Mashed, with Fried Onion, Smash*	½ Pack/269g	191	3.5	71	1.6	13.4	1.3	0.7

P

	Measure INFO/WEIGHT	per Measure KCAL	FAT	Nutrition Values per 100g / 100ml KCAL	PROT	CARB	FAT	FIBRE
POUSSIN								
Meat & Skin, Raw, Average	1oz/28g	57	3.9	202	19.1	0.0	13.9	0.0
Spatchcock, British, Waitrose*	½ Poussin/225g	364	20.2	162	19.0	1.2	9.0	0.0
Spatchcock with Garlic & Herbs, Finest, Tesco*	½ Poussin/235g	348	17.2	148	19.7	1.0	7.3	0.5
POWERADE								
Berry & Tropical Fruit, Coca-Cola*	1 Bottle/500ml	120	0.0	24	0.0	5.6	0.0	0.0
Citrus Charge, Coca-Cola*	1 Bottle/500ml	120	0.0	24	0.0	6.0	0.0	0.0
Gold Rush, Coca-Cola*	1 Bottle/500ml	120	0.0	24	0.0	6.0	0.0	0.0
Ice Storm, Coca-Cola*	1 Bottle/500ml	120	0.0	24	0.0	6.0	0.0	0.0
Isotonic, Sports Drink, Coca-Cola*	1 Bottle/500ml	120	0.0	24	0.0	5.6	0.0	0.0
Zero, Coca-Cola*	1 Bottle/500ml	5	0.0	1	0.0	0.0	0.0	0.0
PRAWN COCKTAIL								
& Orkney Crab, M&S*	1 Serving/90g	180	13.8	200	14.2	1.8	15.3	0.6
20% More Prawns, M&S*	½ Pack/100g	330	31.6	330	8.9	2.2	31.6	0.2
BFY, Morrisons*	1 Serving/100g	149	10.3	149	4.7	9.7	10.3	0.1
BGTY, Sainsbury's*	1 Pack/200g	330	23.4	165	10.1	4.8	11.7	0.9
Delicious, Boots*	1 Pack/250g	285	6.5	114	5.5	17.0	2.6	1.2
HL, Tesco*	1 Pack/170g	305	23.9	180	7.1	5.7	14.1	0.6
King, Sainsbury's*	1 Pack/260g	328	15.1	126	5.8	12.7	5.8	2.3
Light Choices, Tesco*	1 Pot/140g	210	16.0	150	7.5	4.3	11.4	1.3
Reduced Fat, M&S*	1 Pack/200g	260	15.0	130	11.9	3.2	7.5	0.7
Reduced Fat, Tesco*	1 Serving/200g	304	21.2	152	7.6	6.5	10.6	0.4
Sainsbury's*	1 Pot/200g	604	55.8	302	9.4	3.2	27.9	0.8
Tesco*	1 Tub/170g	476	39.1	280	6.6	10.2	23.0	1.0
TTD, Sainsbury's*	1 Serving/100g	333	30.6	333	11.5	2.9	30.6	0.5
PRAWN CRACKERS								
Asda*	1 Serving/25g	134	8.8	535	2.0	53.0	35.0	0.0
Cooked in Sunflower Oil, Sharwood's*	1 Cracker/2g	10	0.5	479	0.7	68.3	22.6	0.8
Food to Go, Sainsbury's*	1 Bag/40g	214	12.5	534	2.9	60.2	31.3	0.4
Green Thai Curry, M&S*	1 Pack/50g	250	12.9	500	3.2	62.2	25.8	1.6
M & S*	1 Bag/50g	262	15.6	525	2.8	57.4	31.3	0.8
Ready to Eat, Sharwood's*	1 Bag/60g	316	18.5	527	0.5	62.0	30.8	1.2
Red Mill*	1 Bag/50g	282	18.8	563	2.8	53.1	37.7	0.7
Sainsbury's*	1 Cracker/3g	16	1.0	537	2.4	60.4	31.7	0.8
Tesco*	1/3 Pack/20g	114	7.4	570	2.5	56.5	37.1	0.9
Uncooked, Sharwood's*	1oz/28g	136	8.3	487	0.7	52.7	29.7	1.7
Waitrose*	1 Pack/50g	266	16.0	533	2.4	58.6	32.1	1.6
PRAWN TOAST								
Baguette from Selection, Modern Asian, M&S*	1 Toast/23g	60	3.3	270	11.0	21.3	14.9	2.1
Chinese Selection, Tesco*	1 Toast/10g	36	2.7	362	8.2	20.7	27.5	1.7
Chinese Snack Selection, Morrisons*	1 Toast/13g	41	2.6	328	11.3	23.1	21.2	6.6
Dim Sum Selection, Sainsbury's*	1 Toast/8g	23	1.5	283	9.9	19.2	18.5	2.0
Mini, Oriental Selection, Party, Iceland*	1 Toast/15g	52	3.6	345	10.5	22.0	23.9	2.1
Oriental Selection, Waitrose*	1 Toast/14g	38	2.4	272	11.1	18.3	17.2	2.1
Sesame, Occasions, Sainsbury's*	1 Toast/12g	34	2.2	283	9.9	19.2	18.5	2.0
Sesame, Oriental Snack Selection, Sainsbury's*	1 Toast/12g	40	2.7	335	9.3	23.0	22.9	5.1
Sesame Prawn, Toasted Triangles, M&S*	1 Pack/220g	616	39.6	280	12.4	17.3	18.0	2.0
PRAWNS								
Boiled	1 Prawn/3g	3	0.0	99	22.6	0.0	0.9	0.0
Cooked & Peeled, Average	1oz/28g	21	0.2	77	17.6	0.2	0.6	0.0
Dried, Average	1 Prawn/3g	8	0.1	281	62.4	0.0	3.5	0.0
Hot & Spicy, Average	1 Serving/170g	461	26.9	271	9.4	22.8	15.8	2.2
Icelandic, Raw, Average	1oz/28g	30	0.4	106	22.7	0.0	1.6	0.0
in Brine, John West*	½ Can/60g	58	0.6	97	21.0	1.0	1.0	0.0

	Measure INFO/WEIGHT	per Measure		Nutrition Values per 100g / 100ml				
		KCAL	FAT	KCAL	PROT	CARB	FAT	FIBRE
PRAWNS								
King, Raw, Average	*1 Bag/200g*	*145*	*1.9*	*72*	*15.8*	*0.2*	*1.0*	*0.1*
King, Sweet Chilli, Skewers, BBQ Favourites, Asda*	1 Skewer/48g	48	0.5	100	16.6	5.4	1.1	1.0
King, Tandoori, Average	1 Prawn/59g	33	0.6	55	5.7	5.9	1.1	0.7
North Atlantic, Peeled, Cooked, Average	*1oz/28g*	*22*	*0.3*	*80*	*17.5*	*0.0*	*1.1*	*0.0*
North Atlantic, Raw, Average	*1oz/28g*	*17*	*0.1*	*62*	*14.4*	*0.0*	*0.4*	*0.0*
Raw, Average	*1oz/28g*	*22*	*0.2*	*79*	*17.8*	*0.2*	*0.7*	*0.0*
Sweet Chilli, Skewers, Tesco*	1 Skewer/22g	26	0.2	120	20.4	6.9	0.9	0.5
Tempura, Finest, Tesco*	1 Prawn/18g	31	1.6	175	11.5	11.0	9.1	4.0
Tiger, Cooked & Peeled, Average	*1 Pack/180g*	*151*	*2.0*	*84*	*18.4*	*0.1*	*1.1*	*0.0*
Tiger, Jumbo, Average	*1 Serving/50g*	*39*	*0.2*	*78*	*18.2*	*0.3*	*0.5*	*0.0*
Tiger, Raw, Average	*1 Prawn/30g*	*19*	*0.2*	*64*	*14.2*	*0.0*	*0.7*	*0.0*
Tiger, Wrapped, M&S*	1 Pack/190g	477	25.8	251	11.3	20.7	13.6	1.3
PRAWNS CHILLI								
& Coriander, King, Honduran, M&S*	½ Pack/70g	70	2.2	100	17.2	0.1	3.2	0.4
& Coriander, King, M&S*	1 Pack/140g	147	5.6	105	17.1	0.5	4.0	0.5
& Coriander, King, Sainsbury's*	1 Pack/140g	112	1.8	80	16.6	0.4	1.3	0.5
Coriander & Lime, King, Waitrose*	1 Pack/140g	143	3.2	102	19.9	0.5	2.3	0.6
Sweet, Asda*	1 Pack/360g	500	24.8	139	4.1	15.0	6.9	0.3
Sweet, Crispy, Dipping Sauce, M&S*	1 Pack/240g	515	27.8	215	7.5	19.9	11.6	2.3
Sweet, King, Simply, Birds Eye*	1 Serving/140g	258	17.2	184	11.9	6.4	12.3	0.1
Sweet, Thai, King, Sainsbury's*	1 Serving/150g	177	6.2	118	6.4	13.9	4.1	1.9
with Noodles, & Lemon Grass, BGTY, Sainsbury's*	1 Pack/400g	328	2.8	82	5.0	13.8	0.7	1.3
with Spicy Chilli Dip, King, Sainsbury's*	½ Pack/150g	282	10.8	188	8.6	22.2	7.2	1.0
PRAWNS CREOLE								
with Vegetable Rice, King, COU, M&S*	1 Pack/400g	300	2.4	75	4.5	13.3	0.6	0.7
PRAWNS IN								
Batter Crisp, Lyons*	1 Pack/160g	350	20.3	219	8.0	18.2	12.7	1.1
Creamy Garlic Sauce, Youngs*	1 Serving/158g	261	22.9	165	8.5	0.3	14.5	0.0
Filo, & Breaded, Wrapped, M&S*	1 Serving/19g	45	2.5	235	9.5	20.4	13.0	1.4
Filo, King, Finest, Tesco*	1 Prawn/20g	38	0.6	189	13.0	27.8	2.9	1.6
PRAWNS SZECHUAN								
Spicy, COU, M&S*	1 Pack/400g	380	3.6	95	4.5	16.9	0.9	1.5
PRAWNS WITH								
Cocktail Sauce Dipper, Honduran, M&S*	1 Pack/120g	258	21.6	215	13.6	0.0	18.0	1.1
Garlic, Parsley & Lemon Butter, King, COOK!, M&S*	½ Pack/110g	160	11.3	145	12.9	0.8	10.2	0.5
Garlic & Herb Butter, King, Fresh, M&S*	1 Serving/200g	330	18.0	165	12.5	9.1	9.0	0.5
Garlic Butter, King, M&S*	1 Serving/100g	165	9.0	165	12.5	9.1	9.0	0.5
Ginger & Spring Onion, King, Budgens*	1 Pack/350g	150	4.2	43	5.9	2.1	1.2	0.7
Ginger & Spring Onion, Waitrose*	1 Pack/300g	207	5.1	69	6.4	7.1	1.7	1.9
Green Thai Sauce, Tiger, Waitrose*	½ Pack/117g	108	2.7	92	16.1	0.8	2.3	0.1
Lemon & Pepper, Honduran, King, M&S*	1 Pack/140g	133	3.6	95	17.4	0.4	2.6	0.7
Rice, Sweet Chilli, Tesco*	1 Pack/460g	488	10.1	106	2.4	19.2	2.2	0.5
with Creamy Lime Dip, King, Waitrose*	1 Pot/230g	518	40.7	225	15.8	0.8	17.7	0.2
PRETZELS								
American Style, Salted, Sainsbury's*	1 Serving/50g	202	2.2	403	10.8	79.7	4.5	1.8
Cheddar Cheese, Penn State Pretzels*	1 Bag/30g	124	2.8	412	10.0	71.6	9.3	3.8
Choc Full Of, Cadbury*	½ Bag/55g	250	10.4	455	7.7	62.0	19.0	2.9
Giant, Penn State Pretzels*	1 Pretzel/18g	66	0.7	374	10.5	74.7	3.7	4.1
Giant, Salted, Tesco*	1 Serving/25g	99	1.1	395	12.2	75.8	4.3	3.4
Jumbo, Tesco*	1 Serving/50g	194	3.4	388	9.7	71.9	6.8	5.4
Lightly Salted, Tesco*	1 Serving/25g	99	1.8	395	9.3	73.4	7.1	5.5
Mini, 99% Fat Free, Free Natural*	1 Serving/50g	188	0.5	376	10.1	81.7	1.0	0.0
Mini, M&S*	1 Pack/45g	194	6.0	430	10.4	66.6	13.4	4.9

INFO/WEIGHT	Measure	per Measure KCAL	FAT	Nutrition Values per 100g / 100ml KCAL	PROT	CARB	FAT	FIBRE

PRETZELS

	Measure INFO/WEIGHT	per Measure KCAL	FAT	KCAL	PROT	CARB	FAT	FIBRE
Salt & Cracked Black Pepper, COU, M&S*	1 Pack/25g	95	0.6	380	9.7	83.3	2.4	2.7
Salted, Average	1 Serving/30g	114	0.8	380	10.3	79.8	2.6	3.0
Salted, Mini, M&S*	1 Pack/25g	94	0.5	375	10.0	79.0	2.1	4.2
Salted, Sainsbury's*	1 Serving/50g	200	1.8	401	9.8	82.4	3.6	3.4
Sea Salt & Black Pepper, Penn State Pretzels*	1 Serving/25g	94	1.0	375	10.4	73.7	4.2	4.7
Sea Salt & Black Pepper, Tesco*	1 Serving/50g	190	1.3	379	10.0	79.0	2.6	4.1
Soft, Cinnamon Sugar, Auntie Anne's*	1 Pretzel/112g	380	1.0	339	7.1	75.0	0.9	1.8
Soft, Salted, Original, Auntie Anne's*	1 Pretzel/112g	310	1.0	277	7.1	58.0	0.9	1.8
Soft, Sesame, Auntie Anne's*	1 Pretzel/112g	360	6.0	321	8.9	59.8	5.4	2.7
Sour Cream & Chive, Penn State Pretzels*	1 Serving/25g	111	3.2	443	8.9	71.8	12.9	2.0
Sour Cream & Onion, M&S*	1 Serving/30g	136	4.4	455	11.0	70.9	14.5	0.7
Spicy Salsa, Penn State Pretzels*	1 Serving/25g	105	2.6	420	9.5	72.4	10.4	1.3
Sweet Thai Chilli Twists, Penn State Pretzels*	1 Serving/25g	98	2.0	393	9.8	70.1	8.2	6.8
Wheat, GF, Trufree*	1 Bag/60g	282	12.0	470	0.5	72.0	20.0	0.7
with Sea Salt, Giant, M&S*	1 Pretzel/8g	31	0.5	390	9.7	77.3	6.8	5.4

PRINGLES*

	Measure INFO/WEIGHT	per Measure KCAL	FAT	KCAL	PROT	CARB	FAT	FIBRE
Barbecue, Pringles*	1 Serving/50g	266	18.0	533	4.9	48.0	36.0	5.1
BBQ Spare Rib, Rice Infusions, Pringles*	1 Pack/23g	108	5.3	469	5.1	60.0	23.0	2.6
Cheese & Onion, Pringles*	1 Serving/25g	132	8.5	528	4.1	50.0	34.0	3.4
Hot & Spicy, Pringles*	1 Serving/25g	132	8.5	530	4.6	49.0	34.0	3.7
Light, Original, Pringles*	1 Serving/25g	121	6.2	484	4.3	59.0	25.0	3.6
Light, Sour Cream & Onion, Pringles*	1 Serving/25g	122	6.2	487	4.7	57.0	25.0	3.6
Margarita Pizza, Classic Takeaways, Pringles*	1 Serving/25g	134	8.0	538	3.9	53.0	32.0	2.6
Minis, Original, Pringles*	1 Pack/23g	118	6.9	514	5.1	55.0	30.0	3.7
Minis, Salt & Vinegar, Pringles*	1 Pack/23g	115	6.4	502	4.5	55.0	28.0	3.6
Minis, Sour Cream & Onion, Pringles*	1 Pack/23g	118	6.7	511	5.2	56.0	29.0	3.5
Original, Pringles*	1 Serving/25g	130	8.5	522	3.8	51.0	34.0	2.6
Paprika, Pringles*	1 Serving/25g	132	8.5	529	4.9	49.0	34.0	6.5
Prawn Cocktail, Pringles*	1 Serving/25g	130	8.0	518	4.1	53.0	32.0	2.5
Salt & Vinegar, Pringles*	1 Serving/25g	128	8.0	512	3.9	52.0	32.0	2.4
Sour Cream & Onion, Big Sharing Pack, Pringles*	1 Tube/190g	982	62.7	517	4.1	52.0	33.0	2.5
Sour Cream & Onion, Pringles*	1 Serving/25g	133	8.8	531	4.5	49.0	35.0	3.6
Texas BBQ Sauce, Pringles*	1 Serving/25g	132	8.5	527	4.2	50.0	34.0	3.5

PROBIOTIC DRINK

	Measure INFO/WEIGHT	per Measure KCAL	FAT	KCAL	PROT	CARB	FAT	FIBRE
Orange, Health, Tesco*	1 Serving/100g	67	0.9	67	1.5	13.4	0.9	1.3
Peach, Dairy, Asda*	1 Bottle/100ml	68	0.8	68	2.3	13.0	0.8	2.3
Yoghurt, Original, Tesco*	1 Bottle/100g	68	1.0	68	1.7	13.1	1.0	1.4

PROFITEROLES

	Measure INFO/WEIGHT	per Measure KCAL	FAT	KCAL	PROT	CARB	FAT	FIBRE
Asda*	1 Serving/64g	218	17.2	343	5.0	20.0	27.0	0.0
Chocolate, 8 Pack, Co-Op*	¼ Pack/112g	330	17.9	295	6.0	31.0	16.0	2.0
Chocolate, Sainsbury's*	1/6 Pot/95g	192	8.5	202	5.4	25.1	8.9	0.8
Chocolate, Stack, Sainsbury's*	¼ Pack/76g	311	19.5	409	5.3	39.3	25.6	2.0
Chocolate, Tesco*	1 Serving/76g	293	21.8	386	5.1	26.9	28.7	0.5
Chocolate Covered, Tesco*	1 Serving/72g	295	21.2	410	5.7	29.3	29.5	2.0
Choux & Chocolate Sauce, Tesco*	1 Serving/77g	295	22.0	386	5.1	26.9	28.7	0.5
Filled with Cream, Stack, Fresh, M&S*	1 Serving/75g	281	21.4	375	5.3	23.6	28.5	1.9
in a Pot, Waitrose*	1 Pot/80g	207	11.3	259	6.3	25.6	14.1	2.9
Waitrose*	4 Profiteroles/75g	269	17.9	359	4.8	31.1	23.9	0.7

PRUNES

	Measure INFO/WEIGHT	per Measure KCAL	FAT	KCAL	PROT	CARB	FAT	FIBRE
Average	1 Serving/50g	79	0.2	158	2.5	36.4	0.4	5.8
in Apple Juice, Average	1 Serving/90g	76	0.1	84	0.8	19.8	0.1	1.4
in Fruit Juice, Average	1oz/28g	25	0.0	88	0.9	21.4	0.2	3.0
in Syrup, Average	1oz/28g	26	0.0	92	1.0	22.1	0.2	2.6

	Measure INFO/WEIGHT	per Measure		Nutrition Values per 100g / 100ml				
		KCAL	FAT	KCAL	PROT	CARB	FAT	FIBRE
PRUNES								
Stewed with Sugar	1oz/28g	29	0.1	103	1.3	25.5	0.2	3.1
Stewed without Sugar	1oz/28g	23	0.1	81	1.4	19.5	0.3	3.3
Stoned, Dried Ready to Eat, CBY, Asda*	1 Serving/24g	48	0.1	204	2.5	33.9	0.4	5.7
PUDDING								
Apple & Sultana, Steamed, BGTY, Sainsbury's*	1 Pudding/110g	294	3.2	267	2.9	57.4	2.9	0.8
Bread, Retail Average	1 Slice/120g	301	8.0	251	8.4	41.8	6.7	0.5
Brilliant Black Forest, Graze*	1 Punnet/37g	97	3.3	262	4.0	40.0	9.0	2.0
Cherry Cobbler, GFY, Asda*	1 Pudding/100g	158	2.0	158	2.1	33.0	2.0	0.9
Chocolate, Gu*	1 Pack/240g	780	27.4	325	3.9	51.8	11.4	1.6
Chocolate, M&S*	¼ Pudding/76g	265	12.0	350	4.1	48.0	15.8	2.1
Chocolate, Melting Middle, M&S*	1 Pudding/155g	510	27.8	330	5.8	36.2	18.0	3.1
Chocolate, Tesco*	1 Serving/110g	348	21.0	316	3.1	32.9	19.1	1.9
Chocolate & Vanilla Swirls, Sugar Free, Jell-O*	1 Pot/106g	60	1.5	57	0.9	12.3	1.4	0.0
Chocolate Bombe, Cooked, Fox's*	½ Pudding/114g	435	16.9	383	4.3	57.0	14.9	1.7
Chocolate Ganache, Mini Pot, Gu*	1 Pot/45g	199	16.6	442	3.3	26.4	36.8	2.3
Chocolate Sponge with Rich Caramel Sauce, Cadbury*	1 Pudding/110g	352	16.6	320	4.0	41.1	15.1	1.2
Chocolate with Cream, Delice, Campina*	1 Pot/100g	136	5.4	136	2.5	18.9	5.4	0.0
Crumble, Fruit, Hot, Weight Watchers*	1 Crumble/90g	163	4.1	181	2.2	35.0	4.6	2.4
Eve's, Average	1oz/28g	67	3.7	241	3.5	28.9	13.1	1.4
Hot Chocolate Melting Middle Puds, Gu*	1 Pud/100g	409	26.9	409	6.0	36.0	26.9	2.7
Jam Roly Poly, & Custard, Co-Op*	1 Serving/105g	262	7.4	250	3.0	44.0	7.0	0.8
Jam Roly Poly, Aunt Bessie's*	1 Serving/75g	290	10.4	387	3.4	62.2	13.8	0.9
Jam Roly Poly, Sainsbury's*	¼ Pack/81g	291	11.5	359	4.4	53.3	14.2	0.5
Jam Roly Poly, Tesco*	1 Serving/90g	320	10.9	356	4.3	59.0	12.1	13.9
Queen of Puddings	1oz/28g	60	2.2	213	4.8	33.1	7.8	0.2
Raspberry, Jam Sponge Puddings, M&S*	1 Pot/119g	400	14.0	335	4.0	53.1	11.7	1.4
Sticky Toffee, & Sticky Toffee Sauce, BGTY, Sainsbury's*	1 Serving/130g	318	5.3	245	5.0	49.3	4.1	2.2
Sticky Toffee, Bistro, M Kitchen, Morrisons*	¼ Pack/100g	361	15.6	361	2.7	51.4	15.6	2.0
Sticky Toffee, Co-Op*	¼ Pudding/100g	355	20.0	355	3.0	40.0	20.0	0.7
Sticky Toffee, Extra Special, Asda*	¼ Pudding/100g	378	18.0	378	1.9	52.0	18.0	1.8
Sticky Toffee, Individual, Mr Kipling*	1 Pudding/85g	266	7.2	312	2.7	56.1	8.4	0.9
Sticky Toffee, Steamed, Aunty's*	1 Pudding/110g	331	5.3	301	2.6	58.4	4.8	1.2
Sticky Toffee, Tesco*	1 Serving/110g	287	14.7	261	3.3	31.8	13.4	0.7
Sticky Toffee, Weight Watchers*	1 Pudding/100g	172	1.1	172	3.0	27.2	1.1	20.5
Sticky Toffee, with Custard, Somerfield*	1 Pack/245g	576	19.6	235	3.0	38.0	8.0	0.0
Summer Fruits, Co-Op*	1 Pack/260g	273	0.5	105	1.0	25.0	0.2	1.0
Summer Fruits, Eat Well, M&S*	1 Pudding/135g	128	0.7	95	1.7	20.8	0.5	3.0
Summer Pudding, BGTY, Sainsbury's*	1 Pot/110g	223	5.1	203	3.2	40.9	4.6	2.4
Summer Pudding, Waitrose*	1 Pot/120g	125	0.5	104	2.0	23.1	0.4	1.4
Syrup, Golden, Steamed, Aunty's*	1 Pudding/110g	324	4.5	295	2.9	58.6	4.1	0.7
PUMPKIN								
Boiled in Salted Water	1oz/28g	4	0.1	13	0.6	2.1	0.3	1.1
Solid Pack, 100% Pure, Canned, Libby's*	1 Can/425g	139	1.7	33	1.6	7.4	0.4	4.1

Measure INFO/WEIGHT	per Measure KCAL	FAT	Nutrition Values per 100g / 100ml KCAL	PROT	CARB	FAT	FIBRE

QUAVERS

	Measure INFO/WEIGHT	per Measure KCAL	FAT	KCAL	PROT	CARB	FAT	FIBRE
Cheese, Walkers*	1 Bag/20g	109	6.1	534	2.7	62.5	30.1	1.1
Prawn Cocktail, Walkers*	1 Bag/16g	88	5.1	537	2.1	62.0	31.0	1.2
Salt & Vinegar, Walkers*	1 Bag/16g	86	4.9	527	1.9	62.0	30.0	1.2

QUICHE

	Measure INFO/WEIGHT	per Measure KCAL	FAT	KCAL	PROT	CARB	FAT	FIBRE
Asparagus, & Cheddar, New Covent Garden Food Co*	¼ Quiche/100g	275	18.1	275	7.1	19.8	18.1	2.3
Asparagus, & Feta, Little, Higgidy*	1 Portion/155g	369	23.4	238	8.1	17.3	15.1	1.4
Asparagus, & Herby Summer Vegetable, Higgidy*	1 Quiche/400g	848	50.0	212	5.9	18.9	12.5	2.7
Asparagus, & Mushroom, Tesco*	½ Quiche/200g	474	32.8	237	5.1	17.2	16.4	1.2
Bacon & Brie, Smoked, Asda*	¼ Quiche/90g	249	17.0	277	8.9	17.8	18.9	1.0
Bacon & Cheese, Smoked, Cheddar, Little, Higgidy*	1 Quiche/155g	485	33.8	313	11.5	17.6	21.8	1.0
Bacon & Leek, & Cheese, Weight Watchers*	1 Quiche/165g	327	15.7	198	8.2	18.0	9.5	1.8
Bacon & Leek, & Mushroom, M&S*	¼ Quiche/100g	245	16.4	245	6.9	17.2	16.4	1.3
Bacon & Leek, Asda*	¼ Quiche/100g	252	15.9	252	8.4	18.9	15.9	1.5
Bacon & Leek, Individual, Tesco*	1 Quiche/175g	485	32.4	277	8.3	19.4	18.5	0.9
Bacon & Tomato, Asda*	1 Serving/107g	201	8.6	188	8.0	21.0	8.0	1.1
Bacon & Tomato, Good Intentions, Somerfield*	1 Serving/145g	255	21.5	176	5.7	5.1	14.8	0.1
Broccoli, & Cheese, Morrisons*	1/3 Quiche/134g	338	22.4	253	7.1	18.4	16.8	1.7
Broccoli, Tesco*	1 Serving/100g	249	17.2	249	6.0	17.6	17.2	1.4
Broccoli, Tomato & Cheese, BGTY, Sainsbury's*	1 Quiche/390g	632	32.0	162	6.4	15.7	8.2	1.3
Broccoli, Tomato & Cheese, Deep Filled, Sainsbury's*	¼ Quiche/100g	203	12.9	203	5.2	16.9	12.9	2.3
Broccoli & Stilton, Mini, Sainsbury's*	1 Quiche/14g	52	3.0	369	8.8	35.2	21.4	3.3
Broccoli & Stilton, with Cheddar Crumb, Higgidy*	½ Quiche/200g	558	38.6	279	9.2	17.2	19.3	1.4
Cheese & Bacon, Crustless, Tesco*	1 Serving/85g	170	11.7	200	8.8	9.6	13.8	3.3
Cheese & Bacon, Pork Farms*	1 Pack/120g	378	24.0	315	11.1	20.8	20.0	0.0
Cheese & Bacon, Smart Price, Asda*	¼ Quiche/82g	211	13.9	257	6.0	20.0	17.0	0.7
Cheese & Bacon, Smoked, Mature Cheddar, Higgidy*	1 Quiche/400g	1096	74.0	274	8.4	18.6	18.5	1.5
Cheese & Egg	1oz/28g	88	6.2	314	12.5	17.3	22.2	0.6
Cheese & Ham, & Chive, GFY, Asda*	1 Serving/78g	173	7.8	222	9.0	24.0	10.0	1.5
Cheese & Ham, Basics, Somerfield*	¼ Quiche/81g	187	11.0	231	7.0	20.1	13.6	0.7
Cheese & Ham, Sainsbury's*	1 Serving/100g	266	19.0	266	9.3	14.4	19.0	1.2
Cheese & Ham, Soft Cheese, Tesco*	¼ Quiche/100g	280	20.1	280	7.4	17.5	20.1	1.9
Cheese & Ham, Somerfield*	1 Quiche/325g	835	58.5	257	7.0	18.0	18.0	0.0
Cheese & Mushroom, Budgens*	½ Quiche/170g	474	32.8	279	7.8	18.4	19.3	1.4
Cheese & Onion, Caramelised, Cheddar, Asda*	1/3 Quiche/117g	367	26.8	315	7.0	20.0	23.0	1.0
Cheese & Onion, Cheddar, Crustless, Love Life, Waitrose*	1 Quiche/160g	277	13.4	173	8.0	16.0	8.4	0.7
Cheese & Onion, Crustless, Asda*	1 Quiche/160g	277	15.2	173	7.6	14.3	9.5	1.3
Cheese & Onion, Crustless, Weight Watchers*	1 Quiche/160g	267	12.3	167	11.3	11.1	7.7	4.3
Cheese & Onion, Deep Filled, Sainsbury's*	¼ Quiche/100g	254	17.2	254	7.3	17.2	17.2	2.2
Cheese & Onion, Farmhouse Cheddar, Waitrose*	¼ Quiche/100g	257	18.1	257	8.1	15.4	18.1	1.3
Cheese & Onion, Finest, Tesco*	1 Serving/130g	346	24.3	266	9.1	15.3	18.7	2.5
Cheese & Onion, Retail, Average	¼ Quiche/100g	262	17.8	262	8.4	17.1	17.8	1.3
Cheese & Onion, VLH Kitchens	1 Serving/80g	134	7.5	167	9.6	18.1	6.0	1.8
Cheese & Onion, Weight Watchers*	1 Quiche/165g	325	15.3	197	7.0	21.2	9.3	1.6
Cheese & Tomato, Retail, Average	¼ Quiche/100g	268	17.1	268	8.0	20.2	17.1	1.1
Ham & Tomato, M&S*	½ Pack/200g	440	31.0	220	8.1	12.4	15.5	2.9
Leek, Cheese & Chive, Sainsbury's*	1/3 Quiche/125g	292	20.2	234	7.1	14.9	16.2	1.3
Leek & Sweet Potato, Waitrose*	½ Quiche/200g	440	29.0	220	5.3	17.0	14.5	2.3
Lorraine, Crustless, Asda*	1 Quiche/160g	259	12.6	162	9.3	13.5	7.9	1.1
Lorraine, Crustless, LC, Tesco*	1 Pack/160g	280	13.4	175	12.6	11.8	8.4	2.5
Lorraine, Crustless, You Count, Love Life, Waitrose*	1 Quiche/160g	295	15.4	185	8.9	15.2	9.6	0.9
Lorraine, Extra Special, Asda*	¼ Quiche/100g	270	18.0	270	8.0	19.0	18.0	2.3
Lorraine, Finest, Tesco*	1 Serving/100g	330	25.1	330	8.4	17.5	25.1	1.5
Lorraine, LC, Tesco*	¼ Pack/100g	170	6.4	170	12.3	15.5	6.4	3.2

QUICHE

	Measure INFO/WEIGHT	per Measure KCAL	FAT	Nutrition Values per 100g / 100ml KCAL	PROT	CARB	FAT	FIBRE
Lorraine, Quiche Selection, M&S*	1 Slice/56g	160	11.5	285	12.8	12.3	20.6	2.1
Lorraine, Retail, Average	¼ Quiche/100g	280	19.5	280	9.0	16.8	19.5	2.0
Lorraine, Smoked Bacon & Cheese, M&S*	¼ Quiche/100g	270	18.4	270	9.7	16.4	18.4	1.6
Lorraine, Snack, Morrisons*	1 Serving/50g	142	9.4	285	10.2	19.0	18.7	2.0
Lorraine, TTD, Sainsbury's*	1/3 Quiche/158g	402	28.3	254	10.9	12.3	17.9	2.5
Lorraine, Weight Watchers*	1 Quiche/165g	292	13.2	177	8.7	17.5	8.0	3.2
Mushroom	1oz/28g	80	5.5	284	10.0	18.3	19.5	0.9
Salmon & Broccoli, Asda*	¼ Quiche/106g	289	18.0	273	10.0	20.0	17.0	2.6
Salmon & Broccoli, Tesco*	1 Serving/133g	311	20.1	234	7.9	16.6	15.1	0.9
Salmon & Spinach, Sainsbury's*	1/3 Quiche/125g	318	21.9	254	8.2	15.9	17.5	1.0
Spinach, Feta & Roasted Red Pepper, Higgidy*	1 Quiche/400g	888	53.2	222	5.8	19.9	13.3	2.2
Spinach, Red Pepper, & Goats Cheese, Waitrose*	1 Serving/100g	218	14.3	218	6.5	15.8	14.3	2.6
Spinach & Gruyere, Baby, Sainsbury's*	¼ Quiche/93g	228	16.0	245	7.4	15.1	17.2	1.0
Spinach & Gruyere, Sainsbury's*	¼ Quiche/100g	258	19.1	258	7.7	13.9	19.1	1.0
Spinach & Ricotta, Gruyere, Slice, Somerfield*	1 Serving/130g	348	26.0	268	7.0	15.0	20.0	0.0
Spinach & Ricotta, Tesco*	¼ Quiche/100g	237	14.9	237	5.8	19.9	14.9	1.0
Spinach & Roast Red Pepper, Little, Higgidy*	1 Quiche/155g	397	27.3	256	9.1	15.2	17.6	1.2
Sweet Cherry Pepper & Fontal Cheese, Finest, Tesco*	¼ Quiche/100g	293	22.1	293	6.7	16.9	22.1	0.9
Sweetfire Pepper, Feta & Olive, Waitrose*	¼ Quiche/100g	238	16.9	238	5.7	15.7	16.9	1.4
Tomato, Mozzarella, & Basil, Weight Watchers*	1 Quiche/165g	300	12.2	182	6.1	22.8	7.4	1.3
Tomato, Pesto & Mozzarella, TTD, Sainsbury's*	1/3 Quiche/158g	370	25.6	234	5.5	16.5	16.2	2.1
Tomato & Cheese, Sainsbury's*	1/3 Quiche/133g	374	24.5	281	7.9	20.9	18.4	1.5
Tuna, Tomato & Basil, Asda*	1 Serving/125g	305	20.0	244	9.0	16.0	16.0	1.5
Vegetable, Garden, Crustless, Tesco*	½ Quiche/170g	270	13.8	160	6.5	12.2	8.2	3.5
Vegetable, Mediterranean, Style, Classic, Sainsbury's*	1 Quiche/400g	868	50.4	217	6.2	19.8	12.6	2.2
Vegetable, Mediterranean, Weight Watchers*	1 Quiche/165g	285	13.5	173	3.8	21.1	8.2	4.0
Vegetable, Tesco*	1 Serving/100g	257	17.7	257	6.9	17.5	17.7	1.5

QUINCE

Average	*1 Fruit/209g*	*54*	*0.2*	*26*	*0.3*	*6.3*	*0.1*	*1.9*

QUINOA

Cooked, Love Life, Waitrose*	1 Serving/180g	216	3.5	120	9.9	4.4	1.9	2.8
Dry Weight, Average	*1 Serving/70g*	*258*	*4.2*	*368*	*14.1*	*64.2*	*6.1*	*7.0*
Organic, Dry Weight, Love Life, Waitrose*	1 Serving/40g	154	2.3	384	13.1	68.9	5.8	5.9
Red	1 Serving/100g	358	6.0	358	12.9	62.2	6.0	9.7

QUORN*

Bacon Style, Rashers, Deli	1 Rasher/15g	30	2.3	199	11.8	3.0	15.5	5.0
Bacon Style, Rashers, Streaky, Frozen	3 Strips/38g	74	5.8	198	11.0	3.5	15.5	5.0
Bacon Style, Slices, Smoky, Frozen	¼ Pack/38g	45	1.0	121	16.9	7.5	2.6	4.5
Balls, Swedish Style, Frozen	¼ Pack/75g	88	1.9	117	12.0	9.0	2.5	5.2
Beef Style, Pieces	½ Pack/75g	69	1.6	92	13.5	4.5	2.2	5.0
Biryani, Chicken Style, Lunch Pot	1 Pot/300g	300	13.0	100	3.5	10.9	4.4	1.7
Bites	½ Pack/70g	77	1.8	110	13.8	8.0	2.5	5.0
Bites, Lamb Style Kofta	1 Bite/25g	47	2.4	186	5.0	20.0	9.5	3.0
Burgers, Chicken, Southern Style	1 Burger/63g	119	6.2	189	10.7	14.5	9.8	3.1
Burgers, Chicken Style	1 Burger/70g	136	6.7	194	11.0	16.0	9.6	4.6
Burgers, Frozen	1 Burger/50g	80	3.6	160	14.1	8.1	7.3	2.4
Burgers, Original	1 Burger/50g	73	2.4	146	18.9	6.7	4.8	3.0
Burgers, Quarter Pounder	1 Burger/114g	158	5.1	139	18.0	6.5	4.5	4.5
Burgers, Quarter Pounder, Mexican Style	1 Burger/113g	180	6.3	159	18.3	8.9	5.6	3.8
Burgers, Sizzling	1 Burger/80g	123	4.8	154	18.0	7.0	6.0	3.0
Burgers, Smoked Chilli & Lime, Chef's Selection	1 Burger/90g	147	6.3	163	17.0	6.6	7.0	3.0
Casserole	1oz/28g	46	3.1	165	11.9	5.1	10.9	0.9
Chicken Style, Dippers	1 Dipper/19g	32	2.0	167	11.0	7.2	10.5	4.0

QUORN*

	Measure INFO/WEIGHT	per Measure KCAL	per Measure FAT	100g KCAL	PROT	CARB	FAT	FIBRE
Chicken Style, Pieces, Frozen or Chilled	1 Serving/87g	77	1.2	89	14.0	1.0	1.4	8.3
Chicken Style, Tikka Pieces	1 Pack/175g	201	5.2	115	12.5	7.0	3.0	6.0
Chilli, Mexican, Chef's Selection	½ Pack/170g	143	4.3	84	6.6	6.5	2.5	4.5
Chilli, Vegetarian, Tesco*	1 Pack/400g	340	3.2	85	4.4	15.0	0.8	2.1
Cottage Pie	1 Pack/500g	365	10.0	73	2.5	10.0	2.0	2.5
Crispbake, Tuna & Sweetcorn Style	1 Crispbake/100g	176	6.2	176	6.6	22.0	6.2	3.0
Crispy Bites, with Sweet & Sour Sauce	½ Pack/125g	222	9.4	178	8.5	16.0	7.5	3.2
Curry, Red Thai	1 Pack/400g	464	15.6	116	4.6	15.5	3.9	4.0
Curry & Rice	1 Pack/400g	412	8.0	103	3.8	17.5	2.0	1.5
Dippers, Sticky Chilli	½ Pack/130g	230	8.4	177	10.5	19.0	6.5	4.0
Enchiladas	1 Pack/401g	405	14.8	101	5.3	11.7	3.7	1.9
Escalopes, Cheese & Leek	1 Escalope/120g	256	13.2	213	9.0	17.0	11.0	5.0
Escalopes, Creamy Garlic & Mushroom	1 Escalope/120g	266	15.0	222	7.9	19.4	12.5	3.1
Escalopes, Creamy Peppercorn	1 Escalope/120g	252	15.2	210	7.8	16.0	12.7	4.0
Escalopes, Garlic & Herb	1 Escalope/140g	293	16.5	209	8.9	16.9	11.8	3.8
Escalopes, Goats Cheese & Cranberry	1 Escalope/120g	281	16.8	234	10.0	17.0	14.0	4.0
Escalopes, Gruyere Cheese	1 Escalope/110g	262	15.4	238	10.0	18.0	14.0	2.6
Escalopes, Lemon & Black Pepper	1 Escalope/110g	256	12.9	233	9.6	20.5	11.7	2.1
Escalopes, Mozzarella & Pesto	1 Escalope/120g	260	15.6	217	10.0	15.0	13.0	4.5
Escalopes, Sweet Pepper & Mozzarella	1 Escalope/120g	231	12.4	193	8.7	16.1	10.4	3.8
Fajita Meal Kit	½ Pack/214g	268	5.4	125	7.0	18.5	2.5	3.5
Fajita Strips	½ Pack/70g	69	1.0	98	14.0	7.0	1.5	5.0
Fillets, Barbecue, Sliced	½ Pack/70g	65	0.7	93	13.0	8.0	1.0	5.0
Fillets, Breaded, Mini	1 Fillet/30g	59	2.9	196	10.2	15.0	9.6	4.5
Fillets, Cajun Spice	1 Serving/100g	176	8.2	176	10.9	14.7	8.2	3.4
Fillets, Chicken Style, Plain	1 Fillet/64g	68	1.0	106	13.0	5.0	1.5	5.0
Fillets, Chinese Style Chargrilled, Mini	1 Serving/85g	115	2.3	135	12.1	15.6	2.7	4.7
Fillets, Crispy	1 Fillet/100g	184	8.5	184	12.5	14.2	8.5	4.0
Fillets, Garlic & Herb	1 Fillet/100g	208	9.8	208	13.9	16.1	9.8	4.1
Fillets, Lemon & Pepper	1 Fillet/100g	195	8.5	195	13.3	16.2	8.5	3.5
Fishless Fingers	1 Finger/28g	66	3.0	233	10.0	22.0	10.5	5.0
Goujons	1 Goujon/31g	57	2.9	187	10.2	15.0	9.6	4.5
Grills, Lamb Style	1 Grill/89g	116	5.3	130	10.0	9.0	6.0	4.0
Jalfrezi, Chicken Style, Lunch Pot	1 Pot/300g	267	9.0	89	3.5	11.0	3.0	2.0
Kievs, Mini	1 Kiev/20g	41	2.2	207	14.0	13.0	11.0	6.5
Lamb Style, Strips	¼ Pack/75g	74	1.1	99	14.8	3.5	1.5	6.0
Lasagne, Frozen or Chilled	1 Pack/300g	291	8.1	97	4.8	12.5	2.7	1.6
Mince, Frozen & Chilled	1 Serving/87g	91	1.7	105	14.5	4.5	2.0	5.5
Moussaka	1 Pack/400g	364	16.4	91	3.6	9.8	4.1	1.2
Nuggets, Crispy, Chicken Style	1 Nugget/17g	31	1.8	182	12.0	9.9	10.5	4.0
Ocean Pie, Fish Less	1 Pack/324g	424	24.3	131	5.8	9.0	7.5	2.0
Pasta Bolognese, Lunch Pot	1 Pot/300g	285	6.0	95	5.2	13.0	2.0	2.0
Pasty, Cornish Style	1 Pasty/150g	399	24.0	266	5.5	25.0	16.0	3.0
Pie, & Vegetable	1oz/28g	52	3.2	186	6.9	14.7	11.5	2.0
Pie, Chicken Style & Mushroom	1 Pie/150g	268	15.0	179	6.0	14.0	10.0	4.3
Pie, Creamy Mushroom	1 Pie/142g	359	20.6	253	4.5	26.0	14.5	2.0
Pie, Mince & Onion	1 Pie/142g	360	19.8	254	5.0	27.0	14.0	1.5
Pie, Mince & Potato	1 Pie/200g	388	16.0	194	6.5	22.5	8.0	3.0
Pie, Quorn & Mushroom	1 Pie/141g	378	23.7	268	5.3	23.8	16.8	1.3
Roast, Chicken Style	1/5 Roast/91g	96	1.8	106	15.0	4.5	2.0	4.9
Sausage Roll, Chilled	1 Roll/75g	194	9.6	258	12.0	24.0	12.7	4.0
Sausages	1 Sausage/43g	70	2.9	165	12.6	11.6	6.8	3.5
Sausages, & Mash	1 Pack/400g	332	9.2	83	4.6	9.5	2.3	2.7

QUORN*

Measure INFO/WEIGHT	per Measure KCAL	per Measure FAT	Nutrition Values per 100g / 100ml KCAL	PROT	CARB	FAT	FIBRE

	Measure INFO/WEIGHT	per Measure KCAL	per Measure FAT	KCAL	PROT	CARB	FAT	FIBRE
Sausages, Bangers	1 Sausage/50g	58	2.4	116	11.7	6.6	4.8	3.0
Sausages, Bangers, Bbq, Sizzling	1 Banger/50g	98	5.5	195	12.0	9.5	11.0	5.0
Sausages, Bangers, Bramley Apple	1 Sausage/50g	59	2.3	117	11.5	7.5	4.6	3.0
Sausages, Bangers, Sizzling	1 Sausage/50g	86	5.5	171	13.0	5.0	11.0	5.0
Sausages, Best of British, Chef's Selection	1 Sausage/60g	111	5.7	185	11.0	12.0	9.5	3.5
Sausages, Cocktail	1 Sausage/15g	33	1.8	218	11.2	13.9	12.2	3.9
Sausages, Cumberland	1 Sausage/50g	86	3.5	172	13.5	12.0	7.0	3.5
Sausages, Frankfurter	1 Frankfurter/45g	82	5.8	183	12.5	4.0	13.0	3.0
Sausages, Leek & Pork Style	1 Sausage/44g	56	2.2	127	15.1	5.5	4.9	4.3
Sausages, Pork & Apple Style	1 Sausage/50g	58	2.3	117	11.5	7.5	4.6	3.0
Sausages, Red Leicester & Onion	1 Sausage/50g	82	2.9	164	18.0	10.0	5.8	3.4
Sausages, Tomato & Basil	1 Sausage/50g	51	1.2	102	14.3	6.0	2.3	2.8
Sausages, Wild Garlic & Parsley, Chef's Selection	1 Sausage/60g	104	5.4	174	12.0	9.0	9.0	4.5
Savoury Eggs, Mini	1 Egg/20g	50	2.3	248	15.0	21.0	11.5	4.6
Slices, Chicken Style, Deli	1 Slice/13g	13	0.3	107	16.3	4.5	2.6	6.0
Slices, Chicken Style, Wafer Thin, Deli	1/3 Pack/60g	64	1.6	107	16.3	4.5	2.6	5.9
Slices, Ham Style, Deli	1 Slice/13g	14	0.3	110	16.0	6.5	2.2	5.8
Slices, Ham Style, Smoky	½ Pack/50g	55	1.2	110	16.5	5.7	2.4	5.0
Slices, Ham Style, Wafer Thin, Deli	1/3 Pack/60g	66	1.3	110	16.0	6.5	2.2	5.8
Slices, Peppered Beef Style	1 Slice/13g	13	0.3	107	14.5	7.6	2.1	4.0
Slices, Pepperoni Style	1 Slice/5g	11	0.8	217	12.0	6.5	15.0	4.0
Slices, Roast Chicken Style	½ Pack/50g	54	1.1	109	16.0	6.4	2.2	5.6
Slices, Turkey Style & Cranberry	½ Pack/50g	56	1.2	113	14.5	8.0	2.5	4.0
Slices, Turkey Style with Stuffing, Deli	½ Pack/50g	60	1.2	120	16.0	8.9	2.3	4.0
Spaghetti & Balls	1 Pack/400g	302	3.2	76	4.3	11.9	0.8	1.8
Spaghetti Bolognese	1 Pack/400g	240	3.6	60	3.7	9.2	0.9	1.6
Spaghetti Bolognese, Sainsbury's*	1 Pack/450g	346	5.0	77	4.9	11.9	1.1	1.8
Spring Rolls, Mini	1 Roll/20g	41	2.1	205	4.5	23.0	10.5	2.4
Steak, Strips, Frozen	¼ Pack/77g	83	1.8	108	14.3	4.3	2.4	6.0
Steak, Strips, Seasoned	½ Pack/70g	76	0.9	109	14.0	7.5	1.3	5.5
Steaks, Peppered	1 Steak/98g	123	3.9	126	13.6	5.7	4.0	6.9
Stir Fry, Spicy Chilli with Vegetables & Rice	½ Pack/170g	162	1.7	95	5.9	15.6	1.0	1.8
Stir Fry, Strips, Sweet Chilli	1 Pack/175g	247	4.9	141	12.0	14.5	2.8	5.0
Strips, Southern Style, Fried	1 Strip/31g	62	2.9	200	9.5	19.0	9.5	3.5
Tikka Masala, Chef's Selection	½ Pack/170g	274	17.0	161	6.0	10.0	10.0	3.5

Measure INFO/WEIGHT	per Measure KCAL	per Measure FAT	Nutrition Values per 100g / 100ml KCAL	PROT	CARB	FAT	FIBRE
RABBIT							
Meat Only, Raw	1oz/28g	38	1.5	137	21.9	0.0	5.5	0.0
Meat Only, Raw, Weighed with Bone	1 Serving/200g	274	11.0	137	21.9	0.0	5.5	0.0
Meat Only, Stewed	1oz/28g	32	0.9	114	21.2	0.0	3.2	0.0
Meat Only, Stewed, Weighed with Bone	1oz/28g	19	0.5	68	12.7	0.0	1.9	0.0
RADDICCIO							
Raw	1oz/28g	4	0.1	14	1.4	1.7	0.2	1.8
RADISH							
Red, Unprepared, Average	1 Radish/8g	1	0.0	12	0.7	1.9	0.2	0.9
White, Mooli, Raw	1oz/28g	4	0.0	15	0.8	2.9	0.1	0.0
RAISINS							
& Apricots, The Fruit Factory*	1 Box/14g	41	0.1	290	3.5	67.9	0.5	6.3
& Sultanas, Jumbo, M&S*	1 Serving/80g	212	0.4	265	2.4	62.4	0.5	2.6
& Sultanas, The Fruit Factory*	1 Box/14g	43	0.1	305	3.0	72.3	0.5	4.0
Cherry Infused, Nak'd*	1 Pack/25g	68	0.0	272	2.1	79.0	0.0	2.0
Crazy Cola Infused, Nak'd*	1 Pack/25g	68	0.1	272	2.1	69.3	0.4	2.0
Lemon Infused, Nak'd*	1 Serving/25g	68	0.1	272	2.1	69.3	0.4	2.0
Lime Infused, Tangy, Nak'd*	1 Pack/25g	68	0.0	272	2.1	69.3	0.0	0.0
Orange Infused, Nak'd*	1 Bag/25g	68	0.1	272	2.1	69.3	0.4	1.0
Pineapple Infused, Nak'd*	1 Pack/25g	68	0.0	272	3.0	79.0	0.0	4.0
Seedless, Average	1 Serving/75g	215	0.4	287	2.2	68.5	0.5	3.2
Sunny, Whitworths*	1 Box/43g	116	0.2	272	2.4	65.0	0.4	4.9
Yoghurt Coated, Graze*	1 Pack/40g	182	8.5	456	2.9	64.1	21.3	0.0
Yoghurt Covered, Blueberry, Boots*	1 Pack/75g	322	13.5	429	2.7	64.0	18.0	0.7
RAITA							
Cucumber & Mint, Patak's*	1oz/28g	18	0.5	64	3.4	8.4	1.8	0.0
Plain, Average	1oz/28g	16	0.6	57	4.2	5.8	2.2	0.0
RASPBERRIES							
Dried, Graze*	1 Pack/30g	85	0.8	284	3.2	62.0	2.6	0.0
Fresh, Raw, Average	1 Serving/80g	20	0.2	25	1.3	4.7	0.3	6.5
Frozen, Average	1 Serving/100g	27	0.3	27	1.3	4.7	0.3	5.2
in Fruit Juice, Average	1oz/28g	9	0.0	32	0.8	6.7	0.2	1.7
in Syrup, Canned	1oz/28g	25	0.0	88	0.6	22.5	0.1	1.5
RATATOUILLE							
Average	1oz/28g	23	2.0	82	1.3	3.8	7.0	1.8
Chicken, Finest, Tesco*	1 Pack/550g	407	11.6	74	7.8	5.9	2.1	0.0
Princes*	1 Can/360g	86	1.4	24	1.0	4.2	0.4	0.0
Provencale, French Style Mixed Vegetables, Tesco*	½ Can/195g	76	3.9	39	1.1	4.2	2.0	1.9
Roasted Vegetable, Sainsbury's*	1 Pack/300g	134	3.0	45	1.4	7.5	1.0	2.3
Sainsbury's*	1 Pack/300g	99	1.8	33	1.5	5.5	0.6	1.6
RAVIOLI							
Asparagus, Waitrose*	1 Serving/150g	303	9.0	202	10.5	26.4	6.0	2.0
Basil & Parmesan, Organic, Sainsbury's*	½ Pack/192g	290	10.0	151	7.4	21.1	5.2	2.1
Beef	1 Serving/300g	501	13.7	167	6.4	25.0	4.6	1.4
Beef, & Red Wine, Italiano, Tesco*	½ Pack/150g	315	9.8	210	7.3	30.0	6.5	2.3
Beef, & Red Wine, Rich, Morrisons*	1 Pack/300g	813	20.7	271	12.0	42.8	6.9	2.6
Beef, & Shiraz, Finest, Tesco*	½ Pack/200g	358	9.0	179	8.4	26.1	4.5	1.8
Beef, in Rich Tomato Sauce, Minced, Corale, Aldi*	½ Can/200g	172	2.0	86	2.8	16.4	1.0	0.5
Beef, in Tomato Sauce, Canned, Asda*	1 Can/400g	352	8.0	88	3.6	14.0	2.0	3.0
Beef, in Tomato Sauce, Canned, Great Stuff, Asda*	1 Can/200g	146	3.0	73	2.2	12.7	1.5	1.4
Beef, Weight Watchers*	1 Pack/300g	258	6.3	86	4.3	12.1	2.1	0.8
Butternut Squash & Goats Cheese, M&S*	1 Pack/359g	305	11.5	85	2.7	9.8	3.2	2.9
Cheese, & Asparagus, Waitrose*	1 Serving/100g	242	7.2	242	12.6	31.7	7.2	2.4
Cheese, & Tomato, Fresh, Organic, Tesco*	1 Serving/125g	342	14.0	274	12.5	30.8	11.2	1.1

R

	Measure INFO/WEIGHT	per Measure KCAL	FAT	Nutrition Values per 100g / 100ml KCAL	PROT	CARB	FAT	FIBRE
RAVIOLI								
Cheese, & Tomato, Heinz*	1 Can/400g	340	8.4	85	2.4	13.9	2.1	0.9
Cheese, Garlic & Herb, Fresh, Organic, Tesco*	1 Serving/125g	382	19.5	306	11.3	30.1	15.6	0.9
Cheese, Tomato & Basil, Italiano, Tesco*	½ Pack/125g	309	11.0	247	13.1	28.5	8.8	2.1
Chicken, & Bacon, Cooked, Sainsbury's*	½ Pack/211g	335	11.4	159	5.5	22.2	5.4	2.0
Chicken, & Mushroom, Finest, Tesco*	½ Pack/125g	268	8.9	214	11.6	25.8	7.1	1.1
Chicken, & Tomato, PB, Waitrose*	1 Serving/125g	265	3.4	212	13.5	33.4	2.7	2.8
Chicken, Tomato & Basil, Finest, Tesco*	1 Serving/200g	358	12.0	179	9.6	21.7	6.0	1.0
Feta Cheese, M&S*	1 Serving/100g	195	8.5	195	9.1	20.5	8.5	1.3
Florentine, Weight Watchers*	1 Serving/241g	220	5.0	91	3.7	14.1	2.1	1.2
Four Cheese, in Tomato Sauce, COU, M&S*	1 Pack/345g	345	7.6	100	7.5	12.3	2.2	1.5
Four Cheese, Italian Choice, Asda*	1 Pack/449g	467	26.9	104	3.4	9.0	6.0	2.1
Fresh, Pasta Reale*	1 Serving/150g	459	8.8	306	13.1	53.3	5.9	0.0
Goat's Cheese, & Pesto, Asda*	½ Pack/150g	204	5.4	136	6.0	20.0	3.6	0.0
Goat's Cheese, & Roasted Red Pepper, Finest, Tesco*	½ Pack/125g	308	9.6	246	11.4	32.8	7.7	1.8
in Tomato Sauce, Heinz*	1 Can/400g	308	6.8	77	2.4	13.2	1.7	0.9
Meat, Italian, Fresh, Asda*	½ Pack/150g	261	6.3	174	8.0	26.0	4.2	0.0
Mozzarella, Tomato & Basil, Tesco*	1 Serving/125g	304	12.8	243	13.6	24.1	10.2	0.5
Mushroom, Fresh, Sainsbury's*	½ Pack/125g	196	5.1	157	7.4	22.6	4.1	1.9
Mushroom, Garlic, Finest, Tesco*	1 Serving/250g	552	18.2	221	8.9	30.0	7.3	2.0
Mushroom, Italian, Fresh, Somerfield*	½ Pack/125g	336	12.2	269	10.8	34.4	9.8	1.8
Mushroom, Wild, Finest, Tesco*	1 Serving/200g	472	12.2	236	10.8	34.4	6.1	1.9
Pancetta & Mozzarella, Finest, Tesco*	1 Serving/125g	344	13.2	275	12.2	32.8	10.6	1.8
Salmon, & Dill, Sainsbury's*	1 Pack/300g	615	21.3	205	8.7	26.5	7.1	3.0
Spinach & Ricotta, Waitrose*	1 Serving/125g	309	9.0	247	10.5	35.0	7.2	1.9
Vegetable, Canned, Sainsbury's*	1 Can/400g	328	2.8	82	2.6	16.3	0.7	0.7
Vegetable, Roasted, Asda*	½ Pack/150g	218	0.8	145	6.0	29.0	0.5	0.0
RED BULL*								
Energy Shot, Red Bull*	1 Can/60ml	27	0.0	45	0.0	10.7	0.0	0.0
Regular, Red Bull*	1 Can/250ml	112	0.0	45	0.0	11.3	0.0	0.0
REDCURRANTS								
Raw, Average	*1oz/28g*	*6*	*0.0*	*21*	*1.1*	*4.4*	*0.0*	*3.4*
REFRESHERS								
Bassett's*	1oz/28g	106	0.0	377	4.3	78.1	0.0	0.0
RELISH								
Barbeque, Sainsbury's*	1 Serving/50g	50	1.0	100	1.0	19.3	2.1	1.1
Burger, Juicy, Asda*	1 Tbsp/15g	17	0.1	113	1.2	25.4	0.7	0.7
Caramelised Onion & Chilli, M&S*	1 Serving/20g	47	0.2	235	1.4	55.1	1.1	1.0
Caramelised Red Onion, Tesco*	1 Serving/10g	28	0.0	280	0.6	69.1	0.1	0.7
Hamburger, Bick's*	1oz/28g	27	0.1	96	1.3	22.3	0.2	0.0
Mango & Chilli, Levi Roots*	1 Serving/100g	110	0.2	110	0.7	25.0	0.2	1.1
Onion, M&S*	1oz/28g	46	0.8	165	1.0	32.1	3.0	1.1
Onion & Garlic, Spicy, Waitrose*	1 Tbsp/15g	35	0.2	232	0.8	54.2	1.1	1.7
Sweet Chilli & Ginger, Branston*	1 Serving/20g	33	0.1	163	1.5	38.2	0.4	0.5
Sweet Onion, Branston*	1 Serving/10g	15	0.0	153	1.0	36.3	0.4	0.7
Sweetcorn, & Red Pepper, Branston*	1 Serving/10g	17	0.1	171	1.3	39.9	0.6	0.6
Sweetcorn, American Style, Maryland, Tesco*	1 Serving/15g	15	0.0	101	1.1	23.9	0.1	0.9
Sweetcorn, Bick's*	1 Tbsp/22g	23	0.0	103	1.3	24.3	0.2	0.0
Tomato, & Chilli Texan Style, Tesco*	1 Tbsp/14g	20	0.0	140	1.7	32.0	0.1	1.1
Tomato, & Red Pepper, Branston*	1 Serving/15g	24	0.1	160	1.3	37.4	0.4	0.7
Tomato, M&S*	1oz/28g	36	0.1	130	1.8	30.2	0.3	1.5
Tomato, Spicy, Bick's*	1 Serving/28g	28	0.1	99	1.3	23.2	0.2	0.0
Tomato, Sweet, Heinz*	1 Serving/25g	34	0.0	136	0.9	32.6	0.2	0.9

R

	Measure INFO/WEIGHT	per Measure KCAL	FAT	Nutrition Values per 100g / 100ml KCAL	PROT	CARB	FAT	FIBRE
REVELS								
Mars*	1 Pack/35g	168	7.3	480	5.1	68.0	20.9	0.0
RHUBARB								
In Juice, Canned, Drained, Average	1 Serving/100g	46	0.0	46	0.5	10.8	0.0	0.8
Raw, Average	*1 Stalk/51g*	*11*	*0.1*	*21*	*0.9*	*4.5*	*0.2*	*1.8*
Stewed with Sugar, Average	*1oz/28g*	*32*	*0.0*	*116*	*0.4*	*31.2*	*0.0*	*2.0*
RIBENA*								
Apple & Peach, Immunity Support, Plus, Ribena*	1 Carton/200ml	2	0.0	1	0.0	0.2	0.0	0.0
Blackcurrant, Carton, Plus, Ribena*	1 Carton/200ml	6	0.0	3	0.0	0.6	0.0	0.0
Blackcurrant, Diluted with Water, Ribena*	1 Serving/100ml	46	0.0	46	0.0	11.4	0.0	0.0
Blackcurrant, No Added Sugar, Diluted, Ribena*	1 Serving/250ml	11	0.0	4	0.0	0.6	0.0	0.0
Blackcurrant, Original, Undiluted, Ribena*	1 Serving/50ml	108	0.0	216	0.0	53.0	0.0	0.0
Blackcurrant, Ready Made, Juice Drink, Ribena*	1 Carton/200ml	86	0.0	43	0.0	10.6	0.0	0.0
Blackcurrant, Really Light, No Added Sugar, Ribena*	1 Carton/250ml	8	0.0	3	0.0	0.8	0.0	0.0
Blackcurrant & Cranberry, Ribena*	1 Bottle/500ml	205	0.0	41	0.0	9.9	0.0	0.0
Light, Ribena*	1 Carton/288ml	26	0.0	9	0.1	2.1	0.0	0.0
Orange, Juice Drink, Ribena*	1 Serving/288ml	98	0.0	34	0.1	8.1	0.0	0.0
Really Light, Undiluted, Ribena*	1 Serving/25ml	20	0.0	80	0.0	2.5	0.0	0.0
Strawberry, Juice Drink, Ribena*	1 Carton/288ml	130	0.0	45	0.0	10.9	0.0	0.0
RIBS								
in a Chinese Style Coating, Tesco*	1 Serving/250g	420	21.8	168	19.5	5.3	8.7	2.5
Pork, Barbecue, Average	1 Serving/100g	275	17.9	275	21.4	7.2	17.9	0.3
Pork, Chinese Style, Average	1 Serving/300g	736	44.7	245	17.9	10.0	14.9	0.7
Pork, Full Rack, Sainsbury's*	1 Serving/225g	567	38.7	252	18.0	6.5	17.2	0.9
Spare, Barbecue, Chinese Style, Farmfoods*	1 Pack/400g	464	25.2	116	9.3	5.6	6.3	0.1
Spare, Cantonese, Mini, Sainsbury's*	1 Rib/38g	97	5.0	259	17.2	17.3	13.4	1.0
Spare, Chinese Style, Meal Solutions, Co-Op*	1 Serving/165g	214	14.8	130	8.0	4.0	9.0	0.2
Spare, Chinese Style, Summer Eating, Asda*	1 Serving/116g	334	18.6	288	32.0	4.1	16.0	0.8
Spare, Sweet, Sticky, Mini, M&S*	1 Pack/300g	615	34.5	205	16.6	8.6	11.5	0.2
RICE								
Arborio, Dry, Average	*1 Serving/80g*	*279*	*0.6*	*348*	*7.1*	*78.3*	*0.8*	*0.8*
Balti Style, Quick, Sainsbury's*	1 Serving/228g	192	1.1	84	4.3	15.7	0.5	2.0
Basmati, & Wild, Cooked, Sainsbury's*	½ Pack/125g	150	0.8	120	3.1	25.7	0.6	1.3
Basmati, & Wild, Dry Weight, Tilda*	1 Serving/70g	244	0.3	349	9.4	77.0	0.5	1.0
Basmati, Boil in the Bag, Dry, Average	1 Serving/50g	176	0.4	352	8.4	77.8	0.8	0.4
Basmati, Brown, Dry, Average	*1 Serving/50g*	*177*	*1.5*	*353*	*9.5*	*71.8*	*3.0*	*2.2*
Basmati, Cooked, Average	*1 Serving/140g*	*189*	*1.0*	*135*	*3.1*	*29.0*	*0.7*	*0.4*
Basmati, Cooked, Tilda*	1 Serving/200g	214	0.2	107	2.4	24.0	0.1	1.2
Basmati, Dry Weight, Average	*1 Serving/60g*	*212*	*0.6*	*353*	*8.1*	*77.9*	*1.0*	*0.6*
Basmati, Indian, Dry, Average	*1 Serving/75g*	*260*	*0.7*	*346*	*8.4*	*76.1*	*0.9*	*0.1*
Basmati, Microwave, Cooked, Average	1 Serving/125g	182	2.3	146	2.7	30.0	1.8	0.0
Basmati, Uncooked, TTD, Sainsbury's*	1 Serving/50g	174	0.5	349	8.8	76.2	1.0	1.7
Basmati, White, Dry, Average	*1 Serving/75g*	*262*	*0.4*	*349*	*8.1*	*77.1*	*0.6*	*2.2*
Basmati, Wholegrain, Cooked, Tilda*	1 Portion/180g	203	1.6	113	3.3	23.0	0.9	3.2
Basmati, with Mushroom, Dine In, Veetee*	1 Pack/280g	372	6.4	133	3.3	24.4	2.3	1.2
Beef, Savoury, Batchelors*	1 Pack/120g	431	2.8	359	8.9	75.7	2.3	2.5
Broccoli, Sweetcorn & Peas, SteamFresh, Birds Eye*	1 Bag/170g	192	5.6	113	3.5	17.3	3.3	2.1
Brown, Cooked, Average	*1 Serving/140g*	*173*	*1.5*	*123*	*2.6*	*26.6*	*1.1*	*0.9*
Brown, Dry, Average	*1 Serving/75g*	*266*	*2.3*	*355*	*7.5*	*76.2*	*3.0*	*1.4*
Brown, Long Grain, Dry, Average	*1 Serving/50g*	*182*	*1.4*	*364*	*7.6*	*76.8*	*2.8*	*2.0*
Brown, Short Grain, Dry, Average	*1 Serving/50g*	*176*	*1.4*	*351*	*6.8*	*77.6*	*2.8*	*1.0*
Brown, Whole Grain, Cooked, Average	*1 Serving/170g*	*223*	*1.9*	*132*	*2.6*	*27.8*	*1.1*	*1.2*
Brown, Whole Grain, Dry, Average	*1 Serving/40g*	*138*	*1.2*	*344*	*7.4*	*71.6*	*2.9*	*3.0*
Chicken, Fried, Chinese Takeaway, Iceland*	1 Pack/340g	510	15.6	150	6.5	20.7	4.6	0.6

RICE

INFO/WEIGHT	Measure per Measure KCAL	FAT	Nutrition Values per 100g / 100ml KCAL	PROT	CARB	FAT	FIBRE
Chicken, Savoury, Batchelors*	1 Pack/124g	455	1.9	367	8.9	79.4	1.5	2.6
Chicken, Savoury, Smart Price, Asda*	½ Pack/168g	210	1.5	125	3.2	26.0	0.9	2.4
Chicken, Savoury, Tesco*	1 Serving/87g	177	1.9	204	6.4	39.4	2.2	6.7
Chilli & Coriander, TTD, Sainsbury's*	1 Pack/446g	522	12.5	117	6.5	16.5	2.8	2.2
Chinese, Savoury, Batchelors*	1 Serving/50g	177	1.2	354	9.9	73.1	2.4	2.8
Chinese Style, Express, Uncle Ben's*	1 Pack/250g	392	5.5	157	3.4	30.9	2.2	0.4
Coconut, & Lime, Asda*	1 Pack/360g	695	17.6	193	4.5	32.7	4.9	0.9
Coconut, M&S*	½ Pack/124g	217	5.0	175	3.1	31.8	4.0	0.3
Coconut, Thai, Sainsbury's*	½ Pack/100g	178	9.1	178	2.6	21.3	9.1	1.9
Coriander & Herb, Packet, Cooked, Sainsbury's*	¼ Pack/150g	204	0.8	136	2.5	30.4	0.5	1.5
Curry, Mild, Savoury, Batchelors*	1 Pack/120g	426	2.5	355	8.0	76.1	2.1	1.6
Egg Fried, 2 Minute Meals, Sainsbury's*	1 Pack/250g	342	1.5	137	3.8	29.2	0.6	0.8
Egg Fried, Average	1 Serving/300g	624	31.8	208	4.2	25.7	10.6	0.4
Egg Fried, Chinese Style, Tesco*	1 Portion/250g	418	10.5	167	4.4	27.9	4.2	0.7
Egg Fried, Chinese Takeaway, Iceland*	1 Pack/340g	374	7.8	110	4.2	18.1	2.3	1.1
Egg Fried, Chinese Takeaway, Tesco*	1 Serving/200g	250	3.0	125	4.7	23.3	1.5	1.8
Egg Fried, Express, Uncle Ben's*	½ Pack/125g	216	5.2	173	4.0	29.9	4.2	0.3
Egg Fried, Micro, Tesco*	1 Pack/250g	312	9.2	125	4.6	18.3	3.7	6.4
Egg Fried, Sainsbury's*	1 Pack/250g	432	9.5	173	4.5	30.3	3.8	0.8
Golden Savoury, Dry Weight, Batchelors*	1 Pack/120g	437	3.4	364	10.1	74.7	2.8	2.4
Golden Savoury, Nirvana*	1 Pack/120g	142	0.8	118	2.5	25.4	0.7	2.9
Ground, Whitworths*	1 Serving/28g	98	0.2	349	7.7	77.7	0.8	0.7
Long Grain, & Wild, Dry, Average	*1 Serving/75g*	*254*	*1.5*	*338*	*7.6*	*72.6*	*2.0*	*1.7*
Long Grain, American, Cooked, Average	*1 Serving/160g*	*229*	*2.8*	*143*	*3.0*	*28.8*	*1.8*	*0.2*
Long Grain, American, Dry, Average	*1 Serving/50g*	*175*	*0.5*	*350*	*7.2*	*77.8*	*1.1*	*0.6*
Long Grain, Brown, Micro Rice, Asda*	1 Portion/100g	153	1.4	153	3.8	30.2	1.4	2.4
Long Grain, Cooked, Value, Tesco*	1 Portion/50g	175	0.4	350	7.7	78.0	0.8	0.4
Long Grain, Dry, Average	*1 Serving/50g*	*169*	*0.5*	*337*	*7.4*	*75.5*	*1.0*	*1.7*
Long Grain, Microwavable, Cooked, Average	1 Serving/150g	180	0.9	120	2.7	25.8	0.6	0.7
Mexican Style, Ainsley Harriott*	1 Pack/170g	206	1.5	121	1.7	26.5	0.9	2.3
Mexican Style, Cooked, Express, Uncle Ben's*	1 Pack/250g	385	4.8	154	3.2	31.1	1.9	0.7
Mexican Style, Old El Paso*	1 Serving/75g	268	0.8	357	9.0	78.0	1.0	0.0
Mexican Style, Spicy, Savoury, Made Up, Tesco*	1 Serving/164g	213	2.5	130	2.9	26.3	1.5	2.4
Microwave, Express, Uncle Ben's*	1 Serving/250g	370	4.2	148	3.2	30.0	1.7	0.0
Mushroom Pilau, Bombay Brasserie, Sainsbury's*	1 Pack/400g	672	17.2	168	3.7	28.6	4.3	0.7
Mushroom Savoury, Batchelors*	½ Pack/61g	217	1.3	356	10.7	73.6	2.1	2.8
Paella, Savoury, Tesco*	1 Serving/60g	220	2.8	367	8.4	72.7	4.7	4.5
Pilau, Cooked, Average	*1 Serving/140g*	*244*	*6.2*	*174*	*3.5*	*30.3*	*4.4*	*0.8*
Pilau, Dry, Average	*1oz/28g*	*101*	*0.7*	*362*	*8.4*	*78.2*	*2.4*	*3.4*
Pilau, Indian Mushroom, Sainsbury's*	1 Serving/100g	119	2.4	119	3.0	21.3	2.4	1.9
Pilau, Mushroom, Sainsbury's*	1 Pack/250g	400	13.8	160	3.4	24.1	5.5	2.4
Pilau, Spinach, Bombay Brasserie, Sainsbury's*	1 Pack/401g	642	17.3	160	3.5	26.9	4.3	0.8
Pilau, Spinach & Carrot, Waitrose*	1 Pack/350g	466	8.4	133	3.1	24.8	2.4	1.2
Pilau, Waitrose*	½ Pack/175g	308	7.4	176	4.2	30.4	4.2	1.2
Pudding, Dry Weight, Average	1 Serving/100g	356	1.1	356	6.9	82.0	1.1	0.4
Quinoa & Basmati, Chilli & Lime, Cooked, Ainsley Harriott*	1 Serving/203g	256	2.2	126	4.3	24.7	1.1	2.9
Risotto, Dry, Average	*1 Serving/50g*	*174*	*0.6*	*348*	*7.8*	*76.2*	*1.3*	*2.4*
Saffron, Cooked, Average	*1 Serving/150g*	*208*	*4.7*	*139*	*2.6*	*25.3*	*3.2*	*0.5*
Special Fried, Cantonese, Sainsbury's*	½ Pack/250g	442	10.0	177	4.9	30.4	4.0	1.2
Special Fried, Chinese, Tesco*	1 Serving/300g	618	33.3	206	6.5	19.9	11.1	0.8
Special Fried, Chinese Takeaway, Iceland*	1 Pack/350g	630	17.5	180	5.5	28.2	5.0	1.2
Special Fried, M&S*	1 Pack/450g	922	35.1	205	6.2	27.2	7.8	0.5
Special Fried, Sainsbury's*	1 Serving/166g	272	7.6	164	5.1	25.5	4.6	0.7

R

RICE

INFO/WEIGHT	Measure KCAL	FAT	per 100g KCAL	PROT	CARB	FAT	FIBRE
RICE							
Special Fried, Waitrose*	1 Serving/350g	532	22.4	152	6.1	17.6	6.4	3.2
Sweet & Spicy, Express, Uncle Ben's*	1 Pack/250g	418	10.0	167	2.7	30.1	4.0	0.0
Thai, Cooked, Average	*1 Serving/100g*	*136*	*1.8*	*136*	*2.5*	*27.4*	*1.8*	*0.3*
Thai, Dry, Average	*1 Serving/50g*	*174*	*0.2*	*348*	*7.1*	*78.9*	*0.4*	*0.9*
Thai, Fragrant, Dry, Average	*1 Serving/75g*	*272*	*0.5*	*363*	*7.2*	*82.0*	*0.7*	*0.3*
Thai, Glutinous, Sticky, White, Dry, Raw	1 Serving/100g	370	0.6	370	6.8	81.7	0.6	2.8
Thai, Sticky, Tesco*	1 Serving/250g	358	6.2	143	2.5	27.6	2.5	0.4
Vegetable, Golden, Freshly Frozen, Asda*	1 Sachet/200g	238	2.6	119	3.2	23.6	1.3	1.3
Vegetable, Golden, Savoury, Morrisons*	1 Serving/50g	70	0.4	141	3.4	30.1	0.8	1.1
Vegetable, Golden, Savoury, Sainsbury's*	¼ Pack/100g	122	1.0	122	2.9	25.4	1.0	0.3
Vegetable, Mixed, Savoury, Dry Weight, Tesco*	1 Pack/120g	450	3.2	375	7.8	79.1	2.7	2.9
Vegetable, Savoury, Co-Op*	½ Pack/60g	210	0.6	350	9.0	76.0	1.0	3.0
White, Cooked, Average	*1 Serving/140g*	*182*	*1.1*	*130*	*2.6*	*28.7*	*0.8*	*0.2*
White, Cooked, Frozen, Average	*1 Serving/150g*	*168*	*0.8*	*112*	*2.9*	*23.8*	*0.6*	*1.2*
White, Flaked, Dry Weight, Average	*1oz/28g*	*97*	*0.3*	*346*	*6.6*	*77.5*	*1.2*	*0.0*
White, Fried	1oz/28g	37	0.9	131	2.2	25.0	3.2	0.6
White, Long Grain, Dry Weight, Average	*1 Serving/50g*	*181*	*1.0*	*362*	*7.1*	*79.1*	*1.9*	*0.4*
White, Microwave, Cooked, Average	½ Pack/125g	185	2.4	148	3.3	29.4	1.9	1.4
Whole Grain, Dry, Average	*1 Serving/50g*	*171*	*1.2*	*342*	*8.2*	*72.0*	*2.3*	*4.0*
Wholegrain, Microwave, Eat Well, M&S*	½ Pack/125g	181	1.5	145	2.5	31.0	1.2	2.2
Wild, Coronation, Sainsbury's*	¼ Pot/75g	140	4.8	186	3.1	29.1	6.4	0.9
With Red Kidney Beans, Average	1oz/28g	49	1.0	175	5.6	32.4	3.5	2.5
RICE CAKES							
& Corn, Salt & Vinegar Flavour, M&S*	1 Pack/22g	80	1.3	365	6.7	71.7	5.9	0.7
Apple & Cinnamon Flavour, Kallo*	1 Cake/11g	41	0.2	376	6.2	83.1	2.2	3.9
Asda*	1 Cake/8g	31	0.2	386	8.7	81.1	3.0	2.8
Barbeque, Tesco*	1 Cake/9g	28	0.2	328	9.6	66.8	2.5	6.2
Black & White Sesame, Clearspring*	1 Cake/8g	31	0.2	385	7.4	82.2	2.9	0.0
Brink*	1 Cake/15g	56	0.3	370	8.8	78.8	2.2	0.0
Caramel, Jumbo, Tesco*	1 Cake/10g	34	0.3	340	7.0	74.0	3.0	5.0
Caramel, Kallo*	1 Cake/10g	38	0.5	383	6.2	78.9	4.8	3.9
Caramel, Large, Tesco*	1 Cake/10g	34	0.2	344	6.5	73.9	2.5	5.1
Caramel, Less Than 3% Fat, Sainsbury's*	1 Pack/35g	134	0.6	382	5.6	86.4	1.6	1.8
Caramel, Snack Size, Tesco*	1 Pack/35g	133	1.0	379	5.5	82.7	2.9	0.9
Cheese, Jumbo, Free From, Tesco*	1 Serving/10g	44	1.8	439	8.1	62.1	17.6	3.8
Cheese & Chive, Mature, Kallo*	1 Cake/9g	32	0.4	374	8.2	75.2	4.5	3.1
Chilli, Mini, M&S*	1 Pack/22g	88	1.7	400	6.9	74.9	7.9	3.5
Chocolate, Dark, Organic, Kallo*	1 Cake/12g	57	2.9	471	6.8	57.2	24.1	7.4
Chocolate, Fabulous Bakin' Boys*	1 Biscuit/17g	83	3.7	490	6.4	66.7	22.0	1.6
Chocolate, Happy Shopper*	2 Portions/33g	156	6.3	469	5.1	69.9	18.8	2.4
Chocolate, Milk, Organic, Kallo*	1 Cake/11g	57	3.2	509	6.5	56.2	28.7	3.5
Co-Op*	1 Cake/20g	80	0.6	402	8.0	84.0	3.1	0.0
Low Fat, Kallo*	1 Cake/10g	38	0.2	375	6.2	83.1	2.2	3.9
Multigrain, Ryvita*	3 Cakes/11g	43	0.5	384	9.1	76.2	4.7	5.3
Oat & Rice, Salted, High Fibre, Thick Slice, Kallo*	1 Cake/8g	27	0.4	356	10.6	75.0	5.5	9.0
Organic, Tesco*	1 Cake/8g	29	0.2	380	7.2	80.7	2.9	3.4
Paprika, Good Food*	1 Cake/12g	50	1.1	414	7.9	73.0	9.3	3.1
Salt & Vinegar, Jumbo, Tesco*	1 Cake/9g	31	0.2	347	8.4	72.7	2.5	6.0
Salt & Vinegar, Sainsbury's*	1 Pack/30g	121	2.5	403	8.3	73.3	8.3	2.7
Salt & Vinegar, Snack, Tesco*	1 Pack/35g	116	0.6	332	7.5	71.5	1.8	1.1
Salt & Vinegar Flavour, Morrisons*	1 Bag/30g	122	2.6	407	6.7	75.8	8.6	1.2
Salted, Lightly, Thick Slice, Low Fat, Kallo*	1 Cake/8g	28	0.2	372	8.0	78.7	2.8	5.1
Salted, Sea Salt & Balsamic Vinegar, Kallo*	1 Cake/9g	32	0.2	361	6.5	78.1	2.5	3.0

RICE CAKES

	Measure INFO/WEIGHT	per Measure KCAL	FAT	Nutrition Values per 100g / 100ml KCAL	PROT	CARB	FAT	FIBRE
Salted, Slightly, Mrs Crimble's*	1 Slice/6g	21	0.2	380	7.6	80.4	3.1	3.2
Salted, Slightly, Organic, Thin Slice, Kallo*	1 Cake/5g	17	0.1	372	8.0	78.7	2.8	5.1
Salted, Slightly, Thick Slice, Organic, Kallo*	1 Cake/8g	28	0.2	372	8.0	78.7	2.8	5.1
Salted, Slightly, with Cracked Pepper, Snack Size, Kallo*	1 Cake/2g	8	0.1	372	8.0	78.7	2.8	5.1
Sesame, No Added Salt, Thick Sliced, Organic, Kallo*	1 Cake/10g	37	0.3	373	8.0	78.0	3.2	5.4
Sesame, Slightly Salted, Thick Slice, Organic, Kallo*	1 Cake/8g	28	0.2	373	8.0	78.0	3.2	5.4
Sesame, Slightly Salted, Thin Slice, Organic, Kallo*	1 Cake/5g	17	0.1	373	8.0	78.0	3.2	5.4
Sesame, Teriyaki, Clearspring*	1 Cake/7g	28	0.2	377	6.5	82.8	2.2	0.0
Sesame, Toasted, Ryvita*	1 Pack/11g	43	0.5	391	8.4	78.4	4.9	3.5
Sour Cream & Chive, Sainsbury's*	1 Pack/30g	119	2.6	396	7.9	72.0	8.5	2.9
Thin Slice, No Added Salt, Organic, Kallo*	1 Cake/5g	19	0.1	372	8.0	78.7	2.8	5.1
Thin Slice, Organic, Hawkwood*	1 Cake/6g	21	0.2	378	7.6	79.1	3.5	3.4
Thin Slice, Organic, Waitrose*	1 Serving/5g	17	0.1	340	8.0	70.0	2.0	4.0
Wholegrain, Mild Chilli, Tesco*	1 Cake/10g	38	1.4	400	7.2	59.8	14.4	5.8
Wholegrain, No Added Salt, BGTY, Sainsbury's*	1 Cake/8g	30	0.2	372	8.0	78.7	2.8	5.1
Wholegrain, No Added Salt, Thick Slice, Organic, Kallo*	1 Cake/9g	33	0.3	365	7.6	80.0	3.1	3.4
Wholegrain, Salt & Vinegar, Tesco*	1 Cake/9g	28	0.2	314	8.4	61.9	2.6	6.0

RICE CRACKERS

	Measure INFO/WEIGHT	per Measure KCAL	FAT	Nutrition Values per 100g / 100ml KCAL	PROT	CARB	FAT	FIBRE
Authentic Thai Chilli, Tyrrells*	½ Pack/75g	389	20.2	519	5.0	64.0	27.0	1.0
Barbecue, Sakata*	½ Pack/50g	204	1.3	407	7.3	85.2	2.6	1.6
Barbecue, Tesco*	1 Pack/25g	102	1.8	409	6.7	78.8	7.4	1.7
Black Pepperdoms & Mango Chutney, Graze*	1 Punnet/28g	106	3.2	377	3.1	65.5	11.3	1.2
Brown, Wakama*	1 Cracker/5g	19	0.0	375	8.0	84.8	0.4	0.0
Cheddar Gorge, Graze*	1 Punnet/24g	128	8.3	534	10.6	48.3	34.7	2.3
Chilli, Korean, Graze*	1 Pack/19g	98	5.1	519	5.0	64.0	27.0	0.5
Chilli, Temptations, Tesco*	1 Serving/25g	128	7.2	512	4.4	58.0	28.8	0.0
Chilli, Whitworths*	½ Pack/50g	254	12.8	507	5.1	63.9	25.7	0.5
Cracked Pepper, Sakata*	½ Pack/50g	200	1.5	400	7.3	84.4	3.0	2.0
Crispy, Sea Salt & Vinegar, Go Ahead, McVitie's*	1 Serving/25g	102	1.4	408	6.6	80.6	5.4	1.8
Japanese, Apollo*	1 Pack/75g	297	3.5	396	9.6	78.8	4.7	0.9
Japanese, Graze*	1 Pack/40g	159	1.9	397	9.0	79.7	4.7	0.0
Japanese, Julian Graves*	1 Serving/25g	92	0.4	369	8.8	79.5	1.7	3.8
Japanese, Mini, Sunrise*	1 Serving/50g	180	0.0	360	7.0	83.0	0.0	7.0
Japanese, Seaweed, Very Nori-sh, Graze*	1 Punnet/14g	64	1.8	454	5.9	78.8	12.7	1.0
Japanese, Style, Tesco*	1 Serving/25g	101	1.5	405	11.7	75.2	6.1	3.3
Mix, M&S*	½ Pack/63g	225	0.1	360	6.5	82.9	0.1	1.6
Sainsbury's*	1 Serving/20g	87	1.9	433	11.2	74.3	9.4	1.0
Seaweed, Woolworths Homebrand*	12 Crackers/25g	100	0.7	398	7.3	85.0	2.7	0.0
Sour Cream & Chive, Sakata*	1 Serving/25g	107	2.0	430	7.8	80.6	7.9	0.0
Thai, Chilli, Nature's Harvest*	1 Pack/75g	401	22.3	535	4.6	61.5	29.7	4.2
Thai, M&S*	1 Serving/55g	209	1.8	380	7.0	80.2	3.3	1.2
Thai, Sesame & Soy Sauce, M&S*	1 Pack/55g	210	2.6	385	7.6	77.8	4.8	1.4
Thin, Blue Dragon*	3 Crackers/5g	20	0.2	395	6.1	84.4	3.7	0.0
Veggie Sushi Plate, Graze*	1 Punnet/24g	107	3.1	444	11.1	68.4	12.8	3.9

RICE MILK

	Measure INFO/WEIGHT	per Measure KCAL	FAT	Nutrition Values per 100g / 100ml KCAL	PROT	CARB	FAT	FIBRE
Organic, Provamel*	1 Serving/250ml	122	3.8	49	0.1	9.5	1.5	0.0
Original, Rice Dream*	1 Serving/150ml	70	1.5	47	0.1	9.4	1.0	0.1

RICE PUDDING

	Measure INFO/WEIGHT	per Measure KCAL	FAT	Nutrition Values per 100g / 100ml KCAL	PROT	CARB	FAT	FIBRE
50% Less Fat, Asda*	½ Can/212g	180	1.7	85	3.3	16.2	0.8	0.2
Apple, Mini Pot, Muller Rice, Muller*	1 Pot/95g	103	2.2	108	3.2	18.6	2.3	0.0
Apple, Muller Rice, Muller*	1 Pot/190g	205	4.4	108	3.2	18.6	2.3	0.4
Apple & Blackberry, Muller Rice, Muller*	1 Pot/190g	207	4.2	109	3.2	19.0	2.2	0.4
Apple Strudel Flavour Sauce, Muller Rice, Muller*	1 Pot/190g	205	4.4	108	3.2	18.6	2.3	0.4

	Measure INFO/WEIGHT	per Measure		Nutrition Values per 100g / 100ml				
		KCAL	FAT	KCAL	PROT	CARB	FAT	FIBRE
RICE PUDDING								
Banana & Toffee (Limited Edition), Muller Rice, Muller*	1 Pot/190g	207	4.2	109	3.1	19.3	2.2	0.4
Canned, Average	1oz/28g	25	0.7	89	3.4	14.0	2.5	0.2
Canned, Basics, Sainsbury's*	½ Can/213g	157	1.7	74	3.1	13.7	0.8	1.4
Canned, BGTY, Sainsbury's*	1 Can/425g	344	2.6	81	3.3	15.5	0.6	0.4
Caramel, Ambrosia*	1 Pot/150g	149	3.8	99	3.1	16.1	2.5	0.0
Clotted Cream, Cornish, Waitrose*	1 Serving/150g	304	20.1	203	3.0	17.6	13.4	0.5
Clotted Cream, M&S*	1 Pudding/185g	431	30.7	233	3.0	19.2	16.6	0.2
Creamed, Asda*	1 Serving/215g	196	3.4	91	3.2	16.0	1.6	0.0
Creamed, Canned, Ambrosia*	1 Can/425g	382	8.1	90	3.1	15.2	1.9	0.0
Creamed, Canned, Sainsbury's*	½ Can/212g	187	2.8	88	3.0	16.0	1.3	0.3
Creamed, Devon, Low Fat, Ambrosia*	½ Can/213g	193	2.8	91	3.2	16.5	1.3	0.0
Creamed, Luxury, Added Cream, Canned, Sainsbury's*	½ Can/213g	272	12.1	128	3.3	15.9	5.7	0.0
Creamed, Morrisons*	1 Can/212g	189	3.4	89	3.1	15.7	1.6	0.0
Creamed, Pot, Ambrosia*	1 Pot/150g	156	3.8	104	3.3	17.0	2.5	0.1
Creamed, Value, Tesco*	1 Can/425g	348	3.4	82	3.2	15.5	0.8	0.0
Creamed, Weight Watchers*	1 Pot/130g	108	0.9	83	3.2	16.0	0.7	0.3
Creamy, Ambrosia*	½ Can/212g	197	4.0	93	3.2	15.7	1.9	0.0
Low Fat, Tesco*	1 Can/425g	404	5.5	95	3.2	16.9	1.3	0.1
Luxury, Llangadog Creamery*	1 Serving/220g	310	16.9	141	3.1	15.2	7.7	0.0
Organic, Ambrosia*	1 Can/425g	455	15.7	107	3.4	15.1	3.7	0.0
Original, Muller Rice, Muller*	1 Pot/190g	196	4.9	103	3.6	16.3	2.6	0.3
Raspberry, Mini Pot, Muller Rice, Muller*	1 Pot/95g	101	2.2	106	3.2	18.2	2.3	0.5
Raspberry, Mullerice, Muller*	1 Pot/190g	201	4.4	106	3.2	18.2	2.3	0.5
Rhubarb, Muller*	1 Pot/200g	226	4.4	113	3.2	20.0	2.2	0.0
Strawberry, Mini Pot, Muller Rice, Muller*	1 Pot/95g	102	2.2	107	3.2	18.4	2.3	0.4
Strawberry, Mullerrice, Muller*	1 Pot/200g	220	4.4	110	3.2	19.3	2.2	0.4
Thick & Creamy, Co-Op*	1 Can/425g	531	25.5	125	3.0	16.0	6.0	0.0
Toffee, Smooth, Muller Rice, Muller*	1 Pot/190g	201	4.4	106	3.3	18.0	2.3	0.3
Vanilla Custard, Mullerrice, Muller*	1 Pot/200g	230	5.0	115	3.4	19.8	2.5	0.3
with Strawberry Sauce, Ambrosia*	1 Pot/160g	174	3.2	109	2.7	19.8	2.0	0.1
with Sultanas & Nutmeg, Ambrosia*	1 Pack/425g	446	12.3	105	3.2	16.6	2.9	0.1
RICE SALAD								
Indian Style, with Chickpeas & Yoghurt Dressing, M&S*	1 Pack/220g	264	7.0	120	3.7	19.3	3.2	3.4
Mexican, with Beans, COU, M&S*	1 Serving/250g	250	3.5	100	6.0	15.6	1.4	1.2
Rainbow, M&S*	1 Serving/262g	340	8.4	130	2.5	23.3	3.2	1.5
Rainbow, Waitrose*	1/3 Pack/60g	70	1.6	117	3.2	18.1	2.7	3.6
Spanish Style, with Chicken, M&S*	1 Serving/220g	319	12.8	145	5.8	17.4	5.8	0.5
RICE WINE								
Sake, Average	*1oz/28g*	*38*	*0.0*	*134*	*0.5*	*5.0*	*0.0*	*0.0*
Shaoxing, Waitrose*	1 Tbsp/15ml	21	0.0	138	1.6	3.9	0.0	0.2
RIGATONI								
Carbonara, Tesco*	1 Serving/205g	236	11.9	115	5.2	10.6	5.8	1.2
Dry, Average	*1 Serving/80g*	*272*	*1.2*	*340*	*11.4*	*68.4*	*1.5*	*2.7*
RISOTTO								
Balls, Mushroom, Occasions, Sainsbury's*	1 Ball/25g	76	3.4	304	3.8	41.2	13.8	1.7
Balls, Sun Dried Tomato, Occasions, Sainsbury's*	1 Ball/25g	71	3.8	285	6.8	30.8	15.0	2.9
Beef, Vesta*	1 Serving/100g	346	5.9	346	15.3	57.8	5.9	5.6
Beetroot & Goats Cheese, Lovely Vegetables, M&S*	1 Pack/379g	530	17.0	140	4.4	20.7	4.5	3.6
Caramelised Onion & Gruyere Cheese, M&S*	1 Pack/200g	350	20.6	175	3.0	17.8	10.3	1.7
Cheese, Onion & Wine, Rice & Simple, Ainsley Harriott*	1 Pack/140g	253	7.0	181	3.1	31.0	5.0	1.6
Cherry Tomato, COU, M&S*	1 Pack/360g	324	8.3	90	2.0	15.4	2.3	1.8
Chicken	1 Serving/380g	494	17.4	130	7.2	15.2	4.6	1.3
Chicken, Chargrilled, Ready Meal, M&S*	1 Pack/365g	493	25.2	135	6.4	11.6	6.9	0.7

RISOTTO	Measure INFO/WEIGHT	per Measure KCAL	FAT	Nutrition Values per 100g / 100ml KCAL	PROT	CARB	FAT	FIBRE
Chicken, Lemon & Wild Rocket, Sainsbury's*	1 Pack/360g	683	41.0	190	16.2	5.6	11.4	0.1
Chicken, Little Dish*	1 Pack/200g	209	9.2	104	7.1	9.1	4.6	0.6
Chicken, Ready Meal, M&S*	1 Pack/360g	450	15.8	125	6.7	14.4	4.4	0.9
Chicken & Bacon, Italiano, Tesco*	1 Pack/450g	652	20.2	145	5.9	20.2	4.5	1.5
Chicken & Lemon, Weight Watchers*	1 Pack/330g	327	6.9	99	6.3	13.7	2.1	0.5
Chicken & Mushroom, Creamy, Italian, CBY, Asda*	1 Pack/350g	374	11.9	107	6.6	11.9	3.4	1.3
Chicken & Mushroom, Finest, Tesco*	1 Pack/400g	496	11.2	124	7.4	17.2	2.8	0.5
Chicken & Mushroom, Waitrose*	1 Pack/350g	364	16.1	104	6.0	9.7	4.6	0.8
Chicken & Mushroom, Weight Watchers*	1 Pack/320g	310	4.5	97	6.5	14.5	1.4	0.3
Green Bean, Asparagus & Pecorino, Finest, Tesco*	1 Pack/400g	460	15.6	115	4.4	15.0	3.9	1.5
Haddock, Smoked, Italian, Tesco*	½ Pack/350g	400	15.1	114	4.2	14.3	4.3	0.8
King Prawn, & Snow Crab, M&S*	1 Pack/365g	402	16.4	110	4.1	12.7	4.5	0.5
King Prawn, Pea & Mint, M&S*	½ Pack/300g	405	18.6	135	3.8	15.9	6.2	0.9
Mushroom, & Chestnut, Waitrose*	1 Pack/400g	496	90.0	124	14.6	58.4	22.5	7.2
Mushroom, & Garlic, Wild, Tesco*	1 Pack/320g	522	14.1	163	3.6	27.2	4.4	1.6
Mushroom, Asda*	1 Pack/340g	340	11.6	100	2.3	15.0	3.4	0.6
Mushroom, BGTY, Sainsbury's*	1 Pack/400g	387	8.7	102	2.7	17.6	2.3	1.0
Mushroom, COU, M&S*	1 Pack/375g	338	5.6	90	3.0	16.1	1.5	1.5
Mushroom, Italiano, Tesco*	1 Pack/340g	367	6.8	108	2.4	20.0	2.0	4.6
Mushroom, Low Saturated Fat, Waitrose*	1 Pack/400g	440	9.6	110	4.6	15.1	2.4	1.5
Mushroom, PB, Waitrose*	1 Pack/400g	384	6.4	96	4.3	16.1	1.6	2.1
Mushroom, Wild, Made Up, Ainsley Harriott*	1 Sachet/140g	785	21.7	561	12.0	93.3	15.5	14.7
Mushroom, Wild, Weight-Away*	1 Pack/250g	320	9.8	128	3.1	18.0	3.9	1.0
Pea, Broad Bean & Asparagus, M&S*	1 Pack/380g	418	9.9	110	4.5	15.1	2.6	2.9
Primavera, with Asparagus, Spinach & Peas, COU, M&S*	1 Pack/375g	340	7.2	90	3.6	15.0	1.9	1.0
Roasted Red Pepper & Italian Cheese, M&S*	1 Pack/400g	500	13.2	125	2.9	20.4	3.3	1.0
Roasted Vegetable & Sunblush Tomato, Finest, Tesco*	½ Pack/200g	306	18.0	153	3.7	14.5	9.0	1.4
Salmon, Weight Watchers*	1 Pack/320g	261	2.5	82	4.7	13.8	0.8	0.3
Salmon & Spinach, Hot Smoked, M&S*	½ Pack/300g	420	24.0	140	6.4	11.0	8.0	0.6
Seafood, with Spinach & Tomatoes, Fuller Longer, M&S*	1 Pack/420g	420	9.2	100	8.8	10.8	2.2	1.7
Seafood, Youngs*	1 Pack/350g	424	13.0	121	4.5	17.4	3.7	0.1
Spring Vegetable, M&S*	1 Serving/330g	330	13.2	100	2.0	14.2	4.0	0.9
Tomato & Chilli, Solo Slim, Rosemary Conley*	1 Pack/300g	240	8.7	80	6.8	6.7	2.9	3.5
Tomato & Mascarpone, Cooked, Ainsley Harriott*	1 Serving/346g	553	18.7	160	2.5	25.3	5.4	1.6
Vegetable, Average	1oz/28g	41	1.8	147	4.2	19.2	6.5	2.2
Vegetable, Brown Rice, Average	1oz/28g	40	1.8	143	4.1	18.6	6.4	2.4
RISSOLES								
Lentil, Fried in Vegetable Oil, Average	1oz/28g	59	2.9	211	8.9	22.0	10.5	3.6
ROCK SALMON								
Raw, Flesh Only, Average	*1oz/28g*	*43*	*2.7*	*154*	*16.6*	*0.0*	*9.7*	*0.0*
ROCKET								
Fresh, Raw, Average	*1 Serving/80g*	*12*	*0.4*	*16*	*0.8*	*1.7*	*0.5*	*1.2*
ROE								
Cod, Average	*1 Can/100g*	*96*	*2.8*	*96*	*17.1*	*0.5*	*2.8*	*0.0*
Cod, Hard, Coated in Batter, Fried	1oz/28g	53	3.3	189	12.4	8.9	11.8	0.2
Herring, Soft, Fried in Blended Oil	1oz/28g	74	4.4	265	26.3	4.7	15.8	0.2
Herring, Soft, Raw	*1oz/28g*	*25*	*0.7*	*91*	*16.8*	*0.0*	*2.6*	*0.0*
ROGAN JOSH								
Chicken, & Rice, Sainsbury's*	1 Pack/500g	675	27.0	135	6.7	14.1	5.4	2.4
Chicken, Breast, Chunks, Hot, Sainsbury's*	½ Pack/114g	143	2.0	126	23.6	3.9	1.8	1.0
Chicken, with Pilau Rice, Farmfoods*	1 Pack/325g	354	6.8	109	5.3	17.1	2.1	0.4
Lamb, & Pilau Rice, Indian Takeaway, Asda*	1 Pack/569g	888	27.9	156	7.0	21.0	4.9	1.7
Lamb, & Pilau Rice, Tesco*	1 Pack/550g	770	29.2	140	6.0	16.9	5.3	1.0

R

	Measure INFO/WEIGHT	per Measure KCAL	FAT	Nutrition Values per 100g / 100ml KCAL	PROT	CARB	FAT	FIBRE
ROGAN JOSH								
Lamb, Asda*	1 Pack/450g	688	40.5	153	13.0	5.0	9.0	3.1
Lamb, Indian Takeaway, M Kitchen, Morrisons*	½ Pack/175g	224	9.5	128	0.0	4.5	5.4	0.0
Lamb, Sainsbury's*	1 Pack/400g	660	44.4	165	11.3	4.9	11.1	1.9
Lamb, Tesco*	1 Pack/350g	402	20.3	115	10.2	5.0	5.8	1.3
Lamb, Waitrose*	½ Pack/175g	242	13.3	138	12.4	5.0	7.6	1.3
Lamb, with Pilau Rice, Eastern Classics*	1 Pack/400g	604	21.6	151	5.6	19.9	5.4	1.0
Prawn, & Pilau Rice, BGTY, Sainsbury's*	1 Pack/401g	353	3.2	88	4.8	15.3	0.8	1.9
Prawn, COU, M&S*	1 Pack/400g	360	2.4	90	4.9	16.2	0.6	0.8
ROLL								
Bacon, & Mushroom, Crusty, M&S*	1 Roll/160g	424	20.2	265	8.7	29.0	12.6	2.3
Cheese, & Chutney, M&S*	1 Roll/165g	256	1.2	155	13.9	23.1	0.7	1.2
Cheese, & Mustard, Chunky, Finest, Tesco*	1 Roll/88g	260	9.0	295	10.9	40.0	10.2	2.4
Cheese, & Onion, Asda*	1 Serving/67g	199	12.0	298	7.0	27.0	18.0	2.0
Cheese, & Onion, Co-Op*	1 Roll/66g	195	11.9	295	7.0	26.0	18.0	2.0
Cheese, & Onion, Iceland*	1 Roll/67g	222	13.6	332	7.5	29.6	20.4	1.5
Cheese, & Onion, King Size, Pork Farms*	1 Serving/130g	443	28.6	341	7.4	28.4	22.0	0.0
Cheese, & Onion, M&S*	1 Roll/25g	80	5.1	320	9.6	24.7	20.5	1.3
Cheese, & Onion, Sainsbury's*	1 Roll/67g	205	13.6	306	8.0	22.9	20.3	1.9
Cheese, & Onion, Tesco*	1 Roll/67g	203	12.1	305	7.3	28.0	18.1	1.9
Cheese, & Pickle, Sainsbury's*	1 Roll/136g	359	13.6	264	10.6	35.1	10.0	0.0
Cheese, Ploughman's, Malted Wheat, BGTY, Sainsbury's*	1 Roll/172g	309	3.6	180	10.9	29.3	2.1	3.8
Cheese, Tomato & Onion, Sainsbury's*	1 Pack/100g	518	28.1	518	18.4	47.9	28.1	0.0
Chicken, & Herb, Shapers, Boots*	1 Roll/168g	290	4.7	173	12.0	25.0	2.8	1.7
Chicken, Salad, Mini, Selection Pack, British, M&S*	1 Roll/61g	134	4.1	220	11.9	28.1	6.8	2.1
Chicken, Spicy, Crusty, M&S*	1 Roll/150g	382	16.6	255	12.8	25.8	11.1	2.0
Egg, & Tomato, Shapers, Boots*	1 Roll/166g	301	5.3	181	8.0	30.0	3.2	2.6
Egg Mayonnaise, & Cress, Fullfillers*	1 Roll/125g	266	11.8	213	10.0	25.7	9.4	0.0
Egg Mayonnaise, & Cress, Sub, Delicious, Boots*	1 Pack/205g	399	14.1	195	10.0	23.0	6.9	2.4
Egg Mayonnaise, & Cress, White, Soft, Somerfield*	1 Serving/211g	475	17.3	225	9.4	28.2	8.2	2.1
Ham, & Cheese in Pastry, Pork Farms*	1 Roll/70g	216	12.5	308	8.0	28.8	17.9	0.0
Ham, & Tomato, Taste!*	1 Serving/112g	211	4.8	188	10.4	27.0	4.3	0.0
Ham, Darwins Deli*	1 Serving/125g	298	7.5	238	11.0	37.4	6.0	0.0
Ham Salad, BGTY, Sainsbury's*	1 Roll/178g	292	3.4	164	10.8	25.9	1.9	0.0
Ham Salad, Good Intentions, Somerfield*	1 Pack/214g	325	4.7	152	8.7	24.3	2.2	1.6
Pork, Stuffing, & Apple Sauce, Roast, Boots*	1 Roll/218g	602	26.2	276	10.0	32.0	12.0	1.8
Salmon, Oak Smoked, M&S*	1 Roll/55g	139	6.2	252	14.6	23.1	11.3	1.2
Sausage, Lincolnshire, COU, M&S*	1 Roll/175g	280	4.7	160	10.0	23.2	2.7	2.6
Steak, & Onion, M&S*	1 Serving/150g	308	10.5	205	11.0	24.5	7.0	3.8
Tuna, & Sweetcorn with Mayonnaise, Shell*	1 Pack/180g	536	26.3	298	13.1	28.6	14.6	0.0
Tuna, Cheese Melt, Boots*	1 Roll/199g	612	35.8	308	13.0	23.0	18.0	1.2
Tuna Mayonnaise, & Cucumber, Taste!*	1 Serving/111g	274	12.5	247	9.0	27.3	11.3	0.0
Tuna Mayonnaise, with Cucumber, Yummies*	1 Serving/132g	340	18.6	257	10.4	22.5	14.0	0.0
Turkey Salad, Northern Bites*	1 Roll/231g	323	8.3	140	8.6	19.6	3.6	3.0
ROLO								
Chocolate, Nestle*	2 Pieces/20g	102	5.3	509	4.1	62.6	26.6	1.3
Giant, Nestle*	1 Sweet/9g	42	1.8	470	3.1	70.1	19.7	0.3
Little, Nestle*	1 Pack/40g	196	9.4	491	4.0	65.5	23.5	0.5
Nestle*	1 Sweet/5g	24	1.0	481	3.9	73.1	19.2	1.9
ROOT BEER								
Average	1 Can/330ml	135	0.0	41	0.0	10.6	0.0	0.0
ROSE WATER								
The English Provender Co.*	1 Tsp/5g	0	0.0	2	0.1	0.6	0.1	0.1

	Measure INFO/WEIGHT	per Measure KCAL	FAT	Nutrition Values per 100g / 100ml KCAL	PROT	CARB	FAT	FIBRE
ROSEHIP								
Wild	1 Serving/100g	162	0.3	162	1.6	38.2	0.3	24.1
ROSEMARY								
Dried	*1 Tsp/1g*	*3*	*0.2*	*331*	*4.9*	*46.4*	*15.2*	*0.0*
Fresh	*1 Tsp/0.7g*	*1*	*0.0*	*99*	*1.4*	*13.5*	*4.4*	*0.0*
ROSTI								
Oven Baked, McCain*	1 Rosti/100g	194	9.3	194	2.6	25.0	9.3	2.3
Potato, Baby, M&S*	1 Rosti/23g	40	1.5	175	3.5	25.1	6.7	1.6
Potato, Chicken & Sweetcorn Bake, Asda*	1 Serving/400g	440	18.8	110	7.0	10.0	4.7	0.6
Potato, McCain*	1 Rosti/95g	161	8.6	169	2.2	19.6	9.1	0.0
Potato, Mini, Party Bites, Sainsbury's*	1 Serving/100g	218	11.5	218	2.5	26.2	11.5	3.0
Potato, Mini, Party Range, Tesco*	1 Rosti/17g	32	1.9	193	2.1	20.6	11.4	3.3
Potato, Onion & Gruyere, Finest, Tesco*	½ Pack/200g	206	10.6	103	3.2	10.5	5.3	2.0
Potato, Spinach & Mozzarella, Tesco*	1 Serving/140g	228	7.7	163	3.8	24.5	5.5	2.0
Potato & Leek, Sainsbury's*	½ Pack/190g	296	20.9	156	4.5	9.8	11.0	0.3
Potato & Root Vegetable, COU, M&S*	1 Rosti/100g	85	2.7	85	1.6	13.3	2.7	1.5
Vegetable, Waitrose*	1 Pack/400g	248	9.2	62	1.4	8.8	2.3	1.3
Waitrose*	1 Rosti/45g	112	7.2	248	3.8	22.5	15.9	2.7
ROULADE								
Chocolate, Finest, Tesco*	1 Serving/80g	222	4.5	277	3.4	53.2	5.6	2.3
Chocolate, Sainsbury's*	1 Serving/72g	264	15.7	367	5.7	36.9	21.8	1.8
Lemon, Asda*	1 Serving/100g	343	12.0	343	2.7	56.0	12.0	0.0
Mini, M&S*	1 Serving/63g	201	19.1	321	8.5	3.0	30.5	0.0
Orange & Lemon Meringue, Co-Op*	1 Serving/82g	287	9.8	350	3.0	57.0	12.0	0.3
Raspberry, Finest, Tesco*	1/6 Roulade/75g	220	9.2	295	2.7	41.5	12.4	2.7
Salmon & Spinach, Smoked, Finest, Tesco*	1 Serving/60g	91	6.1	152	11.5	3.6	10.2	0.6
Toffee Pecan, Finest, Tesco*	1 Serving/60g	218	8.9	363	3.6	53.8	14.8	0.5
RUM								
37.5% Volume	*1 Pub Shot/35ml*	*72*	*0.0*	*207*	*0.0*	*0.0*	*0.0*	*0.0*
40% Volume	*1 Pub Shot/35ml*	*78*	*0.0*	*222*	*0.0*	*0.0*	*0.0*	*0.0*
Captain Morgans & Cola, Premixed, Canned, Diageo*	1 Can/250ml	180	0.0	72	0.0	9.1	0.0	0.0
*Malibu, 21% Volume, Pernod Ricard**	*1 Pub Shot/35ml*	*70*	*0.0*	*200*	*0.0*	*29.0*	*0.0*	*0.0*
White	*1 Pub Shot/35ml*	*72*	*0.0*	*207*	*0.0*	*0.0*	*0.0*	*0.0*
RUSKS								
Banana, Farleys*	1 Serving/17g	70	1.5	409	7.3	75.1	8.8	2.9
Mini, Farleys*	1 Serving/30g	122	2.2	405	7.0	77.7	7.3	2.1
Original, Farleys*	1 Rusk/17g	69	1.2	406	7.1	77.6	7.1	2.4

R

	Measure INFO/WEIGHT	per Measure KCAL	FAT	Nutrition Values per 100g / 100ml KCAL	PROT	CARB	FAT	FIBRE
SAAG								
Aloo, Fresh, Sainsbury's*	1 Pack/400g	388	13.2	97	2.0	14.7	3.3	4.8
Aloo, North Indian, Sainsbury's*	1 Pack/300g	354	24.0	118	2.4	9.0	8.0	1.6
Aloo, Sainsbury's*	1 Pack/300g	441	31.8	147	2.1	10.7	10.6	3.5
Aloo, Tesco*	1 Serving/200g	144	7.0	72	2.1	8.0	3.5	2.0
Aloo Gobi, Indian, Tesco*	1 Pack/225g	225	16.4	100	2.1	6.5	7.3	1.8
Aloo Gobi, Indian Takeaway, Sainsbury's*	1 Pack/334g	164	3.7	49	1.7	8.0	1.1	1.5
Aloo Gobi, M Kitchen, Morrisons*	1 Pack/225g	130	6.1	58	2.0	4.6	2.7	3.8
Aloo Gobi, M&S*	1 Pack/225g	270	19.1	120	1.9	9.3	8.5	2.4
Aloo Gobi, Tesco*	1 Serving/175g	166	8.9	95	2.1	9.5	5.1	1.9
Aloo Gobi, Waitrose*	½ Pack/150g	147	7.5	98	2.1	9.0	5.0	3.9
Chicken, Aloo, Lemon & Coriander Rice, Weight Watchers*	1 Pack/400g	372	4.4	93	6.7	13.4	1.1	1.1
Chicken, Masala, M&S*	½ Pack/175g	228	12.4	130	13.3	3.1	7.1	5.2
Chicken, Masala, Waitrose*	1 Pack/400g	452	20.9	113	11.7	3.8	5.2	1.8
Chicken, with Pilau Rice, Love Life, Waitrose*	1 Pack/400g	436	6.8	109	6.8	15.4	1.7	2.2
Paneer, Sainsbury's*	1 Pack/300g	441	32.7	147	7.1	3.9	10.9	2.5
SAFFRON								
Average	*1 Tsp/1g*	*2*	*0.0*	*310*	*11.4*	*61.5*	*5.9*	*0.0*
SAGE								
Dried, Ground	*1 Tsp/1g*	*3*	*0.1*	*315*	*10.6*	*42.7*	*12.7*	*0.0*
Fresh	*1oz/28g*	*33*	*1.3*	*119*	*3.9*	*15.6*	*4.6*	*0.0*
SAGO								
Raw	*1oz/28g*	*99*	*0.1*	*355*	*0.2*	*94.0*	*0.2*	*0.5*
SALAD								
Adzuki & Edamame Bean, Aromatic, Waitrose*	1/3 Pack/67g	62	1.5	93	7.5	5.7	2.2	10.3
Alfresco Style, Tesco*	1 Serving/200g	40	0.6	20	0.9	3.3	0.3	2.1
American Ranch, Asda*	1 Serving/220g	253	19.8	115	2.5	6.0	9.0	2.0
American Style, Sweet & Crispy, Morrisons*	1 Serving/25g	7	0.1	28	1.2	4.2	0.3	2.0
Aromatic Herb, Waitrose*	¼ Pack/27g	4	0.1	15	0.9	1.7	0.5	1.0
Assorted, Asda*	1 Serving/100g	22	0.6	22	2.4	1.7	0.6	0.0
Avocado & Feta, Gourmet To Go, M&S*	1 Pack/320g	512	32.0	160	5.4	12.1	10.0	3.1
Baby Leaf, & Beetroot, Bistro, M&S*	1 Pack/165g	41	0.0	25	2.0	3.6	0.0	2.4
Baby Leaf, & Herb, Asda*	1 Serving/50g	7	0.1	14	2.3	0.7	0.2	2.4
Baby Leaf, Aldi*	1 Serving/50g	11	0.0	22	3.5	1.0	0.1	1.5
Baby Leaf, Asda*	1 Serving/80g	10	0.2	12	2.1	0.2	0.3	1.7
Baby Leaf, Florette*	1 Serving/40g	5	0.1	12	2.0	0.4	0.3	1.0
Baby Leaf, Fully Prepared, Sainsbury's*	½ Bag/63g	10	0.3	16	1.3	1.9	0.4	1.5
Baby Leaf, Italian Style, M&S*	1 Serving/55g	11	0.3	20	1.3	2.3	0.5	1.3
Baby Leaf, M&S*	1 Pack/100g	20	0.2	20	3.0	1.7	0.2	0.5
Baby Leaf, Mild, Seasonal, Tesco*	½ Pack/42g	9	0.3	21	1.5	1.6	0.6	1.8
Baby Leaf, Organic, Sainsbury's*	1 Serving/20g	3	0.1	14	1.5	1.4	0.3	1.1
Baby Leaf, Sainsbury's*	1 Serving/60g	12	1.1	20	2.8	1.1	1.9	1.9
Baby Leaf, Seasonal, Organic, Sainsbury's*	1 Serving/30g	3	0.1	10	1.6	0.4	0.3	1.2
Baby Leaf, Seasonal, Sainsbury's*	¼ Bag/63g	11	0.3	17	2.8	0.5	0.5	2.7
Baby Leaf, Sweet, Seasonal, M&S*	½ Bag/60g	9	0.2	15	2.4	0.6	0.4	1.8
Baby Leaf, with Purple Basil, Finest, Tesco*	½ Pack/43g	7	0.1	17	2.9	0.9	0.2	1.8
Baby Leaf, with Watercress, Tesco*	1 Serving/30g	6	0.2	19	1.8	1.3	0.7	1.8
Bean, & Chorizo, Tapas Selection, Sainsbury's*	1 Serving/22g	29	1.4	132	8.1	10.7	6.3	1.9
Bean, & Sweetcorn, Side, M&S*	1 Serving/125g	131	9.0	105	2.5	7.0	7.2	1.3
Bean, Cannellini, & Tuna, M&S*	1 Serving/255g	215	11.6	84	5.3	5.4	4.5	2.1
Bean, Five, & Mint, Asda*	1 Pack/340g	408	12.9	120	6.2	12.7	3.8	5.3
Bean, Lentil, & Chargrilled Halloumi, Love Life, Waitrose*	1 Pack/400g	352	12.0	88	5.1	8.5	3.0	3.3
Bean, M&S*	1 Serving/80g	72	0.7	90	6.4	14.3	0.9	3.9
Bean, Mexican, Sainsbury's*	1 Pot/260g	291	8.1	112	5.2	12.9	3.1	5.8

SALAD

	Measure INFO/WEIGHT	per Measure KCAL	per Measure FAT	Nutrition Values per 100g / 100ml KCAL	PROT	CARB	FAT	FIBRE
Bean, Mixed, in Water, Essential, Waitrose*	1 Serving/80g	68	0.6	85	6.5	12.9	0.8	6.2
Bean, Mixed, Vinaigrette, Tesco*	1 Can/400g	280	2.0	70	3.2	13.1	0.5	1.9
Bean, Retail	1oz/28g	41	2.6	147	4.2	12.8	9.3	3.0
Bean, Three, & Mint, Finest, Tesco*	½ Pack/115g	155	6.9	135	6.8	7.7	6.0	11.5
Bean, Three, in Water, Drained, Wholefoods, Tesco*	½ Can/123g	135	1.2	110	7.7	17.6	1.0	5.3
Bean, Three, Sainsbury's*	1 Tub/270g	281	6.2	104	7.1	13.6	2.3	5.9
Bean, Three, Sainsbury's*	1 Serving/125g	108	6.3	86	4.2	6.0	5.0	0.0
Bean, Three, Tinned, Tesco*	1 Tin/160g	176	1.6	110	7.7	17.6	1.0	5.3
Bean, Three, with Mint Vinaigrette, M&S*	1 Pack/250g	250	6.0	100	5.9	8.2	2.4	11.1
Beetroot	1oz/28g	28	1.9	100	2.0	8.4	6.8	1.7
Beetroot, & Carrot, Continental, Iceland*	1 Serving/100g	24	0.2	24	1.2	4.3	0.2	2.1
Beetroot, & Cherry Tomato, & Lemon Dressing, M&S*	1 Pack/215g	129	8.2	60	1.3	5.2	3.8	1.5
Beetroot, & Goats Cheese, Shaker, Good to Go, Waitrose*	1 Pack/240g	357	11.0	149	6.2	17.9	4.6	5.0
Beetroot, & Lettuce, Asda*	1 Serving/30g	5	0.0	16	1.4	2.7	0.0	2.5
Beetroot, 1% Fat, M&S*	1 Serving/225g	130	6.1	58	1.1	7.7	2.7	1.7
Beetroot, Asda*	1 Carton/270g	119	1.1	44	1.3	8.8	0.4	2.4
Beetroot, Co-Op*	1 Pack/250g	100	0.8	40	0.9	8.0	0.3	2.0
Beetroot, Cous Cous & Quinoa, Tesco*	1 Serving/100g	70	0.6	70	2.3	12.9	0.6	2.3
Beetroot, Freshly Prepared, Tesco*	1 Pack/240g	58	0.7	24	1.9	3.3	0.3	2.7
Beetroot, Lentil & Goats Cheese, Roasted, M&S*	1 Pack/295g	354	8.6	120	4.9	16.6	2.9	3.3
Beetroot, M&S*	1 Serving/225g	124	0.7	55	1.0	12.0	0.3	3.0
Beetroot, Morrisons*	1 Pot/250g	138	1.0	55	1.2	11.6	0.4	1.6
Beetroot, Roast with Quinoa & Feta, Tesco*	1 Pack/400g	452	19.6	113	4.8	12.4	4.9	2.3
Beetroot, Sainsbury's*	1 Tub/200g	148	2.4	74	1.7	14.1	1.2	1.7
Beetroot, Shredded, Asda*	1 Serving/140g	29	0.4	21	1.1	3.5	0.3	1.5
Beetroot, with Balsamic Dressing, Finest, Tesco*	1 Portion/75g	49	1.1	65	1.1	11.9	1.5	2.4
Beetroot, with Lemon Mayonnaise Dressing, Sainsbury's*	½ Pack/115g	104	9.2	90	1.0	3.3	8.0	1.4
Bistro, Asda*	1 Serving/180g	29	0.0	16	1.4	2.7	0.0	2.5
Bistro, Morrisons*	1 Serving/20g	5	0.0	23	1.2	4.2	0.2	2.0
Bistro, Sainsbury's*	1 Pack/150g	26	0.3	17	1.9	2.0	0.2	2.0
Bistro, Washed Ready to Eat, Tesco*	1 Pack/140g	22	0.7	16	1.1	1.7	0.5	1.0
Black Bean Salsa, Salad Bar, Waitrose*	1 Serving/100g	118	5.8	118	0.0	0.0	5.8	0.0
Bulgar Wheat, & Carrot, Sainsbury's*	½ Pot/125g	167	6.7	134	2.8	16.1	5.4	4.8
Bulgar Wheat, Lentil & Edamame Shaker, Waitrose*	1 Pack/190g	217	10.6	114	4.7	11.1	5.6	4.4
Butternut Squash & Fennel, Roast, TTD, Sainsbury's*	1 Pack/165g	214	7.6	130	3.4	15.2	4.6	6.9
Cabbage, Beetroot & Carrot, Mix, Florette*	½ Pack/100g	30	0.2	30	1.3	4.4	0.2	0.0
Cabbage & Leek, Crunchy Mix, Sainsbury's*	½ Pack/126g	24	0.8	19	1.2	2.1	0.6	1.9
Caesar	1 Serving/200g	352	27.8	176	4.8	8.1	13.9	0.7
Caesar, Bacon, M&S*	1 Serving/250g	400	31.2	160	7.1	4.1	12.5	1.3
Caesar, Chicken, Asda*	1 Pack/273g	535	43.7	196	10.0	3.0	16.0	1.9
Caesar, Chicken, Bistro, M&S*	½ Pack/135g	189	14.3	140	5.0	6.5	10.6	0.6
Caesar, Chicken, Eat Well, M&S*	1 Pack/397g	595	24.6	150	9.9	18.7	6.2	2.1
Caesar, Chicken, M&S*	½ Pack/140g	266	20.0	190	6.7	8.7	14.3	0.8
Caesar, Chicken, Shapers, Boots*	1 Pack/200g	205	5.8	102	8.2	10.0	2.9	1.0
Caesar, Chicken, Tesco*	1 Pack/300g	330	13.5	110	6.8	10.6	4.5	0.8
Caesar, Chicken & Bacon, Gourmet, M&S*	1 Salad/250g	550	43.5	220	9.0	7.3	17.4	0.7
Caesar, Chicken & Bacon, Tesco*	1 Pack/200g	506	40.2	253	6.6	11.4	20.1	1.0
Caesar, Classic, M&S*	½ Pack/112g	174	14.2	155	2.9	6.8	12.7	0.5
Caesar, Classic, Reduced Fat, M&S*	1 Serving/115g	132	5.6	115	4.8	12.7	4.9	0.5
Caesar, Finest, Tesco*	1 Bowl/220g	374	30.6	170	4.9	5.1	13.9	1.6
Caesar, M&S*	1 Pack/268g	510	40.5	190	5.7	8.3	15.1	1.3
Caesar, Morrisons*	1 Serving/115g	194	18.1	169	3.6	5.9	15.7	0.3
Caesar, with Dressing, Croutons & Parmesan, M&S*	1 Serving/115g	190	15.5	165	4.3	6.4	13.5	1.4

SALAD

Measure INFO/WEIGHT	per Measure		Nutrition Values per 100g / 100ml				
	KCAL	FAT	KCAL	PROT	CARB	FAT	FIBRE
Caesar, with Parmigiano Reggiano, Tesco* 1 Bag/275g	552	49.0	201	4.1	5.8	17.8	1.3
Caesar, with Romaine Lettuce, Kit, BGTY, Sainsbury's* ½ Pack/130g	139	7.9	107	3.7	9.2	6.1	1.4
Caponata, Organic, Florentin* 1 Serving/100g	111	12.3	111	1.5	3.7	12.3	0.0
Carrot, Courgette & Coriander, Salad Bar, Waitrose* 1 Serving/100g	92	7.9	92	0.0	0.0	7.9	0.0
Carrot, M&S* 1 Pack/215g	280	7.3	130	3.1	22.4	3.4	2.7
Carrot, Orange & Ginger, Good Intentions, Somerfield* 1 Serving/250g	275	3.5	110	2.0	22.4	1.4	1.4
Carrot, with Fresh Coriander Vinaigrette, M&S* ½ Pack/105g	126	3.6	120	3.7	19.1	3.4	6.5
Carrot & Beetroot, Classic, Tesco* ½ Pack/83g	17	0.2	20	0.9	3.7	0.2	1.6
Carrot & Beetroot, with a Balsamic Dressing, Asda* 1 Pack/160g	101	6.6	63	0.9	5.6	4.1	1.0
Carrot & Beetroot, with Balsamic Dressing, Eat Well, M&S* ½ Pack/200g	80	3.5	40	1.0	6.2	1.8	1.6
Carrot & Nut, with French Dressing, Average 1oz/28g	61	4.9	218	2.1	13.7	17.6	2.4
Carrot & Sultana, BGTY, Sainsbury's* ½ Pack/100g	55	0.3	55	0.6	12.4	0.3	0.0
Celery & Apple, Salad Bar, Waitrose* 1 Serving/100g	136	12.9	136	0.0	0.0	12.9	0.0
Cheese, Layered, M&S* ½ Pack/230g	300	20.5	130	4.6	9.3	8.9	1.2
Cheese, Layered, Tesco* 1 Serving/225g	437	32.0	194	5.8	10.8	14.2	0.8
Cheese & Coleslaw, Tesco* 1 Serving/125g	135	10.9	108	3.4	3.4	8.7	1.1
Cherry Tomato, All Good Things* 1 Pack/185g	31	0.6	17	0.8	2.8	0.3	1.4
Cherry Tomato, Salad Bar, Waitrose* 1 Serving/100g	77	5.3	77	0.0	0.0	5.3	0.0
Cherry Tomato, Tesco* 1 Pack/210g	136	9.4	65	0.9	4.2	4.5	1.1
Chick Pea & Cous Cous, Tesco* 1 Serving/250g	245	6.5	98	3.2	15.5	2.6	0.0
Chick Pea & Spinach, M&S* 1 Serving/260g	299	10.7	115	7.3	12.5	4.1	2.7
Chick Pea & Sweet Potato, Salad Bar, Sainsbury's* 1 Serving/100g	99	1.9	99	0.0	9.6	1.9	0.0
Chicken, & Quinoa, Chargrilled, Shapers, Boots* 1 Pack/185g	139	1.8	75	6.2	10.0	1.0	1.8
Chicken, Avocado & Bacon, M&S* 1 Serving/235g	235	13.6	100	8.5	2.8	5.8	2.8
Chicken, Cajun, David Lloyd Leisure* 1 Pack/300g	429	10.0	143	11.7	17.7	3.3	1.0
Chicken, Caribbean, Shapers, Boots* 1 Pack/220g	222	5.1	101	5.8	14.0	2.3	1.2
Chicken, Chargrilled, Tesco* 1 Serving/300g	384	14.4	128	6.1	15.0	4.8	2.4
Chicken, Chargrilled, Wholefood, M&S* 1 Pot/219g	230	4.2	105	10.1	11.6	1.9	4.8
Chicken, Fajita, Shapers, Boots* 1 Pack/258g	181	3.4	70	7.0	7.4	1.3	2.7
Chicken, Roast, & Coleslaw, Boots* 1 Serving/245g	392	34.3	160	4.5	3.9	14.0	1.3
Chicken, Roast, Tesco* 1 Salad/300g	348	22.2	116	5.3	7.0	7.4	1.0
Chicken, Sweet Chilli, & Noodle, COU, M&S* 1 Pack/340g	408	7.8	120	6.8	17.4	2.3	1.2
Chicken, Tesco* 1 Serving/300g	348	22.2	116	5.3	7.0	7.4	1.0
Chicken, Thai Style, & Noodles, M&S* ½ Pot/145g	160	7.1	110	5.2	11.6	4.9	1.4
Chicken, Thai Style, M&S* 1 Serving/195g	205	3.7	105	6.7	15.1	1.9	1.9
Chicken, with Mayonnaise, Waitrose* 1 Pack/208g	406	19.8	195	10.3	17.1	9.5	2.5
Chicken & Bacon, Asda* 1 Pack/381g	480	22.9	126	7.0	11.0	6.0	0.0
Chicken & Bacon, Layered, Asda* 1 Serving/375g	472	22.5	126	7.0	11.0	6.0	1.6
Chicken & Bacon Layered, Tesco* 1 Pack/360g	600	39.6	167	4.6	12.1	11.0	1.8
Chicken & Bacon Ranch, Sainsbury's* 1 Pack/210g	315	15.8	150	8.4	12.1	7.5	0.9
Chicken & Moroccan Cous Cous, Tesco* 1 Pack/210g	252	4.2	120	7.8	16.9	2.0	3.5
Chicken Noodle, & Sweet Chilli, Shapers, Boots* 1 Pack/197g	266	5.1	135	12.0	16.0	2.6	0.9
Chicken Noodle, Thai Style, Sainsbury's* 1 Pack/260g	283	7.5	109	6.6	14.2	2.9	1.3
Chickpea, & Halloumi, Spicy, Cranks* 1 Pack/238g	295	11.2	124	5.0	15.5	4.7	2.6
Chickpea, Spicy, BGTY, Sainsbury's* ½ Pack/125g	119	2.1	95	4.7	15.3	1.7	5.5
Chickpea & Bean, Salad Bar, Waitrose* 1 Serving/100g	165	10.2	165	0.0	2.2	10.2	0.0
Chilli, Tomato, Chick Pea & Butterbean, Tesco* 1 Pack/130g	146	6.0	112	3.4	14.3	4.6	0.5
Classic, Complete Salad, Sainsbury's* 1 Pack/220g	112	8.4	51	1.0	3.3	3.8	1.4
Classic, Co-Op* ½ Pack/80g	16	0.2	20	0.8	2.9	0.3	2.2
Continental, Budgens* 1 Serving/55g	8	0.2	14	1.2	1.4	0.4	2.1
Continental, Co-Op* 1 Serving/80g	12	0.3	15	1.0	2.0	0.4	1.0
Continental, Four Leaf, Sainsbury's* ½ Pack/100g	13	0.2	13	1.2	1.7	0.2	1.9
Coronation Rice, Tesco* 1 Serving/50g	104	7.6	207	2.0	15.9	15.1	0.8

SALAD

	Measure INFO/WEIGHT	per Measure KCAL	per Measure FAT	Nutrition Values per 100g / 100ml KCAL	PROT	CARB	FAT	FIBRE
Cosmopolitan, Fresh, Sainsbury's*	1 Bag/135g	20	0.5	15	1.2	1.6	0.4	1.9
Cous Cous, & Roast Vegetable, GFY, Asda*	1 Serving/100g	120	1.6	120	3.5	23.0	1.6	2.7
Cous Cous, & Roasted Vegetable, Waitrose*	1 Pack/220g	396	13.4	180	5.1	26.1	6.1	1.2
Cous Cous, & Wheatberry, Love Life, Waitrose*	1 Pot/200g	290	11.6	145	5.0	18.1	5.8	3.5
Cous Cous, BFY, Morrisons*	½ Pot/113g	164	4.0	145	4.6	23.8	3.5	0.5
Cous Cous, BGTY, Sainsbury's*	1 Pot/200g	236	4.4	118	4.7	19.7	2.2	2.8
Cous Cous, Tesco*	1 Serving/25g	35	0.4	141	4.8	26.9	1.6	0.6
Cous Cous, with Chargrilled Chicken, Sainsbury's*	1 Pack/240g	446	20.9	186	7.4	19.6	8.7	0.0
Cous Cous, with Mixed Peppers & Cucumber, GFY, Asda*	¼ Pot/56g	66	0.1	117	3.9	25.0	0.2	1.5
Crisp, Mix, Somerfield*	1 Pack/215g	34	0.6	16	0.9	2.4	0.3	1.6
Crisp & Crunchy, Asda*	1 Pack/250g	55	1.5	22	0.8	3.3	0.6	1.4
Crispy, Co-Op*	1 Serving/80g	13	0.2	16	0.8	3.0	0.3	1.0
Crispy, Crunch, Lasting Leaf*	1 Serving/75g	14	0.3	18	1.1	1.5	0.4	1.9
Crispy, Florette*	1 Portion/100g	22	0.3	22	1.5	3.4	0.3	3.0
Crispy, Medley, Waitrose*	1 Serving/50g	8	0.2	15	0.8	1.7	0.5	0.9
Crunchy, Basics, Sainsbury's*	1 Pack/200g	50	0.4	25	1.3	3.4	0.2	2.2
Crunchy, Fully Prepared, Sainsbury's*	½ Pack/150g	24	0.2	16	1.1	3.0	0.1	1.7
Crunchy, Layered, Tesco*	1 Serving/54g	15	0.2	27	1.1	4.9	0.3	1.7
Crunchy, Mini, Co-Op*	1 Pack/80g	16	0.4	20	1.0	2.5	0.5	1.7
Crunchy, Mix, Co-Op*	1 Bag/200g	20	0.4	10	0.9	1.7	0.2	1.5
Crunchy, Simple, M&S*	1 Serving/50g	8	0.2	15	1.0	1.6	0.5	1.8
Crunchy, Value, Tesco*	1 Serving/56g	11	0.2	19	1.2	2.8	0.3	2.1
Crunchy, Waitrose*	½ Pack/100g	18	0.4	18	1.0	2.6	0.4	1.5
Cucumber & Cherry Tomato, Fresh Tastes, Asda*	1 Serving/100g	22	0.3	22	1.6	2.4	0.3	0.0
Duck & Herb, Crispy, M&S*	½ Pack/140g	378	25.6	270	20.7	3.7	18.3	1.4
Edamame & Butterbean, TTD, Sainsbury's*	1/3 Pack/62g	70	2.5	113	6.6	9.9	4.1	4.9
Edamame Bean, Oriental Style, Asda*	1 Pack/220g	183	8.4	83	4.8	7.3	3.8	4.0
Egg, & Baby Spinach, Waitrose*	1 Pack/215g	167	13.5	78	3.5	1.8	6.3	1.0
Egg, & Ham with Salad Cream Dressing, M&S*	1 Pack/240g	145	7.2	60	4.9	3.2	3.0	1.2
Egg, & Potato, Fresh, M&S*	1 Serving/250g	150	7.2	60	3.0	4.6	2.9	0.9
Endive & Radicchio, Somerfield*	1 Pack/150g	20	0.0	13	2.0	1.0	0.0	0.0
Exotic, with Mango & Chilli Dressing, Co-Op*	½ Pack/65g	25	0.4	38	0.6	7.7	0.6	0.8
Feta, & Butternut Squash, Tesco*	1 Pot/245g	404	19.1	165	6.5	14.9	7.8	3.1
Feta Cheese & Sunblushed Tomato, M&S*	1 Serving/190g	361	21.1	190	5.5	17.2	11.1	2.1
Fine Cut, Asda*	1 Serving/100g	24	0.3	24	1.2	4.3	0.3	2.3
Florida, Retail, Average	1oz/28g	63	5.7	224	0.9	9.7	20.5	1.0
Four Bean, Finest, Tesco*	1 Pack/225g	259	9.4	115	5.0	14.2	4.2	4.6
Four Bean, Sainsbury's*	½ Pot/113g	114	2.5	101	6.7	6.2	2.2	15.0
Four Leaf, M&S*	1 Serving/130g	20	0.4	15	0.9	2.0	0.3	1.4
Fresh & Crispy, Tesco*	1 Serving/230g	30	0.7	13	0.7	1.9	0.3	1.3
Garden, Classic, Morrisons*	1 Tray/175g	33	0.5	19	0.8	3.2	0.3	2.8
Garden, English, Tesco*	1 Serving/180g	22	0.4	12	0.7	1.8	0.2	0.7
Garden, Side, Asda*	1 Pack/175g	32	0.5	18	0.9	2.8	0.3	1.3
Garden, Side with Dressing, Waitrose*	1 Pack/184g	101	8.1	55	12.0	2.6	4.4	13.0
Garden, Sweet & Crispy, Tesco*	1 Bag/225g	54	0.9	24	1.0	4.2	0.4	1.4
Garden, Sweet & Crunchy, Tesco*	1 Pack/225g	54	0.9	24	1.0	4.2	0.4	1.4
Garden, Tesco*	1 Serving/225g	34	0.7	15	1.0	2.0	0.3	0.9
Garden, with Cherry Tomatoes, Side, Waitrose*	1 Pack/170g	25	0.7	15	0.8	2.0	0.4	1.3
Garden, with Yoghurt & Mint Dressing, GFY, Asda*	1 Serving/195g	51	2.0	26	1.1	3.2	1.0	0.0
Goat's Cheese, French, Extra Fine, Asda*	1 Pack/185g	462	35.2	250	8.4	11.4	19.0	0.8
Goat's Cheese, Sainsbury's*	1 Pack/192g	242	12.9	126	5.0	10.6	6.7	1.7
Greek	1oz/28g	36	3.5	130	2.7	1.9	12.5	0.8
Greek, Classic, Tesco*	1 Pack/255g	293	23.7	115	2.6	5.2	9.3	1.2

SALAD

Measure INFO/WEIGHT		per Measure		Nutrition Values per 100g / 100ml				
		KCAL	FAT	KCAL	PROT	CARB	FAT	FIBRE
Greek, Feta & Pepper with Cous Cous, Asda*	1 Pack/316g	262	10.4	83	3.2	10.2	3.3	0.0
Greek, Salad Bar, Waitrose*	1 Serving/100g	103	7.8	103	0.0	0.0	7.8	0.0
Greek, Side, Waitrose*	1 Pack/175g	175	15.8	100	2.1	2.2	9.0	1.1
Greek, Style, Fresh, Food Counter, Sainsbury's*	1 Serving/166g	247	23.2	149	1.9	2.7	14.0	0.0
Greek, Style, Waitrose*	½ Pack/125g	54	2.8	43	1.9	4.0	2.2	1.2
Greek, Style Feta, Tip & Mix, M&S*	1 Pack/195g	214	18.3	110	4.0	2.5	9.4	1.6
Greek, Style with Herb Dressing, Tesco*	1 Pack/240g	305	28.3	127	3.2	2.0	11.8	0.0
Greek, Style with Houmous Dip & Pitta, Sainsbury's*	1 Bowl/195g	296	17.4	152	5.4	12.5	8.9	2.6
Greek, with Basil & Mint Oil Dressing, M&S*	1 Pack/200g	220	19.6	110	3.6	2.2	9.8	1.5
Green, Average	1oz/28g	4	0.1	13	0.8	1.8	0.3	0.9
Green, Complete, Sainsbury's*	1/3 Pack/55g	92	6.7	168	4.2	10.3	12.2	1.4
Green, Crispy, Fresh, Sainsbury's*	1 Serving/40g	5	0.1	12	0.9	1.6	0.2	0.8
Green, Crispy, Sainsbury's*	1 Serving/70g	8	0.1	12	0.9	1.6	0.2	0.8
Green, Mixed, Average	1 Serving/100g	12	0.3	12	0.7	1.8	0.3	1.0
Green, Side, M&S*	1 Serving/200g	30	0.4	15	0.9	2.5	0.2	0.0
Green, Side, Sainsbury's*	1 Pack/200g	28	0.2	14	1.2	2.1	0.1	1.4
Green, Side, Tesco*	1 Serving/100g	12	0.3	12	0.7	1.6	0.3	1.3
Green, with Chives, Tesco*	½ Pack/90g	13	0.4	14	1.0	1.6	0.4	1.7
Green, with Honey & Mustard Dressing, M&S*	1 Pack/200g	120	9.6	60	0.9	2.7	4.8	0.8
Green Butterhead & Peppercress, Duo, Florette*	1 Portion/30g	7	0.1	23	2.3	1.3	0.3	2.0
Ham, & Free Range Egg, Fresh Tastes, Asda*	1 Bowl/265g	167	9.3	63	5.7	2.2	3.5	0.8
Ham, Antony Worrall Thompson's*	1 Pack/202g	257	2.6	127	9.8	19.1	1.3	2.7
Ham, Smoked, Weight Watchers*	1 Pack/181g	233	3.6	129	11.0	16.6	2.0	3.0
Ham & Free Range Egg, British, M&S*	1 Pack/280g	182	6.4	65	6.1	5.3	2.3	1.0
Ham Hock, Waitrose*	1 Pack/350g	245	9.5	70	6.6	4.8	2.7	2.0
Herb, Asda*	1 Serving/20g	2	0.1	12	1.8	0.6	0.3	2.0
Herb, Garden, Morrisons*	1 Serving/28g	4	0.1	14	0.9	1.7	0.5	0.0
Herb, M&S*	1 Pack/100g	20	0.4	20	2.9	1.4	0.4	1.9
Herb, Sainsbury's*	1 Pack/120g	22	0.6	18	2.7	0.8	0.5	2.2
Italian Style, Asda*	1 Serving/20g	3	0.1	15	1.1	1.6	0.5	1.2
Italian Style, Tesco*	1/3 Pack/40g	6	0.2	16	1.0	1.9	0.5	1.2
King Prawn, & Mango, Layered, Love Life, Waitrose*	1 Pack/300g	195	4.2	65	3.9	9.2	1.4	1.7
King Prawn, & Noodle, PB, Waitrose*	1 Pack/225g	223	2.2	99	5.0	17.4	1.0	1.0
King Prawn, & Noodle, Watercress & Sweet Chilli, M&S*	1 Pack/370g	314	2.6	85	5.0	14.1	0.7	1.6
King Prawn, & Pasta, COU, M&S*	1 Pack/270g	284	6.5	105	5.9	15.1	2.4	2.7
King Prawn, GFY, Asda*	1 Serving/175g	112	2.6	64	4.7	8.0	1.5	1.3
King Prawn, Salmon & Cous Cous, Fuller Longer, M&S*	1 Pack/320g	320	8.6	100	10.1	8.3	2.7	7.0
King Prawn, Thai Style, M&S*	1 Pack/295g	266	7.4	90	4.4	12.6	2.5	1.3
King Prawn, with Rice & Lentils, Fuller Longer, M&S*	1 Pack/230g	276	6.2	120	11.8	12.1	2.7	6.0
Lambs Lettuce & Ruby Chard, Duo, Florette*	1 Serving/35g	7	0.1	21	2.0	1.0	0.4	2.9
Leaf, Crispy, Asda*	1 Serving/80g	11	0.4	14	0.8	1.6	0.5	0.9
Leaf, Crispy, Sainsbury's*	½ Pack/68g	9	0.3	14	1.0	1.7	0.4	1.7
Leafy, Organic, Sainsbury's*	½ Pack/50g	8	0.2	15	1.7	1.3	0.3	1.8
Leafy Mixed, Co-Op*	1 Bag/200g	40	0.6	20	1.0	4.0	0.3	1.0
Leaves, Oriental Mix, Waitrose*	1 Bag/100g	18	0.6	18	1.5	1.7	0.6	1.9
Lentil, Red Pepper & Spinach, Green, Waitrose*	1 Pack/250g	485	20.0	194	8.6	22.0	8.0	2.9
Lentils, Cous Cous & Goats Cheese, Eat Well, M&S*	1 Pack/215g	312	10.3	145	6.9	17.4	4.8	3.3
Lettuce Leaves, Crisp & Sweet, Florette*	¼ Pack/70g	10	0.4	14	0.8	1.7	0.5	0.9
Lettuce Leaves, Mix, Crisp & Sweet, Florette*	1 Portion/67g	12	0.2	18	1.5	1.2	0.3	2.5
Lovely Summer, Jamie Oliver*	½ Bag/60g	48	4.0	80	1.7	4.0	6.6	1.2
Mediterranean, Orzo Pasta, Love Life, Waitrose*	1 Pack/220g	299	10.8	136	3.9	19.0	4.9	3.2
Mediterranean, Side, Sainsbury's*	1 Pack/170g	44	2.2	26	0.9	2.7	1.3	1.3
Mediterranean, Style, Asda*	½ Pack/135g	22	0.0	16	1.0	3.0	0.0	0.0

SALAD

INFO/WEIGHT	Measure	per Measure KCAL	FAT	Nutrition Values per 100g / 100ml KCAL	PROT	CARB	FAT	FIBRE
Mediterranean, Style, Tray, Morrisons*	1 Tray/100g	26	0.3	26	1.2	3.6	0.3	1.8
Mixed, Crisp, Mild, Tesco*	½ Pack/145g	29	0.4	20	1.2	3.0	0.3	2.1
Mixed, Crisp, Morrisons*	1 Pack/230g	39	0.7	17	1.0	2.8	0.3	0.0
Mixed, Crisp, Tesco*	1 Pack/200g	40	0.6	20	1.1	3.2	0.3	2.0
Mixed, Florette*	1 Serving/100g	20	0.2	20	1.3	3.4	0.2	3.0
Mixed, Green Leaf, Lasting Leaf*	1 Serving/69g	12	0.3	17	0.8	1.8	0.4	1.5
Mixed, Iceland*	1 Serving/50g	12	0.1	24	1.2	4.3	0.2	2.1
Mixed, Sainsbury's*	1 Serving/100g	21	0.2	21	1.4	3.4	0.2	2.1
Mixed, Sweet & Crispy, Tesco*	1 Serving/200g	48	0.6	24	1.0	4.2	0.3	2.0
Mixed, Sweet & Crunchy, Lasting Leaf*	1 Serving/62g	15	0.2	24	0.8	3.6	0.3	1.9
Mixed, Tesco*	1 Serving/100g	24	0.3	24	1.0	4.2	0.3	2.0
Mixed Bean, Asda*	½ Can/145g	126	3.6	87	5.0	11.0	2.5	6.0
Mixed Bean, Canned, Sainsbury's*	1 Can/270g	227	2.4	84	5.4	13.5	0.9	3.8
Mixed Bean, Tesco*	1 Serving/70g	49	0.4	70	3.2	13.1	0.5	1.9
Mixed Leaf, & Baby Basil, A Taste of Italy, Florette*	1 Pack/155g	143	8.2	92	2.7	8.5	5.3	1.0
Mixed Leaf, Asda*	1 Serving/100g	21	0.2	21	1.5	3.2	0.2	2.1
Mixed Leaf, Medley, Waitrose*	1 Serving/25g	4	0.1	15	0.8	1.7	0.5	1.4
Mixed Leaf, Tomato, Feta, Boots*	1 Pack/179g	218	17.0	122	3.7	5.4	9.5	1.0
Mixed Leaf, Tomato & Olive, Tesco*	1 Serving/170g	150	13.3	88	1.0	3.4	7.8	2.0
Mixed Leaf, with Olive Oil, Supermarket, Pizza Express*	1 Pack/240g	326	33.8	136	0.9	2.1	14.1	0.7
Mixed Leaves, Tesco*	1 Serving/20g	3	0.1	14	0.9	1.6	0.4	0.9
Mixed Leaves, with Beetroot, Earthy, Waitrose*	1 Bag/140g	34	0.6	24	1.5	3.6	0.4	2.1
Mixed Pepper, Asda*	½ Pack/100g	24	0.3	24	1.0	4.3	0.3	1.7
Mixed Vegetable, Aldi*	1 Serving/200g	120	4.0	60	0.6	10.0	2.0	0.0
Mixed with Peppers & Iceberg Lettuce, Somerfield*	1 Pack/200g	50	0.0	25	1.0	5.0	0.0	0.0
Moroccan Cous Cous, Fruity, Waitrose*	1 Pack/90g	139	3.2	154	5.0	25.6	3.6	4.6
Moroccan Styles, COU, M&S*	½ Pack/100g	160	1.2	160	5.0	32.8	1.2	4.8
Mozzarella, with Sun Ripened Tomato, Bocconcini, M&S*	½ Pack/100g	250	21.4	250	9.8	4.9	21.4	2.0
Mozzarella & Sunkissed Tomato, Tesco*	1 Bag/160g	270	22.9	169	4.6	4.3	14.3	2.1
Mozzarella & Tomato, M&S*	1 Serving/310g	400	14.8	129	5.5	15.5	4.8	0.9
Mozzarella & Tomato (no dressing)	1 Serving/105g	190	14.5	182	8.0	5.9	13.8	3.3
Nicoise, Style, Layered, Waitrose*	1 Bowl/275g	129	3.8	47	2.7	5.8	1.4	1.0
Nicoise, Tesco*	1 Pack/260g	286	21.8	110	3.2	5.3	8.4	1.4
Noodle, & Sesame, Salad Bar, Waitrose*	1 Serving/100g	178	11.5	178	0.0	0.0	11.5	0.0
Noodle, Thai Style, BGTY, Sainsbury's*	1 Pack/185g	150	3.5	81	2.7	13.5	1.9	0.0
Nutty Rice, Love Life, Waitrose*	1 Portion/200g	368	14.4	184	4.5	25.3	7.2	3.1
Nutty Super Wholefood, M&S*	½ Pack/115g	150	5.9	130	5.3	12.8	5.1	6.1
Oriental Slaw, Crunchy, Salad Bar, Waitrose*	1 Serving/100g	68	2.8	68	0.0	0.0	2.8	0.0
Orzo & Sunbaked Tomato, BGTY, Sainsbury's*	1 Tub/276g	292	6.1	106	3.1	18.5	2.2	2.5
Pancetta, Express, Pizza Express*	1 Salad/90g	200	17.9	223	7.4	3.3	20.0	0.0
Pea & Bean, Sprouted, Mint Dressing, Eat Well, M&S*	1 Pot/165g	182	8.7	110	7.3	8.7	5.3	7.4
Pea Shoot, Baby Cos & Batavia Lettuce, Bagged, M&S*	1 Bag/120g	24	0.6	20	2.6	0.8	0.5	2.3
Pea Shoots & Baby Leaves, Steve's Leaves*	1 Pack/60g	14	0.4	24	2.7	2.0	0.6	2.0
Pepper, with Cous Cous, Chargrilled, Asda*	1 Pack/325g	426	10.7	131	4.3	21.0	3.3	0.0
Potato, & Cheese, Pasta & Mixed Leaf, Waitrose*	1 Serving/205g	266	17.4	130	3.2	10.1	8.5	1.1
Potato, & Egg with Mayonnaise, Tesco*	½ Tub/150g	115	8.5	77	2.9	3.1	5.7	1.2
Potato, & Free Range Egg, M&S*	1 Pack/305g	214	11.6	70	2.5	7.0	3.8	0.8
Potato, & Free Range Egg, Side, Baby, Asda*	1 Pack/305g	168	6.7	55	2.6	5.5	2.2	1.3
Potato, & Free Range Egg, Side, Sainsbury's*	1 Pack/290g	174	12.2	60	2.5	3.1	4.2	1.4
Potato, & Sweet Chilli Prawn, M&S*	1 Pack/210g	147	1.0	70	2.8	14.0	0.5	0.7
Potato, & Tuna Sweetcorn, Eat Well, M&S*	1 Pack/190g	133	3.4	70	5.4	8.4	1.8	1.9
Potato, 30% Less Fat, BGTY, Sainsbury's*	1 Serving/60g	64	3.7	106	1.7	11.1	6.1	1.1
Potato, Asda*	¼ Pot/57g	67	4.0	117	0.9	12.5	7.0	1.1

S

SALAD

INFO/WEIGHT	Measure	per Measure		Nutrition Values per 100g / 100ml				
		KCAL	FAT	KCAL	PROT	CARB	FAT	FIBRE
Potato, Creamy, Asda*	½ Tub/150g	226	16.0	151	1.1	11.3	10.7	2.5
Potato, Creamy, Waitrose*	1 Serving/100g	163	11.9	163	1.3	12.7	11.9	1.1
Potato, Finest, Tesco*	1 Tub/250g	588	51.5	235	2.4	9.7	20.6	1.2
Potato, From Salad Selection, Sainsbury's*	1 Serving/50g	102	8.8	204	1.0	10.5	17.5	1.3
Potato, GFY, Asda*	½ Pack/125g	145	8.8	116	1.3	12.0	7.0	0.0
Potato, LC, Tesco*	1 Pack/100g	110	5.9	110	1.3	12.5	5.9	0.9
Potato, New, Co-Op*	1 Serving/50g	98	8.0	195	1.0	10.0	16.0	2.0
Potato, New, Less Than 5% Fat, M&S*	1 Serving/110g	88	3.4	80	1.3	12.1	3.1	1.5
Potato, New, Luxury, Morrisons*	½ Tub/125g	341	30.8	273	1.7	11.2	24.6	0.0
Potato, New, M&S*	1 Serving/60g	114	9.8	190	0.9	9.9	16.3	1.3
Potato, Reduced Calorie, Pre Packed	1oz/28g	27	1.1	97	1.3	14.8	4.1	0.8
Potato, Side, Waitrose*	1 Pack/250g	181	11.0	72	3.0	5.2	4.4	1.0
Potato, Tesco*	1 Serving/100g	165	13.5	165	1.3	9.5	13.5	1.3
Potato, Tomato & Egg with Salad Cream, M&S*	1 Pack/300g	165	7.2	55	2.9	5.4	2.4	1.3
Potato, Tuna & Egg, M&S*	1 Pack/340g	255	12.9	75	3.8	6.7	3.8	0.7
Potato, with Mayonnaise, Pre Packed	1oz/28g	67	5.8	239	1.6	12.2	20.8	0.9
Potato, with Mayonnaise, Retail	1oz/28g	80	7.4	287	1.5	11.4	26.5	0.8
Potato, with Onions & Chives, Co-Op*	1 Serving/50g	80	6.0	160	1.0	12.0	12.0	1.0
Prawn, & Avocado, M&S*	1 Serving/220g	176	15.0	80	3.0	2.0	6.8	3.1
Prawn, King & Rice Noodle, M&S*	1 Pack/320g	208	2.6	65	2.9	11.6	0.8	0.9
Prawn, Layer, Eat Well, M&S*	1 Pack/220g	143	4.6	65	4.3	6.9	2.1	1.4
Prawn, Layered, Co-Op*	1 Pack/300g	375	18.0	125	4.0	14.0	6.0	2.0
Prawn, Layered, M&S*	1 Pack/455g	410	17.7	90	4.5	8.9	3.9	1.2
Prawn, Layered, Single Size, Asda*	1 Serving/197g	217	9.8	110	4.3	12.0	5.0	1.0
Prawn, Layered, Tesco*	1 Pack/180g	243	13.0	135	4.2	13.1	7.2	2.0
Prawn Cocktail, Shapers, Boots*	1 Pack/245g	120	5.9	49	4.7	2.2	2.4	0.7
Prawn Cocktail, Tesco*	1 Pack/300g	360	18.0	120	5.7	10.9	6.0	0.8
Rainbow, Crunchy, Super Bowl, M&S*	1 Bowl/165g	107	5.3	65	1.6	6.0	3.2	2.9
Rainbow, Sainsbury's*	1 Pack/215g	300	14.8	140	5.5	13.8	6.9	3.9
Red Cabbage & Sweetcorn, Crunchy, M&S*	1 Serving/80g	28	0.4	35	1.3	6.6	0.5	1.2
Rice, Courgette & Pine Nut, BGTY, Sainsbury's*	1/3 Pot/65g	68	1.0	105	2.7	20.0	1.6	1.5
Rice, Spicy, Waitrose*	1 Serving/200g	318	13.2	159	3.2	21.7	6.6	0.9
Rice, Wild, Salad Bar, Waitrose*	1 Serving/100g	159	6.6	159	0.0	0.0	6.6	0.0
Richly Dressed Coleslaw, Salad Bar, Waitrose*	1 Serving/100g	134	11.8	134	0.0	0.0	11.8	0.0
Rocket, & Chard, Wild, Waitrose*	½ Bag/53g	8	0.3	15	0.8	1.7	0.5	1.4
Rocket, Leafy, Asda*	1 Serving/75g	10	0.1	13	1.5	1.4	0.1	1.8
Rocket, Morrisons*	1 Serving/100g	14	0.5	14	0.8	1.7	0.5	0.0
Rocket, Spinach & Watercress, Wild, Asda*	1 Serving/100g	21	0.6	21	2.8	1.2	0.6	1.9
Rocket & Lambs Lettuce, Italian Style, M&S*	½ Bag/60g	12	0.3	20	1.3	2.3	0.5	1.3
Salad, Bistro, Somerfield*	½ Pack/50g	7	0.2	14	0.8	1.6	0.5	1.4
Salmon, & New Potato, Honey Smoked, M&S*	1 Pack/270g	270	14.3	100	5.5	7.5	5.3	1.5
Salmon, & Roquette, M&S*	1 Serving/255g	306	20.4	120	3.9	8.5	8.0	1.0
Salmon, Hot Smoked with Potato Salad, M&S*	1 Pack/338g	270	7.4	80	4.5	10.3	2.2	1.3
Salmon, Moroccan Style, Light Lunch, John West*	1 Pack/220g	299	11.7	136	11.7	8.8	5.3	3.4
Santa Tomato, Side, M&S*	1 Pack/225g	146	12.4	65	0.8	3.3	5.5	0.9
Santini, Side, M&S*	1 Pack/195g	127	11.1	65	1.0	3.0	5.7	2.0
Seafood, Marinated, Waitrose*	1 Tub/160g	235	10.6	147	16.3	5.5	6.6	0.0
Seafood, Prawn & Calamari, Deli, M&S*	1 Pack/120g	132	6.1	110	14.7	1.2	5.1	0.8
Seasonal, Organic, Waitrose*	¼ Pack/25g	4	0.1	15	0.8	1.7	0.5	0.9
Side, Fresh & Crispy, Tesco*	1 Salad/230g	30	0.7	13	0.7	1.9	0.3	1.3
Side, Spring, Crunchy, M&S*	1 Serving/160g	32	0.3	20	0.9	4.1	0.2	1.3
Spinach, Rocket & Watercress, Asda*	1 Serving/100g	21	0.6	21	2.8	1.2	0.6	1.9
Spinach, Waitrose*	1 Pack/100g	25	0.8	25	2.8	1.6	0.8	2.1

SALAD

	Measure INFO/WEIGHT	per Measure KCAL	FAT	Nutrition Values per 100g / 100ml KCAL	PROT	CARB	FAT	FIBRE
Super Wholefood with Blueberries & Mango, M&S*	1 Pack/215g	260	7.7	121	4.4	17.0	3.6	8.7
Sweet & Crispy, Side, Sainsbury's*	¼ Bag/93g	23	0.2	25	1.3	4.4	0.2	2.2
Sweet & Crispy, Somerfield*	1 Pack/100g	25	0.0	25	1.0	5.0	0.0	0.0
Sweet & Crunchy, Mixed, Prepared, Co-Op*	1 Serving/120g	42	0.4	35	1.1	5.9	0.3	1.8
Sweet & Crunchy, Morrisons*	1 Serving/100g	23	0.3	23	0.8	3.4	0.3	1.8
Sweet & Crunchy, Sainsbury's*	1 Pack/150g	22	0.2	15	0.9	2.6	0.1	1.8
Sweet Green, M&S*	1 Serving/150g	22	0.4	15	1.5	1.3	0.3	2.0
Sweet Leaf, Fully Prepared, Fresh, Sainsbury's*	¼ Pack/75g	12	0.1	16	0.8	3.0	0.1	2.1
Sweet Leaf, Sainsbury's*	1 Serving/80g	19	0.2	24	0.8	3.6	0.3	1.9
Sweet Leaf & Carrot, Asda*	½ Pack/164g	34	0.5	21	0.9	3.6	0.3	1.4
Sweet Leaf & Carrot, Lasting Leaf*	1 Serving/70g	16	0.3	23	1.0	2.8	0.4	2.2
Sweet Pepper, Medley, Waitrose*	½ Pack/100g	22	0.4	22	0.9	3.8	0.4	1.5
Sweet Pepper, Side, Tesco*	1 Serving/54g	22	0.2	41	1.3	8.0	0.4	2.1
Tabbouleh, & Feta, Tesco*	1 Pack/225g	302	11.2	134	5.4	16.7	5.0	0.6
Tabbouleh, Feta, Finest, Tesco*	1 Pack/225g	266	11.7	118	4.2	13.7	5.2	0.6
Tabbouleh, Fruity, Salad Bar, Waitrose*	1 Serving/100g	184	6.6	184	0.0	0.0	6.6	0.0
Tabbouleh, Salad Bar, Waitrose*	1 Serving/100g	94	1.7	94	0.0	0.0	1.7	0.0
Tabbouleh, Style, PB, Waitrose*	1 Pack/225g	234	8.8	104	2.8	14.3	3.9	2.6
Tender Leaf, Waitrose*	1 Serving/200g	30	1.0	15	0.9	1.6	0.5	1.1
Tender Leaf, with Mizuna, Tesco*	1 Serving/30g	4	0.1	15	1.6	1.4	0.3	1.7
Tomato, Avocado & Rocket, M&S*	1 Pack/350g	508	46.9	145	1.7	4.1	13.4	0.2
Tomato, Baby, Tesco*	1 Pack/205g	35	0.6	17	0.8	2.8	0.3	0.9
Tomato, Lettuce & Cucumber, Classics, M&S*	1 Serving/275g	151	11.6	55	0.9	3.3	4.2	1.6
Tomato & Cucumber, Ready to Eat, Morrisons*	¼ Pack/81g	17	0.2	21	0.9	3.7	0.3	2.0
Tomato & Mozzarella, Finest, Tesco*	1 Pack/175g	254	21.4	145	5.6	3.3	12.2	0.7
Tomato & Mozzarella, M&S*	1 Pack/220g	264	16.5	120	9.8	2.8	7.5	1.1
Tomato & Onion	1oz/28g	20	1.7	72	0.8	4.0	6.1	1.0
Trio Leaf, Lettuce, Asda*	1 Portion/80g	12	0.4	15	0.8	1.7	0.5	0.9
Tuna, & Mixed Bean	1 Serving/220g	287	14.4	131	9.5	11.2	6.6	3.7
Tuna, & Three Bean, Healthily Balanced, M&S*	1 Serving/350g	332	10.2	95	8.7	8.8	2.9	4.6
Tuna, & Tomato, Boots*	1 Pack/171g	150	10.3	88	6.5	2.0	6.0	1.0
Tuna, French Style, Light Lunch, John West*	1 Pack/220g	218	6.2	99	7.5	9.8	2.8	2.5
Tuna, Italian Style, Light Lunch, John West*	1 Pack/220g	205	5.7	93	7.3	9.8	2.6	0.5
Tuna, Layer, COU, M&S*	1 Pack/340g	272	8.8	80	6.2	7.5	2.6	1.5
Tuna, Layered, Tesco*	1 Serving/370g	466	29.2	126	4.4	9.4	7.9	1.0
Tuna, Mediterranean Style, Light Lunch, John West*	1 Pack/220g	211	4.2	96	8.5	10.0	1.9	2.4
Tuna, Pasta, Layered, Asda*	1 Serving/100g	98	2.8	98	5.4	12.7	2.8	1.9
Tuna, Skipjack, John West*	1 Can/192g	190	11.7	99	7.3	3.7	6.1	0.0
Tuna, Tomato Salsa Style, Light Lunch, John West*	1 Pack/220g	187	2.9	85	7.6	10.8	1.3	0.8
Tuna Nicoise, BGTY, Sainsbury's*	1 Pack/300g	315	6.0	105	6.3	15.5	2.0	2.5
Tuna Nicoise, Finest, Tesco*	1 Serving/250g	430	23.5	172	8.5	13.3	9.4	0.8
Tuna Nicoise, No Mayonnaise, Shapers, Boots*	1 Pack/276g	133	3.6	48	4.0	5.0	1.3	0.8
Vegetable, & Cous Cous, Roasted, Sainsbury's*	1 Pot/225g	378	24.1	168	5.3	12.6	10.7	1.9
Vegetable, Chargrilled, M&S*	1 Tub/165g	91	5.4	55	1.4	5.3	3.3	2.6
Vegetable, Feta & Cous Cous, Roasted, Somerfield*	1 Pack/299g	491	17.4	164	5.0	22.9	5.8	1.6
Vegetable, Heinz*	1 Can/195g	259	16.6	133	1.5	12.6	8.5	1.3
Vegetable, Nutty Grain, Eat Well, M&S*	1 Pack/230g	299	11.7	130	5.3	12.8	5.1	6.1
Waldorf, Average	1 Serving/100g	193	17.7	193	1.4	7.5	17.7	1.3
Waldorf, TTD, Sainsbury's*	¼ Pot/69g	203	19.5	296	1.9	8.1	28.4	4.7
Watercress, Baby Spinach & Rocket, Somerfield*	1 Serving/100g	25	0.9	25	3.0	1.2	0.9	1.7
Watercress, Spinach & Rocket, Tesco*	1 Serving/30g	7	0.2	22	3.0	0.8	0.8	1.9
Watercress, Spinach & Rocket, Waitrose*	1 Bag/145g	30	1.2	21	2.2	1.2	0.8	1.5
Wheatberry & Bean Refreshing, Waitrose*	1 Pack/220g	297	13.2	135	4.7	11.9	6.0	7.2

S

	Measure INFO/WEIGHT	per Measure KCAL	per Measure FAT	Nutrition Values per 100g / 100ml KCAL	PROT	CARB	FAT	FIBRE
SALAD								
Wholefood, Super, Nutritionally Balanced, M&S*	1 Pack/285g	271	8.0	95	2.6	14.7	2.8	3.5
Wild Rocket & Parmesan, Italian, Sainsbury's*	1 Serving/50g	88	7.4	177	7.5	3.4	14.8	0.5
with Chive Dressing, Classic, M&S*	½ Pack/138g	76	5.8	55	0.9	3.3	4.2	1.6
with Green Herb Dressing, Classic, Co-Op*	1 Serving/90g	86	8.1	95	1.0	2.0	9.0	1.0
with Sweetcorn, Side, Tesco*	1 Serving/135g	51	0.7	38	1.3	7.2	0.5	1.5
SALAD BOWL								
Coleslaw, M&S*	1 Pack/325g	292	24.0	90	1.3	4.9	7.4	1.3
Crispy, M&S*	1 Serving/250g	88	1.2	35	1.3	6.6	0.5	1.2
Egg Layered, Tesco*	1 Pack/410g	726	57.8	177	4.2	8.4	14.1	1.3
Frisee, Radicchio & Green Oak Leaf Lettuce, M&S*	1 Bowl/150g	30	0.6	20	1.1	2.6	0.4	1.1
Goats Cheese, Sainsbury's*	1 Serving/100g	161	11.9	161	5.8	7.6	11.9	1.3
Greek Style, M&S*	1 Bowl/223g	212	18.3	95	2.5	2.4	8.2	0.7
Greek Style, Somerfield*	1 Bowl/225g	178	14.0	79	2.2	3.5	6.2	1.1
Honey & Mustard Chicken, Fresh, Sainsbury's*	1 Serving/300g	408	23.7	136	5.9	10.3	7.9	1.7
Italian Avocado & Tomato, Sainsbury's*	1 Bowl/180g	97	4.7	54	1.0	6.7	2.6	1.3
Large, Sainsbury's*	1/6 Pack/52g	12	0.2	23	0.9	4.3	0.3	1.1
Mixed, Medley, Waitrose*	¼ Pack/60g	9	0.3	15	0.9	1.7	0.5	1.0
Mixed, Waitrose*	¼ Pack/64g	9	0.3	14	0.8	1.6	0.5	1.4
Prawn, Sainsbury's*	1 Bowl/400g	632	46.8	158	3.7	9.4	11.7	1.2
Tomato, Sainsbury's*	½ Bowl/150g	93	6.8	62	0.9	4.4	4.5	1.6
Tomato & Basil, M&S*	1 Serving/225g	225	22.7	100	0.8	3.7	10.1	1.1
Tuna, BGTY, Sainsbury's*	½ Pack/175g	180	2.6	103	7.0	15.4	1.5	1.7
Tuna, Fresh, Asda*	1 Serving/160g	184	11.2	115	8.0	5.0	7.0	0.0
Tuna, Sainsbury's*	1 Serving/200g	336	21.4	168	6.1	11.7	10.7	1.5
SALAD CREAM								
Average	*1 Tsp/5g*	*17*	*1.4*	*335*	*1.7*	*18.6*	*27.8*	*0.1*
Heinz*	1 Tbsp/15g	50	4.0	332	1.4	20.0	26.8	0.0
Reduced Calorie, Average	*1 Tsp/5g*	*6*	*0.4*	*130*	*1.0*	*12.9*	*7.9*	*0.2*
Weight Watchers*	1 Serving/14g	16	0.6	115	1.5	16.2	4.4	0.0
SALAD KIT								
Caesar, Asda*	½ Pack/113g	154	9.0	136	5.0	11.0	8.0	1.4
Caesar, Tesco*	½ Pack/138g	279	25.3	202	4.7	4.5	18.3	1.3
Caesar, Waitrose*	1 Bag/250g	436	36.1	174	4.4	6.1	14.4	1.3
SALAMI								
Ardennes Pepper, Waitrose*	1 Serving/7g	30	2.7	429	18.6	1.9	38.5	1.1
Average	*1 Slice/5g*	*18*	*1.3*	*360*	*28.4*	*1.8*	*26.2*	*0.0*
Danish, Average	*1 Serving/17g*	*89*	*8.8*	*524*	*13.2*	*1.3*	*51.7*	*0.0*
Emiliano, Sainsbury's*	1 Serving/70g	209	14.2	298	28.8	0.1	20.3	0.0
German, Average	*1 Serving/60g*	*200*	*16.4*	*333*	*20.3*	*1.6*	*27.3*	*0.1*
German, Peppered, Average	*3 Slices/25g*	*86*	*6.8*	*342*	*22.2*	*2.5*	*27.1*	*0.2*
Giganti, Sliced, TTD, Sainsbury's*	1 Slice/5g	21	1.8	411	25.0	0.1	34.4	0.6
Healthy Range, Average	*4 Slices/25g*	*55*	*3.6*	*220*	*22.4*	*0.6*	*14.3*	*0.0*
Milano, Average	*1 Serving/70g*	*278*	*22.6*	*397*	*25.9*	*0.9*	*32.2*	*0.0*
Napoli, Average	*1 Slice/5g*	*17*	*1.3*	*342*	*27.1*	*0.8*	*25.5*	*0.0*
Pepperoni, Italian, Morrisons*	1 Slice/6g	23	1.9	406	24.0	0.9	34.0	0.0
Spanish, Wafer Thin, Tesco*	1 Pack/80g	273	18.8	341	25.5	6.8	23.5	0.0
SALMON								
Alaskan, Pink, Canned, Crown Prince*	¼ Cup/55g	90	4.0	164	20.0	0.0	7.3	0.0
Alaskan, Wild, TTD, Sainsbury's*	1 Fillet/115g	173	8.3	150	21.2	0.1	7.2	0.1
Cooked, Prepacked, Average	1 Fillet/93g	180	11.1	194	21.8	0.0	11.9	0.0
Crunchies, Tesco*	1 Serving/112g	211	11.0	188	9.0	15.9	9.8	1.3
Fillets, Cajun, Waitrose*	1 Serving/150g	214	9.8	143	20.6	0.4	6.5	0.0
Fillets, Chargrilled, Sainsbury's*	1 Serving/270g	270	19.5	243	20.9	0.2	17.6	0.0

SALMON

Measure INFO/WEIGHT	per Measure KCAL	FAT	Nutrition Values per 100g / 100ml KCAL	PROT	CARB	FAT	FIBRE
Fillets, Fresh, Value, Tesco*	1 Slice/85g	153	9.4	180	21.6	0.0	11.0	0.0
Fillets, Herb & Pink Peppercorn Crust, Waitrose*	1 Fillet/145g	393	30.0	271	16.6	4.6	20.7	0.8
Fillets, Honey Roast, Co-Op*	1 Fillet/100g	250	13.8	250	26.7	4.7	13.8	0.1
Fillets, Lightly Smoked, TTD, Sainsbury's*	1 Serving/100g	201	13.2	201	20.2	0.3	13.2	0.6
Fillets, Lime & Coriander, Tesco*	1 Pack/250g	282	5.2	113	18.2	5.4	2.1	0.0
Fillets, Lime & Coriander Marinade, Pacific, Sainsbury's*	1 Serving/100g	139	4.1	139	24.4	1.3	4.1	0.9
Fillets, Raw, Average	*1 Fillet/120g*	*227*	*14.0*	*189*	*20.9*	*0.1*	*11.7*	*0.1*
Fillets, Red Thai Marinade, Harbour Salmon Co*	1 Fillet/110g	176	10.3	160	18.5	0.3	9.4	0.5
Fillets, Select, Farm Prime, 4 Pack, Waitrose*	1 Pack/550g	979	57.8	178	20.2	0.0	10.5	0.0
Fillets, Skin On, TTD, Sainsbury's*	1 Fillet/126g	249	14.3	197	23.5	0.2	11.3	0.0
Fillets, Sunblush Tomato Dressing, The Saucy Fish Co.*	2 Fillets/270g	483	29.4	179	19.9	0.1	10.9	0.0
Fillets, Watercress & Creme Fraiche, The Saucy Fish Co*	2 Fillets/230g	428	26.9	186	20.1	0.1	11.7	0.0
Fillets, Wild Alaskan, Keta, Love Life, Waitrose*	1 Fillet/110g	170	6.2	155	25.9	0.2	5.6	0.3
Fillets, Wild Alaskan, Keta, Sainsbury's*	1 Fillet/115g	178	6.4	155	25.9	0.2	5.6	0.3
Fillets, with Lemon & Herb Butter, Asda*	1 Fillet/125g	305	22.5	244	20.0	0.4	18.0	0.0
Fillets, with Orange & Dill Dressing, Tesco*	1 Serving/300g	540	30.9	180	17.7	4.1	10.3	0.0
Fillets, with Sicilian Citrus Glaze, Sainsbury's*	1 Fillet/145g	371	25.8	256	21.9	2.3	17.8	0.7
Flakes, Honey Roast, Average	*1oz/28g*	*56*	*3.0*	*198*	*24.0*	*1.9*	*10.7*	*0.2*
Flakes, Honey Roast, Sainsbury's*	½ Pack/68g	166	9.5	244	25.9	3.6	14.0	0.0
Flaky, Smoked, Salar, Loch Duart Ltd*	1 Serving/150g	198	6.2	132	23.6	0.3	4.1	0.3
Goujons, Average	1 Pack/150g	321	16.4	214	16.4	12.4	11.0	1.1
Gravadlax, Finest, Tesco*	1 Serving/70g	125	6.9	178	22.1	0.2	9.9	0.0
Gravadlax, M&S*	1 Serving/140g	294	16.0	210	18.4	5.3	11.4	0.5
Gravadlax, Scottish, M&S*	1 Serving/70g	147	8.0	210	18.4	5.3	11.4	0.5
Gravadlax, Smoked, Limoncello, Wild Waters*	1 Pack/150g	362	12.0	241	19.9	2.5	8.0	0.5
Gravadlax, with Mustard Sauce, Waitrose*	1 Pack/200g	382	22.2	191	21.8	1.0	11.1	0.4
Grilled	*1oz/28g*	*60*	*3.7*	*215*	*24.2*	*0.0*	*13.1*	*0.0*
Hot Smoked, Average	*1 Serving/62g*	*103*	*4.4*	*166*	*24.0*	*0.9*	*7.2*	*0.1*
Hot Smoked, Kiln Baked, TTD, Sainsbury's*	½ Pack/63g	121	6.4	193	24.6	0.7	10.2	0.5
Hot Smoked, Ready Meal, Sainsbury's*	1 Pack/370g	363	12.8	105	8.0	8.2	3.7	3.4
Juniper & Birch Smoked, TTD, Sainsbury's*	½ Pack/60g	132	8.4	220	23.3	0.3	14.0	0.1
Lime & Coriander, Tesco*	1 Serving/120g	176	4.4	147	21.4	7.0	3.7	0.7
Mild Oak Smoked, Average	*1 Slice/25g*	*46*	*2.5*	*182*	*22.6*	*0.1*	*10.2*	*0.0*
Mousse, Tesco*	1 Mousse/57g	100	7.0	177	13.5	2.9	12.4	0.2
Pink, Canned, Average	*1 Serving/125g*	*162*	*7.2*	*130*	*19.5*	*0.1*	*5.8*	*0.1*
Pink, in Brine, Average	*1 Can/105g*	*161*	*6.9*	*153*	*23.5*	*0.0*	*6.6*	*0.0*
Poached, Average	*1 Serving/90g*	*176*	*10.5*	*195*	*22.5*	*0.2*	*11.7*	*0.3*
Potted, M&S*	1 Serving/75g	184	14.6	245	17.1	0.5	19.4	1.2
Red, Average	*½ Can/90g*	*141*	*7.4*	*156*	*20.4*	*0.1*	*8.2*	*0.1*
Red, in Brine, Average	*1oz/28g*	*47*	*2.5*	*169*	*22.4*	*0.0*	*8.9*	*0.0*
Sashimi, Smoked, Scottish Lochmuir, M&S*	1 Pack/130g	214	11.0	165	18.6	3.3	8.5	0.5
Slices, Roasted, Tesco*	1 Slice/33g	71	3.5	215	26.7	2.7	10.5	1.9
Smoked, Appetisers, Tesco*	1/3 Pack/33g	80	6.2	240	16.3	1.1	18.5	0.0
Smoked, Average	*1 Serving/70g*	*126*	*7.0*	*179*	*21.9*	*0.5*	*10.0*	*0.1*
Smoked, Lemon & Pepper, Hot, Roasties, Scottish, Asda*	1 Pack/100g	195	7.7	195	26.0	5.5	7.7	0.5
Smoked, Parcels, TTD, Sainsbury's*	1 Serving/58g	144	11.1	250	13.4	5.7	19.3	1.0
Smoked, Sockeye, Wild, TTD, Sainsbury's*	½ Pack/60g	82	1.9	137	26.3	0.7	3.2	0.6
Smoked, Trimmings, Average	*1 Serving/55g*	*101*	*5.7*	*184*	*22.8*	*0.2*	*10.3*	*0.0*
Smoked, Trimmings, Value, Tesco*	1 Serving/50g	89	5.0	178	22.1	0.2	9.9	0.0
Smoked, Wild Alaskan, TTD, Sainsbury's*	¼ Pack/25g	34	0.8	137	26.3	0.7	3.2	0.6
Soy & Ginger, Scottish Lochmuir, Fuller Longer, M&S*	1 Pack/360g	415	18.0	115	8.0	7.8	5.0	3.1
Steaks	*1 Serving/100g*	*180*	*11.0*	*180*	*20.2*	*0.0*	*11.0*	*0.0*
Steamed	*1oz/28g*	*55*	*3.6*	*197*	*20.1*	*0.0*	*13.0*	*0.0*

	Measure INFO/WEIGHT	per Measure KCAL	FAT	Nutrition Values per 100g / 100ml KCAL	PROT	CARB	FAT	FIBRE
SALMON								
Whole, Raw, Average	1 Serving/100g	228	13.9	228	25.6	0.0	13.9	0.0
SALMON &								
Spinach, Roulade, Tesco*	1 Serving/60g	155	14.2	258	9.5	1.7	23.7	0.2
SALMON EN CROUTE								
Frozen, Tesco*	1 Serving/166g	365	18.4	220	10.1	19.1	11.1	1.1
Iceland*	1 Serving/170g	476	31.3	280	8.5	20.1	18.4	1.0
M & S*	½ Pack/185g	574	40.5	310	10.4	17.3	21.9	0.6
Retail, Average	1oz/28g	81	5.3	288	11.8	18.0	19.1	0.0
Wild Alaskan, Inspired To Cook, Sainsbury's*	1 Parcel/173g	476	24.4	275	12.5	24.7	14.1	10.8
with Lemon & Dill, Easy to Cook, Waitrose*	½ Pack/185g	487	31.5	263	10.7	16.9	17.0	2.7
SALMON IN								
Chilli Lime & Ginger Dressing, The Saucy Fish Co.*	1 Fillet/140g	273	15.8	195	16.7	5.5	11.3	0.0
Creamy Horseradish Sauce, Fillets, Wonnemeyer*	1 Serving/300g	459	31.5	153	9.4	5.3	10.5	0.0
Creamy Watercress Sauce, Fillets, Scottish, Seafresh*	1 Pack/300g	528	38.7	176	13.7	1.2	12.9	0.1
Lime & Coriander, Fillets, Good Choice, Iceland*	½ Pack/150g	189	4.4	126	19.8	5.1	2.9	0.8
Tomato & Mascarpone Sauce, Fillets, Asda*	½ Pack/181g	279	19.9	154	13.0	0.8	11.0	0.6
White Wine & Cream Sauce, Tesco*	1 Serving/170g	279	19.2	164	13.5	2.0	11.3	1.2
White Wine & Parsley Dressing, Fillets, Tesco*	1 Fillet/150g	291	20.4	194	17.5	0.3	13.6	0.6
SALMON WELLINGTON								
with Prawn & White Wine Sauce, Northern Catch, Aldi*	¼ Wellington/175g	457	27.8	261	13.3	15.6	15.9	1.2
SALMON WITH								
Cream Sauce, Fillets, Scottish, M&S*	1 Serving/200g	360	26.0	180	13.8	1.0	13.0	0.1
Crushed Minted Peas & Lemon, Love Life, Waitrose*	½ Pack/205g	287	16.6	140	12.7	4.0	8.1	2.4
Fillets, Sweet Chilli, Kiln Roasted, Tesco*	1 Fillet/93g	167	10.7	260	23.3	3.4	16.6	1.4
Garlic & Herb Butter, Tesco*	1 Fillet/112g	291	23.1	260	17.6	0.0	20.6	0.0
Penne Pasta & Dill Sauce, SteamFresh, Birds Eye*	1 Pack/424g	335	6.4	79	6.4	9.9	1.5	1.1
Rice, Oriental Style, M&S*	1 Pot/210g	252	6.9	120	5.9	16.5	3.3	3.3
Spinach & Pasta, Smoked, Milson's Kitchen (Aldi)*	1 Pack/400g	472	16.0	118	5.6	15.0	4.0	1.7
Sweet Chilli, Hot Smoked, Scottish, Tesco*	1 Fillet/120g	252	12.7	210	26.1	1.7	10.6	0.6
Sweet Chilli, Lime & Ginger, Simply Fish, Tesco*	½ Pack/98g	235	17.2	240	17.4	3.2	17.5	0.0
Sweet Soy Sauce, Fillets, Inspired To Cook, Sainsbury's*	1 Fillet/142g	278	16.5	196	17.5	5.3	11.6	0.4
SALSA								
Bottled, M&S*	½ Jar/136g	95	3.3	70	1.2	12.0	2.4	1.5
Chunky, Sainsbury's*	½ Pot/84g	43	1.4	51	1.1	7.8	1.7	1.2
Cool, Sainsbury's*	1 Serving/100g	31	0.3	31	1.0	6.1	0.3	1.2
Extra Hot, Fresh, Somerfield*	1oz/28g	13	0.3	47	1.0	8.0	1.0	0.0
Fresh, Asda*	1oz/28g	10	0.2	35	1.2	6.2	0.6	2.0
Fresh, Sainsbury's*	1oz/28g	15	0.6	54	1.7	7.0	2.1	0.9
GFY, Asda*	½ Pot/236g	85	0.9	36	1.1	7.0	0.4	0.7
Hot, Fresh, Chilled, Tesco*	1 Tub/200g	120	4.8	60	1.4	7.5	2.4	1.2
Medium Hot, Discovery*	1 Serving/30g	17	0.1	56	1.4	11.7	0.4	0.8
Original, from Dinner Kit, Old El Paso*	1 Jar/226g	71	0.7	32	1.2	6.0	0.3	0.0
Original, Mild, Old El Paso*	1 Sachet/144g	60	0.7	42	1.6	9.0	0.5	0.0
Red Onion & Tomato, Tapas Selection, Sainsbury's*	1 Serving/22g	17	1.0	77	3.0	6.0	4.5	0.9
Red Pepper, Sainsbury's*	1 Serving/85g	31	1.4	37	1.7	3.8	1.7	1.5
Spiced Mango, Ginger & Chilli, Weight Watchers*	½ Pot/50g	42	0.1	85	1.0	19.9	0.2	2.6
Spicy, Less Than 3% Fat, M&S*	½ Pot/85g	30	0.7	35	1.3	5.6	0.8	0.8
Spicy Bean, CBY, Asda*	½ Pot/100g	71	1.2	71	3.1	10.6	1.2	2.5
Spicy Mango & Lime, Morrisons*	½ Pot/85g	62	0.3	73	1.0	15.9	0.4	1.3
Spicy Red Pepper, Fresh, Waitrose*	½ Pot/85g	27	0.8	32	1.9	4.1	0.9	1.6
Spicy Red Pepper, Sainsbury's*	1 Pot/170g	54	2.4	32	1.4	3.2	1.4	1.3
Sweetcorn, Fresh, Sainsbury's*	¼ Pot/51g	32	0.9	63	1.1	10.5	1.8	1.3
Tomato, & Avocado, Chunky, COU, M&S*	½ Pack/86g	30	1.2	35	0.8	5.4	1.4	1.4

	Measure INFO/WEIGHT	per Measure KCAL	FAT	Nutrition Values per 100g / 100ml KCAL	PROT	CARB	FAT	FIBRE
SALSA								
Tomato, & Jalapeno, Vine Ripened, Sainsbury's*	¼ Tub/50g	34	1.8	68	1.1	8.0	3.5	1.2
Tomato, Chunky, Tesco*	1 Pot/170g	68	2.2	40	1.1	5.9	1.3	1.1
Tomato, Chunky, Tex Mex, Tesco*	1 Serving/50g	26	1.2	52	1.0	6.4	2.5	1.0
Tomato, Mexican Style, Dip, Morrisons*	½ Pack/50g	26	0.9	51	1.2	7.6	1.8	0.8
Tomato, Onion, Coriander & Chilli, Fresh, Waitrose*	1 Tub/170g	110	5.3	65	1.3	8.0	3.1	1.2
Tomato, Spicy, Worldwide Sauces*	1 Serving/25g	8	0.0	30	1.2	5.9	0.2	1.2
Tomato, Vine Ripened, Tesco*	½ Tub/100g	47	1.8	47	1.0	6.7	1.8	1.1
SALT								
Alternative, Reduced Sodium, Losalt*	10g	0	0.0	0	0.0	0.0	0.0	0.0
Rock, Average	¼ Tsp/1g	0	0.0	0	0.0	0.0	0.0	0.0
Table, Average	**1 Tsp/5g**	**0**	**0.0**	**0**	**0.0**	**0.0**	**0.0**	**0.0**
SAMBUCA								
Average	**1 Pub Shot/35ml**	**122**	**0.0**	**348**	**0.0**	**37.2**	**0.0**	**0.0**
SAMOSAS								
Chicken, Mumtaz*	1 Serving/105g	177	8.3	169	19.6	4.9	7.9	0.0
Chicken Tikka, Sainsbury's*	1 Samosa/50g	120	6.4	239	8.3	22.5	12.9	3.1
Indian Style Selection, Co-Op*	1 Samosa/21g	50	2.7	240	5.0	27.0	13.0	3.0
Lamb, Morrisons*	1 Samosa/50g	144	7.8	288	9.8	15.7	15.7	1.5
Vegetable, Indian, Takeaway, CBY, Asda*	1 Samosa/50g	126	5.2	250	5.2	32.5	10.3	3.3
Vegetable, Indian Starter Selection, M&S*	1 Samosa/21g	60	3.5	290	5.0	29.0	16.9	3.3
Vegetable, Large, Individual, Sainsbury's*	1 Samosa/110g	254	16.5	231	3.3	20.7	15.0	2.1
Vegetable, Large, Tesco*	1 Samosa/64g	148	7.9	231	4.8	25.2	12.4	3.4
Vegetable, Lightly Spiced, Sainsbury's*	1 Samosa/50g	112	6.3	223	4.0	23.5	12.5	1.2
Vegetable, M&S*	1 Samosa/45g	115	6.9	255	5.1	24.8	15.3	2.8
Vegetable, Mini, Asda*	1 Samosa/23g	52	2.0	233	6.0	32.0	9.0	2.6
Vegetable, Mini, Indian, Party Selection, Tesco*	1 Samosa/30g	58	1.5	195	3.6	33.9	5.0	2.2
Vegetable, Mini, Indian, Somerfield*	1 Samosa/25g	64	3.3	253	5.7	28.1	13.1	3.4
Vegetable, Mini, Indian Snack Selection, Sainsbury's*	1 Samosa/25g	70	4.0	280	4.7	29.8	15.8	3.2
Vegetable, Mini, Indian Snack Selection, Tesco*	1 Samosa/32g	76	4.2	238	4.7	25.5	13.0	3.3
Vegetable, Mini, Waitrose*	1 Samosa/29g	70	3.8	242	3.6	27.1	13.2	3.1
Vegetable, Morrisons*	1 Samosa/60g	101	3.5	169	4.9	24.1	5.8	2.0
Vegetable, Northern Indian, Sainsbury's*	1 Samosa/50g	126	5.9	252	5.8	30.6	11.8	2.6
Vegetable, Retail, Average	1 Samosa/110g	239	10.2	217	5.1	30.0	9.3	2.5
Vegetable, Waitrose*	1 Samosa/50g	118	7.2	236	3.7	23.1	14.3	2.7
SANDWICH								
All Day Breakfast, BGTY, Sainsbury's*	1 Pack/188g	294	4.5	156	9.6	22.7	2.4	0.0
All Day Breakfast, Deep Fill, Ginsters*	1 Sandwich/215g	514	19.8	239	11.4	27.6	9.2	1.5
All Day Breakfast, Finest, Tesco*	1 Pack/275g	660	41.5	240	9.7	16.4	15.1	1.6
All Day Breakfast, Shapers, Boots*	1 Pack/207g	323	5.2	156	11.0	23.0	2.5	2.2
Avocado, Mozzarella & Tomato, M&S*	1 Pack/273g	655	36.0	240	8.8	21.7	13.2	2.3
Bacon, Cheese & Chicken, Triple, BGTY, Sainsbury's*	1 Serving/266g	506	16.8	190	12.7	20.7	6.3	2.6
Bacon & Brie, Asda*	1 Pack/181g	603	38.2	333	13.3	22.9	21.1	1.3
Bacon & Brie, Finest, Tesco*	1 Pack/201g	571	33.6	284	14.1	19.4	16.7	2.1
Bacon & Egg, Boots*	1 Pack/179g	480	28.6	268	12.0	19.0	16.0	1.4
Bacon & Egg, Co-Op*	1 Pack/188g	536	32.0	285	13.0	20.0	17.0	2.0
Bacon & Egg, on Malted Whole Grain Bread, Budgens*	1 Pack/175g	593	37.4	339	12.3	21.4	21.4	1.6
Bacon & Egg, Sainsbury's*	1 Pack/160g	384	17.8	240	13.0	22.0	11.1	1.8
Bacon & Egg, Taste!*	1 Pack/187g	495	28.6	265	12.8	19.1	15.3	0.0
Bacon & Egg, Tesco*	1 Pack/188g	481	24.2	256	14.1	21.0	12.9	1.9
Beef, Roast, Daily Bread*	1 Pack/199g	281	5.4	141	8.7	20.0	2.7	0.0
Beef, Roast, Finest, Tesco*	1 Sandwich/222g	455	15.1	205	13.2	22.3	6.8	2.5
Beef, Roast, Handmade, Tesco*	1 Pack/223g	439	15.8	197	12.5	20.7	7.1	1.6
Beef, Roast, Plain, From Restaurant, Average	1 Sandwich/139g	346	13.8	249	15.5	24.1	9.9	0.0

S

SANDWICH

INFO/WEIGHT	Measure		per Measure		Nutrition Values per 100g / 100ml				
			KCAL	FAT	KCAL	PROT	CARB	FAT	FIBRE
Beef, Roast, Sainsbury's*	1 Pack/174g		426	17.4	245	9.4	29.3	10.0	0.0
Beef, Salt with Gherkins & Mustard Mayo, Sainsbury's*	1 Pack/242g		486	18.2	201	9.3	24.1	7.5	3.1
Beef & Horseradish, Deep Filled, BGTY, Sainsbury's*	1 Pack/202g		313	4.8	155	11.4	22.0	2.4	2.4
Beef & Horseradish, Mayo, Roast, Rare, Waitrose*	1 Pack/197g		415	15.3	211	12.2	23.1	7.8	2.0
Beef & Horseradish, Rare, Roast, Eat Well, M&S*	1 Serving/200g		360	9.2	180	13.1	21.9	4.6	2.7
Beef & Horseradish, Roast, So Good, Somerfield*	1 Pack/188g		404	11.5	215	12.4	27.6	6.1	1.8
Beef & Horseradish, Sainsbury's*	1 Pack/187g		389	13.3	208	12.0	24.1	7.1	0.0
Beef & Onion, Co-Op*	1 Pack/221g		530	24.3	240	11.0	24.0	11.0	1.0
Beef & Pate, M&S*	1 Pack/188g		310	7.3	165	11.2	21.6	3.9	2.4
Beef & Salad, Deep Fill, Iceland*	1 Pack/188g		317	9.2	169	11.1	20.1	4.9	2.7
Beef & Salad, Gibsons*	1 Pack/185g		348	10.6	188	10.6	23.5	5.7	0.0
Beef & Salad, Roast, Daily Bread*	1 Pack/202g		319	8.3	158	9.0	21.4	4.1	0.0
Beef & Stilton, Roast, on White, Fuller Longer, M&S*	1 Pack/204g		337	10.0	165	12.9	17.2	4.9	2.2
BLT, & Chicken Salad, Co-Op*	1 Pack/230g		472	20.7	205	10.0	21.0	9.0	2.0
BLT, Asda*	1 Sandwich/172g		325	11.9	189	9.9	21.8	6.9	4.6
BLT, Bacon, Lettuce & Tomato, LC, Tesco*	1 Pack/155g		310	7.9	200	9.9	26.5	5.1	2.2
BLT, BGTY, Sainsbury's*	1 Pack/196g		331	4.4	169	10.4	27.0	2.2	0.0
BLT, Bloomer, Freshly Prepared, M&S*	1 Pack/210g		430	19.5	205	8.2	21.8	9.3	1.8
BLT, Classic, Taste!*	1 Serving/150g		345	14.8	230	9.3	25.2	9.9	0.0
BLT, COU, M&S*	1 Pack/174g		278	4.7	160	9.5	25.6	2.7	2.5
BLT, Deep Fill, Ginsters*	1 Pack/197g		439	18.1	223	10.3	24.7	9.2	2.7
BLT, Deep Fill, Tesco*	1 Pack/231g		635	38.1	275	11.8	19.8	16.5	1.2
BLT, M&S*	1 Serving/181g		381	14.7	210	10.7	23.8	8.1	1.8
BLT, Shapers, Boots*	1 Pack/175g		272	7.5	155	11.0	18.0	4.3	5.9
BLT, Tesco*	1 Pack/203g		520	29.2	256	11.9	19.5	14.4	1.5
BLT, Waitrose*	1 Pack/184g		398	16.4	216	9.5	24.5	8.9	2.3
BLT, with Mayo, Seeded Malted Bread, Deep Fill, Heinz*	1 Pack/182g		444	19.8	244	10.3	26.2	10.9	3.0
Breakfast, Mega Triple, Co-Op*	1 Pack/267g		750	40.0	281	11.6	25.5	15.0	3.4
Brie, LT, Cranks*	1 Pack/192g		383	16.9	199	7.7	21.5	8.8	1.7
Brie, with Apple & Grapes, Sainsbury's*	1 Pack/220g		473	24.2	215	8.2	20.8	11.0	0.0
Brie & Grape, Finest, Tesco*	1 Pack/209g		527	31.6	252	8.5	20.6	15.1	1.5
Cheddar, Gorge, Cranks*	1 Pack/190g		454	23.2	239	11.5	19.4	12.2	3.0
Cheddar, Oldfields*	1 Pack/121g		384	17.3	317	12.8	33.2	14.3	1.5
Cheddar, Red Leicester & Onion, Tesco*	1 Pack/182g		604	38.9	332	11.0	23.8	21.4	2.5
Cheddar & Celery, M&S*	1 Pack/200g		540	31.8	270	9.7	22.4	15.9	1.5
Cheddar & Coleslaw, Simply, Boots*	1 Pack/185g		538	33.3	291	9.2	23.0	18.0	1.8
Cheddar & Ham, British, M&S*	1 Serving/165g		395	18.6	240	15.1	20.0	11.3	1.7
Cheddar & Ham, M&S*	1 Pack/165g		396	18.6	240	15.1	20.0	11.3	1.7
Cheddar & Ham, Oldfields*	1 Pack/246g		674	39.6	274	11.7	20.5	16.1	2.0
Cheddar & Ham, Smoked, Deep Filled, Tesco*	1 Serving/203g		573	33.1	282	14.3	19.5	16.3	1.2
Cheddar & Ham, with Pickle, Smoked, Finest, Tesco*	1 Pack/217g		532	24.7	245	11.9	23.7	11.4	3.9
Cheddar & Pickle, Mature, Sainsbury's*	1 Pack/171g		588	27.0	344	14.3	38.7	15.8	7.0
Cheddar & Salad, Mature, Upper Crust*	1 Pack/225g		466	22.1	207	9.5	20.3	9.8	0.0
Cheddar & Tomato, Mature, Big, Sainsbury's*	1 Pack/233g		596	25.6	256	12.9	26.3	11.0	0.0
Cheddar & Tomato, Red, Tesco*	1 Pack/182g		526	31.7	289	9.2	24.0	17.4	1.1
Cheese, Asda*	1 Pack/262g		618	31.4	236	12.2	20.3	12.0	3.0
Cheese, Savoury, Northern Bites*	1 Serving/210g		212	4.0	101	3.6	18.5	1.9	0.0
Cheese, Savoury, Sandwich King*	1 Pack/135g		328	11.2	243	11.6	30.2	8.3	0.0
Cheese & Celery, Shapers, Boots*	1 Pack/181g		288	4.2	159	11.0	24.0	2.3	3.0
Cheese & Coleslaw, Asda*	1 Pack/262g		799	51.4	305	10.1	22.1	19.6	3.3
Cheese & Coleslaw, Classic, Somerfield*	1 Pack/201g		642	40.5	320	11.2	23.4	20.2	3.7
Cheese & Coleslaw, M&S*	1 Pack/186g		498	32.4	268	10.2	17.6	17.4	3.2
Cheese & Coleslaw, Shapers, Boots*	1 Pack/224g		338	4.7	151	11.0	22.0	2.1	3.2

SANDWICH

	Measure INFO/WEIGHT	per Measure KCAL	per Measure FAT	Nutrition Values per 100g / 100ml KCAL	PROT	CARB	FAT	FIBRE
Cheese & Coleslaw, Sutherland*	1 Pack/185g	376	8.3	203	10.7	29.9	4.5	0.0
Cheese & Ham, & Pickle, Co-Op*	1 Serving/185g	370	7.4	200	13.0	27.0	4.0	3.0
Cheese & Ham, & Pickle, Healthy Range, Average	1 Pack/185g	299	5.1	162	13.6	20.6	2.8	2.5
Cheese & Ham, & Pickle, Shapers, Boots*	1 Pack/184g	318	8.5	173	13.0	20.0	4.6	2.5
Cheese & Ham, & Pickle, Simply, Boots*	1 Pack/225g	551	29.2	245	11.0	21.0	13.0	2.4
Cheese & Ham, & Pickle, Tesco*	1 Serving/215g	497	24.7	231	11.7	20.3	11.5	1.8
Cheese & Ham, Baxter & Platts*	1 Pack/168g	408	21.8	243	11.3	20.5	13.0	1.7
Cheese & Ham, Smoked, Co-Op*	1 Pack/167g	334	8.4	200	15.0	24.0	5.0	2.0
Cheese & Marmite, No Mayonnaise, Boots*	1 Pack/156g	420	20.0	269	12.2	26.3	12.8	1.7
Cheese & Onion, Deep Fill, Tesco*	1 Pack/212g	742	51.9	350	12.3	20.2	24.5	1.3
Cheese & Onion, GFY, Asda*	1 Pack/156g	317	4.1	203	14.0	31.0	2.6	2.7
Cheese & Onion, Ginsters*	1 Pack/172g	491	26.8	286	11.1	25.4	15.6	1.8
Cheese & Onion, LC, Tesco*	1 Pack/144g	310	9.4	215	12.7	26.5	6.5	3.6
Cheese & Onion, M&S*	1 Serving/188g	460	24.2	245	11.2	21.3	12.9	2.9
Cheese & Onion, Morrisons*	1 Pack/142g	260	2.4	183	14.1	27.8	1.7	2.9
Cheese & Onion, Reduced Fat, NUME, Morrisons*	1 Pack/142g	348	13.6	245	11.8	26.1	9.6	3.5
Cheese & Onion, Tesco*	1 Pack/178g	573	37.9	322	11.6	21.0	21.3	3.5
Cheese & Onion, Waitrose*	1 Pack/176g	579	38.7	329	12.5	20.2	22.0	2.8
Cheese & Pickle, Shapers, Boots*	1 Pack/165g	342	8.1	207	9.8	31.0	4.9	2.3
Cheese & Pickle, Tesco*	1 Pack/140g	400	19.3	286	12.7	27.8	13.8	1.4
Cheese & Salad, & Reduced Fat Mayo, Waitrose*	1 Pack/180g	301	9.0	167	9.8	20.8	5.0	3.1
Cheese & Salad, Budgens*	1 Pack/169g	250	3.0	148	10.9	21.9	1.8	1.6
Cheese & Salad, COU, M&S*	1 Pack/188g	244	3.0	130	12.1	17.0	1.6	2.4
Cheese & Salad, Shapers, Boots*	1 Pack/205g	308	5.1	150	9.7	22.0	2.5	2.2
Cheese & Salad, Tesco*	1 Serving/188g	429	22.4	228	10.1	20.2	11.9	2.1
Cheese & Spring Onion, Asda*	1 Pack/160g	576	39.9	361	13.0	21.0	25.0	1.9
Cheese & Spring Onion, Co-Op*	1 Pack/164g	607	42.6	370	12.0	21.0	26.0	3.0
Cheese & Spring Onion, Sainsbury's*	1 Serving/177g	605	39.5	342	11.4	24.0	22.3	1.1
Cheese & Tomato, Asda*	1 Pack/154g	388	19.7	252	11.0	23.2	12.8	3.7
Cheese & Tomato, Co-Op*	1 Pack/155g	365	18.5	235	10.6	21.8	11.9	1.9
Cheese & Tomato, Freshmans*	1 Pack/111g	248	18.6	223	11.0	8.0	16.8	0.0
Cheese & Tomato, Organic, M&S*	1 Pack/165g	559	35.3	339	11.8	24.8	21.4	1.9
Cheese & Tomato, Sainsbury's*	1 Pack/216g	542	26.3	251	12.9	22.8	12.2	0.0
Cheese & Tomato, Spar*	1 Pack/124g	294	13.0	237	11.1	24.4	10.5	0.0
Cheese & Tomato, Tesco*	1 Pack/182g	582	38.9	320	9.2	22.6	21.4	1.1
Chicken, & Chorizo, British, Finest, Tesco*	1 Pack/186g	391	12.6	210	15.7	21.2	6.8	2.7
Chicken, & Pesto, Flatbread, Deep, Fuller Longer, M&S*	1 Pack/208g	312	10.2	150	11.9	15.0	4.9	1.4
Chicken, & Salad, Roast, Shapers, Boots*	1 Pack/183g	274	4.4	150	12.0	20.0	2.4	3.4
Chicken, BLT, Taste!*	1 Pack/239g	458	19.8	192	10.3	19.0	8.3	0.0
Chicken, Chargrilled, Malted Bap, Co-Op*	1 Bap/201g	492	26.1	245	9.0	23.0	13.0	2.0
Chicken, Chargrilled, Pitta Pocket, M&S*	1 Pack/208g	279	7.3	134	11.2	14.5	3.5	1.6
Chicken, Coronation, Indulgence, Taste!*	1 Pack/159g	396	18.8	249	9.1	26.5	11.8	0.0
Chicken, Coronation, M&S*	1 Pack/210g	420	20.4	200	11.2	20.2	9.7	3.1
Chicken, Coronation, on Onion Bread, M&S*	1 Pack/260g	520	21.3	200	10.7	20.0	8.2	1.9
Chicken, Coronation, Taste!*	1 Pack/178g	367	13.4	206	10.6	24.0	7.5	0.0
Chicken, Curry, Lifestyle*	1 Serving/160g	211	9.6	132	13.0	6.0	6.0	0.0
Chicken, Mexican, Healthy Choices, Shell*	1 Serving/168g	376	11.8	224	12.2	28.1	7.0	0.0
Chicken, No Mayo, Just Chicken, Tesco*	1 Pack/120g	246	3.8	205	15.9	28.1	3.2	3.8
Chicken, No Mayo, M&S*	1 Pack/142g	248	3.3	175	16.6	20.6	2.3	3.2
Chicken, No Mayo, on Wholemeal, COU, M&S*	1 Pack/153g	260	3.5	170	16.6	20.6	2.3	3.2
Chicken, No Mayonnaise, Waitrose*	1 Pack/173g	332	9.5	192	11.6	24.0	5.5	2.1
Chicken, Roast, Breast, BGTY, Sainsbury's*	1 Pack/174g	275	4.4	158	14.8	20.9	2.5	1.8
Chicken, Roast, Ginsters*	1 Pack/160g	313	10.1	196	13.6	21.2	6.3	2.6

SANDWICH

	Measure INFO/WEIGHT	per Measure KCAL	FAT	Nutrition Values per 100g / 100ml KCAL	PROT	CARB	FAT	FIBRE
Chicken, Roast, Shapers, Boots*	1 Pack/163g	259	2.1	159	16.0	21.0	1.3	2.5
Chicken, Roast, Tesco*	1 Pack/158g	412	19.8	261	13.1	23.9	12.5	1.5
Chicken, Rustlers*	1 Pack/150g	346	14.2	231	16.3	20.1	9.5	0.0
Chicken, Southern Fried, Tesco*	1 Pack/174g	365	13.9	210	9.8	24.2	8.0	1.6
Chicken, Sweet Chilli, Special Edition, Ginsters*	1 Pack/172g	351	9.5	204	12.5	26.3	5.5	2.3
Chicken, Thai, BGTY, Sainsbury's*	1 Pack/196g	280	5.1	143	10.2	19.6	2.6	0.6
Chicken, Tikka, Asda*	1 Pack/186g	316	8.7	170	11.0	21.0	4.7	1.5
Chicken, Tikka, COU, M&S*	1 Pack/185g	268	3.3	145	12.1	20.5	1.8	3.2
Chicken, Tikka, M&S*	1 Pack/180g	391	19.6	217	10.4	19.5	10.9	2.0
Chicken, Tikka, on Pepper Chilli Bread, Shapers, Boots*	1 Pack/172g	296	4.5	172	13.0	25.0	2.6	2.5
Chicken, Triple, Shapers, Boots*	1 Serving/228g	440	12.3	193	13.0	23.0	5.4	2.3
Chicken, with a Mayo Free Dressing, British, COU, M&S*	1 Pack/153g	260	4.1	170	13.4	22.2	2.7	3.0
Chicken, with Mayonnaise, on Thick Softgrain, Tasties*	1 Pack/192g	338	15.2	176	9.5	16.1	7.9	0.0
Chicken & Bacon, & Avocado, M&S*	1 Pack/242g	508	28.3	210	10.7	15.8	11.7	3.2
Chicken & Bacon, & Cheese, Club, M&S*	1 Pack/383g	805	37.2	210	11.9	18.5	9.7	1.9
Chicken & Bacon, & Guacamole, Darwins Deli*	1 Pack/198g	340	16.4	172	3.6	15.9	8.3	1.7
Chicken & Bacon, & Lettuce, No Mayo, LC, Tesco*	1 Pack/186g	326	6.9	175	15.2	19.6	3.7	2.5
Chicken & Bacon, & Salad, Big, Sainsbury's*	1 Pack/249g	610	31.6	245	11.1	21.7	12.7	0.0
Chicken & Bacon, & Tomato, BGTY, Sainsbury's*	1 Pack/190g	270	4.4	142	11.4	19.0	2.3	0.0
Chicken & Bacon, BGTY, Sainsbury's*	1 Pack/211g	315	4.9	149	11.7	20.8	2.3	0.0
Chicken & Bacon, Club, Fully Loaded, Tesco*	1 Pack/257g	580	21.1	225	12.1	24.3	8.2	2.3
Chicken & Bacon, COU, M&S*	1 Pack/179g	250	3.6	140	13.5	15.8	2.0	3.8
Chicken & Bacon, Deep Fill, Ginsters*	1 Pack/200g	435	15.7	224	12.4	25.3	8.1	2.4
Chicken & Bacon, Deep Filled, Co-Op*	1 Pack/166g	556	33.2	335	16.0	23.0	20.0	3.0
Chicken & Bacon, M&S*	1 Pack/185g	509	27.2	275	15.9	20.2	14.7	2.1
Chicken & Bacon, on Oatmeal, Fuller Longer, M&S*	1 Pack/228g	274	10.0	120	10.3	10.3	4.4	6.1
Chicken & Bacon, Roast, Boots*	1 Pack/175g	413	14.0	236	15.4	26.3	8.0	2.2
Chicken & Bacon, Tesco*	1 Pack/195g	486	24.2	249	14.3	20.0	12.4	2.7
Chicken & Bacon, Waitrose*	1 Serving/191g	495	23.5	259	11.8	25.3	12.3	2.2
Chicken & Bacon, with Mayo, Malted Brown, Mattessons*	1 Pack/182g	467	18.5	257	15.1	26.4	10.2	2.2
Chicken & Balsamic Roasted Tomatoes, COU, M&S*	1 Pack/200g	280	4.6	140	11.6	18.1	2.3	2.6
Chicken & Chorizo, & Chipotle Mayonaise, Tesco*	1 Pack/174g	365	13.4	210	12.1	22.7	7.7	2.3
Chicken & Coleslaw, Tesco*	1 Pack/160g	305	7.1	191	12.0	25.7	4.4	2.4
Chicken & Coriander, with Lime, BGTY, Sainsbury's*	1 Pack/168g	282	5.9	168	10.6	23.5	3.5	0.0
Chicken & Ham, & Pepperoni, Meat Feast, Tesco*	1 Pack/196g	470	22.5	240	14.7	19.4	11.5	1.5
Chicken & Ham, Oak Smoked, Big, Sainsbury's*	1 Pack/244g	461	17.6	189	12.3	18.8	7.2	0.0
Chicken & Mayonnaise, Country Harvest*	1 Pack/120g	268	9.0	223	13.1	27.6	7.5	0.0
Chicken & Mayonnaise, Simply, Oldfields*	1 Pack/128g	357	16.4	279	12.8	30.2	12.8	2.1
Chicken & Mayonnaise, The Sandwich Company*	1 Pack/72g	251	10.7	348	17.8	35.9	14.8	0.0
Chicken & Mayonnaise, Wholemeal, Sodhexo*	1 Pack/128g	346	17.4	270	13.1	24.0	13.6	3.6
Chicken & Pesto, Shapers, Boots*	1 Pack/181g	311	4.2	172	12.0	26.0	2.3	1.7
Chicken & Salad, Choice*	1 Pack/174g	285	5.0	164	11.5	22.9	2.9	1.7
Chicken & Salad, Co-Op*	1 Pack/195g	448	21.4	230	10.0	24.0	11.0	2.0
Chicken & Salad, COU, M&S*	1 Pack/194g	262	3.7	135	9.8	19.0	1.9	1.6
Chicken & Salad, Deep Fill, Ginsters*	1 Pack/203g	364	12.4	179	10.3	20.8	6.1	2.1
Chicken & Salad, Deep Filled, Co-Op*	1 Pack/213g	437	19.2	205	10.0	20.0	9.0	1.0
Chicken & Salad, Deep Filled, Tesco*	1 Pack/238g	440	19.5	185	13.1	14.6	8.2	2.8
Chicken & Salad, GFY, Asda*	1 Pack/194g	252	2.9	130	12.0	17.0	1.5	2.6
Chicken & Salad, Ham & Cheese, Twin, Tesco*	1 Pack/189g	434	21.5	230	10.8	21.1	11.4	2.3
Chicken & Salad, Healthy Living, Co-Op*	1 Pack/196g	265	3.5	135	10.4	19.1	1.8	3.9
Chicken & Salad, LC, Tesco*	1 Pack/207g	290	3.9	140	13.9	16.8	1.9	2.7
Chicken & Salad, Low Fat, Waitrose*	1 Pack/188g	291	8.1	155	10.4	18.6	4.3	2.1
Chicken & Salad, M&S*	1 Pack/226g	350	9.3	155	10.6	18.8	4.1	3.0

SANDWICH

INFO/WEIGHT	Measure	per Measure KCAL	FAT	Nutrition Values per 100g / 100ml KCAL	PROT	CARB	FAT	FIBRE
Chicken & Salad, Malted Brown, Wild Bean Cafe*	1 Serving/222g	377	8.4	170	11.7	22.2	3.8	2.0
Chicken & Salad, Roast, BGTY, Sainsbury's*	1 Pack/182g	268	4.0	147	11.9	19.9	2.2	2.7
Chicken & Salad, Roast, COU, M&S*	1 Pack/196g	265	4.5	135	8.9	19.6	2.3	2.2
Chicken & Salad, Roast, LC, Tesco*	1 Pack/194g	300	4.3	155	11.2	22.0	2.2	1.2
Chicken & Salad, Roast, Pick of the Pantry, On A Roll*	1 Pack/225g	293	6.8	130	9.7	16.2	3.0	1.4
Chicken & Salad, Roast, Waitrose*	1 Pack/217g	482	24.1	222	9.4	21.1	11.1	2.0
Chicken & Salad, Sainsbury's*	1 Pack/240g	425	14.2	177	12.1	18.8	5.9	0.0
Chicken & Salad, Tesco*	1 Pack/193g	386	17.6	200	11.9	17.6	9.1	1.5
Chicken & Salad, Waitrose*	1 Pack/208g	406	19.8	195	10.3	17.1	9.5	2.5
Chicken & Salad, with Mayonnaise, BGTY, Sainsbury's*	1 Serving/200g	314	4.8	157	12.0	21.9	2.4	0.0
Chicken & Salad, with Mayonnaise, Woolworths*	1 Serving/183g	337	12.4	184	11.3	19.3	6.8	0.0
Chicken & Salad with Mayo, Roast, Big, Sainsbury's*	1 Pack/269g	559	23.9	208	11.0	20.9	8.9	9.0
Chicken & Stuffing, LC, Tesco*	1 Pack/172g	275	4.8	160	14.4	18.7	2.8	6.9
Chicken & Stuffing, M&S*	1 Pack/166g	398	17.1	240	13.9	23.1	10.3	5.6
Chicken & Stuffing, M&S*	1 Pack/182g	400	12.6	220	13.9	24.5	6.9	2.5
Chicken & Stuffing, Pork Sage & Onion, Tesco*	1 Pack/136g	376	17.0	276	12.1	28.1	12.5	1.4
Chicken & Stuffing, Roast, Boots*	1 Pack/235g	669	39.9	285	12.0	22.0	17.0	1.9
Chicken & Stuffing, Roast, LC, Tesco*	1 Pack/169g	304	3.4	180	14.9	24.6	2.0	1.9
Chicken & Stuffing, Roast, Tesco*	1 Sandwich/200g	450	14.4	225	15.0	24.8	7.2	1.9
Chicken & Stuffing, Shapers, Boots*	1 Serving/185g	327	5.2	177	13.0	25.0	2.8	2.2
Chicken & Stuffing, Tesco*	1 Pack/323g	1043	58.8	323	10.4	29.4	18.2	1.0
Chicken & Stuffing, Waitrose*	1 Pack/183g	450	18.8	246	12.8	25.6	10.3	1.5
Chicken & Sweet Chilli, Flora Light, Flora*	1 Pack/154g	296	5.7	192	13.1	27.0	3.7	1.9
Chicken & Sweetcorn, Eat Well, M&S*	1 Pack/194g	340	10.5	175	11.4	19.6	5.4	3.1
Chicken & Sweetcorn, Shapers, Boots*	1 Pack/180g	324	6.3	180	12.0	25.0	3.5	2.0
Chicken & Sweetcorn, with Mayonnaise, Benedicts*	1 Pack/185g	437	19.8	236	12.2	20.6	10.7	0.0
Chicken & Watercress, COU, M&S*	1 Pack/164g	266	2.8	162	12.8	23.9	1.7	2.1
Chicken Caesar, Malted Brown Bread, Tesco*	1 Pack/186g	410	18.6	220	14.0	17.8	10.0	1.8
Club, New York Style, Sainsbury's*	1 Serving/212g	608	33.5	287	13.3	22.8	15.8	2.7
Corned Beef, on White, Simply, Brambles*	1 Pack/126g	325	10.8	258	14.2	30.8	8.6	1.4
Corned Beef, Tomato & Onion, Salad Garden*	1 Pack/137g	338	14.8	247	14.2	23.0	10.8	0.0
Corned Beef & Onion, White Bap, Open Choice Foods*	1 Bap/144g	331	8.8	230	12.7	30.7	6.1	0.0
Crab, Marie Rose, Brown, Royal London Hospital*	1 Pack/158g	293	11.2	185	9.7	22.0	7.1	0.0
Crayfish & Rocket, Bistro, Waitrose*	1 Pack/193g	422	19.5	219	11.5	20.4	10.1	2.4
Cream Cheese, & Ham, Tesco*	1 Pack/212g	655	36.7	309	11.0	27.2	17.3	1.2
Cream Cheese, & Salad, Choice*	1 Serving/156g	294	7.4	188	7.8	28.1	4.7	0.0
Cumberland Sausage, Ginsters*	1 Pack/210g	564	29.5	268	9.3	26.0	14.0	2.4
Duck, Peking, No Mayo, Boots*	1 Pack/222g	399	10.2	180	7.7	27.0	4.6	1.7
Egg, Co-Op*	1 Pack/190g	285	7.0	150	6.8	22.1	3.7	3.7
Egg & Bacon, & Mayo, Delifresh*	1 Pack/129g	310	12.6	240	10.1	29.7	9.8	2.1
Egg & Bacon, Deep Fill, Ginsters*	1 Pack/216g	503	21.8	233	14.5	21.0	10.1	2.3
Egg & Bacon, Handmade, Tesco*	1 Pack/217g	489	20.4	225	13.4	20.8	9.4	2.0
Egg & Cress, BGTY, Sainsbury's*	1 Pack/145g	268	7.5	185	9.1	25.4	5.2	2.7
Egg & Cress, Co-Op*	1 Pack/159g	398	23.8	250	9.0	21.0	15.0	2.0
Egg & Cress, COU, M&S*	1 Pack/192g	240	5.2	125	9.8	15.5	2.7	2.8
Egg & Cress, Free Range, Co-Op*	1 Pack/154g	370	18.5	240	8.0	25.0	12.0	3.0
Egg & Cress, Free Range, M&S*	1 Pack/192g	307	9.0	160	10.7	17.8	4.7	3.0
Egg & Cress, Free Range, Sainsbury's*	1 Pack/204g	404	16.9	198	10.5	20.3	8.3	3.3
Egg & Cress, Healthy Choice, Somerfield*	1 Pack/150g	234	5.4	156	8.9	22.0	3.6	3.3
Egg & Cress, M&S*	1 Pack/182g	331	17.7	182	10.1	13.6	9.7	3.2
Egg & Cress, No Mayo, LC, Tesco*	1 Pack/160g	280	7.2	175	9.4	23.7	4.5	3.0
Egg & Cress, on Wheat Germ Bread, Tesco*	1 Pack/174g	365	15.8	210	11.0	20.5	9.1	2.1
Egg & Cress, Reduced Fat, Asda*	1 Pack/164g	290	8.7	177	9.8	22.4	5.3	0.0

S

SANDWICH

	Measure INFO/WEIGHT	per Measure KCAL	FAT	Nutrition Values per 100g / 100ml KCAL	PROT	CARB	FAT	FIBRE
Egg & Cress, Reduced Fat, Waitrose*	1 Pack/162g	262	10.4	162	9.7	16.5	6.4	6.4
Egg & Cress, with Mayo, Oatmeal Bread, Heinz*	1 Pack/150g	304	10.8	203	9.6	25.0	7.2	2.7
Egg & Salad, Co-Op*	1 Pack/190g	285	7.6	150	7.0	22.0	4.0	4.0
Egg & Salad, Deep Filled, Asda*	1 Pack/231g	395	16.2	171	8.0	19.0	7.0	1.0
Egg & Salad, Free Range, Sainsbury's*	1 Pack/225g	449	16.8	200	8.5	24.5	7.5	0.0
Egg & Salad, Free Range, Waitrose*	1 Pack/180g	281	11.5	156	7.6	16.9	6.4	3.3
Egg & Salad, GFY, Asda*	1 Pack/157g	229	4.5	146	8.0	22.0	2.9	2.9
Egg & Salad, Shapers, Boots*	1 Pack/184g	304	8.5	165	6.9	24.0	4.6	1.1
Egg & Salad, with Mayonnaise, Wholemeal, Waitrose*	1 Pack/180g	257	8.8	143	8.3	16.5	4.9	3.6
Egg & Tomato, & Salad Cream, M&S*	1 Pack/216g	400	14.9	185	7.4	21.7	6.9	2.3
Egg & Tomato, Delicious, Boots*	1 Pack/218g	362	10.0	166	8.2	22.0	4.6	2.0
Egg & Tomato, Tesco*	1 Pack/172g	311	10.8	181	8.5	22.6	6.3	2.3
Egg & Tomato, with Salad Cream, Big, Sainsbury's*	1 Pack/266g	463	15.4	174	9.1	21.3	5.8	0.0
Egg & Watercress, Bloomer, Freshly Prepared, M&S*	1 Pack/221g	465	26.1	210	10.2	15.3	11.8	3.0
Egg Mayonnaise, & Cress, BHS*	1 Serving/188g	462	23.9	246	10.0	24.7	12.7	1.9
Egg Mayonnaise, & Cress, Co-Op*	1 Serving/159g	405	23.8	255	9.0	21.0	15.0	2.0
Egg Mayonnaise, & Cress, Delicious, Boots*	1 Pack/195g	343	12.3	176	8.7	21.0	6.3	3.9
Egg Mayonnaise, & Cress, Go Simple, Asda*	1 Pack/169g	370	18.6	219	10.0	20.0	11.0	1.7
Egg Mayonnaise, & Cress, on Oatmeal, Somerfield*	1 Pack/149g	346	16.6	232	9.5	23.6	11.1	2.0
Egg Mayonnaise, & Cress, Reduced Fat, Waitrose*	1 Pack/162g	300	12.8	185	10.4	18.1	7.9	3.4
Egg Mayonnaise, & Cress, Shapers, Boots*	1 Pack/156g	292	7.6	187	11.0	25.0	4.9	2.6
Egg Mayonnaise, & Cress, Weight Watchers*	1 Pack/126g	238	4.2	189	8.8	31.1	3.3	3.3
Egg Mayonnaise, & Cress, Wheatgerm Bread, Asda*	1 Pack/158g	371	19.6	235	9.7	21.3	12.4	1.9
Egg Mayonnaise, & Cress, Wholemeal Bread, Oldfields*	1 Pack/128g	301	14.3	235	9.7	24.0	11.2	3.6
Egg Mayonnaise, & Salad, You Count, Love Life, Waitrose*	1 Pack/205g	337	12.5	164	8.4	17.2	6.1	3.0
Egg Mayonnaise, Boots*	1 Pack/184g	448	23.9	244	9.7	22.0	13.0	2.3
Egg Mayonnaise, Deep Fill, Benedicts*	1 Pack/195g	560	21.6	287	9.6	36.3	11.1	0.0
Egg Mayonnaise, Free Range, Asda*	1 Sandwich/178g	311	10.1	175	9.3	21.5	5.7	2.1
Egg Mayonnaise, Free Range, Finest, Tesco*	1 Pack/217g	412	19.1	190	10.9	16.8	8.8	2.3
Egg Mayonnaise, Free Range, on Oatmeal Bread, M&S*	1 Pack/180g	315	12.2	175	9.4	18.2	6.8	2.8
Egg Mayonnaise, on Malted Wheatgrain, Taste!*	1 Serving/169g	394	20.8	233	10.6	20.0	12.3	0.0
Egg Mayonnaise, Simply, Boots*	1 Pack/181g	449	27.2	248	9.2	19.0	15.0	2.9
Egg Mayonnaise, Simply, Ginsters*	1 Serving/163g	365	15.9	224	10.1	24.0	9.8	3.1
Egg Mayonnaise, Waitrose*	1 Pack/180g	396	20.5	220	10.1	19.1	11.4	3.4
Feta Cheese, & Salad, Tastte*	1 Pack/178g	367	13.4	206	10.6	24.0	7.5	0.0
Gammon, & Salad, Tasties*	1 Pack/172g	261	6.0	152	9.6	20.6	3.5	0.0
Goat's Cheese, & Cranberry, Shapers, Boots*	1 Pack/150g	323	6.3	216	8.4	36.0	4.2	2.6
Goat's Cheese, Sunblush Tomato, Deli Continental*	1 Pack/179g	480	29.4	268	9.5	20.5	16.4	0.0
Ham, Just Ham, Shoprite*	1 Pack/148g	286	7.1	193	12.4	25.0	4.8	0.0
Ham, M&S*	1 Pack/200g	220	5.2	110	17.2	3.2	2.6	0.0
Ham, No Mayo, Just Ham, Tesco*	1 Pack/122g	250	4.9	205	11.6	30.4	4.0	2.1
Ham & Cheese, & Mayo, Brown Bread, Mattessons*	1 Pack/172g	439	18.1	255	13.8	27.0	10.5	2.2
Ham & Cheese, & Pickle, Average	1 Pack/220g	524	25.1	238	12.2	21.6	11.4	2.5
Ham & Cheese, & Pickle, BGTY, Sainsbury's*	1 Sandwich/198g	325	5.0	164	14.0	21.3	2.5	2.1
Ham & Cheese, & Pickle, Deep Fill, Tesco*	1 Pack/225g	495	20.7	220	14.6	19.4	9.2	2.4
Ham & Cheese, & Pickle, in a Soft Wrap, Sainsbury's*	1 Pack/195g	503	23.2	258	10.9	26.8	11.9	0.9
Ham & Cheese, & Pickle, Leicester, Waitrose*	1 Pack/205g	512	24.4	250	11.9	23.7	11.9	2.1
Ham & Cheese, & Pickle, Platter, M&S*	1 Sandwich/224g	582	33.4	260	11.9	19.3	14.9	5.3
Ham & Cheese, & Salad, Pick of the Pantry, On A Roll*	1 Pack/228g	431	22.6	189	10.9	13.5	9.9	2.6
Ham & Cheese, Ginsters*	1 Sandwich/170g	434	20.9	256	14.1	22.1	12.3	2.5
Ham & Cheese, LC, Tesco*	1 Pack/158g	284	5.1	180	14.5	22.8	3.2	5.0
Ham & Cheese, Morrisons*	1 Serving/183g	273	4.6	149	12.5	19.2	2.5	4.1
Ham & Cheese, Pickle & Lettuce, No Mayo, Tesco*	1 Pack/207g	435	16.2	210	12.2	23.0	7.8	2.7

SANDWICH

INFO/WEIGHT	Measure	per Measure		Nutrition Values per 100g / 100ml				
		KCAL	FAT	KCAL	PROT	CARB	FAT	FIBRE
Ham & Coleslaw, Smoked, Brambles*	1 Pack/166g	283	4.1	171	8.2	28.8	2.5	1.8
Ham & Mustard, Dijon, Healthy Selection, Budgens*	1 Pack/120g	190	3.0	158	9.7	21.9	2.5	2.0
Ham & Mustard, Ginsters*	1 Pack/140g	307	9.4	219	11.8	28.0	6.7	2.5
Ham & Mustard, Heinz*	1 Pack/180g	460	20.7	255	11.8	25.6	11.5	5.0
Ham & Mustard, Mayo, on White, Urban Eat*	1 Pack/130g	299	11.2	230	11.0	27.2	8.6	1.4
Ham & Mustard, Salad, BGTY, Sainsbury's*	1 Pack/183g	261	3.8	143	8.7	22.4	2.1	2.6
Ham & Mustard, Smoked, on Oatmeal, Sainsbury's*	1 Pack/154g	275	8.1	179	11.9	20.8	5.3	3.0
Ham & Mustard, Smoked, Tesco*	1 Pack/131g	315	11.4	240	11.5	28.0	8.7	1.4
Ham & Mustard, Somerfield*	1 Pack/144g	301	11.7	209	10.9	24.8	8.1	1.9
Ham & Mustard, Tesco*	1 Pack/147g	437	27.9	297	10.6	20.8	19.0	1.2
Ham & Mustard, Wiltshire, The Ultimate, M&S*	1 Sandwich/246g	344	11.8	140	9.8	15.0	4.8	1.4
Ham & Philadelphia Light, Dry Cured, Boots*	1 Pack/172g	339	9.3	197	12.8	24.4	5.4	2.5
Ham & Pickle, Simple, EAT*	1 Pack/233g	354	11.6	152	7.3	20.5	5.0	1.6
Ham & Salad, Bap, Co-Op*	1 Bap/164g	295	4.9	180	8.0	30.0	3.0	2.0
Ham & Salad, British, COU, M&S*	1 Pack/204g	255	4.3	125	6.7	19.9	2.1	2.9
Ham & Salad, Foo-Go*	1 Pack/178g	297	7.1	167	9.8	22.9	4.0	0.0
Ham & Salad, Fulfilled*	1 Serving/183g	288	6.4	157	11.8	19.6	3.5	0.0
Ham & Salad, Ginsters*	1 Pack/179g	287	6.2	160	8.8	23.6	3.4	0.0
Ham & Salad, Healthy, Spar*	1 Serving/181g	286	6.7	158	8.4	22.7	3.7	0.0
Ham & Salad, Leicester, Waitrose*	1 Serving/187g	325	9.0	174	8.6	24.0	4.8	1.6
Ham & Salad, Select*	1 Serving/180g	266	4.7	148	8.0	23.2	2.6	0.0
Ham & Salad, Shapers, Boots*	1 Pack/195g	269	2.7	138	9.4	22.0	1.4	1.8
Ham & Salad, Smoked, Taste!*	1 Serving/188g	309	9.7	164	9.8	19.8	5.2	0.0
Ham & Salad, Wild Bean Cafe*	1 Pack/212g	301	5.5	142	10.7	18.8	2.6	2.0
Ham & Salad, with Mustard, Finest, Tesco*	1 Pack/200g	466	21.0	233	15.3	19.3	10.5	1.3
Ham & Soft Cheese, Tesco*	1 Serving/164g	333	12.1	203	11.6	22.5	7.4	2.2
Ham & Swiss Cheese, M&S*	1 Pack/159g	393	20.0	247	14.7	18.9	12.6	3.3
Ham & Tomato, & Lettuce, Oldfields*	1 Pack/216g	393	17.5	182	12.3	19.0	8.1	3.5
Ham & Tomato, Brambles*	1 Pack/159g	288	7.3	181	11.1	24.1	4.6	3.3
Ham & Tomato, GFY, Asda*	1 Pack/173g	254	2.9	147	10.0	23.0	1.7	1.4
Ham & Tomato, Honey Roast, Feel Good, Shell*	1 Pack/171g	388	18.8	227	9.8	22.1	11.0	0.0
Ham & Turkey, & Salad, Sutherland*	1 Pack/185g	303	4.8	164	9.8	25.2	2.6	0.0
Ham & Turkey, Asda*	1 Pack/190g	393	19.4	207	12.9	15.8	10.2	2.3
Ham & Turkey, with Salad, Co-Op*	1 Serving/181g	290	5.4	160	10.0	24.0	3.0	3.0
Houmous, & Carrot, Shapers, Boots*	1 Pack/204g	323	10.2	158	7.5	21.0	5.0	5.2
Houmous, & Crunchy Salad, Oldfields*	1 Pack/180g	256	7.6	142	6.3	20.0	4.2	0.0
Houmous, Salad, in Flatbread, Sainsbury's*	1 Pack/177g	313	11.0	177	5.5	24.7	6.2	3.3
Houmungously Crunchy, Cranks*	1 Pack/199g	353	14.2	177	5.6	21.3	7.1	2.8
It's The Slaw, Cranks*	1 Pack/155g	465	26.2	300	8.6	27.4	16.9	1.9
King Prawn, & Avocado, Finest, Tesco*	1 Pack/185g	370	16.6	200	9.1	19.6	9.0	2.5
King Prawn, & Wild Rocket, Honduran, M&S*	1 Serving/196g	450	23.9	230	9.4	20.3	12.2	1.4
King Prawn, Sainsbury's*	1 Pack/204g	424	16.3	208	11.6	22.3	8.0	0.0
Mozzarella, & Roast Vegetables, Felix Van Den Berghe*	1 Pack/158g	330	13.3	209	9.5	23.8	8.4	0.0
Mozzarella, & Tomato, Waitrose*	1 Pack/193g	359	18.1	186	9.7	15.7	9.4	2.3
Mozzarella, & Tomato Calzone, Waitrose*	1 Pack/175g	410	19.4	234	10.8	22.7	11.1	2.2
Mozzarella, Tomato, & Basil, Healthy Options, Oldfields*	1 Pack/175g	285	8.4	163	8.1	22.1	4.8	3.3
New York Deli, Extra Special, Asda*	1 Pack/201g	403	15.4	201	12.4	20.6	7.7	3.8
Philadelphia Light, with Roasted Peppers, LC, Tesco*	1 Pack/179g	304	7.0	170	6.4	27.2	3.9	2.8
Pitta, Falafel, Houmous & Salad, Benedicts*	1 Pack/220g	405	13.0	184	6.8	26.1	5.9	0.0
Ploughman's, Cheddar, Mature Vintage, Sainsbury's*	1 Pack/204g	439	20.2	215	9.3	22.3	9.9	0.0
Ploughman's, Cheddar Cheese, Deep Fill, Asda*	1 Pack/229g	471	22.9	206	9.0	20.0	10.0	4.3
Ploughman's, Cheese, Deep Fill, Ginsters*	1 Pack/213g	491	24.2	231	8.4	23.8	11.4	2.2
Ploughman's, Wiltshire Ham & Cheddar, Bloomer, M&S*	1 Pack/185g	490	22.9	265	12.7	25.4	12.4	1.7

S

SANDWICH

INFO/WEIGHT	Measure KCAL	FAT	KCAL	PROT	CARB	FAT	FIBRE
Pork, & Apple Sauce, Bells*	1 Pack/180g	341	8.1	190	11.5	26.1	4.5	0.0
Prawn, Crayfish & Rocket, Tesco*	1 Pack/193g	425	17.4	220	11.4	22.3	9.0	2.0
Prawn, Marie Rose, Waitrose*	1 Pack/164g	226	5.6	138	8.8	18.0	3.4	1.9
Prawn, Salad, COU, M&S*	1 Pack/200g	230	3.6	115	8.0	16.6	1.8	3.8
Prawn & Salmon, Waitrose*	1 Pack/154g	345	14.6	224	12.5	22.0	9.5	2.8
Prawn Cocktail, Classic, Heinz*	1 Pack/193g	409	16.8	212	8.4	25.0	8.7	2.5
Prawn Cocktail, Platter, M&S*	1 Sandwich/200g	460	25.6	230	8.1	22.3	12.8	2.2
Prawn Cocktail, Waitrose*	1 Pack/196g	300	8.0	153	8.3	20.7	4.1	2.5
Prawn Mayonnaise, Co-Op*	1 Pack/154g	285	6.0	185	9.7	27.3	3.9	3.2
Prawn Mayonnaise, COU, M&S*	1 Pack/155g	240	3.6	155	10.2	22.9	2.3	2.8
Prawn Mayonnaise, GFY, Asda*	1 Pack/160g	251	4.5	157	10.0	23.0	2.8	2.8
Prawn Mayonnaise, Ginsters*	1 Pack/160g	397	21.1	248	9.1	23.3	13.2	2.4
Prawn Mayonnaise, Healthy Living, Co-Op*	1 Pack/154g	246	3.5	160	10.0	24.0	2.3	3.0
Prawn Mayonnaise, M&S*	1 Pack/156g	328	12.0	210	10.0	24.7	7.7	2.2
Prawn Mayonnaise, Morrisons*	1 Pack/157g	234	3.9	149	9.0	22.7	2.5	3.0
Prawn Mayonnaise, Nutritionally Balanced, M&S*	1 Pack/162g	300	10.7	185	10.2	21.2	6.6	1.9
Prawn Mayonnaise, Oatmeal Bread, Co-Op*	1 Pack/159g	445	22.3	280	11.0	28.0	14.0	2.0
Prawn Mayonnaise, Oatmeal Bread, Waitrose*	1 Pack/180g	463	27.0	257	10.2	20.4	15.0	3.2
Prawn Mayonnaise, Sainsbury's*	1 Pack/151g	323	14.0	214	11.6	20.9	9.3	0.0
Prawn Mayonnaise, Shapers, Boots*	1 Pack/160g	293	7.5	183	9.4	25.6	4.7	2.5
Prawn Mayonnaise, Tesco*	1 Pack/143g	300	9.7	210	11.6	25.3	6.8	1.8
Prawn Mayonnaise, Triple, Asda*	1 Pack/248g	635	39.7	256	9.0	19.0	16.0	3.4
Prawn Mayonnaise on Oatmeal Bread, Fulfilled*	1 Pack/144g	393	19.9	273	12.7	24.3	13.8	0.0
Prawn Mayonnaise on Oatmeal Bread, Sainsbury's*	1 Pack/150g	285	9.3	190	10.1	22.3	6.2	2.4
Rib, BBQ, Pork, Rustlers*	1 Pack/170g	459	22.1	270	14.3	22.9	13.0	2.0
Rokafeta, Cranks*	1 Pack/185g	377	18.1	204	6.9	21.1	9.8	1.9
Salad, Simply, Shapers, Boots*	1 Pack/216g	300	6.3	139	5.2	23.0	2.9	1.8
Salad, Taste!*	1 Serving/200g	246	6.5	123	4.4	18.9	3.2	0.0
Salmon, Poached, Prawn & Rocket, Waitrose*	1 Pack/166g	308	8.6	186	11.2	23.5	5.2	2.1
Salmon, Smoked, Daily Bread*	1 Pack/122g	296	10.6	243	13.5	28.0	8.7	0.0
Salmon & Black Pepper, Smoked, Fulfilled*	1 Pack/120g	293	10.3	244	13.8	29.0	8.6	0.0
Salmon & Cream Cheese, Smoked, M&S*	1 Pack/184g	450	22.4	245	12.7	20.8	12.2	1.8
Salmon & Cucumber, Brown Bread, Waitrose*	1 Pack/150g	296	10.6	197	10.5	22.7	7.1	1.4
Salmon & Cucumber, LC, Tesco*	1 Pack/178g	330	5.7	185	10.1	26.8	3.2	2.3
Salmon & Cucumber, M&S*	1 Pack/168g	329	13.9	196	11.0	19.5	8.3	2.6
Salmon & Cucumber, Malted Bread, BGTY, Sainsbury's*	1 Pack/189g	305	5.7	161	9.2	24.3	3.0	2.3
Salmon & Cucumber, Red, BGTY, Sainsbury's*	1 Pack/192g	278	4.4	145	9.4	21.7	2.3	2.4
Salmon & Cucumber, Red, Tesco*	1 Pack/144g	284	9.2	197	11.1	23.8	6.4	1.9
Salmon & Cucumber, Red, Wild, Eat Well, M&S*	1 Pack/208g	385	14.4	185	10.7	18.0	6.9	3.3
Salmon & Cucumber, White Bread, Waitrose*	1 Pack/161g	305	8.6	189	9.8	25.5	5.3	1.7
Salmon & Cucumber, with Dill, Pick of the Pantry, On A Roll*	1 Pack/185g	320	12.0	173	9.9	18.5	6.5	1.7
Salmon & Rocket, Poached, M&S*	1 Pack/180g	495	26.8	275	13.5	21.2	14.9	2.1
Salmon & Soft Cheese, Smoked, Sainsbury's*	1 Pack/165g	383	15.2	232	11.9	25.1	9.2	2.4
Salmon & Soft Cheese, Smoked, Waitrose*	1 Pack/154g	300	10.0	195	14.8	19.2	6.5	4.2
Salmon & Spinach, Poached, Shapers, Boots*	1 Pack/168g	284	7.6	169	9.2	23.0	4.5	3.1
Salmon & Watercress, Poached, Lochmuir, M&S*	1 Pack/192g	355	11.7	185	10.3	22.3	6.1	1.6
Sausage, Speedy Snacks*	1 Serving/93g	258	9.4	279	11.6	35.2	10.2	0.0
Sausage & Egg, Wedge, Tesco*	1 Pack/269g	699	38.7	260	9.1	23.6	14.4	1.1
Seafood Cocktail, Asda*	1 Pack/190g	486	30.0	256	6.7	21.3	15.8	1.6
Seafood Cocktail, Waitrose*	1 Pack/210g	267	6.3	127	7.3	17.6	3.0	8.1
Spicy Falafel & Houmous Salad, Delifresh*	1 Pack/209g	429	19.7	205	6.1	24.0	9.4	2.6
Spinach Feta, Amy's Kitchen*	1 Roll/128g	262	9.0	205	8.6	27.0	7.0	2.3
Steak, Hot, M&S*	1 Roll/190g	513	15.2	270	11.9	37.0	8.0	3.2

SANDWICH

INFO/WEIGHT	Measure KCAL	FAT	KCAL	PROT	CARB	FAT	FIBRE
Sub, Beef & Onion, M&S*							
1 Pack/207g	611	31.7	295	13.3	25.6	15.3	1.5
Sub, Beef & Onion, Roast, Sainsbury's*							
1 Serving/174g	426	17.4	245	9.4	29.3	10.0	0.0
Sub, Chicken, & Salad, Asda*							
1 Sub/200g	460	27.2	230	9.4	17.4	13.6	0.9
Sub, Chicken & Bacon, Sainsbury's*							
1 Pack/190g	554	27.0	291	13.4	27.4	14.2	0.8
Tuna, Healthy Options, Spar*							
1 Pack/150g	268	3.6	179	14.3	24.9	2.4	0.0
Tuna, Mediterranean, COU, M&S*							
1 Pack/260g	364	5.7	140	10.3	19.6	2.2	1.6
Tuna, Nicoise, Taste!*							
1 Pack/218g	404	14.4	185	11.3	20.1	6.6	0.0
Tuna & Cucumber, BGTY, Sainsbury's*							
1 Pack/178g	268	3.2	151	11.3	22.3	1.8	3.1
Tuna & Cucumber, Co-Op*							
1 Serving/268g	510	13.4	190	12.0	25.0	5.0	2.0
Tuna & Cucumber, Finest, Tesco*							
1 Pack/169g	380	16.7	225	10.2	23.4	9.9	2.7
Tuna & Cucumber, Healthy Living, Co-Op*							
1 Pack/192g	250	3.5	130	10.9	17.9	1.8	3.0
Tuna & Cucumber, Less Than 350 Cals, Ginsters*							
1 Serving/193g	298	7.5	154	10.8	19.0	3.9	3.1
Tuna & Cucumber, on a Roll, M&S*							
1 Roll/160g	320	12.0	200	11.8	21.6	7.5	3.2
Tuna & Cucumber, on Malted Wheatgrain, Ginsters*							
1 Pack/175g	318	7.5	182	14.1	21.8	4.3	0.0
Tuna & Cucumber, On Oatmeal Bread, Ginsters*							
1 Pack/175g	290	7.2	166	11.7	20.7	4.1	2.4
Tuna & Cucumber, PB, Waitrose*							
1 Pack/178g	240	3.6	135	11.0	18.3	2.0	3.6
Tuna & Cucumber, Weight Watchers*							
1 Pack/173g	279	2.9	161	11.4	25.1	1.7	1.4
Tuna & Cucumber, You Count, Love Life, Waitrose*							
1 Pack/195g	321	5.3	165	13.0	21.4	2.7	1.4
Tuna & Lemon Mayo, Shapers, Boots*							
1 Pack/206g	318	9.7	154	10.0	18.0	4.7	1.7
Tuna & Salad, Classic*							
1 Pack/230g	449	15.9	195	8.7	27.3	6.9	2.1
Tuna & Sweetcorn, BGTY, Sainsbury's*							
1 Pack/187g	309	5.1	165	10.8	24.7	2.7	2.8
Tuna & Sweetcorn, COU, M&S*							
1 Pack/180g	270	4.3	150	12.6	19.0	2.4	3.8
Tuna & Sweetcorn, Ginsters*							
1 Pack/169g	348	11.4	205	9.6	26.4	6.7	2.4
Tuna & Sweetcorn, Malted Bap, Co-Op*							
1 Bap/212g	530	27.6	250	9.0	24.0	13.0	2.0
Tuna & Sweetcorn, on Malt Bread, Tesco*							
1 Pack/175g	350	8.2	200	11.6	27.5	4.7	2.2
Tuna & Sweetcorn, Sainsbury's*							
1 Pack/183g	392	15.6	214	12.1	22.3	8.5	0.0
Tuna & Tomato, & Onion, COU, M&S*							
1 Pack/177g	250	4.2	141	11.1	18.8	2.4	2.2
Tuna Mayonnaise, & Cucumber, Classic*							
1 Serving/185g	429	22.8	232	10.6	19.8	12.3	0.0
Tuna Mayonnaise, & Cucumber, Daily Bread*							
1 Pack/190g	392	16.6	206	12.1	19.8	8.7	0.0
Tuna Mayonnaise, & Cucumber, Darwins Deli*							
1 Pack/155g	370	14.6	239	9.6	21.9	9.4	0.0
Tuna Mayonnaise, & Cucumber, Finest, Tesco*							
1 Pack/225g	484	19.1	215	11.6	23.1	8.5	1.7
Tuna Mayonnaise, & Cucumber, Simply, Boots*							
1 Pack/200g	498	26.0	249	12.0	21.0	13.0	2.4
Tuna Mayonnaise, & Salad, Serious About Sandwiches*							
1 Pack/192g	305	9.0	159	8.6	20.5	4.7	2.9
Tuna Mayonnaise, & Sweetcorn, Whistlestop*							
1 Pack/140g	378	17.7	271	13.6	25.5	12.7	0.0
Tuna Mayonnaise, Menu, Boots*							
1 Pack/182g	451	20.0	248	13.0	23.0	11.0	1.1
Tuna Mayonnaise, on White Bread, Oldfields*							
1 Pack/142g	394	18.1	278	15.2	27.4	12.8	2.0
Tuna Mayonnaise, White Bread, Open Choice Foods*							
1 Pack/120g	298	10.1	248	12.0	29.6	8.4	0.0
Turkey, Gibsons*							
1 Pack/138g	260	5.3	188	12.5	26.0	3.8	0.0
Turkey, Just Turkey, White Bread, Sandwich King*							
1 Serving/135g	317	7.0	235	17.3	29.7	5.2	0.0
Turkey, Lettuce & Tomato, Shapers, Boots*							
1 Pack/217g	310	4.8	143	9.8	21.0	2.2	2.9
Turkey, with All the Christmas Trimmings, Tesco*							
1 Pack/189g	425	14.2	225	10.8	28.0	7.5	1.9
Turkey & Bacon, COU, M&S*							
1 Pack/165g	256	4.0	155	12.0	21.0	2.4	1.7
Turkey & Cranberry, COU, M&S*							
1 Pack/180g	279	3.1	155	12.1	22.8	1.7	2.9
Turkey & Cranberry Salad, Fullfillers*							
1 Serving/180g	319	5.8	177	13.0	23.3	3.2	0.0
Turkey & Salad, Brambles*							
1 Pack/170g	248	2.0	146	9.3	24.5	1.2	2.0
Turkey & Salad, Fullfillers*							
1 Serving/218g	320	7.0	147	10.3	18.6	3.2	0.0
Turkey & Salad, Healthy Eating, Wild Bean Cafe*							
1 Serving/230g	315	2.5	137	10.0	21.5	1.1	1.8
Turkey & Stuffing, & Cranberry, Boots*							
1 Pack/192g	328	2.1	171	12.0	28.0	1.1	2.5
Turkey & Stuffing, M&S*							
1 Pack/190g	352	9.3	185	12.3	23.1	4.9	1.9
Veggie Threesome, Cranks*							
1 Pack/227g	500	20.5	220	9.0	24.3	9.0	3.0
Wensleydale & Carmelised Carrot Chutney, Brambles*							
1 Pack/181g	445	21.5	246	10.8	24.4	11.9	1.9
Wensleydale & Carrot, M&S*							
1 Pack/183g	430	22.5	235	9.9	21.4	12.3	2.8

SANDWICH FILLER

Food	Measure INFO/WEIGHT	per Measure KCAL	per Measure FAT	Nutrition Values per 100g / 100ml KCAL	PROT	CARB	FAT	FIBRE
Beef & Onion, Deli, Asda*	1 Serving/50g	78	6.5	157	10.0	0.1	13.0	1.1
Big Breakfast, Asda*	1 Serving/125g	314	26.2	251	12.0	3.5	21.0	0.5
Cajun Chicken, Sainsbury's*	1 Serving/60g	109	8.1	182	13.4	1.8	13.5	1.8
Cheese & Ham, Sainsbury's*	1 Serving/25g	124	12.3	497	12.4	0.8	49.3	0.3
Cheese & Onion, 35% Less Fat, CBY, Asda*	1 Serving/50g	122	9.8	244	12.8	3.5	19.6	1.2
Cheese & Onion, CBY, Asda*	1 Serving/60g	214	19.7	356	11.3	3.0	32.8	1.8
Cheese & Onion, Deli, Asda*	1 Serving/57g	217	21.1	381	10.0	2.0	37.0	2.0
Cheese & Onion, Reduced Fat, Supermarket, Average	1 Serving/100g	227	18.1	227	11.8	4.4	18.1	1.7
Cheese & Onion, Sainsbury's*	1 Tub/200g	632	59.6	316	8.7	3.2	29.8	2.2
Cheese & Onion, Supermarket, Average	1 Serving/100g	405	38.6	405	10.2	4.1	38.6	1.3
Cheese & Onion, Tesco*	1 Pack/170g	721	72.4	424	10.0	0.2	42.6	1.5
Cheese & Spring Onion, M&S*	1 Serving/56g	199	18.8	355	8.5	5.0	33.6	0.2
Chicken, Bacon & Sweetcorn, BGTY, Sainsbury's*	1 Tub/300g	399	18.3	133	14.0	5.5	6.1	0.5
Chicken, Stuffing & Bacon, COU, M&S*	1 Pack/170g	170	3.7	100	13.1	6.2	2.2	1.3
Chicken, Sweetcorn & Bacon, Tesco*	1 Serving/50g	167	14.8	334	12.3	4.3	29.7	1.6
Chicken, Tomato & Sweetcure Bacon, M&S*	1 Pot/170g	502	44.9	295	11.4	2.8	26.4	0.7
Chicken & Bacon with Sweetcorn, Sainsbury's*	1 Serving/60g	123	9.4	205	12.0	4.0	15.7	0.9
Chicken & Stuffing, Sainsbury's*	½ Tub/120g	397	37.8	331	6.5	5.3	31.5	1.7
Chicken & Sweetcorn, Sainsbury's*	1 Tub/170g	396	33.7	233	11.0	2.7	19.8	1.9
Chicken Caesar, BGTY, Sainsbury's*	½ Jar/85g	117	6.1	137	15.6	2.5	7.2	2.2
Chicken Fajita, Tesco*	1 Serving/50g	78	4.2	155	13.8	5.9	8.5	1.4
Chicken Tikka, BGTY, Sainsbury's*	½ Pot/85g	99	2.6	117	16.5	6.0	3.0	1.0
Chicken Tikka, Mild, Heinz*	1 Serving/52g	102	7.3	196	5.2	12.3	14.0	0.7
Chunky Egg & Smoked Ham, Tesco*	1 Serving/100g	234	20.7	234	11.8	0.2	20.7	0.3
Chunky Seafood Cocktail, Tesco*	1 Serving/100g	308	27.8	308	6.0	8.3	27.8	2.0
Coronation Chicken, 50 % Less Fat, Tesco*	1 Serving/50g	102	6.3	205	11.5	9.7	12.6	2.7
Coronation Chicken, BGTY, Sainsbury's*	1 Portion/50g	73	3.5	146	11.9	8.9	7.0	1.4
Coronation Chicken, Sainsbury's*	¼ Tub/60g	183	14.8	305	12.1	8.9	24.6	1.2
Coronation Chicken, Somerfield*	1 Serving/85g	326	29.3	383	8.4	9.7	34.5	0.8
Coronation Chicken, Tesco*	1 Tbsp/30g	84	6.5	279	14.7	6.1	21.8	0.7
Coronation Tuna, BGTY, Sainsbury's*	1 Can/80g	90	2.1	112	16.5	5.7	2.6	1.0
Egg & Bacon, Fresh, Tesco*	1 Serving/45g	112	9.0	248	12.7	4.2	20.1	0.6
Egg Mayonnaise, & Bacon, Free Range, Co-Op*	1 Pot/200g	500	44.0	250	13.0	0.9	22.0	0.6
Egg Mayonnaise, 50% Less Fat, CBY, Asda*	1 Serving/50g	67	4.2	134	10.3	4.2	8.3	0.5
Egg Mayonnaise, 50% Less Fat, Tesco*	1 Serving/50g	65	3.8	130	10.2	3.8	7.6	0.5
Egg Mayonnaise, BGTY, Sainsbury's*	1 Serving/63g	71	4.1	113	10.2	3.4	6.5	0.1
Egg Mayonnaise, Chunky Free Range, Tesco*	1 Serving/50g	104	8.9	209	11.3	0.9	17.8	1.6
Egg Mayonnaise, Country Fresh, Aldi*	¼ Pack/50g	106	8.9	211	9.8	2.9	17.8	0.0
Egg Mayonnaise, Deli, Asda*	1 Serving/50g	114	10.0	227	11.0	0.8	20.0	0.3
Egg Mayonnaise, Deli, Somerfield*	1 Serving/40g	120	11.7	301	9.7	0.2	29.2	0.0
Egg Mayonnaise, Free Range, Co-Op*	1 Pack/200g	260	17.6	130	10.1	2.4	8.8	0.5
Egg Mayonnaise, M&S*	1oz/28g	62	5.5	220	10.1	0.8	19.7	1.1
Egg Mayonnaise, Morrisons*	1 Serving/50g	71	5.3	142	10.0	1.7	10.6	0.0
Egg Mayonnaise, Tesco*	1 Serving/50g	100	7.8	199	10.9	3.5	15.6	0.5
Peppered Mackerel, Creamy, Shippam*	1 Serving/15g	27	2.8	177	7.8	6.5	18.6	0.0
Poached Salmon & Cucumber, Deli, M&S*	1 Pot/170g	348	27.7	205	14.0	1.0	16.3	0.5
Prawn Marie Rose, Sainsbury's*	1 Serving/60g	121	10.6	201	8.1	2.5	17.6	0.9
Prawn Mayonnaise, Deli, Asda*	1 Serving/50g	170	16.5	339	9.0	1.6	33.0	0.4
Prawn Mayonnaise, GFY, Asda*	1 Serving/57g	101	7.4	177	12.0	3.0	13.0	0.1
Prawn Mayonnaise, M&S*	½ Pack/170g	502	47.6	295	10.6	0.6	28.0	0.3
Prawn Mayonnaise, Waitrose*	1 Pot/170g	537	52.9	316	8.9	0.2	31.1	0.0
Roast Beef, Onion & Horseradish, Sainsbury's*	1 Serving/100g	372	36.8	372	6.4	3.7	36.8	1.2
Roast Chicken & Stuffing, Sainsbury's*	1 Serving/100g	424	41.5	424	10.8	1.9	41.5	1.2

SANDWICH FILLER	Measure INFO/WEIGHT	per Measure KCAL	FAT	Nutrition Values per 100g / 100ml KCAL	PROT	CARB	FAT	FIBRE
Seafood Cocktail, M&S*	1oz/28g	76	6.7	272	6.4	8.2	23.8	0.2
Seafood Cocktail, Sainsbury's*	½ Tub/120g	314	27.6	262	5.7	8.1	23.0	1.0
Smoked Salmon & Soft Cheese, M&S*	1 Pack/170g	450	40.6	265	11.1	4.9	23.9	0.0
Tex-Mex Chicken, Tesco*	1 Pack/250g	255	2.2	102	12.3	11.2	0.9	1.2
Tuna & Sweetcorn, 30% Less Fat, CBY, Asda*	1 Serving/100g	131	7.1	131	10.3	6.0	7.1	0.7
Tuna & Sweetcorn, Deli, Asda*	1 Serving/50g	148	13.0	296	12.0	3.4	26.0	1.4
Tuna & Sweetcorn, Deli Filler, Sainsbury's*	¼ Pack/58g	105	7.5	183	9.7	6.1	13.1	1.2
Tuna & Sweetcorn, M&S*	1oz/28g	70	5.8	250	14.2	2.3	20.7	1.3
Tuna & Sweetcorn, Morrisons*	1 Tub/170g	382	28.4	225	15.3	7.0	16.7	3.4
Tuna & Sweetcorn, Reduced Fat, Supermarket, Average	1 Serving/100g	119	5.4	119	11.5	5.8	5.4	1.2
Tuna & Sweetcorn, Reduced Fat, Tesco*	1 Serving/100g	140	6.3	140	11.4	8.0	6.3	0.8
Tuna & Sweetcorn, Supermarket, Average	1 Serving/100g	228	17.8	228	11.6	5.7	17.8	1.4
Tuna & Sweetcorn, Tesco*	1 Serving/54g	127	9.8	235	8.6	8.1	18.1	0.6
Tuna & Sweetcorn with Salad Vegetables, Heinz*	1oz/28g	53	3.7	191	5.8	12.1	13.2	0.7
Tuna Mayonnaise, BGTY, Sainsbury's*	1 Serving/100g	114	3.4	114	17.6	3.5	3.4	0.1
Tuna Mayonnaise & Cucumber, Choice, Tesco*	1 Serving/200g	463	22.8	232	12.8	23.2	11.4	1.6
SANDWICH FILLING								
Baked Beans, Paste, British Classics, Princes*	1 Jar/75g	82	0.3	110	5.0	21.6	0.4	0.0
Cheese & Onion, Co-Op*	1 Serving/56g	269	26.3	480	10.0	4.0	47.0	0.5
Cheese & Onion, GFY, Asda*	1 Serving/80g	206	16.8	257	11.0	6.0	21.0	0.8
Chicken & Bacon, Asda*	1 Serving/100g	341	29.0	341	17.0	3.0	29.0	0.5
Chicken & Sweetcorn, Asda*	1 Serving/60g	187	16.8	312	11.0	4.0	28.0	2.0
Chicken Tikka, Asda*	1 Serving/28g	80	5.6	284	13.0	13.0	20.0	0.7
Chicken Tikka, Less Than 5% Fat, Asda*	1 Serving/56g	65	2.6	116	11.0	7.3	4.7	1.2
Crab, BGTY, Sainsbury's*	1oz/28g	36	2.0	128	8.7	7.6	7.0	0.5
Egg Mayonnaise, Asda*	1oz/28g	72	6.5	258	10.3	1.9	23.3	0.7
Egg Mayonnaise, Co-Op*	1oz/28g	66	5.9	235	10.0	1.0	21.0	1.0
Egg Mayonnaise, with Chives, Asda*	1oz/28g	92	8.9	327	9.1	1.1	31.8	0.0
Prawns with Seafood Sauce, Asda*	1oz/28g	107	10.3	382	11.7	1.4	36.8	0.0
Sausage & Tomato, Paste, British Classics, Princes*	1 Jar/75g	163	11.1	217	14.6	6.3	14.8	0.0
Tuna & Sweetcorn, Asda*	1oz/28g	83	7.4	295	8.2	6.0	26.5	0.6
Tuna & Sweetcorn, Reduced Fat, Co-Op*	1 Serving/50g	102	7.0	205	13.0	7.0	14.0	0.9
Tuna & Sweetcorn, Reduced Fat, Morrisons*	1oz/28g	48	2.9	172	13.2	6.9	10.2	0.0
SANDWICH SPREAD								
Beef, Classic, Shippam*	1 Pot/75g	133	8.8	177	15.5	2.2	11.8	0.0
Chicken, Classic, Shippam*	1 Serving/35g	64	4.4	182	15.5	1.8	12.5	0.0
Chicken & Bacon, Asda*	¼ Jar/43g	153	13.2	359	18.0	2.0	31.0	1.0
Chicken Tikka, Asda*	1 Serving/50g	77	5.0	154	7.0	9.0	10.0	0.2
Crab, Classic, Shippam*	1 Jar/35g	60	3.8	170	13.1	4.6	10.9	0.0
Heinz*	1 Tbsp/10ml	22	1.3	220	1.0	24.0	13.0	1.0
Light, Heinz*	1 Tbsp/10g	16	0.9	161	1.1	18.2	9.2	0.9
Salmon, Classic, Shippam*	1 Serving/35g	70	4.9	200	14.7	4.2	14.1	0.0
Tuna & Mayonnaise, Shippam*	1 Pot/75g	189	13.9	252	18.3	3.1	18.5	0.0
SARDINES								
Grilled	**1oz/28g**	**55**	**2.9**	**195**	**25.3**	**0.0**	**10.4**	**0.0**
in BBQ Sauce, John West*	1 Tin/121g	177	7.7	146	16.1	6.2	6.4	0.0
in Brine, Canned, Drained	**1oz/28g**	**48**	**2.7**	**172**	**21.5**	**0.0**	**9.6**	**0.0**
in Oil, Canned, Drained	**1oz/28g**	**62**	**3.9**	**220**	**23.3**	**0.0**	**14.1**	**0.0**
in Olive Oil, Canned, Ambrosia*	1 Can/100g	320	13.7	320	22.3	0.7	13.7	0.0
in Peri Peri Sauce, John West*	1 Can/120g	181	12.3	150	12.3	2.3	10.2	0.3
in Spring Water, Portuguese, Sainsbury's*	1 Can/90g	165	9.3	183	22.4	0.0	10.3	0.0
in Tomato Sauce, Canned	1oz/28g	45	2.8	162	17.0	1.4	9.9	0.0
Raw, Whole with Head	**1oz/28g**	**46**	**2.6**	**165**	**20.6**	**0.0**	**9.2**	**0.0**

	INFO/WEIGHT	per Measure KCAL	FAT	Nutrition Values per 100g / 100ml KCAL	PROT	CARB	FAT	FIBRE
SATAY								
Chicken, Breast, Iceland*	1 Satay/10g	15	0.1	155	34.1	2.7	0.9	0.1
Chicken, Breast, Party Bites, Sainsbury's*	1 Stick/10g	16	0.1	157	34.1	2.7	0.9	0.1
Chicken, GFY, Asda*	1 Serving/168g	242	6.1	144	22.0	6.0	3.6	0.8
Chicken, Indonesian, Bighams*	1 Serving/240g	314	15.4	131	12.2	6.2	6.4	0.6
Chicken, Indonesian, Mini, Sainsbury's*	1 Stick/10g	17	0.7	171	23.0	4.0	7.0	0.7
Chicken, Kebab, Waitrose*	½ Pack/125g	246	13.5	197	18.9	6.0	10.8	0.5
Chicken, M&S*	1 Satay/43g	90	5.5	210	19.1	4.4	12.7	0.7
Chicken, Mini, Iceland*	1 Satay/8g	19	1.1	236	23.0	4.5	14.0	0.7
Chicken, Morrisons*	1 Satay/10g	17	0.7	171	23.5	3.5	7.0	0.7
Chicken, Occasions, Sainsbury's*	1 Satay/10g	15	0.6	150	22.0	2.0	6.0	0.7
Chicken, Oriental, Tesco*	1 Serving/100g	160	5.0	160	23.6	5.1	5.0	0.4
Chicken, Party, Mini, Tesco*	1 Satay/10g	13	0.3	133	23.7	3.4	2.8	1.0
Chicken, Sticks, Asda*	1 Stick/20g	43	2.8	216	18.0	4.5	14.0	0.0
Chicken, Taste Original*	1 Stick/20g	33	1.3	164	23.0	2.5	6.5	0.7
Chicken & Turkey, Co-Op*	1 Pack/120g	264	16.8	220	20.0	4.0	14.0	0.0
Chicken & Turkey, Sainsbury's*	1 Stick/20g	44	2.8	222	20.0	4.0	14.0	1.9
Chicken with Peanut Sauce, Waitrose*	1 Pack/250g	492	27.0	197	18.9	6.0	10.8	0.5
SATSUMAS								
Fresh, Raw, Flesh Only, Average	*1 Sm/56g*	*21*	*0.0*	*37*	*0.9*	*8.6*	*0.1*	*1.3*
Weighed with Peel, Average	*1 Sm/60g*	*22*	*0.1*	*37*	*0.9*	*8.6*	*0.1*	*0.9*
SAUCE								
Apple, & Brandy, Asda*	1 Serving/125g	56	0.0	45	0.2	11.0	0.0	0.0
Apple, Baxters*	1 Tsp/15g	7	0.1	49	0.1	11.1	0.4	0.7
Apple, Bramley, Colman's*	1 Tbsp/15ml	16	0.0	107	0.2	26.5	0.0	1.3
Apple, Bramley, M&S*	1 Tbsp/15g	21	0.0	140	0.2	32.6	0.3	0.4
Apple, Bramley, Sainsbury's*	1 Tsp/15g	17	0.0	111	0.2	27.2	0.1	1.8
Apple, Everyday Value, Tesco*	1 Tbsp/15g	15	0.0	105	0.1	24.8	0.1	0.5
Apple, Heinz*	1 Tsp/15g	8	0.0	56	0.3	13.4	0.2	1.5
Apple, Smart Price, Asda*	1 Tsp/5g	5	0.0	101	0.3	25.0	0.0	0.9
Arrabbiata, Fresh, Waitrose*	1 Serving/100g	52	2.5	52	1.4	5.9	2.5	2.0
Arrabbiata, Italian, Tesco*	½ Pot/175g	72	0.5	41	1.3	8.3	0.3	1.1
Bacon & Tomato, Smoked, Stir in, Dolmio*	½ Tub/75g	74	4.2	98	4.6	7.2	5.6	1.3
Balti, Cooking, Sharwood's*	¼ Jar/140g	120	8.3	86	1.2	7.1	5.9	1.4
Balti, Cooking, Tesco*	1 Serving/500g	395	20.0	79	1.5	9.2	4.0	2.2
Balti, Ready Made, Average	1 Serving/100g	98	6.1	98	2.0	8.3	6.1	1.8
Balti, Reduced Fat, Healthy Living, Cook in, Co-Op*	½ Jar/225g	135	5.4	60	2.0	7.5	2.4	2.3
Balti, Tomato & Coriander, Canned, Patak's*	1 Can/283g	235	17.0	83	0.8	6.5	6.0	1.2
Balti Curry, Tesco*	1 Serving/200g	126	9.2	63	1.7	4.3	4.6	1.7
Barbecue, Chicken Tonight, Knorr*	¼ Jar/125g	76	0.5	61	2.0	12.4	0.4	0.9
Barbeque, Cook in, Homepride*	1 Can/500g	375	7.5	75	0.7	14.6	1.5	0.6
BBQ, Bick's*	1 Serving/100g	119	0.3	119	1.6	27.5	0.3	0.0
BBQ, Heinz*	1 Serving/20g	28	0.1	139	1.1	31.7	0.3	0.5
BBQ, HP*	1 Serving/20ml	29	0.0	143	0.8	33.1	0.2	0.0
BBQ, Sticky, Spread & Bake, Heinz*	¼ Jar/78g	131	0.5	168	1.0	39.6	0.6	1.2
Bearnaise, Mary Berry*	1 Serving/100g	435	39.8	435	1.7	17.3	39.8	0.4
Bearnaise, Sainsbury's*	1 Tbsp/15g	59	6.2	393	0.6	5.0	41.0	0.0
Bechamel, for Lasagne, Loyd Grossman*	1 Jar/400g	396	33.2	99	0.6	5.4	8.3	0.1
Beef in Ale, Cooking, Asda*	1 Jar/500g	160	1.0	32	1.6	6.0	0.2	0.0
Bhuna, Cooking, Sharwood's*	1/3 Jar/140g	116	7.6	83	1.2	7.6	5.4	1.6
Black Bean, & Chilli, Stir Fry, Asda*	½ Jar/97g	158	11.6	163	3.7	10.0	12.0	0.8
Black Bean, & Green Pepper, Stir Fry, Sharwood's*	1 Serving/150g	82	0.4	55	2.0	11.0	0.3	0.5
Black Bean, & Red Pepper, Sharwood's*	½ Jar/213g	132	3.0	62	1.9	10.5	1.4	1.2
Black Bean, Asda*	1 Serving/55g	55	0.8	100	2.9	19.0	1.4	0.0

S

SAUCE

INFO/WEIGHT	Measure	per Measure		Nutrition Values per 100g / 100ml				
		KCAL	FAT	KCAL	PROT	CARB	FAT	FIBRE
Black Bean, Canton, Stir Fry, Blue Dragon*	½ Pack/60g	53	1.2	88	2.8	14.8	2.0	1.5
Black Bean, Cantonese, Sharwood's*	½ Jar/212g	131	3.0	62	1.9	10.5	1.4	1.2
Black Bean, Crushed, Stir Fry Sensations, Amoy*	1 Pouch/150g	150	4.4	100	2.4	16.9	2.9	1.0
Black Bean, Fresh, Sainsbury's*	1 Sachet/50ml	78	1.3	156	6.7	27.5	2.6	1.7
Black Bean, Ready to Stir Fry, M&S*	1 Sachet/120g	78	1.1	65	2.5	11.5	0.9	1.4
Black Bean, Stir Fry, Fresh, M&S*	1 Pot/120g	120	0.7	100	2.6	20.3	0.6	1.4
Black Bean, Stir Fry, Fresh Ideas, Tesco*	½ Sachet/25g	33	0.7	132	4.2	22.6	2.8	0.8
Black Bean, Stir Fry, Fresh Tastes, Asda*	1 Pack/180ml	149	5.2	83	3.7	10.4	2.9	1.4
Black Bean, Stir Fry, Morrisons*	1 Serving/50g	92	5.4	185	4.1	17.3	10.8	1.5
Black Bean, Stir Fry, Sainsbury's*	½ Pack/75ml	91	3.2	121	3.3	17.6	4.3	1.7
Black Bean, Stir Fry, Sharwood's*	1 Jar/195g	127	0.6	65	2.3	12.9	0.3	0.0
Black Bean, Stir Fry, Tesco*	½ Jar/220g	297	10.8	135	3.4	18.1	4.9	2.5
Black Bean, Stir Fry Additions, Tesco*	1 Sachet/50g	69	1.5	138	4.1	23.6	3.0	0.0
Black Pepper, Stir Fry, Blue Dragon*	½ Sachet/60g	47	2.6	79	1.6	8.4	4.4	0.1
Bolognese, Italiano, Tesco*	1 Serving/175g	194	13.1	111	5.9	4.8	7.5	0.8
Bolognese, Loyd Grossman*	¼ Jar/106g	80	3.1	75	2.0	10.2	2.9	1.4
Bolognese, Waitrose*	1 Serving/175g	150	8.6	86	5.4	5.3	4.9	2.0
Bread, Luxury, M&S*	1 Serving/115g	196	16.2	170	3.2	8.1	14.1	2.2
Bread, M&S*	1 Serving/85g	153	12.4	180	3.1	8.7	14.6	0.2
Bread, Made with Semi-Skimmed Milk	1 Serving/45g	42	1.4	93	4.3	12.8	3.1	0.3
Brown, Asda*	1 Serving/10g	10	0.0	97	0.7	23.0	0.2	0.4
Brown, Bottled	1 Tsp/6g	6	0.0	99	1.1	25.2	0.0	0.7
Brown, Branston, Crosse & Blackwell*	1 Serving/15g	18	0.0	121	0.7	29.0	0.2	0.7
Brown, HP*	1 Tbsp/15g	18	0.0	122	0.9	28.3	0.1	0.4
Brown, Iceland*	1 Serving/20g	16	0.0	82	0.7	19.3	0.2	1.1
Brown, Reduced Salt & Sugar, HP*	1 Tbsp/15g	13	0.0	87	0.7	20.0	0.1	0.3
Brown, Tesco*	1 Tsp/10g	10	0.0	104	0.7	25.1	0.1	0.6
Brown, Tiptree, Wilkin & Sons*	1 Serving/100g	104	0.0	104	1.1	42.0	0.0	0.0
Brown, Value, Value, Tesco*	1 Serving/15g	13	0.0	86	0.7	18.8	0.1	0.3
Burger, Hellmann's*	1 Tbsp/15g	36	3.2	240	1.1	12.0	21.0	0.0
Butter & Tarragon, Chicken Tonight, Knorr*	¼ Jar/125g	132	13.0	106	1.0	2.1	10.4	0.7
Butter Chicken, Patak's*	1 Jar/500g	725	60.0	145	1.2	7.6	12.0	1.4
Butter Chicken, TTD, Sainsbury's*	½ Pack/174g	272	23.5	156	1.8	6.7	13.5	0.9
Caramelised Onion & Red Wine, M&S*	1 Serving/52g	31	1.6	60	1.9	6.7	3.1	0.6
Carbonara, TTD, Sainsbury's*	½ Pot/175g	347	31.0	198	5.2	4.5	17.7	0.5
Caribbean Curry, Levi Roots*	½ Jar/175g	182	14.2	104	0.4	7.2	8.1	0.3
Chasseur, Classic, Chicken Tonight, Knorr*	¼ Jar/125g	61	3.6	49	0.6	5.3	2.9	0.7
Chasseur, Cook in, Homepride*	1 Can/390g	160	0.4	41	0.7	9.2	0.1	0.4
Cheese, Basics, Sainsbury's*	¼ Pot/124g	71	3.1	57	2.5	6.1	2.5	0.5
Cheese, Cheddar, Made Up, Colman's*	1 Serving/85ml	348	13.1	410	19.2	48.5	15.4	1.9
Cheese, Dry, Asda*	1 Serving/27g	101	3.0	373	4.4	64.0	11.0	7.0
Cheese, Fresh, Italiano, Tesco*	½ Tub/175g	236	16.1	135	6.8	6.2	9.2	0.0
Cheese, Fresh, Waitrose*	1 Pot/350g	458	34.3	131	5.1	5.7	9.8	0.0
Cheese, Instant, Morrisons*	1 Serving/14g	38	2.8	272	7.9	14.3	20.3	0.0
Cheese, Made with Semi-Skimmed Milk	1 Serving/60g	107	7.6	179	8.1	9.1	12.6	0.2
Cheese, Made with Whole Milk	1 Serving/60g	118	8.8	197	8.0	9.0	14.6	0.2
Cherry Tomato, & Fresh Basil, M&S*	1 Serving/175g	131	9.3	75	1.2	5.5	5.3	1.1
Cherry Tomato, Finest, Tesco*	½ Pot/171g	120	4.4	70	1.5	9.4	2.6	1.1
Chilli, & Jalapeno Peppers, Mexican, Seeds of Change*	½ Jar/175g	131	2.4	75	2.1	12.0	1.4	2.1
Chilli, Amoy*	1 Tsp/6g	2	0.0	25	1.0	5.2	0.0	1.0
Chilli, Barbeque, Encona*	1 Tbsp/15ml	19	0.0	129	1.3	30.7	0.1	0.0
Chilli, Hot, Asda*	1 Jar/570g	319	2.3	56	2.1	11.0	0.4	1.9
Chilli, Hot, Blue Dragon*	1 Tbsp/15ml	14	0.0	96	0.5	23.0	0.2	0.0

SAUCE	Measure INFO/WEIGHT	per Measure KCAL	FAT	Nutrition Values per 100g / 100ml KCAL	PROT	CARB	FAT	FIBRE
Chilli, Hot, Co-Op*	1 Jar/440g	242	2.2	55	2.0	10.0	0.5	2.0
Chilli, Hot, Heinz*	1 Portion/10g	8	0.0	80	1.4	18.0	0.0	0.0
Chilli, Hot, Mexican, Morrisons*	¼ Jar/125g	72	0.6	58	2.2	11.2	0.5	2.0
Chilli, Hot, Sharwood's*	1 fl oz/30ml	36	0.2	120	0.5	29.4	0.6	1.3
Chilli, HP*	1 Tsp/6g	8	0.0	134	1.2	32.3	0.0	0.0
Chilli, Linghams*	1 Tsp/5g	4	0.0	79	0.0	17.3	0.8	0.0
Chilli, Medium, Deliciously Good, Homepride*	1 Jar/460g	258	2.3	56	2.3	10.4	0.5	1.2
Chilli, Mild, Tesco*	1 Jar/550g	302	1.6	55	2.3	10.0	0.3	3.4
Chilli, Seeds of Change*	1 Jar/400g	408	6.0	102	4.0	18.2	1.5	2.2
Chilli, Sweet, Thai, Dipping, Original, Blue Dragon*	1 Serving/30ml	69	0.2	229	0.6	55.1	0.7	1.6
Chilli, Tesco*	1 Tsp/5ml	4	0.2	90	1.3	14.0	3.2	1.1
Chilli, Tomato Based, Bottled, Average	*1 Tbsp/15g*	*16*	*0.0*	*104*	*2.5*	*19.8*	*0.3*	*5.9*
Chilli, with Kidney Beans, Old El Paso*	1 Serving/115g	92	0.5	80	4.3	14.8	0.4	0.0
Chilli & Garlic, Blue Dragon*	1 Serving/30ml	26	0.1	85	1.1	19.7	0.2	0.0
Chilli & Garlic, Lee Kum Kee*	1 Tsp/15g	16	0.0	110	2.1	24.7	0.3	4.3
Chilli & Garlic, Stir Fry, M&S*	1 Serving/83g	120	1.0	145	0.7	32.4	1.2	1.1
Chilli Con Carne, Classic, Loyd Grossman*	1 Jar/350g	242	10.5	69	2.2	7.6	3.0	1.3
Chilli Con Carne, Cook in, BGTY, Sainsbury's*	¼ Jar/125g	69	0.6	55	1.7	11.0	0.5	2.5
Chilli Con Carne, Cook in, Homepride*	1 Can/390g	234	2.3	60	2.5	11.2	0.6	0.0
Chilli Con Carne, Hot, Uncle Ben's*	1 Jar/500g	295	3.0	59	2.3	10.9	0.6	1.7
Chilli Men, Spicy, Wagamama*	½ Jar/125g	138	5.9	110	2.0	14.9	4.7	0.6
Chilli Soy, Amoy*	1 Tbsp/15g	8	0.0	55	4.6	9.1	0.0	0.0
Chinese, Curry, Farmfoods*	1 Sachet/200g	220	17.6	110	0.6	7.1	8.8	0.7
Chinese, Stir Fry, Sachet, Fresh, Sainsbury's*	½ Sachet/51ml	83	5.7	163	1.7	14.1	11.1	1.8
Chinese, Stir Fry, Sainsbury's*	½ Sachet/75g	61	1.9	81	0.4	14.1	2.5	1.0
Chinese, Stir Fry, Tesco*	1 Serving/90g	86	3.2	95	1.3	14.3	3.5	0.6
Chinese, Style, Curry, Cooking, CBY, Asda*	1 Serving/140g	89	4.3	64	1.5	7.4	3.1	3.5
Chinese, Style, Stir Fry, Fresh, Asda*	½ Sachet/50ml	93	6.0	186	1.5	18.0	12.0	0.0
Chinese, with Soy, Ginger & Garlic, Stir Fry, Tesco*	1 Pack/150g	180	8.4	120	2.1	14.2	5.6	0.8
Chocolate, Dessert, Belgian Chocolate, Finest, Tesco*	1 Tbsp/15g	56	2.2	370	3.3	54.9	14.9	1.3
Chocolate, Sainsbury's*	1 Serving/25g	81	1.6	323	1.8	64.7	6.3	2.7
Chop Suey, Stir Fry, Sharwood's*	1 Jar/160g	120	2.4	75	0.7	14.6	1.5	0.2
Chow Mein, Cantonese, Stir Fry, Sainsbury's*	½ Jar/100g	67	1.9	67	0.4	12.1	1.9	0.8
Chow Mein, Sainsbury's*	1 Serving/50g	36	1.2	71	1.8	10.5	2.4	0.0
Chow Mein, Stir Fry, Asda*	½ Jar/98g	97	1.0	99	1.6	21.0	1.0	0.1
Chow Mein, Stir Fry, Blue Dragon*	1 Sachet/120g	110	3.5	92	1.1	15.4	2.9	0.4
Chow Mein, Stir Fry, Straight to Wok, Amoy*	1 Pack/120g	172	7.0	143	0.9	21.9	5.8	0.5
Chow Mein Stir Fry, Morrisons*	½ Sachet/50g	85	2.6	170	1.3	29.0	5.1	0.7
Coconut, Ginger & Lemon Grass, Stir Fry, Wagamama*	½ Jar/125g	144	7.1	115	1.2	14.7	5.7	0.4
Coconut, Lime & Coriander, Cooking, Nando's*	1 Serving/65g	88	6.5	135	1.5	12.2	10.0	1.2
Coconut, Thai Style, Stir Fry, Waitrose*	½ Pack/50ml	52	4.3	105	1.5	5.5	8.6	1.8
Coronation, Heinz*	1 Tbsp/10g	33	3.1	334	0.8	13.1	31.0	0.9
Country French, Chicken Tonight, Knorr*	¼ Jar/125g	110	8.8	89	0.4	5.3	7.1	0.8
Cranberry, Sainsbury's*	1 Tsp/15g	23	0.0	154	0.8	37.1	0.3	1.3
Cranberry, Tesco*	1 Tsp/15g	23	0.0	156	0.1	38.8	0.0	0.9
Cranberry, Waitrose*	1 Tbsp/20g	31	0.0	156	0.2	38.5	0.2	14.0
Cranberry & Port, M&S*	1 Serving/75g	71	0.3	95	2.3	20.2	0.4	2.1
Cranberry Jelly, Baxters*	1 Tsp/15g	40	0.0	268	0.0	67.0	0.0	0.0
Cranberry Jelly, Morrisons*	1 Tsp/12g	23	0.0	189	0.2	47.0	0.0	0.1
Cranberry with Brandy & Orange Zest, Finest, Tesco*	1 Serving/10g	24	0.1	235	0.3	57.2	0.6	1.3
Cream, Graddsås, Ikea*	1 Serving/60ml	72	6.6	120	1.0	4.0	11.0	0.0
Creole, & Spice Mix, Two Step, Soulful, Discovery*	1 Jar/370g	314	6.7	85	1.7	18.0	1.8	3.3
Curry, Chip Shop Style, Knorr*	1 Sachet/150ml	146	6.9	97	1.7	12.4	4.6	0.7

SAUCE

	Measure INFO/WEIGHT	per Measure KCAL	FAT	Nutrition Values per 100g / 100ml KCAL	PROT	CARB	FAT	FIBRE
Curry, Cook in, Homepride*	½ Can/250g	140	4.8	56	1.1	8.6	1.9	0.5
Curry, Creamy, Chicken Tonight, Knorr*	½ Jar/250g	208	18.5	83	0.6	3.6	7.4	0.8
Curry, Deliciously Good, Homepride*	1/3 Jar/149g	91	2.7	61	1.1	10.0	1.8	0.5
Curry, Green Thai, Finest, Tesco*	1 Serving/350g	420	37.1	120	1.4	4.8	10.6	0.7
Curry, Green Thai, Sharwood's*	1 Serving/403g	431	30.6	107	1.1	8.4	7.6	0.1
Curry, Kashmiri, Bibijis*	¼ Pack/119g	51	1.7	43	2.1	7.1	1.4	1.5
Curry, Mild, Tesco*	1 Jar/500g	420	14.0	84	1.1	13.4	2.8	0.8
Curry, Red Thai, Sainsbury's*	½ Pouch/250g	390	35.8	156	1.7	5.0	14.3	1.5
Curry, Red Thai, Sharwood's*	1 Serving/138g	150	11.0	109	1.2	7.9	8.0	0.2
Curry, Sri Lanken, Seasoned Pioneers*	½ Pack/200g	194	16.8	97	1.8	3.4	8.4	0.8
Curry, Sweet	1 Serving/115g	105	6.4	91	1.2	9.6	5.6	1.4
Curry, Thai Coconut, Uncle Ben's*	1 Serving/125g	128	6.0	102	1.4	13.2	4.8	0.0
Curry, Value, Tesco*	1 Can/390g	355	17.6	91	1.6	11.0	4.5	1.3
Dark Soy, Sesame & Ginger, for Fish, Schwartz*	1 Pack/300g	279	4.2	93	1.3	18.8	1.4	0.5
Dill & Lemon, Delicate for Fish, Schwartz*	1 Pack/300g	387	34.2	129	1.1	5.6	11.4	0.5
Dill & Mustard for Gravadlax, Dry, Waitrose*	1 Sachet/35g	123	9.0	352	2.5	27.8	25.7	0.6
Dopiaza, Cooking, Tesco*	1 Serving/166g	176	11.0	106	2.2	9.4	6.6	1.9
Dopiaza, Medium, Cook in, Sharwood's*	½ Bottle/210g	193	10.7	92	1.4	10.2	5.1	0.6
Dopiaza, Tomato & Onion, Original, Patak's*	1 Jar/540g	605	39.4	112	1.6	9.8	7.3	1.2
Enchilada, Medium, Old El Paso*	1 Can/270g	92	4.6	34	0.0	5.0	1.7	0.0
Fennel & Apricot, Tagine, Moroccan, Seasoned Pioneers*	½ Pouch/200g	136	10.0	68	0.9	4.6	5.0	1.2
Fiery Guava, Dipping, Levi Roots*	1 Serving/20g	26	0.0	128	0.4	31.5	0.0	0.1
Fiesta, Chilli, Cooking, Aldi*	¼ Jar/124g	87	0.6	70	2.5	12.5	0.5	2.6
Fish, Nuoc Mam, Thai, Blue Dragon*	1 Tsp/5ml	7	0.0	145	5.9	30.9	0.1	0.0
Fish, Thai, Nuoc Mam, Amoy*	1 Tbsp/15ml	12	0.0	80	13.4	6.7	0.0	0.0
Four Cheese for Pasta, Waitrose*	1 Pot/300g	392	24.8	112	6.6	5.5	7.1	0.5
Fruit Squirt, Passionfruit, Topping, Easiyo*	1 Serving/20g	34	0.0	172	1.0	38.9	0.1	6.3
Fruity, HP*	1 Tsp/6g	8	0.0	141	1.2	35.1	0.1	0.0
Garlic, Heinz*	1 Serving/10ml	32	3.0	323	1.0	12.1	29.9	1.2
Garlic, Lea & Perrins*	1 Tsp/6g	20	1.7	337	1.8	17.8	29.0	0.0
Garlic & Chive, Heinz*	1 Serving/10ml	35	3.3	350	1.0	11.3	33.2	0.1
Garlic & Chive, Table & Dip, Heinz*	1 Serving/10ml	32	3.0	323	1.0	12.1	29.9	0.2
Garlic & Herb, Cooking, Simply Stir, Philadelphia *	1 Serving/60g	81	7.2	135	2.5	4.6	12.0	0.4
Green Thai, Loyd Grossman*	½ Jar/175g	182	11.2	104	1.6	10.0	6.4	0.8
Green Thai, Stir Fry, Sainsbury's*	½ Pack/75g	112	8.0	149	1.2	11.9	10.7	1.0
Hoi Sin, & Garlic, Blue Dragon*	1 Serving/60g	80	1.6	133	1.2	26.1	2.6	0.0
Hoi Sin, & Plum, Dipping, Finest, Tesco*	1 Serving/50g	78	1.4	156	2.3	35.3	0.6	1.4
Hoi Sin, & Plum, Sweet & Fruity, Stir Fry, Sharwood's*	1 Serving/136g	128	1.8	94	0.7	19.9	1.3	0.9
Hoi Sin, & Spring Onion, Stir Fry, Sharwood's*	1 Jar/165g	196	1.5	119	1.3	26.5	0.9	0.8
Hoi Sin, CBY, Asda*	1 Jar/210g	309	2.3	147	0.8	31.3	1.1	1.4
Hoi Sin, Lee Kum Kee*	1 Serving/35g	80	0.5	230	1.2	53.3	1.3	0.0
Hoi Sin, Sharwood's*	1 Tbsp/15g	32	0.0	211	2.7	49.5	0.3	0.1
Hoi Sin, Stir Fry, CBY, Asda*	1 Jar/210g	296	2.3	141	0.8	31.3	1.1	1.4
Hoi Sin, Stir Fry, Rich, Straight to Wok, Amoy*	½ Sachet/60g	68	1.4	114	1.8	21.4	2.3	0.7
Hoi Sin, Stir Fry, Tesco*	½ Sachet/60g	87	2.9	145	1.1	23.9	4.9	0.5
Hoi Sin, with Garlic & Spring Onion, Stir Fry, Tesco*	¼ Pack/38g	46	0.4	120	2.2	25.2	1.1	0.5
Hollandaise, Classic, for Fish, Schwartz*	1 Sachet/300g	456	49.2	152	0.7	0.4	16.4	2.0
Hollandaise, Dry, Maille*	1 Serving/30g	148	15.2	495	1.0	10.8	50.6	0.0
Hollandaise, Finest, Tesco*	1 Serving/98g	473	44.5	485	1.4	17.2	45.6	0.3
Hollandaise, Fresh, Average	1 Pack/150g	342	32.4	228	2.4	6.1	21.6	0.0
Hollandaise, Homemade, Average	1oz/28g	198	21.3	707	4.8	0.0	76.2	0.0
Hollandaise, M&S*	1 Serving/10g	41	4.4	410	0.9	3.6	43.6	0.5
Hollandaise, Mary Berry*	1 Serving/100g	472	43.8	472	1.4	17.8	43.8	0.3

SAUCE

INFO/WEIGHT	Measure		Nutrition Values per 100g / 100ml				
	KCAL	FAT	KCAL	PROT	CARB	FAT	FIBRE
Hollandaise, Sainsbury's*	1 Tbsp/15g	72	7.6	478	0.2	5.9	50.4	0.4
Honey & Mustard, Chicken Tonight, Knorr*	¼ Jar/125g	132	6.6	106	1.0	12.6	5.3	1.8
Honey & Mustard, Low Fat, Chicken Tonight, Knorr*	¼ Jar/131g	105	3.0	80	1.0	13.8	2.3	0.8
Horseradish, Colman's*	1 Tbsp/15ml	17	0.9	112	1.9	9.8	6.2	2.6
Horseradish, Creamed, Colman's*	1 Tsp/16g	37	2.1	229	4.3	21.4	13.3	0.0
Horseradish, Creamed, M&S*	1 Tsp/5g	16	1.5	325	2.4	12.1	29.3	2.5
Horseradish, Creamed, Waitrose*	1 Tbsp/16g	30	1.6	185	2.4	19.6	9.9	2.3
Horseradish, Creamy, Sainsbury's*	1 Tsp/5g	11	0.6	223	2.8	28.9	11.8	1.6
Horseradish, Hot, Morrisons*	1 Serving/20g	22	1.1	110	1.6	10.9	5.6	1.1
Horseradish, Hot, Tesco*	1 Tsp/5g	9	0.5	185	2.3	19.7	10.6	2.3
Horseradish, Mustard, Sainsbury's*	1 Tsp/5g	8	0.3	163	7.9	18.2	6.6	3.5
Horseradish, Sainsbury's*	1 Dtsp/10g	14	0.7	145	1.5	17.8	6.6	2.4
Horseradish Cream, Tesco*	1 Serving/15g	29	1.8	195	2.3	18.7	11.9	2.1
Hot Pepper	1 Tsp/5g	1	0.1	26	1.6	1.7	1.5	0.0
Hot Pepper, Encona*	1 Tsp/5ml	3	0.1	52	0.5	10.5	1.2	0.0
Hunters Chicken, Cooking, Tesco*	1/3 Jar/163g	155	0.3	95	1.2	20.6	0.2	0.8
Jalfrezi, Cooking, Asda*	1 Jar/570g	519	35.9	91	1.2	7.4	6.3	1.7
Jalfrezi, Cooking, Sainsbury's*	1 Serving/250g	160	6.0	64	1.0	9.6	2.4	1.7
Jalfrezi, Spice & Stir, Geeta's*	½ Jar/175g	156	11.2	89	1.4	6.5	6.4	1.4
Jalfrezi, Stir Fry, Patak's*	1 Jar/250g	260	18.8	104	1.4	7.6	7.5	1.4
Jalfrezi, Sweet Pepper & Coconut, in Glass Jar, Patak's*	1 Jar/540g	626	37.8	116	1.7	11.3	7.0	1.4
Jalfrezi, TTD, Sainsbury's*	½ Jar/175g	205	16.8	117	1.3	6.4	9.6	1.5
Jerk/Bbq, Levi Roots*	¼ Bottle/78g	94	0.1	121	1.1	28.8	0.1	0.5
Korma, Asda*	1 Serving/225g	434	33.8	193	2.5	12.0	15.0	2.2
Korma, Authentic, VLH Kitchens	1 Serving/118g	180	11.0	153	1.9	6.7	13.0	0.8
Korma, Coconut & Cream, Mild in Glass Jar, Patak's*	1 Jar/540g	940	79.4	174	1.3	9.1	14.7	0.8
Korma, Cooking, GFY, Asda*	¼ Jar/143g	110	4.4	77	2.0	10.2	3.1	0.6
Korma, Cooking, LC, Tesco*	¼ Jar/125g	100	4.0	80	1.6	10.2	3.2	1.6
Korma, Cooking, Patak's*	¼ Jar/125g	211	17.5	169	1.3	9.3	14.0	2.4
Korma, Cooking, Sharwood's*	1 Jar/420g	680	42.8	162	1.7	15.9	10.2	2.2
Korma, Tesco*	¼ Jar/125g	192	14.6	154	2.4	9.9	11.7	1.3
Korma, with Flaked Almonds, Weight Watchers*	1 Serving/175g	107	3.7	61	2.0	8.5	2.1	1.6
Lemon, Peking, Stir Fry, Blue Dragon*	1 Serving/35g	47	0.2	134	0.0	31.6	0.7	0.5
Lime & Coriander, Tangy for Fish, Schwartz*	1 Pack/300g	381	37.2	127	1.1	2.7	12.4	1.3
Marie Rose, Fresh, The Saucy Fish Co.*	1 Pack/150g	590	59.7	393	1.6	7.0	39.8	0.0
Mediterranean Vegetable, Chargrilled, Italiano, Tesco*	1 Pot/350g	175	3.9	50	1.6	8.4	1.1	1.3
Mint, Baxters*	1oz/28g	17	0.1	62	1.7	13.2	0.3	0.0
Mint, Garden, Fresh, Tesco*	1 Tsp/5g	2	0.0	40	2.6	3.6	0.4	1.5
Mint, Sainsbury's*	1 Dtsp/10g	13	0.0	126	2.5	28.7	0.1	4.0
Mint, Smart Price, Asda*	1 Serving/5g	3	0.0	52	0.1	13.0	0.0	1.2
Mint, Value, Tesco*	1 Serving/10g	4	0.0	41	1.1	9.0	0.1	1.8
Mornay, Cheese, Asda*	¼ Pot/71g	114	9.0	161	6.8	6.6	12.7	0.4
Moroccan Chicken, Chicken Tonight, Knorr*	¼ Jar/125g	91	1.6	73	0.4	14.7	1.3	1.4
Mushroom, & White Wine, Knorr*	1 Serving/100ml	99	8.0	99	1.0	4.0	8.0	0.6
Mushroom, Creamy, Asda*	1 Serving/125g	76	4.6	61	0.8	6.0	3.7	0.5
Mushroom, Creamy, Chicken Tonight, Knorr*	¼ Jar/125g	99	7.1	79	0.5	6.0	5.7	1.0
Mushroom, Creamy, Cooking, M&S*	1 Jar/510g	663	57.6	130	1.3	5.4	11.3	0.5
Mushroom, Creamy, Homepride*	1 Portion/100g	76	5.6	76	1.1	5.2	5.6	0.3
Mushroom, Creamy, Knorr*	1 Serving/125g	111	9.6	89	0.4	4.5	7.7	0.4
Mushroom, Creamy, Tesco*	½ Pot/175g	142	10.2	81	1.5	5.6	5.8	0.4
Mushroom, Wild, Finest, Tesco*	½ Pack/175g	158	11.9	90	1.9	5.2	6.8	0.4
Mushroom & White Wine, Risotto, Sacla*	1 Serving/95g	151	12.4	159	3.7	6.9	13.0	0.0
Napoletana, Italian, Tesco*	1 Pot/350g	178	4.2	51	1.5	8.5	1.2	1.0

SAUCE

INFO/WEIGHT	Measure KCAL	FAT	Nutrition Values per 100g / 100ml KCAL	PROT	CARB	FAT	FIBRE
Napoletana, Waitrose*	1 Pot/600g	252	8.4	42	1.8	5.5	1.4	1.7
Onion, Made with Semi-Skimmed Milk	1 Serving/60g	52	3.0	86	2.9	8.4	5.0	0.4
Onion, Made with Skimmed Milk	1 Serving/60g	46	2.4	77	2.9	8.4	4.0	0.4
Orange & Dill for Fish, Zesty, Schwartz*	1 Pack/300g	180	1.5	60	0.4	13.5	0.5	0.5
Oriental, Cantonese, Uncle Ben's*	¼ Jar/125g	108	0.2	86	0.8	20.3	0.2	1.2
Oyster, & Spring Onion, Stir Fry, Blue Dragon*	1 Sachet/120g	122	0.1	102	1.4	23.5	0.1	0.1
Oyster, Amoy*	1 Tsp/5ml	5	0.0	108	2.0	25.0	0.0	0.0
Oyster, Blue Dragon*	1 Tsp/5ml	6	0.0	121	3.4	26.9	0.0	0.0
Oyster, Lee Kum Kee*	1 Serving/100g	138	0.1	138	5.0	29.3	0.1	0.0
Oyster, Stir Fry, Sainsbury's*	1 Tbsp/15g	9	0.0	61	1.6	13.3	0.1	0.2
Pad Thai, Stir Fry, Amoy*	1 Pack/120g	179	5.4	149	2.5	24.7	4.5	1.3
Pad Thai, Stir Fry, Tesco*	1 Pack/125g	112	2.9	90	1.3	15.8	2.3	0.8
Parsley, Fresh, Sainsbury's*	½ Pot/150g	117	7.6	78	2.0	5.9	5.1	0.5
Parsley, Instant, Dry, Asda*	1 Serving/23g	82	1.6	355	7.0	66.0	7.0	4.4
Parsley, Lemon Caper, New Covent Garden Food Co*	¼ Carton/65ml	137	12.1	211	2.5	8.7	18.6	0.8
Parsley, Made Up, Bisto*	1 Serving/50ml	41	2.4	82	0.6	9.2	4.8	0.0
Parsley, Tesco*	½ Pack/89g	85	5.1	95	2.8	8.1	5.7	1.1
Peanut, Sainsbury's*	1 Sachet/70g	185	9.2	264	1.9	34.7	13.1	1.6
Peanut Satay, Roast, Stir Fry, Straight to Wok, Amoy*	½ Pack/60g	106	6.4	176	4.0	16.3	10.6	1.3
Peanut Satay, Roast, Stir Fry Sensations, Amoy*	1 Pouch/160g	354	19.8	221	4.7	21.9	12.4	1.0
Pepper, Creamy, Schwartz*	1 Pack/170g	116	9.2	68	1.5	3.4	5.4	1.0
Pepper, Creamy, Tesco*	1 Serving/85ml	128	11.4	151	1.2	6.4	13.4	0.5
Pepper & Tomato, Spicy, Stir Through, M&S*	½ Jar/95g	166	14.6	175	1.6	7.5	15.4	0.0
Peppercorn, Creamy, Asda*	¼ Jar/137g	137	11.0	100	1.1	6.0	8.0	0.2
Peppercorn, Creamy, Chicken Tonight, Knorr*	¼ Jar/125g	110	9.8	88	0.3	3.8	7.8	0.4
Peppercorn & Whisky, Creamy, Baxters*	1 Pack/320g	422	34.6	132	1.9	6.7	10.8	0.2
Pepperoni & Tomato, Spicy, Stir in, Dolmio*	½ Pack/75g	116	8.7	154	3.3	9.3	11.6	0.8
Peri Peri, Garlic, Nando's*	1 Serving/15g	9	0.5	59	0.5	6.6	3.4	0.8
Peri-Peri, Extra Hot, Nando's*	1 Serving/5g	4	0.2	71	0.7	8.8	3.7	1.4
Peri-Peri, Hot, Nando's*	1 Serving/5g	4	0.2	75	0.6	9.6	3.8	1.3
Peri-Peri, Sweet, Nando's*	1 Tbsp/25g	36	0.5	142	0.5	30.7	2.1	0.0
Pesto, Green, Asda*	1 Tsp/5g	21	2.2	429	4.7	3.5	44.0	1.4
Plum, & Mandarin, Sichuan, Seasoned Pioneers*	1 Pouch/400g	328	17.2	82	0.7	12.4	4.3	2.3
Plum, Spiced, Heinz*	1 Serving/25g	32	0.0	128	0.5	31.1	0.1	1.0
Plum, Sticky, Stir Fry, Blue Dragon*	1 Serving/60g	145	0.2	242	0.1	35.6	0.3	0.0
Prawn Cocktail, Frank Cooper*	1 Tbsp/15g	47	4.0	316	0.8	18.3	26.7	0.1
Prawn Cocktail, Morrisons*	1 Portion/15ml	81	8.5	540	1.4	5.5	56.9	1.1
Puttanesca, Fresh, Waitrose*	½ Pot/176g	118	7.7	67	1.8	6.2	4.4	1.2
Red Thai, Loyd Grossman*	1 Jar/350g	438	22.8	125	2.8	13.7	6.5	1.5
Red Wine, Cook in, Homepride*	¼ Can/98g	47	0.6	48	0.5	10.1	0.6	0.0
Red Wine, Cooking, Homepride*	1 Serving/250ml	115	1.5	46	0.4	9.8	0.6	0.0
Redcurrant, Colman's*	1 Tsp/12g	44	0.0	368	0.7	90.0	0.0	0.0
Reggae Reggae, Cooking, Levi Roots*	½ Jar/175g	215	0.9	123	1.3	28.5	0.5	0.7
Reggae Reggae, Jerk Bbq, Levi Roots*	1 Jar/310g	375	0.3	121	1.1	28.8	0.1	0.5
Rich & Fruity, Branston, Crosse & Blackwell*	1 Serving/15g	20	0.0	130	0.0	31.5	0.0	1.6
Rogan Josh, Curry, The Curry Sauce Company*	1 Serving/235g	310	23.7	132	1.9	8.4	10.1	1.5
Rogan Josh, Medium, Sharwood's*	½ Jar/210g	151	7.6	72	1.4	8.6	3.6	0.5
Rogan Josh, Sharwood's*	½ Jar/210g	220	16.8	105	1.2	7.0	8.0	1.5
Rogan Josh, Tesco*	½ Can/220g	156	10.3	71	1.3	5.9	4.7	1.4
Satay, Stir Fry & Dipping, Finest, Tesco*	1 Tsp/5g	22	1.7	432	9.0	20.7	34.8	2.7
Satay, Thai, Taylor's *	1 Serving/50ml	122	8.4	245	4.8	31.6	16.9	2.0
Satay, with Peanuts & Chillies, Cooking, Blue Dragon*	1 Serving/110g	198	10.7	180	4.3	18.0	9.7	1.5
Sausage Casserole, Cook in, Homepride*	½ Jar/250g	92	0.5	37	0.7	8.0	0.2	0.6

SAUCE

INFO/WEIGHT	Measure		per Measure		Nutrition Values per 100g / 100ml				
			KCAL	FAT	KCAL	PROT	CARB	FAT	FIBRE
Seafood, 25% Less Fat, Tesco*	1 Tsp/5g		17	1.4	344	2.7	18.2	28.5	0.3
Seafood, Asda*	1 Serving/10g		45	4.2	448	1.6	16.0	42.0	0.2
Seafood, Average	1 Tsp/5g		20	1.9	410	1.4	15.4	38.0	0.2
Seafood, Colman's*	1 Tbsp/15g		44	3.4	296	0.9	21.5	22.9	0.4
Seafood, GFY, Asda*	1 Dtsp/10ml		31	2.7	313	0.6	17.0	27.0	0.0
Seafood, Sainsbury's*	1 Tbsp/15g		50	4.2	330	0.7	17.6	28.2	0.1
Seafood, Tesco*	1 Serving/10g		46	4.4	465	1.8	15.6	43.5	0.3
Smoky BBQ, Original, for Fajitas, Cooking, Old El Paso*	1 Jar/395g		222	5.1	56	1.5	9.6	1.3	0.0
Soy, & Garlic, Stir Fry, Fresh Tastes, Asda*	1 Pack/180g		175	6.7	97	1.7	14.1	3.7	0.5
Soy, & Plum, Stir Fry Additions, COOK!, M&S*	½ Sachet/60g		48	0.2	80	1.5	17.5	0.3	1.5
Soy, Average	1 Tsp/5ml		3	0.0	64	8.7	8.3	0.0	0.0
Soy, Dark, Amoy*	1 Tsp/5ml		5	0.0	106	0.9	25.6	0.0	0.0
Soy, Dark, Average	1 Tsp/5g		4	0.0	84	4.0	16.7	0.1	0.2
Soy, Light, Amoy*	1 Tsp/5ml		3	0.0	52	2.5	10.5	0.0	0.0
Soy, Light, Asda*	1 Tbsp/15ml		7	0.0	47	0.8	11.0	0.0	0.0
Soy, Light, Sharwood's*	1 Tsp/5ml		2	0.0	37	2.7	6.4	0.2	0.0
Soy, Naturally Brewed, Kikkoman*	1 Tbsp/15g		11	0.0	74	10.3	8.1	0.0	0.0
Soy, Reduced Salt, Amoy*	1 Tsp/5ml		3	0.0	56	4.0	10.0	0.0	0.0
Soy, Rich, Sharwood's*	1 Tsp/5ml		4	0.0	79	3.1	16.6	0.4	0.0
Soy & Roasted Red Chilli, Sweet, Stir Fry, Blue Dragon*	1 Pack/120g		122	0.1	102	1.3	24.0	0.1	0.2
Soy with Ginger & Garlic, Sweet, Stri Fry, Blue Dragon*	½ Pack/60g		52	0.0	87	0.8	20.6	0.0	0.1
Soya, Japanese, Waitrose*	1 Tbsp/15ml		11	0.1	74	7.7	9.4	0.6	0.8
Spaghetti Bolognese, Dolmio*	1 Serving/100g		33	0.2	33	1.5	6.3	0.2	1.3
Spanish Chicken, Chicken Tonight, Knorr*	¼ Jar/125g		68	2.0	55	1.6	7.3	1.6	2.3
Stroganoff, Mushroom, Creamy, M&S*	1 Serving/75g		86	6.9	115	3.3	4.8	9.2	0.6
Sweet & Sour, Aromatic, Stir Fry Sensations, Amoy*	1 Pack/160g		312	0.5	195	0.4	46.8	0.3	0.8
Sweet & Sour, Basics, Sainsbury's*	¼ Jar/110g		59	0.3	54	0.3	12.4	0.3	0.4
Sweet & Sour, Chinese, Sainsbury's*	½ Jar/150g		222	0.2	148	0.2	36.6	0.1	0.1
Sweet & Sour, Classic, Canned, Homepride*	1 Can/500g		510	0.5	102	0.4	24.9	0.1	0.5
Sweet & Sour, Cook In, Glass Jar, Homepride*	1 Jar/500g		335	0.5	67	0.3	16.2	0.1	0.5
Sweet & Sour, Cooking, Chinese, Sainsbury's*	¼ Jar/125g		155	0.1	124	0.6	30.1	0.1	0.7
Sweet & Sour, Cooking, LC, Tesco*	1 Jar/510g		357	0.5	70	0.3	16.1	0.1	0.5
Sweet & Sour, Extra Pineapple, Uncle Ben's*	1 Serving/165g		147	0.3	89	0.3	21.2	0.2	0.7
Sweet & Sour, Fresh, Sainsbury's*	1 Sachet/50ml		102	4.3	205	0.8	31.2	8.6	0.3
Sweet & Sour, Fresh Ideas, Tesco*	1 Serving/50ml		77	0.7	154	1.1	34.3	1.4	0.5
Sweet & Sour, GFY, Asda*	½ Jar/164g		77	0.3	47	0.4	11.0	0.2	0.3
Sweet & Sour, Light, Uncle Ben's*	¼ Jar/125g		71	0.1	57	0.4	12.6	0.1	0.9
Sweet & Sour, Organic, Seeds of Change*	1 Jar/350g		350	0.4	100	0.4	24.4	0.1	0.6
Sweet & Sour, Oriental, Express, Uncle Ben's*	1 Serving/170g		221	3.2	130	0.8	27.5	1.9	0.0
Sweet & Sour, Original, Uncle Ben's*	1 Pack/300g		264	0.6	88	0.4	21.9	0.2	0.8
Sweet & Sour, Peking Style, Finest, Tesco*	1 Serving/175g		147	0.2	84	0.6	20.1	0.1	0.5
Sweet & Sour, Spicy, Sharwood's*	1 Serving/138g		142	0.7	103	0.7	23.8	0.5	0.4
Sweet & Sour, Spicy, Stir Fry, Sainsbury's*	1 Jar/500g		430	0.5	86	0.7	20.0	0.1	0.7
Sweet & Sour, Spicy, Uncle Ben's*	1 Jar/400g		364	0.4	91	0.6	22.1	0.1	0.0
Sweet & Sour, Stir Fry, Asda*	1 Serving/63g		146	3.2	232	0.8	46.0	5.0	0.0
Sweet & Sour, Stir Fry, M&S*	1 Pack/120g		150	0.5	125	0.7	29.8	0.4	1.3
Sweet & Sour, Stir Fry, Pouch, Average	1 Serving/100g		124	1.9	124	0.8	25.7	1.9	1.0
Sweet & Sour, Stir Fry, Sachet, Blue Dragon*	1 Sachet/120g		100	1.2	84	0.4	17.8	1.0	0.4
Sweet & Sour, Stir Fry, Sharwood's*	1 Jar/160g		168	0.8	105	0.6	24.5	0.5	0.8
Sweet & Sour, Stir Fry, Tesco*	½ Jar/222g		164	0.4	74	0.6	17.0	0.2	0.4
Sweet & Sour, Stir Fry Additions, Tesco*	1 Sachet/50g		84	0.5	167	0.8	38.7	1.0	0.5
Sweet & Sour, Take-Away	1oz/28g		44	1.0	157	0.2	32.8	3.4	0.0
Sweet & Sour, Value, Tesco*	1 Serving/100g		83	0.2	83	0.3	20.0	0.2	1.0

SAUCE

	Measure INFO/WEIGHT	per Measure KCAL	FAT	Nutrition Values per 100g / 100ml KCAL	PROT	CARB	FAT	FIBRE
Sweet Chilli, & Garlic, Stir Fry & Dipping, Tesco*	½ Jar/95ml	78	0.0	82	0.3	20.1	0.0	0.1
Sweet Chilli, & Lemon Grass, Stir Fry, Sharwood's*	1 Serving/155g	127	0.2	82	0.3	19.7	0.1	0.3
Sweet Chilli, Dipping, M&S*	1 Tbsp/15g	34	0.1	225	0.9	53.2	0.7	0.6
Sweet Chilli, Dipping, Sharwood's*	1 Bottle/150ml	339	3.9	226	0.6	51.5	2.6	1.6
Sweet Chilli, Dipping, Thai, Amoy*	1 Serving/10g	14	0.3	142	0.5	34.2	2.8	0.3
Sweet Chilli, Garlic, Stir Fry, Blue Dragon*	1 Pack/120g	142	0.1	118	0.2	28.8	0.1	0.3
Sweet Chilli, Heinz*	1 Serving/25g	38	0.1	150	0.3	36.5	0.4	6.4
Sweet Chilli, Stir Fry, Additions, Tesco*	1 Serving/50g	106	3.8	211	0.3	35.2	7.6	0.6
Sweet Chilli, Stir Fry, BGTY, Sainsbury's*	1 Pack/150ml	178	2.8	119	0.6	25.0	1.9	1.1
Sweet Chilli, Thai, Blue Dragon*	1 Serving/15g	28	0.1	188	0.5	45.5	0.6	0.0
Sweet Pepper, Stir in, Dolmio*	½ Pot/75g	103	7.7	137	1.5	9.7	10.3	0.0
Szechuan, Spicy Tomato, Stir Fry, Blue Dragon*	½ Sachet/60g	59	1.8	98	1.3	15.8	3.0	0.9
Szechuan, Stir Fry, Sharwood's*	1 Jar/150g	126	1.6	84	3.0	15.5	1.1	0.4
Szechuan, Style, Stir Fry, Fresh Ideas, Tesco*	1 Sachet/50g	114	4.8	228	1.9	33.4	9.7	0.1
Szechuan, Tomato, Stir Fry Sensations, Amoy*	1 Serving/64g	71	0.6	111	1.4	23.7	1.0	1.6
Tabasco, Tabasco*	1 Tsp/5ml	1	0.0	12	1.3	0.8	0.8	0.6
Tamarind & Lime, Stir Fry, Sainsbury's*	1 Serving/75g	88	5.6	117	1.1	11.4	7.4	0.8
Tartare	1oz/28g	84	6.9	299	1.3	17.9	24.6	0.0
Tartare, Colman's*	1 Tbsp/15g	45	3.7	290	1.5	17.0	24.0	0.6
Tartare, Rich, Colman's*	1 Tsp/5ml	14	1.2	284	1.2	17.0	23.0	0.6
Tartare, Sainsbury's*	1 Serving/20ml	94	9.8	469	0.4	5.8	49.0	1.0
Tartare, Tesco*	1 Tbsp/15g	43	3.3	287	1.5	19.6	21.8	0.3
Tartare, with Olives, The English Provender Co.*	1 Tbsp/15g	64	6.6	425	2.2	5.7	43.7	0.7
Teriyaki, Asda*	1 Serving/98g	99	0.1	101	2.1	23.0	0.1	0.0
Teriyaki, Fresh, The Saucy Fish Co.*	1 Pack/150g	318	2.8	212	2.8	45.8	1.9	0.0
Teriyaki, Japanese Grill, Kikkoman*	1 Serving/15ml	24	0.0	158	4.5	30.8	0.1	0.0
Teriyaki, Sticky, Oven Cook, Blue Dragon*	1 Jar/310g	391	0.3	126	0.7	30.4	0.1	0.0
Teriyaki, Stir Fry, Blue Dragon*	1 Sachet/120g	124	0.0	103	0.5	25.0	0.0	0.0
Teriyaki, Stir Fry, Fresh Ideas, Tesco*	1 Serving/25g	33	0.6	133	1.1	26.9	2.3	0.0
Teriyaki, Stir Fry, Sharwood's*	1 Jar/150g	144	0.4	96	0.9	22.5	0.3	0.3
Thai Chilli, Sweet, Stir Fry, Straight to Wok, Amoy*	1 Serving/60g	68	1.1	113	0.3	23.8	1.8	0.3
Tikka, Cooking, BGTY, Sainsbury's*	1 Jar/500g	370	9.5	74	1.2	12.9	1.9	0.3
Tikka Masala, Hot & Spicy in Glass Jar, Patak's*	1 Jar/350g	332	23.8	95	1.7	6.5	6.8	1.7
Tikka Masala, LC, Tesco*	¼ Jar/125g	100	3.4	80	2.0	11.1	2.7	1.2
Tikka Masala, Medium, Cooking, Sharwood's*	1/3 Jar/140g	150	9.7	107	1.3	9.7	6.9	0.5
Tikka Masala, PB, Waitrose*	½ Jar/175g	107	1.4	61	2.7	10.7	0.8	1.5
Tikka Masala, with Coriander, Weight Watchers*	½ Jar/175g	130	3.7	74	2.6	11.2	2.1	0.7
Toffee, GFY, Asda*	1 Serving/5g	15	0.1	306	2.2	68.0	2.8	0.0
Toffee, Luxury, Rowse*	1 Serving/20g	67	0.7	336	1.9	73.9	3.7	0.4
Toffee Fudge, Sainsbury's*	1 Serving/40g	134	1.5	336	1.9	73.9	3.7	0.4
Tomato, Heinz*	1 Tbsp/17g	18	0.0	103	0.9	24.1	0.1	0.7
Tomato, Pizza Topping, Napolina*	1 Serving/70g	34	1.5	49	0.8	6.3	2.2	0.6
Tomato, Spicy, Fresh, Somerfield*	1/3 Pot/100g	41	1.3	41	0.8	6.4	1.3	1.1
Tomato & Basil, for Meatballs, Dolmio*	¼ Jar/125g	48	0.2	38	1.5	6.9	0.2	1.3
Tomato & Basil, Fresh, Asda*	½ Tub/175g	100	3.7	57	1.5	7.9	2.1	0.5
Tomato & Basil, Fresh, Organic, Waitrose*	¼ Pot/175g	77	3.0	44	1.0	6.2	1.7	0.8
Tomato & Basil, Italian, Sainsbury's*	½ Pot/175g	80	3.7	46	1.6	5.1	2.1	2.5
Tomato & Basil, Sun Dried, Seeds of Change*	1 Serving/100g	169	13.2	169	1.8	9.3	13.2	0.0
Tomato & Basil, Tesco*	½ Jar/175g	84	5.8	48	0.7	3.8	3.3	0.8
Tomato & Basil Sauce, Fresh, Tesco*	1 Pot/500g	245	9.0	49	1.5	6.8	1.8	0.8
Tomato & Chilli, Table & Dip, Heinz*	1 Tsp/10ml	8	0.0	76	1.4	16.6	0.2	0.8
Tomato & Chilli, Waitrose*	1 Pot/350g	182	9.1	52	10.0	6.2	2.6	3.2
Tomato & Garlic, for Pasta, Asda*	¼ Jar/125g	80	2.9	64	2.7	8.0	2.3	1.1

	Measure INFO/WEIGHT	per Measure KCAL	FAT	Nutrition Values per 100g / 100ml KCAL	PROT	CARB	FAT	FIBRE
SAUCE								
Tomato & Garlic, Roasted, Stir in, Dolmio*	½ Pack/75g	94	7.6	125	1.2	7.7	10.2	0.0
Tomato & Marscapone, Finest, Tesco*	1 Serving/350g	270	17.5	77	2.7	5.4	5.0	0.8
Tomato & Marscapone, Italian, Somerfield*	½ Pot/150g	159	12.3	106	1.6	6.5	8.2	0.9
Tomato & Marscapone, Italiano, Tesco*	1 Serving/175g	194	15.2	111	2.8	5.4	8.7	0.6
Tomato & Mascarpone, Asda*	½ Tub/175g	152	10.2	87	1.8	7.0	5.8	0.5
Tomato & Mascarpone, Italian, Sainsbury's*	½ Tub/175g	158	10.2	90	2.6	6.8	5.8	1.2
Tomato & Mascarpone, Italian, Tesco*	½ Tub/175g	159	11.0	91	2.7	5.9	6.3	0.7
Tomato & Mozzarella, Finest, Tesco*	1 Serving/175g	89	5.6	51	1.6	4.1	3.2	0.6
Tomato & Worcester, Table, Lea & Perrins*	1 Serving/10g	10	0.0	102	0.8	23.0	0.5	0.7
Vegetable, Roast, with Basil & Tomato, M&S*	1 Serving/100g	85	4.1	85	2.0	9.5	4.1	1.2
Vongole, Sainsbury's*	½ Pot/150g	106	4.5	71	3.1	7.8	3.0	1.9
Watercress, & Creme Fraiche, COU, M&S*	½ Pack/154g	100	2.8	65	3.2	9.2	1.8	0.5
Watercress, & Stilton, Creamy for Fish, Schwartz*	1 Pack/300g	141	12.3	47	0.6	2.0	4.1	0.7
Watercress, Fresh, The Saucy Fish Co.*	1 Pack/150g	170	14.6	113	2.2	5.8	9.7	0.0
White, for Lasagne, Dolmio*	1 Jar/470g	451	34.3	96	0.6	7.0	7.3	0.0
White, for Lasagne, Tesco*	1 Jar/430g	452	35.7	105	2.2	5.3	8.3	0.6
White, Savoury, Made with Semi-Skimmed Milk	1oz/28g	36	2.2	128	4.2	11.1	7.8	0.2
White, Savoury, Made with Whole Milk	1oz/28g	42	2.9	150	4.1	10.9	10.3	0.2
White Wine, & Cream, Cook in, Classic, Homepride*	¼ Can/125g	101	5.1	81	1.0	8.0	4.1	0.4
White Wine, & Mushroom, BGTY, Sainsbury's*	¼ Jar/125g	81	2.5	65	2.8	9.0	2.0	0.3
White Wine, & Tarragon, French for Fish, Schwartz*	1 Pack/300g	372	33.3	124	1.1	5.0	11.1	0.8
Worcestershire, Average	*1 Tsp/5g*	*3*	*0.0*	*65*	*1.4*	*15.5*	*0.1*	*0.0*
Worcestershire, Lea & Perrins*	1 Tsp/5ml	4	0.0	88	1.1	22.0	0.0	0.0
Worcestershire, Sainsbury's*	1 Tbsp/15ml	16	0.0	107	0.7	23.3	0.1	0.3
Yellow Bean & Cashew, Tesco*	½ Jar/210g	170	6.1	81	1.6	11.9	2.9	0.3
SAUCE MIX								
Beef Bourguignon, Colman's*	1 Pack/40g	123	0.6	308	4.9	68.6	1.6	2.2
Bombay Potatoes, Schwartz*	1 Pack/33g	84	4.0	254	16.1	20.1	12.1	31.1
Bread, As Sold, Knorr*	1 Pack/46g	179	5.1	390	12.0	59.0	11.0	4.0
Bread, Colman's*	1 Pack/40g	131	0.4	327	11.4	67.9	1.1	3.2
Bread, Luxury as Sold, Schwartz*	1 Pack/40g	148	1.5	369	11.5	70.3	3.8	3.7
Bread, Made Up, Colman's*	1 Serving/80ml	66	1.3	82	0.0	5.4	1.6	0.0
Cajun Chicken, Schwartz*	1 Pack/38g	108	0.5	285	6.4	61.9	1.3	0.5
Chargrilled Chicken Pasta, Schwartz*	1 Pack/35g	119	3.1	341	8.6	56.8	8.8	6.1
Cheddar Cheese, Colman's*	1 Pack/40g	163	6.2	407	18.3	48.8	15.4	1.2
Cheddar Cheese, Dry Mix, Schwartz*	1 Pack/40g	144	3.0	361	18.4	55.1	7.4	2.3
Cheese, Knorr*	1 Pack/58g	132	2.8	227	7.8	38.0	4.9	1.8
Cheese, Made Up, Crosse & Blackwell*	1 Pack/30g	26	1.0	86	5.1	9.2	3.2	0.7
Cheese, Made Up with Skimmed Milk	1 Serving/60g	47	1.4	78	5.4	9.5	2.3	0.0
Chicken Chasseur, Colman's*	1 Pack/45g	128	0.7	284	8.0	59.2	1.6	3.8
Chicken Chasseur, Schwartz*	1 Pack/40g	126	1.8	316	9.6	59.1	4.6	6.8
Chicken Curry for Slow Cookers, as Sold, Schwartz*	1 Pack/33g	89	2.3	270	12.5	25.7	7.0	27.3
Chicken Supreme, Colman's*	1 Pack/40g	143	3.7	358	12.1	56.7	9.2	2.4
Chilli Con Carne, Asda*	1 Sachet/50g	157	0.8	314	7.0	68.0	1.6	2.5
Chilli Con Carne, Hot, Colman's*	1 Pack/40g	127	1.2	317	10.4	62.4	2.9	7.0
Chilli Con Carne, Schwartz*	1 Pack/41g	120	1.5	293	7.9	57.2	3.6	9.5
Coq Au Vin, Colman's*	1 Pack/50g	150	0.9	301	5.6	65.6	1.8	3.3
Cream, for Meatballs, Ikea*	1 Pack/40g	179	9.4	448	9.6	49.2	23.6	0.0
Curry, Chip Shop Style, Dry Weight, Bisto*	1 Dtsp/9g	38	1.6	427	3.4	63.5	17.7	1.3
Curry, Creamy Chicken, Colman's*	1 Sachet/50g	192	8.6	385	11.0	46.4	17.3	7.9
Curry, Dinaclass, Kerry Group*	1 Bag/382g	1282	32.0	336	17.2	47.1	8.4	1.6
Four Cheese, Colman's*	1 Pack/35g	127	3.9	362	17.1	48.4	11.1	1.8
Garlic Mushrooms, Creamy, Schwartz*	1 Pack/35g	109	1.6	311	7.6	59.7	4.7	4.2

SAUCE MIX	Measure INFO/WEIGHT	per Measure KCAL	FAT	Nutrition Values per 100g / 100ml KCAL	PROT	CARB	FAT	FIBRE
Hollandaise, Colman's*	1 Pack/28g	104	3.1	372	6.4	61.6	11.1	1.8
Hollandaise, Schwartz*	1 Pack/25g	98	3.2	394	10.6	59.2	12.8	3.7
Lamb Hotpot, Colman's*	1 Pack/40g	119	0.7	297	6.9	63.3	1.7	2.1
Lasagne, Schwartz*	1 Pack/36g	106	0.5	294	7.0	63.4	1.4	7.0
Lemon Butter for Fish, Schwartz*	1 Pack/38g	136	3.0	357	6.1	65.3	8.0	5.8
Mexican Chilli Chicken, Schwartz*	1 Pack/35g	105	2.0	299	7.0	55.1	5.6	12.0
Mixed Herbs for Chicken, So Juicy, Maggi*	1 Pack/34g	97	1.0	285	8.3	53.8	2.8	5.5
Paprika For Chicken, So Juicy, Maggi*	1 Pack/34g	91	1.4	267	8.8	45.5	4.0	7.1
Parsley, Creamy, Made Up, Schwartz*	1 Serving/79g	59	2.0	75	4.2	8.7	2.5	0.3
Parsley, Dry, Colman's*	1 Pack/20g	63	0.3	313	7.2	67.9	1.4	3.8
Parsley, Knorr*	1 Sachet/48g	210	11.6	437	4.2	50.6	24.2	0.8
Parsley & Chive for Fish, Schwartz*	1 Pack/38g	132	3.2	348	9.0	58.9	8.5	7.7
Pepper, Creamy, Colman's*	1 Pack/25g	88	2.8	352	13.0	50.0	11.0	0.0
Pepper, Creamy, Schwartz*	1 Pack/25g	86	1.7	342	17.9	52.0	6.9	7.0
Pepper & Mushroom, Creamy, Colman's*	1 Pack/25g	83	1.0	332	9.6	64.6	3.8	3.0
Peppercorn, Mild, Creamy, Schwartz*	1 Pack/25g	88	2.2	352	13.8	55.0	8.6	5.0
Savoury Mince, Schwartz*	1 Pack/35g	108	0.7	310	14.6	58.3	2.0	1.8
Shepherd's Pie, Bramwells*	1 Pack/50g	168	3.0	336	8.6	62.0	6.0	6.9
Shepherd's Pie, Schwartz*	1 Pack/38g	104	1.0	273	7.9	54.4	2.6	11.1
Spaghetti Bolognese, Colman's*	1 Pack/40g	120	0.4	300	8.9	64.1	0.9	5.2
Spaghetti Bolognese, Schwartz*	1 Pack/40g	114	0.6	285	9.2	59.0	1.6	7.0
Spaghetti Carbonara, Schwartz*	1 Pack/32g	135	6.4	421	10.4	49.4	20.1	7.2
Stroganoff, Beef, Colman's*	1 Pack/40g	140	3.6	350	11.6	56.1	8.9	2.7
Stroganoff, Beef, Schwartz*	1 Pack/35g	125	3.6	358	15.6	50.8	10.3	4.4
Stroganoff, Mushroom, Schwartz*	1 Pack/35g	113	1.9	324	10.0	59.2	5.3	9.6
Sweet & Sour, for Chicken, So Juicy, Maggi*	½ Pack/15g	42	0.3	279	7.1	55.8	2.3	3.5
Tuna & Mushroom Pasta Melt, Schwartz*	1 Pack/40g	122	2.8	304	10.2	49.7	7.1	7.7
Tuna Napolitana, Schwartz*	1 Pack/30g	107	3.9	357	10.3	49.6	13.1	0.5
Tuna Pasta Bake, Colman's*	1 Pack/45g	144	2.4	319	10.4	57.1	5.4	5.2
White, Dry Weight, Bisto*	1 Dtsp/9g	45	2.5	496	3.2	57.4	28.2	0.4
White, Instant, Made Up, Sainsbury's*	1 Serving/90ml	65	2.5	72	0.8	10.9	2.8	0.1
White, Made Up with Semi-Skimmed Milk	1oz/28g	20	0.7	73	4.0	9.6	2.4	0.0
White, Made Up with Skimmed Milk	1oz/28g	17	0.3	59	4.0	9.6	0.9	0.0
White, Savoury, Colman's*	1 Pack/25g	105	3.8	420	9.0	63.0	15.0	2.0
White, Savoury, Knorr*	½ Pack/16g	46	0.9	290	7.8	52.2	5.6	5.2
White, Savoury, Schwartz*	1 Pack/25g	108	5.7	434	11.5	45.6	22.9	5.9
White Wine with Herbs, Creamy, Schwartz*	1 Pack/26g	86	1.7	330	8.0	60.0	6.5	9.1
Wholegrain Mustard, Creamy, Schwartz*	1 Pack/25g	92	2.8	370	12.9	54.4	11.2	7.5
SAUERKRAUT								
Average	*1oz/28g*	*4*	*0.0*	*13*	*1.3*	*1.9*	*0.0*	*1.1*
SAUSAGE								
Beef, Average	*1 Sausage/60g*	*151*	*11.1*	*252*	*14.5*	*7.0*	*18.5*	*0.6*
Beef, with Onion & Red Wine, Finest, Tesco*	1 Sausage/63g	117	6.9	185	13.2	8.5	10.9	1.2
Billy Bear, Kids, Tesco*	1 Slice/20g	37	2.2	185	13.7	7.5	11.2	0.4
Bockwurst, Average	*1 Sausage/45g*	*114*	*10.4*	*253*	*10.8*	*0.8*	*23.0*	*0.0*
Bratwurst, Frozen, Lidl*	1 Sausage/80g	235	21.4	294	12.8	0.5	26.8	0.0
Buffalo & Smoked Bacon, Laverstoke Park Farm*	1 Sausage/67g	187	15.3	281	17.3	1.3	23.0	0.7
Cambridge GF, Waitrose*	1 Sausage/57g	121	9.3	213	14.6	1.9	16.3	1.3
Chicken, & Tarragon, Butchers Choice, Sainsbury's*	1 Sausage/47g	106	6.8	225	18.1	5.8	14.4	0.2
Chicken, Manor Farm*	1 Sausage/65g	126	8.1	194	13.7	6.6	12.5	1.2
Chilli & Coriander, TTD, Sainsbury's*	1 Sausage/44g	136	10.7	310	18.5	4.2	24.4	1.2
Chipolata, Average	*1 Sausage/28g*	*81*	*6.5*	*291*	*12.1*	*8.7*	*23.1*	*0.7*
Chipolata, Lamb & Rosemary, Tesco*	1 Sausage/32g	69	4.9	218	11.3	8.3	15.5	0.0

	Measure INFO/WEIGHT	per Measure KCAL	FAT	Nutrition Values per 100g / 100ml KCAL	PROT	CARB	FAT	FIBRE
SAUSAGE								
Chipolata, Pork, Extra Lean, BGTY, Sainsbury's*	1 Sausage/24g	46	2.1	189	16.9	10.9	8.6	0.5
Chipolata, Pork, Free Range, Cooked, Duchy Originals*	2 Chipolatas/46g	104	6.4	227	21.7	3.5	14.0	0.1
Chipolata, Premium, Average	*1 Serving/80g*	*187*	*13.8*	*234*	*14.8*	*4.7*	*17.3*	*1.2*
Chipolata, TTD, Sainsbury's*	1 Sausage/27g	79	6.0	294	20.3	3.0	22.3	0.6
Chorizo, Average	*1 Serving/80g*	*250*	*19.4*	*313*	*21.1*	*2.6*	*24.2*	*0.2*
Chorizo, Lean, Average	*1 Sausage/67g*	*131*	*9.2*	*195*	*15.7*	*2.3*	*13.7*	*0.8*
Cocktail, Average	*1 Sausage/7g*	*23*	*1.9*	*323*	*12.1*	*8.6*	*26.7*	*0.9*
Cumberland, Average	*1 Sausage/57g*	*167*	*13.0*	*293*	*13.8*	*8.6*	*22.8*	*0.8*
Cumberland, Healthy Range, Average	*1 Sausage/53g*	*75*	*2.1*	*142*	*17.4*	*9.0*	*4.0*	*0.9*
Cumberland, Weight Watchers*	1 Sausage/39g	55	1.3	140	18.6	8.3	3.4	1.1
Cumberland, with Cracked Black Pepper & Herbs, Asda*	1 Sausage/56g	127	8.0	225	13.6	10.8	14.2	2.2
Debrecziner, Spicy Smoked, Gebirgsjager*	1 Sausage/37g	118	10.4	320	16.0	1.0	28.0	0.0
Extrawurst, German, Waitrose*	1 Slice/28g	80	7.1	281	13.0	1.0	25.0	0.0
French Saucisson, Tesco*	1 Slice/5g	19	1.4	379	26.7	4.1	28.4	0.0
Garlic, Average	*1 Slice/11g*	*25*	*2.0*	*227*	*15.7*	*0.8*	*18.2*	*0.0*
German, Bierwurst, Selection, Sainsbury's*	1 Slice/4g	8	0.6	224	15.0	1.0	17.8	0.1
German, Extrawurst, Selection, Sainsbury's*	1 Slice/3g	9	0.8	279	13.1	0.5	25.0	0.1
German, Schinkenwurst, Selection, Sainsbury's*	1 Slice/3g	8	0.7	251	13.1	0.3	21.9	0.1
Irish, Average	*1 Sausage/40g*	*119*	*8.3*	*298*	*10.7*	*17.2*	*20.7*	*0.7*
Irish Recipe, Asda*	1 Sausage/57g	120	6.8	212	12.1	14.0	12.0	2.7
Lamb, Spiced & Mint, Morrisons*	1 Sausage/34g	79	4.5	233	22.9	5.1	13.2	1.1
Lincolnshire, Average	*1 Sausage/42g*	*122*	*9.1*	*291*	*14.6*	*9.2*	*21.8*	*0.6*
Lincolnshire, Healthy Range, Average	*1 Sausage/50g*	*89*	*4.3*	*177*	*15.8*	*9.0*	*8.6*	*0.8*
Lorne, Average	*1 Sausage/25g*	*78*	*5.8*	*312*	*10.8*	*16.0*	*23.1*	*0.6*
Merguez	1 Sausage/55g	165	14.3	300	16.0	0.6	26.0	0.0
Mortadella, Sainsbury's*	1 Slice/13g	34	2.8	261	17.3	0.1	21.2	0.1
Pigs in Blankets, Cooked, Morrisons*	1 Roll/22g	52	2.9	235	22.9	5.2	13.3	1.5
Polish Kabanos, Sainsbury's*	1 Sausage/25g	92	7.6	366	23.0	0.1	30.4	0.1
Polony, Slicing, Value, Tesco*	1 Serving/25g	54	3.5	215	10.9	10.2	14.1	0.7
Pork, 30% Less Fat, Butcher's Choice, Sainsbury's*	1 Sausage/50g	99	5.4	198	15.9	9.5	10.7	0.5
Pork, and Fresh Herb, Uncooked, TTD, Sainsbury's*	1 Sausage/67g	180	13.7	269	20.0	1.1	20.4	0.5
Pork, Apricot & Herb, Waitrose*	1 Sausage/67g	165	11.1	246	11.2	12.9	16.6	1.3
Pork, Average	*1 Sausage/45g*	*139*	*11.2*	*309*	*11.9*	*9.8*	*25.0*	*0.8*
Pork, Battered, Thick, Average	1oz/28g	126	10.2	448	17.3	21.7	36.3	2.0
Pork, Breakfast, Grilled, Wall's*	1 Sausage/22g	65	4.0	294	12.2	12.8	18.0	1.8
Pork, Cocktail, Hot & Spicy, Cooked, Asda*	1 Sausage/10g	31	2.4	312	13.0	11.0	24.0	1.3
Pork, Extra Lean, Average	*1 Sausage/54g*	*84*	*3.7*	*155*	*17.3*	*6.1*	*6.8*	*0.8*
Pork, Free From, Tesco*	1 Sausage/57g	124	8.6	218	12.1	8.5	15.0	2.2
Pork, Frozen, Fried	*1oz/28g*	*88*	*6.9*	*316*	*13.8*	*10.0*	*24.8*	*0.0*
Pork, Frozen, Grilled	*1oz/28g*	*81*	*5.9*	*289*	*14.8*	*10.5*	*21.2*	*0.0*
Pork, Garden Herb, 97%, Debbie & Andrews*	1 Sausage/67g	141	5.1	211	21.3	0.5	7.6	1.0
Pork, Garlic & Herb, Average	*1 Sausage/76g*	*203*	*16.5*	*268*	*12.0*	*6.0*	*21.8*	*1.2*
Pork, GF, Premium, The Black Farmer's Daughter*	2 Sausage/133g	321	26.2	241	14.8	1.0	19.7	0.6
Pork, Low Fat, Skinny Lizzie*	1 Sausage/66g	87	0.9	132	16.9	13.1	1.3	1.6
Pork, Premium, Average	*1 Sausage/74g*	*191*	*13.6*	*258*	*14.9*	*8.3*	*18.4*	*1.0*
Pork, Reduced Fat, Chilled, Grilled	*1oz/28g*	*64*	*3.9*	*230*	*16.2*	*10.8*	*13.8*	*1.5*
Pork, Reduced Fat, Healthy Range, Average	*1 Sausage/57g*	*86*	*3.4*	*151*	*15.6*	*9.0*	*6.0*	*0.9*
Pork, Skinless, Average	*1oz/28g*	*81*	*6.6*	*291*	*11.7*	*8.2*	*23.6*	*0.6*
Pork, Smoked, Reduced Fat, Mattessons*	½ Pack/113g	288	21.5	255	14.0	7.0	19.0	0.9
Pork, Thick, Average	*1 Sausage/39g*	*115*	*8.7*	*296*	*13.3*	*10.0*	*22.4*	*1.0*
Pork, Thick, Reduced Fat, Healthy Range, Average	*1 Sausage/52g*	*90*	*3.8*	*172*	*14.0*	*12.3*	*7.4*	*0.8*
Pork & Apple, Average	*1 Sausage/57g*	*146*	*10.7*	*256*	*14.5*	*7.5*	*18.8*	*1.9*
Pork & Beef, Average	*1 Sausage/45g*	*133*	*10.2*	*295*	*8.7*	*13.6*	*22.7*	*0.5*

SAUSAGE	Measure INFO/WEIGHT	per Measure KCAL	FAT	Nutrition Values per 100g / 100ml KCAL	PROT	CARB	FAT	FIBRE
Pork & Caramelised Onion, Thick, Cooked, Morrisons*	1 Sausage/45g	125	8.3	279	20.1	7.1	18.6	0.9
Pork & Chilli, Grilled, Finest, Tesco*	2 Sausage/108g	275	17.3	255	19.9	7.2	16.0	1.3
Pork & Herb, Average	*1 Sausage/75g*	*231*	*19.5*	*308*	*13.2*	*5.4*	*26.0*	*0.4*
Pork & Herb, Healthy Range, Average	*1 Sausage/59g*	*75*	*1.4*	*126*	*16.0*	*10.8*	*2.4*	*1.1*
Pork & Leek, Average	*1oz/28g*	*73*	*5.6*	*262*	*14.6*	*6.0*	*20.0*	*1.1*
Pork & Stilton, Average	*1 Sausage/57g*	*180*	*15.2*	*316*	*13.2*	*5.8*	*26.7*	*0.3*
Pork & Sweet Chilli, Waitrose*	1 Sausage/67g	151	10.1	226	15.5	6.9	15.1	2.7
Pork & Tomato, Grilled, Average	*1 Sausage/47g*	*127*	*9.7*	*273*	*13.9*	*7.5*	*20.8*	*0.4*
Premium, Chilled, Fried	*1oz/28g*	*77*	*5.8*	*275*	*15.8*	*6.7*	*20.7*	*0.0*
Premium, Chilled, Grilled	*1oz/28g*	*82*	*6.3*	*292*	*16.8*	*6.3*	*22.4*	*0.0*
Red Onion & Rosemary, Linda McCartney*	2 Sausages/100g	128	3.7	128	14.2	9.7	3.7	5.8
Saucisson Montagne, Waitrose*	1 Slice/5g	21	1.8	421	20.7	1.9	36.7	0.0
Saveloy, The Delicatessen, Tesco*	1 Saveloy/65g	185	14.9	285	9.5	8.3	23.0	2.3
Schinkenwurst, German, Waitrose*	1 Slice/13g	28	2.2	224	16.0	0.8	17.6	0.0
Sicilian Style, TTD, Sainsbury's*	1 Sausage/50g	146	12.2	293	17.6	0.7	24.4	0.9
Smoked, Average	*1 Sausage/174g*	*588*	*52.2*	*338*	*13.0*	*4.0*	*30.0*	*0.0*
Toulouse, M&S*	1 Sausage/57g	123	8.9	215	12.4	5.8	15.6	1.3
Toulouse, So Good, Somerfield*	1 Sausage/67g	197	15.3	296	15.2	7.2	22.9	0.8
Toulouse, TTD, Sainsbury's*	1 Sausage/45g	146	11.5	324	21.4	2.3	25.5	0.8
Turkey, Average	*1 Sausage/57g*	*90*	*4.6*	*157*	*15.7*	*6.3*	*8.0*	*0.0*
Turkey & Chicken, Average	*1 Sausage/57g*	*126*	*8.2*	*222*	*14.4*	*8.2*	*14.6*	*1.8*
Tuscan, M&S*	1 Sausage/66g	145	10.6	220	14.9	4.6	16.0	0.6
Venison, & Pork, Waitrose*	1 Sausage/64g	93	4.0	146	16.5	5.3	6.3	1.1
Venison, & Red Wine, TTD, Sainsbury's*	1 Sausage/58g	130	7.7	226	19.7	6.8	13.3	1.7
Venison, Grilled, Finest, Tesco*	1 Sausage/41g	86	5.5	215	16.6	6.3	13.7	0.6
Venison, Oisin, M&S*	1 Serving/25g	41	2.3	165	16.8	3.8	9.3	0.7
Wiejska, Polish, Sainsbury's*	1/8 Pack/50g	78	4.5	157	18.7	0.4	9.0	0.5
Wild Boar	1 Sausage/85g	220	17.0	259	16.5	1.2	20.0	0.0
SAUSAGE & MASH								
& Rich Onion Gravy, British Pork, M&S*	1 Pack/400g	340	6.8	85	5.7	12.2	1.7	1.3
British Classic, Tesco*	1 Pack/450g	675	42.8	150	5.1	11.1	9.5	0.9
GFY, Asda*	1 Pack/400g	330	10.0	82	4.2	10.8	2.5	1.8
in Cider Gravy with Apple & Onion, Weight Watchers*	1 Pack/400g	332	11.6	83	5.5	7.5	2.9	2.2
Light Choices, Tesco*	1 Pack/400g	360	8.8	90	4.4	11.8	2.2	1.4
Onion, M&S*	1 Pack/300g	315	17.1	105	4.1	9.0	5.7	1.5
Vegetarian, Tesco*	1 Pack/410g	398	15.6	97	4.6	11.1	3.8	2.0
Waitrose*	1 Pack/420g	517	31.1	123	4.2	9.9	7.4	0.1
with Onion Gravy, Tesco*	1 Pack/500g	525	27.0	105	3.0	11.1	5.4	1.6
with Red Wine & Onion Gravy, BGTY, Sainsbury's*	1 Pack/380g	315	7.2	83	5.0	11.4	1.9	2.0
SAUSAGE MEAT								
Pork, Average	*1oz/28g*	*96*	*8.2*	*344*	*9.9*	*10.2*	*29.4*	*0.6*
SAUSAGE MEAT FREE								
Cheese & Sundried Tomato, Tesco*	1 Sausage/50g	82	3.4	165	17.4	7.7	6.8	6.5
Chorizo Style Chunks, The Redwood Co*	1 Serving/50g	176	10.4	351	25.1	5.3	20.9	0.8
SAUSAGE ROLL								
Basics, Party Size, Somerfield*	1 Roll/13g	45	2.9	343	7.0	29.0	22.0	0.0
Cocktail, Average	1 Roll/15g	57	3.7	378	8.9	29.4	24.9	1.9
Cumberland, CBY, Asda*	1 Roll/66g	201	10.9	304	8.3	28.9	16.5	3.1
Frozen, Greggs Iceland*	1 Roll/103g	371	26.3	360	8.0	22.0	25.5	1.5
Go Large, Asda*	1 Roll/170g	660	47.6	388	9.0	25.0	28.0	0.9
Jumbo, Sainsbury's*	1 Roll/145g	492	34.4	339	8.2	23.2	23.7	1.5
Kingsize, Pork Farms*	½ Roll/50g	241	15.9	483	10.5	39.9	31.8	0.0
Large, Freshbake*	1 Roll/52g	153	9.5	294	6.6	25.9	18.3	4.6

INFO/WEIGHT	Measure	per Measure		Nutrition Values per 100g / 100ml				
		KCAL	FAT	KCAL	PROT	CARB	FAT	FIBRE
SAUSAGE ROLL								
Large, Frozen, Tesco*	1 Roll/50g	182	11.9	365	6.0	31.0	23.8	0.9
Mini, 40 Pack, Tesco*	1 Roll/16g	60	4.0	375	8.4	28.5	25.1	2.5
Mini, Tesco*	1 Roll/15g	53	3.7	356	9.0	23.9	24.9	1.5
Mini, Waitrose*	1 Roll/35g	124	9.2	353	13.0	16.1	26.3	1.0
Party, Sainsbury's*	1 Roll/13g	54	4.0	422	8.7	26.7	31.1	1.2
Party, Size, Tesco*	1 Roll/14g	49	3.5	350	5.9	25.0	24.9	1.1
Party, Size, Value, Tesco*	1 Roll/12g	40	2.7	335	6.6	26.0	22.5	1.5
Pork, 2 Pack, CBY, Asda*	1 Roll/65g	266	18.8	409	9.0	28.0	29.0	1.0
Pork, 30% Less fat, CBY, Asda*	1 Roll/66g	207	12.3	313	9.8	26.4	18.7	1.2
Pork, Morrisons*	1 Roll/70g	195	9.0	278	9.6	31.2	12.8	1.5
Pork, Snack, 30% Less Fat, CBY, Asda*	1 Serving/33g	85	4.2	258	11.1	22.5	12.8	4.0
Pork Farms*	1 Roll/54g	196	12.9	363	7.9	30.0	23.9	0.0
Puff Pastry	1 Med/60g	230	16.6	383	9.9	25.4	27.6	1.0
Snack, GFY, Asda*	1 Roll/34g	112	7.0	329	9.4	26.5	20.6	0.9
Snack, Sainsbury's*	1 Roll/34g	130	8.5	383	9.7	29.9	25.0	2.1
Snack, Size, Tesco*	1 Roll/32g	118	8.8	369	9.1	21.7	27.4	2.3
TTD, Sainsbury's*	1 Roll/115g	440	31.9	383	11.9	21.3	27.8	2.0
SAUSAGE ROLL VEGETARIAN								
Linda McCartney*	1 Roll/52g	145	7.1	278	13.1	26.0	13.7	1.6
Mini, Linda McCartney*	1 Roll/14g	41	2.2	293	11.3	23.7	15.8	5.2
SAUSAGE VEGETARIAN								
Asda*	1 Sausage/43g	81	3.9	189	20.0	7.0	9.0	2.9
Braai Flavour, Fry's Special Vegetarian*	1 Sausage/63g	86	4.4	138	16.5	10.0	7.0	4.0
Cumberland, Cauldron Foods*	1 Sausage/46g	75	4.0	163	14.0	6.5	8.6	2.0
Cumberland, Waitrose*	1 Sausage/50g	80	3.4	160	12.6	12.3	6.7	2.4
Glamorgan, Asda*	1 Sausage/50g	100	5.1	199	4.6	22.4	10.1	2.0
Glamorgan, Leek & Cheese, Goodlife*	1 Sausage/50g	94	4.9	188	4.9	20.0	9.8	2.3
Glamorgan, Organic, Cauldron Foods*	1 Sausage/41g	67	3.8	162	12.5	7.3	9.2	1.7
Glamorgan, Organic, Waitrose*	1 Sausage/42g	81	4.2	194	14.5	11.2	10.1	1.7
Glamorgan Leek & Cheese, Sainsbury's*	1 Sausage/50g	98	5.2	197	4.3	21.3	10.5	2.7
Granose*	1oz/28g	63	3.8	226	8.5	17.5	13.5	0.0
Italian, Linda McCartney*	1 Sausage/50g	76	2.8	152	16.8	6.9	5.6	3.4
Leek & Cheese, Organic, Cauldron Foods*	1 Sausage/41g	80	4.1	194	14.4	11.3	10.1	1.7
Lincolnshire, Asda*	1 Sausage/56g	96	4.5	172	17.0	8.0	8.0	1.4
Lincolnshire, Chilled, Cauldron Foods*	1 Sausage/46g	76	4.1	165	14.0	6.5	8.8	2.0
Lincolnshire, Frozen, Tesco*	1 Sausage/50g	78	2.5	155	15.5	10.8	5.0	3.0
Linda McCartney*	1 Sausage/50g	101	4.4	202	22.5	8.3	8.8	1.6
Morrisons*	1 Serving/90g	149	8.8	165	17.2	2.0	9.8	8.1
Realeat*	1 Sausage/40g	66	3.9	165	17.2	2.0	9.8	8.1
Spinach, Leek & Cheese, Gourmet, Wicken Fen*	1 Sausage/46g	92	4.7	201	10.3	17.0	10.2	1.9
Sun Dried Tomato & Black Olive, Cauldron Foods*	1 Sausage/50g	71	3.8	142	8.7	9.4	7.7	2.6
Sun Dried Tomato & Herb, Linda McCartney*	1 Sausage/35g	93	5.4	266	21.8	10.1	15.4	1.7
SAVOURY EGGS								
Bites, Mini, Sainsbury's*	1 Egg/12g	35	2.2	288	9.4	21.7	17.8	1.6
Mini, Iceland*	1 Egg/20g	66	4.8	327	11.0	17.5	23.7	1.1
Mini, Tesco*	1 Egg/20g	55	3.5	274	9.2	20.2	17.4	2.3
Snack, Tesco*	1 Egg/45g	133	8.9	295	9.0	19.6	19.7	1.8
SCALLOPS								
Breaded, Thai Style with Plum Sauce, Finest, Tesco*	1 Serving/210g	401	14.7	191	11.5	20.6	7.0	0.8
Canadian, Finest, Tesco*	½ Pack/100g	80	0.2	80	16.4	2.6	0.2	0.1
Hotbake Shells, Sainsbury's*	1 Serving/140g	241	15.7	172	9.5	8.4	11.2	0.8
Lemon Grass & Ginger, Tesco*	½ Pack/112g	90	1.1	80	15.2	2.5	1.0	0.6
Raw, Bay or Sea with Roe, Average	*1 Scallop/15g*	*13*	*0.1*	*88*	*16.8*	*2.4*	*0.8*	*0.0*

	Measure INFO/WEIGHT	per Measure KCAL	per Measure FAT	Nutrition Values per 100g / 100ml KCAL	PROT	CARB	FAT	FIBRE
SCALLOPS								
Steamed, Average	1oz/28g	33	0.4	118	23.2	3.4	1.4	0.0
with Roasted Garlic Butter, Finest, Tesco*	1 Serving/100g	201	14.3	201	16.2	1.8	14.3	0.4
SCAMPI								
Bites, Everyday, Value, Tesco*	½ Pack/125g	262	10.0	210	9.4	23.4	8.0	1.2
Breaded, Baked, Average	½ Pack/255g	565	27.4	222	10.7	20.5	10.7	1.0
Breaded, Fried in Oil, Average	1 Serving/100g	237	13.6	237	9.4	20.5	13.6	0.0
Breaded & Chips, Oakhouse Foods Ltd*	1 Meal/300g	456	16.5	152	4.6	21.5	5.5	2.3
Wholetail, Breaded, Frozen, CBY, Asda*	1 Serving/93g	197	8.7	212	9.7	21.4	9.4	1.3
Wholetail, Premium, Youngs*	1 Serving/125g	256	11.4	205	29.5	21.6	9.1	2.1
Wholetail with a Hint of Lemon, Youngs*	1 Pack/228g	505	20.5	202	9.6	22.4	8.2	1.2
SCAMPI & CHIPS								
Chunky, Finest, Tesco*	1 Pack/280g	420	15.4	150	5.9	18.3	5.5	1.4
with Peas	1 Serving/490g	822	43.6	168	10.1	11.3	8.9	1.2
Youngs*	1oz/28g	42	1.5	150	5.0	20.3	5.4	1.7
SCHNITZEL VEGETARIAN								
Breaded, Tivall*	1 Schnitzel/100g	172	8.0	172	16.0	9.0	8.0	5.0
SCONE								
3% Fat, M&S*	1 Scone/65g	179	1.6	275	7.2	55.1	2.5	2.3
All Butter, CBY, Asda*	1 Serving/100g	377	14.5	377	7.2	54.3	14.5	1.7
All Butter, Sultana, Duchy Originals*	1 Scone/78g	276	9.8	353	7.3	52.9	12.5	2.6
All Butter, Tesco*	1 Scone/41g	126	3.2	308	7.2	52.3	7.8	1.6
Cheese, Average	1 Scone/40g	145	7.1	363	10.1	43.2	17.8	1.6
Cheese, Cornish, TTD, Sainsbury's*	1 Scone/74g	267	13.8	361	12.3	36.1	18.6	2.3
Cheese, Double Butter, Genesis Crafty*	1 Scone/60g	180	7.0	300	12.2	36.7	11.6	0.0
Cheese, Extra Special, CBY, Asda*	1 Serving/100g	315	8.7	315	0.0	18.9	8.7	0.0
Cheese, Sainsbury's*	1 Scone/70g	250	13.0	357	10.6	36.9	18.6	2.0
Cheese & Black Pepper, Mini, M&S*	1 Scone/18g	67	3.3	370	10.2	41.1	18.3	1.7
Cherry, Double Butter, Genesis Crafty*	1 Scone/63g	198	4.8	314	6.8	54.5	7.6	1.4
Cherry, Genesis Crafty*	1 Scone/81g	226	5.8	279	4.9	50.5	7.1	0.0
Cherry, M&S*	1 Scone/60g	202	7.3	337	6.9	49.7	12.2	1.9
Cream, Cornish Clotted, TTD, Sainsbury's*	1 Scone/70g	269	12.7	384	8.4	46.6	18.2	2.1
Cream, Fresh, Finest, Tesco*	1 Serving/133g	469	23.2	354	4.6	44.5	17.5	1.7
Cream, Fresh, Tesco*	1 Scone/80g	242	9.9	304	15.8	32.3	12.5	0.9
Cream, Sainsbury's*	1 Scone/50g	172	8.7	345	4.6	42.5	17.4	3.1
Cream, with Strawberry Jam, Fresh, Tesco*	1 Scone/83g	290	15.6	352	4.7	40.7	18.9	1.1
Derby, Asda*	1 Scone/59g	202	5.9	342	7.0	56.0	10.0	0.0
Derby, CBY, Asda*	1 Serving/100g	342	10.0	342	7.0	56.0	10.0	0.0
Derby, Tesco*	1 Scone/60g	201	6.1	335	7.2	53.7	10.2	2.0
Devon, Asda*	1 Scone/59g	208	6.3	353	7.3	55.5	10.6	3.0
Devon, M&S*	1 Scone/59g	225	9.6	380	7.1	50.8	16.2	1.5
Devon, Sainsbury's*	1 Scone/54g	201	8.4	372	7.1	51.1	15.5	1.6
Devon, Waitrose*	1 Scone/72g	268	9.5	373	7.5	56.0	13.2	2.3
Fruit, Average	1 Scone/40g	126	3.9	316	7.3	52.9	9.8	0.0
Fruit, Breakfast Griddle, Genesis Crafty*	1 Scone/65g	192	5.5	296	6.2	50.7	8.5	1.9
Fruit, Economy, Sainsbury's*	1 Scone/34g	111	3.2	326	7.9	52.5	9.4	1.7
Fruit, Genesis Crafty*	1 Scone/78g	231	6.6	296	6.2	50.7	8.5	0.0
Fruit, Smart Price, Asda*	1 Scone/41g	139	4.1	338	7.0	55.0	10.0	3.0
Fruit, Somerfield*	1 Scone/35g	116	3.5	332	8.0	53.0	10.0	0.0
Fruit, Waitrose*	1 Scone/59g	190	4.8	325	6.3	56.5	8.2	2.2
Plain, Average	1 Scone/40g	145	5.8	362	7.2	53.8	14.6	1.9
Plain, CBY, Asda*	1 Serving/100g	364	14.8	364	0.0	5.9	14.8	0.0
Plain, Genesis Crafty*	1 Scone/74g	227	7.4	307	6.8	49.1	10.0	0.0
Potato, Average	1 Scone/40g	118	5.7	296	5.1	39.1	14.3	1.6

S

INFO/WEIGHT	Measure	per Measure KCAL	FAT	Nutrition Values per 100g / 100ml KCAL	PROT	CARB	FAT	FIBRE
SCONE								
Potato, Mother's Pride*	1 Scone/37g	77	0.8	207	4.7	42.0	2.2	4.3
Strawberry, Fresh Cream, BGTY, Sainsbury's*	1 Scone/50g	154	5.6	309	5.1	47.0	11.2	1.1
Strawberry, Fresh Cream, Sainsbury's*	1 Scone/60g	218	11.2	363	6.5	42.5	18.6	1.4
Strawberry Jam with Cream, CBY, Asda*	1 Serving/100g	332	16.7	332	5.2	40.1	16.7	2.8
Sultana, BGTY, Sainsbury's*	1 Scone/63g	178	1.8	283	7.7	56.7	2.8	2.4
Sultana, Finest, Tesco*	1 Scone/70g	238	7.6	340	8.9	50.9	10.9	2.1
Sultana, M&S*	1 Scone/66g	231	8.2	350	6.5	53.0	12.5	2.0
Sultana, Reduced Fat, Waitrose*	1 Scone/65g	187	3.4	287	6.6	53.2	5.3	2.6
Sultana, Sainsbury's*	1 Scone/54g	176	5.9	327	6.9	50.2	11.0	6.5
Sultana, Tesco*	1 Scone/60g	189	5.0	315	7.1	52.5	8.4	2.6
Sultana, TTD, Sainsbury's*	1 Scone/70g	239	8.1	341	6.5	52.9	11.5	2.6
Sultana, Value, Tesco*	1 Scone/40g	134	4.0	335	6.5	53.8	10.1	2.7
Tattie, Scottish, Nick Nairn's*	1 Scone/21g	42	0.3	199	4.0	34.7	1.6	0.7
Wholemeal	1 Scone/40g	130	5.8	326	8.7	43.1	14.4	5.2
Wholemeal, Fruit	1 Scone/40g	130	5.1	324	8.1	47.2	12.8	4.9
SCONE MIX								
Fruit, Asda*	1 Scone/48g	143	2.4	301	7.0	57.0	5.0	3.7
SCOTCH EGGS								
Asda*	1 Egg/114g	286	19.2	251	11.2	13.7	16.8	1.4
Budgens*	1 Egg/113g	294	19.9	260	11.4	13.8	17.6	0.0
Cumberland, Waitrose*	1 Egg/114g	243	14.3	214	13.0	12.1	12.6	1.6
Finest, Tesco*	1 Egg/114g	280	20.1	247	11.6	10.4	17.7	1.1
Free Range, Sainsbury's*	1 Egg/113g	284	19.0	252	12.4	12.5	16.9	2.5
Ginsters*	1 Egg/95g	228	15.1	240	15.3	9.7	15.9	0.6
Morrisons*	1 Egg/114g	286	19.1	251	11.2	13.7	16.8	1.4
Retail	1 Egg/120g	301	20.5	251	12.0	13.1	17.1	0.0
Sainsbury's*	1 Egg/113g	311	21.8	275	11.1	14.2	19.3	1.3
Savoury, M&S*	1 Egg/21g	63	4.5	305	11.0	15.7	21.8	1.3
Super Mini, Asda*	1 Egg/13g	38	2.6	305	10.0	19.0	21.0	2.1
SEA BASS								
Cooked, Dry Heat, Average	**1 Fillet/101g**	**125**	**2.6**	**124**	**23.6**	**0.0**	**2.6**	**0.0**
Fillets, Aromatic Fennel Butter, Easy to Cook, Waitrose*	½ Pack/103g	274	23.4	266	16.1	0.1	22.7	0.6
Fillets, Beurre Blanc & Dill Sauce, The Saucy Fish Co.*	2 Fillets/230g	354	21.2	154	17.8	0.0	9.2	0.0
Fillets, Caramelised Ginger & Lime Butter, Sainsbury's*	1 Fillet/115g	235	14.2	204	22.7	0.6	12.3	0.8
Fillets, Corsican, TTD, Sainsbury's*	1 Fillet/130g	211	3.2	162	23.8	0.1	2.5	0.0
Fillets, Pan Fried, CBY, Asda*	½ Pack/90g	173	11.2	192	18.1	1.3	12.5	1.0
Fillets, Raw, Average	**1 Fillet/95g**	**108**	**3.4**	**113**	**20.3**	**0.0**	**3.5**	**0.1**
Fillets, with Lemon & Parsley Butter, Iceland*	½ Pack/110g	197	13.2	179	17.6	0.1	12.0	0.1
SEA BREAM								
Fillets, Raw, Average	**1oz/28g**	**27**	**0.8**	**96**	**17.5**	**0.0**	**2.9**	**0.0**
SEAFOOD COCKTAIL								
Average	1oz/28g	24	0.4	87	15.6	2.9	1.5	0.0
SEAFOOD SELECTION								
Asda*	1 Pack/240g	173	1.9	72	13.4	2.9	0.8	0.0
Fresh, Tesco*	1 Pack/234g	187	2.3	80	17.7	0.1	1.0	0.0
M & S*	1 Serving/200g	170	2.0	85	17.4	1.6	1.0	0.5
Mussels, King Prawns & Squid, Frozen, Tesco*	½ Pack/200g	140	3.0	70	13.7	0.1	1.5	0.0
Sainsbury's*	½ Pack/125g	85	1.2	68	14.6	0.8	1.0	2.5
SEAFOOD STICKS								
Average	1 Stick/15g	16	0.0	106	8.0	18.4	0.2	0.2
SEASONING MIX								
Aromat, Knorr*	1oz/28g	45	1.0	161	11.7	15.1	3.7	0.9
Beef Taco, Colman's*	1 Pack/30g	76	3.6	252	9.1	26.9	12.0	14.0

SEASONING MIX	Measure INFO/WEIGHT	KCAL	FAT	KCAL	PROT	CARB	FAT	FIBRE
		per Measure		Nutrition Values per 100g / 100ml				
Cajun, Perfect Shake, As Sold, Schwartz*	1 Tbsp/1g	2	0.1	249	9.9	27.2	7.0	19.0
Cajun, Sizzle & Grill, Schwartz*	1 Tsp/4g	7	0.2	182	9.8	23.0	5.6	24.4
Chicken, Chargrilled, Grill & Sizzle, Schwartz*	1 Tsp/5g	12	0.2	232	8.2	40.8	4.0	13.1
Chicken, Piri Piri, Tray Bake, Maggi*	1 Pack/40g	120	2.0	300	9.6	49.5	4.9	9.6
Chicken, Simply Shake, Schwartz*	1 Serving/100g	273	8.1	273	12.3	67.9	8.1	29.1
Chicken & Chorizo Gratin, Schwartz*	1 Pack/35g	108	0.5	310	5.8	63.4	1.4	10.4
Chicken Fajitas, Schwartz*	1 Pack/35g	99	0.9	283	10.9	54.1	2.5	10.8
Chilli, Old El Paso*	1 Pack/39g	117	2.0	301	7.0	57.0	5.0	0.0
Chinese Curry, Youngs*	1 Serving/22g	109	6.8	495	8.3	46.4	30.7	0.0
Fajita, Asda*	1 Serving/8g	20	0.6	251	6.0	41.0	7.0	0.9
Fajita, Chicken, Colman's*	1 Pack/40g	138	2.5	344	9.4	62.5	6.3	4.8
Garlic, for Chicken, Cook in Bag, Average	1 Bag/36g	108	0.7	300	9.6	58.3	2.0	5.9
Garlic, Papyrus Sheets, SoTender, Maggi*	1 Sheet/6g	25	1.9	438	6.3	24.4	32.5	11.4
Garlic & Herb Mash, Perfect Shake, Schwartz*	1 Serving/10g	29	2.2	290	7.6	43.0	21.9	20.2
Italian Herb, Schwartz*	1 Tsp/1g	3	0.0	338	11.0	64.5	4.0	0.0
Italian Herbs, Papyrus Sheets, SoTender, Maggi*	1 Sheet/6g	26	2.0	440	7.3	22.1	34.1	7.7
Jamaican Jerk Chicken, Recipe, Schwartz*	1 Pack/27g	75	0.8	276	9.8	69.8	3.0	17.2
Lamb, Simply Shake, Schwartz*	1oz/28g	54	0.9	193	12.1	53.1	3.1	23.9
Lemon & Herb, for Chicken, Cook in Bag, Average	1 Bag/34g	121	1.9	356	10.8	63.7	5.5	4.1
Mediterranean, for Chicken, Cook in Bag, Average	1 Bag/33g	99	0.7	302	10.6	56.6	2.0	7.0
Mediterranean Chicken, Season & Shake, Colman's*	1 Pack/33g	99	0.7	300	10.3	56.8	2.1	5.9
Mediterranean Roasted Vegetable, Schwartz*	1 Pack/30g	86	1.2	288	6.9	56.1	4.0	10.3
One Pan Rice Meal, for Chicken, Old El Paso*	¼ Pack/89g	203	4.3	228	4.4	40.9	4.8	1.7
Paprika, for Chicken, Cook in Bag, Average	1 Bag/34g	96	1.3	283	12.3	45.8	4.0	8.1
Paprika, Papyrus Sheets, SoTender, Maggi*	1 Sheet/6g	25	2.0	431	9.1	12.2	35.2	14.5
Potato Roasties, Rosemary & Garlic, Crispy, Schwartz*	1 Pack/33g	88	2.6	267	13.0	36.1	7.8	21.1
Potato Roasties, Southern Fried, Crispy, Schwartz*	1 Pack/35g	78	1.5	222	9.2	36.2	4.4	25.1
Potato Wedges, Cajun, Schwartz*	1 Pack/38g	112	2.9	295	9.1	47.6	7.6	14.3
Potato Wedges, Garlic & Herb, Schwartz*	1 Pack/38g	106	1.9	278	11.4	47.1	4.9	11.7
Potato Wedges, Nacho Cheese, Schwartz*	1 Pack/38g	114	3.7	299	13.6	39.3	9.7	7.7
Potato Wedges, Onion & Chive, Schwartz*	1 Pack/38g	113	0.7	297	10.9	59.4	1.8	6.5
Season-All, Schwartz*	1 Tsp/6g	4	0.1	72	2.3	11.6	1.8	0.0
Shepherd's Pie, Colman's*	1 Pack/50g	141	0.7	282	12.5	54.7	1.4	4.3
Shotz, Cajun Chicken Seasoning, Schwartz*	1 Pack/3g	8	0.2	268	9.9	45.6	5.2	0.0
Shotz, Chargrilled Chicken Seasoning, Schwartz*	1 Pack/3g	8	0.1	283	7.5	52.0	4.9	0.0
Shotz, Garlic Pepper Steak Seasoning, Schwartz*	1 Pack/3g	11	0.2	370	14.0	67.0	5.0	0.0
Shotz, Moroccan Chicken Seasoning, Schwartz*	1 Pack/3g	9	0.2	312	9.7	56.7	5.2	0.0
Shotz, Seven Pepper Steak Seasoning, Schwartz*	1 Pack/3g	7	0.1	246	8.2	47.8	2.4	0.0
Shotz, Smoky BBQ Pork, Seasoning, Schwartz*	1oz/28g	64	0.3	228	1.0	53.8	1.0	0.0
Spanish Roasted Vegetables, Schwartz*	1 Pack/15g	22	0.9	147	9.1	14.1	6.0	22.6
Sticky Spare Ribs, Season & Shake, Colman's*	1 Pack/52g	179	1.5	344	5.1	72.7	2.8	4.0
Taco, Old El Paso*	¼ Pack/9g	30	0.4	334	5.5	69.0	4.0	0.0
Thai Seven Spice, Schwartz*	1 Serving/10g	24	0.4	243	7.5	44.1	4.1	0.0
Whole Grain Mustard & Herb Potato Mash, Colman's*	1 Pack/30g	153	13.2	510	9.7	19.1	44.1	0.0
SEAWEED								
Chuka Wakame, Daiwa*	1 Serving/100g	70	3.3	70	1.3	8.8	3.3	1.4
Crispy, Average	*1oz/28g*	*182*	*17.3*	*651*	*7.5*	*15.6*	*61.9*	*7.0*
Irish Moss, Raw	*1oz/28g*	*2*	*0.1*	*8*	*1.5*	*0.0*	*0.2*	*12.3*
Kombu, Dried, Raw	*1oz/28g*	*12*	*0.4*	*43*	*7.1*	*0.0*	*1.6*	*58.7*
Nori, Dried, Raw	*1oz/28g*	*38*	*0.4*	*136*	*30.7*	*0.0*	*1.5*	*44.4*
Wakame, Dried, Raw	*1oz/28g*	*20*	*0.7*	*71*	*12.4*	*0.0*	*2.4*	*47.1*
SEEDS								
Chia, Black, The Chia Company*	1 Tbsp/15g	69	4.6	458	20.4	37.0	30.4	36.0

S

	Measure INFO/WEIGHT	per Measure KCAL	FAT	Nutrition Values per 100g / 100ml KCAL	PROT	CARB	FAT	FIBRE
SEEDS								
Chia, White, The Chia Company*	1 Tbsp/15g	69	5.1	458	20.4	37.0	34.0	36.0
Chocolate Covered, Munchy Seeds*	1 Pack/50g	275	14.2	550	15.2	37.2	28.4	14.2
Fenugreek, Average	*1 Tsp/4g*	*12*	*0.2*	*323*	*23.0*	*58.4*	*6.4*	*24.6*
Fiery, Graze*	1 Pack/34g	173	14.8	510	21.8	17.3	43.5	7.9
Flaxseed, Sunflower & Pumpkin, Milled, Linwoods*	1 Scoop/10g	54	4.9	542	22.7	2.4	49.1	16.2
Hemp, Raw, Organic, Navitas Naturals*	1 Serving/15g	80	7.0	533	33.3	20.0	46.7	6.7
Hemp, Shelled, Linwoods*	2 Tbsps/30g	178	14.8	593	35.1	7.6	49.5	5.9
Melon, Average	*1 Tbsp/15g*	*87*	*7.2*	*583*	*28.5*	*9.9*	*47.7*	*0.0*
Mixed, Cajun, Graze*	1 Pack/43g	246	21.1	573	26.5	18.1	49.0	11.5
Mixed, Chilli, Graze*	1 Pack/25g	152	11.8	606	30.4	6.1	47.2	5.2
Mixed, Fennel Seed & Honey Peanuts, Graze*	1 Punnet/35g	184	12.2	526	16.6	44.9	34.8	5.6
Mixed, Granola, Graze*	1 Pack/25g	122	7.4	490	12.0	43.7	29.7	0.0
Mixed, Omega, Graze*	1 Pack/25g	153	12.4	613	28.4	13.1	49.7	0.0
Mixed, Omega, Morrisons*	¼ Pack/25g	138	11.4	554	20.9	15.0	45.6	6.4
Mixed, Omega, Munchy Seeds*	1 Bag/30g	184	14.9	613	28.4	13.1	49.7	2.2
Mixed, Original, The Food Doctor*	1 Serving/30g	157	13.3	522	28.2	3.7	44.4	17.7
Mixed, Roasted, Graze*	1 Pack/25g	160	12.9	640	27.1	4.8	51.5	0.0
Mixed, Salad Sprinkle, Nature's Harvest*	1 Serving/8g	48	4.1	598	20.0	14.6	51.1	4.9
Mixed, Savoury Roasted Seeds, Graze*	1 Pack/34g	203	16.2	595	21.4	17.8	47.5	5.5
Mixed, Seedsational, Graze*	1 Punnet/34g	203	16.2	593	20.5	20.8	47.3	6.5
Mixed, Snacking, CBY, Asda*	1 Serving/25g	145	10.9	581	33.1	10.9	43.5	6.7
Mixed, Toasted, Asda*	1 Serving/28g	132	9.0	470	34.4	10.6	32.2	11.6
Mixed, Wholesome, Love Life, Waitrose*	1 Serving/30g	166	13.6	554	21.3	15.5	45.2	8.0
Mustard, Average	*1 Tsp/3g*	*15*	*0.9*	*469*	*34.9*	*34.9*	*28.8*	*14.7*
Nigella, Average	*1 Tsp/5g*	*20*	*1.7*	*392*	*21.3*	*1.9*	*33.3*	*8.4*
Poppy, Average	*1 Tbsp/9g*	*47*	*3.9*	*533*	*18.0*	*23.7*	*44.7*	*10.0*
Pumpkin, Average	*1 Tbsp/10g*	*57*	*4.6*	*568*	*27.9*	*13.0*	*45.9*	*3.8*
Pumpkin, Love Life, Waitrose*	1 Serve/30g	171	13.7	569	24.4	15.2	45.6	5.3
Pumpkin, Sainsbury's*	1 Pack/90g	490	37.6	545	36.7	5.5	41.8	5.7
Pumpkin, Whole, Roasted, Salted, Average	*1 Serving/50g*	*261*	*21.1*	*522*	*33.0*	*13.4*	*42.1*	*3.9*
Sesame, Average	1oz/28g	171	15.8	610	22.3	3.6	56.4	7.8
Sesame, Love Life, Waitrose*	1 Serving/100g	598	58.0	598	18.2	0.9	58.0	11.8
Sesame, Tesco*	1 Tsp/4g	24	2.3	598	18.2	0.9	58.0	7.9
Sunflower, Average	*1 Tbsp/10g*	*59*	*4.9*	*585*	*23.4*	*15.0*	*48.7*	*5.7*
SEMOLINA								
Average	*1oz/28g*	*98*	*0.5*	*348*	*11.0*	*75.2*	*1.8*	*2.1*
Pudding, Creamed, Ambrosia*	1 Can/425g	344	7.2	81	3.3	13.1	1.7	0.2
Pudding, Creamed, Co-Op*	1 Can/425g	382	8.5	90	4.0	15.0	2.0	0.0
SHALLOTS								
Pickled in Hot & Spicy Vinegar, Tesco*	1 Onion/18g	14	0.0	77	1.0	18.0	0.1	1.9
Raw, Average	*1 Serving/80g*	*16*	*0.2*	*20*	*1.5*	*3.3*	*0.2*	*1.4*
SHANDY								
Bavaria*	1 Can/300ml	109	0.0	36	0.0	0.0	0.0	0.0
Bitter, Original, Ben Shaws*	1 Can/330ml	89	0.0	27	0.0	6.0	0.0	0.0
Canned, Morrisons*	1 Can/330ml	36	0.0	11	0.0	1.8	0.0	0.0
Homemade, Average	1 Pint/568ml	148	0.0	26	0.2	2.9	0.0	0.0
Lemonade, Schweppes*	1 Can/330ml	76	0.0	23	0.0	5.1	0.0	0.0
Lemonade, Traditional Style, Tesco*	1 Can/330ml	63	0.0	19	0.0	4.7	0.0	0.0
Traditional, Fentiman's*	1 Bottle/275ml	102	0.0	37	0.4	8.7	0.0	0.0
SHARK								
Raw	*1oz/28g*	*29*	*0.3*	*102*	*23.0*	*0.0*	*1.1*	*0.0*
SHARON FRUIT								
Average	*1oz/28g*	*20*	*0.0*	*73*	*0.8*	*18.6*	*0.0*	*1.6*

	Measure INFO/WEIGHT	per Measure KCAL	FAT	Nutrition Values per 100g / 100ml KCAL	PROT	CARB	FAT	FIBRE
SHERBET LEMONS								
M & S*	1oz/28g	107	0.0	382	0.0	93.9	0.0	0.0
SHERRY								
Dry, Average	*1 Glass/120ml*	*139*	*0.0*	*116*	*0.2*	*1.4*	*0.0*	*0.0*
Medium	*1 Serving/50ml*	*58*	*0.0*	*116*	*0.1*	*5.9*	*0.0*	*0.0*
Sweet	*1 Serving/50ml*	*68*	*0.0*	*136*	*0.3*	*6.9*	*0.0*	*0.0*
SHORTBREAD								
All Butter, Deans*	1 Biscuit/15g	77	3.8	511	4.9	65.7	25.4	1.2
All Butter, Fingers, Highland, Sainsbury's*	2 Biscuits/40g	208	11.5	521	4.8	59.4	28.8	2.7
All Butter, Fingers, McVitie's*	1 Finger/20g	106	5.4	530	6.5	64.7	27.2	0.0
All Butter, Fingers, Royal Edinburgh Bakery*	1 Biscuit/17g	88	4.8	519	5.8	60.3	28.3	1.8
All Butter, Fingers, Scottish, M&S*	1 Finger/18g	90	4.9	510	5.7	58.9	27.8	4.7
All Butter, Petticoat Tails, Co-Op*	1 Biscuit/13g	68	3.8	520	5.0	60.0	29.0	2.0
All Butter, Petticoat Tails, Gardiners of Scotland*	1 Biscuit/12g	64	3.4	514	5.2	62.1	27.2	0.0
All Butter, Round, Luxury, M&S*	1 Biscuit/20g	105	5.8	525	6.2	60.0	29.0	2.0
All Butter, Royal Edinburgh, Asda*	1 Biscuit/18g	93	5.1	519	5.8	60.3	28.3	1.8
All Butter, Scottish, M&S*	1 Biscuit/34g	173	9.5	510	5.7	58.9	27.8	2.3
All Butter, Thins, M&S*	1 Biscuit/10g	50	2.2	485	5.8	68.4	21.1	3.5
All Butter, Trufree*	1 Biscuit/11g	58	3.1	524	2.0	66.0	28.0	0.9
Assortment, Parkside*	1 Serving/30g	155	8.6	517	5.4	59.8	28.5	2.0
Average	1oz/28g	139	7.3	498	5.9	63.9	26.1	1.9
Bites, Murray*	1 Bar/21g	80	3.5	381	4.8	76.2	16.7	14.3
Butter, Extra Special, Asda*	1 Serving/19g	101	5.9	531	7.0	56.0	31.0	1.8
Caramel, Millionaires, Fox's*	1 Serving/16g	75	3.9	483	6.1	57.9	25.3	0.1
Chocolate, Waitrose*	1oz/28g	144	7.8	516	5.5	61.2	27.7	1.8
Chocolate Chip, Fair Trade, Co-Op*	1 Biscuit/19g	100	6.0	526	5.3	57.9	31.6	2.6
Chocolate Chip, Jacob's*	1 Biscuit/17g	87	4.7	513	5.2	61.2	27.5	1.8
Chocolate Chip, Tesco*	1 Serving/20g	105	6.1	525	7.5	55.0	30.6	3.0
Chocolate Chunk, Belgian, Asda*	1 Biscuit/20g	106	6.2	531	7.0	56.0	31.0	1.8
Chocolate Chunk, Belgian, TTD, Sainsbury's*	1 Biscuit/19g	101	5.7	521	5.1	59.1	29.4	2.0
Clotted Cream, Finest, Tesco*	1 Biscuit/20g	109	6.4	543	5.2	58.0	32.2	1.7
Crawfords*	1 Biscuit/13g	67	3.4	533	6.6	65.0	27.4	2.0
Demerara, Rounds, TTD, Sainsbury's*	1 Biscuit/22g	113	5.9	508	5.1	62.2	26.5	1.8
Double Choc Chip, Petit Four, Scottish, Tesco*	1 Serving/50g	266	15.0	531	5.1	60.4	30.0	1.7
Dutch, M&S*	1 Biscuit/17g	90	5.2	530	5.7	58.2	30.6	0.9
Fingers, Asda*	1 Finger/18g	93	5.1	519	5.8	60.3	28.3	18.0
Fingers, Cornish Cookie*	1 Finger/25g	124	6.4	498	6.4	61.0	25.5	0.0
Fingers, Deans*	1 Finger/24g	115	5.9	488	5.1	60.1	24.8	1.4
Fingers, Highland, Organic, Sainsbury's*	1 Serving/16g	84	4.8	527	5.8	58.7	29.9	1.9
Fingers, Light & Buttery, TTD, Sainsbury's*	1 Biscuit/20g	106	5.8	528	5.1	61.6	29.0	1.7
Fingers, Scottish, Finest, Tesco*	1 Biscuit/21g	104	5.0	498	5.1	65.5	23.9	2.0
Free From, Sainsbury's*	1 Biscuit/20g	98	5.2	490	6.0	58.0	26.0	6.0
Hearts, with Milk Chocolate, M&S*	1 Biscuit/25g	125	6.4	500	7.2	59.5	25.8	3.0
Highland, Organic, Duchy Originals*	1 Biscuit/16g	80	4.2	515	5.2	61.8	27.4	1.7
Mini Bites, Co-Op*	1 Biscuit/10g	53	3.0	530	7.0	59.0	30.0	2.0
Mini Bites, Country Table*	1 Biscuit/10g	52	3.0	525	7.1	59.3	29.5	1.5
Organic, Waitrose*	1 Biscuit/13g	62	3.0	495	5.8	63.0	24.4	1.8
Petticoat Tails, All Butter, Highland, Sainsbury's*	1 Biscuit/13g	64	3.6	516	6.3	58.0	28.8	2.2
Pure Butter, Jacob's*	1 Biscuit/20g	105	5.9	525	5.7	58.6	29.7	1.8
Rings, Handbaked, Border*	1 Biscuit/17g	86	4.9	520	6.2	61.2	29.5	0.0
Stem Ginger, Waitrose*	1 Biscuit/15g	71	3.3	487	4.7	66.0	22.7	1.6
Wheat & GF, Free From Range, Tesco*	1 Biscuit/20g	98	5.2	490	6.0	58.0	26.0	6.0
SHRIMP								
Boiled, Average	*1 Serving/60g*	*70*	*1.4*	*117*	*23.8*	*0.0*	*2.4*	*0.0*

S

	Measure INFO/WEIGHT	per Measure		Nutrition Values per 100g / 100ml				
		KCAL	FAT	KCAL	PROT	CARB	FAT	FIBRE
SHRIMP								
Dried, Average	1oz/28g	69	0.7	245	55.8	0.0	2.4	0.0
Frozen, Average	1oz/28g	20	0.2	73	16.5	0.0	0.8	0.0
in Brine, Canned, Drained, Average	1oz/28g	26	0.3	94	20.8	0.0	1.2	0.0
SKATE								
Grilled	1oz/28g	22	0.1	79	18.9	0.0	0.5	0.0
in Batter, Fried in Blended Oil	1oz/28g	47	2.8	168	14.7	4.9	10.1	0.2
Raw, Edible Portion	1oz/28g	18	0.1	64	15.1	0.0	0.4	0.0
SKIPS								
Bacon, KP Snacks*	1 Bag/17g	81	3.8	474	6.5	62.1	22.2	2.3
Cheesy, KP Snacks*	1 Bag/17g	89	5.0	524	6.2	58.5	29.5	1.0
Pickled Onion, KP Snacks*	1 Bag/13g	67	4.0	512	3.4	56.4	30.3	1.4
Prawn Cocktail, KP Snacks*	1 Bag/15g	82	4.7	532	6.0	58.7	30.1	1.0
SKITTLES								
Mars*	1 Pack/55g	223	2.4	406	0.0	90.6	4.4	0.0
SLICES								
Apple & Raisin, Asda*	3 Slices/43g	173	3.3	400	6.5	74.7	7.7	2.8
Bacon & Cheese, Pastry, Tesco*	1 Slice/165g	480	32.0	291	7.4	21.7	19.4	1.0
Bacon & Cheese, Savoury, Pastry, Somerfield*	1 Slice/165g	490	33.5	297	7.4	21.2	20.3	1.5
Beef, Minced, Morrisons*	1 Slice/143g	457	29.6	320	8.8	24.6	20.7	1.0
Beef, Minced, Steak & Onion, Tesco*	1 Slice/150g	424	27.2	283	8.7	21.3	18.1	1.6
Beef, Minced, with Onion, Sainsbury's*	1 Slice/120g	328	19.7	273	6.8	24.5	16.4	1.1
Cheese, Leek & Red Onion Plait, Linda McCartney*	1 Plait/170g	473	28.1	278	6.7	25.9	16.5	2.4
Cheese & Ham, Pastry, Sainsbury's*	1 Slice/118g	352	23.2	298	7.8	22.5	19.7	1.8
Cheese & Ham, Savoury, Pastry, Somerfield*	1 Slice/150g	399	24.0	266	7.0	23.0	16.0	0.0
Cheese & Onion, Cheddar, Ginsters*	1 Slice/180g	583	40.9	324	7.1	22.8	22.7	1.0
Cheese & Onion, Pastry, Tesco*	1 Slice/150g	502	37.0	335	8.0	20.1	24.7	1.4
Chicken & Mushroom, Ginsters*	1 Slice/180g	439	26.8	244	8.3	19.1	14.9	1.8
Chicken & Mushroom, Sainsbury's*	1 Slice/164g	427	26.5	259	7.3	21.3	16.1	1.0
Chicken & Mushroom, Tesco*	1 Slice/165g	457	28.9	277	9.2	20.6	17.5	0.9
Chocolate, Belgian, Weight Watchers*	1 Slice/30g	99	2.0	329	5.9	61.3	6.7	2.3
Custard, Pastry, Tesco*	1 Slice/108g	275	11.1	255	2.8	37.2	10.3	1.3
Fresh Cream, Tesco*	1 Slice/75g	311	21.0	414	3.5	37.4	27.9	1.0
Iced Lemon, GFY, Asda*	1 Serving/30g	97	0.7	327	3.0	73.6	2.3	1.1
Meat Feast, Ginsters*	1 Slice/180g	468	32.0	260	8.0	17.2	17.8	2.2
Peppered Steak, Asda*	1 Slice/164g	483	31.1	295	9.0	22.0	19.0	1.2
Pork & Egg, Gala, Tesco*	1 Slice/105g	333	24.2	317	10.3	17.2	23.0	3.4
Raisin, Crispy, LC, Tesco*	1 Biscuit/15g	56	0.6	370	6.0	76.6	3.9	5.5
Steak, Peppered, Deep Fill, Ginsters*	1 Slice/180g	513	36.2	285	9.4	16.1	20.1	3.1
Steak, Peppered, Ginsters*	1 Slice/180g	457	27.0	254	8.4	21.3	15.0	1.6
Steak & Onion, Aberdeen Angus, Tesco*	1 Slice/165g	444	27.7	269	8.7	20.7	16.8	1.3
SLIMFAST*								
Cafe Latte, Ready To Drink, Slim Fast*	1 Bottle/325ml	230	6.5	71	4.5	7.0	2.0	1.0
Meal Bar, Fruits of the Forest, Slim Fast*	1 Bar/60g	211	6.1	351	23.7	42.1	10.1	7.3
Meal Bar, Yoghurt & Muesli, Slim Fast*	1 Bar/60g	208	6.5	347	23.9	42.2	10.8	7.4
Milk Shake, Banana, Canned, Slim Fast*	1 Can/325ml	214	8.4	66	4.2	10.6	2.6	4.9
Milk Shake, Chocolate, Ready to Drink, Slim Fast*	1 Bottle/325ml	211	5.2	65	4.6	8.0	1.6	1.5
Shake, Blissful Banana, Ready To Drink, Slim Fast*	1 Bottle/325ml	230	6.6	70	4.5	7.0	2.0	1.5
Shake, Chocolate, Powder, Dry, Slim Fast*	2 Scoops/38g	136	2.8	363	13.9	59.0	7.5	10.9
Shake, Summer Strawberry, Ready to Drink, Slim Fast*	1 Bottle/325ml	230	6.6	70	4.5	7.0	2.0	1.0
Shake, Vanilla, Powder, Dry, Slim Fast*	2 Scoops/37g	131	2.4	360	13.4	60.9	6.5	11.0
Snacks, Chocolate Caramel Bar, Slim Fast*	1 Bar/26g	99	3.2	382	3.4	69.6	12.4	1.2
Snacks, Sour Cream & Chive Pretzels, Slim Fast*	1 Pack/23g	96	2.0	416	9.5	75.2	8.6	3.4

	Measure INFO/WEIGHT	per Measure KCAL	per Measure FAT	Nutrition Values per 100g / 100ml KCAL	PROT	CARB	FAT	FIBRE
SMARTIES								
Biscuits, Nestle*	1 Biscuit/5g	26	1.4	519	7.7	57.6	28.6	0.0
Giants, Nestle*	1 Pack/186g	882	35.9	474	4.6	70.4	19.3	0.7
Mini Cones, Nestle*	1 Serving/44g	145	5.8	330	4.5	45.0	13.1	0.0
Mini Eggs, Nestle*	1 Bag/100g	488	20.3	488	3.9	72.5	20.3	1.2
Nestle*	1 Tube/40g	188	7.1	469	3.9	72.5	17.7	2.4
Tree Decoration, Nestle*	1 Chocolate/18g	95	5.4	529	5.6	58.9	30.1	0.8
SMIRNOFF*								
Ice, Smirnoff*	1 Bottle/275ml	188	0.0	68	1.8	12.0	0.0	0.0
SMOOTHIE								
Apples & Blackcurrants for Kids, Innocent*	1 Carton/180ml	104	0.2	58	0.3	14.1	0.1	0.1
Banana, M&S*	1 Bottle/500ml	400	2.0	80	1.8	16.8	0.4	1.2
Banana & Mango, Juice, Calypso*	1 Carton/200ml	106	0.0	53	0.0	12.8	0.0	1.0
Berry, Prepacked, Average	1 Serving/250ml	133	0.5	53	0.7	11.6	0.2	0.9
Blackberries, Strawberries & Blackcurrants, Innocent*	1 Serving/200ml	108	0.0	54	0.6	11.9	0.0	1.5
Blackberries, Strawberries & Boysenberries, Innocent*	1 Serving/250ml	130	0.2	52	0.6	11.8	0.0	1.3
Blackberries & Blueberries, Innocent*	1 Bottle/250ml	120	0.2	48	0.5	12.0	0.1	2.1
Blackberry, Strawberry, Raspberry, Prepacked, Average	1 Serving/250ml	122	1.0	49	1.2	9.6	0.4	1.1
Blueberry, Blackcurrant & Beetroot, Love Life, Waitrose*	1 Serving/250ml	90	0.2	36	0.2	8.5	0.1	0.8
Cherries & Strawberries, Innocent*	1 Bottle/250ml	122	0.2	49	0.6	12.6	0.1	0.0
Cranberries, Yumberries & Blackcurrants, Innocent*	1 Bottle/250ml	130	0.2	52	0.5	14.2	0.1	1.5
Fruit, The Green One, Ella's Kitchen*	1 Pack/90g	52	0.0	58	0.4	13.4	0.0	1.8
Fruit, The Red One, Ella's Kitchen*	1 Pack/90g	48	0.1	53	0.6	11.6	0.1	1.9
Fruit, Tropical, Free From, Tesco*	1 Pouch/90g	72	1.8	80	0.7	13.4	2.0	1.1
Fruit Kick, Orange, Mango & Pineapple, PJ Smoothies*	1 Carton/100ml	54	0.0	54	0.6	12.2	0.0	0.0
Fruits, The Yellow One, Ella's Kitchen*	1 Pack/90g	63	0.2	70	0.7	15.3	0.2	2.1
Guavas, Mangoes & Goji Berries, Innocent*	1 Bottle/250ml	112	0.2	45	0.6	12.0	0.1	2.1
Kiwi, Apples & Limes, Innocent*	1 Bottle/250ml	125	0.2	50	0.5	11.0	0.1	1.8
Mango & Passionfruit, Prepacked, Average	1 Serving/250ml	145	0.3	58	0.6	12.7	0.1	1.5
Mango & Passionfruit, Tesco*	1 Glass/250ml	150	0.2	60	0.5	12.7	0.1	1.8
Mangoes & Passion Fruits, Pure Fruit, Innocent*	1 Bottle/250ml	142	0.5	57	0.6	12.5	0.2	1.6
Mixed Berry, CBY, Asda*	1 Glass/250ml	143	0.0	57	0.6	12.6	0.0	1.6
Orange, Banana & Pineapple, Innocent*	1 Bottle/250ml	120	1.0	48	0.6	10.8	0.4	0.0
Orange, Mango, Banana & Passion Fruit, Asda*	1 Serving/100ml	55	0.2	55	0.8	12.0	0.2	1.1
Orange, Mango & Pineapple, Prepacked, Average	1 Serving/250ml	131	0.2	52	0.6	11.9	0.1	0.7
Orange & Mango, Fruit, Morrisons*	1 Bottle/250ml	145	0.0	58	0.5	14.0	0.0	0.7
Orange & Mango, Prepacked, Average	1 Serving/250ml	138	0.4	55	0.6	12.4	0.2	0.4
Oranges, Bananas & Pineapples, Innocent*	1 Bottle/250ml	142	0.2	57	0.6	14.1	0.1	0.0
Oranges, Mangoes & Pineapples For Kids, Innocent*	1 Carton/180ml	94	0.2	52	0.7	11.7	0.1	0.9
Peaches & Passion Fruits, Innocent*	1 Bottle/250ml	120	0.2	48	0.5	10.7	0.1	1.7
Peaches & Passionfruit, for Kids, Innocent*	1 Carton/180ml	95	0.0	53	0.6	14.7	0.0	0.9
Peaches & Passionfruits, Innocent For Kids*	1 Carton/180ml	95	0.0	53	0.6	14.7	0.0	0.9
Pineapple, Banana & Coconut, CBY, Asda*	1 Glass/250ml	178	2.8	71	0.7	13.6	1.1	1.0
Pineapples, Bananas & Coconuts, Innocent*	1 Bottle/250ml	172	2.8	69	0.7	13.6	1.1	1.0
Pomegranates, Blueberries & Acai, Special, Innocent*	1 Serving/250ml	170	0.5	68	0.6	15.6	0.2	0.8
Pomegranates & Raspberries, Innocent*	1 Bottle/250ml	150	0.2	60	0.6	15.4	0.1	2.0
Raspberry & Blueberry, Plus, Tesco*	1 Serving/100ml	59	0.3	59	2.6	11.6	0.3	0.5
Strawberries, Blackberries, Raspberries, Kids, Innocent*	1 Carton/180ml	81	0.2	45	0.5	9.9	0.1	1.3
Strawberries & Bananas, PJ Smoothies*	1 Bottle/250ml	118	0.2	47	0.4	11.0	0.1	0.0
Strawberries & Bananas, Pure Fruit, Innocent*	1 Bottle/250ml	132	0.2	53	0.7	13.1	0.1	1.3
Strawberry, Raspberry & Banana, Waitrose*	1 Bottle/250ml	122	0.2	49	0.7	10.8	0.1	0.8
Strawberry & Banana, Fruit, Serious Food Company*	1 Bottle/250ml	135	0.0	54	0.5	12.7	0.0	1.3
Strawberry & Banana, Morrisons*	1 Bottle/250ml	135	0.0	54	0.5	13.0	0.0	0.6
Strawberry & Banana, Prepacked, Average	1 Serving/250ml	131	0.2	53	0.6	11.9	0.1	0.9

S

	Measure INFO/WEIGHT	per Measure KCAL	FAT	Nutrition Values per 100g / 100ml KCAL	PROT	CARB	FAT	FIBRE
SMOOTHIE								
Strawberry & Banana, Tesco*	1 Bottle/250ml	112	0.5	45	0.6	10.1	0.2	0.8
Summer Fruits, Tesco*	1 Bottle/250ml	140	0.0	56	0.2	13.8	0.0	0.5
Super Berry, M&S*	1 Bottle/250ml	150	1.0	60	0.9	13.0	0.4	1.2
Vanilla Bean, M&S*	1 Bottle/500ml	450	13.0	90	3.3	13.9	2.6	0.0
SNACK-A-JACKS								
Barbecue, Jumbo, Quaker Oats*	1 Cake/10g	38	0.2	380	8.0	83.0	2.0	1.7
Barbecue, Snack, Quaker Oats*	1 Bag/30g	123	1.8	410	7.5	81.0	6.0	1.0
Barbeque, Quaker Oats*	1 Pack/26g	106	1.6	408	7.3	81.1	6.1	0.9
Caramel, Jumbo, Quaker Oats*	1 Cake/13g	51	0.3	390	5.5	87.0	2.1	1.4
Caramel, Snack, Quaker Oats*	1 Bag/30g	122	0.9	405	6.0	88.0	3.0	0.8
Cheese, Jumbo, Quaker Oats*	1 Cake/10g	38	0.2	380	8.5	81.0	2.5	1.7
Cheese, Snack, Quaker Oats*	1 Bag/26g	108	2.1	415	8.5	77.0	8.0	0.9
Cheese & Onion, Snack, Quaker Oats*	1 Bag/30g	120	2.2	400	6.7	77.0	7.5	1.5
Chocolate & Caramel, Delights, Quaker Oats*	1 Cake/15g	62	0.9	415	6.0	83.0	6.0	1.6
Chocolate Chip, Jumbo, Quaker Oats*	1 Cake/15g	62	1.0	410	6.0	81.0	7.0	1.7
Hot Tomato, Quaker Oats*	1 Bag/26g	105	2.0	405	7.3	77.1	7.5	1.2
Mini Bagels, Cream Cheese & Chive, Quaker Oats*	1 Bag/35g	145	3.4	415	10.6	71.0	9.7	3.4
Mini Bites, Sour Cream & Sweet Chilli, Quaker Oats*	1 Bag/28g	115	2.2	410	6.5	78.0	8.0	2.0
Mini Breadsticks, Cheese & Onion, Quaker Oats*	1 Bag/35g	145	3.1	414	12.9	71.1	8.9	3.7
Prawn Cocktail, Quaker Oats*	1 Bag/26g	106	2.0	408	6.9	78.3	7.5	0.9
Prawn Cocktail, Snack, Quaker Oats*	1 Bag/30g	123	2.2	410	7.0	78.0	7.5	0.8
Salt & Vinegar, Jumbo Quaker Oats*	1 Cake/10g	41	0.6	391	7.4	75.4	5.7	1.6
Sour Cream & Chive, Quaker Oats*	1 Bag/22g	92	1.7	418	7.7	78.2	7.7	1.4
Sweet Chilli, Quaker Oats*	1 Pack/26g	108	2.0	414	7.3	78.9	7.5	1.1
SNAILS								
in Garlic Butter, Average	6 Snails/50g	219	20.8	438	9.7	8.0	41.5	1.0
Raw, Average	1 Snail/5g	4	0.1	90	16.1	2.0	1.4	0.0
SNAPPER								
Red, Fried in Blended Oil	*1oz/28g*	*35*	*0.9*	*126*	*24.5*	*0.0*	*3.1*	*0.0*
Red, Weighed with Bone, Raw	*1oz/28g*	*25*	*0.4*	*90*	*19.6*	*0.0*	*1.3*	*0.0*
SNICKERS								
Cruncher, Mars*	1 Bar/40g	209	12.0	523	9.0	57.0	30.0	2.3
Mars*	1 Snacksize/41g	208	11.5	511	9.4	54.3	28.2	1.3
SORBET								
Blackcurrant, Del Monte*	1oz/28g	30	0.0	106	0.4	27.1	0.1	0.0
Blackcurrant, Iceland*	¼ Pot/100g	100	0.0	100	0.0	25.0	0.0	0.0
Exotic Fruit, Sainsbury's*	1 Serving/75g	90	1.5	120	1.2	24.1	2.0	0.0
Jamaican Me Crazy, Ben & Jerry's*	1 Serving/100g	130	0.0	130	0.2	32.0	0.0	0.4
Lemon	1 Scoop/60g	79	0.0	131	0.9	34.2	0.0	0.0
Lemon, Organic, Evernat*	1oz/28g	27	0.1	96	0.1	22.8	0.5	0.0
Lemon, Sainsbury's*	¼ Pot/89g	100	0.0	112	0.0	28.1	0.0	0.1
Lemon, Sicilian, Seriously Fruity, Waitrose*	1/5 Pot/100ml	77	0.1	77	18.8	13.5	0.1	0.2
Lemon, Tesco*	1 Serving/75g	80	0.0	106	0.0	26.2	0.0	0.4
Mango, Del Monte*	1 Sorbet/500g	575	0.5	115	0.2	29.6	0.1	0.0
Mango, Organic, M&S*	1 Serving/100g	99	0.1	99	0.3	24.1	0.1	0.9
Mango, Tesco*	1 Serving/100g	107	0.0	107	0.1	26.5	0.0	0.3
Mango, Waitrose*	1 Pot/100g	90	0.0	90	0.1	22.1	0.0	0.6
Mango Berry Swirl, Ben & Jerry's*	1 Serving/100g	100	0.0	100	0.2	25.0	0.0	1.5
Orange, Del Monte*	1 Sorbet/500g	625	0.5	125	0.2	32.1	0.1	0.0
Passion Fruit, Fat Free, M&S*	1 Sorbet/125g	129	0.0	103	0.4	25.0	0.0	0.4
Pear, Organic, Evernat*	1oz/28g	33	0.2	119	0.0	28.3	0.6	0.0
Pineapple, Del Monte*	1 Sorbet/500g	600	0.5	120	0.3	30.6	0.1	0.0
Raspberry, Haagen-Dazs*	½ Cup/105g	120	0.0	114	0.0	28.6	0.0	1.9

	Measure INFO/WEIGHT	per Measure KCAL	FAT	Nutrition Values per 100g / 100ml KCAL	PROT	CARB	FAT	FIBRE
SORBET								
Raspberry, Sticks, Haagen-Dazs*	1oz/28g	28	0.0	99	0.2	24.2	0.1	0.0
Raspberry, Tesco*	1 Serving/70ml	97	0.0	138	0.5	34.0	0.0	0.0
Raspberry, Waitrose*	1 Pot/750ml	690	0.8	92	0.5	22.2	0.1	1.1
Strawberry, & Champagne, Sainsbury's*	¼ Pot/89g	95	0.0	107	0.2	25.5	0.0	0.6
Strawberry, M&S*	1oz/28g	27	0.0	95	0.3	23.4	0.1	0.5
Summer Berry, Swirl, Asda*	¼ Pack/89g	97	0.4	109	3.0	26.0	0.4	0.0
SOUFFLE								
Cheese	1oz/28g	71	5.4	253	11.4	9.3	19.2	0.3
Cheese, Alizonne*	1 Serving/33g	129	3.4	392	60.5	14.5	10.2	0.2
Cheese, Mini, Waitrose*	1 Souffle/14g	32	2.4	232	16.0	2.9	17.4	2.4
Chocolate, Gu*	1 Pot/70g	307	24.9	439	6.3	24.4	35.6	2.9
Hot Chocolate, Gu*	1 Pot/65g	298	23.5	458	6.0	24.1	36.2	2.5
Lemon, Finest, Tesco*	1 Pot/80g	270	20.5	338	2.9	24.1	25.6	0.2
Plain	1oz/28g	56	4.1	201	7.6	10.4	14.7	0.3
Raspberry & Amaretto, M&S*	1oz/28g	83	4.7	298	2.8	33.1	16.7	0.1
Strawberry, M&S*	1 Serving/95g	171	10.1	180	1.6	19.5	10.6	0.9
SOUP								
Asparagus, & Chicken, Waitrose*	1 Can/415g	166	4.6	40	2.1	5.3	1.1	0.7
Asparagus, Fresh, Finest, Tesco*	½ Pot/300g	153	8.1	51	1.6	5.0	2.7	1.0
Asparagus, Fresh, M&S*	1 Serving/300g	135	10.8	45	1.1	2.5	3.6	0.9
Asparagus, in a Cup, You Count, Love Life, Waitrose*	1 Serving/200ml	57	1.6	28	0.5	4.8	0.8	0.3
Asparagus, New Covent Garden Food Co*	½ Carton/300g	132	7.2	44	1.5	4.1	2.4	0.9
Asparagus, Slimline, Cup, Made Up, Waitrose*	1 Serving/204ml	51	1.4	25	0.4	4.3	0.7	0.7
Bacon, Leek & Potato, Big Soup, Canned, Heinz*	1 Can/515g	278	10.8	54	1.9	6.6	2.1	0.6
Bacon & Bean, Smoked, Diet Chef Ltd*	1 Pack/300g	162	3.3	54	2.8	8.2	1.1	2.1
Bacon & Lentil, CBY, Asda*	1 Pot/600g	348	7.2	58	3.3	7.7	1.2	1.6
Bacon & Three Bean, Smoked, Chunky, Baxters*	1 Can/400g	232	4.8	58	2.9	8.8	1.2	1.8
Bean, Italian, Fresh, Love Life, Waitrose*	½ Pot/300g	165	7.2	55	1.6	6.0	2.4	1.7
Bean, Spicy, Mexican, Weight Watchers*	1 Can/295g	112	1.5	38	1.2	6.8	0.5	0.9
Bean, Three, & Vegetable, LC, Tesco*	½ Can/200g	110	0.6	55	2.6	9.7	0.3	1.9
Bean, Three, Spicy, Tesco*	½ Carton/300g	165	4.5	55	2.8	7.3	1.5	2.1
Bean, Tuscan, Chunky, Love Life, Waitrose*	½ Can/200g	90	1.0	45	2.6	7.6	0.5	2.3
Bean, Tuscan, GFY, Asda*	1 Carton/400ml	224	3.6	56	2.9	9.0	0.9	0.8
Bean, Tuscan, New Covent Garden Food Co*	½ Carton/300g	84	2.4	28	1.6	3.7	0.8	1.0
Bean & Ham, Boston, New Covent Garden Food Co*	½ Carton/300g	171	0.6	57	2.4	7.8	0.2	1.6
Bean & Pancetta, White, Finest, Tesco*	1 Pot/600g	450	19.8	75	3.5	6.2	3.3	2.2
Bean & Pasta, Italian, Healthy, Baxters*	1 Can/415g	208	1.2	50	2.1	8.6	0.3	2.4
Bean & Sausage, Tuscan Style, Chunky, M&S*	1 Can/415g	249	9.1	60	2.4	7.7	2.2	1.0
Bean & Vegetable, Chunky, CBY, Asda*	1 Can/400g	224	1.2	56	2.6	9.7	0.3	1.9
Beef, Spicy, & Tomato, Diet Chef Ltd*	1 Pack/300g	165	5.7	55	2.3	7.3	1.9	1.9
Beef & Ale, Canned, M&S*	1 Can/400g	150	4.0	38	1.0	5.4	1.0	1.4
Beef & Black Bean, Brazilian, Glorious!*	½ Pot/300g	144	6.9	48	2.0	4.8	2.3	0.8
Beef & Tomato, Cup a Soup, Made Up, Batchelors*	1 Serving/252g	83	1.6	33	0.6	6.3	0.6	0.4
Beef & Tomato, in a Cup, Made Up, Sainsbury's*	1 Serving/210ml	61	1.1	29	0.6	5.6	0.5	0.2
Beef & Vegetable, Big Soup, Heinz*	1 Can/400g	212	4.0	53	3.5	7.5	1.0	0.9
Beef & Vegetable, Broth, Chunky, Canned, M&S*	1 Can/415g	166	3.3	40	1.9	6.4	0.8	0.6
Beef & Vegetable, Chunky, Asda*	1 Can/400g	212	8.4	53	1.7	5.7	2.1	2.2
Beef & Vegetable, Chunky, Canned, Sainsbury's*	1 Can/400g	188	3.2	47	3.2	6.7	0.8	1.3
Beef Broth, Big Soup, Heinz*	1 Can/400g	184	2.8	46	2.5	7.0	0.7	0.9
Beef Broth, CBY, Asda*	1 Pot/300g	174	3.6	58	2.6	8.6	1.2	1.3
Beef Broth, Classic, Heinz*	1 Can/400g	180	2.0	45	1.9	7.6	0.5	0.8
Beef Goulash, & Paprika Potatoes, Eat Live Enjoy, Tesco*	1 Pack/300g	229	3.9	76	9.1	6.7	1.3	0.7
Beef Stew & Dumplings, Taste of Home, Heinz*	1 Pot/430g	378	13.8	88	3.7	11.1	3.2	0.8

SOUP

INFO/WEIGHT	Measure	per Measure		Nutrition Values per 100g / 100ml				
		KCAL	FAT	KCAL	PROT	CARB	FAT	FIBRE
Beetroot, & Smokey Bacon, Daylesford Organics*	½ Carton/250ml	312	24.0	125	3.2	6.4	9.6	1.2
Beetroot, Tomato & Buckwheat, Stay Full, Baxters*	1 Can/400g	264	4.8	66	3.4	8.7	1.2	2.9
Beetroot, with Chopped Dill, Duchy Originals*	½ Pot/298g	152	7.4	51	1.1	5.9	2.5	0.9
Black Bean, Corn & Chipotle, Fresh, Finest, Tesco*	½ Pot/300g	165	4.8	55	2.2	7.0	1.6	1.9
Broccoli, Pea & Mint, Love Life, Waitrose*	1 Pot/400g	200	9.6	50	2.7	4.3	2.4	2.1
Broccoli, Salmon & Watercress, Stay Full, Baxters*	1 Can/400g	244	8.8	61	3.3	5.8	2.2	2.4
Broccoli & Cauliflower, Cup, BFY, Morrisons*	1 Sachet/15g	56	2.1	376	4.9	57.2	14.2	4.9
Broccoli & Cauliflower, Cup-A-Soup, Made Up, Batchelors*	1 Serving/255g	107	5.1	42	0.6	5.3	2.0	1.1
Broccoli & Stilton, Canned, Sainsbury's*	½ Can/200g	108	7.0	54	2.0	3.7	3.5	0.6
Broccoli & Stilton, Canned, Tesco*	1 Can/400g	240	14.0	60	1.7	5.0	3.5	0.4
Broccoli & Stilton, Classics, Fresh, Tesco*	½ Pot/300g	180	8.4	60	2.9	5.8	2.8	1.1
Broccoli & Stilton, Cup Soup, Made Up, Ainsley Harriott*	1 Serving/229ml	87	1.8	38	1.0	7.0	0.8	1.3
Broccoli & Stilton, English, Dry, Knorr*	1 Pack/65g	331	24.6	509	11.7	30.3	37.9	1.6
Broccoli & Stilton, Farmers Market, Heinz*	½ Can/200g	108	7.4	54	1.5	3.2	3.7	0.9
Broccoli & Stilton, Fresh, Sainsbury's*	½ Pot/300ml	141	9.9	47	2.7	1.8	3.3	1.5
Broccoli & Stilton, New Covent Garden Food Co*	1 Carton/600ml	240	14.4	40	2.2	1.9	2.4	1.1
Broccoli & Stilton, Somerfield*	½ Pack/250g	140	9.8	56	1.6	3.5	3.9	1.5
Broccoli & Stilton, Tesco*	1 Can/400g	192	10.4	48	1.9	4.2	2.6	1.2
Butter Bean, & Chorizo, Meal, Sainsbury's*	1 Pot/400g	257	9.6	64	3.9	5.6	2.4	2.3
Butternut Squash, & Edamame Bean, Stay Full, Baxters*	1 Can/400g	272	4.0	68	3.5	9.5	1.0	3.6
Butternut Squash, & Red Pepper, Vegetarian, Baxters*	1 Can/415g	149	2.5	36	0.9	6.6	0.6	0.5
Butternut Squash, & Sage, New Covent Garden Food Co*	½ Carton/300g	153	6.9	51	0.9	6.6	2.3	0.7
Butternut Squash, & Tarragon, Waitrose*	½ Pot/300g	123	6.6	41	0.8	4.5	2.2	1.0
Butternut Squash, Creamy, New Covent Garden Food Co*	½ Carton/300g	153	7.5	51	0.8	6.4	2.5	0.9
Butternut Squash, Curried, & Lentil, Seeds of Change*	1 Pack/400g	164	1.2	41	2.3	7.2	0.3	1.9
Butternut Squash, Diet Chef Ltd*	1 Pack/300g	135	5.4	45	0.8	6.5	1.8	1.6
Butternut Squash, Fresh, Waitrose*	½ Pot/300g	153	8.7	51	0.5	5.8	2.9	0.8
Butternut Squash, Skinny Soup, Glorious!*	½ Pot/300g	103	3.6	34	0.6	5.9	1.2	0.7
Butternut Squash & Ginger, Waitrose*	½ Pot/300g	210	17.4	70	0.9	3.5	5.8	1.0
Carrot, Honey & Coriander, Cully And Sully*	1 Bowl/200g	56	3.2	28	0.5	3.3	1.6	1.0
Carrot, Onion & Chickpea, Healthy, Baxters*	1 Can/415g	170	0.8	41	1.9	8.0	0.2	1.2
Carrot, Orange & Coriander, COU, M&S*	1 Pack/415g	145	2.5	35	0.6	6.9	0.6	1.2
Carrot, Red Lentil & Cumin, Organic, Waitrose*	1 Pack/350g	175	8.8	50	0.2	6.7	2.5	0.5
Carrot, Thai, Fragrant, Skinny Soup, Glorious!*	½ Tub/298g	119	5.4	40	0.3	3.5	1.8	1.6
Carrot & Butterbean, & Coriander Soup, Chunky, Baxters*	1 Can/415g	220	2.5	53	2.1	9.9	0.6	2.2
Carrot & Butterbean, Diet Chef Ltd*	1 Pack/300g	174	2.1	58	2.7	10.3	0.7	2.8
Carrot & Butterbean, Vegetarian, Baxters*	1 Can/415g	237	7.9	57	1.5	7.2	1.9	2.2
Carrot & Coriander, & Ginger, So Organic, Sainsbury's*	½ Can/197g	75	3.3	38	0.3	5.3	1.7	0.7
Carrot & Coriander, 'A' Meal, Feeling Great, Findus*	1 Serving/371g	130	3.7	35	1.5	5.5	1.0	1.5
Carrot & Coriander, Average	1 Serving/200g	83	4.3	42	0.6	4.8	2.2	1.0
Carrot & Coriander, Blended, Heinz*	½ Can/200g	104	5.4	52	0.7	6.2	2.7	0.6
Carrot & Coriander, Canned, BGTY, Sainsbury's*	½ Can/200g	62	2.0	31	0.8	4.8	1.0	0.9
Carrot & Coriander, Canned, GFY, Asda*	1 Can/400g	116	2.4	29	0.7	5.3	0.6	0.6
Carrot & Coriander, Canned, M&S*	½ Can/210g	94	5.0	45	0.4	5.9	2.4	0.9
Carrot & Coriander, Canned, Tesco*	1 Can/400g	220	11.6	55	0.7	5.7	2.9	0.8
Carrot & Coriander, Carton, Campbell's*	1 Serving/250ml	110	5.5	44	0.7	5.4	2.2	0.0
Carrot & Coriander, Classic, Classic, Heinz*	1 Can/400g	164	6.4	41	0.4	5.8	1.6	0.9
Carrot & Coriander, Classic Homestyle, M&S*	1 Can/425g	170	8.5	40	0.6	5.6	2.0	0.7
Carrot & Coriander, Fresh, Healthy Living, Co-Op*	1 Pot/600g	180	6.0	30	0.6	4.7	1.0	1.0
Carrot & Coriander, Fresh, Love Life, Waitrose*	½ Pot/300g	141	9.6	47	0.7	3.6	3.2	1.0
Carrot & Coriander, Fresh, M&S*	½ Pot/300g	90	4.5	30	0.4	4.2	1.5	0.5
Carrot & Coriander, Fresh, Morrisons*	½ Pot/300g	117	7.2	39	1.1	3.2	2.4	0.9
Carrot & Coriander, Fresh, Organic, Simply Organic*	1 Pot/600g	276	18.0	46	0.5	4.5	3.0	1.3

SOUP

	Measure INFO/WEIGHT	per Measure KCAL	FAT	Nutrition Values per 100g / 100ml KCAL	PROT	CARB	FAT	FIBRE
Carrot & Coriander, In A Mug, Made Up, LC, Tesco*	1 Serving/219ml	63	1.5	29	0.5	5.1	0.7	1.2
Carrot & Coriander, Less Than 5% Fat, Asda*	1 Serving/300g	96	0.9	32	1.0	6.0	0.3	0.8
Carrot & Coriander, Low Calorie, Average	1 Serving/200g	45	1.3	22	0.6	3.5	0.6	1.1
Carrot & Coriander, New Covent Garden Food Co*	½ Carton/300g	108	4.5	36	0.6	4.2	1.5	1.4
Carrot & Coriander, Weight Watchers*	1 Pouch/300g	102	3.9	34	0.4	5.1	1.3	0.6
Carrot & Ginger, Fresh, Sainsbury's*	1 Pot/600g	150	5.4	25	0.4	3.9	0.9	1.0
Carrot & Lentil, Microwave, Heinz*	1 Can/303g	94	0.3	31	1.5	6.1	0.1	0.8
Carrot & Lentil, Weight Watchers*	1 Can/295g	87	0.3	29	1.3	5.5	0.1	0.7
Carrot & Orange	1oz/28g	6	0.1	20	0.4	3.7	0.5	1.0
Carrot & Orange, Fresh, Finest, Tesco*	½ Tub/300g	150	5.7	50	0.7	7.5	1.9	1.1
Carrot & Parsnip, Fresh, Extra Special, Asda*	½ Pot/300g	153	8.4	51	1.2	4.8	2.8	0.8
Celeriac, & Root Veg, New Covent Garden Food Co*	1 Serving/300g	126	7.5	42	0.7	3.1	2.5	2.1
Celeriac & Truffle, New Covent Garden Food Co*	1 Serving/300g	225	17.7	75	1.1	4.3	5.9	0.7
Chick Pea & Chorizo, Truly Irresistible, Co-Op*	½ Pack/300g	170	5.3	55	2.7	7.0	1.7	1.2
Chicken, & Orzo, Tuscan, Glorious!*	½ Pot/300g	120	1.2	40	2.8	6.2	0.4	0.7
Chicken, & Pasta, Big, Heinz*	½ Can/200g	68	0.8	34	1.8	5.9	0.4	0.8
Chicken, Broth, Organic, Low Sodium, Pacific Foods*	1 Serving/250ml	10	0.1	4	0.4	0.4	0.0	0.0
Chicken, Condensed, 99% Fat Free, Campbell's*	1 Can/295g	77	2.1	26	1.0	3.8	0.7	0.1
Chicken, Cream of, Canned, Tesco*	1 Can/400g	260	15.2	65	1.2	5.5	3.8	0.0
Chicken, Cream of, Reduced Salt, Heinz*	1 Can/400g	216	12.0	54	1.7	4.9	3.0	0.1
Chicken, Cream of, Thai Spices, Black Label, Heinz*	1 Can/400g	260	13.6	65	1.6	6.9	3.4	0.1
Chicken, Cream of, Twist of Sage, Special Edition, Heinz*	½ Can/200g	108	6.0	54	1.7	4.9	3.0	0.1
Chicken, Cup, Calorie Counter, Dry, Co-Op*	1 Sachet/13g	40	1.4	320	6.0	49.0	11.0	7.0
Chicken, Fresh, Sainsbury's*	½ Carton/300g	126	5.7	42	2.2	4.0	1.9	0.3
Chicken, Green Thai, Sainsbury's*	1 Pot/600g	366	19.8	61	1.9	5.8	3.3	0.3
Chicken, Green Thai, Spiced, M&S*	½ Pot/300g	195	11.4	65	2.0	6.3	3.8	0.6
Chicken, Green Thai, Waitrose*	1 Pot/600g	462	30.0	77	4.4	3.5	5.0	1.6
Chicken, Indian, Glorious!*	½ Pot/300g	201	7.5	67	3.4	7.6	2.5	0.7
Chicken, Jamaican Jerk & Pumpkin, Sainsbury's*	½ Pot/300g	141	5.1	47	2.7	5.1	1.7	0.2
Chicken, Keralan Spiced, Waitrose*	½ Pot/300g	222	14.1	74	3.9	4.0	4.7	2.2
Chicken, Low Fat, Condensed, Batchelors*	1 Can/295g	148	4.1	50	1.9	7.5	1.4	0.2
Chicken, Moroccan, Finest, Tesco*	½ Pot/300g	180	5.1	60	3.6	6.8	1.7	1.2
Chicken, Moroccan, New Covent Garden Food Co*	1 Serving/300g	108	5.7	36	2.1	2.7	1.9	0.4
Chicken, Moroccan Inspired, Sainsbury's*	1 Bowl/342g	202	3.1	59	2.6	10.2	0.9	7.5
Chicken, Moroccan Style, Spiced, Eat Well, M&S*	1 Portion/300g	195	9.9	65	4.0	5.3	3.3	4.4
Chicken, New Covent Garden Food Co*	1 Carton/600g	510	32.4	85	3.8	5.4	5.4	0.6
Chicken, Packet, Knorr*	1 Pack/85g	423	27.5	498	7.7	44.3	32.3	0.2
Chicken, Potato, & Lentil, Weight Watchers*	1 Can/400g	136	3.6	34	1.2	5.3	0.9	0.3
Chicken, Potato & Bacon, Big Soup, Heinz*	1 Can/515g	294	11.3	57	3.0	6.1	2.2	0.5
Chicken, Potato & Leek, Weight Watchers*	1 Can/295g	97	2.4	33	1.1	5.1	0.8	0.3
Chicken, Roast, Celebrity Slim*	1 Pack/55g	210	3.1	382	28.6	52.6	5.6	0.9
Chicken, Scrumpy, New Covent Garden Food Co*	½ Carton/300g	144	5.1	48	3.3	4.3	1.7	1.2
Chicken, Spicy Cajun Style, Whole & Hearty, CBY, Asda*	1 Pot/400g	220	4.8	55	4.1	6.4	1.2	1.1
Chicken, Spicy Thai, Nupo*	1 Serving/32g	114	2.4	356	38.0	39.0	7.6	9.3
Chicken, Thai, Cully & Sully*	1 Pack/400g	204	7.2	51	2.7	6.4	1.8	0.6
Chicken, Thai, Fresh, Finest, Tesco*	½ Tub/300g	255	16.2	85	4.1	4.2	5.4	1.1
Chicken, Thai, GFY, Asda*	1 Serving/200g	85	3.0	42	1.7	5.5	1.5	0.5
Chicken, Thai, New Covent Garden Food Co*	½ Carton/300g	174	10.5	58	2.6	4.1	3.5	0.8
Chicken, Thai, Sunny, Glorious!*	½ Pot/300g	201	6.6	67	3.6	8.3	2.2	1.0
Chicken, Thai, Whole & Hearty, CBY, Asda*	1 Pot/400g	265	8.4	66	4.3	7.1	2.1	0.9
Chicken, Thai Style, GFY, Asda*	½ Can/200g	66	2.2	33	1.3	4.4	1.1	0.8
Chicken, Thai Style, Morrisons*	1 Serving/250g	240	15.5	96	4.6	5.5	6.2	1.2
Chicken, Thai Style, Thick & Creamy, in a Mug, Tesco*	1 Sachet/28g	107	4.0	390	3.7	61.3	14.5	5.1

SOUP

INFO/WEIGHT	Measure	per Measure KCAL	per Measure FAT	Nutrition Values per 100g / 100ml KCAL	PROT	CARB	FAT	FIBRE
Chicken, Tomato & Red Pepper, Italian, Big Soup, Heinz*	½ Can/200g	78	1.8	39	1.6	6.2	0.9	0.7
Chicken, Weight Watchers*	1 Can/295g	97	3.0	33	1.6	4.4	1.0	0.0
Chicken, West Indian, Bowl, Waitrose*	1 Bowl/400g	240	4.8	60	2.4	8.1	1.2	1.4
Chicken, with Thai Herbs, Deli Inspired, Baxters*	1 Can/415g	349	25.7	84	1.8	5.1	6.2	0.8
Chicken, with Tomato & Rosemary, Farmers Market, Heinz*	1 Can/400g	164	4.0	41	2.0	5.8	1.0	0.5
Chicken & Bacon, with Vegetables, Organic, Tideford*	½ Pot/300g	225	3.6	75	3.6	6.5	1.2	2.4
Chicken & Barley, & Vegetable, Fuller Longer, M&S*	1 Pack/400g	200	6.0	50	4.9	4.5	1.5	1.6
Chicken & Barley, Broth, Heinz*	1 Can/400g	128	1.2	32	1.3	5.9	0.3	0.8
Chicken & Chickpea, Moroccan, TTD, Sainsbury's*	½ Pot/300g	207	3.9	69	4.2	9.4	1.3	1.6
Chicken & Country Vegetable, Farmers Market, Heinz*	½ Can/200g	106	4.6	53	2.2	5.3	2.3	1.3
Chicken & Country Vegetable, Soupfulls, Batchelors*	1 Serving/400g	164	3.6	41	5.1	3.0	0.9	1.3
Chicken & Ham, Big, Heinz*	½ Can/200g	92	2.0	46	2.3	6.9	1.0	0.7
Chicken & Leek, & Potato, Canned, BGTY, Sainsbury's*	½ Can/200g	62	0.8	31	1.6	5.3	0.4	0.4
Chicken & Leek, & Potato Soup, Weight Watchers*	1 Tin/295g	80	1.2	27	0.9	5.0	0.4	0.3
Chicken & Leek, & White Wine, Fresh, Finest, Tesco*	1 Pack/300g	216	12.6	72	2.8	5.7	4.2	0.3
Chicken & Leek, Big Soup, Heinz*	½ Can/258g	162	5.2	63	3.0	8.2	2.0	0.6
Chicken & Leek, Cup, Co-Op*	1 Serving/18g	64	2.5	355	3.0	55.0	14.0	8.0
Chicken & Leek, Cup a Soup, Made Up, Batchelors*	1 Serving/259g	96	4.7	37	0.5	4.7	1.8	0.7
Chicken & Leek, Farmhouse, Dry, Knorr*	1 Pack/54g	248	15.7	459	10.3	39.3	29.0	1.5
Chicken & Leek, Instant, Cup, Average	1 Pack/19g	73	2.7	382	5.0	58.2	14.4	8.5
Chicken & Leek, Knorr*	1 Serving/300ml	82	5.2	27	0.6	2.4	1.7	0.1
Chicken & Mushroom, & Rice, Chilled, M&S*	½ Pot/300g	225	10.2	75	3.2	7.3	3.4	1.8
Chicken & Mushroom, Canned, Tesco*	½ Can/200g	130	7.6	65	1.4	5.6	3.8	0.1
Chicken & Mushroom, Creamy, Very Special, Heinz*	1 Serving/260g	130	6.2	50	1.9	5.3	2.4	0.0
Chicken & Mushroom, Extra, Slim a Soup, Batchelors*	1 Serving/257g	90	1.5	35	1.4	5.9	0.6	0.3
Chicken & Mushroom, in a Cup, Made Up, Sainsbury's*	1 Serving/223ml	107	4.2	48	0.7	7.1	1.9	0.1
Chicken & Mushroom, Slim A Soup, Made Up, Batchelors*	1 Serving/203g	63	2.0	31	0.7	4.7	1.0	0.3
Chicken & Mushroom, Soup-A-Slim, Asda*	1 Sachet/14g	51	1.4	362	10.0	58.0	10.0	4.2
Chicken & Sweetcorn, & Potato, Heinz*	1 Can/400g	204	11.2	51	1.2	5.4	2.8	0.3
Chicken & Sweetcorn, Asda*	1 Pot/600g	246	8.4	41	2.2	4.9	1.4	1.6
Chicken & Sweetcorn, Canned, Tesco*	1 Can/400ml	240	6.0	60	1.6	8.2	1.5	0.7
Chicken & Sweetcorn, Cantonese, Fresh, Sainsbury's*	½ Pot/300ml	135	1.5	45	2.1	7.9	0.5	0.5
Chicken & Sweetcorn, CBY, Asda*	1 Pot/600g	294	9.6	49	4.4	4.1	1.6	0.5
Chicken & Sweetcorn, Chinese, Soups of the World, Heinz*	½ Can/260g	117	3.6	45	1.9	6.2	1.4	0.3
Chicken & Sweetcorn, Classic, Heinz*	1 Can/400g	240	11.6	60	2.0	6.3	2.9	0.2
Chicken & Sweetcorn, Fresh, Asda*	1 Pack/500g	260	9.5	52	2.6	6.0	1.9	0.0
Chicken & Sweetcorn, Fresh, Average	1 Serving/300g	146	3.1	48	2.4	7.3	1.0	0.6
Chicken & Sweetcorn, In A Cup, BGTY, Sainsbury's*	1 Sachet/15g	57	1.3	379	7.6	68.3	9.0	1.4
Chicken & Sweetcorn, Light Choice, Tesco*	½ Can 200g	84	0.8	42	1.7	7.9	0.4	0.2
Chicken & Sweetcorn, New Covent Garden Food Co*	1 Carton/600g	282	5.4	47	1.0	8.7	0.9	0.5
Chicken & Thyme, Diet Chef Ltd*	1 Pack/300g	147	9.0	49	2.2	3.4	3.0	0.7
Chicken & Vegetable, Big Soup, Heinz*	½ Can/200g	104	2.8	52	3.3	6.7	1.4	0.8
Chicken & Vegetable, Canned, Average	1 Can/400g	192	8.5	48	2.5	4.6	2.1	0.8
Chicken & Vegetable, Chunky, Asda*	1 Tin/400g	168	2.8	42	2.8	5.4	0.7	1.5
Chicken & Vegetable, Chunky, Canned, Eat Well, M&S*	½ Can/213g	138	4.0	65	4.6	6.9	1.9	1.0
Chicken & Vegetable, Chunky, Meal Soup, Tesco*	1 Can/400g	184	7.2	46	2.5	4.6	1.8	1.0
Chicken & Vegetable, Classic, Heinz*	1 Can/400g	132	1.6	33	1.2	6.2	0.4	0.6
Chicken & Vegetable, Crouton, Cup, Made Up, Campbell's*	1 Serving/222ml	100	4.0	45	0.7	5.9	1.8	0.9
Chicken & Vegetable, Cully & Sully*	½ Pot/200g	98	6.8	49	1.9	3.0	3.4	0.8
Chicken & Vegetable, Fresh, M&S*	½ Pot/300g	120	4.2	40	3.0	2.9	1.4	0.8
Chicken & Vegetable, Fresh, Somerfield*	½ Pot/300g	177	8.4	59	2.9	5.6	2.8	3.0
Chicken & Vegetable, Healthy, Baxters*	1 Can/415g	170	2.1	41	1.9	6.3	0.5	1.8
Chicken & Vegetable, Loyd Grossman*	1 Pack/400g	272	15.2	68	0.5	8.0	3.8	0.6

SOUP

	Measure INFO/WEIGHT	per Measure KCAL	FAT	KCAL	PROT	CARB	FAT	FIBRE
Chicken & Vegetable, Moroccan, Love Life, Waitrose*	½ Pot/300g	192	5.7	64	3.7	7.9	1.9	1.9
Chicken & Vegetable, New Covent Garden Food Co*	1 Carton/600g	288	9.6	48	2.8	5.1	1.6	1.0
Chicken & Vegetable, Soup in a Mug, Value, Tesco*	1 Serving/19g	75	2.5	395	4.4	64.1	13.4	1.6
Chicken & Vegetable, Soup to Go, Asda*	1 Pot/330g	145	5.0	44	2.4	5.1	1.5	0.7
Chicken & Vegetable, Squeeze & Stir, Made Up, Heinz*	1 Serving/249g	102	6.7	41	1.4	2.6	2.7	0.1
Chicken & Vegetable Broth, M Kitchen, Morrisons*	½ Pot/298g	131	4.5	44	2.8	4.0	1.5	1.6
Chicken & Vegetable Casserole, Chunky, Baxters*	1 Can/415g	195	2.9	47	2.4	7.8	0.7	1.1
Chicken & Vegetable Casserole, Taste of Home, Heinz*	1 Pot/430g	331	16.8	77	3.9	6.7	3.9	0.8
Chicken & Wild Garlic, Fresh, Finest, Tesco*	½ Pot/300g	195	12.0	65	4.3	2.6	4.0	0.6
Chicken &Vegetable, Chunky, Love Life, Waitrose*	1 Can/400g	229	5.2	57	4.0	7.3	1.3	1.6
Chicken Arrabbiata, Meal, Fresh, Sainsbury's*	1 Pot/400g	232	6.0	58	4.1	5.3	1.5	1.5
Chicken Balti, Meal, Sainsbury's*	1 Pack/400g	242	7.1	61	3.9	6.3	1.8	1.8
Chicken Broth, Favourites, Baxters*	1 Can/400g	128	0.8	32	1.4	5.7	0.2	0.8
Chicken Curry, & Brown Rice, Sainsbury's*	1 Can/400g	208	4.4	52	3.1	6.3	1.1	2.1
Chicken Curry, CBY, Asda*	½ Pot/300g	216	5.4	72	5.0	8.6	1.8	0.5
Chicken Hotpot, Chunky, Big Soup, Heinz*	½ Can/258g	126	3.1	49	2.3	7.4	1.2	0.8
Chicken Miso, CBY, Asda*	1 Pack/350g	266	6.6	76	9.0	5.0	1.9	1.6
Chicken Miso, Noodle, Waitrose*	1 Pot/400g	268	8.8	67	5.9	5.9	2.2	0.9
Chicken Mulligatawny, Chunky, Meal, Weight Watchers*	1 Pack/340g	163	4.4	48	2.2	6.8	1.3	1.5
Chicken Mulligatawny, Finest, Tesco*	½ Pot/300g	240	12.0	80	4.0	7.0	4.0	0.8
Chicken Mulligatawny, PB, Waitrose*	1 Serving/300g	138	6.0	46	1.7	5.3	2.0	0.4
Chicken Noodle, & Red Pepper, Fresh, Tesco*	1 Serving/400ml	200	1.2	50	3.6	8.5	0.3	0.4
Chicken Noodle, & Vegetable, Slim a Soup, Batchelors*	1 Serving/203g	55	1.0	27	0.8	4.8	0.5	0.6
Chicken Noodle, Batchelors*	1 Pack/284g	71	0.6	25	1.6	4.2	0.2	0.3
Chicken Noodle, Canned, Asda*	1 Can/400g	148	4.4	37	1.7	5.1	1.1	0.7
Chicken Noodle, Canned, Sainsbury's*	½ Can/217g	78	0.7	36	1.7	7.4	0.3	0.7
Chicken Noodle, Chinese, Dry, Knorr*	1 Pack/45g	138	2.0	307	15.1	51.8	4.4	2.9
Chicken Noodle, Chinese, Slim a Soup Extra, Batchelors*	1 Sachet/246g	69	0.7	28	1.0	5.3	0.3	0.4
Chicken Noodle, Chunky, Campbell's*	½ Can/200g	86	1.2	43	2.8	6.5	0.6	0.0
Chicken Noodle, Classic, Heinz*	1 Can/400g	124	1.2	31	1.2	6.0	0.3	0.2
Chicken Noodle, Clear, Weight Watchers*	1 Can/295g	51	0.6	17	0.8	3.1	0.2	0.2
Chicken Noodle, Cup, Dry, Heinz*	1 Sachet/20g	48	0.5	240	8.0	46.0	2.5	1.5
Chicken Noodle, Cup, Made Up, Eat Smart, Morrisons*	1 Serving/216g	41	0.2	19	0.6	4.1	0.1	0.2
Chicken Noodle, Cup, Made Up, GFY, Asda*	1 Serving/215ml	43	0.2	20	0.6	4.2	0.1	0.1
Chicken Noodle, Dry, Nissin*	1 Pack/85g	364	14.1	428	9.5	62.0	16.6	3.3
Chicken Noodle, in a Cup, Love Life, Waitrose*	1 Cup/205ml	43	0.2	21	0.7	4.5	0.1	0.1
Chicken Noodle, in Seconds, Super, Dry, Knorr*	1 Pack/37g	111	1.7	299	17.9	46.1	4.7	0.3
Chicken Noodle, Jeremy's Soups Ltd*	1 Serving/300g	132	5.7	44	3.5	3.3	1.9	0.7
Chicken Noodle, Laksa, Fuller Longer, M&S*	1 Pot/385g	289	7.7	75	7.0	7.1	2.0	0.9
Chicken Noodle, Simmer & Serve, Dried, Sainsbury's*	1 Pack/600ml	102	1.2	17	0.8	2.9	0.2	0.0
Chicken Noodle, Soup in a Cup, Made Up, Sainsbury's*	1 Serving/200ml	44	0.2	22	0.7	4.7	0.1	0.2
Chicken Noodle, Super, Dry, Knorr*	1 Pack/56g	182	2.7	325	14.3	56.0	4.9	1.8
Chickpea, Spiced, & Fresh Red Pepper, M&S*	1 Serving/300g	165	6.9	55	2.2	5.8	2.3	2.5
Chilli, Meal, Chunky, Canned, Tesco*	½ Can/200g	120	2.4	60	5.0	6.3	1.2	1.6
Chilli Bean, CBY, Asda*	1 Pot/600g	258	1.8	43	2.1	6.8	0.3	2.2
Chilli Bean, M&S*	½ Carton/300g	150	7.5	50	2.5	4.7	2.5	2.7
Chilli Bean, Mexican, Tesco*	1 Carton/600g	270	6.6	45	2.2	6.4	1.1	1.9
Chilli Beef, Chunky, Asda*	1 Can/400g	212	4.0	53	4.2	5.7	1.0	2.4
Chilli Beef with Lentils & Buckwheat, Deli Inspired, Baxters*	1 Can/415g	237	2.1	57	3.7	9.3	0.5	1.2
Chilli Pumpkin, Fresh, Sainsbury's*	½ Carton/300g	120	7.2	40	0.6	4.0	2.4	1.3
Chilli Tomato & Pasta, COU, M&S*	1 Serving/300g	150	5.7	50	1.3	7.2	1.9	0.9
Chipotle Chicken, New Covent Garden Food Co*	½ Carton/300g	186	3.3	62	3.9	8.0	1.1	2.3
Chorizo & Bean, TTD, Sainsbury's*	1 Pack/298g	161	2.4	54	4.0	7.6	0.8	5.8

SOUP

Measure INFO/WEIGHT		per Measure		Nutrition Values per 100g / 100ml				
		KCAL	FAT	KCAL	PROT	CARB	FAT	FIBRE
Chowder, Bacon & Corn, M&S*	½ Pot/300g	195	10.8	65	2.5	6.0	3.6	1.8
Chowder, Clam, New England, Select, Campbell's*	1 Cup/240ml	221	14.4	92	2.5	6.0	6.0	0.8
Chowder, Corn, Spicy, New Covent Garden Food Co*	½ Carton/300g	132	5.4	44	1.6	4.3	1.8	2.2
Chowder, Haddock, New Covent Garden Food Co*	½ Carton/300g	125	4.2	42	1.9	4.8	1.4	1.4
Chowder, Haddock, Smoked, Asda*	1 Serving/300g	462	12.0	154	1.6	28.0	4.0	0.5
Chowder, Ham & Sweetcorn, Diet Chef Ltd*	1 Pack/300g	165	3.6	55	1.9	9.2	1.2	0.9
Chowder, Ham & Sweetcorn, Wiltshire, Deli, Baxters*	1 Can/415g	261	12.4	63	1.8	7.1	3.0	0.7
Chowder, Seafood, Waitrose*	1 Can/404g	226	11.3	56	2.2	5.6	2.8	0.6
Chowder, Smoked Haddock, M&S*	½ Pot/300g	180	7.2	60	3.1	6.4	2.4	0.8
Chowder, Sweetcorn & Chicken, Heinz*	1 Serving/200g	148	5.6	74	3.3	9.1	2.8	0.6
Chowder, Vegetable, New Covent Garden Food Co*	½ Carton/300g	159	5.1	53	2.9	6.6	1.7	1.1
Cock-A-Leekie, Favourites, Baxters*	1 Can/400g	116	2.4	29	1.1	4.7	0.6	0.3
Country Garden, Canned, Vegetarian, Baxters*	1 Can/400g	144	2.0	36	1.0	6.2	0.5	1.0
Courgette & Parmesan, Fresh, Sainsbury's*	1 Pack/300ml	198	16.8	66	1.5	2.5	5.6	0.4
Cumberland Sausage & Vegetable, Big Soup, Heinz*	1 Can/515g	221	4.1	43	1.9	6.7	0.8	0.8
Fire Roasted Tomato & Red Pepper, Asda*	½ Tub/265g	114	6.9	43	0.7	4.1	2.6	1.0
Fish, Frozen, Findus*	1 Serving/85g	128	4.7	150	11.0	13.0	5.5	0.0
Fish, Mediterranean, Waitrose*	½ Pot/300g	108	2.7	36	3.4	3.5	0.9	0.7
French Onion	1oz/28g	11	0.6	40	0.2	5.7	2.1	1.0
French Onion, & Cider, Waitrose*	1 Can/425g	94	0.4	22	0.5	4.8	0.1	0.4
French Onion, & Gruyere Cheese, Fresh, Finest, Tesco*	½ Pot/300g	210	15.3	70	1.4	4.7	5.1	0.5
French Onion, Chilled, M&S*	½ Pot/300g	150	4.5	50	2.0	7.2	1.5	1.0
French Onion, Favourites, Baxters*	½ Can/200g	68	1.2	34	0.6	6.0	0.6	0.6
French Onion, Fresh, Sainsbury's*	½ Pot/300g	134	3.6	45	0.9	6.2	1.2	1.2
French Onion, Knorr*	1 Pack/40g	118	1.0	296	6.0	62.5	2.5	6.6
Gazpacho, Canned, Average	1 Can/400g	76	0.4	19	2.9	1.8	0.1	0.2
Gazpacho, New Covent Garden Food Co*	1 Carton/600g	276	17.4	46	1.0	3.3	2.9	1.2
Green Thai Curry, Chicken Noodle, M&S*	1 Pack/256g	333	9.0	130	5.3	18.9	3.5	1.1
Ham Hock & Maple, Creamy, New York Soup Co*	½ Pot/300g	135	5.4	45	2.0	5.0	1.8	0.3
Highlander's Broth, Favourites, Baxters*	1 Can/400g	192	5.6	48	1.7	6.3	1.4	0.9
Hot & Sour, Cup Soup, Made Up, Ainsley Harriott*	1 Serving/221ml	62	0.0	28	0.5	5.9	0.0	1.1
Hot & Sour Noodle, Cantonese, Baxters*	1 Serving/215g	133	2.8	62	1.4	11.1	1.3	0.5
Italian Wedding, Deli Inspired, Baxters*	1 Can/400g	199	5.4	48	2.1	6.9	1.3	0.9
Lamb & Vegetable, Big Soup, Heinz*	½ Can/200g	120	2.6	60	3.0	9.1	1.3	1.3
Lamb Casserole, Chunky, Baxters*	1 Can/415g	232	3.3	56	2.4	9.0	0.8	1.6
Lancashire Lamb Hotpot, Taste of Home, Heinz*	1 Pot/430g	299	11.1	70	2.6	8.9	2.6	1.1
Leek, Cream of, Favourites, Baxters*	1 Can/400g	228	16.8	57	1.1	3.8	4.2	0.7
Leek & Potato	1oz/28g	15	0.7	52	1.5	6.2	2.6	0.8
Leek & Potato, & Bacon, Fresh, Baxters*	½ Pot/300g	249	16.8	83	2.0	6.1	5.6	0.7
Leek & Potato, & Thyme, Farmers Market, Heinz*	1 Can/515g	294	15.4	57	0.9	6.7	3.0	0.6
Leek & Potato, Chunky, Meal, Canned, Tesco*	½ Can/200g	60	2.6	30	1.0	3.5	1.3	1.0
Leek & Potato, Classics, Canned, Heinz*	1 Can/400g	184	7.2	46	0.8	6.7	1.8	0.6
Leek & Potato, Creamy, Fresh, Asda*	1 Serving/300g	106	2.4	35	1.0	5.4	0.8	1.2
Leek & Potato, Cup a Soup, Batchelors*	1 Sachet/28g	121	4.9	432	5.2	63.2	17.6	1.8
Leek & Potato, Favourites, Baxters*	1 Can/400g	192	7.2	48	1.0	6.6	1.8	0.9
Leek & Potato, Fresh, Chilled, CBY, Asda*	½ Pot/300g	105	2.4	35	1.0	5.4	0.8	1.2
Leek & Potato, Fresh, Sainsbury's*	½ Pot/300ml	141	7.2	47	1.0	5.3	2.4	0.4
Leek & Potato, Fresh, Sainsbury's*	½ Pot/300g	114	3.6	38	0.7	6.1	1.2	1.3
Leek & Potato, Fresh, Waitrose*	½ Pot/300g	108	5.1	36	0.7	4.6	1.7	0.9
Leek & Potato, Fresh with Cream, Tesco*	½ Tub/300g	180	7.2	60	1.5	8.0	2.4	0.9
Leek & Potato, in a Cup, BGTY, Made Up, Sainsbury's*	1 Serving/218ml	59	1.5	27	0.3	4.9	0.7	0.2
Leek & Potato, in a Mug, Made Up, LC, Tesco*	1 Serving/220g	55	0.9	25	0.5	4.9	0.4	0.6
Leek & Potato, Instant, Cup, Average	1 Pack/22g	83	1.9	379	5.0	70.0	8.7	4.0

SOUP

INFO/WEIGHT	Measure INFO/WEIGHT	per Measure KCAL	FAT	Nutrition Values per 100g / 100ml KCAL	PROT	CARB	FAT	FIBRE
Leek & Potato, Maris Piper, Chilled, M&S*	1 Serving/300g	165	11.4	55	0.6	4.5	3.8	0.9
Leek & Potato, Mix, Made Up, Sainsbury's*	½ Pack/204g	39	0.4	19	0.6	3.6	0.2	0.5
Leek & Potato, Slim a Soup, Batchelors*	1 Serving/204g	57	1.4	28	0.4	5.0	0.7	0.2
Leek & Potato, Smooth, Vie, Knorr*	1 Pack/500ml	155	4.5	31	0.9	4.8	0.9	1.0
Leek & Potato, Solo Slim, Rosemary Conley*	1 Pack/300g	156	6.6	52	0.9	7.2	2.2	1.1
Leek & Potato, Weight Watchers*	1 Serving/215ml	58	1.1	27	0.5	5.1	0.5	0.1
Lemon Rasam, Love Life, Waitrose*	½ Pot/300g	147	4.2	49	3.7	5.3	1.4	1.8
Lentil, & Chilli, Red, Fresh, Love Life, Waitrose*	½ Pot/300g	138	4.5	46	1.7	6.4	1.5	1.3
Lentil, & Ham, Red, Waitrose*	½ Pot/300g	147	3.3	49	3.9	5.8	1.1	2.0
Lentil, & Smoked Bacon, Red, M&S*	½ Pot/300g	225	9.6	75	4.3	6.6	3.2	1.9
Lentil, & Vegetable, Red, Favourites, Baxters*	1 Can/400g	192	2.0	48	2.6	8.3	0.5	1.2
Lentil, & Vine Ripened Tomato, Puy, Finest, Tesco*	1 Pot/600g	360	7.8	60	2.8	9.2	1.3	1.5
Lentil, Asda*	½ Can/202g	89	0.4	44	2.6	8.0	0.2	0.7
Lentil, Average	1 Carton/600g	594	22.8	99	4.4	12.7	3.8	1.1
Lentil, Canned	1 Serving/220g	86	0.4	39	3.1	6.5	0.2	1.2
Lentil, Carrot & Cumin, Canned, BGTY, Sainsbury's*	1 Can/400g	204	3.6	51	2.3	8.4	0.9	0.1
Lentil, Classic, Heinz*	1 Can/400g	192	0.8	48	2.3	8.7	0.2	0.8
Lentil, Farmfoods*	1 Can/225g	304	8.3	135	8.4	16.9	3.7	3.2
Lentil, Low Fat, Solo Slim, Rosemary Conley*	1 Pack/300g	102	0.9	34	2.0	5.8	0.3	0.3
Lentil, Spicy, Chilled, Morrisons*	1 Serving/300ml	271	8.6	90	3.9	12.3	2.9	4.0
Lentil, Spicy, Cup, Made Up, Ainsley Harriott*	1 Serving/226ml	86	1.1	38	1.1	7.3	0.5	0.4
Lentil, Spicy, in a Mug, Made Up, LC, Tesco*	1 Serving/221ml	62	0.0	28	1.1	5.9	0.0	0.0
Lentil, Spicy, Morrisons*	1 Pot/330g	198	5.6	60	2.1	9.0	1.7	0.8
Lentil, Tomato & Vegetable, M&S*	1 Can/415g	170	3.4	41	2.0	6.3	0.8	1.4
Lentil, with Red Lentils, Carrots, Potato & Onion, Asda*	1 Can/400g	192	0.8	48	1.4	10.2	0.2	1.2
Lentil & Bacon, Canned, Tesco*	1 Serving/200g	96	1.4	48	3.2	7.2	0.7	0.5
Lentil & Bacon, Chunky, Canned, M&S*	1 Can/400g	180	2.4	45	3.3	5.8	0.6	2.1
Lentil & Bacon, Classic, Heinz*	1 Can/400g	232	5.6	58	2.7	8.4	1.4	0.7
Lentil & Bacon, Favourites, Baxters*	1 Can/400g	216	4.4	54	3.3	7.4	1.1	0.8
Lentil & Bacon, Morrisons*	1 Can/400g	188	2.0	47	3.1	7.4	0.5	1.1
Lentil & Bacon, Sainsbury's*	½ Pot/300g	199	5.4	66	4.3	8.2	1.8	1.3
Lentil & Bacon, Somerfield*	1 Can/400g	240	4.4	60	3.0	9.5	1.1	2.2
Lentil & Barley, Superbean, M&S*	1 Pack/400g	180	6.0	45	1.8	5.1	1.5	2.1
Lentil & Bean, Spicy, Canned, Organic, Asda*	1 Can/400g	212	3.2	53	2.8	8.6	0.8	3.0
Lentil & Chick Pea, Fresh, Organic, Tesco*	1 Serving/300ml	117	2.4	39	1.9	6.1	0.8	0.5
Lentil & Parsley, Simply Organic*	1 Pot/600g	390	1.8	65	4.4	11.8	0.3	1.4
Lentil & Red Pepper, Sainsbury's*	½ Pot/300g	162	3.6	54	3.5	7.4	1.2	1.6
Lentil & Smoked Bacon, Fresh, Tesco*	1 Pack/600g	420	11.4	70	3.9	8.5	1.9	1.6
Lentil & Smoked Bacon, New Covent Garden Food Co*	½ Carton/300g	201	3.6	67	4.4	8.6	1.2	2.0
Lentil & Tomato, New Covent Garden Food Co*	½ Pack/284g	162	3.1	57	3.6	8.1	1.1	0.7
Lentil & Tomato, Spicy, Chunky, Fresh, Tesco*	½ Pot/300g	195	5.4	65	2.6	9.7	1.8	1.3
Lentil & Vegetable, Healthy, Baxters*	1 Can/415g	174	1.2	42	1.9	7.4	0.3	1.2
Lentil & Vegetable, LC, Tesco*	1 Can/400g	188	0.8	47	2.5	8.8	0.2	1.1
Lentil & Vegetable, Spicy, CBY, Asda*	1 Pot/330g	178	3.3	54	2.4	8.5	1.0	0.7
Lentil & Vegetable, Spicy, Chilled, M&S*	½ Serving/300g	150	2.4	50	2.7	8.0	0.8	1.1
Lentil & Vegetable, with Bacon, Organic, Baxters*	½ Can/211g	93	1.5	44	1.9	7.6	0.7	1.0
Lincolnshire Sausage Hotpot, Taste of Home, Heinz*	1 Pot/430g	301	13.3	70	2.4	7.9	3.1	1.0
Lobster Bisque, Luxury, with Brandy & Cream, Baxters*	1 Can/415g	282	17.8	68	2.6	4.8	4.3	0.2
Lobster Bisque, New Covent Garden Food Co*	½ Carton/300g	108	1.8	36	3.2	4.4	0.6	0.4
Lobster Bisque, Waitrose*	½ Carton/300g	201	13.8	67	0.9	5.5	4.6	0.6
Luxury Game, Baxters*	1 Can/415g	245	4.6	59	6.2	6.0	1.1	0.5
Masala Dhal, Moorish, Tesco*	1 Pot/400g	276	10.8	69	3.2	7.9	2.7	1.7
Meal, Toulouse Inspired, Sausage & Lentil, Sainsbury's*	1 Pot/400g	249	7.2	62	3.6	6.7	1.8	2.4

S

SOUP

INFO/WEIGHT	Measure	per Measure		Nutrition Values per 100g / 100ml				
		KCAL	FAT	KCAL	PROT	CARB	FAT	FIBRE
Meatball & Pasta, Italian, New Covent Garden Food Co*	½ Pot/225g	122	3.2	54	2.3	7.5	1.4	1.3
Meatball & Tomato, Italian, Soups of the World, Heinz*	1 Can/515g	319	14.9	62	2.5	6.4	2.9	1.8
Minestrone, Calorie Counter, Low Calorie Cup, Co-Op*	1 Sachet/13g	40	0.3	310	7.0	66.0	2.0	3.0
Minestrone, Canned	1oz/28g	9	0.2	32	1.4	5.1	0.8	0.6
Minestrone, Canned, Average	1 Can/400g	252	12.0	63	1.8	7.6	3.0	0.9
Minestrone, Carton, Tesco*	½ Carton/300g	114	2.1	38	1.5	6.5	0.7	1.3
Minestrone, CBY, Asda*	½ Can/200g	70	1.0	35	0.4	6.4	0.5	1.6
Minestrone, Chilled, M&S*	½ Pot/300g	135	3.9	45	2.0	5.8	1.3	1.9
Minestrone, Chunky, Asda*	½ Tub/300g	111	4.2	37	1.4	4.7	1.4	1.8
Minestrone, Chunky, Big Soup, Heinz*	½ Can/200g	74	1.6	37	1.3	6.2	0.8	1.1
Minestrone, Chunky, Classic, Fresh, Tesco*	½ Pot/300g	126	2.1	42	1.2	7.8	0.7	1.2
Minestrone, Chunky, Classic, Meal, Canned, Tesco*	½ Can/200g	92	1.2	46	2.0	8.3	0.6	1.2
Minestrone, Chunky, Fresh, Sainsbury's*	½ Pot/300g	93	0.6	31	1.4	6.1	0.2	2.3
Minestrone, Chunky, Love Life, Waitrose*	1 Can/400g	166	0.4	42	1.3	8.7	0.1	1.9
Minestrone, Chunky, Waitrose*	1 Can/415g	195	3.3	47	1.6	8.3	0.8	1.1
Minestrone, Classic, Heinz*	1 Can/400g	128	0.8	32	1.0	6.2	0.2	0.8
Minestrone, Croutons, Cup a Soup, Made Up, Batchelors*	1 Serving/251g	93	1.3	37	0.7	7.3	0.5	0.3
Minestrone, Croutons, in a Cup, Made Up, Sainsbury's*	1 Serving/225ml	72	0.9	32	0.9	6.3	0.4	0.5
Minestrone, Diet Chef Ltd*	1 Pack/300g	123	1.8	41	1.4	7.5	0.6	1.2
Minestrone, Favourites, Baxters*	1 Can/400g	156	2.4	39	1.5	5.5	0.6	1.3
Minestrone, Fresh, Asda*	½ Pot/300g	138	2.1	46	1.8	8.2	0.7	1.2
Minestrone, Fresh, Average	1 Carton/600g	244	4.9	41	1.7	6.8	0.8	1.2
Minestrone, Fresh, Waitrose*	1 Pack/600g	240	8.4	40	1.1	5.8	1.4	1.2
Minestrone, in a Cup, BGTY, Sainsbury's*	1 Serving/200ml	54	0.2	27	0.8	6.0	0.1	0.6
Minestrone, Instant, Cup, Average	1 Pack/23g	79	0.7	351	7.7	72.1	3.3	3.4
Minestrone, Italian, Dry, Knorr*	1 Pack/62g	193	2.5	311	11.5	57.1	4.1	7.8
Minestrone, Italian, M&S*	1 Can/425g	191	2.1	45	2.2	9.0	0.5	0.8
Minestrone, Mediterranean, Campbell's*	½ Carton/250ml	95	2.8	38	0.9	6.1	1.1	0.6
Minestrone, Mix, Made Up, Sainsbury's*	1 Serving/200ml	44	0.0	22	0.3	6.0	0.0	0.3
Minestrone, Packet, Dry, Knorr*	1 Pack/61g	178	2.7	292	9.2	53.9	4.4	6.5
Minestrone, Sainsbury's*	½ Can/200g	66	0.8	33	1.1	6.3	0.4	0.9
Minestrone, Simmer, Dry, Asda*	1 Pack/50g	131	0.6	262	6.0	57.0	1.1	15.0
Minestrone, Squeeze & Stir, Heinz*	1 Made up/196g	59	1.4	30	0.8	5.0	0.7	0.4
Minestrone, Tuscan, Weight Watchers*	1 Can/295g	121	3.2	41	1.0	6.9	1.1	0.8
Minestrone, Verde, New Covent Garden Food Co*	½ Carton/300g	123	2.4	41	1.8	6.1	0.8	1.2
Minestrone, with Basil & Parmesan, Stay Full, Baxters*	1 Can/400g	276	5.2	69	3.5	9.2	1.3	2.6
Minestrone, with Croutons, Dry, Soupreme*	1 Serving/27g	94	1.7	349	7.6	65.3	6.4	4.4
Minestrone, with Croutons, Slim a Soup, Batchelors*	1 Serving/203g	55	1.2	27	0.6	4.8	0.6	0.6
Minestrone, with Croutons in a Mug, Tesco*	1 Sachet/23g	83	1.9	360	9.0	62.6	8.1	2.7
Minestrone, with Pasta, Chunky, Co-Op*	1 Pack/400g	140	2.4	35	1.0	6.0	0.6	0.7
Minestrone, with Pasta, New Covent Garden Food Co*	½ Carton/300g	102	2.1	34	1.2	5.3	0.7	1.0
Minted Lamb Hot Pot, Big Soup, Heinz*	1 Can/400g	228	5.2	57	2.9	8.1	1.3	1.0
Miso, Instant, Blue Dragon*	1 Sachet/18g	25	0.7	139	10.0	14.4	3.9	0.0
Miso, Instant, Dry, Sanchi*	1 Sachet/8g	27	0.6	336	18.4	48.6	7.6	0.0
Miso, Japanese, Made Up, Yutaka*	1 Serving/250ml	24	0.7	10	0.6	1.1	0.3	0.0
Miso, Organic, Instant, Sanchi*	1 Sachet/10g	27	0.3	270	14.0	47.0	3.0	0.0
Miso, Wakama*	1 Sachet/8g	27	0.6	336	18.7	48.6	7.6	0.0
Miso, with Sea Vegetables, Clearspring*	1 Sachet/10g	26	0.9	260	20.0	26.0	9.0	11.0
Miso, with Sea Vegetables, Instant, Clearspring*	1 Sachet/10g	28	1.3	283	27.1	15.2	12.6	13.7
Miso, with Tofu, Instant, Kikkoman*	1 Sachet/10g	35	1.0	350	30.0	30.0	10.0	0.0
Miso, with Tofu, Instant, Wakama*	1 Serving/8g	27	0.6	338	17.0	51.0	7.3	0.0
Mulligatawny	1 Serving/220g	213	15.0	97	1.4	8.2	6.8	0.9
Mulligatawny, Asda*	1 Can/400g	172	4.4	43	2.2	6.0	1.1	0.3

SOUP

INFO/WEIGHT	Measure	per Measure KCAL	FAT	Nutrition Values per 100g / 100ml KCAL	PROT	CARB	FAT	FIBRE
Mulligatawny, Canned, Tesco*	1 Can/400g	188	4.0	47	1.3	8.1	1.0	0.3
Mulligatawny, Classic, Heinz*	1 Can/400g	208	7.2	52	2.0	7.1	1.8	0.6
Mulligatawny, Cup, Made Up, Ainsley Harriott*	1 Serving/228ml	105	1.4	46	0.7	9.6	0.6	0.7
Mushroom, & Chestnut, Fresh, Finest, Tesco*	1 Serving/250g	130	8.2	52	1.1	4.7	3.3	0.7
Mushroom, & Crouton, Cup Soup, Made Up, Heinz*	1 Cup/200ml	80	4.2	40	0.7	4.5	2.1	0.0
Mushroom, & Parsley, Made Up, Squeeze & Stir, Heinz*	1 Serving/249g	92	6.0	37	0.8	2.9	2.4	0.1
Mushroom, 98% Fat Free, Baxters*	1 Can/425g	170	6.8	40	0.9	5.6	1.6	0.3
Mushroom, CBY, Asda*	½ Pot/300g	108	5.1	36	1.0	3.8	1.7	0.9
Mushroom, Country, Selection, Campbell's*	1 Serving/250ml	80	4.5	32	0.6	3.4	1.8	0.5
Mushroom, Cream of, Canned	1 Serving/220g	101	6.6	46	1.1	3.9	3.0	0.1
Mushroom, Cream of, Canned, Tesco*	½ Can/200g	94	5.8	47	0.7	4.8	2.9	0.2
Mushroom, Cream of, Classics, Heinz*	1 Can/400g	208	11.2	52	1.5	5.2	2.8	0.1
Mushroom, Cream of, Crosse & Blackwell*	1 Can/400g	186	9.9	47	1.3	4.7	2.5	0.0
Mushroom, Cream of, Favourites, Baxters*	1 Can/400g	244	15.2	61	1.0	5.6	3.8	0.2
Mushroom, Cream of, Fresh, Tesco*	½ Tub/300g	96	2.4	32	1.4	4.8	0.8	0.5
Mushroom, Cream of, with a Hint of Garlic, Heinz*	1 Can/400g	220	11.2	55	1.8	5.6	2.8	0.2
Mushroom, Creamy, Asda*	1 Pot/500g	228	14.0	46	1.1	4.0	2.8	1.3
Mushroom, Cully & Sully*	1 Carton/400g	192	17.6	48	0.8	1.3	4.4	1.0
Mushroom, Diet Chef Ltd*	1 Pack/300g	105	5.1	35	1.9	3.2	1.7	0.9
Mushroom, for One, Heinz*	1 Can/290g	148	7.8	51	1.4	5.1	2.7	0.1
Mushroom, Four, Loyd Grossman*	1 Pack/420g	202	16.4	48	0.8	2.5	3.9	0.2
Mushroom, Fresh, Average	1 Serving/300g	146	9.3	49	1.3	4.0	3.1	0.8
Mushroom, Fresh, M&S*	½ Pack/300g	165	11.7	55	1.8	3.5	3.9	0.9
Mushroom, in a Cup, Sainsbury's*	1 Serving/200ml	96	3.8	48	0.5	7.0	1.9	0.2
Mushroom, Low Fat, Fresh, Sainsbury's*	½ Pot/300g	132	8.7	44	0.7	3.7	2.9	0.6
Mushroom, Moreish, New Covent Garden Food Co*	1 Carton/300g	90	3.0	30	1.3	2.9	1.0	1.4
Mushroom, Morrisons*	1 Serving/500g	250	18.0	50	1.3	3.2	3.6	0.3
Mushroom, Potage, Woodland Mushrooms, Baxters*	1 Can/415g	328	20.8	79	1.6	6.9	5.0	0.3
Mushroom, Squeeze & Stir, Made Up, Heinz*	1 Serving/250g	89	6.8	36	0.6	2.3	2.7	0.0
Mushroom, Wild, & Maderia, Fresh, Finest, Tesco*	½ Tub/300g	250	16.8	85	2.1	5.2	5.7	0.7
Mushroom, Wild, Farmers Market, Heinz*	½ Carton/300g	93	3.3	31	0.9	4.4	1.1	0.5
Mushroom, Wild, in a Cup, BGTY, Sainsbury's*	1 Serving/200ml	56	1.8	28	0.4	4.5	0.9	0.2
Mushroom, Wild, New Covent Garden Food Co*	1 Carton/600g	222	7.2	37	1.5	4.1	1.2	0.9
Mushroom, Wild, Tesco*	1 Pot/400g	360	30.4	90	0.8	4.3	7.6	0.2
Mushroom, with Croutons, in a Cup, Made Up, Waitrose*	1 Serving/212g	102	4.2	48	0.6	6.8	2.0	0.5
Mushroom, with Croutons, Soup in a Mug, Tesco*	1 Pack/26g	113	4.6	435	6.1	63.3	17.5	2.9
Mushroom, Woodland, Farmers Market, Heinz*	1 Can/515g	227	12.4	44	0.9	4.7	2.4	0.3
Oxtail, Average	1 Can/400g	163	4.5	41	2.0	5.8	1.1	0.4
Oxtail, Canned	1 Serving/220g	97	3.7	44	2.4	5.1	1.7	0.1
Oxtail, Classic, Heinz*	1 Can/400g	168	2.0	42	1.9	7.3	0.5	0.3
Oxtail, Favourites, Baxters*	1 Can/400g	192	4.4	48	1.8	6.8	1.1	0.5
Oxtail, For One, Heinz*	1 Can/300g	126	1.5	42	1.9	7.3	0.5	0.3
Parsnip, & Apple, COU, M&S*	1 Can/415g	187	10.4	45	0.7	5.4	2.5	1.2
Parsnip, & Apple, Spicy, NUME, Morrisons*	½ Can/200g	98	1.6	49	1.6	8.4	0.8	1.0
Parsnip, & Butternut Squash, The Best, Morrisons*	1 Can/400g	244	8.4	61	2.4	8.1	2.1	1.6
Parsnip, & Chilli, Diet Chef Ltd*	1 Serving/300g	102	4.2	34	0.8	4.6	1.4	1.3
Parsnip, & Honey, Fresh, Sainsbury's*	½ Carton/300g	192	12.6	64	1.1	5.4	4.2	1.5
Parsnip, & Orchard Apple, Duchy Originals*	1 Pack/350g	116	3.2	33	0.7	5.4	0.9	1.0
Parsnip, Creamy, New Covent Garden Food Co*	½ Carton/300g	174	9.0	58	1.2	6.6	3.0	1.6
Parsnip, Fresh, Morrisons*	½ Pot/250g	100	3.8	40	0.9	5.8	1.5	1.4
Parsnip, Leek & Ginger, New Covent Garden Food Co*	1 Carton/600g	162	1.8	27	1.2	4.9	0.3	1.3
Parsnip, Spicy, Aldi*	1 Serving/250g	132	8.5	53	0.6	4.9	3.4	1.4
Parsnip, Spicy, Average	1 Serving/400g	212	11.2	53	0.9	6.0	2.8	1.6

SOUP

INFO/WEIGHT	Measure	per Measure		Nutrition Values per 100g / 100ml				
		KCAL	FAT	KCAL	PROT	CARB	FAT	FIBRE
Parsnip, Spicy, Fresh, Tesco*	1 Serving/300g	123	6.3	41	0.8	4.6	2.1	1.9
Parsnip, Spicy, New Covent Garden Food Co*	½ Box/297g	116	3.9	39	0.9	5.8	1.3	1.8
Parsnip, Spicy, Vegetarian, Baxters*	1 Can/425g	212	10.6	50	0.7	5.3	2.5	1.7
Pea, Artichoke & Parmesan, The Best, Morrisons*	½ Pot/300g	171	7.8	57	2.8	5.6	2.6	1.0
Pea, Cream of, Garden, Jeremy's Soups Ltd*	1 Serving/300g	138	9.3	46	1.6	2.9	3.1	1.2
Pea, Organic, Suma*	1 Can/400g	272	8.8	68	2.7	9.4	2.2	0.7
Pea, Perfect, New Covent Garden Food Co*	1 Carton/300g	93	0.9	31	1.7	4.6	0.3	1.7
Pea & Ham	1 Serving/220g	154	4.6	70	4.0	9.2	2.1	1.4
Pea & Ham, Campbell's*	1 Can/500g	310	4.5	62	4.6	7.4	0.9	2.8
Pea & Ham, Canned, Favourites, Baxters*	1 Can/400g	218	4.0	55	3.3	7.1	1.0	2.0
Pea & Ham, Canned, Tesco*	1 Can/400g	240	4.4	60	2.6	9.0	1.1	0.8
Pea & Ham, CBY, Asda*	1 Pot/600g	282	6.6	47	2.9	5.6	1.1	1.4
Pea & Ham, Classic, Heinz*	1 Can/400g	252	3.2	63	2.8	10.1	0.8	1.1
Pea & Ham, Diet Chef Ltd*	1 Pack/300g	138	3.3	46	3.2	5.8	1.1	2.6
Pea & Ham, Eat Well, M&S*	½ Can/207g	93	2.1	45	3.7	5.1	1.0	2.2
Pea & Ham, Extra Thick, in a Cup, Made Up, Sainsbury's*	1 Serving/224ml	85	1.8	38	1.1	6.7	0.8	0.4
Pea & Ham, Fresh, Sainsbury's*	½ Pack/300ml	120	1.5	40	1.9	7.0	0.5	0.3
Pea & Ham, Fresh, Waitrose*	1 Serving/300g	196	10.0	65	2.9	6.2	3.3	1.6
Pea & Ham, Mix, Traditional, King	1 Serving/200ml	66	0.4	33	2.2	5.9	0.2	0.0
Pea & Ham, Morrisons*	1 Serving/250g	92	2.8	37	2.0	4.8	1.1	1.2
Pea & Ham, Smoked, Farmers Market, Heinz*	½ Can/258g	103	1.0	40	3.5	5.6	0.4	0.8
Pea & Ham, Split, Asda*	1 Serving/300g	129	0.6	43	3.5	6.9	0.2	0.7
Pea & Ham, TTD, Sainsbury's*	1 Bowl/300g	188	7.2	63	3.7	6.0	2.4	1.2
Pea & Mint, Baxters*	1 Serving/300g	186	9.6	62	2.3	6.1	3.2	1.5
Pea & Mint, Fresh, Finest, Tesco*	1 Serving/300g	165	7.2	55	1.3	6.0	2.4	1.5
Pea & Mint, Fresh, M&S*	1 Serving/164g	49	0.2	30	1.8	6.3	0.1	1.5
Pea & Mint, Fresh, Sainsbury's*	½ Pot/300g	102	2.7	34	1.4	5.0	0.9	1.9
Pea & Mint, Garden, Vegetarian, Baxters*	½ Can/200g	100	1.6	50	2.5	7.3	0.8	1.9
Pea & Mint, Tinned, Tesco*	1 Can/400g	180	2.8	45	2.0	7.8	0.7	1.3
Pea & Mint, with Leek, Fresh, Waitrose*	1 Serving/300g	123	4.5	41	1.7	4.4	1.5	1.5
Pea Souper, Londoner's, New Covent Garden Food Co*	½ Carton/300g	153	6.0	51	4.3	4.1	2.0	1.1
Plum Tomato & Basil, Farmers Market, Heinz*	1 Can/515g	247	13.9	48	0.7	5.3	2.7	0.7
Plum Tomato & Basil, Italian, PB, Waitrose*	½ Pot/300g	69	1.5	23	0.9	3.8	0.5	0.9
Plum Tomato & Basil, New Covent Garden Food Co*	½ Carton/300g	132	6.0	44	1.3	5.2	2.0	1.3
Plum Tomato & Mascarpone, Italian, Finest, Tesco*	1 Pot/600g	360	13.8	60	1.3	7.2	2.3	0.6
Pork, Chinese Dumpling, New Cultural Revolution*	1 Serving/250ml	156	4.0	62	6.4	6.0	1.6	0.4
Pork & Orzo, Slow Cooked, CBY, Asda*	1 Pot/400g	160	3.6	40	2.4	4.8	0.9	1.4
Pork & Stuffing, Taste of Home, Heinz*	1 Pot/410g	241	5.7	59	3.0	8.6	1.4	1.0
Potato, Bacon & Onion, Cup a Soup, Made Up, Batchelors*	1 Serving/280ml	106	2.8	38	0.9	7.3	1.0	0.5
Prawn Laksa, Waitrose*	1 Pot/400g	388	25.2	97	2.5	9.7	6.3	0.6
Pumpkin, & Apple, New Covent Garden Food Co*	½ Carton/300g	99	1.8	33	1.1	5.9	0.6	0.8
Pumpkin, Creamy, Very Special, Heinz*	1 Can/290g	188	5.5	65	1.3	9.9	1.9	1.1
Pumpkin, Ghoulash, New Covent Garden Food Co*	1 Carton/600g	186	1.2	31	1.3	5.2	0.2	1.2
Pumpkin, Spicy, Fresh, Sainsbury's*	½ Pot/300g	87	3.0	29	0.9	4.2	1.0	1.3
Pumpkin, Sweet Potato & Red Pepper, SO, Sainsbury's*	½ Pot/300g	111	3.9	37	0.8	5.6	1.3	0.8
Pumpkin & Coconut, Thai, New Covent Garden Food Co*	1 Carton/568ml	182	7.4	32	1.3	3.5	1.3	1.1
Red Pepper, & Tomato, Canned, Sainsbury's*	1 Can/400g	120	4.4	30	0.9	4.1	1.1	1.6
Red Pepper, & Tomato, Canned, Weight Watchers*	1 Can/295g	35	0.2	12	0.4	2.4	0.1	0.4
Red Pepper, & Tomato, Roasted, M&S*	1 Serving/150g	105	7.4	70	1.4	5.0	4.9	0.6
Red Pepper, & Tomato, Roasted, Weight Watchers*	1 Can/400g	136	0.4	34	0.7	7.7	0.1	0.6
Red Pepper, & Wensleydale, Asda*	1 Carton/600g	306	12.6	51	2.5	5.0	2.1	0.8
Red Pepper, Roasted, Finest, Tesco*	1 Pot/600g	290	12.6	48	1.4	5.4	2.1	1.1
Red Pepper, Roasted, Fresh, Waitrose*	1 Pack/600g	172	9.0	29	0.8	3.0	1.5	1.0

SOUP

	Measure INFO/WEIGHT	per Measure KCAL	FAT	Nutrition Values per 100g / 100ml KCAL	PROT	CARB	FAT	FIBRE
Red Pepper, Tomato & Basil, M&S*	1 Can/415g	83	1.2	20	1.3	2.7	0.3	0.8
Root Vegetable, & Butternut Squash, Baxters*	1 Can/415g	195	1.2	47	1.7	8.3	0.3	1.9
Root Vegetable & Barley, Broth, Special, Heinz*	1 Can/400g	188	6.0	47	0.9	7.4	1.5	1.1
Root Vegetable & Sweet Potato, Farmers Market, Heinz*	1 Can/515g	278	9.8	54	0.9	8.5	1.9	1.1
Royal Game, Favourites, Baxters*	1 Can/400g	152	0.8	38	1.8	6.9	0.2	0.3
Salmon & Dill, Smoked, Fresh, Finest, Tesco*	½ Carton/300g	240	16.5	80	2.2	5.3	5.5	0.6
San Marzano Tomato & Mascarpone, Finest, Tesco*	½ Pot/300g	225	13.5	75	1.3	6.7	4.5	0.7
Sausage, Toulouse, Terrific, Tesco*	1 Pot/400g	248	8.8	62	3.7	6.9	2.2	2.0
Sausage & Bean, Spicy, Meal, Canned, Tesco*	1 Can/500g	265	7.0	53	2.8	6.4	1.4	1.2
Scotch Broth, Canned, Tesco*	½ Can/200g	72	1.8	36	1.4	6.4	0.9	0.8
Scotch Broth, Classic, Heinz*	1 Can/400g	156	2.4	39	1.4	6.7	0.6	0.6
Scotch Broth, Co-Op*	1 Can/400g	220	5.2	55	2.7	7.9	1.3	2.3
Scotch Broth, Favourites, Baxters*	1 Can/400g	196	6.0	49	1.8	6.2	1.5	1.5
Scotch Broth, Fresh, Baxters*	1 Serving/300g	108	2.1	36	1.6	5.9	0.7	0.6
Scotch Broth, Fresh, Tesco*	½ Pack/300g	129	5.4	43	1.7	5.0	1.8	1.4
Scotch Broth, M&S*	1 Serving/300g	150	7.2	50	2.1	5.1	2.4	1.1
Scotch Broth, Mix, Made Up, Sainsbury's*	1 Serving/175g	32	0.4	18	0.2	3.8	0.2	0.6
Soup & Broth Mix, Dry, Wholefoods, Tesco*	¼ Pack/125g	456	2.4	365	14.7	71.4	1.9	7.3
Spinach & Green Lentil, Spiced, Asda*	½ Pot/250g	122	5.0	49	2.7	5.0	2.0	0.0
Spinach & Nutmeg, New Covent Garden Food Co*	½ Carton/300g	147	6.6	49	1.9	5.3	2.2	1.0
Spinach & Watercress, New Covent Garden Food Co*	½ Carton/298g	60	1.2	20	1.3	2.8	0.4	0.8
Split Peas, Yellow, Simply Organic*	1 Pot/600g	354	3.0	59	4.3	10.4	0.5	2.6
Steak & Onion, Angus, Big Soup, Heinz*	½ Can/250g	135	2.1	54	3.3	7.7	0.8	0.9
Steak & Potato, Angus, Big Soup, Heinz*	½ Can/250g	120	2.0	48	3.1	6.8	0.8	0.6
Stilton, Celery & Watercress, Morrisons*	1 Serving/250g	272	23.0	109	3.9	3.1	9.2	0.3
Summer Garden, English, New Covent Garden Food Co*	½ Carton/300g	72	1.8	24	1.0	3.4	0.6	0.8
Super Green, Fresh, M&S*	½ Pot/300g	120	5.7	40	1.5	3.7	1.9	1.7
Sweet Potato, Chickpea & Coriander, BGTY, Sainsbury's*	1 Can/400g	188	2.0	47	1.4	9.3	0.5	1.3
Sweet Potato & Coconut, COU, M&S*	1 Can/415g	166	5.4	40	0.7	6.7	1.3	0.8
Sweet Potato & Coconut, Diet Chef Ltd*	1 Pouch/300g	147	8.7	49	0.8	4.9	2.9	0.9
Sweetcorn, & Chilli Chowder, Simply Organic*	½ Pot/300g	126	2.7	42	2.2	6.1	0.9	3.8
Sweetcorn, Carrot, Pepper, New Covent Garden Food Co*	1 Carton/600g	372	16.2	62	1.4	7.6	2.7	1.0
Sweetcorn, Spicy, Fresh, New Covent Garden Food Co*	½ Carton/300g	159	4.8	53	1.4	7.8	1.6	0.7
Sweetcorn, Spicy, Super, Fresh, Tesco*	½ Pack/300g	160	5.2	55	1.0	7.7	1.8	0.6
Tomato, & Balsamic, Rustic, Skinny Soup, Glorious!*	½ Pot/300g	105	1.8	35	0.9	6.6	0.6	0.6
Tomato, Big Red, Heinz*	½ Can/210g	63	0.8	30	0.5	6.4	0.4	0.0
Tomato, Canned, LC, Tesco*	½ Can/200g	90	3.8	45	0.9	5.9	1.9	0.4
Tomato, Cannellini & Borlotti Bean, M&S*	½ Pot/300g	195	9.9	65	2.1	6.7	3.3	2.5
Tomato, Chunky, Organic, Canned, Amy's Kitchen*	1 Can/400g	212	5.6	53	1.2	8.6	1.4	1.2
Tomato, Co-Op*	½ Can/200g	80	2.6	40	0.7	6.9	1.3	0.2
Tomato, Cream of, Asda*	½ Can/200g	122	6.4	61	0.7	7.3	3.2	0.7
Tomato, Cream of, Canned, Average	1 Can/400g	208	12.0	52	0.8	5.9	3.0	0.7
Tomato, Cream of, Canned, Crosse & Blackwell*	1 Can/400g	228	10.0	57	0.9	7.4	2.5	0.8
Tomato, Cream of, Canned, Tesco*	½ Can/192g	115	4.8	60	0.9	7.4	2.5	0.8
Tomato, Cream of, Classic, Heinz*	½ Can/200g	118	6.0	59	0.9	6.7	3.0	0.4
Tomato, Cream of, Condensed, Batchelors*	1 Can/295g	454	19.5	154	1.7	21.9	6.6	0.6
Tomato, Cream of, Condensed, Prepared, Batchelors*	1 Serving/295g	227	9.7	77	0.9	11.0	3.3	0.3
Tomato, Cream of, for One, Heinz*	1 Can/300g	189	10.8	63	0.8	6.9	3.6	0.4
Tomato, Cream of, Fresh, Sainsbury's*	1 Pot/600g	318	19.2	53	0.8	5.2	3.2	1.3
Tomato, Cream of, Fresh, Tesco*	½ Tub/300g	168	5.7	56	1.4	8.4	1.9	0.4
Tomato, Cream of, Fresh, Waitrose*	½ Pot/300g	99	2.1	33	1.1	5.6	0.7	1.5
Tomato, Cream of, Kick Of Chilli, Black Label, Heinz*	1 Can/400g	232	12.0	58	0.9	6.6	3.0	0.4
Tomato, Cream of, Mexican Spices, Black Label, Heinz*	1 Can/400g	244	12.0	61	1.0	7.1	3.0	0.5

SOUP

INFO/WEIGHT	Measure	per Measure		Nutrition Values per 100g / 100ml				
		KCAL	FAT	KCAL	PROT	CARB	FAT	FIBRE
Tomato, Cream of, Microwaveable Cup, Heinz*	1 Cup/275ml	169	9.4	61	0.8	6.9	3.4	0.4
Tomato, Cream of, Morrisons*	1 Serving/205g	141	6.2	69	1.2	9.4	3.0	0.6
Tomato, Cream of, Organic, Heinz*	1 Can/400g	220	10.4	55	1.0	7.0	2.6	0.4
Tomato, Cream of, Prepared, Campbell's*	½ Can/295g	195	9.4	66	0.8	8.5	3.2	0.0
Tomato, Cream of, Sainsbury's*	1 Can/400g	244	12.8	61	0.7	7.3	3.2	0.7
Tomato, Cream of, Soup & Go, Heinz*	1 Cup/293ml	161	8.5	55	0.9	6.4	2.9	0.4
Tomato, Cream of with a Hint of Basil, Heinz*	½ Can/200g	114	6.0	57	0.9	6.6	3.0	0.4
Tomato, Cream of with Red Pepper, Classic, Heinz*	1 Can/400g	232	11.6	58	0.9	7.0	2.9	0.6
Tomato, Creamy, CBY, Asda*	1 Pack/600g	288	12.0	48	1.2	5.5	2.0	1.4
Tomato, Creamy, Very Special, Heinz*	1 Serving/290g	148	6.4	51	0.7	6.5	2.2	0.0
Tomato, Cup a Soup, Made Up, Batchelors*	1 Serving/256g	92	2.3	36	0.3	6.7	0.9	0.3
Tomato, Diet Chef Ltd*	1 Pack/300g	159	5.4	53	1.3	7.7	1.8	1.2
Tomato, Fresh, Tesco*	1 Serving/100g	44	2.3	44	0.7	5.2	2.3	0.4
Tomato, in a Cup, Tesco*	1 Serving/23g	75	0.7	328	6.4	68.5	3.2	0.1
Tomato, Mediterranean, Campbell's*	1 Can/295g	83	0.0	28	0.6	6.4	0.0	0.0
Tomato, Mediterranean, Fresh, Organic, Sainsbury's*	1 Serving/250ml	78	3.5	31	1.3	3.3	1.4	1.0
Tomato, Mediterranean, in a Cup, Waitrose*	1 Sachet/18g	52	1.5	289	8.3	45.6	8.3	10.0
Tomato, Mediterranean, Instant, Weight Watchers*	1 Serving/200ml	50	0.2	25	0.7	5.2	0.1	0.1
Tomato, Mediterranean, Rich, Fresh, Baxters*	1 Carton/600g	318	10.2	53	1.8	7.7	1.7	1.1
Tomato, Mediterranean, Slim a Soup, Cup, Batchelors*	1 Serving/208g	56	1.2	27	0.5	4.8	0.6	0.4
Tomato, Mediterranean, Vegetarian, Baxters*	1 Can/400g	126	0.4	32	0.9	5.6	0.1	0.8
Tomato, Onion & Basil, GFY, Asda*	1 Can/400g	96	2.8	24	1.0	3.4	0.7	1.7
Tomato, Oriental Spiced, Skinny Soup, Glorious!*	1 Pot/600g	258	10.8	43	1.0	5.8	1.8	1.1
Tomato, Original, Cup a Soup, Batchelors*	1 Sachet/24g	90	2.1	387	3.9	70.5	9.0	3.4
Tomato, Red Lentil & Pepper, CBY, Asda*	½ Pot/300g	177	3.3	59	3.0	8.8	1.1	0.9
Tomato, Red Pepper & Basil, Thick & Creamy, Asda*	1 Sachet/24g	89	2.3	370	5.6	65.7	9.4	5.5
Tomato, Simmer & Serve, Dried, Sainsbury's*	1 Serving/200ml	70	2.2	35	0.3	6.0	1.1	0.4
Tomato, Smart Price, Asda*	1 Can/400g	184	7.6	46	0.6	6.5	1.9	0.9
Tomato, Spicy, Cup a Soup, Batchelors*	1 Sachet/23g	74	0.7	322	7.6	65.8	3.2	3.2
Tomato, Squeeze & Stir, Heinz*	1 Made Up/248g	144	7.2	58	0.9	6.8	2.9	0.4
Tomato, Sweet Chilli, & Pasta, Classic, Heinz*	½ Can/200g	74	0.2	37	0.8	8.0	0.1	0.3
Tomato, Tangy, Extra, Slim a Soup, Batchelors*	1 Pack/253g	121	2.0	48	1.2	9.0	0.8	0.4
Tomato, Tangy, Slim a Soup, Made Up, Batchelors*	1 Serving/230ml	81	1.0	35	1.1	6.7	0.4	0.5
Tomato, Weight Watchers*	1 Can/295g	76	1.5	26	0.7	4.6	0.5	0.3
Tomato & Basil, Campbell's*	1 Pack/500ml	205	6.5	41	0.7	6.7	1.3	1.1
Tomato & Basil, Canned, M&S*	1 Can/400g	140	2.8	35	0.7	5.8	0.7	0.5
Tomato & Basil, CBY, Asda*	½ Pot/297g	89	2.4	30	1.0	4.3	0.8	0.7
Tomato & Basil, Cream Of, Somerfield*	1 Pack/450g	279	18.0	62	1.0	5.0	4.0	0.0
Tomato & Basil, Creamy, Cully & Sully*	1 Pack/400g	216	18.5	54	0.8	2.5	4.6	0.5
Tomato & Basil, Cup a Soup, Made Up, GFY, Asda*	1 Serving/250ml	50	0.2	20	0.4	4.4	0.1	0.2
Tomato & Basil, Fresh, Avonmore*	1 Carton/250g	135	7.5	54	1.2	5.5	3.0	0.2
Tomato & Basil, Fresh, Finest, Tesco*	½ Pot/300g	219	14.7	73	1.0	6.3	4.9	0.6
Tomato & Basil, Fresh, Low Fat, Sainsbury's*	½ Carton/300ml	75	1.8	25	1.1	4.1	0.6	0.7
Tomato & Basil, Fresh, M&S*	½ Pot/300g	120	5.1	40	1.0	5.0	1.7	1.3
Tomato & Basil, Fresh, Morrisons*	½ Pot/300g	117	2.1	39	1.5	6.6	0.7	1.0
Tomato & Basil, Fresh, Sainsbury's*	½ Pot/300g	114	3.0	38	1.1	5.9	1.0	0.7
Tomato & Basil, Fresh, So Organic, Sainsbury's*	½ Carton/200g	100	4.0	50	0.5	7.5	2.0	0.2
Tomato & Basil, Fresh, Somerfield*	1 Serving/295g	83	2.4	28	0.7	4.5	0.8	0.8
Tomato & Basil, Fresh, Tesco*	½ Pack/300g	138	4.8	46	0.9	6.9	1.6	0.6
Tomato & Basil, Fresh, The Fresh Soup Company*	½ Pot/250g	85	2.2	34	1.3	5.1	0.9	0.6
Tomato & Basil, GFY, Asda*	1 Serving/250ml	100	3.5	40	0.9	6.0	1.4	1.6
Tomato & Basil, Instant, Cup, Average	1 Pack/22g	76	1.2	346	6.1	67.8	5.4	4.2
Tomato & Basil, Italian, 99% Fat Free, Baxters*	½ Can/208g	119	2.1	57	2.6	9.3	1.0	1.1

SOUP

	Measure INFO/WEIGHT	KCAL	FAT	KCAL	PROT	CARB	FAT	FIBRE
Tomato & Basil, Italian, Go Organic*	1 Jar/495g	183	10.4	37	1.2	3.3	2.1	0.8
Tomato & Basil, Italian, Vegetarian, Baxters*	1 Can/415g	170	3.7	41	1.4	5.7	0.9	0.6
Tomato & Basil, Italian Style, Co-Op*	1 Pack/500g	200	10.0	40	1.0	4.0	2.0	0.6
Tomato & Basil, Squeeze & Stir, Heinz*	1 Made Up/196g	114	5.7	58	0.9	6.8	2.9	0.4
Tomato & Basil, Sundried, Heinz*	1 Serving/275ml	124	5.2	45	0.6	6.5	1.9	0.1
Tomato & Basil, Vie, Knorr*	1 Pack/500ml	145	2.0	29	0.8	5.5	0.4	0.9
Tomato & Basil, Vine Ripened, Fresh, Avonmore*	1 Serving/300g	141	8.1	47	1.0	4.7	2.7	0.3
Tomato & Basil, Weight Watchers*	1 Serving/295g	77	1.8	26	0.6	4.4	0.6	0.5
Tomato & Basil, with Pasta, Bertolli*	1 Serving/100g	47	1.1	47	1.5	7.9	1.1	1.6
Tomato & Basil with Onion, Crosse & Blackwell*	1 Serving/300g	87	1.8	29	0.9	5.1	0.6	0.3
Tomato & Black Bean, New Covent Garden Food Co*	½ Carton/302g	124	1.8	41	2.0	7.0	0.6	1.7
Tomato & Butterbean, Classic, Heinz*	½ Can/200g	92	1.4	46	1.3	8.1	0.7	0.8
Tomato & Lentil, Brown, Healthy, Baxters*	1 Can/415g	199	0.8	48	2.6	9.0	0.2	2.7
Tomato & Lentil, Goan Spiced, Skinny Soup, Glorious!*	½ Pot/300g	153	3.3	51	2.1	8.1	1.1	1.2
Tomato & Lentil, M&S*	½ Can/211g	95	0.4	45	2.3	8.4	0.2	1.5
Tomato & Lentil, Organic, Tideford*	1 Carton/300g	120	2.7	40	2.3	8.1	0.9	0.9
Tomato & Lentil, Spicy, Canned, Tesco*	1 Can/400g	180	0.8	45	2.1	8.7	0.2	0.8
Tomato & Lentil, Truly Irresistible, Co-Op*	½ Pot/300g	165	2.1	55	3.1	8.0	0.7	1.2
Tomato & Red Pepper, & Basil, Farmers Market, Heinz*	½ Carton/300g	117	4.2	39	1.3	5.2	1.4	0.5
Tomato & Red Pepper, Campbell's*	1 Can/590g	366	19.5	62	0.5	7.7	3.3	0.0
Tomato & Red Pepper, to Go, Asda*	1 Pot/330g	102	4.3	31	0.6	4.3	1.3	0.6
Tomato & Rice, with Sweetcorn, Spicy, Healthy, Baxters*	1 Can/414g	211	0.8	51	1.6	9.2	0.2	1.0
Tomato & Spinach, Organic, Waitrose*	1 Serving/300g	126	5.7	42	1.4	4.9	1.9	0.7
Tomato & Three Bean, Canned, BGTY, Sainsbury's*	½ Can/200g	118	1.8	59	3.7	9.1	0.9	1.7
Tomato & Three Bean, Co-Op*	½ Can/200g	130	1.8	65	3.7	10.2	0.9	2.0
Tomato & Vegetable, Cup a Soup, Batchelors*	1 Serving/218g	107	2.6	49	1.1	8.5	1.2	0.6
Tomato & Vegetable, Instant, Cup, Average	1 Pack/22g	80	1.5	364	6.2	69.9	6.6	3.0
Tomato & Vegetable, Mediterranean, Fresh, Tesco*	½ Pot/300g	105	2.1	35	1.0	6.2	0.7	0.7
Tomato & Vegetable, Organic, Baxters*	1 Can/400g	200	3.2	50	1.6	9.2	0.8	0.8
Tomato & Vegetable, Spicy, Healthy Living, Co-Op*	1 Can/400g	180	3.2	45	2.0	8.0	0.8	2.0
Turkey Broth, Canned, Baxters*	½ Can/208g	79	1.5	38	1.3	6.5	0.7	0.7
Turkey Broth, Favourites, Baxters*	1 Can/400g	152	2.8	38	1.3	6.5	0.7	0.7
Vegetable, & Lentil, Autumn, Heinz*	1 Can/400g	184	1.2	46	2.3	8.6	0.3	1.0
Vegetable, Asda*	1 Can/400g	144	1.6	36	1.1	7.0	0.4	0.8
Vegetable, Autumn, Blended, Heinz*	½ Can/200g	114	6.0	57	1.2	6.4	3.0	0.7
Vegetable, Autumn, Vie, Knorr*	1 Pack/500ml	190	10.0	38	0.7	4.3	2.0	0.7
Vegetable, Basics, Sainsbury's*	½ Can/200g	76	0.4	38	1.5	7.5	0.2	0.4
Vegetable, Batchelors*	1 Can/400g	168	3.6	42	1.0	5.3	0.9	4.4
Vegetable, Bean & Pasta, Organic, Baxters*	1 Can/415g	212	3.3	51	2.2	8.7	0.8	1.4
Vegetable, Broth, Country Kitchen, Avondale Foods*	1 Bowl/250g	105	0.8	42	1.3	8.5	0.3	1.2
Vegetable, Broth, Hearty, Weight Watchers*	1 Can/295g	135	0.6	46	2.0	8.2	0.2	1.4
Vegetable, Broth, M&S*	1 Pack/213g	85	3.0	40	1.0	6.3	1.4	0.8
Vegetable, Broth, Ten, Veg, Morrisons*	1 Pot/600g	240	7.8	40	1.7	5.8	1.3	1.1
Vegetable, Broth, Winter, Classic, Heinz*	1 Serving/200g	56	0.2	28	0.8	5.3	0.1	0.8
Vegetable, Canned	1oz/28g	13	0.2	48	1.4	9.9	0.6	1.5
Vegetable, Canned, Average	1 Can/400g	208	16.0	52	0.9	3.2	4.0	0.9
Vegetable, Canned, Tesco*	½ Can/200g	84	0.6	42	0.7	9.2	0.3	0.7
Vegetable, Chunky, Canned, Sainsbury's*	1 Can/400g	184	2.8	46	1.5	8.3	0.7	1.2
Vegetable, Chunky, Diet Chef Ltd*	1 Pack/300g	114	0.9	38	1.4	7.4	0.3	1.3
Vegetable, Chunky, Fresh, CBY, Asda*	½ Pot/300g	117	2.1	39	1.6	5.9	0.7	1.1
Vegetable, Chunky, Fresh, Tesco*	1 Serving/300g	123	5.7	41	0.6	5.5	1.9	1.0
Vegetable, Chunky, Fresh, Waitrose*	½ Pot/300g	117	5.4	39	1.3	4.5	1.8	2.1
Vegetable, Chunky, Low Fat, Solo Slim, Rosemary Conley*	1 Pack/300g	144	2.4	48	1.4	6.4	0.8	1.9

S

SOUP

	Measure INFO/WEIGHT	per Measure KCAL	per Measure FAT	Nutrition Values per 100g / 100ml KCAL	PROT	CARB	FAT	FIBRE
Vegetable, Chunky, Organic, Tesco*	½ Pot/300g	150	3.6	50	1.7	8.0	1.2	2.1
Vegetable, Chunky, Tesco*	1 Pot/600g	288	17.4	48	0.8	5.0	2.9	1.3
Vegetable, Classic, Heinz*	1 Can/400g	188	3.2	47	1.1	8.3	0.8	0.9
Vegetable, Condensed, Campbell's*	1 Can/295g	103	2.4	35	0.8	6.2	0.8	0.0
Vegetable, Condensed, Classic, Campbell's*	1 Can/295g	221	5.0	75	1.7	13.2	1.7	1.7
Vegetable, Country, & Herb, Farmers Market, Heinz*	½ Carton/300g	114	3.6	38	1.2	5.7	1.2	0.9
Vegetable, Country, Asda*	1 Serving/125g	59	3.6	47	0.6	4.5	2.9	0.8
Vegetable, Country, Canned, Heinz, Weight Watchers*	1 Can/295g	97	0.6	33	1.2	5.9	0.2	1.0
Vegetable, Country, Casserole, Taste of Home, Heinz*	1 Pot/430g	206	6.0	48	1.3	7.6	1.4	1.3
Vegetable, Country, Chunky, Asda*	½ Pot/300g	138	1.8	46	2.0	8.2	0.6	0.5
Vegetable, Country, Chunky, Baxters*	1 Can/400g	188	2.4	47	1.6	7.2	0.6	2.0
Vegetable, Country, Fresh, Asda*	1 Carton/500g	195	2.0	39	1.9	7.0	0.4	0.0
Vegetable, Country, Fresh, Chilled, Eat Well, M&S*	½ Pot/300g	135	6.0	45	1.0	5.2	2.0	1.4
Vegetable, Country, Fresh, Sainsbury's*	½ Pot/300g	123	2.7	41	1.6	6.6	0.9	2.5
Vegetable, Country, Fresh, Somerfield*	½ Pack/300g	123	6.0	41	1.1	4.6	2.0	1.2
Vegetable, Country, Knorr*	1 Pack/500ml	160	3.5	32	0.9	5.5	0.7	1.2
Vegetable, Country, Weight Watchers*	1 Can/295g	97	0.3	33	1.2	6.3	0.1	1.0
Vegetable, Cream of, Cup a Soup, Batchelors*	1 Sachet/33g	134	5.3	406	5.8	59.8	16.0	6.2
Vegetable, Cream of, Cup a Soup, Soupreme*	1 Pack/21g	73	2.2	356	4.9	59.5	10.7	6.3
Vegetable, Cream of, Fresh, Sainsbury's*	1 Pot/600g	216	12.6	36	0.5	3.8	2.1	1.2
Vegetable, Cream of, Jeremy's Soups Ltd*	1 Serving/300g	99	8.1	33	0.6	1.6	2.7	0.7
Vegetable, Cream of, Velouté De Légumes, Liebig*	1 Portion/200ml	84	4.0	42	0.7	5.3	2.0	1.0
Vegetable, Cully & Sully*	1 Pack/400g	204	14.4	51	0.6	4.2	3.6	0.9
Vegetable, Cup Soup, Made Up, Eat Smart, Morrisons*	1 Pack/213ml	51	1.1	24	0.4	4.4	0.5	0.4
Vegetable, Cup Soup, Made Up, Heinz*	1 Cup/200g	50	1.0	25	0.4	4.7	0.5	0.2
Vegetable, Extra Thick, Canned, Sainsbury's*	1 Can/400g	184	2.4	46	1.5	8.6	0.6	1.4
Vegetable, Farmhouse, Fresh, Avonmore*	½ Carton/250g	138	5.0	55	1.9	7.4	2.0	0.8
Vegetable, Farmhouse, Soup-A-Cup, Made Up, GFY, Asda*	1 Serving/219ml	59	1.1	27	0.6	4.9	0.5	0.4
Vegetable, Farmhouse, Thick, Co-Op*	1 Can/400g	140	1.6	35	1.0	7.0	0.4	0.3
Vegetable, for One, Heinz*	1 Can/300g	129	2.1	43	1.1	8.1	0.7	0.9
Vegetable, Fresh, Average	1 Serving/300g	118	4.1	40	1.4	5.4	1.4	1.3
Vegetable, Fresh, Co-Op*	1 Pack/600g	150	6.0	25	0.6	4.0	1.0	1.0
Vegetable, Fresh, Somerfield*	1 Serving/600g	150	4.8	25	0.7	3.7	0.8	1.1
Vegetable, From Heinz, Canned, Weight Watchers*	1 Can/295g	86	0.9	29	0.9	5.6	0.3	0.8
Vegetable, Garden, Celebrity Slim*	1 Pack/55g	211	3.0	384	25.6	56.4	5.4	1.4
Vegetable, Garden, Heinz*	1 Can/400g	160	3.2	40	0.9	7.2	0.8	0.9
Vegetable, Garden, with Barley, Co-Op*	1 Pot/600g	240	0.6	40	2.1	7.4	0.1	0.7
Vegetable, Golden, Cup, Calorie Counter, Co-Op*	1 Sachet/11g	35	1.1	320	7.0	50.0	10.0	9.0
Vegetable, Golden, Cup, Made Up, GFY, Asda*	1 Serving/217ml	52	1.1	24	0.5	4.4	0.5	0.2
Vegetable, Golden, in a Mug, Tesco*	1 Sachet/17g	60	1.3	351	8.2	62.0	7.8	3.7
Vegetable, Golden, Slim a Soup, Made Up, Batchelors*	1 Serving/207g	58	1.7	28	0.5	4.7	0.8	0.7
Vegetable, in a Cup, BGTY, Sainsbury's*	1 Sachet/200g	52	1.6	26	0.5	4.4	0.8	0.9
Vegetable, in a Cup, Weight Watchers*	1 Serving/100g	57	1.2	57	1.2	10.4	1.2	0.5
Vegetable, Instant, Cup, Average	1 Pack/19g	69	2.0	362	8.7	57.1	10.5	5.5
Vegetable, Mediterranean, Aldi*	1 Serving/250g	78	0.5	31	5.2	2.0	0.2	0.9
Vegetable, Mediterranean, GFY, Asda*	½ Pot/250g	80	4.2	32	0.5	3.6	1.7	1.6
Vegetable, Mediterranean, Squeeze&Stir, Made Up, Heinz*	1 Serving/196g	114	8.1	58	1.3	4.1	4.1	0.4
Vegetable, Moroccan, Harira, Meal Soup, Glorious!*	1 Pot/600g	288	3.6	48	2.0	8.7	0.6	1.1
Vegetable, Nupo*	1 Serving/32g	111	2.1	347	37.0	39.0	6.7	9.8
Vegetable, Roasted, Chunky, M&S*	1 Can/400g	140	2.4	35	1.3	5.8	0.6	1.1
Vegetable, Roasted, Fresh, Sainsbury's*	½ Pot/300ml	78	1.5	26	0.5	4.8	0.5	1.2
Vegetable, Root, Medley, New Covent Garden Food Co*	1 Carton/600g	168	4.8	28	0.7	4.9	0.8	1.1
Vegetable, Scotch, Baxters*	1 Can/425g	183	2.6	43	1.9	7.4	0.6	1.2

	Measure INFO/WEIGHT	per Measure KCAL	FAT	Nutrition Values per 100g / 100ml KCAL	PROT	CARB	FAT	FIBRE
SOUP								
Vegetable, Spring, Classic, Heinz*	1 Can/400g	136	1.6	34	0.8	6.8	0.4	0.7
Vegetable, Spring, Sainsbury's*	½ Can/200g	72	0.8	36	0.8	7.4	0.4	0.6
Vegetable, Summer, New Covent Garden Food Co*	1 Carton/600g	336	14.4	56	1.7	6.5	2.4	0.7
Vegetable, Super, M&S*	½ Pot/300g	120	4.2	40	1.0	5.0	1.4	1.2
Vegetable, Tesco*	½ Carton/200g	78	2.6	39	0.9	5.8	1.3	1.0
Vegetable, Thick & Creamy, Soup in a Mug, Tesco*	1 Serving/26g	104	4.3	399	5.2	57.4	16.5	7.5
Vegetable, Traditional, Knorr*	1 Serving/200ml	42	0.2	21	1.0	3.2	0.1	1.0
Vegetable, Tuscan, Organic, Tideford*	1 Carton/300g	144	3.3	48	2.2	6.2	1.1	2.4
Vegetable, Winter, Chunky, M&S*	1 Can/400g	140	0.8	35	1.2	6.3	0.2	1.5
Vegetable, Winter, New Covent Garden Food Co*	½ Pack/300g	117	2.1	39	2.0	5.1	0.7	2.3
Vegetable, Winter, White, Cully Ans Sully*	1 Pot/400g	172	10.8	43	0.8	4.2	2.7	1.1
Vegetable, with Croutons, Soup in a Mug, Tesco*	1 Pack/23g	90	3.7	392	6.2	55.2	16.3	8.0
Vegetable, with Lamb, Scotch, Favourites, Baxters*	1 Can/400g	172	2.0	43	2.0	7.6	0.5	1.7
Vegetable, with Lentils & Beef, Scottish, Heinz*	1 Can/404g	210	2.8	52	3.4	8.2	0.7	1.2
Vegetable, with Lentils & Pearl Barley, Chunky, Waitrose*	½ Pot/298g	131	5.4	44	1.3	4.5	1.8	2.1
Vegetable, with Mild Spices, Autumn, Healthy, Baxters*	1 Can/415g	191	1.2	46	1.7	8.0	0.3	2.0
Vegetable & Barley Broth, Canned, Sainsbury's*	½ Can/200g	48	0.8	24	1.4	3.7	0.4	0.9
Vegetable & Lentil, Green, Lima*	1 Serving/300g	96	3.6	32	1.6	3.7	1.2	0.5
Vegetable & Lentil, Waitrose*	½ Pot/300g	138	4.5	46	2.9	5.2	1.5	3.5
Vegetable Curry, CBY, Asda*	½ Pot/300g	240	2.1	80	4.5	13.3	0.7	1.1
Vegetable Mulligatawny, Tesco*	½ Pack/300g	210	7.5	70	1.9	9.0	2.5	1.1
Vegetable Pho Noodle, Broth, Heat to Eat, Tesco*	1 Pot/165g	43	0.3	26	1.3	4.5	0.2	0.6
Watercress, M&S*	½ Pot/300g	75	5.1	25	1.3	1.5	1.7	0.6
Watercress & Cream, Soup Chef*	1 Jar/780g	413	22.6	53	0.8	5.9	2.9	0.3
Wonton, Blue Dragon*	1 Can/410g	102	5.3	25	1.2	2.0	1.3	0.2
SOUTHERN COMFORT								
37.5% Volume	**1 Pub Shot/35ml**	**72**	**0.0**	**207**	**0.0**	**0.0**	**0.0**	**0.0**
SOYA								
Chunks, Protein, Natural, Nature's Harvest*	1 Serving/50g	172	0.5	345	50.0	35.0	1.0	4.0
Mince, Dry Weight, Sainsbury's*	1 Serving/50g	164	0.4	328	47.2	33.2	0.8	3.6
Mince, Granules	**1oz/28g**	**74**	**1.5**	**263**	**43.2**	**11.0**	**5.4**	**0.0**
Mince, Prepared, Sainsbury's*	1 Serving/200g	164	0.4	82	11.8	8.3	0.2	0.9
Mince with Onion, Cooked, Sainsbury's*	½ Pack/180g	122	2.9	68	5.4	8.0	1.6	1.8
SOYA MILK								
Choco Flavour, Provamel*	1 Serving/250ml	208	6.0	83	3.8	11.1	2.4	1.1
Flavoured, Average	1 fl oz/30ml	12	0.5	40	2.8	3.6	1.7	0.0
Original, Fat Free, So Good Beverages*	1 Serving/250ml	100	0.2	40	3.6	6.4	0.1	0.0
Plain, Organic, Kirkland*	1 Glass/250ml	118	5.5	47	4.0	3.7	2.2	0.5
Sweetened, Average	**1 Glass/200ml**	**94**	**4.2**	**47**	**3.4**	**3.7**	**2.1**	**0.4**
Sweetened, Calcium Enriched, Average	1 Glass/200ml	91	3.9	46	3.4	3.7	2.0	0.3
Sweetened, Light, with Multivitamins, Alpro*	1 Serving/250ml	78	3.0	31	2.1	2.0	1.2	1.2
Unsweetened, No Added Sugar, Average	**1 Serving/250ml**	**85**	**4.8**	**34**	**3.3**	**0.9**	**1.9**	**0.4**
Unsweetened, Organic, Waitrose*	1 Serving/60ml	19	1.1	31	3.3	0.2	1.9	0.0
Unsweetened, Uht, Organic, Tesco*	1 Serving/150ml	46	2.8	31	3.4	0.1	1.9	0.6
Vanilla, Omega, So Good Beverages*	1 Serving/250ml	130	3.0	52	3.6	7.6	1.2	0.0
SPAGHETTI								
Brown Rice, GF, Organic, Dove's Farm*	1 Serving/70g	237	1.0	338	7.9	70.3	1.5	4.1
Cooked, Average	**1oz/28g**	**33**	**0.2**	**119**	**4.1**	**24.8**	**0.6**	**1.1**
Dry, Average	**1oz/28g**	**98**	**0.4**	**350**	**12.1**	**72.1**	**1.5**	**2.4**
Durum Wheat, Dry, Average	**1oz/28g**	**97**	**0.1**	**348**	**12.4**	**71.8**	**0.4**	**1.4**
Fresh, Chilled, Average	**1 Serving/100g**	**278**	**3.0**	**278**	**10.8**	**53.0**	**3.0**	**2.2**
Fresh, Cooked, Average	**1 Serving/125g**	**182**	**2.2**	**146**	**6.1**	**26.9**	**1.7**	**1.8**
in Tomato Sauce, Canned	1oz/28g	18	0.1	64	1.9	14.1	0.4	0.7

S

	Measure INFO/WEIGHT	per Measure		Nutrition Values per 100g / 100ml				
		KCAL	FAT	KCAL	PROT	CARB	FAT	FIBRE
SPAGHETTI								
in Tomato Sauce, Heinz*	½ Can/200g	120	0.6	60	1.7	12.7	0.3	2.4
In Tomato Sauce, Multigrain, Heinz*	½ Can/200g	120	0.6	60	1.7	12.7	0.3	2.4
in Tomato Sauce, with Parsley, Weight Watchers*	1 Can/200g	100	0.4	50	1.8	9.9	0.2	0.6
in Tomato Sauce, with Sausages, Heinz*	1 Can/400g	352	14.0	88	3.4	10.8	3.5	0.5
Marinara	1 Serving/450g	675	18.9	150	8.0	19.0	4.2	0.9
Whole Wheat, Cooked, Average	***1oz/28g***	***32***	***0.3***	***113***	***4.7***	***23.2***	***0.9***	***3.5***
Whole Wheat, Dry, Average	***1 Serving/100g***	***324***	***2.6***	***324***	***13.5***	***62.2***	***2.6***	***8.0***
SPAGHETTI & MEATBALLS								
Chicken, in Tomato Sauce, Heinz*	1 Can/400g	332	9.2	83	4.2	11.3	2.3	0.5
COU, M&S*	1 Pack/400g	360	8.0	90	6.0	12.3	2.0	2.6
GFY, Asda*	1 Pack/400g	344	6.0	86	7.0	11.0	1.5	1.5
Healthy Range, Average	1 Serving/400g	375	8.3	94	5.7	12.9	2.1	1.7
Italian, Sainsbury's*	1 Pack/450g	495	21.2	110	5.0	11.9	4.7	2.7
Pork & Beef, in Rich Tomato Sauce, BGTY, Sainsbury's*	1 Pack/385g	358	7.3	93	5.8	12.2	1.9	1.8
Tesco*	1 Serving/475g	641	30.9	135	5.1	14.1	6.5	0.9
SPAGHETTI BOLOGNESE								
Al Forno, Sainsbury's*	1 Pack/400g	460	19.6	115	7.8	10.0	4.9	1.1
BGTY, Sainsbury's*	1 Pack/400g	416	9.2	104	6.3	14.4	2.3	1.1
Canned, Asda*	½ Can/205g	174	5.7	85	4.2	10.7	2.8	0.6
CBY, Asda*	1 Pack/100g	108	2.0	108	6.0	15.6	2.0	2.0
GFY, Asda*	1 Pack/400g	352	6.4	88	4.9	13.4	1.6	2.2
Hidden Veg, Heinz*	1 Can/400g	312	6.4	78	3.4	12.6	1.6	0.9
in Rich Beef Sauce, Egg Pasta, Waitrose*	1 Pack/400g	404	10.4	101	7.6	11.7	2.6	1.0
in Tomato & Beef Sauce, Canned, Carlini*	1 Can/410g	324	10.7	79	3.7	10.2	2.6	1.2
Italian, Chilled, Tesco*	1 Pack/400g	520	17.2	130	6.5	15.9	4.3	1.5
M & S*	1 Pack/400g	380	8.4	95	7.5	11.7	2.1	1.7
PB, Waitrose*	1 Pack/400g	380	6.8	95	6.7	13.4	1.7	1.1
Sainsbury's*	1 Pack/400g	525	18.8	131	6.1	16.0	4.7	2.2
Weight Watchers*	1 Pack/320g	293	6.1	91	5.7	12.6	1.9	0.8
SPAGHETTI CARBONARA								
Chicken, Mushroom & Ham, Asda*	1 Pack/700g	686	14.0	98	10.0	10.0	2.0	1.5
City Kitchen, Tesco*	1 Pack/385g	578	29.6	150	4.8	15.5	7.7	1.5
COU, M&S*	1 Pack/330g	346	7.2	105	6.1	15.7	2.2	0.8
GFY, Asda*	1 Pack/400g	406	7.6	102	5.5	15.3	1.9	0.7
Italian, Chilled, Sainsbury's*	1 Pack/400g	492	15.6	123	5.5	16.1	3.9	1.4
Italian, Tesco*	1 Pack/450g	608	26.6	135	5.4	14.1	5.9	0.6
Italian Express*	1 Pack/320g	310	11.8	97	4.3	11.6	3.7	1.1
M & S*	1 Pack/400g	560	27.2	140	5.2	14.0	6.8	0.9
Ready Meal, Average	1 Pack/400g	524	21.5	131	5.9	14.4	5.4	1.1
Reduced Calorie, CBY, Asda*	1 Pack/378g	363	7.2	96	5.5	13.8	1.9	0.7
SPAGHETTI HOOPS								
Canned, Smart Price, Asda*	½ Can/205g	127	0.6	62	1.7	13.0	0.3	0.4
in Tomato Sauce, Heinz*	½ Can/200g	106	0.4	53	1.7	11.1	0.2	0.5
in Tomato Sauce, Hidden Veg, Heinz*	1 Can/400g	244	2.0	61	1.7	12.4	0.5	1.1
in Tomato Sauce, Multigrain, Snap Pot, Heinz*	1 Pot/190g	112	0.6	59	1.6	12.7	0.3	1.5
in Tomato Sauce, Snap Pot, Heinz*	1 Pot/192g	113	0.6	59	1.6	12.7	0.3	1.5
Tesco*	½ Can/205g	123	0.4	60	1.6	12.9	0.2	0.5
SPAGHETTI RINGS								
in Tomato Sauce, Canned, Sainsbury's*	1 Serving/213g	136	0.8	64	1.9	13.3	0.4	0.5
SPAGHETTI WITH								
King Prawn, Italian, Cooked, Finest, Tesco*	1 Pack/390g	485	22.9	125	5.0	12.2	5.9	1.3
SPAM*								
Fritters, Hormel Foods*	1 Fritter/80g	221	14.5	276	10.2	18.1	18.1	2.2

	Measure INFO/WEIGHT	per Measure KCAL	FAT	Nutrition Values per 100g / 100ml KCAL	PROT	CARB	FAT	FIBRE
SPAM*								
Pork & Ham, Chopped, Spam*	1 Serving/100g	296	24.2	296	14.5	3.2	24.2	0.0
SPELT								
Organic, Easy Grain, The Food Doctor*	1 Pack/225g	326	4.0	145	5.2	26.6	1.8	5.9
Pearled, Sharpham Park*	1 Portion/100g	314	1.8	314	12.0	68.4	1.8	6.0
SPICE MIX								
for Burritos, Old El Paso*	½ Pack/23g	68	0.9	304	13.0	54.0	4.0	0.0
for Fajitas, Old El Paso*	1 Pack/35g	107	2.1	306	9.0	54.0	6.0	0.0
for Mexican Fajitas, Discovery*	½ Pack/15g	34	1.0	230	8.0	35.0	6.5	17.5
Ras El Hanout, Al'fez*	1 Tsp/2g	4	0.2	217	9.8	25.7	8.3	17.5
Tikka, Blend, Sharwood's*	1 Pack/260g	263	14.0	101	2.7	10.2	5.4	1.7
SPINACH								
Baby, Average	*1 Serving/90g*	*22*	*0.7*	*25*	*2.8*	*1.6*	*0.8*	*2.1*
Canned, Average	*1 Serving/80g*	*18*	*0.4*	*22*	*3.0*	*1.4*	*0.5*	*3.0*
Chopped, Frozen, Fresh, Somerfield*	1 Serving/90g	22	0.7	24	2.8	1.5	0.8	2.7
Chopped, Frozen, Waitrose*	1 Serving/80g	20	0.6	25	2.8	1.6	0.8	2.7
Creamed, Frozen, Weight Watchers*	1 Portion/112g	48	1.1	43	2.5	5.0	1.0	1.5
Creamed with Marscarpone Sauce, Sainsbury's*	½ Pack/147g	110	6.3	75	4.2	5.0	4.3	3.4
Leaf, Frozen, GutBio*	1 Portion/50g	13	0.2	26	3.0	1.0	0.5	2.8
Leaf, Frozen, Organic, Waitrose*	1 Serving/80g	20	0.6	25	2.8	1.6	0.8	2.1
Raw, Average	*1 Serving/80g*	*19*	*0.6*	*24*	*2.9*	*1.4*	*0.7*	*2.2*
SPIRALI								
Dry, Average	*1 Serving/50g*	*176*	*0.8*	*352*	*12.2*	*72.6*	*1.6*	*2.8*
SPIRITS								
37.5% Volume	*1 Pub Shot/35ml*	*72*	*0.0*	*207*	*0.0*	*0.0*	*0.0*	*0.0*
40% Volume	*1 Shot/35ml*	*78*	*0.0*	*222*	*0.0*	*0.0*	*0.0*	*0.0*
SPLIT PEAS								
Dried, Average	*1oz/28g*	*89*	*0.5*	*319*	*22.1*	*57.4*	*1.7*	*3.2*
Green, Dried, Boiled, Average	*1 Tbsp/35g*	*40*	*0.2*	*115*	*8.3*	*19.8*	*0.6*	*3.9*
Yellow, Morrisons*	1 Serving/120g	338	1.4	282	21.3	62.2	1.2	15.6
Yellow, Wholefoods, Tesco*	1 Serving/15g	52	0.4	345	22.1	58.2	2.4	6.3
SPONGE FINGERS								
Boudoir, Sainsbury's*	1 Finger/5g	20	0.2	396	8.1	82.8	3.6	0.4
Tesco*	1 Finger/5g	19	0.2	386	7.6	80.6	3.7	1.0
SPONGE PUDDING								
Average	1 Portion/170g	578	27.7	340	5.8	45.3	16.3	1.1
Banoffee, Heinz*	¼ Can/78g	239	9.5	307	2.8	46.6	12.2	0.6
Blackcurrant, BGTY, Sainsbury's*	1 Serving/110g	155	1.0	141	2.5	30.7	0.9	3.2
Canned, Average	1 Serving/75g	214	8.6	285	3.1	45.4	11.4	0.8
Cherry, Very Fruity, M&S*	1 Pot/110g	286	11.3	260	3.5	38.6	10.3	1.8
Cherry & Almond, Sainsbury's*	¼ Pudding/110g	334	15.7	304	3.5	40.3	14.3	0.7
Chocolate, & Caramel, Bistro, M Kitchen, Morrisons*	1 Pudding/110g	431	24.1	392	3.7	44.1	21.9	1.7
Chocolate, & Sauce, Co-Op*	1 Pack/225g	608	29.2	270	5.0	34.0	13.0	0.6
Chocolate, Free From, Sainsbury's*	1 Pudding/110g	388	10.2	353	5.2	62.0	9.3	0.3
Chocolate, Heinz*	¼ Pudding/77g	229	8.9	298	4.6	44.0	11.5	1.2
Chocolate, M&S*	¼ Pudding/131g	524	32.2	400	6.1	38.6	24.6	1.8
Chocolate, Sainsbury's*	¼ Pudding/110g	464	28.3	422	5.4	42.3	25.7	0.8
Chocolate, Tesco*	1 Pudding/115g	196	4.7	170	4.7	28.3	4.1	2.8
Chocolate, Waitrose*	1 Pudding/110g	400	22.5	363	3.6	41.4	20.4	1.7
Chocolate, with Chocolate Sauce, Individual, Mr Kipling*	1 Pudding/85g	306	13.1	360	3.4	51.2	15.4	1.2
Fruits of the Forest, Asda*	1 Pudding/115g	323	4.4	281	2.8	59.0	3.8	1.3
Ginger with Plum Sauce, Waitrose*	1 Pudding/120g	424	17.9	353	3.1	51.7	14.9	0.7
Jam, Raspberry, Individual, Mr Kipling*	1 Pudding/85g	307	12.2	361	3.0	54.9	14.3	0.5
Jam & Custard, Co-Op*	1 Pack/244g	598	22.0	245	3.0	37.0	9.0	0.3

	Measure INFO/WEIGHT	per Measure		Nutrition Values per 100g / 100ml				
		KCAL	FAT	KCAL	PROT	CARB	FAT	FIBRE
SPONGE PUDDING								
Jam & Custard, Somerfield*	¼ Pudding/62g	143	5.0	231	3.0	38.0	8.0	0.0
Jam or Treacle	1oz/28g	93	4.0	333	5.1	48.7	14.4	1.0
Lemon, COU, M&S*	1 Pudding/100g	157	2.3	157	2.0	32.1	2.3	1.9
Lemon, M&S*	1 Pudding/105g	326	16.0	310	4.3	39.4	15.2	2.3
Lemon, Waitrose*	1 Serving/105g	212	2.5	202	3.4	41.7	2.4	1.4
Lemon Curd, Heinz*	¼ Can/78g	236	9.1	302	2.6	46.7	11.7	0.6
Pear & Ginger, COU, M&S*	1 Pudding/100g	175	0.7	175	1.9	39.8	0.7	1.1
Raspberry Jam, Asda*	½ Pudding/147g	481	16.2	327	3.1	54.0	11.0	4.1
Sticky Toffee, COU, M&S*	1 Pack/150g	278	2.6	185	2.5	39.3	1.7	1.8
Sticky Toffee, Microwavable, Heinz*	1 Serving/75g	233	9.0	311	3.3	47.4	12.0	0.7
Sticky Toffee, Mini, Somerfield*	1 Pudding/110g	384	14.3	349	3.0	54.0	13.0	0.0
Strawberry Jam, Heinz*	¼ Can/82g	230	6.2	281	2.6	50.4	7.6	0.6
Syrup, Finest, Tesco*	1 Pudding/115g	330	9.0	287	3.1	51.2	7.8	0.6
Syrup, Golden, Co-Op*	1 Can/300g	945	39.0	315	2.0	47.0	13.0	0.6
Syrup, Golden, Individual, Mr Kipling*	1 Pudding/85g	304	12.1	358	2.7	54.4	14.3	0.6
Syrup, Golden, Lyles,Heinz*	½ Pudding/95g	368	14.4	386	3.1	53.3	15.1	0.5
Syrup, Individual, Tesco*	1 Pudding/110g	390	14.5	355	3.1	55.6	13.2	0.5
Syrup, Morrisons*	1 Pot/110g	404	13.8	367	3.4	59.7	12.5	0.8
Syrup, Sainsbury's*	¼ Pudding/110g	408	13.0	371	2.7	63.5	11.8	0.4
Syrup, Value, Tesco*	1 Serving/100g	307	10.2	307	2.1	51.7	10.2	0.6
Syrup & Custard, Morrisons*	1 Serving/125g	290	8.6	232	3.4	39.1	6.9	0.8
Treacle, Heinz*	1 Serving/160g	445	13.0	278	2.5	48.9	8.1	0.6
Treacle, Waitrose*	1 Pudding/105g	385	13.8	367	2.8	59.5	13.1	0.5
Treacle with Custard, Farmfoods*	1 Serving/145g	539	33.1	372	3.2	38.4	22.8	0.8
with Custard	1 Serving/200g	521	24.9	261	4.8	34.1	12.4	0.9
SPOTTED DICK								
Average	1 Serving/105g	343	17.5	327	4.2	42.7	16.7	1.0
Individual, Tesco*	1 Pudding/121g	417	14.5	345	3.2	55.2	12.0	1.2
Sainsbury's*	¼ Pudding/82g	270	9.9	329	4.1	50.9	12.1	1.6
with Custard	1 Serving/210g	438	15.6	209	3.4	31.5	7.4	1.3
SPRATS								
Fried	*1oz/28g*	*116*	*9.8*	*415*	*24.9*	*0.0*	*35.0*	*0.0*
Raw	*1oz/28g*	*48*	*3.1*	*172*	*18.3*	*0.0*	*11.0*	*0.0*
SPREAD								
Butter Me Up, Light, Tesco*	1 Thin Spread/7g	24	2.7	350	0.3	0.5	38.0	0.0
Butter Me Up, Tesco*	1 Thin Spread/7g	38	4.1	540	0.8	1.2	59.0	0.0
Butterlicious, Vegetable, Sainsbury's*	1 Thin Spread/7g	44	4.8	628	0.6	1.1	69.0	0.0
Buttersoft, Light, Reduced Fat, Sainsbury's*	1 Thin Spread/7g	38	4.2	544	0.4	0.5	60.0	0.0
Buttery Gold, Somerfield*	1 Thin Spread/7g	44	4.8	627	0.5	1.0	69.0	0.0
Buttery Taste, Benecol*	1 Thin Spread/7g	40	4.4	575	0.0	0.8	63.3	0.0
Cholesterol Reducing, Heart, Dairygold	1 Thin Spread/7g	24	2.5	338	0.7	2.8	36.0	0.0
Clover, Light, Dairy Crest Ltd*	1 Serving/7g	32	3.4	455	0.7	2.9	49.0	0.0
Dairy Free, Organic, M&S*	1 Thin Spread/7g	37	4.1	531	0.0	0.0	59.0	0.0
Dairy Free, Organic, Pure Spreads*	1 Thin Spread/7g	37	4.1	533	0.5	0.0	59.0	0.0
Gold, Light, Pure, 65% Less Fat, Asda*	1 Thin Spread/7g	17	1.8	239	2.5	1.0	25.0	0.0
Gold, Low Fat, Omega 3, St Ivel*	1 Thin Spread/7g	25	2.7	360	0.5	3.1	38.0	0.0
Irish, Dairy, Original, Low Low*	1 Thin Spread/7g	24	2.7	346	0.4	0.5	38.0	0.0
Light, Benecol*	1 Thin Spread/7g	23	2.4	333	2.5	0.0	35.0	0.0
Lighter Than Light, Flora*	1 Serving/10g	19	1.8	188	5.0	1.6	18.0	0.0
Low Fat, Average	1 Thin Spread/7g	27	2.8	390	5.8	0.5	40.5	0.0
Olive, Enriched, Tesco*	1 Thin Spread/7g	38	4.1	540	0.2	1.2	59.0	0.0
Olive, Gold, Reduced Fat, Co-Op*	1 Thin Spread/7g	37	4.1	535	0.2	1.0	59.0	0.0
Olive, Gold, Reduced Fat, Sainsbury's*	1 Thin Spread/7g	38	4.1	536	0.1	1.2	59.0	0.0

	Measure INFO/WEIGHT	per Measure KCAL	FAT	Nutrition Values per 100g / 100ml KCAL	PROT	CARB	FAT	FIBRE
SPREAD								
Olive, Light, GFY, Asda*	1 Thin Spread/7g	24	2.7	345	0.8	0.0	38.0	0.0
Olive, Light, Low Fat, BGTY, Sainsbury's*	1 Thin Spread/7g	19	2.0	265	0.1	0.8	29.0	0.0
Olive, Light, Sainsbury's*	1 Thin Spread/7g	24	2.7	348	1.5	0.0	38.0	0.0
Olive, Low Fat, Morrisons*	1 Thin Spread/7g	24	2.7	346	0.9	0.0	38.0	0.0
Olive, Oil, 55% Reduced Fat, Benecol*	1 Thin Spread/7g	35	3.8	498	0.3	0.5	55.0	0.0
Olive, Oil, Bertolli*	1 Thin Spread/7g	38	4.1	536	0.2	1.0	59.0	0.0
Olive, Reduced Fat, Asda*	1 Thin Spread/7g	38	4.1	536	0.2	1.1	59.0	0.0
Olive, Reduced Fat, M&S*	1 Thin Spread/7g	38	4.1	536	0.2	1.1	59.0	0.0
Olive, Reduced Fat, Morrisons*	1 Thin Spread/7g	38	4.1	536	0.2	1.1	59.0	0.0
Olive, Waitrose*	1 Thin Spread/7g	38	4.2	537	0.9	0.0	59.3	0.3
Olivite, Low Fat, Weight Watchers*	1 Thin Spread/7g	37	4.1	534	0.2	0.5	59.0	0.0
Soft, Reduced Fat, Basics, Sainsbury's*	1 Thin Spread/7g	25	2.7	351	0.0	0.2	38.9	0.0
Soft, Value, Tesco*	1 Thin Spread/7g	30	3.4	425	0.0	0.0	48.1	0.0
Soya, Dairy Free, Pure Spreads*	1 Thin Spread/7g	30	3.4	433	0.0	0.0	48.1	0.0
Soya, Kallo*	1 Thin Spread/7g	37	4.1	532	0.0	0.0	59.0	0.0
Sunflower, Asda*	1 Thin Spread/7g	27	2.6	380	7.0	6.0	37.0	0.0
Sunflower, Average	1 Thin Spread/7g	44	4.9	635	0.2	1.0	70.0	0.0
Sunflower, Dairy Free, Organic, Pure Spreads*	1 Thin Spread/7g	42	4.6	595	0.1	0.4	65.9	0.4
Sunflower, Enriched, Tesco*	1 Thin Spread/7g	42	4.7	603	0.0	0.0	67.0	0.0
Sunflower, Light, BGTY, Sainsbury's*	1 Thin Spread/7g	37	4.1	535	0.1	0.2	59.0	0.0
Sunflower, Light, Reduced Fat, Asda*	1 Thin Spread/7g	19	2.0	265	0.1	0.8	29.0	0.0
Sunflower, Low Fat, Aldi*	1 Thin Spread/7g	24	2.7	347	0.3	1.0	38.0	0.1
Sunflower, Low Fat, M&S*	1 Thin Spread/7g	26	2.7	366	0.2	5.7	38.0	0.0
Sunflower, M&S*	1 Thin Spread/7g	24	2.7	342	0.0	0.0	38.0	1.0
Sunflower, Morrisons*	1 Thin Spread/7g	44	4.9	630	0.0	0.0	70.0	3.0
Sunflower, Reduced Fat, Suma*	1 Thin Spread/7g	37	4.1	531	0.0	0.2	59.0	0.0
Sunflower, Sainsbury's*	1 Thin Spread/7g	38	4.2	537	0.0	0.4	59.5	0.0
Sunflower, Value, Tesco*	1 Thin Spread/7g	37	4.1	532	0.1	0.2	59.0	0.0
Vegetable, Dairy Free, Free From, Sainsbury's*	1 Thin Spread/7g	31	3.4	439	0.1	0.4	48.6	0.0
Vegetable, with Buttermilk, Beautifully Butterfully*	1 Thin Spread/7g	44	4.9	630	0.0	0.0	70.0	3.0
Vitalite, St Ivel*	1 Serving/10g	49	5.4	488	0.4	0.0	54.0	0.0
	1 Thin Spread/7g	35	3.9	503	0.0	0.0	56.0	0.8
SPRING ROLLS								
Cantonese Selection, Sainsbury's*	1 Serving/35g	68	2.7	193	4.1	26.9	7.7	1.4
Char Sui Pork & Bacon, M&S*	1 Pack/220g	528	20.7	240	4.8	33.9	9.4	0.6
Chicken, & Chilli, Cantonese, Sainsbury's*	1 Roll/51g	85	2.8	166	9.7	19.4	5.5	0.6
Chicken, & Chilli, Sainsbury's*	1 Roll/50g	92	4.6	185	9.6	15.6	9.3	2.8
Chicken, Asda*	1 Roll/58g	115	5.2	199	4.6	25.0	9.0	3.4
Chicken, Finest, Tesco*	1 Roll/60g	118	5.0	196	10.1	20.1	8.3	1.0
Chicken, Oriental, Asda*	1 Roll/60g	106	4.2	178	3.7	25.0	7.0	0.4
Chicken, Oriental Snack Selection, Sainsbury's*	1 Roll/15g	38	1.5	256	11.5	30.3	9.9	1.7
Chicken, Tesco*	1 Roll/50g	116	5.6	231	8.1	24.5	11.2	1.5
Chinese Takeaway, Tesco*	1 Roll/50g	100	4.3	201	4.4	26.4	8.6	1.5
Duck, M&S*	1 Roll/30g	75	3.4	250	9.8	27.7	11.2	1.5
Duck, Mini, Asda*	1 Roll/18g	47	1.9	259	8.7	32.8	10.3	1.9
Duck, Morrisons*	1 Roll/65g	147	6.7	226	6.2	27.2	10.3	1.2
Duck, Party Bites, Sainsbury's*	1 Roll/20g	49	1.8	245	10.1	31.4	8.8	1.0
Duck, Roast, M&S*	1 Roll/31g	85	4.9	275	7.8	26.2	15.7	1.4
Duck, with Sweet Chilli Sauce, Waitrose*	1 Roll/72g	66	1.4	92	5.1	14.0	1.9	0.9
M & S*	1 Pack/180g	333	15.1	185	3.5	24.2	8.4	2.3
Mini, Asda*	1 Roll/20g	35	0.6	175	3.5	33.6	3.0	1.9
Mini, Sainsbury's*	1 Roll/12g	27	1.2	221	4.2	28.7	9.9	1.6
Mini Vegetable, Co-Op*	1 Roll/18g	40	1.6	220	4.1	30.9	9.1	2.7
Prawn, & Coriander, Crispy, from Selection, M&S*	1 Roll/25g	55	2.4	225	6.8	26.2	9.9	2.0

INFO/WEIGHT	per Measure		Nutrition Values per 100g / 100ml				
Measure	KCAL	FAT	KCAL	PROT	CARB	FAT	FIBRE

SPRING ROLLS

	Measure INFO/WEIGHT	per Measure KCAL	FAT	KCAL	PROT	CARB	FAT	FIBRE
Prawn, Cantonese, Sainsbury's*	1 Roll/28g	46	1.7	162	6.8	20.3	6.0	2.5
Prawn, Crispy, M&S*	1 Roll/34g	75	3.4	220	10.0	22.2	9.9	1.3
Prawn, Thai, Waitrose*	1 Roll/50g	110	4.8	219	8.0	25.4	9.5	2.4
Thai, Sainsbury's*	1 Roll/30g	69	3.4	229	2.9	28.8	11.3	3.5
Vegetable, & Chicken, Tesco*	1 Roll/60g	110	4.6	183	6.1	22.2	7.7	2.5
Vegetable, Asda*	1 Roll/62g	126	5.6	203	3.5	27.0	9.0	2.7
Vegetable, Cantonese, Large, Sainsbury's*	1 Roll/63g	130	6.3	205	3.6	25.3	9.9	1.5
Vegetable, Cantonese, Sainsbury's*	1 Roll/36g	84	4.2	233	3.6	28.1	11.7	1.4
Vegetable, Chilled, Tesco*	1 Roll/68g	149	7.6	221	4.0	25.9	11.3	1.6
Vegetable, Chinese, Sainsbury's*	1 Roll/26g	50	2.0	193	4.1	26.9	7.7	1.4
Vegetable, Chinese Takeaway, Sainsbury's*	1 Roll/59g	100	3.7	170	4.0	24.4	6.3	2.8
Vegetable, Cocktail, Tiger Tiger*	1 Roll/15g	38	2.0	254	6.4	26.7	13.4	2.0
Vegetable, Frozen, Tesco*	1 Roll/60g	123	6.4	205	3.5	23.0	10.6	1.3
Vegetable, M&S*	1 Roll/37g	80	3.6	215	4.3	27.8	9.6	2.0
Vegetable, Mini, Nirvana*	1 Roll/26g	54	2.7	208	3.5	25.1	10.4	1.7
Vegetable, Mini, Occasions, Sainsbury's*	1 Roll/24g	52	2.3	216	4.1	28.2	9.6	2.9
Vegetable, Mini, Oriental Selection, Waitrose*	1 Roll/18g	35	1.2	192	4.2	28.6	6.8	1.7
Vegetable, Mini, Party Food, M&S*	1 Roll/20g	40	1.6	200	3.7	26.2	8.1	2.7
Vegetable, Mini, Tesco*	1 Roll/18g	36	1.5	205	4.4	26.4	8.6	1.5
Vegetable, Oriental, Sainsbury's*	1 Roll/61g	137	7.2	224	3.8	24.3	11.8	2.9
Vegetable, Oriental, Tesco*	1 Roll/68g	152	7.6	225	4.0	25.9	11.3	1.6
Vegetable, Oriental Selection, Party, Iceland*	1 Roll/15g	36	1.4	241	4.3	34.1	9.7	2.1
Vegetable, Somerfield*	1 Roll/60g	107	4.0	179	3.8	26.1	6.6	1.6
Vegetable, Tempura, M&S*	1 Pack/140g	280	12.0	200	2.8	27.9	8.6	1.8
Vegetable, Waitrose*	1 Roll/57g	107	5.3	187	3.7	22.1	9.3	3.4
Waitrose*	1 Roll/33g	61	2.8	184	3.6	23.1	8.6	2.5

SPRITE*

	Measure INFO/WEIGHT	per Measure KCAL	FAT	KCAL	PROT	CARB	FAT	FIBRE
Sprite*	1 Bottle/500ml	215	0.0	43	0.0	10.5	0.0	0.0
Zero, Lemon & Lime, Sprite*	1 Bottle/500ml	6	0.0	1	0.0	0.0	0.0	0.0
Zero, Sprite*	1 Can/330ml	3	0.0	1	0.0	0.0	0.0	0.0

SPRITZER

	Measure INFO/WEIGHT	per Measure KCAL	FAT	KCAL	PROT	CARB	FAT	FIBRE
White Wine, Echo Falls*	1 Serving/125ml	78	0.0	39	0.0	0.0	0.0	0.0
with White Zinfadel, Echo Falls*	1 Serving/200ml	216	0.0	108	0.0	0.0	0.0	0.0

SQUASH

	Measure INFO/WEIGHT	per Measure KCAL	FAT	KCAL	PROT	CARB	FAT	FIBRE
Apple, Cherry & Raspberry, High Juice, Robinson's*	1 Serving/25ml	49	0.0	196	0.2	47.6	0.1	0.0
Apple, Hi Juice, Tesco*	1 fl oz/30ml	52	0.0	173	0.0	42.5	0.0	0.0
Apple, No Added Sugar, Morrisons*	1 Serving/40ml	8	0.0	21	0.1	4.1	0.0	0.0
Apple & Blackcurrant, Fruit, Robinson's*	1 Glass/50ml	18	0.0	36	0.1	8.0	0.0	0.0
Apple & Blackcurrant, Low Sugar, Diluted, Sainsbury's*	1 Glass/250ml	5	0.2	2	0.1	0.2	0.1	0.1
Apple & Blackcurrant, No Added Sugar, Tesco*	1 Serving/30ml	4	0.0	15	0.2	2.0	0.0	0.0
Apple & Blackcurrant, Special R, Diluted, Robinson's*	1 fl oz/30ml	2	0.0	8	0.1	1.1	0.1	0.0
Apple & Blackcurrant, Special R, Robinson's*	1 Serving/30ml	2	0.0	8	0.1	1.1	0.0	0.0
Apple & Mango, High Juice, Diluted, Sainsbury's*	1 Serving/250ml	88	0.0	35	0.0	8.5	0.0	0.2
Blackcurrant, High Juice, Tesco*	1 Serving/75ml	215	0.0	287	0.3	70.0	0.0	0.0
Blackcurrant, No Added Sugar, Tesco*	1 Serving/25ml	4	0.0	14	0.4	1.7	0.0	0.0
Butternut, Courgette & Mange Tout, M&S*	1 Pack/80g	24	0.2	30	2.0	5.8	0.2	2.3
Butternut, Moroccan, Parcels, M&S*	1 Parcel/20g	54	2.6	270	4.7	33.7	13.0	2.9
Butternut, Roasted, & Chargrilled Halloumi, M&S*	1 Pack/370g	445	15.5	120	6.2	10.9	4.2	5.3
Cherries & Berries, No Added Sugar, CBY, Asda*	1 Drink/250ml	4	0.0	2	0.0	0.2	0.0	0.0
Cherries & Berries, Sugar Free, Diluted, Tesco*	1 Glass/250ml	5	0.0	2	0.0	0.3	0.0	0.0
Cherries & Berries, Tesco*	1 Serving/25ml	5	0.0	21	0.2	3.2	0.0	0.0
Fruit & Barley, No Added Sugar, Robinson's*	1 fl oz/30ml	4	0.0	14	0.3	2.0	0.0	0.0
Fruit & Barley, Orange, Diluted, Robinson's*	1 Serving/50ml	6	0.0	12	0.2	1.7	0.0	0.1

	Measure INFO/WEIGHT	per Measure KCAL	FAT	Nutrition Values per 100g / 100ml KCAL	PROT	CARB	FAT	FIBRE
SQUASH								
Fruit & Barley, Tropical, No Added Sugar, Robinson's*	1 Serving/60ml	7	0.0	12	0.2	1.6	0.0	0.0
Grape & Passion Fruit, High Juice, Diluted, Sainsbury's*	1 Serving/250ml	100	0.2	40	0.1	9.8	0.1	0.1
Grapefruit, High Juice, No Added Sugar, Sainsbury's*	1 Serving/25ml	2	0.0	6	0.1	1.1	0.0	0.0
Lemon, Barley Water, Made Up, Robinson's*	1 Serving/250ml	48	0.0	19	0.1	4.4	0.0	0.0
Lemon, Double Concentrate, Value, Tesco*	1 Serving/25ml	3	0.0	11	0.2	0.3	0.0	0.0
Lemon, High Juice, Diluted, Sainsbury's*	1 Glass/250ml	98	0.2	39	0.1	9.1	0.1	0.1
Lemon, No Added Sugar, Double Concentrate, Tesco*	1 Serving/25ml	4	0.0	16	0.3	0.7	0.0	0.0
Lemon, No Sugar, Asda*	1 Serving/200ml	5	0.2	2	0.1	0.3	0.1	0.1
Lemon & Lime, Double Strength, No Added Sugar, Asda*	1 Glass/200ml	4	0.0	2	0.0	0.0	0.0	0.0
Mixed Fruit, Diluted, Kia Ora*	1 Serving/250ml	5	0.0	2	0.0	0.3	0.0	0.0
Mixed Fruit, Low Sugar, Sainsbury's*	1 Glass/250ml	5	0.2	2	0.1	0.2	0.1	0.1
Mixed Fruit, Tesco*	1 Serving/75ml	13	0.0	17	0.0	3.5	0.0	0.0
Orange, Fruit & Barley, CBY, Asda*	1 Serving/100ml	2	0.0	2	0.0	0.2	0.0	0.0
Orange, Hi Juice, Tesco*	1 Serving/75ml	140	0.1	187	0.3	45.0	0.1	0.0
Orange, High Juice, Undiluted, Robinson's*	1 Serving/200ml	364	0.2	182	0.3	44.0	0.1	0.0
Orange, No Added Sugar, High Juice, Sainsbury's*	1 Serving/100ml	6	0.1	6	0.1	1.1	0.1	0.1
Orange, Sainsbury's*	1 Glass/250ml	8	0.2	3	0.1	0.5	0.1	0.1
Orange, Special R, Diluted, Robinson's*	1 fl oz/30ml	2	0.0	8	0.2	0.7	0.1	0.0
Orange, Whole, Tesco*	1 Serving/100ml	45	1.0	45	0.2	10.1	1.0	1.0
Orange & Mango, Low Sugar, Sainsbury's*	1 Serving/250ml	5	0.2	2	0.1	0.2	0.1	0.1
Orange & Mango, No Added Sugar, Robinson's*	1 Serving/25ml	2	0.0	8	0.2	0.9	0.0	0.0
Orange & Mango, Special R, Diluted, Robinson's*	1 Serving/250ml	20	0.0	8	0.2	0.9	0.0	0.0
Orange & Pineapple, No Sugar Added, Robinson's*	1 Serving/25ml	2	0.0	8	0.2	0.7	0.0	0.2
Orange & Pineapple, Original, Undiluted, Robinson's*	1 Serving/250ml	138	0.0	55	1.0	13.0	0.0	0.0
Peach, High Juice, Undiluted, Robinson's*	1 fl oz/30ml	54	0.0	181	0.5	43.0	0.1	0.0
Peach & Apricot, Fruit & Barley (Diluted), CBY, Asda*	1 Serving/250ml	5	0.0	2	0.0	0.2	0.0	0.1
Pink Grapefruit, High Juice, Diluted, Sainsbury's*	1 Serving/250ml	85	0.0	34	0.0	8.1	0.0	0.0
Pink Grapefruit, High Juice, Low Sugar, Tesco*	1 Serving/75ml	12	0.1	16	0.2	3.7	0.1	0.0
Red Apple, No Added Sugar, Diluted, Ribena*	1 Serving/250ml	12	0.0	5	0.0	0.9	0.0	0.0
Spaghetti, Baked	*1oz/28g*	**6**	*0.1*	**23**	*0.7*	*4.3*	*0.3*	*2.1*
Spaghetti, Including Pips & Rind, Raw	*1oz/28g*	**7**	*0.2*	**26**	*0.6*	*4.6*	*0.6*	*2.3*
Summer, All Varieties	1 Small/118g	19	0.2	16	1.2	3.4	0.2	1.1
Summer Fruits, No Added Sugar, Double Strength, Asda*	1 Serving/50ml	1	0.0	2	0.0	0.2	0.0	0.0
Summer Fruits, No Added Sugar, Made Up, Morrisons*	1 Glass/200ml	3	0.0	2	0.0	0.2	0.0	0.0
Summer Fruits, No Added Sugar, Sainsbury's*	1 Serving/250ml	5	0.2	2	0.1	0.2	0.1	0.1
Summer Fruits, Robinson's*	1 Serving/25ml	14	0.0	56	0.1	13.0	0.0	0.0
Summer Fruits & Barley, no Added Sugar, Tesco*	1 Serving/50ml	6	0.0	11	0.2	1.7	0.0	0.0
Winter, Acorn, Baked, Average	*1oz/28g*	**16**	*0.0*	**56**	*1.1*	*12.6*	*0.1*	*3.2*
Winter, Acorn, Raw, Average	*1oz/28g*	**11**	*0.0*	**40**	*0.8*	*9.0*	*0.1*	*2.3*
Winter, All Varieties, Flesh Only, Raw, Average	*1oz/28g*	**10**	*0.0*	**34**	*1.0*	*8.6*	*0.1*	*1.5*
Winter, Butternut, Baked, Average	*1oz/28g*	**9**	*0.0*	**32**	*0.9*	*7.4*	*0.1*	*1.4*
Winter, Butternut, Organic, Tesco*	1 Serving/100g	39	0.1	39	1.1	8.3	0.1	1.6
Winter, Butternut, Raw, Prepared, Average	1 Serving/80g	29	0.1	36	1.1	8.3	0.1	1.6
Winter, Butternut, Raw, Unprepared, Average	*1 Serving/80g*	**29**	*0.1*	**36**	*1.1*	*8.3*	*0.1*	*1.6*
SQUID								
Battered, Fried in Blended Oil, Average	1oz/28g	55	2.8	195	11.5	15.7	10.0	0.5
Calamari, Battered with Tartar Sauce Dip, Tesco*	1 Pack/210g	573	41.0	273	8.9	15.4	19.5	0.6
Pieces in Squid Ink, Palacio De Oriente*	1 Can/120g	274	21.6	228	13.0	3.6	18.0	0.0
Raw, Average	*1oz/28g*	**23**	*0.5*	**81**	*15.4*	*1.2*	*1.7*	*0.0*
with Sweet Chilli Sauce, Pan Fried, CBY, Asda*	1 Serving/125g	229	9.3	183	9.6	19.0	7.4	0.9
STAR FRUIT								
Average, Tesco	*1oz/28g*	**9**	*0.1*	**32**	*0.5*	*7.3*	*0.3*	*1.3*

	Measure INFO/WEIGHT	per Measure		Nutrition Values per 100g / 100ml				
		KCAL	FAT	KCAL	PROT	CARB	FAT	FIBRE
STARBAR								
Cadbury*	1 Bar/53g	260	14.8	491	10.7	49.0	27.9	0.0
STARBURST								
Fruit Chews, Tropical, Mars*	1 Tube/45g	168	3.3	373	0.0	76.9	7.3	0.0
Joosters, Mars*	1 Pack/45g	160	0.0	356	0.0	88.8	0.1	0.0
Juicy Gums, Mars*	1 Pack/45g	139	1.8	309	5.9	71.0	4.1	0.0
Mars*	1 Pack/45g	185	3.4	411	0.3	85.3	7.6	0.0
STEAK & KIDNEY PUDDING								
Fray Bentos*	1 Tin/213g	477	26.8	224	7.8	19.8	12.6	0.0
M & S*	1 Pudding/121g	260	13.4	215	9.2	19.4	11.1	3.2
Tesco*	1 Serving/190g	437	22.6	230	10.0	20.7	11.9	1.2
Waitrose*	1 Pudding/223g	497	26.1	223	8.9	20.4	11.7	1.2
STEW								
Bean, Tuscan, Tasty Veg Pot, Innocent*	1 Pot/400g	320	7.6	80	3.1	12.5	1.9	3.6
Beef, & Dumplings	1 Serving/652g	766	32.7	117	7.4	10.7	5.0	0.8
Beef, Asda*	½ Can/196g	178	4.9	91	10.0	7.0	2.5	1.5
Beef, Meal for One, M&S*	1 Pack/440g	350	8.4	80	7.0	8.7	1.9	2.0
Beef, Value, Tesco*	1 Serving/200g	170	9.8	85	4.0	6.2	4.9	1.0
Beef & Dumplings, British Classics, Tesco*	1 Pack/450g	563	29.7	125	7.9	8.6	6.6	0.5
Beef & Dumplings, Classic British, Sainsbury's*	1 Pack/450g	531	23.4	118	7.7	10.2	5.2	0.5
Beef & Dumplings, COU, M&S*	1 Pack/454g	431	11.8	95	8.9	9.1	2.6	0.8
Beef & Dumplings, Morrisons*	1 Pack/400g	440	18.4	110	6.0	11.1	4.6	1.5
Beef & Dumplings, Sainsbury's*	1 Pack/450g	603	27.4	134	9.3	10.5	6.1	0.7
Beef & Dumplings, Weight Watchers*	1 Pack/327g	262	6.9	80	5.2	10.0	2.1	0.8
Chicken, Morrisons*	1 Pack/400g	492	7.6	123	17.6	8.9	1.9	0.5
Chicken & Chorizo with Patatas Bravas, Co-Op*	1 Pack/400g	380	12.8	95	8.0	8.6	3.2	1.6
Chicken & Dumplings, Tesco*	1 Serving/450g	567	29.7	126	7.6	9.1	6.6	0.7
Chickpea, Roast Sweet Potato, & Feta, Stewed!*	½ Pot/250g	188	7.2	75	3.3	8.8	2.9	2.7
Irish, Asda*	¼ Can/196g	172	7.8	88	6.0	7.0	4.0	1.0
Irish, Morrisons*	1 Can/392g	243	4.7	62	3.8	8.9	1.2	0.0
Irish, Sainsbury's*	1 Pack/450g	274	9.4	61	5.7	4.8	2.1	0.5
Irish, Tesco*	1 Can/400g	308	11.2	77	7.0	5.9	2.8	0.8
Lentil & Vegetable, Organic, Simply Organic*	1 Pack/400g	284	6.0	71	3.5	11.0	1.5	1.3
Lentil & Vegetable, Winter, Organic, Pure & Pronto*	1 Pack/400g	364	9.6	91	3.6	14.0	2.4	4.0
Mutton, Barley & Vegetables, Look What We Found*	1 Pack/300g	252	8.1	84	8.7	6.3	2.7	1.7
Vegetable, Mixed, Topped with Herb Dumplings, Tesco*	1 Pack/420g	508	26.0	121	1.9	14.5	6.2	1.3
STIR FRY								
Baby Vegetable & Pak Choi, Two Step, Tesco*	½ Pack/95g	29	0.8	31	2.1	4.0	0.8	2.3
Bean Sprout, & Noodles, Tesco*	½ Pack/125g	131	2.6	105	4.2	16.1	2.1	0.7
Bean Sprout, & Vegetable with Red Peppers, Asda*	1 Pack/350g	126	3.9	36	1.8	4.7	1.1	2.3
Bean Sprout, & Vegetables, Asda*	½ Pack/173g	107	6.9	62	2.0	4.5	4.0	1.8
Bean Sprout, Asda*	½ Pack/175g	56	0.9	32	2.9	4.0	0.5	1.5
Bean Sprout, Chinese, Sainsbury's*	1 Pack/300g	144	8.4	48	1.9	5.1	2.8	1.5
Bean Sprout, Morrisons*	1 Serving/150g	46	0.6	31	2.0	4.8	0.4	1.8
Bean Sprout, Ready to Eat, Washed, Sainsbury's*	1 Serving/150g	82	5.8	55	1.5	3.3	3.9	1.8
Beef, BGTY, Sainsbury's*	½ Pack/125g	156	5.1	125	22.0	0.1	4.1	0.0
Beef, Less Than 10% Fat, Asda*	1 Pack/227g	275	6.4	121	24.0	0.0	2.8	0.8
Beef, Less Than 3% Fat, BGTY, Sainsbury's*	½ Pack/125g	134	2.6	107	22.1	0.0	2.1	0.0
Cabbage, Carrot, Broccoli & Onion, Vegetable, Tesco*	1 Serving/100g	31	0.4	31	1.9	4.9	0.4	2.6
Chicken, & Noodle, GFY, Asda*	1 Pack/330g	403	10.9	122	7.0	16.0	3.3	2.4
Chicken, Chinese, Iceland*	1 Pack/298g	262	4.2	88	6.2	12.7	1.4	2.9
Chicken, Chinese, Sizzling, Oriental Express*	1 Pack/400g	400	8.0	100	6.6	13.8	2.0	1.7
Chicken, Chow Mein, Orient Express, Oriental Express*	1 Pack/400g	384	10.8	96	7.3	10.7	2.7	2.2
Chinese, Family, Sainsbury's*	1 Serving/150g	60	3.0	40	2.3	3.3	2.0	3.6

STIR FRY

INFO/WEIGHT	Measure		per Measure		Nutrition Values per 100g / 100ml				
			KCAL	FAT	KCAL	PROT	CARB	FAT	FIBRE
Chinese, with Oriental Sauce, Tesco*	1 Pack/530g		180	2.1	34	2.3	5.4	0.4	1.5
Chinese, with Soy, Garlic & Ginger, Tesco*	1 Pack/150g		90	0.2	60	1.5	12.6	0.1	0.5
Chinese Style, Co-Op*	1 Pack/300g		105	1.2	35	3.0	6.0	0.4	2.0
Classic Medley, Veg Cuisine*	½ Pack/150g		45	0.6	30	2.5	4.1	0.4	2.1
Edamame Bean, Morrisons*	½ Pack/175g		220	8.4	126	10.9	7.7	4.8	5.2
Hot & Spicy, & Red Chillies, Fresh Tastes, Asda*	½ Pack/125g		60	2.5	48	1.8	4.2	2.0	0.0
Mixed Pepper, & Sweet Chilli Sauce, Asda*	1 Pack/300g		180	6.0	60	1.6	9.0	2.0	2.6
Mixed Pepper, & Vegetable, Asda*	½ Pack/150g		42	1.5	28	1.6	3.2	1.0	2.6
Mixed Pepper, Crisp & Sweet, Waitrose*	½ Pack/150g		51	0.6	34	1.9	4.8	0.4	1.9
Mixed Pepper, Fresh Tastes, Asda*	½ Pack/160g		75	4.2	47	1.4	4.6	2.6	2.0
Mixed Pepper, Sainsbury's*	1 Pack/300g		188	12.9	70	1.5	4.6	4.8	1.2
Mixed Pepper, Tesco*	1 Serving/34g		12	0.1	34	2.0	4.6	0.4	2.0
Mushroom, Chinese, Sainsbury's*	1 Serving/175g		66	4.2	38	1.7	2.4	2.4	1.7
Mushroom, Just Stir Fry, Sainsbury's*	1 Pack/350g		172	9.5	49	2.8	3.3	2.7	2.8
Mushroom, Tesco*	1 Portion/100g		34	0.5	34	2.6	3.9	0.5	2.0
Mushroom, Waitrose*	½ Pack/165g		43	0.7	26	2.3	3.3	0.4	1.6
Pak Choi, Oriantal Style, M&S*	1 Pack/220g		165	12.5	75	2.2	3.5	5.7	2.4
Pepper & Butternut Squash, Chunky, Finest, Tesco*	1 Pack/220g		68	0.9	31	1.6	4.2	0.4	2.0
Prawn, Chinese Style, GFY, Asda*	1 Pack/400g		324	6.4	81	3.6	13.0	1.6	1.6
Rainbow, Fresh Tastes, Asda*	1 Serving/225g		119	5.0	53	1.8	4.6	2.2	3.8
Rice & Vegetables, Chinese, Style, Tesco*	1 Serving/550g		495	13.8	90	2.2	14.8	2.5	0.3
Thai Style, M&S*	1 Serving/150g		44	0.5	29	1.0	4.4	0.3	2.0
Thai Style, Tesco*	1 Pack/350g		301	17.8	86	3.9	6.2	5.1	1.9
Vegetable, & Bean Sprout, M&S*	1 Pack/350g		105	1.4	30	1.8	4.6	0.4	2.0
Vegetable, & Beansprout, Tesco*	1 Pack/380g		129	1.9	34	2.0	5.4	0.5	2.2
Vegetable, & Beansprout, Waitrose*	1 Pack/300g		78	0.9	26	1.4	4.5	0.3	2.1
Vegetable, & Beansprouts, Family, Fresh, Tesco*	1 Pack/600g		108	0.6	18	2.0	2.2	0.1	2.1
Vegetable, & Broccoli, Fresh Tastes, Asda*	½ Bag/175g		88	3.5	50	2.5	3.7	2.0	3.7
Vegetable, & Mushroom, Asda*	½ Pack/160g		59	2.4	37	2.4	3.4	1.5	3.4
Vegetable, & Noodle, Asda*	1 Pack/330g		465	14.8	141	4.0	21.0	4.5	3.0
Vegetable, & Noodles, BGTY, Sainsbury's*	1 Pack/455g		391	9.1	86	3.2	14.0	2.0	1.4
Vegetable, & Oyster Sauce, Chinese, Asda*	1 Serving/150g		93	3.8	62	1.9	8.0	2.5	0.0
Vegetable, & Oyster Sauce, Chinese, Tesco*	1 Pack/350g		98	0.7	28	2.0	4.6	0.2	1.1
Vegetable, & Peashoot, Mixed, Tesco*	1 Serving/100g		36	0.5	36	2.1	4.7	0.5	2.0
Vegetable, Basics, Sainsbury's*	½ Bag/325g		101	2.9	31	2.1	3.5	0.9	2.2
Vegetable, Cantonese, Sainsbury's*	1 Serving/150g		90	5.2	60	2.8	4.2	3.5	2.7
Vegetable, Chinese, Tesco*	1 Serving/175g		93	0.7	53	1.6	10.8	0.4	1.3
Vegetable, Chinese Style, Asda*	1 Pack/300g		81	2.1	27	1.6	3.6	0.7	2.8
Vegetable, Crunchy, Sainsbury's*	½ Pack/150g		86	5.8	57	1.4	4.1	3.9	2.1
Vegetable, Crunchy, Waitrose*	1 Pack/300g		81	0.3	27	1.6	4.8	0.1	2.4
Vegetable, Exotic, Chinese, Sainsbury's*	1 Pack/350g		133	7.7	38	1.7	2.8	2.2	1.8
Vegetable, Family Pack, Co-Op*	½ Pack/300g		90	1.2	30	2.0	5.0	0.4	2.0
Vegetable, Frozen, Farm Foods*	1 Pack/650g		208	3.2	32	1.9	4.9	0.5	2.2
Vegetable, Green, M&S*	1 Pack/220g		165	13.0	75	3.1	2.5	5.9	2.2
Vegetable, Mixed, Asda*	1 Serving/200g		96	5.0	48	1.7	4.7	2.5	3.0
Vegetable, Mixed Pepper, M&S*	½ Pack/150g		52	0.6	35	1.9	4.9	0.4	1.9
Vegetable, Mixed with Slices of Pepper, Tesco*	1 Pack/300g		102	1.2	34	2.0	4.6	0.4	2.0
Vegetable, Oriental, Frozen, Asda*	1 Serving/150g		116	6.8	77	2.1	7.0	4.5	1.7
Vegetable, Oriental, Frozen, Freshly, Asda*	1 Serving/100g		25	0.3	25	2.2	3.4	0.3	2.0
Vegetable, Oriental, Just Stir Fry, Sainsbury's*	½ Pack/135g		94	7.2	70	2.2	3.4	5.3	1.3
Vegetable, Oriental Style, Sainsbury's*	1 Pack/300g		195	14.4	65	1.5	4.1	4.8	2.1
Vegetable, Ready Prepared, M&S*	½ Pack/150g		38	0.4	25	2.2	3.5	0.3	2.2
Vegetable, Sweet & Crunchy, Waitrose*	1 Pack/300g		69	0.3	23	1.8	3.6	0.1	1.4

S

	Measure INFO/WEIGHT	per Measure		Nutrition Values per 100g / 100ml				
		KCAL	FAT	KCAL	PROT	CARB	FAT	FIBRE
STIR FRY								
Vegetable, Tesco*	¼ Bag/100g	35	0.4	35	1.8	4.7	0.4	2.5
Vegetable, Thai Style, Tesco*	½ Pack/135g	42	0.7	31	2.3	4.2	0.5	2.1
Water Chestnut & Bamboo Shoot, Fresh Tastes, Asda*	½ Pack/210g	82	2.9	39	1.4	4.3	1.4	1.7
STOCK								
Beef, Cooks' Ingredients, Waitrose*	1 Jar/500g	74	0.5	15	3.0	0.3	0.1	0.8
Beef, Fresh, Tesco*	1 Serving/300ml	54	0.9	18	2.1	1.6	0.3	0.5
Beef, Made Up, Stock Pot, Knorr*	1 Serving/100ml	10	0.4	10	0.2	1.0	0.4	0.0
Beef, Pots, Unprepared, Sainsbury's*	1 Pot/28g	31	1.7	112	4.1	8.5	6.2	2.9
Beef, Signature, Sainsbury's*	1 Pack/500g	65	1.0	13	2.7	0.0	0.2	0.0
Beef, Simply Stock, Knorr*	1 Serving/100ml	6	0.0	6	1.4	0.1	0.0	0.0
Beef, Slowly Prepared, Sainsbury's*	1 Serving/100g	7	0.3	7	0.7	0.3	0.3	0.5
Chicken, As Sold, Stock Pot, Knorr*	1 Serving/100ml	5	0.4	95	2.4	4.9	7.3	0.8
Chicken, Asda*	½ Pot/150g	26	1.4	17	1.8	0.7	0.9	0.2
Chicken, Cooks' Ingredients, Waitrose*	1 Pack/500ml	75	0.5	15	3.2	0.3	0.1	0.2
Chicken, Fresh, Sainsbury's*	½ Pot/142ml	23	0.1	16	3.7	0.1	0.1	0.3
Chicken, Fresh, Tesco*	1 Serving/300ml	27	0.3	9	1.6	0.5	0.1	0.5
Chicken, Granules, Knorr*	1 Tsp/5g	10	0.2	232	13.1	36.5	3.7	0.4
Chicken, Home Prepared, Average	*1 fl oz/30ml*	*7*	*0.3*	*24*	*3.8*	*0.7*	*0.9*	*0.3*
Chicken, Made Up, Stock Pot, Knorr*	1 fl oz/30ml	2	0.1	5	0.1	0.3	0.4	0.0
Chicken, Prepared, Tesco*	1 Serving/300ml	54	0.3	18	2.4	1.8	0.1	0.5
Chicken, Simply Stock, Knorr*	1 Pack/450ml	27	0.0	6	1.5	0.1	0.0	0.1
Chicken, Slowly Prepared, Sainsbury's*	1 Pot/300g	27	0.3	9	0.6	1.3	0.1	0.5
Fish, Fresh, Finest, Tesco*	1 Serving/100g	10	0.0	10	0.6	1.8	0.0	0.5
Fish, Home Prepared, Average	*1 Serving/250ml*	*42*	*2.0*	*17*	*2.3*	*0.0*	*0.8*	*0.0*
Vegetable, As Sold, Stock Pot, Knorr*	1 Serving/100ml	9	0.5	180	6.0	19.0	9.0	1.5
Vegetable, Campbell's*	1 Serving/250ml	38	1.8	15	0.3	2.0	0.7	0.0
Vegetable, Cooks Ingredients, Waitrose*	1 Pouch/500ml	15	0.5	3	0.2	0.4	0.1	0.5
Vegetable, Made Up, Stock Pot, Knorr*	1 Serving/100ml	10	0.5	10	0.4	1.0	0.5	0.1
STOCK CUBES								
Beef, Dry Weight, Bovril*	1 Cube/6g	12	0.2	197	10.8	29.3	4.1	0.0
Beef, Dry Weight, Oxo*	1 Cube/6g	15	0.3	265	17.3	38.4	4.7	1.5
Beef, Knorr*	1 Cube/10g	31	2.3	310	5.0	19.0	23.0	0.0
Beef, Organic, Kallo*	1 Cube/12g	25	1.0	208	16.7	16.7	8.3	0.0
Beef Flavour, Made Up, Oxo*	1 Serving/189ml	17	0.4	9	0.6	1.3	0.2	0.1
Chicken	1 Cube/6g	14	0.9	237	15.4	9.9	15.4	0.0
Chicken, Dry, Average	1 Cube/10g	29	1.8	293	7.3	25.5	18.0	0.4
Chicken, Dry, Oxo*	1 Cube/7g	17	0.2	249	10.9	44.0	3.3	0.9
Chicken, Just Bouillon, Kallo*	1 Cube/12g	30	1.3	247	11.8	26.1	10.6	1.0
Chicken, Knorr*	1 Cube/10g	31	2.0	310	4.0	29.0	20.0	0.0
Chicken, Made Up, Average	1 Pint/568ml	43	1.0	8	0.4	1.1	0.2	0.1
Chicken, Made Up, Sainsbury's*	1 Serving/200ml	16	0.2	8	0.3	1.4	0.1	0.1
Chicken, Prepared, Oxo*	1 Serving/100ml	9	0.1	9	0.4	1.5	0.1	0.1
Chicken, Tesco*	1 Cube/11g	32	2.5	290	10.5	11.1	22.6	0.7
Chicken, Value, Tesco*	1 Cube/10g	15	0.6	150	9.4	14.3	5.9	0.8
Fish, Knorr*	1 Cube/10g	32	2.4	321	8.0	18.0	24.0	1.0
Fish, Sainsbury's*	1 Cube/11g	31	2.2	282	19.1	7.3	20.0	0.9
Ham, Knorr*	1 Cube/10g	31	1.9	313	11.8	24.4	18.7	0.0
Italian, Dry Weight, Oxo*	1 Cube/6g	19	0.4	309	11.9	48.9	7.3	4.6
Lamb, Made Up, Knorr*	1 Cube/10g	32	2.5	320	11.0	14.0	25.0	0.0
Parsley & Garlic, Herb Cubes, Knorr*	1 Cube/10g	42	2.7	422	8.6	35.2	27.4	1.8
Vegetable, Average	1 Cube/7g	18	1.2	253	13.5	11.6	17.3	0.0
Vegetable, Dry, Oxo*	1 Cube/6g	17	0.3	251	10.4	41.4	4.9	1.4
Vegetable, Knorr*	1 Cube/10g	33	2.4	330	10.0	25.0	24.0	1.0

	Measure INFO/WEIGHT	per Measure KCAL	FAT	Nutrition Values per 100g / 100ml KCAL	PROT	CARB	FAT	FIBRE
STOCK CUBES								
Vegetable, Low Salt, Organic, Made Up, Kallo*	1 Serving/500ml	50	3.5	10	0.3	0.7	0.7	0.2
Vegetable, Made Up, Organic, Kallo*	1 Serving/100ml	7	0.4	7	0.1	0.5	0.4	0.1
Vegetable, Made up, Oxo*	1 Serving/100ml	9	0.2	9	0.4	1.4	0.2	0.1
Vegetable, Organic, Yeast Free, Dry, Kallo*	1 Cube/11g	37	3.1	334	11.4	8.2	27.8	2.3
Vegetable, Premium, Made Up, Kallo*	1 Serving/125ml	7	0.4	6	0.4	0.4	0.3	0.1
Vegetable, Value, Tesco*	1 Cube/10g	14	0.3	145	10.6	17.4	3.3	3.6
Vegetable, Yeast Free, Made Up, Kallo*	1 Serving/500ml	35	3.0	7	0.3	0.2	0.6	0.1
Vegetable Bouillon, Vegetarian, Amoy*	1 Cube/10g	30	2.0	300	0.0	20.0	20.0	0.0
Vegetable Bouillon, Yeast Free, Made Up, Marigold*	1 Serving/250ml	19	1.6	8	0.0	0.5	0.6	0.0
STOLLEN								
Slices, Average	1 Slice/42g	160	6.3	381	5.5	55.8	15.0	3.1
STORTELLI								
Microwaveable, Dolmio*	1 Serving/220g	299	2.2	136	5.3	26.3	1.0	0.0
STRAWBERRIES								
Dried, Urban Fresh Fruit*	1 Pack/35g	111	0.1	318	1.6	77.0	0.4	5.9
Freeze Dried, Slices, Crunchy in Munchcup, Benjoy*	1 Pot/6g	21	0.2	350	6.6	65.1	2.9	18.6
Fresh, Raw, Average	*1 Strawberry/12g*	*3*	*0.0*	*28*	*0.8*	*6.0*	*0.1*	*1.4*
Frozen, Average	*1 Serving/100g*	*30*	*0.2*	*30*	*0.8*	*6.3*	*0.2*	*1.0*
in Fruit Juice, Canned, Average	*1/3 Can/127g*	*58*	*0.0*	*46*	*0.4*	*11.0*	*0.0*	*1.0*
in Syrup, Canned, Average	1 Serving/100g	63	0.0	63	0.4	15.2	0.0	0.6
STROGANOFF								
Beef, & Rice, TTD, Sainsbury's*	1 Pack/410g	595	20.9	145	9.6	15.2	5.1	1.7
Beef, Asda*	1 Serving/120g	276	20.4	230	16.0	3.3	17.0	0.6
Beef, Finest, Tesco*	½ Pack/200g	330	13.4	165	9.4	16.2	6.7	0.7
Beef, Low Fat with White & Wild Rice, Waitrose*	1 Pack/401g	429	6.4	107	7.9	15.3	1.6	1.0
Beef, with White & Wild Rice, Classic, Tesco*	1 Pack/500g	770	29.6	154	9.5	15.5	5.9	2.3
Beef, with White & Wild Rice, Love Life, Waitrose*	1 Pack/370g	418	9.0	113	6.0	16.3	2.4	1.0
Chicken, & Mushroom, COU, M&S*	1 Serving/400g	400	8.0	100	3.2	16.7	2.0	0.1
Chicken, with Rice, BGTY, Sainsbury's*	1 Pack/415g	448	5.4	108	7.0	17.1	1.3	1.1
Mushroom, Diet Chef Ltd*	1 Pouch/250g	202	14.8	81	2.6	4.5	5.9	1.7
Mushroom, Solo Slim, Rosemary Conley*	1 Pack/251g	193	11.3	77	2.7	6.5	4.5	2.7
Mushroom, with Rice, BGTY, Sainsbury's*	1 Serving/450g	418	6.8	93	3.3	16.6	1.5	1.0
Mushroom, with Rice, Vegetarian, LC, Tesco*	1 Pack/450g	420	7.5	95	2.6	16.4	1.7	1.1
STRUDEL								
Apple, Co-Op*	1 Slice/100g	225	12.0	225	3.0	28.0	12.0	3.0
Apple, Frozen, Sainsbury's*	1 Serving/100g	283	15.4	283	3.2	32.8	15.4	1.9
Apple, Sainsbury's*	1/6 Strudel/90g	255	13.9	283	3.2	32.8	15.4	1.9
Apple, Tesco*	1 Serving/150g	432	21.6	288	3.3	36.4	14.4	2.8
Apple & Mincemeat, Tesco*	1 Serving/100g	322	16.7	322	3.3	39.6	16.7	2.0
Apple with Sultanas, Tesco*	1/6 Strudel/100g	245	12.0	245	2.9	30.9	12.0	0.7
Tesco*	1 Serving/150g	370	19.4	247	2.9	29.8	12.9	4.7
Woodland Fruit, Sainsbury's*	1/6 Strudel/95g	276	14.8	290	3.7	34.0	15.5	2.0
Woodland Fruit, Tesco*	1 Serving/100g	257	13.1	257	3.2	31.5	13.1	1.8
STUFFING								
Apple & Herb, Mix, Special Recipe, Sainsbury's*	1 Serving/41g	68	0.9	165	3.8	32.4	2.2	2.2
Apricot & Walnut, Mix, Made Up, Celebrations, Paxo*	1 Serving/50g	80	1.8	161	4.3	28.0	3.5	2.8
Chestnut, Mix, Morrisons*	1 Serving/20g	33	0.7	165	4.6	29.1	3.4	3.7
Chestnut & Cranberry, Mix, Celebration, Paxo*	1 Serving/25g	35	0.5	141	4.0	26.7	2.0	2.4
Chestnut & Pork, M&S*	1oz/28g	67	4.7	240	6.6	16.3	16.7	2.9
Dry, Mix, Average	1 Serving/25g	84	1.0	338	9.6	70.1	3.8	5.3
Parsley, Thyme & Lemon, Mix, Paxo*	1 Serving/45g	68	0.9	150	4.3	28.4	2.1	2.4
Parsley, Thyme & Lemon, Mix, Sainsbury's*	1 Pack/170g	240	2.2	141	4.2	28.2	1.3	1.3
Parsley & Thyme, Co-Op*	1 Serving/28g	95	0.8	340	10.0	67.0	3.0	6.0

	Measure INFO/WEIGHT	per Measure KCAL	FAT	Nutrition Values per 100g / 100ml KCAL	PROT	CARB	FAT	FIBRE
STUFFING								
Pork, Chestnut & Onion, Cooked, Finest, Tesco*	¼ Pack/98g	230	11.5	235	9.5	21.5	11.7	1.7
Pork & Chestnut, M&S*	1oz/28g	64	4.8	230	5.3	12.6	17.1	3.7
Sage & Onion, for Chicken, Paxo*	1 Serving/50g	62	0.9	123	3.6	23.0	1.8	1.7
Sage & Onion, Mix, Asda*	1 Serving/27g	29	0.2	107	3.4	22.0	0.6	1.3
Sage & Onion, Mix, Co-Op*	1 Serving/28g	94	0.6	335	10.0	68.0	2.0	6.0
Sage & Onion, Mix, Dry Weight, Tesco*	1 Pack/170g	578	4.1	340	10.3	69.3	2.4	6.3
Sage & Onion, Mix, Made Up, Paxo*	1 Serving/50g	72	0.6	143	3.2	29.9	1.2	1.9
Sage & Onion, Mix, Smart Price, Asda*	¼ Pack/75g	262	2.8	349	11.0	68.0	3.7	4.7
Sage & Onion, Mix, Value, Tesco*	1 Ball/38g	133	1.1	350	10.2	70.7	2.9	5.1
Sage & Onion, Somerfield*	1oz/28g	100	1.4	358	6.0	74.0	5.0	0.0
Sage & Onion, with Apple, Mix, Made Up, Paxo*	1 Serving/50g	69	0.8	138	3.8	26.0	1.6	2.2
Sage & Onion with Lemon, Paxo*	1 Serving/50g	61	0.6	122	3.4	24.2	1.2	1.9
Sausage Meat, Morrisons*	1 Serving/20g	35	0.5	174	6.8	30.8	2.6	2.9
Sausagemeat, & Thyme, Made Up, Celebrations, Paxo*	1 Serving/50g	80	1.8	160	6.3	25.8	3.5	4.0
Sausagemeat, Sainsbury's*	1 Serving/100g	175	4.2	175	7.0	27.0	4.2	2.3
STUFFING BALLS								
British Pork, Sage & Onion, Cooked, Finest, Tesco*	2 Balls/49g	110	5.0	224	13.9	17.4	10.2	2.2
Pork, Sausagemeat, Aunt Bessie's*	1 Ball/26g	55	2.1	212	7.2	27.3	8.2	3.0
Sage & Onion, Aunt Bessie's*	1 Ball/26g	63	2.3	243	6.4	34.4	8.9	3.1
Sage & Onion, Meat-Free, Aunt Bessie's*	1 Ball/28g	54	1.9	193	5.4	28.0	6.7	1.7
Sage & Onion, Tesco*	1 Serving/20g	64	4.4	322	10.0	21.1	22.0	1.9
Tesco*	1 Ball/21g	65	4.1	315	9.6	23.5	20.0	1.4
SUET								
Beef, Shredded, Original, Atora*	1 Pack/200g	1592	163.0	796	1.1	14.6	81.5	0.5
Beef, Tesco*	1 Serving/100g	854	91.9	854	0.6	6.2	91.9	0.1
Vegetable, Average	*1oz/28g*	*234*	*24.6*	*836*	*1.2*	*10.1*	*87.9*	*0.0*
SUET PUDDING								
Average	*1oz/28g*	*94*	*5.1*	*335*	*4.4*	*40.5*	*18.3*	*0.9*
SUGAR								
Brown, Soft, Average	*1 Tsp/4g*	*15*	*0.0*	*382*	*0.0*	*96.5*	*0.0*	*0.0*
Brown, Soft, Light, Average	*1 Tsp/5g*	*20*	*0.0*	*393*	*0.2*	*97.8*	*0.1*	*0.0*
Caster, Average	*1 Tsp/5g*	*20*	*0.0*	*399*	*0.0*	*99.8*	*0.0*	*0.0*
Dark Brown, Muscovado, Average	*1 Tsp/7g*	*27*	*0.0*	*380*	*0.2*	*94.8*	*0.0*	*0.0*
Dark Brown, Soft, Average	*1 Tsp/5g*	*18*	*0.0*	*369*	*0.1*	*92.0*	*0.0*	*0.0*
Demerara, Average	*1 Tsp/5g*	*18*	*0.0*	*368*	*0.2*	*99.2*	*0.0*	*0.0*
for Making Jam, Silver Spoon*	1oz/28g	111	0.0	398	0.0	99.5	0.0	0.0
Fructose, Fruit Sugar, Tate & Lyle*	1 Tsp/4g	16	0.0	400	0.0	100.0	0.0	0.0
Golden, Unrefined, Average	*1 Tsp/4g*	*16*	*0.0*	*399*	*0.0*	*99.8*	*0.0*	*0.0*
Granulated, Organic, Average	*1 Tsp/4g*	*16*	*0.0*	*398*	*0.2*	*99.7*	*0.0*	*0.0*
Icing, Average	*1 Tsp/4g*	*16*	*0.0*	*394*	*0.0*	*102.2*	*0.0*	*0.0*
Icing, Golden, Cane, Natural, Unrefined, Billingtons*	1oz/28g	111	0.0	397	0.5	98.7	0.0	0.0
Light Or Diet, Average	*1 Tsp/4g*	*16*	*0.0*	*394*	*0.0*	*98.5*	*0.0*	*0.0*
Maple, Average	1 Tsp/5g	18	0.0	354	0.1	90.9	0.2	0.0
Muscovado, Light, Average	1 Tsp/5g	19	0.0	384	0.0	96.0	0.0	0.0
Vanilla, Fairtrade, Cooks' Ingredients, Waitrose*	1 Serving/100g	399	0.0	399	0.0	99.7	0.0	0.0
White, Granulated, Average	*1 Tsp/5g*	*20*	*0.0*	*398*	*0.0*	*100.0*	*0.0*	*0.0*
White, Plus Stevia Blend, Light at Heart, Tate & Lyle*	1 Serving/2g	8	0.0	398	0.0	99.6	0.0	0.0
SULTANAS								
Average	*1oz/28g*	*82*	*0.1*	*291*	*2.8*	*69.2*	*0.4*	*2.0*
SUMMER FRUITS								
Frozen, Sainsbury's*	1 Serving/80g	43	0.1	54	0.9	6.9	0.1	2.0
Mix, Sainsbury's*	1 Serving/80g	26	0.0	32	0.9	7.4	0.0	2.4

	Measure INFO/WEIGHT	per Measure		Nutrition Values per 100g / 100ml				
		KCAL	FAT	KCAL	PROT	CARB	FAT	FIBRE
SUNDAE								
Blackcurrant, M&S*	1 Sundae/53g	212	10.2	400	3.0	54.2	19.2	1.9
Chocolate, Sainsbury's*	1 Pot/140g	393	29.8	281	2.5	19.3	21.3	0.6
Chocolate Brownie, Finest, Tesco*	1 Serving/215g	778	56.5	362	2.7	28.7	26.3	2.3
Chocolate Nut	1 Serving/70g	195	10.7	278	3.0	34.2	15.3	0.1
Hot Fudge, Two Scoop, Baskin Robbins*	1 Serving/203g	530	29.0	261	3.9	30.5	14.3	0.0
Ice Cream	1 Serving/170g	482	15.4	284	5.9	45.3	9.1	0.3
Strawberry, M&S*	1 Sundae/45g	173	8.0	385	3.4	53.3	17.8	1.0
Strawberry, Tesco*	1 Sundae/48g	194	8.7	408	3.3	57.6	18.3	1.3
Strawberry & Vanilla, Tesco*	1 Serving/68g	120	3.9	177	2.0	29.5	5.7	0.1
Toffee, Asda*	1 Serving/120g	322	19.2	268	2.1	29.0	16.0	0.0
Toffee & Vanilla, Tesco*	1 Serving/70g	133	4.5	189	2.1	30.7	6.4	0.1
SUNNY DELIGHT*								
Californian Style, No Added Sugar, Sunny Delight*	1 Serving/200ml	20	0.4	10	0.1	1.4	0.2	0.1
Florida Style, Sunny Delight*	1 Serving/200ml	70	0.2	35	0.4	7.4	0.1	0.2
Original, Sunny Delight*	1 Glass/200ml	88	0.4	44	0.1	10.0	0.2	0.0
SUSHI								
Aya Set, Waitrose*	1 Pack/110g	200	4.3	182	5.4	31.7	3.9	1.5
California Roll Box, M&S*	1 Pack/230g	391	12.0	170	7.0	22.0	5.2	1.1
California Roll Selection, Classics, M&S*	1 Pack/225g	326	6.1	145	7.0	23.2	2.7	1.1
California Rolls 8 Pack	1 Pack/206g	354	9.3	172	5.1	27.5	4.5	1.4
California Set, Waitrose*	1 Pack/120g	223	9.1	186	3.8	25.2	7.6	1.7
Californian Roll, Nigiri & Maki Selection, M&S*	1 Pack/210g	294	4.4	140	4.4	25.9	2.1	2.2
Californian Roll & Nigiri, Selection, M&S*	1 Pack/215g	355	5.8	165	7.1	28.0	2.7	1.1
Chicken, M&S*	1 Pack/186g	260	4.1	140	6.0	24.4	2.2	1.0
Chicken, Tesco*	1 Pack/147g	243	3.5	165	5.2	30.0	2.4	1.0
Classic, Finest, Tesco*	1 Pack/232g	330	0.9	142	6.6	27.6	0.4	0.6
Fish, Large Pack, Tesco*	1 Pack/284g	469	11.1	165	5.5	27.0	3.9	1.5
Fish, Selection, M&S*	1 Pack/191g	295	4.6	155	5.6	26.8	2.4	0.9
Fish, Selection, Medium, Sainsbury's*	1 Pack/157g	256	3.9	163	5.6	28.6	2.5	1.9
Fish, Snack, Tesco*	1 Pack/104g	159	2.6	153	4.5	28.0	2.5	1.5
Fish & Veg Selection, Tesco*	1 Pack/150g	248	3.4	165	6.7	29.2	2.3	0.4
Fish Nigiri, Adventurous, Tesco*	1 Pack/200g	270	4.4	135	7.1	21.7	2.2	0.5
Fish Roll, Nigiri & Maki Selection, M&S*	1 Pack/210g	315	4.8	150	6.5	25.8	2.3	1.0
Fish Selection, M&S*	1 Pack/191g	315	5.9	165	7.4	26.3	3.1	1.4
Fusion, M&S*	1 Pack/186g	260	3.3	140	5.1	23.8	1.8	2.9
GFY, Asda*	1 Pack/220g	352	3.1	160	4.9	32.0	1.4	0.0
Komachi Set with Salmon, Whiting & Handroll, Waitrose*	1 Pack/257g	447	13.9	174	5.3	25.8	5.4	1.2
Large, Boots*	1 Pack/324g	480	5.8	148	5.0	28.0	1.8	0.7
Maki Rolls Box, Sainsbury's*	1 Pack/127g	197	2.2	155	4.5	30.5	1.7	0.8
Maki Selection, Shapers, Boots*	1 Pack/158g	225	2.1	142	3.5	29.0	1.3	1.1
Medium, Vegetarian, Taiko Foods*	1 Pack/267g	403	5.3	151	4.0	36.0	2.0	1.0
Medium Pack, Tesco*	1 Pack/224g	336	3.8	150	4.0	29.4	1.7	1.0
Mini, Boots*	1 Pack/99g	153	1.9	155	5.5	29.0	1.9	0.8
Mixed Box, Somerfield*	1 Pack/220g	339	2.4	154	4.6	31.4	1.1	0.0
Nigiri, M&S*	1 Serving/190g	303	5.9	159	7.3	25.3	3.1	0.6
Nigiri, Selection, Tesco*	1 Pack/152g	236	1.5	155	4.6	31.2	1.0	0.6
Nigiri Set, Taiko, Salmon & Tuna, Waitrose*	1 Pack/113g	174	2.3	154	6.3	26.0	2.0	0.6
Nigri, Californian Roll, Maki Roll, Sainsbury's*	1 Pack/195g	283	2.9	145	5.3	27.4	1.5	1.9
Oriental Fish Box, M&S*	1 Pack/205g	318	8.4	155	6.1	23.3	4.1	0.9
Prawn & Salmon Selection, M&S*	1 Serving/175g	255	2.9	146	5.5	27.4	1.7	0.6
Prawn Feast, M&S*	1 Pack/219g	350	8.1	160	5.7	25.8	3.7	1.1
Roll Selection, Sainsbury's*	1 Pack/217g	363	8.0	167	5.0	28.4	3.7	0.5
Rolls, Shapers, Boots*	1 Pack/168g	259	4.0	154	4.7	28.0	2.4	0.5

S

INFO/WEIGHT	Measure	per Measure KCAL	FAT	Nutrition Values per 100g / 100ml KCAL	PROT	CARB	FAT	FIBRE

SUSHI

	Measure INFO/WEIGHT	per Measure KCAL	FAT	KCAL	PROT	CARB	FAT	FIBRE
Salmon, Smoked, Snack Pack, Tesco*	1 Pack/69g	114	1.9	165	5.0	29.1	2.7	0.9
Salmon & Roll Set, Sainsbury's*	1 Serving/101g	167	2.6	165	4.9	30.4	2.6	0.8
Salmon Feast Box, M&S*	1 Pack/200g	330	5.8	165	5.6	27.0	2.9	1.0
Selection, Boots*	1 Pack/268g	434	9.6	162	5.5	27.0	3.6	1.6
Selection, Shapers, Boots*	1 Pack/162g	245	2.6	151	5.6	29.0	1.6	1.7
Snack Selection, Eat Well, M&S*	1 Pack/96g	134	0.7	140	5.3	28.7	0.7	0.8
Taiko, Fuji Set, Waitrose*	1 Pack/332g	515	10.0	155	5.0	28.0	3.0	1.0
to Share, Tesco*	1 Pack/385g	616	6.2	160	5.7	30.6	1.6	0.7
Tuna, to Snack Selection, Food to Go, M&S*	1 Serving/150g	225	3.9	150	5.2	26.4	2.6	2.3
Veg Selection, Ichiban *	1 Pack/130g	198	1.7	152	2.7	32.3	1.3	1.2
Vegetable, Mixed, Pick & Mix, Snack Pack, Tesco*	1 Pack/85g	132	2.0	155	3.7	28.6	2.4	1.4
Vegetable Selection Pack, M&S*	1 Pack/154g	215	2.8	140	2.8	28.1	1.8	1.3
Vegetarian, Selection, M&S*	1 Pack/171g	248	2.4	145	3.0	28.5	1.4	2.4
Vegetarian, Snack Selection, Tesco*	1 Pack/85g	106	2.8	125	3.7	20.1	3.3	0.6
Vegetarian with Pickled Vegetables, Waitrose*	1 Pack/135g	244	4.9	181	5.0	27.8	3.6	1.7
Yasai Roll Set, Vegetarian, Wasabi Co Ltd*	1 Pack/498g	398	10.4	80	1.9	13.4	2.1	0.0
Yo!, Bento Box, Sainsbury's*	1 Pack/208g	530	6.2	255	8.4	48.7	3.0	0.9
Yo!, Salmon Lunch Set, Sainsbury's*	1 Pack/150g	242	4.2	161	5.9	28.1	2.8	0.8

SWEDE

	Measure INFO/WEIGHT	per Measure KCAL	FAT	KCAL	PROT	CARB	FAT	FIBRE
Boiled, Average	**1oz/28g**	**3**	**0.0**	**11**	**0.3**	**2.3**	**0.1**	**0.7**
Raw, Flesh Only, Peeled	**1 Serving/100g**	**24**	**0.3**	**24**	**0.7**	**5.0**	**0.3**	**1.6**
Raw, Unprepared, Average	**1oz/28g**	**6**	**0.1**	**21**	**0.8**	**4.4**	**0.3**	**1.9**

SWEET & SOUR

	Measure INFO/WEIGHT	per Measure KCAL	FAT	KCAL	PROT	CARB	FAT	FIBRE
Chicken, & Noodles, Chinese Takeaway, Tesco*	1 Pack/350g	350	0.7	100	5.7	18.8	0.2	0.2
Chicken, & Rice, Chilled, Tesco*	1 Pack/450g	540	5.8	120	4.9	21.9	1.3	0.9
Chicken, Balls, Chinese Takeaway, Iceland*	1 Pack/255g	311	3.3	122	9.9	17.5	1.3	6.0
Chicken, Breasts, Tesco*	1 Serving/185g	172	1.8	93	14.6	6.5	1.0	0.1
Chicken, Cantonese, Chilled, Sainsbury's*	1 Pack/350g	410	4.9	117	8.5	17.6	1.4	1.0
Chicken, Chinese Takeaway, Sainsbury's*	1 Pack/264g	515	16.9	195	13.1	21.3	6.4	1.0
Chicken, Crispy, Chinese, M Kitchen, Morrisons*	½ Pack/192g	315	9.8	164	10.6	19.0	5.1	1.8
Chicken, Crispy, Fillets, Tesco*	1 Pack/350g	508	19.6	145	7.2	15.3	5.6	0.9
Chicken, Crispy, Iceland*	1 Serving/125g	221	6.5	177	18.3	14.2	5.2	1.2
Chicken, in Batter, Cantonese, Chilled, Sainsbury's*	1 Pack/350g	560	21.0	160	8.9	22.4	6.0	0.9
Chicken, in Crispy Batter, Morrisons*	1 Pack/350g	511	13.6	146	10.1	17.6	3.9	1.2
Chicken, M&S*	1 Pack/300g	465	10.8	155	6.6	24.4	3.6	0.8
Chicken, Oriental, Tesco*	1 Pack/350g	340	4.0	97	9.3	12.2	1.1	0.8
Chicken, Take It Away, M&S*	1 Pack/200g	200	1.6	100	9.4	13.2	0.8	1.2
Chicken, Waitrose*	1 Serving/400g	372	3.2	93	9.8	11.7	0.8	1.4
Chicken, with Egg Fried Rice, GFY, Asda*	1 Pack/400g	500	7.6	125	6.0	20.3	1.9	1.8
Chicken, with Egg Fried Rice, Sainsbury's*	1 Pack/450g	617	13.3	137	7.3	19.7	3.0	1.3
Chicken, with Long Grain Rice, Weight Watchers*	1 Pack/330g	300	1.6	91	5.4	15.5	0.5	1.4
Pork	1oz/28g	48	2.5	172	12.7	11.3	8.8	0.6
Pork, Battered, Sainsbury's*	½ Pack/175g	306	8.8	175	7.3	25.1	5.0	0.6
Pork, with Rice, 229, Oakhouse Foods Ltd*	1 Meal/400g	484	12.0	121	5.1	18.4	3.0	0.7
with Long Grain Rice, Rice Time, Uncle Ben's*	1 Pot/300g	393	2.4	131	1.9	28.4	0.8	0.7

SWEET POTATO

	Measure INFO/WEIGHT	per Measure KCAL	FAT	KCAL	PROT	CARB	FAT	FIBRE
Baked, Flesh Only, Average	**1 Med/130g**	**150**	**0.5**	**115**	**1.6**	**27.9**	**0.4**	**3.3**
Boiled in Salted Water, Average	**1 Med/200g**	**168**	**0.6**	**84**	**1.1**	**20.5**	**0.3**	**2.3**
Raw, Peeled, Average	1 Potato/130g	112	0.1	86	1.6	20.1	0.0	3.0
Raw, Unprepared, Average	**1 Potato/200g**	**174**	**0.6**	**87**	**1.2**	**21.3**	**0.3**	**2.4**
Roasted, Rosemary & Chipotle Chilli, TTD, Sainsbury's*	½ Pack/100g	199	1.9	199	2.0	17.0	1.9	4.2
Steamed, Average	**1 Med/200g**	**168**	**0.6**	**84**	**1.1**	**20.4**	**0.3**	**2.3**
with Rosemary & Garlic, Frozen, McCain*	1 Serving/150g	172	5.6	115	2.1	18.4	3.7	2.8

	Measure INFO/WEIGHT	per Measure		Nutrition Values per 100g / 100ml				
		KCAL	FAT	KCAL	PROT	CARB	FAT	FIBRE
SWEETBREAD								
Lamb, Fried	**1oz/28g**	**61**	**3.2**	**217**	**28.7**	**0.0**	**11.4**	**0.0**
SWEETCORN								
Baby, & Mangetout, Somerfield*	1 Pack/150g	42	0.4	28	3.2	3.0	0.3	1.9
Baby, Canned, Drained, Average	1 Serving/80g	18	0.3	23	2.9	2.0	0.4	1.5
Baby, Frozen, Average	*1oz/28g*	*7*	*0.1*	*24*	*2.5*	*2.7*	*0.4*	*1.7*
Boiled, Average	*1oz/28g*	*31*	*0.6*	*111*	*4.2*	*19.6*	*2.3*	*2.2*
Canned, No Sugar & Salt, Average	½ Can/125g	99	1.3	79	2.7	15.0	1.1	1.6
Canned with Sugar & Salt, Average	*1 Can/340g*	*376*	*4.0*	*111*	*3.2*	*21.9*	*1.2*	*1.9*
Frozen, Average	*1 Sachet/115g*	*121*	*2.4*	*105*	*3.8*	*17.9*	*2.1*	*1.8*
with Peppers, Canned, Average	*1 Serving/50g*	*40*	*0.2*	*79*	*2.6*	*16.4*	*0.3*	*0.6*
SWEETENER								
Aspartamo, Artificial Sugar, Zen*	1 Tbsp/2g	8	0.0	383	1.8	94.0	0.0	0.0
Calorie Free, Truvia*	1/3 Tsp/2g	0	0.0	0	0.0	99.0	0.0	0.0
Canderel, Spoonful, Canderel*	1 Tsp/0.5g	2	0.0	384	2.9	93.0	0.0	0.0
Canderel*	1 Tbsp/2g	8	0.0	379	24.7	7.0	0.0	5.3
Granulated, Low Calorie, Splenda*	1 Tsp/0.5g	2	0.0	391	0.0	97.7	0.0	0.0
Granulated, Silver Spoon*	1 Tsp/0.5g	2	0.0	387	1.0	96.8	0.0	0.0
Granulated, Tesco*	1 Tsp/1g	4	0.0	383	1.8	94.0	0.0	0.0
Low Calorie, Somerfield*	1 Tsp/1g	2	0.0	380	3.0	92.0	0.0	0.0
Lucuma Powder, Navitas*	1 Tbsp/15g	60	0.0	400	6.7	86.7	0.0	0.0
Natural, Pure Via*	1 Sachet/2g	3	0.0	149	0.0	95.7	0.0	0.0
Natural Syrup, Fruit, Dark, Sweet Freedom*	1 Tsp/5g	13	0.0	292	0.0	79.0	0.0	0.0
Silver Spoon*	1 Tablet/0.05g	0	0.0	325	10.0	71.0	0.0	0.0
Simply Sweet*	1 Tbsp/2g	8	0.0	375	1.4	92.3	0.0	0.0
Slendasweet, Sainsbury's*	1 Tsp/1g	4	0.0	395	1.8	97.0	0.0	0.1
Slendersweet, Sainsbury's*	1 Tsp/1g	4	0.0	395	1.8	97.0	0.0	0.1
Spoonfull, Low Calorie, SupaSweet*	1 Tsp/1g	4	0.0	392	3.0	95.0	0.0	0.0
Sweet' N Low*	1 Sachet/1g	3	0.0	368	0.0	92.0	0.0	0.0
Sweetex**	1oz/28g	0	0.0	0	0.0	0.0	0.0	0.0
Tablet, Average	1 Tablet/0.1g	0	0.0	355	8.7	73.0	0.0	0.8
Tablets, Low Calorie, Canderel*	1 Tablet/0.1g	0	0.0	342	13.0	72.4	0.0	0.0
Tablets, Splenda*	1 Tablet/0.1g	0	0.0	345	10.0	76.2	0.0	1.6
Tablets, Tesco*	1 Tablet/1g	0	0.0	20	2.0	2.0	0.5	0.0
Tagatesse (Tablet), Damhert*	1 Tablet/0.075g	0	0.0	266	2.7	76.3	0.0	0.0
Xylosweet, Xylitol*	1 Serving/4g	10	0.0	240	0.0	100.0	0.0	0.0
SWEETS								
Almonds, Sugared, Dragee*	1 Sweet/4g	17	0.6	472	10.0	68.3	17.9	2.5
Alphabet Candies, Asda*	1 Pack/80g	306	0.0	382	0.5	95.0	0.0	0.0
Banana, Baby Foam, M&S*	1/3 Pack/34g	131	0.0	385	4.1	92.7	0.0	0.0
Big Purple One, Quality Street, Nestle*	1 Sweet/39g	191	9.9	490	4.7	60.5	25.5	0.7
Black Jacks & Fruit Salad, Bassett's*	1 Serving/190g	760	11.8	400	0.7	84.9	6.2	0.0
Blackcurrant & Liquorice, M&S*	1 Sweet/8g	32	0.3	400	0.6	89.0	4.3	0.0
Body Parts, Rowntree's*	1 Pack/42g	146	0.0	348	4.3	82.9	0.0	0.0
Butter Candies, Original, Werther's*	1 Sweet/5g	21	0.4	424	0.1	85.7	8.9	0.1
Campino, Oranges & Cream, Bendicks*	1oz/28g	116	2.3	416	0.1	85.8	8.1	0.0
Campino, Strawberries & Cream, Bendicks*	1oz/28g	117	2.3	418	0.1	86.2	8.1	0.0
Candy Cane, Average	1oz/28g	100	0.0	357	3.6	85.7	0.0	0.0
Candy Floss, Asda*	1 Tub/75g	292	0.0	390	0.0	100.0	0.0	0.0
Candy Foam Shapes, Fun Fruits, Value, Tesco*	1 Serving/25g	94	0.0	374	3.1	90.3	0.1	0.5
Cappuccino Cream, Sugar Free, Sula*	1 Sweet/3g	8	0.2	269	0.1	91.2	5.5	0.0
Cherry Lips, Chewits*	1 Serving/100g	319	0.2	319	5.6	72.1	0.2	0.0
Chew	1oz/28g	107	1.6	381	1.0	87.0	5.6	1.0
Chewits, Blackcurrant, Leaf*	1 Chew/3g	12	0.1	385	0.2	87.5	3.0	0.0

SWEETS

Measure INFO/WEIGHT	per Measure		Nutrition Values per 100g / 100ml				
	KCAL	FAT	KCAL	PROT	CARB	FAT	FIBRE
Chewits, Cola, Leaf* — 1 Chew/3g	12	0.1	385	0.2	87.5	3.0	0.0
Chewits, Fruit Salad, Leaf* — 1 Chew/3g	12	0.1	385	0.2	87.5	3.0	0.0
Chewits, Strawberry, Leaf* — 1 Chew/3g	12	0.1	385	0.2	87.5	3.0	0.0
Chewitts, Blackcurrant — 1 Pack/33g	125	0.9	378	0.3	86.9	2.7	0.0
Chews, Just Fruit, Fruit-tella* — 1 Serving/43g	170	2.8	400	0.9	79.5	6.5	0.0
Chews, Spearmint, Victoria, Aldi* — 1 Sweet/10g	40	0.8	405	0.3	83.8	7.6	0.0
Chews, Strawberry Mix, Starburst* — 1 Sweet/4g	15	0.3	401	0.0	83.9	7.3	0.0
Choco Toffee, Sula* — 1 Sweet/8g	21	1.2	267	3.3	31.7	15.8	0.0
Chocolate, Milk, Originals, Werther's* — 1 Sweet/6g	35	2.5	593	5.8	47.6	42.2	1.8
Chocolate Caramels, Diabetic, Boots* — 5 Sweets/40g	109	13.2	272	3.2	33.0	33.0	2.0
Chocolate Caramels, Milk, Tesco* — 1 Sweet/3g	15	0.5	444	2.7	72.1	16.1	0.1
Chocolate Eclairs, Cadbury* — 1 Sweet/8g	36	1.4	455	4.5	68.9	17.9	0.0
Chocolate Eclairs, Co-Op* — 1 Sweet/8g	38	1.6	480	3.0	71.0	20.0	0.6
Chocolate Limes, Pascall* — 1 Sweet/8g	27	0.2	333	0.3	77.2	2.5	0.0
Cola Bottles, Asda* — 1 Serving/100g	329	0.2	329	9.0	73.0	0.2	0.0
Cola Bottles, Fizzy, M&S* — 1 Pack/200g	650	0.0	325	6.4	75.0	0.0	0.0
Cola Bottles, Fizzy Wizzy, Woolworths* — 1 Bag/100g	336	0.0	336	3.5	77.2	0.0	0.0
Cough, Herbs, Swiss, Orginal, Ricola* — 1 Pack/37g	148	0.0	400	0.0	98.0	0.0	0.0
Crazy Crocs, Chewits* — 1 Serving/100g	316	0.2	316	3.8	73.9	0.2	0.0
Cream Caramel, Sula* — 1 Sweet/3g	10	0.0	297	0.4	86.1	0.0	0.0
Creme Caramel, Sugar Free, Be Light, Aldi* — 1 Sweet/3g	7	0.2	275	0.2	90.2	6.3	0.1
Dolly Mix, Bassett's* — 1 Bag/45g	171	1.4	380	3.0	85.1	3.1	0.4
Double Lolly, Swizzels Matlow* — 1 Lolly/10g	41	0.3	409	0.0	93.2	3.4	0.0
Drops, Lemon & Orange, M&S* — 1 Pack/42g	97	0.0	230	0.0	61.0	0.0	0.0
Drumstick, Matlow's* — 1 Pack/40g	164	2.2	409	0.4	88.3	5.5	0.0
Edinburgh Rock, Gardiners of Scotland* — 1 Piece/2g	8	0.0	380	0.1	94.4	0.3	0.8
Fizzy Mix, Tesco* — ½ Bag/50g	166	0.0	332	5.2	75.2	0.0	0.0
Flipsters, Starburst* — 1 Pack/37g	145	0.0	392	0.0	98.1	0.0	0.0
Flumps, Bassett's* — 1 Serving/5g	16	0.0	325	4.0	77.0	0.0	0.0
Flumps, Fluffy Mallow Twists, Fat Free, Bassett's* — 1 Twist/13g	30	0.0	230	4.1	77.1	0.0	0.0
Foamy Mushrooms, Chewy, Asda* — 1 Sweet/3g	9	0.0	347	4.2	82.0	0.2	0.0
Fruit, Mentos* — 1 Sweet/3g	10	0.0	333	0.0	100.0	0.0	0.0
Fruit Gums & Jellies — 1 Tube/33g	107	0.0	324	6.5	79.5	0.0	0.0
Fruities, Lemon & Lime, Weight Watchers* — 1 Sweet/2g	3	0.0	134	0.0	54.0	0.0	33.0
Fruity Babies, Bassett's* — 1 Sweet/3g	10	0.0	310	4.6	72.7	0.2	0.0
Fruity Chews, Starburst* — 1 Sweet/8g	34	0.6	404	0.0	83.4	7.4	0.0
Fruity Flutterbies, Chewits* — 1 Serving/100g	316	0.2	316	3.8	73.9	0.2	0.0
Fruity Frogs, Rowntree's* — 1 Serving/40g	128	0.1	321	4.7	74.5	0.2	0.0
Fruity Mallows, Fizzy, Asda* — 1 Pack/400g	1252	0.0	313	4.3	74.0	0.0	0.0
Gobstoppers, Everlasting, Wonka* — 9 Pieces/15g	60	0.0	400	0.0	93.3	0.0	0.0
Gummy Bears — 10 Bears/22g	85	0.0	386	0.0	98.9	0.0	98.9
Gummy Mix, Tesco* — 1 Pack/100g	327	0.1	327	5.9	75.7	0.1	0.0
Gummy Worms — 10 Worms/74g	286	0.0	386	0.0	98.9	0.0	98.9
Jellies, Very Berry, Rowntrees* — 1 Sweet/4g	12	0.0	326	5.0	74.8	0.2	0.1
Jelly Babies, Morrisons* — 1 Serving/227g	781	0.0	344	5.3	80.7	0.0	0.0
Jelly Beans, Tesco* — ¼ Bag/63g	243	0.2	385	0.1	94.5	0.3	0.3
Jelly Squirms, Sour, The Natural Confectionery Co.* — 1 Sweet/6g	20	0.0	325	2.8	78.2	0.1	0.0
Kisses, Almond, Chocolate Coated, Hershey* — 9 Kisses/40g	200	13.0	500	10.0	55.0	32.5	2.5
Kisses, Hershey* — 1 Sweet/5g	28	1.6	561	7.0	59.0	32.0	0.0
Lances, Fizzy, Strawberry, Somerfield* — 1 Sweet/4g	13	0.1	362	2.8	79.8	2.7	1.5
Lances, Strawberry & Cream Flavour, Tesco* — 1 Bag/75g	276	0.9	368	3.2	86.1	1.2	2.1
Lances, Strawberry Flavour, Fizzy, Tesco* — ½ Pack/50g	177	1.3	354	2.8	79.8	2.6	1.8
Lemon Mint Flavour, Herb Drops, Sugar Free, Ricola* — 1 Sweet/3g	7	0.0	235	0.0	96.0	0.0	0.0

SWEETS

INFO/WEIGHT	Measure			Nutrition Values per 100g / 100ml				
		KCAL	FAT	KCAL	PROT	CARB	FAT	FIBRE
Liquorice Torpedoes, Sweets For Life*	1 Serving/100g	368	0.3	368	4.1	87.1	0.3	1.4
Lovehearts, Giant, Swizzels*	1 Pack/42g	165	0.0	393	0.0	100.0	0.0	0.0
Lovehearts, Swizzels*	1oz/28g	100	0.0	359	0.7	88.2	0.0	0.0
Maoam Sour, Haribo*	1 Pack/22g	85	1.4	386	1.2	80.0	6.5	0.1
Maynards Sours, Bassett's*	1 Pack/52g	169	0.0	325	6.1	75.0	0.0	0.0
Midget Gems, Maynards*	1 Sweet/1g	3	0.0	340	8.7	76.2	0.0	0.0
Midget Gems, Value, Tesco*	1 Serving/40g	130	0.1	324	4.5	76.1	0.2	0.0
Milk Chocolate Eclairs, Sainsbury's*	1 Sweet/8g	33	1.1	442	2.1	75.7	14.5	0.5
Milk Chocolate Eclairs, Value, Tesco*	1 Bag/200g	918	32.6	459	2.6	75.2	16.3	1.0
Milk Duds, Hershey*	13 Pieces/33g	170	6.0	510	3.0	84.0	18.0	0.0
Mini Marti, Mushrooms, Asda*	1 Sweet/3g	10	0.0	340	3.8	81.1	0.1	0.0
Original, Chocolate Soft Caramel, Speciality, Werther's*	1 Piece/6g	30	1.5	480	5.1	61.5	23.5	1.0
Parma Violets, Swizzlers*	1 Tube/10g	41	0.0	406	0.9	99.1	0.0	0.0
Percy Pig & Pals, Soft, M&S*	1 Sweet/8g	30	0.0	344	5.8	80.0	0.1	0.0
Pic 'n' Mix, Woolworths*	1 Serving/180g	750	6.0	417	0.0	96.7	3.3	0.0
Randoms, Rowntree's*	1 Pack/50g	164	0.2	328	4.9	75.7	0.3	0.6
Rhubarb & Custard, Sainsbury's*	1 Sweet/8g	28	0.0	351	0.1	87.7	0.0	0.0
Rhubarb & Custards, Tesco*	1 Sweet/9g	36	0.0	396	0.3	97.6	0.5	0.1
Rotella, Haribo*	1 Sweet/13g	43	0.0	343	1.5	84.0	0.2	0.0
Salzige Heringe, Katjes*	1 Serving/50g	172	0.0	345	5.8	80.0	0.1	0.0
Scary Mix, Tesco*	1 Bag/100g	327	0.5	327	9.5	71.1	0.5	0.3
Scary Sours, Rowntree's*	1 Serving/100g	321	0.0	321	3.5	74.7	0.0	0.0
Sherbert Dib Dab with Strawberry Lolly, Barratt*	1 Pack/23g	90	0.0	385	0.1	95.6	0.1	0.0
Sherbert Lemons, M&S*	1 Serving/20g	76	0.0	380	0.0	93.9	0.0	0.0
Sherbert Lemons, Weight Watchers*	1 Box/35g	84	0.2	239	0.0	94.7	0.5	0.0
Sherbet Lemons, Bassett's*	1 Sweet/7g	25	0.0	375	0.0	93.9	0.0	0.0
Shrimps & Bananas, Sainsbury's*	½ Pack/50g	188	0.0	376	2.5	91.3	0.1	0.5
Snakes, Bassett's*	1 Sweet/9g	30	0.0	320	3.5	76.8	0.1	0.0
Soft Fruits, Trebor*	1 Roll/45g	165	0.0	367	0.0	90.9	0.0	0.0
Sour Apple Sticks, Fizzy Wizzy, Woolworths*	1 Sweet/5g	18	0.1	358	2.8	79.8	2.7	0.0
Sour Squirms, Bassett's*	1 Serving/7g	21	0.0	325	3.1	78.1	0.0	0.0
Strawberry & Cream, Sugar Free, Sula*	1 Sweet/3g	9	0.2	267	0.2	90.5	5.4	0.0
Sugar Free, Sula*	1 Sweet/3g	7	0.0	231	0.0	96.1	0.0	0.0
Sweetshop Favourites, Bassett's*	1 Sweet/5g	17	0.0	340	0.0	84.3	0.0	0.0
Tic Tac, Cool Cherry, Ferrero*	1 Pack/18g	69	0.1	382	0.2	92.2	0.7	0.0
Toffees, Value, Tesco*	3 Toffees/23g	101	3.3	450	2.1	77.3	14.8	0.3
Toffo*	1 Tube/43g	194	9.5	451	2.2	69.8	22.0	0.0
Tootsie Roll, Small Midgees, Tootsie*	1 Sweet/7g	23	0.5	350	2.5	70.0	7.5	0.0
Tooty Frooties, Rowntree's*	1 Bag/28g	111	1.0	397	0.1	91.5	3.5	0.0
Wiggly Worms, Sainsbury's*	1 Serving/10g	32	0.0	317	5.6	72.7	0.4	0.2
Wine Gummies, Matlow, Swizzels*	1 Pack/16g	52	0.0	324	0.0	58.7	0.0	0.0
Yo Yo's, All Flavours, 100% Fruit, We Are Bear*	1 Roll/10g	28	0.0	275	1.9	63.4	0.2	12.0
Yo Yo's, Strawberry 100% Fruit, We Are Bear*	1 Roll/10g	28	0.0	275	1.9	63.4	0.2	12.0

SWORDFISH

INFO/WEIGHT	Measure							
Grilled, Average	1oz/28g	39	1.5	139	22.9	0.0	5.2	0.0
Raw, Average	1oz/28g	42	2.0	149	21.1	0.0	7.2	0.0

SYRUP

INFO/WEIGHT	Measure							
Balsamic, Merchant Gourmet*	1 Tsp/5g	12	0.0	232	0.4	60.0	0.1	0.0
Caramel, for Coffee, Lyle's*	2 Tsp/10ml	33	0.0	329	0.0	83.0	0.0	0.0
Cinnamon, Monin*	1 Serving/30ml	100	0.0	333	0.0	80.0	0.0	0.0
Corn, Dark, Average	1 Tbsp/20g	56	0.0	282	0.0	76.6	0.0	0.0
Gingerbread, Monin*	1 Serving/30ml	90	0.0	300	0.0	76.7	0.0	0.0
Golden, Average	1 Tbsp/20g	61	0.0	304	0.4	78.2	0.0	0.0

	Measure INFO/WEIGHT	per Measure		Nutrition Values per 100g / 100ml				
		KCAL	FAT	KCAL	PROT	CARB	FAT	FIBRE
SYRUP								
Hazelnut, Monin*	1 Serving/30ml	90	0.0	300	0.0	73.3	0.0	0.0
Maple, Average	**1 Tbsp/20g**	**52**	**0.0**	**262**	**0.0**	**67.2**	**0.2**	**0.0**
Maple, Flavour, Artificial, Sugar Free, Cary's*	1 Serving/60ml	30	0.0	50	0.0	20.0	0.0	0.5
Peppermint, Monin*	1 Serving/30ml	96	0.0	320	0.0	80.0	0.0	0.0
Rice Malt, Organic, Clearspring*	2 Tbsp/42g	133	0.2	316	1.5	76.8	0.4	0.0
Strawberry, Aardbeien Siroop, Plein Sud, Lidl*	1 Serving/20ml	56	0.0	280	0.0	71.0	0.0	0.0
Sugar	1 Tbsp/20g	64	0.0	319	0.0	83.9	0.0	0.0
Vanilla, Monin*	1 Shot/35ml	119	0.0	340	0.0	84.4	0.0	0.0

	Measure INFO/WEIGHT	per Measure KCAL	FAT	Nutrition Values per 100g / 100ml KCAL	PROT	CARB	FAT	FIBRE
TABOO*								
Average, Taboo*	1 Pub Shot/35ml	80	0.0	230	0.0	33.0	0.0	0.0
TABOULEH								
Average	*1oz/28g*	*33*	*1.3*	*119*	*2.6*	*17.2*	*4.6*	*0.0*
TACO SHELLS								
Corn, Crunchy, Old El Paso*	1 Taco/10g	51	2.6	506	7.0	61.0	26.0	0.0
Old El Paso*	1 Taco/12g	57	2.7	478	7.4	60.8	22.8	0.0
Taco, Crunchy, Taco Bell *	1 Serving/78g	133	7.8	170	8.0	13.0	10.0	1.0
Traditional, Discovery*	1 Taco/11g	55	3.2	489	5.7	53.4	28.1	6.0
TAGLIATELLE								
Basil, M&S*	1 Serving/100g	365	2.8	365	15.1	69.0	2.8	4.0
Chicken & Mushroom, Three, Fuller Longer, M&S*	1 Pack/372g	465	13.0	125	10.0	12.4	3.5	1.4
Dry, Average	*1 Serving/100g*	*356*	*1.8*	*356*	*12.6*	*72.4*	*1.8*	*1.0*
Egg, Dry, Average	*1 Serving/75g*	*272*	*2.5*	*362*	*14.2*	*68.8*	*3.3*	*2.3*
Egg, Fresh, Dry, Average	*1 Serving/125g*	*345*	*3.5*	*276*	*10.6*	*53.0*	*2.8*	*2.1*
Fresh, Dry, Average	*1 Serving/75g*	*211*	*2.0*	*281*	*11.4*	*53.3*	*2.6*	*2.6*
Garlic & Herb, Fresh, Tesco*	1 Serving/125g	361	4.6	289	12.0	51.8	3.7	1.5
Ham & Mushroom, Asda*	1 Pack/340g	469	12.9	138	6.0	20.0	3.8	0.2
Ham & Mushroom, BGTY, Sainsbury's*	1 Pack/400g	368	4.8	92	4.2	15.5	1.2	1.1
Ham & Mushroom, LC, Tesco*	1 Pack/400g	400	8.8	100	6.0	13.8	2.2	1.8
Ham & Mushroom, Roasted, Finest, Tesco*	1 Pack/450g	562	23.8	125	7.3	12.0	5.3	2.4
Multigrain, BGTY, Uncooked, Sainsbury's*	1 Serving/190g	294	4.8	155	7.0	26.0	2.5	3.0
Mushroom & Bacon, BGTY, Sainsbury's*	1 Pack/400g	368	9.6	92	4.0	13.5	2.4	1.0
Mushroom & Bacon, Sainsbury's*	1 Pack/450g	585	23.4	130	7.1	13.8	5.2	0.5
Nests, Dry Weight, Napolina*	1oz/28g	93	0.4	332	11.5	68.0	1.5	3.7
Tricolore, Dry, Waitrose*	½ Pack/125g	351	3.6	281	12.0	51.6	2.9	1.6
Verdi, Fresh, Average	*1 Serving/125g*	*171*	*1.8*	*137*	*5.5*	*25.5*	*1.5*	*1.8*
TAHINI PASTE								
Average	*1 Tsp/6g*	*36*	*3.5*	*607*	*18.5*	*0.9*	*58.9*	*8.0*
TAMARIND								
Pulp	*1oz/28g*	*76*	*0.1*	*273*	*3.2*	*64.5*	*0.3*	*0.0*
Whole, Raw, Weighed with Pod, Average	*1oz/28g*	*67*	*0.2*	*239*	*2.8*	*62.5*	*0.6*	*5.1*
TANGERINES								
Fresh, Raw	*1oz/28g*	*10*	*0.0*	*35*	*0.9*	*8.0*	*0.1*	*1.3*
Fresh, Raw, Weighed with Peel, Average	*1 Med/70g*	*18*	*0.1*	*25*	*0.7*	*5.8*	*0.1*	*0.9*
TANGO*								
Cherry, Britvic*	1 Bottle/500ml	55	0.0	11	0.0	2.4	0.0	0.0
Orange, Britvic*	1 Can/330ml	63	0.0	19	0.1	4.4	0.0	0.0
TAPIOCA								
Creamed, Ambrosia*	½ Can/213g	159	3.4	75	2.6	12.6	1.6	0.2
Raw	*1oz/28g*	*101*	*0.0*	*359*	*0.4*	*95.0*	*0.1*	*0.4*
TARAMASALATA								
Average	1 Tbsp/30g	143	14.4	478	4.2	7.9	47.9	1.1
BGTY, Sainsbury's*	1oz/28g	71	5.7	253	4.3	13.5	20.2	0.7
Salmon, Smoked, Tesco*	1 Serving/95g	474	48.2	499	3.0	7.7	50.7	0.3
TARRAGON								
Dried, Ground	*1 Tsp/2g*	*5*	*0.1*	*295*	*22.8*	*42.8*	*7.2*	*0.0*
Fresh, Average	*1 Tbsp/4g*	*2*	*0.0*	*49*	*3.4*	*6.3*	*1.1*	*0.0*
TART								
Apple & Calvados, Normandy, Finest, Tesco*	1/6 Tart/100g	256	7.6	256	3.2	41.4	7.6	1.9
Apple & Cream, Fresh, Asda*	½ Tart/50g	134	8.0	267	3.4	33.0	16.0	0.8
Apple & Custard, Asda*	1 Tart/84g	227	11.0	270	3.1	35.0	13.1	0.1
Apricot Lattice, Sainsbury's*	1 Slice/125g	321	14.2	257	3.4	35.3	11.4	2.6
Asparagus, Filo, Tartlette, M&S*	1 Serving/15g	45	3.1	300	4.4	25.2	20.4	2.1

T

TART

INFO/WEIGHT	Measure	per Measure		Nutrition Values per 100g / 100ml				
		KCAL	FAT	KCAL	PROT	CARB	FAT	FIBRE
Bakewell, Average	1 Tart/50g	228	14.8	456	6.3	43.5	29.7	1.9
Bakewell, Cherry, Morrisons*	1 Tart/46g	198	9.8	430	4.6	54.9	21.4	1.3
Bakewell, Free From, Tesco*	1 Tart/50g	170	4.6	340	1.6	63.0	9.2	4.8
Bakewell, Large, Tesco*	1 Serving/57g	247	11.2	433	4.3	59.5	19.7	1.7
Bakewell, Lemon, Average	1 Tart/46g	206	9.7	447	3.7	60.9	21.1	0.9
Bakewell, Lyons*	1/6 Tart/52g	205	8.9	397	3.8	56.7	17.2	0.9
Bakewell, Toffee, Morrisons*	1 Tart/47g	201	7.4	422	3.0	67.2	15.5	0.9
Bakewell, Weight Watchers*	1 Tart/43g	156	5.0	363	3.6	65.2	11.7	3.2
Blackcurrant Sundae, Asda*	1 Tart/55g	227	10.4	413	3.5	57.0	19.0	2.3
Cherry Tomato & Mascarpone, Asda*	1 Tart/160g	290	18.0	181	4.4	15.6	11.2	1.1
Cherry Tomato & Mascarpone, Extra Special, Asda*	1 Tart/153g	290	18.3	190	4.6	16.0	12.0	1.1
Chocolate, Co-Op*	1 Tart/22g	102	6.8	465	4.0	42.0	31.0	0.7
Coconut, M&S*	1 Tart/53g	220	9.6	415	5.8	57.8	18.1	3.6
Coconut & Raspberry, Waitrose*	1 Tart/48g	204	11.5	426	5.0	45.0	24.0	3.9
Custard, Individual, Average	1 Tart/94g	260	13.6	277	6.3	32.4	14.5	1.2
Date Pecan & Almond, Sticky, Sainsbury's*	1/8 Tart/75g	298	10.3	397	5.0	63.5	13.7	1.7
Egg Custard, Asda*	1 Tart/80g	215	10.4	269	9.0	29.0	13.0	1.2
Egg Custard, Twin Pack, Tesco*	1 Tart/90g	240	11.4	270	5.6	31.6	12.8	0.9
Feta, Spinach & Red Pepper, Olive Infused, CBY, Asda*	1 Tart/145g	263	12.0	182	6.4	19.0	8.3	2.7
Feta Cheese & Spinach, Puff Pastry, Tesco*	1 Tart/108g	306	19.2	283	7.1	23.5	17.8	0.9
Frangipane, Chocolate & William Pear, Waitrose*	1/6 Pack/80g	219	12.4	274	3.5	29.9	15.5	2.5
Frangipane, Lutowska Cherry Amaretto, Sainsbury's*	1 Serving/66g	264	12.9	400	6.0	50.0	19.5	1.3
Frangipane, Spiced Winter Fruit, Rustic Bake, Waitrose*	1 Slice/87g	315	13.6	363	7.2	48.3	15.7	2.1
Jam, Assorted, Tesco*	1 Tart/35g	123	5.0	351	3.4	51.9	14.4	1.2
Jam, Assorted, VLH Kitchens	1 Serving/34g	44.2	42.4	130	3.4	56.0	14.4	1.3
Jam, Average	1 Slice/90g	342	13.4	380	3.3	62.0	14.9	1.6
Jam, Real Fruit, Mr Kipling*	1 Tart/35g	136	5.2	388	3.8	67.9	14.9	1.7
Leek & Stilton, Morrisons*	1 Serving/125g	392	26.9	314	6.9	23.1	21.5	0.3
Lemon, M&S*	1/6 Tart/50g	208	14.6	415	5.0	32.7	29.3	0.9
Lemon, Sainsbury's*	1/8 Tart/56g	258	15.8	459	4.4	47.0	28.1	0.6
Lemon, Zesty, Tesco*	1/6 Tart/64g	260	15.5	405	5.3	41.0	24.2	0.7
Lemon & Almond, Italian, Sainsbury's*	1 Slice/49g	182	11.6	371	7.4	31.9	23.7	4.1
Lemon & Raspberry, Finest, Tesco*	1 Tart/120g	360	16.8	300	5.2	38.4	14.0	2.9
Lemon Curd, Asda*	1 Tart/30g	121	4.5	402	2.8	64.0	15.0	2.2
Lemon Curd, Lyons*	1 Tart/30g	122	5.1	406	3.7	59.3	17.0	0.0
Mixed Fruit, Waitrose*	1 Tart/146g	318	16.4	218	2.3	27.3	11.2	1.0
Raspberry & Blueberry, Tesco*	1 Serving/85g	168	7.5	198	2.7	27.0	8.8	2.8
Red Pepper, Serrano Ham & Goats Cheese, Waitrose*	1 Serving/100g	293	19.2	293	8.7	21.3	19.2	3.2
Spinach & Ricotta, Individual, TTD, Sainsbury's*	1 Quiche/170g	466	33.7	274	7.5	16.5	19.8	1.4
Strawberry, & Cream, Finest, Tesco*	1/6 Tart/74g	210	13.0	280	3.4	27.2	17.3	1.5
Strawberry, & Fresh Cream, Finest, Tesco*	1 Tart/129g	350	19.1	271	3.3	31.1	14.8	1.2
Strawberry, Custard, Asda*	1 Tart/100g	335	15.0	335	3.1	47.0	15.0	0.0
Strawberry, Fresh, M&S*	1 Tart/120g	305	18.4	255	3.1	26.4	15.4	2.4
Strawberry, Sainsbury's*	1 Serving/206g	521	26.2	253	2.6	32.0	12.7	0.7
Strawberry, Waitrose*	1 Serving/101g	241	12.0	239	3.8	29.2	11.9	1.2
Summer Fruit Crumble, Morrisons*	1 Tart/128g	379	15.1	296	3.6	43.8	11.8	1.3
Toffee Apple, Co-Op*	1 Tart/20g	69	3.2	345	3.0	47.0	16.0	0.7
Toffee Pecan, M&S*	1 Tart/91g	414	24.1	455	6.0	48.5	26.5	2.0
Toffee Pecan, Waitrose*	¼ Tart/133g	564	19.1	423	4.3	69.3	14.3	1.6
Tomato, Mozzarella & Basil Puff, Sainsbury's*	1/3 Tart/120g	318	25.0	265	9.2	10.2	20.8	0.9
Treacle, Average	1 Serving/125g	460	17.6	368	3.7	60.4	14.1	1.1
Treacle, with Custard	1 Serving/251g	586	23.5	233	3.1	36.1	9.4	0.8
Treacle Lattice, Mr Kipling*	1/6 Tart/70g	256	8.5	365	4.4	59.8	12.1	1.1

	Measure INFO/WEIGHT	per Measure KCAL	FAT	Nutrition Values per 100g / 100ml KCAL	PROT	CARB	FAT	FIBRE
TART								
Vegetable, & Feta, Deli, M&S*	½ Tart/115g	315	18.4	274	5.0	20.0	16.0	6.0
Vegetable, Roasted, Finest, Tesco*	¼ Tart/113g	226	13.2	200	3.1	20.6	11.7	2.3
TARTAR								
Cream of, Leavening Agent	**1 Tsp/3g**	**8**	**0.0**	**258**	**0.0**	**61.5**	**0.0**	**0.0**
TARTE								
Au Citron, Frozen, Tesco*	1/6 Tarte/81g	255	11.8	315	5.4	39.4	14.6	0.7
Au Citron, Frozen, TTD, Sainsbury's*	1/6 Tart/80g	232	13.4	290	4.7	40.7	16.8	7.7
Au Citron, Seriously Lemony, Large, Waitrose*	1 Tarte/470g	1589	81.8	338	4.6	40.8	17.4	0.5
Au Citron, Waitrose*	1 Tarte/100g	325	18.1	325	4.9	35.7	18.1	1.0
Bacon, Leek & Roquefort, Bistro, Waitrose*	¼ Tarte/100g	277	18.2	277	8.4	19.8	18.2	0.6
Normande, French Style, M&S*	1/6 Tarte/85g	245	16.1	290	3.3	26.8	19.0	0.7
Spinach & Goats Cheese, Flamme, TTD, Sainsbury's*	1/3 Quiche/77g	227	16.7	296	6.9	18.1	21.8	5.0
Tatin, Sainsbury's*	1 Serving/120g	244	8.0	203	2.9	32.8	6.7	1.9
TARTLETS								
Asparagus & Leek, Linda McCartney*	1 Tartlet/150g	375	21.8	250	8.4	19.8	14.5	3.4
Butternut Squash & Goats Cheese, Linda McCartney*	1 Tartlet/150g	405	25.0	270	6.3	24.2	16.7	1.2
Cheddar, Vintage, Potato & Leek, Waitrose*	1 Tartlet/130g	391	25.0	301	7.7	23.3	19.2	2.2
Cheese & Roast Onion, Asda*	1 Tartlet/50g	135	7.5	270	6.0	28.0	15.0	1.9
Raspberry, Mini, M&S*	1 Tartlet/27g	90	5.4	330	4.3	34.4	19.6	0.5
Red Onion & Goats Cheese, Sainsbury's*	1 Tartlet/113g	335	21.8	297	7.0	23.7	19.3	1.5
Salmon & Watercress, Hot Smoked, Waitrose*	1 Serving/130g	315	19.9	242	8.1	18.0	15.3	3.0
Spinach Ricotta & Sundried Tomato, Filo, Tesco*	1 Tartlet/135g	358	23.1	265	5.2	22.4	17.1	1.9
Tomato & Goats Cheese, Waitrose*	1 Tartlet/130g	295	19.0	227	6.6	17.4	14.6	2.0
TAYBERRY								
Average	1 Serving/100g	25	0.0	25	1.2	12.0	0.0	7.0
TEA								
Assam, Blended, TTD, Sainsbury's*	1 Serving/2g	0	0.0	0	0.0	0.0	0.0	0.0
Blackberry & Nettle, Twinings*	1 Cup/250ml	5	0.0	2	0.0	0.3	0.0	0.0
Camomile, Pure, Classic Herbal, Twinings*	1 Serving/200ml	4	0.0	2	0.0	0.3	0.0	0.0
Camomile, Smile, Tetley*	1oz/28g	1	0.0	2	0.0	0.5	0.0	0.0
Chai, Twinings*	1 Cup/200ml	2	0.0	1	0.1	0.0	0.0	0.0
Damask, Rose, Chinese, Choi Time*	1 Mug/500ml	0	0.3	0	0.0	0.0	0.1	0.0
Decaf, Tetley*	1 Cup/100ml	1	0.0	1	0.0	0.3	0.0	0.0
Earl Grey, Green, Twinings*	1 Cup/200ml	2	0.0	1	0.0	0.2	0.0	0.0
Earl Grey, Infusion with Water, Average	1 Mug/250ml	2	0.0	1	0.0	0.2	0.0	0.0
Fennel, Sweet, Made Up, Twinings*	1 fl oz/30ml	1	0.0	2	0.0	0.3	0.0	0.0
Fennel Seeds & Peppermint, Twinings*	1 Cup/200ml	4	0.0	2	0.0	0.3	0.0	0.0
Fruit, Twinings*	1 Mug/227ml	4	0.0	2	0.0	0.4	0.0	0.0
Fruit Or Herbal, Made with Water, Twinings*	1 Mug/200ml	8	0.0	4	0.0	1.0	0.0	0.0
Green, Pure, Twinings*	1 Serving/100g	1	0.0	1	0.0	0.2	0.0	0.0
Green, with Citrus, Twinings*	1 Serving/200ml	2	0.0	1	1.0	0.2	0.0	0.0
Green, with Jasmine, Twinings*	1 Serving/100ml	1	0.0	1	0.0	0.2	0.0	0.0
Green, with Jasmine, Wellbeing Selection, Flavia*	1 Cup/200ml	0	0.0	0	0.0	0.0	0.0	0.0
Green, with Lemon, Jackson's*	1 Serving/200ml	2	0.0	1	0.0	0.2	0.0	0.0
Green, with Lemon, Light & Delicate, Twinings*	1 Cup/100ml	1	0.1	1	0.1	0.2	0.1	0.1
Green, with Mango, Brewed with Water, Twinings*	1 Cup/200ml	2	0.0	1	0.0	0.2	0.0	0.0
Green, with Mint, Whittards of Chelsea*	1 Cup/100ml	1	0.0	1	0.2	0.1	0.0	0.0
Herbal, Wellbeing Blends, Infusions, Twinings*	1 Serving/200ml	4	0.0	2	0.0	0.3	0.0	0.0
Ice with Lemon, Lipton*	1 Bottle/325ml	91	0.0	28	0.0	6.9	0.0	0.0
Ice with Peach, Lipton*	1 Bottle/500ml	140	0.0	28	0.0	6.8	0.0	0.0
Iced, Pickwick*	1 Serving/250ml	32	0.0	13	0.0	3.3	0.0	0.0
Jasmine, Made Up, Twinings*	1 fl oz/30ml	0	0.0	1	0.0	0.2	0.0	0.0
Lemon, & Ginger, Made Up, Lipton*	1 Cup/200ml	8	0.0	4	0.5	0.5	0.0	0.0

T

INFO/WEIGHT	Measure	per Measure KCAL	per Measure FAT	Nutrition Values per 100g / 100ml KCAL	PROT	CARB	FAT	FIBRE
TEA								
Lemon, Instant, Original, Lift*	1 Serving/15g	53	0.0	352	0.0	87.0	0.0	0.0
Lemon, Instant, Tesco*	1 Serving/7g	23	0.0	326	1.0	80.5	0.0	0.0
Made with Water	1 Mug/227ml	0	0.0	0	0.1	0.0	0.0	0.0
Made with Water with Semi-Skimmed Milk, Average	1 Cup/200ml	14	0.4	7	0.5	0.7	0.2	0.0
Made with Water with Skimmed Milk, Average	1 Mug/270ml	16	0.5	6	0.5	0.7	0.2	0.0
Made with Water with Whole Milk, Average	1 Cup/200ml	16	0.8	8	0.4	0.5	0.4	0.0
Morning Detox, Twinings*	1 Serving/200ml	5	0.0	2	0.0	0.3	0.0	0.0
Nettle & Peppermint, Twinings*	1 Cup/200ml	2	0.0	1	0.0	0.2	0.0	0.0
Nettle & Sweet Fennel, Twinings*	1 Cup/200ml	4	0.0	2	0.0	0.3	0.0	0.0
Peppermint, Made with Water, Average	1 Serving/200ml	3	0.0	2	0.0	0.2	0.0	0.0
Peppermint, Spearmint & Fieldmint, Pukka*	1 Serving/200ml	8	0.0	4	0.0	0.0	0.0	0.0
Red Bush, Made with Water, Tetley*	1 Mug/250ml	2	0.0	1	0.0	0.1	0.0	0.0
TEACAKES								
Average	1 Teacake/60g	178	4.5	296	8.0	52.5	7.5	0.0
Burton's*	1 Teacake/13g	57	2.4	455	3.8	66.9	19.3	1.1
Caramel, Highlights, Mallows, Cadbury*	1 Teacake/15g	61	1.9	408	6.2	69.1	12.4	3.6
Currant, Sainsbury's*	1 Teacake/72g	204	2.9	284	8.2	53.7	4.0	2.5
Fruit, Lidl*	1 Teacake/62g	166	2.7	267	10.6	46.3	4.4	2.2
Fruited, Co-Op*	1 Teacake/62g	160	2.0	258	9.7	46.8	3.2	3.2
Fruited, M&S*	1 Teacake/60g	156	0.6	260	8.9	53.4	1.0	2.0
Fruity, Warburton's*	1 Teacake/63g	160	2.2	256	8.7	48.0	3.5	2.7
G H Sheldon*	1 Teacake/95g	274	2.6	288	8.5	57.4	2.7	0.0
Hovis*	1 Teacake/60g	155	1.5	258	9.0	49.9	2.5	3.0
Jam, Castello*	1 Teacake/13g	60	2.4	470	5.3	70.1	18.4	1.3
Large, Sainsbury's*	1 Teacake/100g	291	6.8	291	8.3	49.1	6.8	3.4
Large, TTD, Sainsbury's*	1 Teacake/90g	264	3.5	293	7.5	57.0	3.9	2.6
Lees*	1 Teacake/19g	81	2.9	426	4.2	67.7	15.4	0.0
Mallow, Tesco*	1 Teacake/14g	63	2.7	450	4.1	65.4	19.1	1.0
Mallow, Value, Tesco*	1 Teacake/14g	60	2.3	425	3.6	65.8	16.2	1.4
Marshmallow, Milk Chocolate, Tunnock's*	1 Teacake/24g	106	4.6	440	4.9	61.9	19.2	2.4
Mini Bites, M&S*	1 Bite/6g	29	1.2	484	3.2	72.6	20.3	2.1
Morrisons*	1 Teacake/64g	172	1.9	268	9.9	50.7	2.9	2.8
Richly Fruited, Waitrose*	1 Teacake/72g	205	2.7	285	7.8	55.0	3.7	2.2
Sainsbury's*	1 Teacake/70g	171	2.5	244	8.0	45.0	3.6	2.6
Tesco*	1 Teacake/61g	163	2.1	267	7.8	51.1	3.5	2.4
Toasted, Average	1 Teacake/60g	197	5.0	329	8.9	58.3	8.3	0.0
Value, Tesco*	1 Teacake/68g	180	2.4	265	9.6	47.8	3.6	4.9
with Fruit, Morning Fresh, Aldi*	1 Teacake/65g	155	2.2	239	7.4	44.6	3.4	2.3
TEMPEH								
Average	*1oz/28g*	*46*	*1.8*	*166*	*20.7*	*6.4*	*6.4*	*4.3*
TEQUILA								
Average	*1 Pub Shot/35ml*	*78*	*0.0*	*224*	*0.0*	*0.0*	*0.0*	*0.0*
THYME								
Dried, Ground, Average	*1 Tsp/1g*	*3*	*0.1*	*276*	*9.1*	*45.3*	*7.4*	*0.0*
Fresh, Average	*1 Tsp/1g*	*1*	*0.0*	*95*	*3.0*	*15.1*	*2.5*	*0.0*
TIA MARIA								
Original	*1 Pub Shot/35ml*	*105*	*0.0*	*300*	*0.0*	*0.0*	*0.0*	*0.0*
TIC TAC								
Extra Strong Mint, Ferrero*	2 Sweets/1g	4	0.0	381	0.0	95.2	0.0	0.0
Fresh Mint, Ferrero*	2 Sweets/1g	4	0.0	390	0.0	97.5	0.0	0.0
Lime & Orange, Ferrero*	2 Sweets/1g	4	0.0	386	0.0	95.5	0.0	0.0
Orange, Ferrero*	2 Sweets/1g	4	0.0	385	0.0	95.5	0.0	0.0
Spearmint, Ferrero*	1 Box/16g	62	0.0	390	0.0	97.5	0.0	0.0

	Measure INFO/WEIGHT	per Measure		Nutrition Values per 100g / 100ml				
		KCAL	FAT	KCAL	PROT	CARB	FAT	FIBRE
TIKKA MASALA								
Chicken, & Pilau Rice, BGTY, Sainsbury's*	1 Pack/400g	380	4.8	95	8.1	13.0	1.2	1.1
Chicken, & Pilau Rice, Takeaway, Asda*	1 Pack/561g	852	27.5	152	7.0	20.0	4.9	1.5
Chicken, & Pilau Rice, Waitrose*	1 Pack/500g	797	34.5	159	8.2	16.1	6.9	0.8
Chicken, & Rice, LC, Tesco*	1 Pack/450g	472	7.2	105	7.9	14.6	1.6	1.3
Chicken, & Rice, M&S*	1 Pack/400g	700	35.2	175	7.4	17.0	8.8	1.0
Chicken, Asda*	1 Pack/340g	388	20.4	114	9.0	6.0	6.0	1.5
Chicken, Breast, GFY, Asda*	1 Pack/380g	486	14.4	128	19.0	4.5	3.8	0.2
Chicken, COU, M&S*	1 Pack/400g	400	6.8	100	7.6	14.1	1.7	1.3
Chicken, Hot, Sainsbury's*	1 Pack/400g	604	37.2	151	13.2	3.6	9.3	1.5
Chicken, Hot, Tesco*	1 Pack/400g	588	34.4	147	8.7	8.6	8.6	1.0
Chicken, Indian, Medium, Sainsbury's*	1 Pack/400g	848	61.2	212	13.2	5.3	15.3	0.1
Chicken, Indian, Tesco*	1 Pack/350g	560	32.6	160	11.6	7.2	9.3	0.6
Chicken, Indian Meal for One, BGTY, Sainsbury's*	1 Serving/241g	200	1.9	83	13.9	5.1	0.8	1.0
Chicken, Indian Takeaway, Tesco*	1 Serving/125g	100	3.2	80	9.4	4.9	2.6	2.1
Chicken, Large, Sainsbury's*	1 Pack/650g	1105	68.9	170	11.7	7.0	10.6	0.3
Chicken, Low Fat, Iceland*	1 Pack/400g	360	4.0	90	7.8	12.5	1.0	0.5
Chicken, Morrisons*	1 Pack/340g	561	34.7	165	12.4	5.9	10.2	1.7
Chicken, The Authentic Food Company*	1 Serving/375g	510	31.5	136	10.6	5.5	8.4	0.9
Chicken, Waitrose*	½ Pack/200g	298	19.4	149	12.8	2.6	9.7	1.6
Chicken, Weight Watchers*	1 Pack/331g	344	4.6	104	7.0	15.8	1.4	0.2
Chicken, with Pilau Rice, Love Life, Waitrose*	1 Pack/400g	445	5.2	111	7.8	15.9	1.3	2.4
Chicken, with Rice, Sainsbury's*	1 Pack/500g	960	41.0	192	8.3	21.2	8.2	0.1
Prawn, COU, M&S*	1 Pack/400g	400	6.4	100	6.9	14.7	1.6	1.9
Prawn, King, & Rice, Finest, Tesco*	1 Pack/475g	618	30.4	130	6.0	16.6	6.4	1.2
Spicy, with Long Grain Rice, Rice Time, Uncle Ben's*	1 Tub/300g	399	11.7	133	2.3	21.7	3.9	0.9
Vegetable, Indian, Tesco*	1 Pack/225g	234	13.5	104	2.4	10.4	6.0	2.4
TILAPIA								
Raw, Average	*100g*	*95*	*1.0*	*95*	*20.0*	*0.0*	*1.0*	*0.0*
TIME OUT								
Break Pack, Cadbury*	1 Serving/20g	108	6.3	530	6.2	58.3	30.7	0.0
Chocolate Fingers, Cadbury*	2 Fingers/35g	186	10.6	530	7.1	57.3	30.3	1.1
Orange, Snack Size, Cadbury*	1 Finger/11g	61	3.6	555	5.0	59.4	32.9	0.0
TIRAMISU								
Asda*	1 Pot/100g	252	11.0	252	4.3	34.0	11.0	0.5
BGTY, Sainsbury's*	1 Pot/90g	140	2.4	156	4.5	28.3	2.7	0.3
Choc & Mascarpone, Tiramigu, Gu*	1 Pud/90g	316	23.3	351	3.3	26.1	25.9	1.0
Dine in Dessert, M&S*	½ Dessert/145g	515	36.7	355	2.6	28.8	25.3	0.7
Family Size, Tesco*	1 Serving/125g	356	18.1	285	4.3	34.5	14.5	0.4
Italian, Co-Op*	1 Pack/90g	230	9.0	255	5.0	37.0	10.0	0.4
Light Choices, Tesco*	1 Pot/90g	162	3.5	180	7.7	27.6	3.9	2.4
Morrisons*	1 Pot/90g	248	9.9	276	4.0	38.0	11.0	0.0
Raspberry, M&S*	1 Serving/84g	197	12.1	235	3.8	22.9	14.4	0.2
Sainsbury's*	1 Serving/100g	263	10.0	263	4.4	40.2	10.0	0.1
Single Size, Tesco*	1 Pot/100g	290	12.9	290	3.8	35.1	12.9	4.5
Trifle, Sainsbury's*	1 Serving/100g	243	15.7	243	2.3	23.2	15.7	0.6
Waitrose*	1 Pot/90g	221	11.2	246	6.4	27.2	12.4	0.0
TOAD IN THE HOLE								
Average	1 Serving/231g	640	40.2	277	11.9	19.5	17.4	1.1
Frozen, Cooked, CBY, Asda*	1 Slice/72g	168	7.5	232	9.2	24.2	10.4	2.6
Vegetarian, Aunt Bessie's*	1 Pack/190g	502	19.4	264	15.6	27.5	10.2	2.7
Vegetarian, Linda McCartney*	1 Pack/190g	359	16.7	189	13.6	13.9	8.8	1.1
TOASTIE								
All Day Breakfast, M&S*	1 Serving/174g	375	13.8	215	11.2	25.0	7.9	1.7

T

INFO/WEIGHT	Measure	per Measure		Nutrition Values per 100g / 100ml				
		KCAL	FAT	KCAL	PROT	CARB	FAT	FIBRE
TOASTIE								
Cheese & Ham, Tayto*	1 Serving/50g	260	14.8	519	6.8	58.0	29.7	0.0
Cheese & Onion, Ginsters*	1 Toastie/122g	330	12.3	269	10.9	33.1	10.0	1.5
Cheese & Pickle, M&S*	1 Toastie/136g	320	9.1	235	10.4	33.5	6.7	2.6
Ham & Cheddar, British, M&S*	1 Pack/128g	269	8.6	210	15.5	22.3	6.7	1.3
Ham & Cheese, Tesco*	1 Serving/138g	388	18.2	281	11.5	29.1	13.2	1.0
Ham & Cheese, White Bread	1 Toastie/150g	409	14.9	273	14.5	31.3	9.9	0.9
TOFFEE APPLE								
Average	1 Apple/141g	188	3.0	133	1.2	29.2	2.1	2.3
TOFFEE CRISP								
Nestle*	1 Original/44g	228	12.1	519	3.7	62.8	27.6	1.4
TOFFEES								
Assorted, Bassett's*	1 Toffee/8g	35	1.1	434	3.8	73.1	14.0	0.0
Assorted, Sainsbury's*	1 Sweet/8g	37	1.3	457	2.2	76.5	15.8	0.2
Brazil Nut, Diabetic, Thorntons*	1 Serving/20g	93	7.0	467	3.2	49.0	35.1	0.5
Butter, Smart Price, Asda*	1 Toffee/8g	37	1.3	440	1.3	75.0	15.0	0.0
Chewy, Werther's*	1 Toffee/5g	22	0.8	436	3.5	71.3	15.2	0.1
Dairy, Smart Price, Asda*	1 Sweet/9g	37	1.3	407	1.3	68.4	14.2	0.0
Dairy, Waitrose*	1 Toffee/8g	37	1.1	458	2.0	80.2	14.3	0.5
Devon Butter, Thorntons*	1 Sweet/9g	40	1.5	444	1.7	72.2	16.7	0.0
English Butter, Co-Op*	1 Toffee/8g	38	1.6	470	2.0	71.0	20.0	0.0
Liquorice, Thorntons*	1 Bag/100g	506	29.4	506	1.9	58.8	29.4	0.0
Milk Chocolate Covered, Thorntons*	1 Bag/215g	1120	66.0	521	4.1	57.2	30.7	0.9
Milk Chocolate Smothered, Thorntons*	1 Pack/125g	655	38.5	524	4.3	57.5	30.8	1.1
Mixed, Average	1oz/28g	119	5.2	426	2.2	66.7	18.6	0.0
Original, Hard Butter Candies, Sugar Free, Werther's*	1 Pack/80g	231	7.0	289	0.2	86.8	8.8	0.1
Original, Thorntons*	1 Bag/100g	514	30.1	514	1.8	59.3	30.1	0.0
TOFU								
Average	**1 Pack/250g**	**297**	**16.5**	**119**	**13.4**	**1.4**	**6.6**	**0.1**
Beech Smoked, Organic, Cauldron Foods*	½ Pack/110g	124	7.8	113	10.9	1.0	7.1	0.5
Firm Silken Style, Blue Dragon*	1 Pack/216g	134	5.8	62	6.9	2.4	2.7	0.0
Fresh, Drained, Kong Nam*	1 Tub/575g	397	21.3	69	7.7	1.3	3.7	0.5
Fried, Average	**1oz/28g**	**75**	**4.0**	**268**	**28.6**	**9.3**	**14.1**	**0.0**
Original, Organic, Cauldron Foods*	¼ Pack/99g	84	4.2	85	10.0	1.9	4.2	0.9
Pieces, Marinated, Organic, Cauldron Foods*	1 Pack/160g	363	27.2	227	17.5	1.0	17.0	2.7
Smoked, Organic, Evernat*	1oz/28g	36	1.8	127	16.3	0.8	6.6	0.0
TOMATILLOS								
Raw	**1 Med/34g**	**11**	**0.3**	**32**	**1.0**	**5.8**	**1.0**	**1.9**
TOMATO PASTE								
Average	**1 Tbsp/20g**	**19**	**0.0**	**96**	**5.0**	**19.2**	**0.2**	**1.5**
Sun Dried, Average	**2 Tsp/10g**	**38**	**3.5**	**385**	**3.2**	**13.8**	**35.2**	**0.0**
TOMATO PUREE								
Average	**1 Tsp/5g**	**4**	**0.0**	**76**	**4.5**	**14.1**	**0.2**	**2.3**
Double Concentrate, Average	**1 Tbsp/15g**	**13**	**0.0**	**85**	**4.9**	**14.9**	**0.2**	**3.6**
Sun Dried, & Olive Oil & Herbs, GIA*	1 Serving/20g	41	4.3	204	2.6	0.5	21.6	0.0
TOMATOES								
Cherry, Average	**1 Tomato/15g**	**3**	**0.0**	**18**	**0.7**	**3.0**	**0.3**	**0.5**
Cherry, on the Vine, Average	**1 Serving/80g**	**15**	**0.3**	**18**	**0.7**	**3.1**	**0.3**	**1.2**
Cherry, Tinned, Napolina*	1 Can/400g	92	2.4	23	1.2	3.3	0.6	0.0
Chopped, Canned, Average	1 Serving/100g	19	0.2	19	1.1	3.3	0.2	0.9
Chopped, Canned, Branded Average	**1 Serving/130g**	**27**	**0.2**	**21**	**1.1**	**3.8**	**0.1**	**0.8**
Chopped, Italian, Average	**½ Can/200g**	**47**	**0.2**	**23**	**1.3**	**4.4**	**0.1**	**0.9**
Chopped, Italian, with Olive Oil & Garlic, Waitrose*	1 Serving/100g	33	1.6	33	1.1	3.6	1.6	0.0
Chopped, with Chilli, Sainsbury's*	½ Can/200g	44	1.0	22	1.0	3.5	0.5	0.9

TOMATOES

	Measure INFO/WEIGHT	per Measure KCAL	FAT	Nutrition Values per 100g / 100ml KCAL	PROT	CARB	FAT	FIBRE
Chopped, with Garlic, Average	*½ Can/200g*	*43*	*0.3*	*21*	*1.2*	*3.8*	*0.1*	*0.8*
Chopped, with Green & Black Olives, Sainsbury's*	1 Pack/390g	183	8.2	47	1.3	5.6	2.1	0.7
Chopped, with Herbs, Average	*½ Can/200g*	*42*	*0.3*	*21*	*1.1*	*3.8*	*0.1*	*0.8*
Fresh, Raw, Average	*1 Med/123g*	*22*	*0.2*	*18*	*0.9*	*3.9*	*0.2*	*1.2*
Fried in Blended Oil	1 Med/85g	77	6.5	91	0.7	5.0	7.7	1.3
Green Tiger, Raw, M&S*	1 Serving/80g	16	0.2	20	0.7	3.1	0.3	1.0
Grilled, Average	1oz/28g	6	0.1	20	0.8	3.5	0.3	1.5
Plum, Baby, Average	*1 Serving/50g*	*9*	*0.2*	*18*	*1.5*	*2.3*	*0.3*	*1.0*
Plum, in Tomato Juice, Average	*1 Can/400g*	*71*	*0.4*	*18*	*1.0*	*3.3*	*0.1*	*0.7*
Plum, in Tomato Juice, Premium, Average	*1 Can/400g*	*93*	*1.2*	*23*	*1.3*	*3.8*	*0.3*	*0.7*
Plum, Pomodori d'Oro, TTD, Sainsbury's*	½ Can/200g	42	0.0	21	1.1	4.1	0.0	0.5
Pomodorino, TTD, Sainsbury's*	1 Tomato/78g	13	0.3	17	0.7	3.1	0.4	1.3
Puglian, Sun Drenched, Waitrose*	½ Pack/100g	190	16.2	190	2.2	8.8	16.2	3.8
Ripened on the Vine, Average	*1 Med/123g*	*22*	*0.4*	*18*	*0.7*	*3.0*	*0.3*	*0.7*
Santini, M&S*	1 Serving/80g	16	0.2	20	0.7	3.1	0.3	1.0
Stuffed with Rice Based Filling, Average	1oz/28g	59	3.8	212	2.1	22.2	13.4	1.1
Sun Dried, Average	*3 Pieces/20g*	*43*	*3.2*	*214*	*4.7*	*13.0*	*15.9*	*3.3*
Sun Dried in Oil	100g	301	24.8	301	5.8	13.5	24.8	7.0
Sunblush, TTD, Sainsbury's*	¼ Pack/30g	42	3.2	140	2.4	8.8	10.6	5.8
Sweet, Aromatico, Extra Special, Extra Special, Asda*	1 Serving/100g	21	0.5	21	0.7	3.1	0.5	1.3

TONGUE

	Measure INFO/WEIGHT	per Measure KCAL	FAT	per 100g KCAL	PROT	CARB	FAT	FIBRE
Lunch, Average	*1oz/28g*	*51*	*3.0*	*181*	*20.1*	*1.8*	*10.6*	*0.0*
Slices, Average	*1oz/28g*	*56*	*3.9*	*201*	*18.7*	*0.0*	*14.0*	*0.0*

TONIC WATER

	Measure INFO/WEIGHT	per Measure KCAL	FAT	per 100ml KCAL	PROT	CARB	FAT	FIBRE
Average	1 Glass/250ml	82	0.0	33	0.0	8.8	0.0	0.0
Diet, Asda*	1 Glass/200ml	2	0.0	1	0.0	0.0	0.0	0.0
Indian, Britvic*	1 Can/150ml	39	0.2	26	0.1	6.2	0.1	0.1
Indian, Diet, Schweppes*	1 Glass/100ml	1	0.0	1	0.0	0.0	0.0	0.0
Indian, Fever Tree*	1 Bottle/200ml	76	0.0	38	0.0	9.0	0.0	0.0
Indian, Sainsbury's*	1 Can/150ml	46	0.0	31	0.0	7.4	0.0	0.0
Indian, Schweppes*	1 Serving/500ml	110	0.0	22	0.0	5.1	0.0	0.0
Indian, Slimline, Schweppes*	1 Serving/188ml	3	0.0	2	0.4	0.0	0.0	0.0
Indian, Sugar Free, Essential, Waitrose*	1 Serving/50ml	1	0.0	2	0.0	0.0	0.0	0.0
Indian, with a Hint of Lemon, Low Calorie, Asda*	1 Serving/300ml	3	0.3	1	0.0	0.0	0.1	0.0
Indian with Lime, Low Calorie, Tesco*	1 Glass/250ml	5	0.0	2	0.0	0.0	0.0	0.0
Low Calorie, Tesco*	1 Serving/200ml	4	0.0	2	0.0	0.5	0.0	0.0
Quinine, Schweppes*	1 Glass/125ml	46	0.0	37	0.0	9.0	0.0	0.0
Soda Stream*	1 Glass/100ml	15	0.0	15	0.0	3.2	0.0	0.0

TOPIC

	Measure INFO/WEIGHT	per Measure KCAL	FAT	per 100g KCAL	PROT	CARB	FAT	FIBRE
Mars*	1 Bar/47g	234	12.3	498	6.2	59.6	26.2	1.7

TORTE

	Measure INFO/WEIGHT	per Measure KCAL	FAT	per 100g KCAL	PROT	CARB	FAT	FIBRE
Chocolate, Cheeky Little, Gu*	1 Pud/50g	211	14.6	422	5.7	31.6	29.1	1.8
Chocolate, Fondant, Gu*	1/8 Tarte/63g	264	18.9	423	5.7	32.0	30.2	1.8
Chocolate, Half Fat, Waitrose*	1/6 Torte/70g	135	4.1	193	5.4	29.7	5.8	2.2
Chocolate, Orange & Almond, Gu*	1 Serving/65g	273	19.8	420	5.0	28.2	30.5	2.7
Chocolate, Tesco*	1 Serving/50g	126	6.0	251	3.6	32.3	11.9	1.0
Chocolate, Truffle, Waitrose*	1 Serving/116g	359	20.1	309	4.6	30.1	17.3	1.4
Chocolate & Pecan Brownie, Gu*	1 1/6 Torte/67g	292	17.7	436	5.3	45.1	26.4	3.1
Fruit Mix, Apricot, Graze*	1 Pack/45g	151	3.6	335	3.3	63.0	8.0	4.0
Lemon, Tesco*	1 Serving/62g	142	6.1	230	2.3	32.9	9.9	0.5

TORTELLINI

	Measure INFO/WEIGHT	per Measure KCAL	FAT	per 100g KCAL	PROT	CARB	FAT	FIBRE
Beef Bolognese, Rich, Italian, Giovanni Rana*	½ Pack/125g	222	9.0	178	7.6	20.6	7.2	4.1
Cheese, Four, Italian, Asda*	1 Serving/150g	296	7.5	197	8.0	30.0	5.0	3.4

INFO/WEIGHT	Measure	per Measure		Nutrition Values per 100g / 100ml				
		KCAL	FAT	KCAL	PROT	CARB	FAT	FIBRE
TORTELLINI								
Cheese, Four, with Tomato & Basil Sauce, Tesco*	1 Pack/400g	500	14.8	125	6.1	16.9	3.7	0.6
Cheese, Fresh, Sainsbury's*	½ Pack/180g	329	9.0	183	7.6	26.8	5.0	1.7
Cheese, Three, Sainsbury's*	1 Serving/50g	196	4.4	391	14.4	63.8	8.7	3.0
Cheese, Tomato & Basil, Tesco*	1 Serving/150g	387	8.1	258	13.0	39.5	5.4	3.3
Cheese & Ham, Italiano, Tesco*	½ Pack/150g	396	12.3	264	12.8	34.8	8.2	3.0
Garlic & Herb, Fresh, Sainsbury's*	½ Pack/150g	364	11.7	243	11.1	32.2	7.8	1.8
Ham & Cheese, Fresh, Asda*	½ Pack/150g	255	9.0	170	6.0	23.0	6.0	1.7
Meat, Italian, Tesco*	1 Serving/125g	332	9.5	266	10.6	38.9	7.6	2.3
Mushroom, Asda*	1 Serving/125g	218	5.2	174	6.0	28.0	4.2	2.3
Pesto & Goats Cheese, Fresh, Sainsbury's*	½ Pack/150g	310	12.2	207	8.9	24.6	8.1	2.6
Ricotta & Spinach, Giovanni Rana*	½ Pack/125g	340	13.6	272	10.1	34.6	10.9	10.0
Sausage & Ham, Italiano, Tesco*	1 Pack/300g	816	27.9	272	13.1	34.0	9.3	3.7
Spinach & Ricotta, Italian, Asda*	½ Pack/150g	189	3.6	126	5.0	21.0	2.4	0.6
Spinach & Ricotta, Verdi, Asda*	1 Serving/125g	186	5.6	149	6.0	21.0	4.5	2.4
Tomato & Mozzarella, Fresh, Asda*	½ Pack/150g	236	4.2	157	8.0	25.0	2.8	0.0
Tomato & Mozzarella, Fresh, Sainsbury's*	½ Pack/150g	291	12.0	194	7.5	23.0	8.0	3.4
TORTELLONI								
Arrabbiata, Sainsbury's*	½ Pack/210g	407	11.8	194	7.1	28.8	5.6	2.6
Beef & Chianti, TTD, Sainsbury's*	½ Pack/125g	300	8.0	240	11.3	34.3	6.4	1.9
Cheese & Smoked Ham, Tesco*	½ Pack/150g	315	10.6	210	8.9	26.5	7.1	1.7
Cheese & Smoked Ham, Waitrose*	1 Serving/250g	625	17.0	250	11.5	35.8	6.8	1.8
Chicken & Bacon, Italiano, Tesco*	1 Pack/300g	660	21.9	220	7.8	29.8	7.3	2.1
Five Cheese, Sainsbury's*	1 Serving/125g	285	11.6	228	10.8	25.2	9.3	2.9
Four Cheese, Asda*	½ Pack/150g	312	13.0	208	7.6	24.9	8.7	1.6
Four Cheese, Tesco*	1 Serving/200g	390	13.4	195	8.0	25.5	6.7	1.8
Fresh, Ham & Cheese, Asda*	½ Pack/150g	315	11.4	210	8.8	26.7	7.6	1.4
Ham & Cheese, M Kitchen, Morrisons*	½ Pack/150g	279	7.0	186	9.6	25.5	4.7	1.4
Mushroom, Basics, Sainsbury's*	¼ Pack/125g	196	6.2	157	6.1	21.8	5.0	3.0
Mushroom, Wild, Italian, Sainsbury's*	½ Pack/150g	309	12.3	206	7.7	25.4	8.2	2.3
Mushroom, Wild, Italian, Tesco*	1 Pack/300g	645	24.0	215	6.5	28.5	8.0	2.5
Pasta, Fresh, Cream Cheese, Garlic & Herb, Morrisons*	1 Serving/150g	400	9.0	267	10.3	46.1	6.0	3.2
Pesto, Italian, Tesco*	1 Pack/300g	885	33.9	295	10.7	36.7	11.3	3.0
Ricotta & Tender Spinach, Cooked, Giovanni Rana*	½ Pack/190g	376	12.3	198	7.8	27.0	6.5	3.1
Sausage & Ham, Italiano, Tesco*	1 Serving/150g	285	10.5	190	8.5	22.5	7.0	1.8
Spinach & Ricotta, Chilled, Italiano, Tesco*	½ Pack/150g	412	12.8	275	10.4	38.1	8.5	3.3
Spinach & Ricotta, Fresh, Waitrose*	½ Pack/150g	239	5.3	159	6.3	24.4	3.5	2.5
Spinach & Ricotta, Sainsbury's*	½ Pack/150g	326	10.8	217	7.8	30.2	7.2	2.4
Spinach & Ricotta Cheese, Co-Op*	½ Pack/126g	315	6.3	250	10.0	41.0	5.0	4.0
Tomato & Mozzarella, Sainsbury's*	1 Serving/175g	340	14.0	194	7.5	23.0	8.0	3.4
TORTIGLIONI								
Dry, Average	**1 Serving/75g**	**266**	**1.4**	**355**	**12.5**	**72.2**	**1.9**	**2.1**
TORTILLA CHIPS								
Blazing BBQ, Sainsbury's*	1 Serving/50g	237	11.8	474	6.8	58.9	23.5	4.6
Blue, Organic, Sainsbury's*	1 Serving/50g	252	11.7	504	7.7	65.8	23.4	5.6
Chilli Flavour, Somerfield*	1 Serving/50g	242	12.0	484	6.8	60.1	24.1	5.3
Classic Mexican, Phileas Fogg*	1 Serving/35g	162	6.7	464	5.9	67.2	19.1	3.8
Cool, BGTY, Sainsbury's*	1 Pack/22g	94	2.7	425	7.1	71.4	12.3	4.5
Cool, Salted, Sainsbury's*	1 Serving/50g	253	13.6	506	6.5	58.6	27.3	4.3
Cool, Tesco*	1 Serving/40g	190	9.9	474	6.3	56.7	24.7	7.8
Cool Flavour, Sainsbury's*	1 Serving/50g	232	9.4	463	5.7	68.1	18.7	3.7
Cool Sour Cream, Love Life, Waitrose*	1 Bag/22g	95	2.7	434	7.1	7.1	12.3	4.5
Honey BBQ, Love Life, Waitrose*	1 Bag/22g	94	2.2	425	6.6	76.0	9.8	3.3
Hot Chilli Flavour, Weight Watchers*	1 Bag/18g	83	3.3	461	4.6	67.7	18.2	4.2

TORTILLA CHIPS

INFO/WEIGHT	Measure KCAL	FAT	KCAL	PROT	CARB	FAT	FIBRE
TORTILLA CHIPS							
Lightly Salted, M&S*	1 Serving/20g	98	4.8	490	7.2	61.5	24.1	4.5
Lightly Salted, Smart Price, Asda*	¼ Bag/50g	251	13.0	502	7.0	60.0	26.0	5.0
Lightly Salted, Tesco*	1 Serving/50g	248	13.8	495	4.8	56.8	27.6	7.5
Lightly Salted, Waitrose*	1 Serving/40g	187	8.6	468	7.1	61.2	21.6	6.5
Lighty Salted, Basics, Sainsbury's*	½ Pack/50g	242	11.9	483	6.5	60.7	23.8	5.3
Mexicana Cheddar, Kettle Chips*	1 Serving/50g	249	13.3	498	7.9	56.7	26.6	5.1
Nacho Cheese Flavour, M&S*	1 Serving/30g	144	6.7	480	7.5	62.0	22.4	4.2
Nacho Cheese Flavour, Morrisons*	1 Serving/25g	126	6.6	504	7.2	59.4	26.4	3.6
Nacho Cheese Flavour, Weight Watchers*	1 Pack/18g	83	3.3	459	5.2	66.6	18.2	4.1
Pita, Multigrain, Stacy's*	9 Chips/28g	140	5.0	500	10.7	67.9	17.9	0.0
Plain	1 Serving/100g	486	21.1	486	6.8	62.0	21.1	4.2
Salsa, M&S*	½ Bag/75g	364	18.8	485	5.7	59.1	25.1	6.1
Taco, Tesco*	1 Serving/50g	248	12.7	495	7.4	59.3	25.4	4.4
with Guacamole	1 Serving/100g	515	30.8	515	6.0	53.0	30.8	6.3
TORTILLAS							
Corn, GF, Discovery*	1 Tortilla/22g	53	0.5	243	5.4	53.8	2.3	3.8
Corn, Soft, Old El Paso*	1 Tortilla/38g	129	2.6	343	10.0	60.0	7.0	0.0
Flour, 10 Pack, Asda*	1 Tortilla/30g	94	2.1	315	9.0	54.0	7.0	0.0
Flour, American Style, Sainsbury's*	1 Tortilla/35g	108	2.4	313	8.6	53.9	7.0	2.5
Flour, Bakery, Asda*	1 Tortilla/43g	129	3.0	303	9.1	50.9	7.1	2.6
Flour, From Dinner Kit, Old El Paso*	1 Tortilla/42g	144	4.9	344	8.7	51.1	11.7	0.0
Flour, Mexican Style, Morrisons*	1 Tortilla/33g	103	2.3	313	8.6	53.9	7.0	2.5
Flour, Salsa, Old El Paso*	1 Tortilla/41g	132	3.7	323	9.0	52.0	9.0	0.0
Flour, Soft, Chilli & Jalapeno, Discovery*	1 Tortilla/40g	131	5.2	328	7.8	44.8	13.1	2.2
Flour, Soft, Discovery*	1 Tortilla/40g	119	2.8	298	8.0	49.6	7.1	2.4
Flour, Soft, Garlic & Coriander, Discovery*	1 Tortilla/40g	116	2.4	289	8.1	50.6	6.0	1.7
Flour, Wheat, Waitrose*	1 Tortilla/62g	203	6.1	327	8.5	51.5	9.8	0.0
Made with Wheat Flour	1oz/28g	73	0.3	262	7.2	59.7	1.0	2.4
Mexican Cheese, Phileas Fogg*	1 Pack/278g	1404	72.3	505	6.5	61.4	26.0	3.0
Plain, Morrisons*	1 Serving/35g	92	0.9	263	8.5	51.2	2.7	2.5
Plain, Wheat, Waitrose*	1 Tortilla/43g	134	3.5	311	8.1	51.5	8.1	3.0
Plain, Wraps, Tesco*	1 Tortilla/64g	192	3.8	300	8.4	52.2	5.9	2.7
White, Wraps, M&S*	1 Tortilla/64g	170	2.4	265	7.9	49.0	3.8	1.6
Wholemeal, Discovery*	1 Wrap/40g	109	3.3	273	9.2	40.4	8.3	6.4
Wholewheat, Asda*	1 Tortilla/35g	88	2.7	252	9.8	35.7	7.8	7.1
Wraps, 8 Pack, Asda*	1 Tortilla/50g	143	3.0	286	8.0	50.0	6.0	1.9
Wraps, 8 Pack, LC, Tesco*	1 Tortilla/50g	135	1.0	270	7.1	53.2	2.1	3.5
Wraps, Deli, Multigrain, Mission Deli*	1 Tortilla/61g	202	6.1	330	7.9	50.5	10.0	3.0
Wraps, Flour, Soft, Old El Paso*	1 Tortilla/58g	200	7.2	343	9.3	48.6	12.4	1.7
Wraps, Garlic & Parsley, Sainsbury's*	1 Tortilla/60g	166	3.7	277	7.2	48.0	6.2	1.8
Wraps, Healthy 'n' White, Wrap 'n' Roll, Discovery*	1 Tortilla/40g	161	3.5	288	8.0	49.7	6.3	2.6
Wraps, Less Than 3% Fat, BGTY, Sainsbury's*	1 Tortilla/51g	128	1.1	250	7.8	50.1	2.2	2.9
Wraps, Low Fat, M&S*	1 Serving/180g	225	4.0	125	6.3	20.6	2.2	1.9
Wraps, Mexican, Asda*	1 Tortilla/34g	100	2.8	295	7.9	47.2	8.3	3.9
Wraps, Morrisons*	1 Serving/60g	132	2.1	220	6.2	42.0	3.5	1.7
Wraps, Multiseed, Discovery*	1 Tortilla/57g	160	2.8	280	8.7	50.1	5.0	3.6
Wraps, Organic, Sainsbury's*	1 Tortilla/56g	167	4.3	298	8.6	48.8	7.7	2.1
Wraps, Organic, Tesco*	1 Tortilla/57g	173	4.4	306	8.1	51.0	7.7	2.0
Wraps, Plain, Mini, Morrisons*	1 Tortilla/34g	91	1.4	267	8.1	48.9	4.0	2.8
Wraps, Plain, Nannak*	1 Wrap/80g	134	3.5	167	8.9	62.2	4.4	0.0
Wraps, Plain, Sainsbury's*	1 Tortilla/56g	167	4.4	299	8.1	49.2	7.8	3.6
Wraps, Spicy Tomato, Morrisons*	1 Tortilla/55g	158	3.1	288	8.6	50.5	5.7	0.7
Wraps, Spicy Tomato, Tesco*	1 Tortilla/63g	175	3.5	278	7.8	49.2	5.6	2.4

T

INFO/WEIGHT	Measure	per Measure KCAL	FAT	Nutrition Values per 100g / 100ml KCAL	PROT	CARB	FAT	FIBRE
TORTILLAS								
Wraps, Weight Watchers*	1 Wrap/42g	107	0.4	254	7.1	50.7	1.0	6.7
Wraps, Whole & White, Mini, Kids, Sainsbury's*	1 Tortilla/26g	67	1.4	258	9.2	42.9	5.5	6.2
TREACLE								
Black, Average	*1 Tbsp/20g*	*51*	*0.0*	*257*	*1.2*	*67.2*	*0.0*	*0.0*
TRIFLE								
Average	1 Portion/170g	272	10.7	160	3.6	22.3	6.3	0.5
Banana & Mandarin, Co-Op*	¼ Trifle/125g	238	13.8	190	2.0	21.0	11.0	0.1
Black Forest, Asda*	1 Serving/100g	237	9.0	237	3.1	36.0	9.0	0.0
Cherry, Finest, Tesco*	¼ Trifle/163g	340	19.3	209	2.6	22.9	11.9	0.3
Chocolate, Asda*	1 Serving/125g	272	16.3	217	4.1	21.0	13.0	0.5
Chocolate, Light, Cadbury*	1 Pot/90g	166	6.8	185	5.5	23.4	7.5	0.0
Chocolate, Tesco*	1 Serving/125g	312	19.0	250	4.3	24.0	15.2	0.7
Fruit, Sainsbury's*	1 Serving/125g	232	12.5	186	2.3	21.7	10.0	0.3
Fruit Cocktail, COU, M&S*	1 Trifle/140g	175	3.2	125	2.8	23.1	2.3	0.5
Fruit Cocktail, Individual, M&S*	1 Pot/135g	205	9.2	150	2.7	19.3	6.7	0.7
Fruit Cocktail, Individual, Tesco*	1 Pot/113g	175	8.8	155	1.7	19.6	7.8	0.6
Fruit Cocktail, M&S*	1 Serving/165g	272	13.7	165	2.4	19.6	8.3	0.9
Fruit Cocktail, Sainsbury's*	1 Trifle/150g	241	9.0	161	1.8	24.8	6.0	0.4
Raspberry, Asda*	1 Serving/100g	175	8.0	175	1.8	24.0	8.0	0.1
Raspberry, Co-Op*	1 Trifle/125g	206	10.0	165	2.0	22.0	8.0	0.3
Raspberry, Sainsbury's*	1 Pot/135g	286	17.7	212	3.2	19.9	13.1	0.7
Raspberry, Somerfield*	1 Trifle/125g	208	10.0	166	2.0	22.0	8.0	0.0
Raspberry, Tesco*	1 Pot/150g	210	9.8	140	1.7	18.5	6.5	1.0
Sainsbury's*	1 Serving/133g	215	10.0	162	2.4	20.1	7.5	0.3
Strawberry, Co-Op*	1 Serving/120g	175	9.1	146	1.7	16.7	7.6	1.4
Strawberry, COU, M&S*	1 Pot/138g	145	2.9	105	2.7	19.2	2.1	1.2
Strawberry, Individual, Somerfield*	1 Trifle/125g	186	8.2	149	1.8	20.5	6.6	0.6
Strawberry, Individual, Waitrose*	1 Pot/150g	206	8.6	137	1.8	19.7	5.7	1.0
Strawberry, Sainsbury's*	¼ Tub/150g	261	15.4	174	2.2	18.1	10.3	1.0
Strawberry, Tesco*	1 Trifle/605g	998	55.7	165	1.5	19.1	9.2	0.8
Strawberry, Value, Tesco*	1/3 Pack/141g	227	10.6	161	2.0	20.4	7.5	0.5
TRIFLE MIX								
Strawberry Flavour, Bird's*	1oz/28g	119	2.9	425	2.7	78.0	10.5	1.2
TRIFLE SPONGES								
Sainsbury's*	1 Sponge/24g	77	0.4	323	5.3	71.9	1.6	1.1
Somerfield*	1 Sponge/24g	81	0.5	339	5.0	76.0	2.0	0.0
Tesco*	1 Sponge/24g	75	0.6	311	5.3	66.6	2.6	1.1
TRIPE &								
Onions, Stewed	1oz/28g	26	0.8	93	8.3	9.5	2.7	0.7
TROUT								
Brown, Steamed, Average	*1 Serving/120g*	*162*	*5.4*	*135*	*23.5*	*0.0*	*4.5*	*0.0*
Fillets, Scottish, Hot Smoked, TTD, Sainsbury's*	½ Pack/63g	85	3.4	136	20.8	1.0	5.4	0.5
Fillets, Skinless, Chunky, TTD, Sainsbury's*	½ Pack/123g	227	13.0	185	22.4	0.1	10.6	0.6
Grilled, Weighed with Bones & Skin	1 Serving/100g	98	3.9	98	15.7	0.0	3.9	0.0
Rainbow, Fillets, with Thyme & Lemon Butter, Asda*	1 Serving/147g	210	10.3	143	20.0	0.9	7.0	0.5
Rainbow, Grilled, Average	*1 Serving/120g*	*162*	*6.5*	*135*	*21.5*	*0.0*	*5.4*	*0.0*
Rainbow, Raw, Average	*1oz/28g*	*36*	*1.4*	*127*	*20.5*	*0.0*	*5.1*	*0.0*
Rainbow, Smoked, Average	*1 Pack/135g*	*190*	*7.6*	*140*	*21.7*	*0.8*	*5.6*	*0.0*
Raw, Average	*1 Serving/120g*	*159*	*6.5*	*132*	*20.6*	*0.0*	*5.4*	*0.0*
Smoked, Average	*2 Fillets/135g*	*187*	*7.1*	*138*	*22.7*	*0.3*	*5.2*	*0.1*
TUMS								
Extra 750, Sugar Free, Tums*	2 Tablets/2g	5	0.0	250	0.0	50.0	0.0	0.0
Extra 750, Tums*	2 Tablets/2g	10	0.0	500	0.0	100.0	0.0	0.0

	Measure INFO/WEIGHT	per Measure KCAL	FAT	Nutrition Values per 100g / 100ml KCAL	PROT	CARB	FAT	FIBRE
TUMS								
Regular, Tums*	1 Tablet/2g	2	0.0	125	0.0	25.0	0.0	0.0
Smoothies, Extra Strength 750, Tums*	2 Tablets/2g	10	0.0	500	0.0	100.0	0.0	0.0
TUNA								
Albacore, in Olive Oil, TTD, Sainsbury's*	1 Serving/80g	162	8.7	203	26.1	0.0	10.9	0.0
Bluefin, Cooked, Dry Heat, Average	*1 Serving/100g*	*184*	*6.3*	*184*	*29.9*	*0.0*	*6.3*	*0.0*
Chunks, in Brine, Average, Drained	*1 Can/130g*	*141*	*0.7*	*108*	*25.9*	*0.0*	*0.5*	*0.0*
Chunks, in Brine, Canned, Drained, Princes*	1oz/28g	29	0.1	105	25.0	0.0	0.5	0.0
Chunks, in Brine, Drained, Average	1 Can/130g	141	0.7	108	25.9	0.0	0.5	0.0
Chunks, in Brine, Drained, Value, Morrisons*	1 Can/120g	122	0.6	102	23.1	1.0	0.5	0.0
Chunks, in Spring Water, Average, Drained	*1 Can/130g*	*140*	*0.8*	*108*	*25.4*	*0.0*	*0.6*	*0.1*
Chunks, in Sunflower Oil, Average, Drained	*1 Can/138g*	*260*	*12.6*	*188*	*26.5*	*0.0*	*9.2*	*0.0*
Chunks, Skipjack, in Brine, Average	*1 Can/138g*	*141*	*0.8*	*102*	*24.3*	*0.0*	*0.6*	*0.0*
Chunks, with a Little Brine, No Drain, 120g, John West*	1 Can/120g	130	1.1	108	25.0	0.0	0.9	0.0
Chunks, with a Little Brine, No Drain, 60g, John West*	1 Can/60g	55	0.5	91	21.0	0.0	0.8	0.0
Chunks, with a Little Sunflower Oil, No Drain, John West*	1 Can/120g	202	9.1	168	25.0	0.0	7.6	0.0
Coronation, BGTY, Sainsbury's*	1 Can/80g	90	2.1	112	16.5	5.7	2.6	1.0
Coronation Style, Canned, Average	1 Can/80g	122	7.6	152	10.2	6.5	9.5	0.6
Fillets, in Tomato Sauce, Princes*	1 Can/120g	131	3.0	109	19.0	2.5	2.5	0.0
Flakes, in Brine, Average	*1oz/28g*	*29*	*0.2*	*104*	*24.8*	*0.0*	*0.6*	*0.0*
in a Light Lemon Mayonnaise, Slimming World, Princes*	1 Can/80g	99	3.8	124	16.8	3.5	4.8	0.0
in a Light Mayonnaise, Slimming World, Princes*	1 Can/80g	96	3.3	120	17.3	3.6	4.1	0.0
in a Red Chilli & Lime Dressing, Princes*	1 Sachet/85g	102	2.8	120	21.5	1.0	3.3	0.0
in Thousand Island Dressing, John West*	1 Can/185g	287	13.0	155	18.0	5.1	7.0	0.2
In Thousand Island Dressing, Weight Watchers*	1 Can/79g	67	1.7	85	8.3	7.8	2.2	0.4
in Water, Average	*1 Serving/120g*	*126*	*1.0*	*105*	*24.0*	*0.1*	*0.8*	*0.0*
Lime & Black Pepper, John West*	1 Serving/85g	133	7.8	156	15.6	2.8	9.2	0.0
Nicoise Style, Light Lunch, John West*	1 Pack/250g	245	5.8	98	10.3	9.0	2.3	2.7
Steak, Yellowfin, Skinless & Boneless, Frozen, Aldi*	1oz/28g	32	0.3	113	25.8	0.0	1.1	0.0
Steaks, Chargrilled, Italian, Sainsbury's*	1 Serving/125g	199	8.0	159	25.1	0.2	6.4	0.5
Steaks, in Brine, Average	*1 Can/99g*	*106*	*0.5*	*107*	*25.6*	*0.0*	*0.6*	*0.0*
Steaks, in Olive Oil, Average	*1 Serving/111g*	*211*	*10.7*	*190*	*25.8*	*0.0*	*9.6*	*0.0*
Steaks, in Sunflower Oil, Average	*1 Can/150g*	*276*	*12.9*	*184*	*26.7*	*0.0*	*8.6*	*0.0*
Steaks, in Sunflower Oil, Canned, Drained, Nixe, Lidl*	1 Can/140g	252	11.2	180	27.0	0.0	8.0	0.0
Steaks, in Water, Average	*1 Serving/200g*	*215*	*0.8*	*107*	*25.6*	*0.0*	*0.4*	*0.0*
Steaks, John West*	1 Can/130g	140	0.4	108	26.2	0.0	0.3	0.0
Steaks, Lemon & Herb Marinade, Seared, Sainsbury's*	½ Pack/119g	191	8.8	161	23.4	0.1	7.4	0.0
Steaks, Marinated, Sainsbury's*	1 Serving/100g	153	5.3	153	25.1	1.3	5.3	0.5
Steaks, Raw, Average	*1 Serving/140g*	*185*	*2.8*	*132*	*28.5*	*0.1*	*2.0*	*0.2*
Steaks, Skipjack, in Brine, Average	*½ Can/75g*	*73*	*0.4*	*98*	*23.2*	*0.0*	*0.6*	*0.2*
Steaks, with a Little Brine, No Drain, John West*	1 Can/130g	140	0.4	108	26.2	0.0	0.3	0.0
Steaks, with a Little Olive Oil, No Drain, John West*	1 Can/130g	209	7.0	161	28.2	0.0	5.4	0.0
Steaks, with a Little Sunflower Oil, No Drain, John West*	1 Can/130g	209	7.0	161	28.2	0.0	5.4	0.0
with a Twist, French Dressing, John West*	1 Pack/85g	135	8.2	159	15.2	2.8	9.7	0.1
with a Twist, Oven Dried Tomato & Herb, John West*	1 Pack/85g	112	5.1	132	18.0	2.0	6.0	0.0
Yellowfin, Cooked, Dry Heat, Average	*1 Serving/100g*	*139*	*1.2*	*139*	*30.0*	*0.0*	*1.2*	*0.0*
TUNA IN								
a Sweet & Sour Sauce, Yellowfin, Asda*	1 Pouch/250g	235	5.8	94	11.6	6.7	2.3	1.4
a Tomato & Herb Dressing, Weight Watchers*	1 Can/80g	79	2.9	99	11.6	5.1	3.6	0.5
Coronation Style Dressing, Weight Watchers*	1 Tin/80g	75	2.0	94	9.3	8.7	2.5	0.4
TUNA MAYONNAISE								
& Sweetcorn, Canned, BGTY, Sainsbury's*	1 Can/80g	78	1.8	97	15.2	4.0	2.3	0.7
Garlic & Herb, John West*	½ Can/92g	243	20.4	264	12.0	4.0	22.2	0.2
Light, Slimming World*	1 Serving/80g	96	3.3	120	17.3	3.6	4.1	0.0

T

	Measure INFO/WEIGHT	per Measure KCAL	FAT	Nutrition Values per 100g / 100ml KCAL	PROT	CARB	FAT	FIBRE
TUNA MAYONNAISE								
with Sweetcorn, & Green Peppers, GFY, Asda*	1 Pack/100g	103	3.0	103	14.0	5.0	3.0	0.8
with Sweetcorn, From Heinz, Weight Watchers*	1 Can/80g	114	6.3	142	11.5	6.2	7.9	0.1
with Sweetcorn, John West*	½ Can/92g	231	19.0	251	12.0	4.5	20.6	0.2
TURBOT								
Grilled	*1oz/28g*	*34*	*1.0*	*122*	*22.7*	*0.0*	*3.5*	*0.0*
Raw	*1oz/28g*	*27*	*0.8*	*95*	*17.7*	*0.0*	*2.7*	*0.0*
TURKEY								
Breast, 3% Fat, Bernard Matthews*	1 Slice/20g	21	0.5	103	19.2	0.9	2.5	0.5
Breast, Butter Basted, Average	*1 Serving/75g*	*110*	*3.6*	*146*	*23.7*	*1.9*	*4.9*	*0.4*
Breast, Canned, Average	*1 Can/200g*	*194*	*4.7*	*97*	*18.3*	*0.7*	*2.4*	*0.0*
Breast, Chunks, Bernard Matthews*	1 Serving/55g	64	0.5	116	26.1	0.9	0.9	1.6
Breast, Diced, Healthy Range, Average	*1oz/28g*	*30*	*0.4*	*108*	*23.8*	*0.0*	*1.3*	*0.0*
Breast, Diced in a Hot & Spicy Marinade, Waitrose*	½ Pack/200g	286	7.0	143	24.1	3.5	3.5	0.5
Breast, Golden Norfolk, Bernard Matthews*	1 Slice/20g	22	0.2	109	23.8	0.9	1.1	0.8
Breast, Honey Roast, Sliced, Average	*1 Serving/50g*	*57*	*0.7*	*114*	*24.0*	*1.6*	*1.4*	*0.2*
Breast, Joint, Butter Basted, Cooked, Braemoor, Lidl*	1 Serving/130g	220	9.9	169	21.0	4.0	7.6	0.5
Breast, Joint, Raw, Average	*1 Serving/125g*	*134*	*2.6*	*108*	*21.3*	*0.7*	*2.1*	*0.6*
Breast, Joint, Ready to Roast, Ovenbaked, CBY, Asda*	1 Serving/150g	278	14.0	185	21.2	3.9	9.3	0.5
Breast, Joint, with Sage & Onion Stuffing, Waitrose*	1 Serving/325g	377	13.3	116	19.2	1.4	4.1	0.1
Breast, Pieces, Raw, Everyday, Value, Tesco*	1 Pack/525g	574	4.7	110	24.4	0.0	0.9	0.0
Breast, Raw, Average	*1oz/28g*	*33*	*0.6*	*117*	*24.1*	*0.5*	*2.0*	*0.1*
Breast, Roast, Wafer Thin, M&S*	½ Pack/50g	52	0.6	105	23.2	0.1	1.2	0.1
Breast, Roasted, Average	*1oz/28g*	*37*	*0.9*	*131*	*24.6*	*0.7*	*3.3*	*0.1*
Breast, Roll, Cooked, Average	*1 Slice/10g*	*9*	*0.1*	*92*	*17.6*	*3.5*	*0.8*	*0.0*
Breast, Slices, Bernard Matthews*	1 Slice/20g	21	0.5	103	19.2	0.9	2.5	0.5
Breast, Slices, Cooked, Average	*1 Slice/20g*	*23*	*0.3*	*114*	*24.0*	*1.2*	*1.4*	*0.3*
Breast, Smoked, Sliced, Average	*1 Slice/20g*	*23*	*0.4*	*113*	*23.4*	*0.7*	*2.0*	*0.0*
Breast, Steaks, in Crumbs, Average	1 Steak/76g	217	14.1	286	13.7	16.4	18.5	0.2
Breast, Steaks, Raw, Average	*1oz/28g*	*30*	*0.3*	*107*	*24.3*	*0.0*	*1.1*	*0.0*
Breast, Strips, for Stir Fry, Average	*1 Serving/175g*	*205*	*2.7*	*117*	*25.6*	*0.1*	*1.6*	*0.0*
Breast, Stuffed, Just Roast, Sainsbury's*	1 Serving/100g	155	6.6	155	21.1	2.9	6.6	0.6
Butter Roast, TTD, Sainsbury's*	1 Slice/28g	36	0.3	127	28.1	0.9	1.2	1.0
Butter Roasted, Carvery, Morrisons*	1 Slice/22g	25	0.3	113	24.0	1.2	1.3	0.0
Dark Meat, Raw, Average	*1oz/28g*	*29*	*0.7*	*104*	*20.4*	*0.0*	*2.5*	*0.0*
Drummers, Golden, Bernard Matthews*	1 Drummer/57g	147	10.3	258	13.1	11.0	18.0	1.1
Drummers, Golden, Grilled, Bernard Matthews*	1 Drummer/50g	147	10.6	294	15.6	10.0	21.2	1.0
Drumsticks, Tesco*	1 Serving/200g	272	12.6	136	19.9	0.0	6.3	0.0
Escalope, Average	*1 Escalope/138g*	*341*	*19.3*	*247*	*13.5*	*16.7*	*14.0*	*0.6*
Escalope, Lemon & Pepper, Average	1 Escalope/143g	371	22.6	260	12.6	16.7	15.8	0.4
Fillets, Tikka Marinated, 93% Fat Free, Bernard Matthews*	1 Pack/200g	310	10.4	155	21.8	5.2	5.2	1.5
Goujons, Cooked, Bernard Matthews*	4 Goujons/128g	355	23.3	277	11.8	16.6	18.2	1.1
Leg, Roast, Uncooked, Bernard Matthews*	1 Serving/283g	317	15.3	112	15.4	0.5	5.4	0.0
Light Meat, Raw, Average	*1oz/28g*	*29*	*0.2*	*105*	*24.4*	*0.0*	*0.8*	*0.0*
Light Meat, Roasted	*1 Cup/140g*	*220*	*4.5*	*157*	*29.9*	*0.0*	*3.2*	*0.0*
Mince, Average	*1oz/28g*	*45*	*2.0*	*161*	*23.9*	*0.0*	*7.2*	*0.0*
Mince, Free Range, TTD, Sainsbury's*	1 Serving/131g	184	5.7	141	25.4	0.0	4.4	0.0
Mince, Lean, Healthy Range, Average	*1oz/28g*	*33*	*1.1*	*118*	*20.3*	*0.0*	*4.1*	*0.0*
Mince, Thigh, Essential, Waitrose*	1 Serving/100g	118	3.5	118	20.9	0.5	3.5	0.5
Rashers, Average	*1 Rasher/26g*	*26*	*0.4*	*101*	*19.1*	*2.3*	*1.6*	*0.0*
Rashers, Smoked, Average	*1 Serving/75g*	*76*	*1.4*	*101*	*19.8*	*1.5*	*1.8*	*0.0*
Ready to Roast, with Stuffing & Bacon, M&S*	1/3 Pack/169g	245	10.5	145	20.2	2.1	6.2	1.1
Roast, Meat & Skin, Average	*1oz/28g*	*48*	*1.8*	*171*	*28.0*	*0.0*	*6.5*	*0.0*
Roast, Meat Only, Average	*1 Serving/100g*	*157*	*3.2*	*157*	*29.9*	*0.0*	*3.2*	*0.0*

	Measure INFO/WEIGHT	per Measure		Nutrition Values per 100g / 100ml				
		KCAL	FAT	KCAL	PROT	CARB	FAT	FIBRE
TURKEY								
Roast, Sugar Marinade, Slices, M&S*	½ Pack/120g	156	1.9	130	29.0	0.2	1.6	0.5
Roll, Dinosaur, Cooked, Bernard Matthews*	1 Slice/10g	17	1.0	170	13.6	6.0	10.2	1.1
Schnitzel, Lidl*	1 Schnitzel/115g	210	8.0	183	19.0	11.0	7.0	0.0
Steaks, Breaded, Bernard Matthews*	1 Steak/110g	319	20.0	290	11.0	20.5	18.2	1.5
Strips, Stir-Fried, Average	1oz/28g	46	1.3	164	31.0	0.0	4.5	0.0
Thigh, Diced, Average	*1oz/28g*	*33*	*1.2*	*117*	*19.6*	*0.0*	*4.3*	*0.0*
Wafer Thin, Cooked, Average	1 Slice/10g	12	0.4	122	19.0	3.2	3.7	0.0
Wafer Thin, Honey Roast, Average	1 Slice/10g	11	0.2	109	19.2	4.2	1.7	0.2
Wafer Thin, Roast, Tesco*	1 Slice/8g	8	0.2	105	20.0	1.5	2.0	0.0
Wafer Thin, Smoked, Average	1 Slice/10g	12	0.4	119	18.1	3.6	3.7	0.0
TURKEY DINNER								
Roast, 105, Oakhouse Foods Ltd*	1 Dinner/430g	624	16.3	145	7.0	9.4	3.8	1.4
Roast, Asda*	1 Pack/400g	344	6.4	86	7.0	11.0	1.6	2.0
Roast, Iceland*	1 Meal/400g	374	7.2	94	8.4	10.9	1.8	1.3
Roast, Meal for One, M&S*	1 Pack/370g	462	16.3	125	9.1	12.4	4.4	2.7
Traditional, Birds Eye*	1 Pack/340g	292	7.8	86	6.1	10.3	2.3	1.7
TURKEY HAM								
Average	*1 Serving/75g*	*81*	*2.9*	*108*	*15.6*	*2.8*	*3.9*	*0.0*
TURKEY IN								
BBQ Marinade, Steaks, Asda*	1 Serving/225g	356	5.2	158	30.0	4.4	2.3	0.9
TURKISH DELIGHT								
Assorted Flavours, Julian Graves*	1 Square/30g	110	0.0	366	0.5	91.1	0.1	0.0
Dark Chocolate Covered, Thorntons*	1 Chocolate/10g	39	1.1	390	2.7	69.0	11.0	2.0
Fry's*	1 Bar/51g	185	3.4	365	1.4	74.6	6.7	1.3
Milk Chocolate, M&S*	1 Pack/55g	220	4.7	400	1.6	79.0	8.5	0.0
Sultans*	1 Serving/16g	58	0.0	360	0.0	90.0	0.0	0.0
with Mixed Nuts, Hazer Baba*	1 Piece/12g	47	0.2	389	1.6	88.5	1.7	0.0
with Rose, Hazer Baba*	1 Square/18g	70	0.3	389	1.6	88.6	1.7	0.0
TURMERIC								
Powder	*1 Tsp/3g*	*11*	*0.3*	*354*	*7.8*	*58.2*	*9.9*	*0.0*
TURNIP								
Boiled, Average	*1oz/28g*	*3*	*0.1*	*12*	*0.6*	*2.0*	*0.2*	*1.9*
Mash, Direct Foods*	½ Pack/190g	49	3.4	26	0.6	2.0	1.8	1.9
Mashed, Mash Direct*	1 Pack/400g	148	2.3	37	0.8	6.0	0.6	2.5
Raw, Unprepared, Average	*1oz/28g*	*6*	*0.1*	*23*	*0.9*	*4.7*	*0.3*	*2.4*
TURNOVER								
Apple, Bramley, Tesco*	1 Turnover/88g	304	22.8	346	2.7	25.4	25.9	0.9
Apple, Co-Op*	1 Turnover/77g	308	20.8	400	4.0	35.0	27.0	1.0
Apple, Dutch, Sainsbury's*	1 Serving/33g	130	5.5	393	3.6	56.9	16.8	1.4
Apple, Fresh Cream, Sainsbury's*	1 Turnover/84g	292	20.9	347	4.1	26.9	24.8	2.5
Apple, Tesco*	1 Turnover/88g	294	19.7	334	3.2	29.8	22.4	0.9
Raspberry, Fresh Cream, Asda*	1 Turnover/100g	411	23.0	411	6.0	45.0	23.0	2.1
Raspberry, Tesco*	1 Turnover/84g	290	20.2	345	4.0	27.2	24.1	2.1
TWIGLETS								
Original, Jacob's*	1 Bag/30g	115	3.5	383	12.7	57.0	11.6	11.8
Tangy, Jacob's*	1 Bag/30g	136	6.6	454	8.1	55.9	22.0	5.4
TWIRL								
Cadbury*	1 Finger/22g	118	6.8	535	7.6	56.0	30.9	0.8
Treat Size, Cadbury*	1 Bar/21g	115	6.6	535	7.6	56.0	30.9	0.8
TWIRLS								
Prawn Cocktail, Bobby's*	1 Pack/26g	116	4.8	445	3.4	65.9	18.6	0.0
Salt & Vinegar, Sainsbury's*	½ Bag/40g	167	5.6	418	3.0	70.1	14.0	3.0
Salt & Vinegar, Tesco*	1 Bag/80g	349	14.0	436	3.9	65.8	17.5	2.4

T

	Measure INFO/WEIGHT	per Measure KCAL	per Measure FAT	Nutrition Values per 100g / 100ml KCAL	PROT	CARB	FAT	FIBRE
TWISTS								
Black Olive & Basil, Finest, Tesco*	¼ Pack/31g	151	7.9	483	11.3	53.1	25.1	3.9
Parmesan, All Butter, TTD, Sainsbury's*	1 Serving/8g	38	2.0	487	13.8	51.0	25.3	2.8
TWIX								
Fun Size, Mars*	1 Bar/21g	103	5.0	492	4.7	65.5	23.7	1.5
Standard, Mars*	1 Pack/58g	284	13.7	490	4.7	65.5	23.7	1.5
Top, Mars*	1 Bar/28g	143	7.8	511	5.2	60.2	27.7	0.0
Twixels, Mars*	1 Finger/6g	31	1.6	513	5.0	64.0	26.1	0.0
Xtra, Mars*	1 Pack/85g	416	20.1	490	4.7	65.5	23.7	1.5
TZATZIKI								
Asda*	1 Serving/50g	54	4.2	108	3.8	4.6	8.5	1.2
Average	1 Tbsp/15g	10	0.7	66	3.7	2.0	4.9	0.2
Fresh, Sainsbury's*	1/5 Pot/46g	59	4.8	129	4.4	4.4	10.4	0.2
Greek, Authentic, Total, Fage*	1 Serving/50g	50	3.5	99	4.9	4.1	7.0	1.0
Morrisons*	½ Pot/85g	82	5.4	97	3.6	6.4	6.3	0.5
Tesco*	¼ Pack/50g	72	6.0	145	4.0	5.1	12.0	0.2
Waitrose*	1 Serving/50g	54	2.6	108	6.7	8.4	5.3	0.8

	Measure INFO/WEIGHT	per Measure KCAL	FAT	Nutrition Values per 100g / 100ml KCAL	PROT	CARB	FAT	FIBRE
VANILLA								
Bean, Average	*1 Pod/2g*	*6*	*0.0*	*288*	*0.0*	*13.0*	*0.0*	*0.0*
Bean Paste, Nielsen Massey Vanillas*	1 Serving/100g	286	2.6	286	0.2	53.7	2.6	2.4
VANILLA EXTRACT								
Average	*1 Tbsp/13g*	*37*	*0.0*	*288*	*0.1*	*12.6*	*0.1*	*0.0*
VEAL								
Chop, Loin, Raw, Weighed with Bone, Average	1 Chop/195g	495	27.8	254	29.5	0.0	14.3	0.0
Escalope, Fried, Average	1oz/28g	55	1.9	196	33.7	0.0	6.8	0.0
Escalopes, Breaded, M&S*	1 Escalope/130g	292	13.9	225	13.6	18.7	10.7	0.4
Mince, Raw, Average	*1oz/28g*	*40*	*2.0*	*144*	*20.3*	*0.0*	*7.0*	*0.0*
Shoulder, Lean & Fat, Roasted, Average	*1oz/28g*	*52*	*2.3*	*183*	*25.5*	*0.0*	*8.2*	*0.0*
Shoulder, Lean Only, Roasted, Average	*1oz/28g*	*46*	*1.6*	*164*	*26.1*	*0.0*	*5.8*	*0.0*
Sirloin, Lean & Fat, Roasted, Average	*1oz/28g*	*57*	*3.0*	*202*	*25.1*	*0.0*	*10.4*	*0.0*
Sirloin, Lean Only, Roasted, Average	*1oz/28g*	*48*	*1.8*	*168*	*26.3*	*0.0*	*6.2*	*0.0*
VEGEMITE								
Australian, Kraft*	1 Tsp/5g	9	0.0	173	23.5	19.7	0.0	0.0
VEGETABLE CHIPS								
Beetroot, Carrot & Parsnips, Hand Fried, Tyrrells*	½ Pack/25g	103	7.0	413	3.9	36.0	28.1	11.5
Cassava, Average	1oz/28g	99	0.1	353	1.8	91.4	0.4	4.0
Mixed Root, Tyrrells*	1oz/28g	133	8.3	476	5.7	35.4	29.8	12.8
Parsnip, Golden, Kettle Chips*	½ Pack/50g	258	18.8	515	4.6	39.5	37.6	8.4
Sweet Potato, Kettle Chips*	½ Pack/50g	242	16.4	483	2.4	44.4	32.8	9.3
VEGETABLE CRISPS								
Pan Fried, Glennans*	1 Bag/20g	98	6.7	490	5.0	42.5	33.5	11.0
VEGETABLE FAT								
Pure, Trex*	1 Tbsp/12g	108	12.0	900	0.0	0.0	100.0	0.0
VEGETABLE FINGERS								
Crispy, Birds Eye*	2 Fingers/60g	107	4.8	179	3.2	23.5	8.0	2.3
Crispy Crunchy, Dalepak*	1 Finger/28g	62	3.1	223	4.2	26.7	11.0	15.0
VEGETABLE MEDLEY								
Asda*	1 Pack/300g	84	0.6	28	2.8	3.9	0.2	2.9
Buttered, Sainsbury's*	½ Pack/175g	122	6.8	70	1.7	7.0	3.9	1.8
Carrot, Courgette, Fine Bean & Baby Corn, Tesco*	1 Serving/100g	36	2.4	36	1.1	2.4	2.4	3.0
Carrots, Broccoli, Baby Corn, Sugar Snap Peas, Co-Op*	1/3 Pack/89g	40	0.7	45	3.0	7.0	0.8	3.0
Crunchy, M&S*	1 Pack/250g	75	2.0	30	3.1	2.8	0.8	2.5
Green, Sainsbury's*	1 Pack/220g	178	14.3	81	3.0	2.5	6.5	2.9
Roast, Four Seasons*	1 Pack/375g	202	12.0	54	2.8	3.5	3.2	2.7
Roasted, Waitrose*	½ Pack/200g	282	15.6	141	1.2	16.4	7.8	3.7
with Herby Butter, M&S*	1 Pack/300g	225	15.0	75	1.5	6.2	5.0	2.6
VEGETABLE SELECTION								
Chefs, M&S*	1 Pack/250g	88	1.2	35	2.6	4.5	0.5	2.9
Lightly Buttered & Seasoned, M&S*	1 Pack/300g	195	10.8	65	1.6	6.3	3.6	2.8
Ready to Cook, Morrisons*	1 Serving/150g	51	0.9	34	2.4	4.8	0.6	2.3
Roast, COU, M&S*	1 Serving/250g	95	2.0	38	1.2	6.1	0.8	0.6
Tenderstem Broccoli & Butternut Squash, Waitrose*	½ Pack/100g	42	0.6	42	2.3	5.4	0.6	2.7
VEGETABLES								
& Bean, Stew Mix, Cooks' Ingredients, Waitrose*	½ Pack/200g	166	3.8	83	4.2	10.2	1.9	4.3
Asparagus & Tenderstem Broccoli, Finest, Tesco*	½ Pack/95g	28	0.4	29	3.7	2.7	0.4	2.7
Bean & Vegetable Layer, M&S*	1 Pack/285g	271	13.7	95	3.6	7.2	4.8	3.7
Broccoli, Leek & Cabbage, Fresh, Love Life, Waitrose*	1 Serving/100g	26	0.4	26	1.5	3.1	0.4	1.8
Butternut Squash, Broccoli & Spinach, Eat Well, M&S*	½ Pack/138g	55	0.7	40	2.3	5.0	0.5	2.3
Butternut Squash & Sweet Potato, Fresh Tastes, Asda*	½ Pack/225g	128	0.4	57	1.0	12.9	0.2	1.8
Cauliflower Florets, Peas & Carrots, Frozen, Asda*	1 Serving/119g	44	0.7	37	3.0	5.0	0.6	2.8
Classic Layered, M&S*	1 Pack/320g	224	12.5	70	1.2	7.3	3.9	1.2

V

	Measure INFO/WEIGHT	per Measure		Nutrition Values per 100g / 100ml				
		KCAL	FAT	KCAL	PROT	CARB	FAT	FIBRE
VEGETABLES								
Crisp & Crunchy, Stir Fry, M&S*	½ Pack/115g	29	0.2	25	1.9	3.9	0.2	1.7
Family Steamer, Field Fresh, Birds Eye*	½ Bag/240g	103	1.4	43	2.0	6.1	0.6	2.4
Farmhouse Mix, Frozen, Asda*	1 Serving/100g	25	0.8	25	2.5	2.2	0.8	0.0
Grilled, Frozen, Sainsbury's*	1 Serving/80g	42	2.9	52	1.2	3.8	3.6	1.5
Grilled Mix, Frozen, Essential, Waitrose*	1 Serving/80g	34	0.2	42	1.8	8.1	0.3	2.4
Julienne, Tesco*	1 Serving/100g	30	0.3	30	1.1	5.7	0.3	1.9
Layered, with Butter, Waitrose*	1 Pack/280g	207	16.2	74	1.7	3.6	5.8	2.4
Mediterranean, Ready To Roast, Sainsbury's*	½ Pack/182g	111	4.2	61	1.8	6.8	2.3	2.8
Mediterranean Roasted, Sainsbury's*	1 Serving/150g	118	5.4	79	2.2	9.5	3.6	3.4
Mediterranean Style, Asda*	½ Pack/205g	113	3.7	55	1.7	7.9	1.8	1.3
Mediterranean Style, M&S*	½ Pack/214g	75	1.9	35	1.2	5.5	0.9	1.0
Mediterranean Style, Ready to Roast, Sainsbury's*	½ Pack/200g	138	4.4	69	2.3	9.9	2.2	2.2
Mediterranean Style, Roasting, Tesco*	1 Serving/200g	72	2.0	36	1.1	5.7	1.0	1.3
Mexican Chilli Bean, Lovely Vegetables, M&S*	1 Pack/300g	270	6.9	90	2.9	11.6	2.3	4.6
Mix, Steamer, Love Life, Waitrose*	1 Bag/160g	83	1.8	52	2.8	7.7	1.1	2.8
Mixed, Carrot, Cauliflower, & Broccoli, Fresh, Tesco*	1 Serving/80g	26	0.2	32	2.6	3.9	0.2	2.8
Roasted, Italian, M&S*	1 Serving/95g	218	20.0	230	1.8	7.1	21.0	1.7
Roasted, Mediterranean, Tesco*	½ Pack/173g	95	3.1	55	1.3	7.6	1.8	2.0
Roasted, Selection, COU, M&S*	1 Pack/250g	88	2.0	35	1.2	6.1	0.8	0.6
Roasted Mediterranean, The Best*	1 Serving/125g	100	5.8	80	2.3	7.0	4.6	3.6
Roasted Root, Extra Special, Asda*	½ Pack/205g	160	3.1	78	1.1	15.0	1.5	6.0
Root, for Mashing, Eat Fresh, Tesco*	1 Pack/600g	246	2.4	41	0.9	7.2	0.4	2.6
Root, Honey Roast, Sainsbury's*	1 Pack/400g	748	34.8	187	0.0	25.8	8.7	5.2
Root, Ready to Roast, Sainsbury's*	½ Pack/200g	188	8.6	94	1.3	13.0	4.3	2.2
Sliced Carrots & Broccoli Florets, Fresh, Morrisons*	1 Portion/100g	37	0.7	37	2.2	4.1	0.7	2.5
Soup Mix, Prepared & Washed, Morrisons*	½ Pack/300g	117	1.2	39	1.1	7.3	0.4	1.1
Stir Fry, Frozen, Market, Value, Tesco*	1 Pack/750g	675	32.2	90	2.3	10.0	4.3	4.7
Stir Fry, Frozen, Sainsbury's*	1 Serving/80g	19	0.2	24	1.3	3.9	0.3	2.0
Summer, Rainbow, Roasting, Fresh Tastes, Asda*	½ Pack/175g	84	4.7	48	1.4	3.5	2.7	0.0
Summer, Roasted, TTD, Sainsbury's*	½ Pack/200g	160	2.2	80	1.8	14.5	1.1	2.6
Winter Soup Mix, Sainsbury's*	1 Portion/149g	61	0.3	41	1.1	7.9	0.2	1.7
VEGETARIAN								
Roast, Linda McCartney*	¼ Roast/114g	222	10.2	196	19.4	9.4	9.0	1.5
Sausage & Mash, 617, Wiltshire Farm Foods*	1 Serving/400g	377	18.5	94	5.1	8.7	4.6	2.0
Slices, Sage & Onion, Vegi Deli, The Redwood Co*	1 Slice/10g	23	1.4	233	21.4	5.0	14.1	0.5
Slices, Vegetable, Tesco*	1 Slice/165g	452	30.5	274	5.6	21.4	18.5	3.3
VEGETARIAN MINCE								
Chicken Style Pieces, Realeat*	¼ Pack/88g	119	1.4	136	29.0	1.5	1.6	4.4
Easy Cook, Linda McCartney*	1oz/28g	35	0.1	126	21.4	9.3	0.4	1.7
Frozen, Meatfree, Improved Recipe, Sainsbury's*	1 Pack/454g	799	31.8	176	18.3	10.7	7.0	6.7
Meat Free, Boiled, CBY, Asda*	1 Serving/75g	83	2.5	111	13.7	6.7	3.3	4.4
Meat Free, Tesco*	1 Serving/76g	113	3.8	150	19.0	7.0	5.0	6.0
Vegemince, Realeat*	1 Serving/125g	218	12.5	174	18.0	3.0	10.0	3.0
VENISON								
Grill Steak, Average	*1 Grillsteak/150g*	*178*	*3.8*	*119*	*19.0*	*5.0*	*2.5*	*1.0*
in Red Wine & Port, Average	1oz/28g	21	0.7	76	9.8	3.5	2.6	0.4
Minced, Cooked, Average	*1 Serving/100g*	*187*	*8.2*	*187*	*26.4*	*0.0*	*8.2*	*0.0*
Minced, Raw, Average	*1 Serving/100g*	*157*	*7.1*	*157*	*21.8*	*0.0*	*7.1*	*0.0*
Raw, Haunch, Meat Only, Average	1 Serving/100g	103	1.6	103	22.2	0.0	1.6	0.0
Roasted, Average	*1oz/28g*	*46*	*0.7*	*165*	*35.6*	*0.0*	*2.5*	*0.0*
Steak, Raw, Average	*1oz/28g*	*30*	*0.5*	*108*	*22.8*	*0.0*	*1.9*	*0.0*
VERMICELLI								
Dry	*1oz/28g*	*99*	*0.1*	*355*	*8.7*	*78.3*	*0.4*	*0.0*

	Measure INFO/WEIGHT	per Measure KCAL	FAT	Nutrition Values per 100g / 100ml KCAL	PROT	CARB	FAT	FIBRE
VERMICELLI								
Egg, Cooked, Average	*1 Serving/185g*	*239*	*2.6*	*129*	*5.0*	*24.0*	*1.4*	*1.0*
VERMOUTH								
Dry	*1 Shot/50ml*	*54*	*0.0*	*109*	*0.1*	*3.0*	*0.0*	*0.0*
Sweet	*1 Shot/50ml*	*76*	*0.0*	*151*	*0.0*	*15.9*	*0.0*	*0.0*
VIMTO*								
Cordial, No Added Sugar, Diluted, Vimto Soft Drinks*	1 Glass/250ml	6	0.2	2	0.1	0.4	0.1	0.0
Cordial, No Added Sugar, Undiluted, Vimto Soft Drinks*	1 Serving/50ml	2	0.0	4	0.0	0.7	0.0	0.0
Cordial, Original, Diluted, Vimto Soft Drinks*	1 Serving/200ml	60	0.0	30	0.0	7.4	0.0	0.0
Cordial, Original, Undiluted, Vimto Soft Drinks*	1 Serving/50ml	49	0.0	98	0.0	23.6	0.0	0.0
Fizzy, Vimto Soft Drinks*	1 Can/330ml	147	0.0	44	0.0	11.0	0.0	0.0
VINAIGRETTE								
Balsamic, Hellmann's*	1 Tbsp/15ml	12	0.4	82	0.1	9.6	2.7	0.6
Blush Wine, Briannas*	2 Tbsp/30ml	100	6.0	333	0.0	40.0	20.0	0.0
Fat Free, Hellmann's*	1 Serving/15ml	7	0.0	49	0.1	10.9	0.0	0.3
Frank Cooper*	1 Pot/28g	46	3.2	163	1.0	14.1	11.4	0.3
French, Real, Briannas*	2 Tbsp/30ml	150	17.0	500	0.0	0.0	56.7	0.0
French Style, Finest, Tesco*	1 Tbsp/15ml	93	9.8	620	0.6	6.3	65.3	0.2
Luxury French, Hellmann's*	1 Tsp/5ml	15	1.3	305	0.8	16.0	26.1	0.4
Olive Oil & Lemon, Amoy*	½ Sachet/15ml	38	3.6	250	0.3	3.0	24.0	0.0
PB, Waitrose*	1 Tsp/5ml	4	0.0	89	0.4	20.9	0.4	0.5
Waistline, 99% Fat Free, Crosse & Blackwell*	1 Tbsp/15ml	1	0.0	9	1.0	0.7	0.2	0.2
with Mustard, Delhaize*	1 Serving/20g	93	10.2	464	0.8	0.7	50.9	0.0
VINE LEAVES								
Preserved in Brine	*1oz/28g*	*4*	*0.0*	*15*	*3.6*	*0.2*	*0.0*	*0.0*
Stuffed, Mediterranean Deli, M&S*	1 Leaf/37g	39	1.5	105	2.6	14.2	4.1	1.2
Stuffed, Sainsbury's*	1 Parcel/38g	46	2.1	124	2.9	15.3	5.7	3.1
Stuffed with Rice	1oz/28g	73	5.0	262	2.8	23.8	18.0	0.0
Stuffed with Rice, Dolmades, M&S*	1 Leaf/38g	40	1.6	105	2.6	14.2	4.1	1.2
Stuffed with Rice & Mixed Herbs, Sainsbury's*	1 Leaf/37g	44	1.8	120	2.6	16.3	4.9	1.2
VINEGAR								
Apple Balsamic, Aspall*	1 Serving/100g	123	0.1	123	0.5	26.1	0.1	0.0
Balsamic, Average	*1 Tsp/5ml*	*6*	*0.0*	*115*	*0.9*	*26.0*	*0.0*	*0.0*
Cider	*1 Tbsp/15ml*	*2*	*0.0*	*14*	*0.0*	*5.9*	*0.0*	*0.0*
Malt, Average	*1 Tbsp/15g*	*1*	*0.0*	*4*	*0.4*	*0.6*	*0.0*	*0.0*
Red Wine, Average	1 Tbsp/15ml	3	0.0	19	0.0	0.3	0.0	0.0
Rice, White, Amoy*	1 Tsp/5ml	0	0.0	4	0.0	1.0	0.0	0.0
VODKA								
37.5% Volume	*1 Pub Shot/35ml*	*72*	*0.0*	*207*	*0.0*	*0.0*	*0.0*	*0.0*
40% Volume	*1 Pub Shot/35ml*	*78*	*0.0*	*222*	*0.0*	*0.0*	*0.0*	*0.0*
Bullett & Cola, Premixed, Canned, Diageo*	1 Can/250ml	218	0.0	87	0.0	10.6	0.0	0.0
Smirnoff & Cola, Premixed, Canned, Diageo*	1 Can/250ml	178	0.0	71	0.0	8.9	0.0	0.0
Smirnoff & Cranberry, Premixed, Canned, Diageo*	1 Can/250ml	175	0.0	70	0.0	8.5	0.0	0.0
Smirnoff & Diet Cola, Premixed, Canned, Diageo*	1 Can/250ml	100	0.0	40	0.0	0.0	0.0	0.0
Smirnoff & Tonic, Premixed, Canned, Diageo*	1 Can/250ml	158	0.0	63	0.0	6.4	0.0	0.0

V

INFO/WEIGHT	Measure	per Measure		Nutrition Values per 100g / 100ml				
		KCAL	FAT	KCAL	PROT	CARB	FAT	FIBRE
WAFERS								
Cafe Curls, Rolled, Askeys*	1 Wafer/5g	21	0.4	422	5.8	80.3	8.6	0.0
Caramel, Dark Chocolate, Tunnock's*	1 Wafer/26g	128	6.6	492	5.2	60.7	25.4	0.0
Caramel, Milk Chocolate Coated, Value, Tesco*	1 Wafer/23g	110	4.7	475	5.6	67.6	20.2	0.6
Caramel, Penguin, McVitie's*	1 Bar/21g	106	5.4	492	5.1	60.7	25.2	1.4
Caramel, Tunnock's*	1 Wafer/26g	116	4.5	448	3.6	69.2	17.4	2.5
Caramel Log, Tunnock's*	1 Wafer/32g	152	7.7	474	4.2	64.3	24.0	0.0
Caramel Mallow, Weight Watchers*	1 Mallow/17g	55	0.4	329	5.5	63.9	2.1	17.8
Cheese Footballs, Jacob's*	1 Serving/25g	139	9.2	556	11.8	43.9	36.7	1.5
for Ice Cream, Askeys*	1 Wafer/2g	6	0.0	388	11.4	79.0	2.9	0.0
Hazelnut, Elledi*	1 Wafer/8g	38	1.9	493	6.3	62.4	24.3	0.0
Milk Chocolate, Sainsbury's*	1 Wafer/10g	51	2.7	506	6.2	60.5	26.7	1.4
WAFFLES								
Belgian, TTD, Sainsbury's*	1 Waffle/25g	122	7.3	490	6.0	50.6	29.3	1.2
Caramel, Asda*	1 Waffle/8g	37	1.8	459	3.3	62.0	22.0	1.1
Milk Chocolate, Tregroes*	1 Waffle/49g	220	20.5	450	4.5	57.0	42.0	0.5
Sweet, American Style, Sainsbury's*	1 Waffle/35g	160	8.9	457	7.2	50.6	25.3	1.1
Toasting, McVitie's*	1 Waffle/25g	118	6.3	474	6.0	52.6	25.5	0.6
Toffee, Tregroes, Aldi*	1 Waffle/35g	160	6.2	463	3.5	71.7	18.0	2.2
WAGON WHEEL								
Chocolate, Burton's*	1 Biscuit/39g	165	5.7	424	5.3	67.4	14.6	1.9
Jammie, Burton's*	1 Biscuit/40g	168	5.6	420	5.1	67.7	14.1	1.9
WALNUT WHIP								
Nestle*	1 Whip/35g	173	8.8	494	5.3	61.3	25.2	0.7
The, Classics, M&S*	1 Whip/26g	127	7.1	490	7.2	54.9	27.4	1.1
Vanilla, Nestle*	1 Whip/34g	165	8.4	486	5.7	60.5	24.6	1.1
WALNUTS								
Average	*1 Nut/7g*	*48*	*4.8*	*691*	*15.6*	*3.2*	*68.5*	*3.5*
Halves, Average	*1 Half/3g*	*23*	*2.3*	*669*	*17.4*	*6.3*	*65.0*	*4.7*
Halves, Wholefoods, Tesco*	1 Pack/250g	1762	171.2	705	17.3	3.1	68.5	3.5
Wholesome, Organic, Kernels, Love Life, Waitrose*	1 Serving/30g	207	20.6	689	14.7	3.3	68.5	6.8
WASABI								
Crispy Seaweed Strips, Khun Film*	1 Serving/10g	68	6.4	680	12.0	8.0	64.0	12.0
Paste, Ready Mixed, Japanese, Yutaka*	1 Tsp/5g	14	0.4	286	2.7	53.0	7.0	0.0
WATER								
Apple & Strawberry Flavoured, Morrisons*	1 Serving/200ml	3	0.0	2	0.2	0.1	0.0	0.0
Aqueo, Lemon & Lime Flavour, Aldi*	1 Bottle/500ml	10	0.0	2	0.0	0.3	0.0	0.0
Aqueo, Peach Flavoured, Still, Aldi*	1 Bottle/500ml	10	0.0	2	0.0	0.3	0.0	0.0
Berry Blast, Revive, Volvic*	1 Bottle/500ml	10	0.0	2	0.3	0.4	0.0	0.0
Cranberries & Raspberries, Juicy, Innocent*	1 Bottle/380ml	118	1.1	31	0.1	6.7	0.3	0.0
Cranberry & Blueberry, Lightly Sparkling, Waitrose*	1 Glass/250ml	10	0.0	4	0.0	0.7	0.0	0.0
Cranberry & Raspberry Flavoured, Morrisons*	1 Serving/200ml	3	0.0	2	0.2	0.1	0.0	0.0
Elderflower Presse, Bottle Green*	1 Serving/250ml	88	0.0	35	0.0	8.9	0.0	0.0
Grapefruit, Slightly Sparkling, Tesco*	1 Serving/200ml	4	0.0	2	0.0	0.2	0.0	0.0
Juicy Spring, Blackcurrant & Apple, Drench*	1 Serving/250ml	98	0.0	39	0.0	9.2	0.0	0.0
Lemon, Vittel*	1 Bottle/500ml	6	0.0	1	0.0	0.0	0.0	0.0
Lemon & Lime, Sparkling, M&S*	1 Bottle/500ml	15	0.0	3	0.0	0.4	0.0	0.0
Lemon & Lime, Still, M&S*	1 Bottle/500ml	5	0.0	1	0.0	0.2	0.0	0.0
Lemon & Lime, Sugar Free, Touch of Fruit, Volvic*	1 Bottle/150ml	2	0.0	1	0.0	0.0	0.0	0.0
Lemon & Lime Flavour Sparkling Spring, Co-Op*	1 Serving/200ml	2	0.0	1	0.0	0.0	0.0	0.0
Lemon & Lime Flavoured, Strathmore*	1 Bottle/500ml	85	0.0	17	0.0	4.0	0.0	0.0
Lemons & Limes, Spring Water, This Juicy Water*	1 Bottle/420ml	143	0.4	34	0.1	8.2	0.1	0.0
Mineral Or Tap	*1 Glass/200ml*	*0*	*0.0*	*0*	*0.0*	*0.0*	*0.0*	*0.0*
Peach, Slightly Sparkling, Tesco*	1 Serving/200ml	4	0.0	2	0.0	0.2	0.0	0.0

	Measure INFO/WEIGHT	per Measure KCAL	per Measure FAT	Nutrition Values per 100g / 100ml KCAL	PROT	CARB	FAT	FIBRE
WATER								
Peach & Orange Flavoured, Morrisons*	1 Serving/200ml	3	0.0	2	0.2	0.1	0.0	0.0
Peach & Raspberry, Still, M&S*	1 Bottle/500ml	10	0.0	2	0.0	0.0	0.0	0.0
Sparkling, Blueberry & Pomegranate, M&S*	1 Glass/250ml	5	0.0	2	0.0	0.4	0.0	0.0
Sparkling, San Pellegrino*	1 Glass/200ml	0	0.0	0	0.0	0.0	0.0	0.0
Sparkling, Smart Price, Asda*	1 Glass/300ml	0	0.0	0	0.0	0.0	0.0	0.0
Spring, Apple & Mango, Sparkling, Asda*	1 Glass/200ml	2	0.0	1	0.0	0.2	0.0	0.0
Spring, Apple & Raspberry, Sparkling, Tesco*	1 Glass/330ml	7	0.0	2	0.0	0.5	0.0	0.0
Spring, Cranberry & Raspberry, Drench*	1 Bottle/440ml	146	0.4	33	0.1	7.7	0.1	0.0
Spring, Lemon & Lime, Slightly Sparkling, Tesco*	1 Serving/200ml	4	0.2	2	0.1	0.2	0.1	0.1
Spring, Orange & Passionfruit, Drench*	1 Serving/250ml	95	0.5	38	0.1	9.0	0.2	0.0
Spring, Strawberry & Kiwi, Still, Shapers, Boots*	1 Glass/250ml	2	0.0	1	0.0	0.1	0.0	0.9
Spring, White Grape & Blackberry, Tesco*	1 Glass/200ml	4	0.0	2	0.0	0.5	0.0	0.0
Spring, with a Hint of Orange, Slightly Sparkling, Tesco*	1 Serving/250ml	5	0.0	2	0.0	0.2	0.0	0.0
Strawberry, Original, Touch of Fruit, Volvic*	1 Bottle/500ml	99	0.0	20	0.0	4.8	0.0	0.0
Strawberry, Sugar Free, Touch of Fruit, Volvic*	1 Bottle/500ml	7	0.0	1	0.0	0.1	0.0	0.0
Vitamin, Xxx, Triple Berry, Glaceau, Coca-Cola*	1 Bottle/500ml	95	0.0	19	0.0	4.6	0.0	0.0
WATER CHESTNUTS								
Raw, Average	*1oz/28g*	*10*	*0.0*	*34*	*1.0*	*7.8*	*0.0*	*0.1*
Whole, in Water, Drained, Sainsbury's*	1 Can/140g	25	0.1	18	0.8	3.4	0.1	0.4
with Bamboo Shoots, Sainsbury's*	1 Serving/50g	29	0.1	58	2.0	12.0	0.2	1.1
WATERCRESS								
Baby, Steve's Leaves*	1 Bag/40g	10	0.2	25	2.6	2.5	0.5	2.1
Morrisons*	1 Pack/85g	19	0.8	22	3.0	0.4	1.0	1.5
Raw, Trimmed, Average	*1 Sprig/3g*	*1*	*0.0*	*22*	*3.0*	*0.4*	*1.0*	*1.5*
WATERMELON								
Flesh Only, Average	*1 Serving/250g*	*75*	*0.8*	*30*	*0.4*	*7.0*	*0.3*	*0.4*
Raw, Weighed with Skin, Average	1 Serving/100g	30	0.3	30	0.4	7.0	0.3	0.4
WHEAT								
Whole Grain, Split, Average	*1 Serving/60g*	*205*	*1.0*	*342*	*11.3*	*75.9*	*1.7*	*12.2*
WHEAT BRAN								
Average	*1 Tbsp/7g*	*14*	*0.4*	*206*	*14.1*	*26.8*	*5.5*	*36.4*
Coarse, Holland & Barrett*	1 Tbsp/4g	8	0.2	206	14.1	26.8	5.5	36.4
Natural, Jordans*	1 Tbsp/7g	13	0.4	188	16.3	17.4	5.9	44.5
WHEAT CRUNCHIES								
Golden Wonder*	1 Pack/35g	172	8.7	491	11.1	55.9	24.8	0.0
Salt & Vinegar, Golden Wonder*	1 Bag/34g	165	8.5	484	10.5	54.5	24.9	2.8
Worcester Sauce, Golden Wonder*	1 Bag/35g	172	8.9	492	9.3	56.4	25.5	3.9
WHEAT GERM								
Average	*1oz/28g*	*100*	*2.6*	*357*	*26.7*	*44.7*	*9.2*	*15.6*
Natural, Jordans*	2 Tbsp/16g	54	1.5	340	28.0	36.0	9.3	13.1
WHELKS								
Boiled, Weighed without Shell	*1oz/28g*	*25*	*0.3*	*89*	*19.5*	*0.0*	*1.2*	*0.0*
WHISKEY								
Irish, Jameson*	1 Shot/25ml	58	0.0	233	0.0	0.0	0.0	0.0
Jack Daniel's*	1 Pub Shot/35ml	78	0.0	222	0.0	0.0	0.0	0.0
WHISKY								
37.5% Volume	*1 Pub Shot/35ml*	*72*	*0.0*	*207*	*0.0*	*0.0*	*0.0*	*0.0*
40% Volume	*1 Pub Shot/35ml*	*78*	*0.0*	*222*	*0.0*	*0.0*	*0.0*	*0.0*
Bells & Ginger Ale, Premixed, Canned, Diageo*	1 Can/250ml	170	0.0	68	0.0	7.6	0.0	0.0
Scots, 37.5% Volume	*1 Pub Shot/35ml*	*72*	*0.0*	*207*	*0.0*	*0.0*	*0.0*	*0.0*
Scots, 40% Volume	*1 Pub Shot/35ml*	*78*	*0.0*	*222*	*0.0*	*0.0*	*0.0*	*0.0*
Teacher's*	1 Pub Shot/35ml	78	0.0	222	0.0	0.0	0.0	0.0

W

	Measure INFO/WEIGHT	per Measure KCAL	FAT	KCAL	PROT	CARB	FAT	FIBRE
WHITE PUDDING								
Average	1oz/28g	126	8.9	450	7.0	36.3	31.8	0.0
WHITEBAIT								
in Flour, Fried	1oz/28g	147	13.3	525	19.5	5.3	47.5	0.2
Raw, Average	1 Serving/100g	172	11.0	172	18.3	0.0	11.0	0.0
WHITECURRANTS								
Raw, Average	1oz/28g	7	0.0	26	1.3	5.6	0.0	3.4
WHITING								
in Crumbs, Fried in Blended Oil	1 Serving/180g	344	18.5	191	18.1	7.0	10.3	0.2
Raw	1oz/28g	23	0.2	81	18.7	0.0	0.7	0.0
Steamed	1 Serving/85g	78	0.8	92	20.9	0.0	0.9	0.0
WIENER SCHNITZEL								
Average	1oz/28g	62	2.8	223	20.9	13.1	10.0	0.4
WINE								
Cherry, Lambrini*	1 Sm Glass/125ml	80	0.0	64	0.0	0.0	0.0	0.0
Diet, Lambrini*	1 Sm Glass/125ml	43	0.0	35	0.0	0.0	0.0	0.0
Elderberry & Lemon, Ame*	1 Sml Glass/125ml	46	0.0	37	0.0	6.4	0.0	0.0
Fruit, Average	1 Sm Glass/125ml	115	0.0	92	0.0	5.5	0.0	0.0
Grape & Apricot, Ame*	1 Sm Glass/125ml	49	1.2	39	1.3	6.7	1.0	0.0
Madeira, Henriques & Henriques*	1 Glass/100ml	130	0.0	130	0.0	0.0	0.0	0.0
Mulled, Homemade, Average	1 Sm Glass/125ml	245	0.0	196	0.1	25.2	0.0	0.0
Mulled, Sainsbury's*	1 Sm Glass/125ml	112	0.0	90	0.0	8.6	0.0	0.0
Original, Lambrini*	1 Glass/125ml	88	0.0	70	0.0	0.0	0.0	0.0
Red, Amarone, Average*	1 Sm Glass/125ml	120	0.0	96	0.1	3.0	0.0	0.0
Red, Average	1 Sm Glass/125ml	104	0.0	83	0.0	2.0	0.0	0.0
Red, Burgundy, 12.9% Abv, Average	1 Sm Glass/125ml	110	0.0	88	0.1	3.7	0.0	0.0
Red, Cabernet Sauvignon, 13.1% Abv, Average	1 Sm Glass/125ml	105	0.0	84	0.1	2.6	0.0	0.0
Red, Cabernet Sauvigon, Non Alcoholic, Ariel*	1 Serving/240ml	50	0.0	21	0.0	4.8	0.0	0.0
Red, California, Blossom Hill*	1 Glass/175ml	132	0.0	75	0.0	0.9	0.0	0.0
Red, Claret, 12.8% Abv, Average	1 Sm Glass/125ml	105	0.0	84	0.1	3.0	0.0	0.0
Red, Gamay, 12.3% Abv, Average	1 Sm Glass/125ml	99	0.0	79	0.1	2.4	0.0	0.0
Red, Merlot, 13.3% Abv, Average	1 Sm Glass/125ml	105	0.0	84	0.1	2.5	0.0	0.0
Red, Non Alcoholic, Ame*	1 Sm Glass/125ml	42	0.0	34	0.0	5.7	0.0	0.0
Red, Petit Sirah, 13.5% Abv, Average	1 Sm Glass/125ml	108	0.0	86	0.1	2.7	0.0	0.0
Red, Pinot Noir, 13% Abv, Average	1 Sm Glass/125ml	104	0.0	83	0.1	2.3	0.0	0.0
Red, Sangiovese, 13.6% Abv, Average	1 Sm Glass/125ml	109	0.0	87	0.1	2.6	0.0	0.0
Red, Smooth, Weight Watchers*	1 Glass/125ml	75	0.1	60	0.1	1.4	0.1	0.1
Red, Syrah, 13.1% Abv, Average	1 Sm Glass/125ml	105	0.0	84	0.1	2.6	0.0	0.0
Red, Zinfandel, 13.9% Abv, Average	1 Sm Glass/125ml	111	0.0	89	0.1	2.9	0.0	0.0
Rose, Medium, Average	1 Sm Glass/125ml	98	0.0	79	0.0	2.1	0.0	0.0
Rose, Refreshing, Weight Watchers*	1 Glass/125ml	80	0.0	64	0.0	1.6	0.0	0.0
Rose, Sparkling, Average	1 Sm Glass/125ml	102	0.0	82	0.0	2.5	0.0	0.0
Rose, The Pink Chill, Co-Op*	1 Glass/125ml	85	0.0	68	0.0	0.0	0.0	0.0
Rose, Vie, Low Alcohol, Blossom Hill*	1 Glass/175ml	93	0.0	53	0.0	3.9	0.0	0.0
Rose, Weight Watchers*	1 Bottle/187ml	112	0.2	60	0.1	1.8	0.1	0.1
Rose, White Grenache, Blossom Hill*	1 Sm Glass/125ml	105	0.0	84	0.0	3.2	0.0	0.0
Rose, White Zinfandel, Ernest & Julio Gallo*	1 Glass/125ml	101	0.0	81	0.2	2.7	0.0	0.0
Sangria, Average	1 Glass/125ml	95	0.0	76	0.1	9.9	0.0	0.1
Strong Ale Barley	1 Can/440ml	290	0.0	66	0.7	6.1	0.0	0.0
White, Average	1 Sm Glass/125ml	95	0.0	76	0.0	2.4	0.0	0.0
White, Californian, Chardonnay, LC, Tesco*	1 Bottle/181ml	96	0.0	53	0.0	1.8	0.0	0.0
White, Chardonnay, Low Alcohol, McGuigan*	1 Glass/125ml	75	0.1	60	0.1	2.2	0.1	0.0
White, Chardonnay, Southern Australia, Kissing Tree*	1 Bottle/185ml	85	0.0	46	0.0	0.0	0.0	0.0
White, Chenin Blanc, 12% Abv, Average	1 Sm Glass/125ml	101	0.0	81	0.1	3.3	0.0	0.0

INFO/WEIGHT	Measure INFO/WEIGHT	per Measure KCAL	per Measure FAT	Nutrition Values per 100g / 100ml KCAL	PROT	CARB	FAT	FIBRE
WINE								
White, Dry, Average	**1 Glass/125ml**	**88**	**0.0**	**70**	**0.1**	**0.6**	**0.0**	**0.0**
White, Fume Blanc, 13.1% Abv, Average	1 Sm Glass/125ml	104	0.0	83	0.1	2.3	0.0	0.0
White, Gewurztraminer, 12.6% Abv, Average	1 Sm Glass/125ml	102	0.0	82	0.1	2.6	0.0	0.0
White, Late Harvest, 10.6% Abv, Average	1 Sm Glass/125ml	141	0.0	113	0.1	13.4	0.0	0.0
White, Medium, Average	**1 Sm Glass/125ml**	**92**	**0.0**	**74**	**0.1**	**3.0**	**0.0**	**0.0**
White, Muller-Thurgau, 11.3% Abv, Average	1 Sm Glass/125ml	96	0.0	77	0.1	3.5	0.0	0.0
White, Muscat, 11% Abv, Average	1 Sm Glass/125ml	104	0.0	83	0.1	5.2	0.0	0.0
White, Non Alcoholic, Ame*	1 Sm Glass/125ml	48	0.0	38	0.0	9.5	0.0	0.0
White, Pinot Blanc, 13.3% Abv, Average	1 Sm Glass/125ml	102	0.0	82	0.1	0.0	0.0	0.0
White, Pinot Grigio, 13.4% Abv, Average	1 Sm Glass/125ml	105	0.0	84	0.1	2.1	0.0	0.0
White, Riesling, 11.9% Abv, Average	1 Sm Glass/125ml	101	0.0	81	0.1	3.7	0.0	0.0
White, Sauvignon Blanc, 13.1% Abv, Average	1 Sm Glass/125ml	102	0.0	82	0.1	2.0	0.0	0.0
White, Semillon, 12.5% Abv, Average	1 Sm Glass/125ml	104	0.0	83	0.1	3.1	0.0	0.0
White, Sparkling, Average	**1 Sm Glass/125ml**	**92**	**0.0**	**74**	**0.3**	**5.1**	**0.0**	**0.0**
White, Sweet, Average	**1 Glass/120ml**	**113**	**0.0**	**94**	**0.2**	**5.9**	**0.0**	**0.0**
WINE GUMS								
Average	1 Sweet/6g	19	0.0	315	5.0	73.4	0.2	0.1
Haribo*	1 Pack/175g	609	0.4	348	0.1	86.4	0.2	0.4
Light, Maynards*	1 Pack/42g	90	0.1	215	4.6	48.0	0.2	27.9
Mini, Rowntree's*	1 Bag/36g	125	0.0	348	6.7	80.5	0.0	0.0
Sour, Bassett's*	¼ Bag/50g	160	0.0	319	3.7	78.0	0.0	0.0
WISPA								
Bite, with Biscuit in Caramel, Cadbury*	1 Bar/47g	240	13.4	510	6.4	56.9	28.6	0.0
Cadbury*	1 Bar/40g	210	12.9	525	6.8	53.0	32.2	0.8
Gold, Cadbury*	1 Bar/52g	265	15.1	510	5.3	56.0	29.0	0.7
WONTON								
Prawn, Crispy from Selection, Modern Asian, M&S*	1 Wonton/25g	65	3.3	250	9.5	23.4	12.7	2.0
Prawn, Dim Sum Selection, Sainsbury's*	1 Wonton/10g	26	1.2	259	11.3	26.8	11.8	1.3
Prawn, Oriental Selection, Waitrose*	1 Wonton/18g	45	2.0	252	9.1	29.2	11.0	1.1
Prawn, Oriental Snack Selection, Sainsbury's*	1 Wonton/20g	53	2.7	265	10.6	25.6	13.4	2.0
WOTSITS								
Baked, Really Cheesy, Walkers*	1 Bag/23g	123	7.4	547	5.5	56.0	33.0	1.1
BBQ, Walkers*	1 Bag/21g	108	6.3	515	4.5	57.0	30.0	1.3
Flamin' Hot, Walkers*	1 Bag/19g	101	5.7	532	5.5	60.0	30.0	1.1
Prawn Cocktail, Walkers*	1 Bag/19g	99	5.7	522	4.5	58.0	30.0	1.1
Really Cheesy, Big Eat, Walkers*	1 Bag/36g	197	11.9	547	5.5	56.0	33.0	1.1
WRAP								
Bean, Mexican, Three, M&S*	1 Pack/188g	405	19.2	215	6.9	24.3	10.2	2.2
Bean & Cheese, Average	1 Pack/200g	365	13.5	182	7.4	22.6	6.8	2.5
Bean & Cheese, Tesco*	1 Pack/105g	235	9.4	224	7.0	28.6	9.0	1.0
Bean & Cheese, Three, Co-Op*	1 Pack/201g	392	11.3	195	8.1	26.7	5.6	3.4
Beef, Chilli, COU, M&S*	1 Pack/179g	268	2.9	150	10.1	23.4	1.6	2.6
Beef, Fajita, Boots*	1 Pack/200g	352	8.4	176	9.5	25.5	4.2	3.2
Beef, in Black Bean, M&S*	1 Pack/150g	338	17.1	225	10.2	20.5	11.4	1.6
Beef & Duck, Mouli with Salad, Eat Well, M&S*	1 Pack/88g	48	0.4	55	4.6	7.8	0.4	1.3
Butternut Squash, COU, M&S*	1 Pack/182g	245	4.7	135	4.3	22.2	2.6	2.9
Chicken, Barbecue, Shapers, Boots*	1 Pack/181g	283	4.9	156	10.0	23.0	2.7	3.3
Chicken, BBQ Steak, Hoisin Duck, Selection, M&S*	1 Pack/334g	685	23.7	205	10.9	24.3	7.1	1.7
Chicken, Cajun, Sandwich King*	1 Pack/138g	386	19.9	279	12.3	25.0	14.4	0.0
Chicken, Cajun, Tesco*	1 Pack/184g	415	16.6	225	9.8	25.1	9.0	1.9
Chicken, Chargrilled, PB, Waitrose*	1 Pack/230g	361	6.7	157	10.3	22.7	2.9	2.9
Chicken, Chilli, BGTY, Sainsbury's*	1 Pack/180g	313	4.3	174	10.2	28.0	2.4	0.0
Chicken, Coronation, Waitrose*	1 Pack/164g	283	8.3	173	10.1	21.3	5.1	2.2

W

WRAP

INFO/WEIGHT	Measure	per Measure		Nutrition Values per 100g / 100ml				
		KCAL	FAT	KCAL	PROT	CARB	FAT	FIBRE
Chicken, M&S*	1 Pack/247g	530	24.9	215	8.2	23.4	10.1	1.6
Chicken, Mediterranean Style, Waitrose*	1 Pack/183g	296	11.0	162	8.3	18.6	6.0	2.3
Chicken, Mexican, M&S*	1 Serving/218g	447	22.5	205	8.6	19.7	10.3	1.3
Chicken, Mexican Style, Co-Op*	1 Pack/163g	367	14.7	225	11.0	26.0	9.0	3.0
Chicken, Moroccan, BGTY, Sainsbury's*	1 Pack/207g	315	3.1	152	9.4	25.3	1.5	0.0
Chicken, Nacho, COU, M&S*	1 Pack/175g	280	4.2	160	10.2	24.4	2.4	2.0
Chicken, Sweet Chilli, Shapers, Boots*	1 Pack/195g	302	3.7	155	10.0	24.0	1.9	3.0
Chicken, Sweet Chilli, Waitrose*	1 Pack/200g	390	14.7	195	10.2	22.0	7.4	2.4
Chicken, Tandoori, GFY, Asda*	1 Pack/167g	281	4.5	168	10.0	26.0	2.7	1.7
Chicken, Tandoori Style, Good Intentions, Somerfield*	1 Pack/175g	299	2.4	171	10.9	28.8	1.4	1.6
Chicken, Tortilla, Asda*	1 Pack/125g	252	2.2	202	9.6	36.9	1.8	3.3
Chicken & Bacon, Caesar, COU, M&S*	1 Pack/170g	260	4.2	153	10.6	22.0	2.5	2.1
Chicken & Bacon, Caesar Salad, Asda*	1 Pack/160g	565	35.2	353	18.0	20.8	22.0	0.9
Chicken & Bacon, Simple Solutions, Tesco*	1 Pack/300g	474	23.4	158	20.7	1.2	7.8	0.5
Chicken & Bacon, with Cheese, Asda*	1 Pack/164g	366	21.3	223	25.0	1.4	13.0	0.0
Chicken Caesar, Ginsters*	1 Pack/180g	440	21.1	244	11.1	23.5	11.7	1.8
Chicken Caesar, Tesco*	1 Pack/215g	516	24.3	240	11.6	23.0	11.3	1.2
Chicken Caesar, Weight Watchers*	1 Pack/173g	298	4.7	172	11.2	24.5	2.7	1.3
Chicken Fajita, Asda*	1 Pack/180g	369	16.9	205	9.4	20.6	9.4	0.4
Chicken Fajita, PB, Waitrose*	1 Serving/218g	368	5.7	169	10.5	26.0	2.6	1.9
Chicken Fajita, Shapers, Boots*	1 Pack/216g	291	5.2	135	14.0	15.0	2.4	3.1
Chicken Fajita, Tesco*	1 Pack/220g	407	11.7	185	10.6	23.2	5.3	1.8
Chicken Fajita, VLH Kitchens	1 Serving/170g	311	3.1	183	10.6	25.0	5.2	0.0
Chicken Salad, Roast, Sainsbury's*	1 Pack/214g	443	19.9	207	10.0	20.9	9.3	2.5
Chicken Tikka, Average	1 Wrap/200g	403	15.1	202	9.5	23.6	7.6	4.4
Chicken Tikka, Masala, Patak's*	1 Pack/150g	252	9.9	168	7.8	19.3	6.6	0.0
Duck, Food to Go, M&S*	1 Pack/257g	475	13.9	185	8.5	25.5	5.4	1.0
Duck, Hoi Sin, Delicious, Boots*	1 Pack/160g	295	4.3	184	11.0	28.0	2.7	2.0
Duck, Hoisin, M&S*	1 Pack/225g	405	8.3	180	8.4	27.7	3.7	1.5
Duck, Hoisin, No Mayo, Triple, Tesco*	1 Pack/270g	620	18.6	230	9.3	30.7	6.9	2.3
Duck, Peking, Asda*	1 Pack/195g	406	11.1	208	10.3	27.9	5.7	2.1
Duck, Peking, Average	1 Serving/183g	356	10.5	194	9.2	26.6	5.7	1.1
Egg Mayonnaise, Tomato & Cress, Sainsbury's*	1 Pack/255g	592	38.2	232	7.3	17.7	15.0	0.0
Feta Salad, Greek, Shapers, Boots*	1 Pack/158g	241	5.7	153	6.4	24.0	3.6	1.2
Goats Cheese, & Grilled Pepper, Asda*	1 Serving/75g	194	11.2	259	5.0	26.0	15.0	2.1
Ham, Cheese & Pickle Tortilla, Weight Watchers*	1 Pack/170g	296	4.8	174	10.9	26.4	2.8	1.2
Houmous & Chargrilled Vegetables, Shapers, Boots*	1 Pack/186g	301	5.0	162	5.8	29.0	2.7	3.2
King Prawn, Shapers, Boots*	1 Pack/154g	227	2.2	147	9.2	24.0	1.4	2.1
Lamb, Minted, Darwins Deli*	1 Pack/250g	287	6.3	115	3.2	19.9	2.5	0.0
Pork, Caribbean Spicy, Ginsters*	1 Pack/150g	396	13.6	264	11.3	34.1	9.1	2.3
Prawn & Rocket, Shapers, Boots*	1 Wrap/159g	218	4.1	137	7.6	19.0	2.6	3.0
Salmon, Smoked, Finest, Tesco*	1 Pack/58g	113	8.4	194	15.5	0.6	14.4	0.3
Steak Fajita, Delicatessen, Waitrose*	1 Pack/232g	489	21.1	211	10.5	22.7	9.1	2.7
Tuna, Sweetcorn & Red Pepper, BGTY, Sainsbury's*	1 Pack/178g	306	8.2	172	11.5	21.2	4.6	2.1
Tuna Nicoise, BGTY, Sainsbury's*	1 Pack/181g	273	7.1	151	11.0	18.0	3.9	0.0
Turkey, Bacon & Cranberry, COU, M&S*	1 Pack/144g	230	2.2	160	9.6	27.1	1.5	2.3
Vegetable, & Feta, Roasted, BGTY, Sainsbury's*	1 Serving/200g	318	8.0	159	5.8	25.0	4.0	0.0

	Measure INFO/WEIGHT	per Measure		Nutrition Values per 100g / 100ml				
		KCAL	FAT	KCAL	PROT	CARB	FAT	FIBRE
YAM								
Baked	1oz/28g	43	0.1	153	2.1	37.5	0.4	1.7
Boiled, Average	1oz/28g	37	0.1	133	1.7	33.0	0.3	1.4
Raw	1oz/28g	32	0.1	114	1.5	28.2	0.3	1.3
YEAST								
Dried, Average	1 Tbsp/6g	10	0.1	169	35.6	3.5	1.5	0.0
Extract	1 Tsp/9g	16	0.0	180	40.7	3.5	0.4	0.0
YOFU								
Natural, Alpro*	1 Pot/500g	230	11.5	46	4.0	2.1	2.3	1.0
YOGHURT								
0.1% Fat, Lidl*	1 Pot/150g	118	0.2	79	4.0	15.6	0.1	0.0
Activia, Danone*	1 Pot/132g	125	4.2	94	3.5	12.8	3.2	2.0
Apple, Bramble, Virtually Fat Free, Longley Farm*	1 Pot/150g	118	0.2	79	5.5	13.9	0.1	0.0
Apple, Light, Muller*	1 Pot/175g	94	0.2	54	4.4	9.0	0.1	0.0
Apple & Berry Pie, Dessert Recipe, Weight Watchers*	1 Pot/120g	58	0.1	49	4.1	6.8	0.1	0.3
Apple & Cinnamon, Dessert, Low Fat, Sainsbury's*	1 Pot/125g	115	2.1	92	4.5	14.7	1.7	0.1
Apple & Cinnamon Farmhouse, Twekkelo*	1 Bowl/125g	142	4.1	114	4.1	17.0	3.3	0.4
Apple & Cranberry, Bio, Fat Free, Shape, Danone*	1 Pot/120g	86	0.1	72	4.2	13.5	0.1	0.0
Apple & Elderflower, Bio Live, Low Fat, Rachel's Organic*	1 Serving/70g	62	1.1	88	4.0	16.0	1.6	0.0
Apple & Peach, Oatie Breakfast, Moma Foods*	1 Pot/234g	309	5.6	132	4.3	24.3	2.4	1.7
Apple & Pear, Low Fat, Sainsbury's*	1 Pot/125g	115	1.9	92	4.3	15.2	1.5	0.2
Apple & Pear Crumble, Dessert Recipe, Weight Watchers*	1 Pot/120g	59	0.1	49	4.1	7.1	0.1	0.2
Apple & Prune, Fat Free, Yeo Valley*	1 Pot/125g	98	0.1	78	5.1	14.1	0.1	0.2
Apple & Spice Bio, Virtually Fat Free, Shape, Danone*	1 Pot/120g	67	0.1	56	5.6	7.3	0.1	0.2
Apple Pie, Simply Desserts, Muller*	1 Pot/175g	278	8.0	159	4.6	24.7	4.6	0.7
Apricot, Bio, Low Fat, Benecol*	1 Pot/125g	98	0.8	78	3.9	14.3	0.6	0.0
Apricot, Bio Activia, Danone*	1 Pot/125g	121	4.0	97	3.7	13.3	3.2	1.7
Apricot, Fat Free, Activ8, Ski, Nestle*	1 Pot/120g	88	0.8	73	4.5	13.6	0.7	0.2
Apricot, Fat Free, Bio Live, Rachel's Organic*	1 Pot/142g	81	0.1	57	3.5	10.5	0.1	0.0
Apricot, Fat Free, Weight Watchers*	1 Pot/150g	62	0.2	42	4.1	4.9	0.1	0.2
Apricot, Fruity, Mullerlight, Muller*	1 Pot/175g	88	0.2	50	4.2	7.5	0.1	0.1
Apricot, Honeyed, Greek Style, Corner, Muller*	1 Pot/150g	168	4.5	112	5.0	15.5	3.0	0.1
Apricot, Light, Fat Free, Muller*	1 Pot/190g	93	0.2	49	4.1	7.3	0.1	0.1
Apricot, Low Fat, Organic, Average	1 Serving/100g	84	1.0	84	5.8	13.3	1.0	0.6
Apricot, Low Fat, Tesco*	1 Pot/125g	112	2.2	90	4.3	14.1	1.8	0.0
Apricot, Pro Activ, Flora*	1 Pot/125g	70	0.6	56	4.0	7.9	0.5	1.8
Apricot, Smooth Set French, Sainsbury's*	1 Pot/125g	100	1.5	80	3.5	13.6	1.2	0.0
Apricot & Mango, 25% Extra Fruit, Low Fat, Asda*	1 Pot/125g	120	1.4	96	4.6	17.0	1.1	0.0
Apricot & Mango, Low Fat, Tesco*	1 Pot/125g	126	2.2	101	4.9	16.3	1.8	0.0
Apricot & Mango, Thick & Creamy, Sainsbury's*	1 Pot/150g	178	5.4	119	4.3	17.3	3.6	0.2
Apricot & Mango, Tropical Fruit, Activ8, Ski, Nestle*	1 Pot/120g	112	2.0	93	4.3	15.1	1.7	0.2
Apricot & Nectarine, Sunshine Selection, Sainsbury's*	1 Pot/125g	115	1.9	92	4.4	15.3	1.5	0.1
Apricot & Passion Fruit, Fat Free, Yeo Valley*	1 Pot/125g	94	0.1	75	5.3	13.2	0.1	0.1
Aux Fruit Mixés, Brassé, Carrefour*	1 Pot/125g	118	2.6	94	4.2	14.6	2.1	0.0
Banana, Custard Style, Asda*	1 Pot/150g	224	9.0	149	3.7	20.0	6.0	0.2
Banana, Low Fat, Average	1 Serving/100g	98	1.4	98	4.6	16.7	1.4	0.1
Banana & Custard, Smooth, Mullerlight, Muller*	1 Pot/175g	94	0.2	54	4.1	8.6	0.1	0.6
Banana & Peach, Probiotic, Goat's Milk, Glenisk*	1 Serving/100g	51	3.6	51	4.0	12.9	3.6	0.0
Banana Choco Flakes, Crunch Corner, Muller*	1 Pot/135g	193	6.9	143	4.3	19.3	5.1	0.3
Banana Smooth, M&S*	1 Pot/150g	165	2.6	110	4.8	19.3	1.7	0.2
Banoffee, Snackpot, Activia, Danone*	1 Pot/155g	116	0.2	75	5.0	13.3	0.1	0.3
Bio, Low Fat, Spelga*	1 Pot/125g	125	2.1	100	3.9	17.0	1.7	0.0
Black Cherry, Average	1 Serving/100g	96	2.2	96	3.4	16.5	2.2	0.1
Black Cherry, Extremely Fruity, Bio, M&S*	1 Pot/150g	165	2.2	110	4.9	18.4	1.5	0.2

Y

YOGHURT

Measure INFO/WEIGHT		per Measure KCAL	per Measure FAT	Nutrition Values per 100g / 100ml KCAL	PROT	CARB	FAT	FIBRE
Black Cherry, Extremely Fruity, Low Fat Probiotic, M&S*	1 Pot/170g	162	1.7	95	4.4	17.2	1.0	0.5
Black Cherry, Extremely Fruity, M&S*	1 Pot/200g	220	3.0	110	4.9	18.4	1.5	0.2
Black Cherry, Fat Free, Benecol*	1 Pot/120g	78	0.6	65	3.0	11.0	0.5	2.1
Black Cherry, Greek Style, Corner, Muller*	1 Pot/150g	172	4.5	115	5.0	16.2	3.0	0.1
Black Cherry, Low Fat, Average	1 Serving/100g	69	0.6	69	3.8	12.2	0.6	0.3
Black Cherry, Low Fat, Value, Tesco*	1 Serving/125g	95	0.9	76	3.0	14.2	0.7	0.6
Black Cherry, Thick & Creamy, Waitrose*	1 Pot/125g	139	3.1	111	3.7	18.3	2.5	0.4
Black Cherry, Virtually Fat Free, Longley Farm Yoghurt*	1 Pot/150g	116	0.2	77	4.5	14.4	0.1	0.0
Black Cherry, VLH Kitchens	1 Serving/150g	188	2.5	125	3.7	19.6	3.7	1.0
Blackberry, Fat Free, Danone, Shape*	1 Pot/120g	74	0.2	62	6.7	8.4	0.2	2.4
Blackberry, Soya, Alpro Soya*	1 Pot/125g	91	2.6	73	3.7	9.2	2.1	1.2
Blackberry, Zero% Fat, No Added Sugar, Shape, Danone*	1 Pot/120g	73	0.2	61	6.0	8.9	0.2	1.0
Blackberry & Raspberry, Fruit Corner, Muller*	1 Pot/150g	158	5.8	105	3.8	13.1	3.9	0.9
Blackcurrant, Bio Live, Rachel's Organic*	1 Serving/225g	166	3.8	74	3.6	11.0	1.7	0.0
Blackcurrant, Extra Special, Asda*	1 Pot/100g	163	9.0	163	2.6	18.0	9.0	0.0
Blackcurrant, Fruity, Mullerlight, Muller*	1 Pot/175g	89	0.2	51	4.1	7.9	0.1	0.8
Blackcurrant, Garden Fruits, Low Fat, Tesco*	1 Pot/125g	120	2.4	95	3.8	15.1	1.9	0.3
Blackcurrant, Longley Farm*	1 Pot/150g	168	5.6	112	4.9	14.7	3.7	0.0
Blackcurrant, Low Fat, CBY, Asda*	1 Pot/125g	104	1.6	83	3.6	14.2	1.3	0.6
Blackcurrant, Low Fat, Sainsbury's*	1 Pot/125g	116	1.8	93	4.2	15.9	1.4	0.6
Blackcurrant, Probiotic, Organic, Yeo Valley*	1 Pot/150g	152	5.8	101	4.1	12.4	3.9	0.2
Blueberry, & Cream, Made Up, Easiyo*	1 Serving/100g	105	4.1	105	3.9	13.7	4.1	0.0
Blueberry, Bio, Co-Op*	1 Pot/125g	141	3.5	113	4.5	16.5	2.8	0.4
Blueberry, Extremely Fruity, Low Fat, Probiotic, M&S*	1 Pot/150g	142	2.1	95	4.7	14.7	1.4	1.5
Blueberry, Fat Free, Probiotic, Organic, Yeo Valley*	1 Serving/100g	73	0.1	73	5.1	12.9	0.1	0.4
Blueberry, Fruit Corner, Muller*	1 Pot/150g	156	5.7	104	3.8	12.9	3.8	0.4
Blueberry, Low Fat, Somerfield*	1 Pot/150g	130	1.5	87	4.0	16.0	1.0	0.0
Boysenberry, Low Fat, Yoplait*	1 Pot/100g	49	0.1	49	5.3	6.7	0.1	0.0
Butterscotch, English, Organic, Duchy Originals, Waitrose*	1 Pot/140g	187	7.3	134	5.2	16.5	5.2	0.0
Caramel, Smooth, Intensely Creamy, Activia, Danone*	1 Pot/165g	168	5.0	102	4.8	13.7	3.0	0.1
Cereals, Fibre, Bio Activia, Danone*	1 Pot/120g	119	4.1	99	3.7	13.5	3.4	3.0
Cherry, & Berry, Probiotic, You Count, Love Life, Waitrose*	1 Pot/130g	90	0.1	69	4.8	11.8	0.1	0.8
Cherry, 0% Fat, Yoplait*	1 Pot/125g	70	0.1	56	3.8	9.8	0.1	0.0
Cherry, 0.1% Fat, Shape, Danone*	1 Pot/120g	56	0.1	47	4.6	6.8	0.1	2.1
Cherry, Bakewell Tart Flavour, Muller*	1 Pot/175g	119	0.4	68	4.8	11.8	0.2	0.2
Cherry, Bio, Low Fat, Benecol*	1 Pot/150g	122	0.9	81	3.8	15.2	0.6	0.0
Cherry, Fat Free, Activia, Danone*	1 Pot/125g	76	0.1	61	4.8	9.8	0.1	0.9
Cherry, Fruit, Biopot, Onken*	1 Serving/100g	107	2.7	107	3.7	16.7	2.7	0.2
Cherry, Fruity, Mullerlight, Muller*	1 Pot/175g	86	0.2	49	4.3	7.0	0.1	0.2
Cherry, Greek Style, Shape, Danone*	1 Pot/125g	143	3.4	114	6.0	16.4	2.7	0.0
Cherry, Light, Fat Free, Muller*	1 Pot/175g	88	0.2	50	3.9	7.9	0.1	0.2
Cherry, Low Fat, Asda*	1 Pot/125g	120	1.4	96	4.6	17.0	1.1	0.0
Cherry, Low Fat, CBY, Asda*	1 Pot/125g	90	1.6	72	3.6	11.4	1.3	0.3
Cherry, Luscious, Intensely Creamy, Activia, Danone*	1 Pot/120g	116	3.6	97	4.8	12.7	3.0	0.2
Cherry, Pots, Probiotic, Yeo Valley*	1 Pot/119g	124	4.4	104	4.9	12.8	3.7	0.1
Chocolate, Seriously Smooth, Waitrose*	1 Pot/125g	158	3.0	126	6.0	20.1	2.4	0.1
Chocolate, Vitaline*	1 Pot/125g	102	0.6	82	3.5	15.8	0.5	0.0
Coconut, Biopot, Onken*	1 Pot/450g	562	23.4	125	3.9	15.6	5.2	0.9
Coconut, Malaysian, Thick & Creamy, Waitrose*	1 Pot/150g	242	15.9	161	3.9	12.6	10.6	0.3
Cranberry, Bio Activia, Danone*	1 Pot/125g	115	4.0	92	3.6	12.3	3.2	1.7
Cranberry & Blackcurrant, Bio, Fat Free, Shape, Danone*	1 Pot/120g	54	0.1	45	4.6	5.7	0.1	0.3
Eton Mess, British Classic, Corner, Muller*	1 Pot/135g	171	3.0	127	2.8	23.5	2.2	0.3
Exotic Fruits, French Set, Wholemilk, Asda*	1 Pot/125g	125	4.0	100	3.6	14.1	3.2	0.0

Y

YOGHURT

Measure INFO/WEIGHT		per Measure		Nutrition Values per 100g / 100ml				
		KCAL	FAT	KCAL	PROT	CARB	FAT	FIBRE
Fig, Bio, Activia, Danone*	1 Pot/125g	121	4.0	97	3.7	13.3	3.2	1.6
Forest Fruits, 0.1% Fat, Shape, Danone*	1 Pot/120g	55	0.1	46	4.6	6.7	0.1	2.1
Forest Fruits, Bio, Fat Free, Activia, Danone*	1 Pot/125g	72	0.1	58	4.5	8.9	0.1	1.1
French Style, Whole Milk, Smooth Set, Tesco*	1 Pot/125g	122	3.8	98	3.6	14.1	3.0	0.0
Fruit, Brooklea*	1 Pot/120g	97	0.1	81	2.7	15.0	0.1	0.0
Fruit, Garden, Wholemilk, Bio Live, Rachel's Organic*	1 Pot/125g	109	4.2	87	3.5	10.5	3.4	0.0
Fruit, Low Fat, Average	1 Pot/125g	112	0.9	90	4.1	17.9	0.7	0.0
Fruit, Luscious, Bio Live, Low Fat, Rachel's Organic*	1 Pot/125g	115	2.0	92	4.0	15.3	1.6	0.0
Fruit, Whole Milk	1 Pot/150g	158	4.2	105	5.1	15.7	2.8	0.0
Fruit, with Cherries, Bio, 0% Fat, Danone*	1 Pot/125g	65	0.1	52	3.6	9.1	0.1	0.0
Fruits of the Forest, Iced, Linessa, Lidl*	1 Pot/170g	168	3.9	99	2.5	17.0	2.3	0.0
Fruits of the Forest, Nestle*	1 Pot/125g	122	2.0	98	3.4	16.7	1.6	0.0
Fruity Favourites, Organic, Yeo Valley*	1 Pot/125g	126	4.9	101	4.1	12.4	3.9	0.2
Fudge, Devonshire Style, Finest, Tesco*	1 Pot/150g	281	13.8	187	3.7	22.4	9.2	0.0
Fudge, Thick & Creamy, Co-Op*	1 Pot/150g	196	7.5	131	3.8	17.6	5.0	0.0
Ginger, Greek Style, Bio Live, Rachel's Organic*	1 Serving/100g	134	7.1	134	3.2	14.3	7.1	0.0
Goats, Whole Milk	**1 Carton/150g**	**94**	**5.7**	**63**	**3.5**	**3.9**	**3.8**	**0.0**
Gooseberry, Bio Live, Rachel's Organic*	1 Pot/450g	450	15.3	100	4.0	13.3	3.4	0.2
Gooseberry, Garden Fruits, Low Fat, Tesco*	1 Pot/125g	115	2.4	90	3.3	14.9	1.9	0.3
Gooseberry, Low Fat, Average	1 Serving/100g	90	1.4	90	4.5	14.5	1.4	0.0
Gooseberry, Low Fat, CBY, Asda*	1 Pot/125g	102	1.8	82	3.6	13.7	1.4	0.0
Gooseberry, Luxury Farmhouse, Stapleton*	1 Yogurt/150g	132	3.8	88	3.3	13.7	2.5	0.7
Gooseberry, Virtually Fat Free, Longley Farm*	1 Pot/150g	122	0.2	81	4.2	15.7	0.1	0.0
Greek, 0% Fat, Strained, Authentic, Total, Fage*	¼ Pot/125g	71	0.0	57	10.3	4.0	0.0	0.0
Greek, 2% Fat, Strained, Authentic, Total, Fage*	1 Pot/170g	124	3.4	73	9.9	3.8	2.0	0.0
Greek, Strained, Authentic, Original, Total, Fage*	1 Pot/170g	163	8.5	96	9.0	3.8	5.0	0.0
Greek, with Blueberries, 0%, Total, Fage*	1 Serving/150g	123	0.0	82	8.3	12.3	0.0	0.0
Greek, with Honey, Strained, Authentic, Total, Fage*	1 Pot/150g	255	12.0	170	5.4	19.0	8.0	0.0
Greek, with Strawberry, 2% Fat, Total, Fage*	1 Pot/150g	140	2.4	93	6.7	12.9	1.6	0.0
Greek & Cranberry, Made Up, Easiyo*	1 Serving/100g	113	4.7	113	4.0	14.1	4.7	0.1
Greek 'n Coconut, Made Up, Easiyo*	1 Serving/100g	113	4.7	113	4.0	14.1	4.7	0.1
Greek Style, & Granola, Sainsbury's*	1 Pot/140g	262	7.6	187	5.8	29.0	5.4	0.6
Greek Style, Creamy, Eridanous, Lidl*	1 Pot/1000g	1260	105.0	126	5.0	2.8	10.5	0.00
Greek Style, Fat Free, Natural, CBY, Asda*	1 Tub/200g	114	0.4	57	7.9	5.8	0.2	0.1
Greek Style, Low Fat, M&S*	1 Serving/100g	75	2.7	75	6.1	6.9	2.7	0.5
Greek Style, Luscious Lemon, Fat Free, Light, Muller*	1 Pot/120g	83	0.2	69	6.3	9.7	0.2	0.0
Greek Style, Luxury, Loseley*	1 Pot/175g	226	17.8	129	4.8	4.5	10.2	0.0
Greek Style, Tempting Toffee, Muller Light *	1 Pot/120g	84	0.1	70	6.3	10.1	0.1	0.0
Greek Style, with Golden Honey, Activia, Danone*	1 Pack/126g	122	3.5	97	5.0	13.0	2.8	0.1
Greek Style with Black Cherry Compote, M&S*	1 Pot/241g	205	3.4	85	3.4	15.0	1.4	0.5
Greek Style with Honey, Asda*	1 Pot/150g	237	12.6	158	3.8	16.9	8.4	0.0
Greek Style with Strawberries, Asda*	1 Pot/125g	159	8.2	127	3.2	13.6	6.6	0.2
Greek Style with Strawberry, Morrisons*	1 Pot/125g	162	8.2	130	3.3	14.4	6.6	0.0
Guava & Orange, Fat Free, Organic, Yeo Valley*	1 Pot/125g	92	0.1	74	5.3	13.0	0.1	0.2
Hazelnut, Longley Farm*	1 Pot/150g	201	8.5	134	5.5	16.0	5.7	0.0
Hazelnut, Sainsbury's*	1 Serving/150g	183	3.4	122	5.0	20.3	2.3	0.2
Honey, Greek Style, Organic, Sainsbury's*	1 Pot/100g	156	8.7	156	4.1	15.3	8.7	0.1
Honey, Layered, Greek Style, Shapers, Boots*	1 Pot/150g	136	3.0	91	4.2	14.0	2.0	0.0
Honey, Low Fat, Asda*	1 Pot/125g	130	1.4	104	4.6	19.0	1.1	0.0
Honey & Ginger, Waitrose*	1 Pot/150g	240	12.9	160	3.8	16.8	8.6	0.1
Honey & Muesli, Breakfast Break, Tesco*	1 Pot/170g	207	4.6	122	3.9	20.5	2.7	0.6
Honey Breakfast Pot, Activia, Danone*	1 Pot/160g	192	4.2	120	4.9	18.8	2.6	0.7
Kiwi, Activia, Danone*	1 Pot/125g	119	4.1	95	3.6	12.7	3.3	0.3

Y

	Measure INFO/WEIGHT	per Measure KCAL	FAT	Nutrition Values per 100g / 100ml KCAL	PROT	CARB	FAT	FIBRE
YOGHURT								
Kiwi, Cereal, Fibre, Bio Activia, Danone*	1 Pot/120g	124	4.0	103	3.8	14.5	3.3	3.0
Lemon, Greek Style, GFY, Asda*	1 Pot/150g	124	4.4	83	4.1	10.0	2.9	0.1
Lemon, Greek Style, Shape, Danone*	1 Pot/125g	140	3.4	112	5.9	15.9	2.7	0.0
Lemon, Italian, Amore Luxury, Muller*	1 Pot/150g	219	11.7	146	2.8	16.2	7.8	0.1
Lemon, Low Fat, Average	1 Serving/100g	95	0.9	95	4.6	17.3	0.9	0.1
Lemon, Thick & Fruity, Citrus Fruits, Weight Watchers*	1 Pot/120g	47	0.1	39	4.1	4.9	0.1	0.9
Lemon, Zesty, Intensely Creamy, Activia, Danone*	1 Pot/120g	119	3.6	99	4.8	13.3	3.0	0.1
Lemon & Lime, BGTY, Sainsbury's*	1 Pot/125g	66	0.1	53	4.6	8.3	0.1	1.1
Lemon & Lime, Fat Free, Shape, Danone*	1 Pot/120g	61	0.1	51	4.5	7.3	0.1	0.1
Lemon Cheesecake, Inspired, Corner, Muller*	1 Pot/135g	201	6.2	149	3.6	22.7	4.6	0.0
Lemon Curd, Indulgent, Dessert, Waitrose*	1 Pot/150g	278	13.8	185	4.1	21.5	9.2	0.0
Lemon Curd, West Country, TTD, Sainsbury's*	1 Pot/150g	243	10.0	162	3.7	21.6	6.7	0.5
Lemon Curd, Whole Milk, Yeo Valley*	1 Pot/120g	153	5.3	128	4.8	17.2	4.4	0.2
Lemon Curd with West Country Cream, Morrisons*	1 Pot/150g	244	12.7	163	3.4	17.9	8.5	0.5
Lemon Lime Mousse, Shapers, Boots*	1 Pot/90g	89	3.8	99	4.2	11.0	4.2	0.1
Mandarin, Fat Free, Mullerlight, Muller*	1 Pot/175g	95	0.2	54	4.2	8.5	0.1	0.0
Mandarin, Longley Farm*	1 Pot/150g	141	5.7	94	4.9	13.3	3.8	0.0
Mandarin, Low Fat, Asda*	1 Pot/125g	101	1.5	81	4.6	13.0	1.2	0.0
Mango, Bio, Fat Free, Snackpot, Activia, Danone*	1 Pot/165g	86	0.2	52	4.8	8.1	0.1	0.2
Mango, Bio Activia, Danone*	1 Pot/125g	121	4.0	97	3.7	13.4	3.2	1.6
Mango, Fat Free, Shape Danone*	1 Pot/120g	74	0.1	62	6.6	8.6	0.1	2.2
Mango, Intensely Creamy, Activia, Danone*	1 Pot/125g	122	3.8	98	4.7	13.0	3.0	0.2
Mango, Light, Muller*	1 Pot/175g	96	0.2	55	4.3	9.2	0.1	0.0
Mango, Papaya & Passion Fruit, Biopot, Onken*	1/5 Pot/90g	92	2.4	102	3.7	15.6	2.7	0.2
Mango, Tropical Fruit, Thick & Fruity, Weight Watchers*	1 Pot/120g	49	0.1	41	3.9	6.0	0.1	1.1
Mango, Zer0% Fat, No Added Sugar, Shape, Danone*	1 Pot/120g	72	0.1	60	6.0	8.8	0.1	0.9
Mango & Apple, Fat Free, Onken*	1 Serving/150g	132	0.2	88	4.4	16.0	0.1	0.2
Mango & Passion Fruit, Creamy, Nom Dairy UK*	1 Pot/175g	189	6.6	108	3.1	15.4	3.8	0.3
Mango & Passionfruit, Fruit Corner, Muller*	1 Yoghurt/150g	160	5.8	107	3.8	13.5	3.9	0.3
Mango 0% Fat, Shape Delights*	1 Pot/120g	80	0.1	67	5.5	10.9	0.1	0.9
Muesli Nut, Low Fat	1 Pot/120g	134	2.6	112	5.0	19.2	2.2	0.0
Natural, 0.1% Fat, Stirred, Biopot, Onken*	1 Serving/100g	48	0.1	48	5.4	6.4	0.1	0.0
Natural, Bio, BFY, Morrisons*	1 Serving/100g	65	0.2	65	6.5	9.4	0.2	0.0
Natural, Bio, Co-Op*	1 Pot/150g	117	5.4	78	4.8	5.5	3.6	0.0
Natural, Bio, LC, Tesco*	1 Serving/100g	55	0.1	55	5.4	7.6	0.1	0.0
Natural, Bio, Low Fat, Sainsbury's*	1 Serving/100g	48	1.5	48	4.0	4.6	1.5	0.0
Natural, Bio Activia, Individual Pots, Danone*	1 Pot/125g	86	4.2	69	4.2	5.5	3.4	0.0
Natural, Bio Life, Easiyo*	1 Pot/150g	95	2.7	63	5.0	6.7	1.8	0.0
Natural, Bio Live, Low Fat, Organic, Waitrose*	1/4 Pot/125g	81	1.2	65	5.8	8.3	1.0	0.0
Natural, Bio Live, Very Low Fat, Ann Forshaw's*	1 Pot/125g	52	0.1	42	5.0	5.5	0.1	0.0
Natural, Bio Set, Low Fat, Sainsbury's*	1 Pot/150g	78	2.2	52	3.9	5.7	1.5	0.0
Natural, Danone*	1 Pot/125g	71	3.6	57	3.2	3.8	2.9	0.0
Natural, Fat Free, Biopot, Dr Oetker*	1/4 Pot/125g	60	0.1	48	5.4	6.4	0.1	0.0
Natural, Fat Free, Eat Smart, Morrisons*	1 Pot/150g	88	0.3	59	7.0	7.2	0.2	0.0
Natural, Fat Free, Onken*	1 Serving/100g	48	0.1	48	5.4	6.3	0.1	0.0
Natural, Fat Free, Probiotic, Essential, Waitrose*	1/4 Pot/125g	68	0.0	54	5.5	7.8	0.0	0.0
Natural, Fat Free, Rachel's Organic*	1 Pot/500g	180	0.5	36	3.9	4.8	0.1	0.0
Natural, Greek Style, Average	1 Serving/100g	138	10.6	138	4.7	6.1	10.6	0.0
Natural, Greek Style, BGTY, Sainsbury's*	1 Serving/50g	39	1.4	78	5.5	7.9	2.7	0.0
Natural, Greek Style, Bio Live, Rachel's Organic*	1 Pot/450g	518	40.5	115	3.6	4.9	9.0	0.0
Natural, Greek Style, Fat Free, Tesco*	1/2 Pot/100g	55	0.2	55	7.5	4.8	0.2	0.4
Natural, Greek Style, Low Fat, Asda*	1 Serving/30g	24	0.8	80	5.7	8.2	2.7	0.0
Natural, Greek Style, Low Fat, Average	1 Serving/100g	77	2.7	77	6.1	7.3	2.7	0.2

YOGHURT

	Measure INFO/WEIGHT	per Measure KCAL	FAT	Nutrition Values per 100g / 100ml KCAL	PROT	CARB	FAT	FIBRE
Natural, Greek Style, Probiotic, Unsweetened, M&S*	1 Serving/150g	195	15.2	130	5.5	4.6	10.1	0.1
Natural, Greek Style, with Cow's Milk, Tesco*	1 Pot/150g	214	16.4	143	4.5	6.6	10.9	0.0
Natural, Irish, Low Fat, Everyday Value, Tesco*	1 Serving/100g	45	0.2	45	5.5	5.0	0.2	0.5
Natural, Longley Farm*	1 Pot/150g	118	5.2	79	4.8	7.0	3.5	0.0
Natural, Low Fat, Average	*1 Pot/125g*	*75*	*1.6*	*60*	*5.4*	*7.0*	*1.3*	*0.0*
Natural, Low Fat, Bio, Co-Op*	1 Pot/150g	98	1.5	65	6.0	8.0	1.0	0.0
Natural, Low Fat, Bio, Sainsbury's*	1 Pot/125g	85	1.9	68	5.6	7.9	1.5	0.0
Natural, Low Fat, Live, Waitrose*	1 Pot/175g	114	1.8	65	5.8	8.2	1.0	0.0
Natural, Low Fat, Organic, Average	1 Serving/100g	87	1.2	87	5.7	7.7	1.2	0.0
Natural, Low Fat, Value, Tesco*	1 Pot/125g	81	1.9	65	5.0	7.2	1.5	0.0
Natural, Luxury, Bio Live, Jersey Dairy*	1 Pot/150g	225	12.0	150	4.6	8.2	8.0	0.0
Natural, Organic, Yeo Valley*	1 Pot/150g	120	5.6	80	4.7	6.9	3.7	0.0
Natural, Pouring, Activia, Danone*	1 Carton/950g	484	16.2	51	4.1	4.9	1.7	0.0
Natural, Probiotic, 0.1% Fat, BGTY, Sainsbury's*	1 Serving/125g	69	0.1	55	5.6	8.0	0.1	0.0
Natural, Probiotic, 2% Fat, Sainsbury's*	¼ Pot/125g	76	1.9	61	4.9	7.0	1.5	0.0
Natural, Probiotic, Crunchy Sultana Granola, M&S*	1 Pack/180g	306	9.9	170	6.6	23.6	5.5	0.7
Natural, Probiotic, Fat Free, Organic, Yeo Valley*	1 Pot/150g	87	0.2	58	5.9	8.4	0.1	0.0
Natural, Probiotic, Organic, Yeo Valley*	1 Pot/150g	124	6.4	82	4.5	6.6	4.2	0.0
Natural, Set, Asda*	1 Pot/450g	256	4.5	57	5.1	6.8	1.0	0.0
Natural, Simply More, M&S*	1 Serving/100g	85	3.4	85	5.3	7.9	3.4	0.5
Natural, Sojasun*	1 Serving/100g	51	2.7	51	4.6	2.0	2.7	0.0
Natural, Soya, Sojade*	1 Serving/100g	50	2.5	50	4.5	2.4	2.5	0.0
Natural, Whole Milk, Set, Biopot, Onken*	1 Serving/125g	85	4.4	68	4.5	4.1	3.5	0.0
Natural, Wholemilk, Live Bio, Organic, Waitrose*	1 Serving/100g	88	4.4	88	5.1	7.1	4.4	0.0
Natural, with Cow's Milk, Greek Style, Sainsbury's*	½ Pot/100g	143	10.9	143	4.5	6.6	10.9	0.0
Natural with Honey, Greek Style, Sainsbury's*	1 Pot/150g	243	14.1	162	4.0	15.4	9.4	0.0
Nectarine, Fat Free, Weight Watchers*	1 Pot/120g	48	0.1	40	4.1	4.7	0.1	0.4
Nectarine & Passion Fruit, 0.1% Fat, Shape, Danone*	1 Pot/120g	55	0.1	46	4.6	6.7	0.1	2.1
Nectarine & Passion Fruit, Low Fat, Stapleton Farm*	1 Pot/150g	120	0.8	80	3.2	16.3	0.5	0.6
Orange, Greek Style, Shape, Danone*	1 Pot/125g	140	3.4	112	6.0	16.0	2.7	0.1
Orange, Low Fat, Tesco*	1 Pot/125g	114	2.2	91	4.3	14.5	1.8	0.0
Orange, Sprinkled with Dark Chocolate, Light, Muller*	1 Pot/165g	91	0.8	55	4.3	7.4	0.5	0.1
Orange, Valencia, Seriously Fruity, Low Fat, Waitrose*	1 Pot/150g	147	1.5	98	4.3	18.0	1.0	0.3
Orange & Mango, Thick & Fruity, Probiotic, COU, M&S*	1 Pot/145g	65	0.1	45	4.2	6.5	0.1	0.5
Orange Chocolate, Crunch, Corner, Muller*	1 Pot/135g	204	6.5	151	3.4	23.1	4.8	0.7
Peach, Bio, Activia, Fat Free, Danone*	1 Pot/125g	71	0.1	57	4.7	9.3	0.1	1.0
Peach, Bio, Fat Free, Snackpot, Activia, Danone*	1 Pot/165g	99	0.2	60	4.6	10.2	0.1	1.0
Peach, Biopot, Wholegrain, Onken*	1 Serving/100g	114	2.8	114	4.0	17.8	2.8	0.5
Peach, Custard Style, Low Fat, Sainsbury's*	1 Pot/125g	110	1.9	88	4.4	14.2	1.5	0.1
Peach, Dairy Free, Organic, Yofu, Soya, Provamel*	1 Serving/125g	100	2.8	80	3.9	10.3	2.2	0.8
Peach, Fat Free, Activ8, Ski, Nestle*	1 Yogurt/120g	89	0.1	74	4.5	13.7	0.1	0.7
Peach, Forbidden Fruits, Rachel's Organic*	1 Pot/125g	156	7.6	125	3.4	14.0	6.1	0.0
Peach, Honeyed, Greek Style, Mullerlight, Muller*	1 Pot/120g	85	0.2	71	6.3	10.3	0.2	0.2
Peach, Low Fat, Average	1 Serving/100g	86	1.1	86	4.5	14.6	1.1	0.2
Peach, Luscious, Low Fat, Rachel's Organic*	1 Pot/125g	112	2.0	90	4.0	14.9	1.6	0.2
Peach, Smooth Style, Mullerlight, Muller*	1 Pot/125g	59	0.1	47	4.1	6.9	0.1	0.2
Peach & Apricot, 0.1% Fat, Shape, Danone*	1 Pot/120g	55	0.1	46	4.6	6.7	0.1	2.1
Peach & Apricot, Fruit Corner, Muller*	1 Pot/150g	160	5.7	107	3.9	13.5	3.8	0.5
Peach & Mango, 0.1% Actimel, Danone*	1 Serving/100g	29	0.1	29	2.7	3.6	0.1	0.1
Peach & Mango, Thick & Creamy, Waitrose*	1 Pot/125g	136	3.1	109	3.7	17.8	2.5	0.3
Peach & Mango, Truly Fruity, Brooklea, Aldi*	1 Pot/200g	162	2.8	81	4.6	12.4	1.4	0.0
Peach & Maracuya, Mullerlight, Muller*	1 Pot/200g	102	0.2	51	4.5	8.1	0.1	0.0
Peach & Nectarine, Bio, Fat Free, Activia, Danone*	1 Pot/125g	70	0.1	56	4.5	9.3	0.1	1.0

Y

YOGHURT

INFO/WEIGHT	Measure	per Measure KCAL	FAT	Nutrition Values per 100g / 100ml KCAL	PROT	CARB	FAT	FIBRE
Peach & Papaya, Fat Free, Yeo Valley*	1 Pot/125g	94	0.1	75	5.3	13.1	0.1	0.1
Peach & Papaya, Waitrose*	1 Pot/150g	129	0.2	86	4.2	17.1	0.1	0.2
Peach & Passion Fruit, 0% Fat, Shape Delights*	1 Pot/120g	80	0.1	67	5.6	10.8	0.1	0.6
Peach & Passion Fruit, Average	1 Serving/100g	66	0.7	66	4.5	10.6	0.7	0.4
Peach & Passion Fruit, BGTY, Sainsbury's*	1 Pot/125g	69	0.1	55	4.9	8.6	0.1	0.1
Peach & Passion Fruit, Fat Free, Shape, Danone*	1 Pot/120g	74	0.1	62	6.6	8.6	0.1	2.3
Peach & Passion Fruit, Layers, Mullerlight, Muller*	1 Pot/175g	94	0.2	54	4.5	15.3	1.0	0.2
Peach & Pear, Seriously Fruity, Low Fat, Waitrose*	1 Pot/125g	110	1.2	88	4.3	7.7	0.1	0.3
Peach & Pineapple, Fat Free, Mullerlight, Muller*	1 Pot/175g	89	0.2	51	4.3	7.7	0.1	0.2
Peach Melba, Low Fat, Average	1 Serving/100g	75	0.7	75	2.6	14.5	0.7	0.0
Peach Melba, Value, Tesco*	1 Pot/125g	100	0.9	80	2.3	16.0	0.7	0.1
Peaches & Cream, Intensely Creamy, Activia, Danone*	1 Pot/120g	118	3.6	98	4.8	13.0	3.0	0.3
Pear, Lidl*	1 Serving/125g	108	0.1	86	4.3	16.1	0.1	0.0
Pear & Vanilla, Thick & Creamy, Weight Watchers*	1 Pot/120g	54	0.6	45	4.2	5.8	0.5	0.2
Pineapple, Average	1 Serving/100g	73	1.1	73	4.4	11.3	1.1	0.5
Pineapple, Bio Activia, Fat Free, Danone*	1 Pot/125g	62	0.1	50	4.7	7.5	0.1	1.7
Pineapple, Low Fat, Average	1 Serving/100g	89	1.2	89	4.6	14.7	1.2	0.0
Pineapple, Tropical Fruit, Thick & Fruity, Weight Watchers*	1 Pot/120g	56	0.1	47	3.9	7.7	0.1	0.9
Pineapple & Passion Fruit, Soya, Light, Alpro*	1 Pot/120g	62	1.3	52	2.1	7.3	1.1	0.8
Pineapple & Peach, Fruity, Mullerlight, Muller*	1 Pot/175g	89	0.2	51	4.2	7.7	0.1	0.2
Plain, Low Fat, Average	*1 Serving/100g*	*63*	*1.6*	*63*	*5.2*	*7.0*	*1.6*	*0.0*
Plain, Natural, Dairy Free, Organic, Yofu, Soya, Provamel*	1 Pot/125g	62	2.9	50	4.0	2.8	2.3	1.0
Plain, Soya, Average	*1oz/28g*	*20*	*1.2*	*72*	*5.0*	*3.9*	*4.2*	*0.0*
Plain, Whole Milk, Average	*1oz/28g*	*22*	*0.8*	*79*	*5.7*	*7.8*	*3.0*	*0.0*
Plum, Probiotic, Summer Selection, Yeo Valley*	1 Pot/125g	126	4.9	101	4.1	12.4	3.9	0.1
Probiotic, Fat Free, Average	1 Tbsp/15g	8	0.0	56	5.4	7.7	0.3	0.6
Prune, Bifidus, Activo, Mercadona*	1 Pot/125g	70	0.1	56	4.5	6.8	0.1	3.0
Prune, Bio Activia, Danone*	1 Pot/125g	110	3.5	88	3.5	12.2	2.8	0.2
Prune, Fat Free, Natural Balance, CBY, Asda*	1 Pot/125g	94	0.5	75	3.6	12.6	0.4	3.4
Prune, Probiotic, Natural Balance, Asda*	1 Pot/125g	105	2.9	84	2.1	13.8	2.3	0.8
Raspberry, Bio, Activia, Danone*	1 Pot/125g	112	3.5	90	3.5	12.8	2.8	2.0
Raspberry, Bio, Activia, Fat Free, Danone*	1 Pot/125g	68	0.1	54	4.7	7.2	0.1	2.6
Raspberry, Bio, Fat Free, Snackpot, Activia, Danone*	1 Pot/165g	91	0.2	54	4.7	7.2	0.1	2.6
Raspberry, Bio, Low Fat, Benecol*	1 Pot/125g	99	0.8	79	3.8	14.5	0.6	0.0
Raspberry, Bio, Low Fat, Sainsbury's*	1 Pot/150g	146	1.6	97	4.7	17.0	1.1	0.7
Raspberry, Bio, Pur Natur*	1 Pot/150g	150	4.6	100	1.4	14.5	3.1	0.0
Raspberry, Bio Live, Low Fat, Rachel's Organic*	1 Pot/125g	114	2.0	91	4.1	15.1	1.6	0.1
Raspberry, Extremely Fruity, M&S*	1 Pot/200g	190	3.0	95	5.0	15.6	1.5	0.5
Raspberry, Fat Free, Average	1 Serving/100g	64	0.1	64	4.9	11.0	0.1	1.7
Raspberry, Fat Free, Probiotic, Organic, Yeo Valley*	1 Pot/125g	98	0.1	78	5.2	14.0	0.1	0.4
Raspberry, Forbidden Fruit, Rachel's Organic*	1 Pot/125g	155	7.6	124	3.4	13.8	6.1	0.1
Raspberry, Juicy, Intensely Creamy, Activia, Danone*	1 Pot/125g	121	3.8	97	4.8	12.7	3.0	0.6
Raspberry, Lactose Free, Lactofree, Arla*	1 Pot/125g	130	3.4	104	3.3	16.5	2.7	0.7
Raspberry, Low Fat, Average	1 Serving/100g	83	1.1	83	4.1	14.1	1.1	0.8
Raspberry, Low Fat, Organic, Sainsbury's*	1 Serving/125g	106	1.2	85	5.1	14.0	1.0	0.2
Raspberry, Low Fat, Stapleton*	1 Serving/150g	105	0.8	70	3.3	13.6	0.5	2.0
Raspberry, Organic, Yeo Valley*	1 Pot/150g	152	5.8	101	4.2	12.3	3.9	0.4
Raspberry, Probiotic, Live, Yeo Valley*	1 Pot/125g	106	1.2	85	5.1	14.0	1.0	0.4
Raspberry, Probiotic, Low Fat, Organic, M&S*	1 Pot/170g	128	2.4	75	4.4	11.5	1.4	0.4
Raspberry, Smooth, Activ8, Ski, Nestle*	1 Pot/120g	113	2.0	94	4.6	14.8	1.7	0.7
Raspberry, Smooth, Mullerlight, Muller*	1 Pot/125g	64	0.1	51	4.2	7.8	0.1	0.6
Raspberry, Soya, Alpro*	1 Pot/125g	99	2.4	79	3.7	10.4	1.9	1.2
Raspberry, Summer, Biopot, Onken*	1/5 Pot/90g	91	2.4	101	3.8	15.0	2.7	0.6

Y

YOGHURT

INFO/WEIGHT	Measure	per Measure KCAL	FAT	Nutrition Values per 100g / 100ml KCAL	PROT	CARB	FAT	FIBRE
Raspberry, Thick & Creamy, Sainsbury's*	1 Pot/150g	178	5.6	119	4.4	17.2	3.7	0.2
Raspberry, Thick & Fruity, Probiotic, COU, M&S*	1 Pot/170g	76	0.2	45	4.2	6.9	0.1	0.6
Raspberry, Value, Tesco*	1 Serving/125g	100	0.9	80	2.3	16.0	0.7	0.1
Raspberry, Vitality, Low Fat, with Omega 3, Muller*	1 Pot/125g	115	2.5	92	4.3	13.4	2.0	1.3
Raspberry, with Fruit Layer, Bio Activia, Danone*	1 Pot/125g	108	3.5	86	3.5	11.6	2.8	2.0
Raspberry, Zero% Fat, No Added Sugar, Shape, Danone*	1 Pot/120g	68	0.1	57	6.0	8.1	0.1	0.3
Raspberry & Blackberry, Thick & Creamy, Co-Op*	1 Pot/150g	188	6.9	125	3.6	17.3	4.6	0.1
Raspberry & Cranberry, Fat Free, Mullerlight, Muller*	1 Pot/175g	90	0.2	51	2.2	8.1	0.1	0.5
Raspberry or Strawberry, Smooth (No Bits), Ski, Nestle*	1 Pot/120g	118	3.2	98	3.9	13.6	2.7	0.0
Red Berry, Healthy Balance, Corner, Muller*	1 Pot/150g	178	4.0	119	5.0	18.0	2.7	0.5
Red Cherry, Dairy Free, Organic, Yofu, Soya, Provamel*	1 Pot/125g	101	2.8	81	3.9	10.5	2.2	0.8
Red Cherry, Fat Free, Ski, Nestle*	1 Pot 120g	97	0.1	81	4.5	15.6	0.1	0.1
Red Cherry, Fruit Corner, Muller*	1 Pot/150g	158	5.8	105	3.8	13.0	3.9	0.5
Red Cherry, Fruit Layered, GFY, Asda*	1 Pot/125g	75	0.1	60	3.7	11.0	0.1	0.0
Rhubarb, Bio Activia, Danone*	1 Pot/125g	112	4.0	90	3.5	11.8	3.2	2.2
Rhubarb, Bio Live, Low Fat, Rachel's Organic*	1 Pot/125g	104	2.0	83	4.0	13.1	1.6	0.1
Rhubarb, Custard Style, Somerfield*	1 Pot/125g	149	6.2	119	3.0	16.0	5.0	0.0
Rhubarb, Extremely Fruity, Probiotic, Low Fat, M&S*	1 Pot/170g	153	1.7	90	4.4	15.5	1.0	0.7
Rhubarb, Fruity, Mullerlight, Muller*	1 Pot/175g	91	0.2	52	4.2	7.9	0.1	0.0
Rhubarb, Greek Style, Corner, Muller*	1 Pot/150g	170	4.5	113	5.0	15.8	3.0	0.1
Rhubarb, Live Bio, Low Fat, PB, Waitrose*	1 Pot/150g	114	0.2	76	4.2	14.5	0.1	0.2
Rhubarb, Longley Farm*	1 Pot/150g	165	5.6	110	4.9	14.3	3.7	0.0
Rhubarb, Low Fat, Average	1 Serving/100g	83	1.2	83	4.6	13.3	1.2	0.2
Rhubarb, Low Fat, Garden Fruits, Tesco*	1 Pot/125g	119	2.4	95	3.0	15.5	1.9	0.3
Rhubarb, Spiced, Thick & Creamy, COU, M&S*	1 Pot/170g	68	0.2	40	4.3	5.8	0.1	0.5
Rhubarb, Timperley, Seriously Fruity, Waitrose*	1 Pot/150g	128	1.5	85	4.6	14.4	1.0	0.0
Rhubarb, Timperley, TTD, Sainsbury's*	1 Pot/150g	168	7.4	112	3.4	13.6	4.9	0.4
Rhubarb & Champagne, Truly Irresistible, Co-Op*	1 Pot/150g	195	8.2	130	3.5	16.6	5.5	0.2
Rhubarb Crumble, Crunch Corner, Muller*	1 Pot/150g	238	8.4	159	3.6	23.5	5.6	0.5
Sheep's Milk, Total, Fage*	1 Pot/200g	180	12.0	90	4.8	4.3	6.0	0.0
Strawberry, & Cream, Finest, Tesco*	1 Pot/150g	206	10.4	137	3.4	15.4	6.9	0.5
Strawberry, Amore for Me, Muller*	1 Pot/150g	216	11.0	144	2.7	16.8	7.3	0.2
Strawberry, Balanced Lifestyle, Aldi*	1 Pot/150g	72	0.4	48	4.1	7.1	0.3	0.5
Strawberry, Bettabuy, Morrisons*	1 Pot/115g	91	1.5	79	4.4	12.8	1.3	0.3
Strawberry, Bio, Co-Op*	1 Pot/125g	142	3.5	114	4.5	16.7	2.8	0.1
Strawberry, Bio, Fat Free, Snackpot, Activia, Danone*	1 Pot/165g	101	0.2	61	5.0	10.0	0.1	0.2
Strawberry, Bio, Granola, Corner, Muller*	1 Pot/135g	161	3.5	119	5.5	17.8	2.6	0.8
Strawberry, Bio, Low Fat, Dale Farm*	1 Pot/125g	125	2.1	100	3.9	17.0	1.7	0.2
Strawberry, Bio Activia, Danone*	1 Pot/125g	118	4.0	94	3.5	12.8	3.2	2.0
Strawberry, Biopot, Wholegrain, Onken*	1 Serving/100g	111	2.9	111	4.1	17.2	2.9	0.5
Strawberry, Breakfast Crunch, Corner, Muller*	1 Pack/135g	163	3.5	121	5.5	0.0	2.6	0.0
Strawberry, Custard Style, Shapers, Boots*	1 Pot/150g	117	1.0	78	3.9	14.0	0.7	0.5
Strawberry, Fat Free, Average	1 Serving/100g	66	0.1	66	4.9	11.1	0.1	0.6
Strawberry, Fat free, Greek Style, Brooklea, Aldi*	1 Pot/125g	72	0.3	57	4.9	8.8	0.2	0.2
Strawberry, Fat Free, Probiotic, Organic, Yeo Valley*	1 Pot/125g	108	1.2	86	5.1	14.1	1.0	0.1
Strawberry, Fruit Corner, Snack Size, Muller*	1 Pot/95g	108	3.8	114	3.9	15.6	4.0	0.4
Strawberry, Fruity, Mullerlight, Muller*	1 Pot/175g	89	0.2	51	4.1	7.9	0.1	0.0
Strawberry, Lactose Free, Lactofree, Arla*	1 Pot/125g	126	3.2	101	3.5	15.9	2.6	0.4
Strawberry, LC, Tesco*	1 Pot/200g	86	0.2	43	4.1	6.3	0.1	0.6
Strawberry, Light, Brooklea, Aldi*	1 Pot/200g	154	0.2	77	6.1	12.9	0.1	0.4
Strawberry, Low Fat, Average	1 Serving/100g	81	1.0	81	4.5	13.6	1.0	0.2
Strawberry, Low Fat, Probiotic, Organic, M&S*	1 Pot/170g	136	2.4	80	4.8	11.6	1.4	0.4
Strawberry, Low Fat, Value, Tesco*	1 Pot/125g	100	0.9	80	2.3	16.0	0.7	0.1

Y

YOGHURT

INFO/WEIGHT	Measure		Nutrition Values per 100g / 100ml				
	KCAL	FAT	KCAL	PROT	CARB	FAT	FIBRE
Strawberry, Luxury, Bio Live, Jersey Dairy* — 1 Pot/150g	159	8.6	106	3.8	10.2	5.7	0.5
Strawberry, Organic, Yeo Valley* — 1 Pot/150g	159	5.7	106	4.7	13.2	3.8	0.1
Strawberry, Pouring, Activia, Danone* — 1 Serving/100g	59	1.6	59	3.9	7.3	1.6	0.1
Strawberry, Probiotic, Natural Balance, Asda* — 1 Pot/125g	109	3.0	87	3.1	13.3	2.4	2.4
Strawberry, Probiotic, Organic, Yeo Valley* — 1 Pot/125g	125	5.0	100	4.4	11.7	4.0	0.1
Strawberry, Smooth, Activ8, Ski, Nestle* — 1 Pot/120g	113	2.0	94	4.6	14.8	1.7	0.7
Strawberry, Smooth Set French, Low Fat, Sainsbury's* — 1 Pot/125g	112	4.0	90	3.7	11.8	3.2	0.0
Strawberry, Swiss, Emmi* — 1 Pot/175g	177	4.4	101	3.5	16.0	2.5	0.3
Strawberry, Thick & Creamy, Waitrose* — 1 Pot/125g	135	3.1	108	3.7	17.6	2.5	0.4
Strawberry, Thick & Fruity, Probiotic, COU, M&S* — 1 Pot/170g	76	0.2	45	4.1	7.3	0.1	0.4
Strawberry, Totally, Low Fat, CBY, Asda* — 1 Pot/125g	104	1.2	83	4.1	14.2	1.0	0.4
Strawberry, Virtually Fat Free, Average — 1 Serving/100g	65	0.2	65	4.7	11.3	0.2	0.2
Strawberry, Vitality, Low Fat, with Omega 3, Muller* — 1 Pot/150g	140	2.8	93	4.3	14.0	1.9	0.8
Strawberry, Yoplait* — 1 Pot/125g	61	0.2	49	4.2	7.6	0.2	0.9
Strawberry, Zero% Fat, No Added Sugar, Shape, Danone* — 1 Pot/120g	71	0.1	59	6.0	8.5	0.1	0.9
Strawberry & Banana, Oatie Breakfast, Moma Foods* — 1 Pot/235g	320	5.6	136	4.3	25.4	2.4	1.7
Strawberry & French Vanilla, Amore Luxury, Muller* — 1 Pot/150g	225	11.7	150	2.9	17.0	7.8	0.1
Strawberry & Raspberry, Low Fat, Asda* — 1 Pot/150g	142	1.5	95	4.6	17.4	1.0	0.2
Strawberry & Raspberry, Low Fat, Sainsbury's* — 1 Pot/125g	109	1.8	87	4.2	14.3	1.4	0.2
Strawberry & Rhubarb, Low Fat, Bio, Rachel's Organic* — 1 Pot/120g	103	2.0	86	4.3	13.3	1.7	0.1
Strawberry & Rhubarb, Low Fat, Sainsbury's* — 1 Pot/125g	108	1.8	86	4.2	14.1	1.4	0.2
Strawberry & Rhubarb, Onken* — 1 Serving/100g	85	0.1	85	4.6	16.2	0.1	0.4
Strawberry Cheesecake, Dessert, Weight Watchers* — 1 Pot/120g	57	0.1	48	4.1	6.6	0.1	0.2
Strawberry Cheesecake, Inspired by, Mullerlight, Muller* — 1 Yogurt/165g	99	0.2	60	4.2	10.0	0.1	0.2
Strawberry Crumble, Crunch Corner, Muller* — 1 Pot/150g	234	8.4	156	3.6	22.9	5.6	0.5
Strawberry Orange Balls, Crunch Corner, Muller* — 1 Pot/150g	222	8.1	148	4.0	20.8	5.4	0.2
Strawberry Rice, Low Fat, Muller* — 1 Pot/190g	203	4.4	107	3.2	18.4	2.3	0.4
Strawberry Shortcake, Crunch Corner, Muller* — 1 Pot/135g	212	8.0	157	4.1	21.2	5.9	0.1
Summer Berries, Fat Free, Mullerlight, Muller* — 1 Pot/175g	88	0.2	50	4.1	7.6	0.1	0.4
Summer Berries, Wholegrain, Biopot, Onken* — 1 Portion/100g	110	2.9	110	4.1	16.9	2.9	0.7
Summer Berry Compote, Greek Style, & Granola, M&S* — 1 Pot/205g	336	16.4	164	5.6	17.3	8.0	0.1
Summer Fruits, Cool Country* — 1 Serving/150g	136	2.2	91	3.0	16.3	1.5	0.0
Summer Fruits, Greek Style, Corner, Muller* — 1 Pot/150g	165	4.5	110	5.1	15.0	3.0	0.5
Summer Fruits, Light, Limited Edition, Muller* — 1 Pot/175g	88	0.2	50	4.1	7.6	0.1	0.4
Summer Selection, Fat Free, Organic, Yeo Valley* — 1 Pot/125g	89	0.1	71	5.2	12.3	0.1	0.2
Summer Selection, Thick & Fruity, COU, M&S* — 1 Pot/145g	75	0.2	52	4.2	7.8	0.1	0.5
Summerfruits, Bio Live, Fat Free, Rachel's Organic* — 1 Pot/125g	120	2.2	96	4.7	15.3	1.8	0.0
Sweet Treat, Low Fat, Tesco* — 1 Pot/125g	131	2.9	105	3.1	18.0	2.3	0.3
Toffee, & Vanilla, Fat Free, Multipack, Weight Watchers* — 1 Yoghurt/120g	53	0.1	45	4.2	6.0	0.1	0.6
Toffee, Benecol* — 1 Pot/125g	124	0.9	99	3.8	19.3	0.7	0.0
Toffee, COU, M&S* — 1 Pot/145g	65	0.3	45	4.2	7.7	0.2	0.0
Toffee, Low Fat, Average — 1 Pot/125g	136	3.1	109	4.3	19.5	2.4	0.1
Toffee, Smooth, Fat Free, Mullerlight, Muller* — 1 Pot/175g	89	0.2	51	4.1	7.9	0.1	0.0
Toffee, Smooth & Creamy, Fat Free, Weight Watchers* — 1 Pot/120g	48	0.1	40	3.9	5.9	0.1	0.8
Toffee, with Chocolate Hoops, Crunch Corner, Muller* — 1 Pot/135g	209	7.8	155	4.2	20.8	5.8	0.2
Tropical, Low Fat, Luscious, Rachel's Organic* — 1 Pot/125g	115	2.0	92	4.0	15.3	1.6	0.0
Tropical Fruit, Bio, Granola, Corner, Muller* — 1 Pot/135g	161	3.2	119	5.4	18.2	2.4	0.6
Tropical Fruit, Greek Style, Shapers, Boots* — 1 Pot/150g	100	2.2	67	3.6	9.8	1.5	0.8
Vanilla, Average — 1 Serving/120g	100	5.4	83	4.5	12.4	4.5	0.8
Vanilla, Bio, Fat Free, Snackpot, Activia, Danone* — 1 Pot/165g	87	0.2	53	5.0	8.1	0.1	0.9
Vanilla, Chocolate, & Black Cherry, Mullerlight, Muller* — 1 Pot/175g	103	0.7	59	3.1	10.3	0.4	0.3
Vanilla, Creamy, Smarties, Nestle* — 1 Pot/120g	200	7.4	167	4.1	23.7	6.2	0.0
Vanilla, Fat Free, Onken* — ½ Pot/225g	166	0.2	74	4.4	12.6	0.1	0.3

Y

YOGHURT

	Measure INFO/WEIGHT	per Measure KCAL	FAT	Nutrition Values per 100g / 100ml KCAL	PROT	CARB	FAT	FIBRE
Vanilla, Live Bio, Low Fat, PB, Waitrose*	1 Pot/150g	114	0.2	76	4.1	14.7	0.1	0.0
Vanilla, Low Fat, Probiotic, Organic, M&S*	1 Serving/100g	85	1.8	85	6.2	10.9	1.8	0.0
Vanilla, Low Fat, Tesco*	1 Pot/125g	125	2.1	100	4.9	16.3	1.7	0.0
Vanilla, Madagascan, Indulgent, Dessert, Waitrose*	1 Pot/150g	240	11.4	160	3.7	19.2	7.6	0.0
Vanilla, Madagascan, West Country, TTD, Sainsbury's*	1 Pot/150g	192	8.4	128	3.9	15.5	5.6	0.0
Vanilla, Onken*	1 Serving/100g	100	2.7	100	3.1	15.9	2.7	0.0
Vanilla, Organic, Probiotic, Fat Free, Yeo Valley*	1 Pot/500g	400	0.5	80	5.4	14.2	0.1	0.0
Vanilla, Pouring, Activia, Danone*	1 Serving/100g	62	1.6	62	3.9	8.1	1.6	0.0
Vanilla, Smooth, Light, Fat Free, Muller*	1 Pot/175g	88	0.2	50	4.3	7.2	0.1	0.0
Vanilla, Smooth & Creamy, Fat Free, Weight Watchers*	1 Pot/120g	50	0.1	42	3.9	6.5	0.1	0.1
Vanilla, Soya, Dairy Free, Organic, Yofu, Provamel*	1 Pot/125g	114	2.8	91	3.8	13.3	2.2	0.7
Vanilla, Thick & Creamy, Probiotic, COU, M&S*	1 Pot/170g	76	0.2	45	4.2	6.9	0.1	0.6
Vanilla, Totally, Low Fat, Asda*	1 Pot/150g	134	1.6	89	4.7	15.1	1.1	0.0
Vanilla, Velvety, Intensely Creamy, Activia, Danone*	1 Pot/120g	116	3.6	97	4.8	12.7	3.0	0.1
Vanilla, Virtually Fat Free, Shapers, Boots*	1 Pot/125g	84	0.6	67	3.6	12.0	0.5	0.0
Vanilla, Virtually Fat Free, Yeo Valley*	1 Pot/150g	122	0.2	81	5.1	15.0	0.1	0.0
Vanilla, Weight Watchers*	1 Pot/120g	47	0.1	39	4.2	5.2	0.1	0.2
Vanilla, with Dark Chocolate Flakes, Light, Brooklea*	1 Pot/180g	104	1.8	58	4.9	7.0	1.0	0.5
Vanilla & Chocolate, Muller*	1 Pot/165g	86	0.8	52	4.0	7.2	0.5	0.1
Vanilla & Chocolate Sprinkles, Delights, Shape, Danone*	1 Pot/120g	88	0.6	74	5.4	11.8	0.5	0.5
Walnut & Greek Honey, Amore Luxury, Muller*	1 Pot/150g	242	13.0	161	3.0	17.6	8.7	0.1
Wild Berry, Oatie Breakfast, Moma Foods*	1 Pot/235g	317	4.2	135	4.3	25.6	1.8	2.7
Wild Blackberry, Seriously Fruity, Waitrose*	1 Pot/125g	120	1.3	96	4.4	17.2	1.0	0.4
Wild Blueberry, Finest, Tesco*	1 Pot/150g	212	10.2	141	3.4	16.6	6.8	0.5
with Reduced Sugar Apricot Jam, Bonne Maman*	1 Pot/125g	141	4.1	113	2.4	16.8	3.3	0.4

YOGHURT BREAK

	Measure INFO/WEIGHT	per Measure KCAL	FAT	Nutrition Values per 100g / 100ml KCAL	PROT	CARB	FAT	FIBRE
Blueberry, Go Ahead, McVitie's*	1 Slice/18g	72	1.8	401	5.5	72.1	10.0	2.2
Plain, Go Ahead, McVitie's*	1 Slice/18g	72	2.1	394	6.5	66.0	11.5	3.3
Strawberry, Go Ahead, McVitie's*	1 Slice/18g	72	2.0	397	5.9	68.0	11.1	2.1
Tropical, Go Ahead, McVitie's*	1 Slice/18g	77	2.0	430	5.9	76.3	11.0	2.3

YOGHURT DRINK

	Measure INFO/WEIGHT	per Measure KCAL	FAT	Nutrition Values per 100g / 100ml KCAL	PROT	CARB	FAT	FIBRE
Average	1 fl oz/30ml	19	0.0	62	3.1	13.1	0.0	0.0
Ayran, Gazi*	1 Can/330ml	34	1.9	10	0.5	0.8	0.6	0.0
Blueberry, Low Fat, Prebiotic & Probiotic, Muller*	1 Pot/100g	66	1.4	66	2.6	10.3	1.4	2.2
Blueberry Shot, Cholesterol Reducing, NUME, Morrisons*	1 Bottle/100g	63	0.4	63	3.3	11.6	0.4	0.0
Cholesterol Lowering, Asda*	1 Bottle/100g	76	1.4	76	2.9	13.0	1.4	1.0
Fruit, Mixed, Actimel, Danone*	1 Bottle/100ml	88	1.5	88	2.7	16.0	1.5	0.0
Light, Benecol*	1 Bottle/68g	40	1.4	60	2.8	7.3	2.1	0.1
Light, Yakult*	1 Bottle/65ml	27	0.0	42	1.4	10.2	0.0	1.8
Multi Fruit, Actimel, Danone*	1 Bottle/100g	85	1.5	85	2.7	14.4	1.5	0.1
Multifruit, Probiotic, Value, Tesco*	1 Serving/100g	75	1.1	75	2.8	12.5	1.1	0.3
Orange, Actimel, Danone*	1 Bottle/100g	74	1.5	74	2.9	11.5	1.5	0.0
Original, 0.1% Fat, Actimel, Danone*	1 Bottle/100g	28	0.1	28	2.8	3.3	0.1	1.9
Original, Actimel, Danone*	1 Bottle/100g	80	1.6	80	2.8	12.8	1.6	0.0
Original, Benecol*	1 Serving/70g	62	1.6	88	2.6	14.2	2.3	0.0
Original, Danacol, Danone*	1 Bottle/100ml	64	1.0	64	3.2	10.0	1.0	0.0
Original, Pro Activ, Cholesterol, Flora*	1 Bottle/100g	45	1.5	45	2.6	4.8	1.5	1.1
Peach & Apricot, Benecol*	1 Bottle/68g	38	1.5	56	2.8	6.2	2.2	0.0
Peach & Mango, Actimel, Danone*	1 Bottle/100g	28	0.1	28	2.7	3.1	0.1	0.4
Pomeganate & Raspberry Pro Active, Mini Drink, Flora*	1 Serving/100g	45	1.5	45	2.6	4.7	1.5	1.1
Strawberry, Actimel, Danone*	1 Bottle/100g	74	1.5	74	2.9	11.5	1.5	0.0
Strawberry, Benecol*	1 Bottle/68g	38	1.4	56	3.2	6.2	2.0	0.0
Strawberry, Danacol, Danone*	1 Bottle/100g	68	1.2	68	3.2	11.2	1.2	0.0

INFO/WEIGHT	Measure	per Measure KCAL	FAT	Nutrition Values per 100g / 100ml KCAL	PROT	CARB	FAT	FIBRE
YOGHURT DRINK								
Strawberry, Low Fat, Pre & Probiotic, Muller*	1 Pot/100g	67	1.4	67	2.5	10.7	1.4	2.4
Strawberry, Pro Activ, Cholesterol, Flora*	1 Bottle/100g	45	1.5	45	2.6	4.7	1.5	0.0
Strawberry, Yop, Yoplait*	1 Bottle/330g	261	4.3	79	2.8	14.0	1.3	0.0
Yakult*	1 Pot/65ml	43	0.1	66	1.3	14.7	0.1	0.0
YORK FRUITS								
Terry's*	1 Sweet/9g	29	0.0	320	0.0	78.5	0.0	0.5
YORKIE								
Honeycomb, Nestle*	1 Bar/65g	331	16.8	509	5.7	63.6	25.8	0.0
King Size, Nestle*	1 Bar/83g	445	26.1	537	6.1	57.3	31.5	0.0
Original, Nestle*	1 Bar/55g	302	17.4	546	6.2	57.9	31.5	1.9
Raisin & Biscuit, Nestle*	1 Bar/67g	331	17.4	497	5.5	59.7	26.2	0.9
YORKSHIRE PUDDING								
& Beef Dripping, M&S*	4 Puddings/100g	410	30.4	410	9.4	25.2	30.4	3.2
3", Baked, Aunt Bessie's*	1 Pudding/36g	91	2.8	252	9.0	36.4	7.9	1.7
4 Minute, Aunt Bessie's*	1 Pudding/18g	52	2.0	291	10.5	36.6	11.3	2.2
7", Baked, Aunt Bessie's*	1 Pudding/110g	290	9.9	264	8.5	37.4	9.0	2.0
Average	1 Pudding/30g	62	3.0	208	6.6	24.7	9.9	0.9
Baked, Frozen, 4 Pack, Morrisons*	1 Pudding/34g	82	2.3	241	8.4	36.7	6.7	1.6
Batters, in Foils, Ready to Bake, Frozen, Aunt Bessie's*	1 Pudding/17g	47	1.8	276	9.1	32.6	10.8	1.4
Filled with Beef, Tesco*	1 Pudding/300g	408	15.6	136	6.1	16.2	5.2	1.1
Filled with Chicken & Vegetable, GFY, Asda*	1 Pack/380g	376	9.9	99	6.0	13.0	2.6	1.1
Frozen, Ovenbaked, Iceland*	1 Pudding/12g	36	1.0	290	9.7	45.1	7.9	4.1
Fully Prepared, M&S*	1 Pudding/22g	63	2.9	285	9.4	31.6	13.2	1.2
Giant, Aunt Bessie's*	1 Pudding/110g	290	9.9	264	8.5	37.4	9.0	2.0
Giant VLH Kitchens	1 Serving/110g	284	9.1	259	8.5	33.6	10.0	2.3
Heat & Serve, Waitrose*	1 Pudding/30g	86	3.5	288	9.5	35.3	11.7	1.7
Home Bake, Rise in 20 Minutes, Baked, Aunt Bessie's*	1 Pudding/25g	43	1.7	174	6.0	20.0	7.0	3.1
Large, Aunt Bessie's*	1 Pudding/40g	111	4.6	277	8.5	35.3	11.4	1.5
Large, Co-Op*	1 Serving/110g	319	18.7	290	8.0	27.0	17.0	4.0
Large, The Real Yorkshire Pudding Co*	1 Pudding/34g	103	4.1	304	11.5	37.3	12.1	2.5
Made From Batter Mix, Sainsbury's*	1 Pudding/100g	248	5.3	248	9.9	40.1	5.3	4.0
Mini, Co-Op*	1 Serving/16g	50	2.0	312	6.2	43.8	12.5	2.5
Mini, Farmfoods*	1 Pudding/3g	8	0.2	281	9.6	43.2	7.7	1.9
Ready Baked, Smart Price, Asda*	1 Pudding/12g	36	1.1	297	10.0	44.0	9.0	2.8
Ready to Bake, Aunt Bessie's*	1 Pudding/17g	42	1.4	246	8.5	35.1	8.0	1.7
Ready to Bake, Sainsbury's*	1 Pudding/18g	48	1.6	263	9.9	35.9	8.9	1.3
Roast Chicken Filled, COU, M&S*	1 Pudding/150g	210	4.0	140	12.6	15.7	2.7	0.9
Sage & Onion, Tesco*	1 Pudding/19g	53	2.3	280	8.0	35.0	12.0	2.6
Sainsbury's*	1 Pudding/14g	43	2.0	309	7.9	37.5	14.1	2.9
Steak Filled, COU, M&S*	1 Serving/150g	188	3.8	125	11.0	14.7	2.5	0.8
The Best, Morrisons*	1 Pudding/22g	60	1.8	271	8.3	43.0	8.0	1.6
Traditional, Giant, Asda*	1 Pudding/110g	310	11.0	282	10.0	38.0	10.0	2.3
Traditional Style, Medium, Asda*	1 Pudding/36g	86	3.2	241	9.0	31.0	9.0	2.4
Traditional Style, Small, Asda*	1 Pudding/20g	52	2.0	262	8.0	35.0	10.0	2.9
Value, Tesco*	1 Pudding/16g	45	1.9	282	9.7	34.3	11.8	1.6
with Beef in Gravy, Asda*	1 Serving/290g	406	10.2	140	7.0	20.0	3.5	0.7
YULE LOG								
Chocolate, Sainsbury's*	1 Slice/35g	153	7.7	432	5.0	51.6	21.8	4.6
Christmas Range, Tesco*	1 Serving/30g	131	6.4	442	4.9	56.8	21.7	2.8
Mini, M&S*	1 Cake/36g	165	8.4	460	5.7	56.9	23.3	1.1

BURGER KING

INFO/WEIGHT	Measure	per Measure		Nutrition Values per 100g / 100ml				
		KCAL	FAT	KCAL	PROT	CARB	FAT	FIBRE
APPLES								
Fries, Burger King*	1 Serving/60g	28	0.1	47	0.1	12.0	0.1	2.0
BITES								
Cheese, Chilli, Burger King*	4 Bites/78g	238	13.3	305	9.0	32.2	17.0	30.7
BURGERS								
Angus, Bacon, Smoked, & Cheddar, Burger King*	1 Burger/270g	683	39.1	253	14.3	16.0	14.5	1.1
Angus, Bacon, Smoked, & Cheddar, Dbl, Burger King*	1 Burger/354g	942	58.0	266	17.1	12.2	16.4	1.0
Angus, Classic, Double, Burger King*	1 Burger/323g	1068	67.0	331	22.6	13.2	20.7	1.1
Angus, Mini, Burger King*	1 Burger/97g	272	10.7	280	14.0	31.0	11.0	1.0
Angus, Mini, with Cheese, Burger King*	1 Burger/110g	321	15.4	292	15.0	27.0	14.0	1.0
Bacon, Double Cheese, Burger King*	1 Burger/181g	497	25.8	275	17.4	18.9	14.3	1.3
Bacon, Double Cheese, XL, Burger King*	1 Burger/302g	957	54.8	317	20.9	17.2	18.2	0.9
Bean Burger, Veggie, Kids, Burger King*	1 Burger/116g	313	10.4	270	6.9	39.0	9.0	2.9
Big King, Burger King*	1 Burger/190g	486	26.6	256	14.6	17.5	14.0	1.1
Big King, XL, Burger King*	1 Burger/338g	902	54.1	267	16.0	14.0	16.0	1.0
BK, Veggie Bean Burger, Burger King*	1 Burger/280g	625	26.7	223	6.5	26.9	9.5	2.4
Cheeseburger, Bacon Double, Burger King*	1 Burger/160g	478	25.6	299	19.0	19.0	16.0	1.0
Cheeseburger, Bacon Double, Xtra Large, Burger King*	1 Burger/302g	927	54.4	307	21.0	15.0	18.0	1.0
Cheeseburger, Burger King*	1 Burger/126g	316	13.2	251	13.7	25.7	10.5	1.4
Cheeseburger, Double, Burger King*	1 Burger/173g	460	13.8	266	16.8	19.1	8.0	1.2
Cheeseburger, Kids, Burger King*	1 Burger/113g	329	14.3	291	15.9	28.0	12.6	1.3
Chicken, Chargrilled, Mini, Burger King*	1 Burger/109g	214	3.3	196	15.0	28.0	3.0	1.0
Chicken, Spicy Tendercrisp, Burger King*	1 Burger/254g	621	32.7	245	11.0	20.1	12.9	1.2
Chicken Royale, Burger King*	1 Burger/210g	476	17.1	227	11.4	26.5	8.1	1.3
Chicken Royale, Sweet Chilli, Burger King*	1 Burger/210g	542	23.7	258	11.4	27.3	11.3	1.3
Chicken Royale, with Cheese, Burger King*	1 Burger/263g	688	39.5	261	11.0	20.2	15.0	1.1
Hamburger, Burger King*	1 Burger/114g	274	9.9	241	13.2	28.1	8.7	1.6
Hamburger, Kids, Burger King*	1 Serving/100g	272	9.7	272	14.8	31.8	9.7	1.7
Ocean Catch, Burger King*	1 Burger/196g	498	27.9	254	8.8	22.2	14.2	1.4
Steakhouse, Burger King*	1 Burger/239g	727	43.1	304	14.8	20.3	18.0	1.2
Whopper, Burger King*	1 Burger/292g	652	35.4	223	10.4	17.6	12.1	1.2
Whopper, Double, Burger King*	1 Burger/355g	894	52.8	252	14.5	14.6	14.9	1.1
Whopper, Double, with Cheese, Burger King*	1 Burger/380g	961	60.8	253	14.0	13.0	16.0	1.0
Whopper, Junior, Burger King*	1 Burger/152g	343	16.9	226	10.0	21.6	11.2	1.2
Whopper, with Cheese, Burger King*	1 Burger/299g	721	41.9	241	11.0	16.0	14.0	1.0
Whopper, with Cheese, Junior, Burger King*	1 Burger/161g	388	19.3	241	10.0	19.0	12.0	1.0
CHICKEN								
Bites, Burger King*	14 Bites/112g	317	15.0	283	16.1	25.0	13.4	0.9
Bites, Kids, Burger King*	1 Serving/56g	158	7.3	282	16.0	25.0	13.0	2.0
Nuggets, with Dip, Burger King*	6 Nuggets/138g	307	13.6	223	12.5	20.2	9.9	1.6
COFFEE								
Black, Large, Burger King*	1 Serving/284ml	6	0.0	2	0.0	0.0	0.0	0.0
Black, Regular, Burger King*	1 Serving/200ml	4	0.0	2	0.0	0.0	0.0	0.0
Cappuccino, Large, Burger King*	1 Serving/59g	81	3.0	137	10.0	15.0	5.0	0.0
Cappuccino, Regular, Burger King*	1 Serving/46g	64	1.8	139	9.0	15.0	4.0	0.0
Latte, Large, Burger King*	1 Serving/45g	60	1.8	133	11.0	13.0	4.0	0.0
Latte, Regular, Burger King*	1 Serving/62g	82	3.1	132	10.0	15.0	5.0	0.0
DIP								
Barbeque Sauce, Heinz, Pot, Burger King*	1 Pot/40g	48	0.0	120	0.1	28.0	0.1	0.1
Sweet Chilli, Heinz, Pot, Burger King*	1 Pot/40g	96	0.0	240	0.0	60.0	0.0	0.0
DRESSING								
French, Burger King*	1 Sachet/40g	7	0.0	18	0.0	2.5	0.0	0.0
Honey & Mustard, Burger King*	1 Sachet/40g	32	1.0	80	2.5	15.0	2.5	0.0

	INFO/WEIGHT	per Measure KCAL	per Measure FAT	Nutrition Values per 100g / 100ml KCAL	PROT	CARB	FAT	FIBRE

BURGER KING

FRIES

	INFO/WEIGHT	KCAL	FAT	KCAL	PROT	CARB	FAT	FIBRE
Medium, Burger King*	1 Serving/116g	277	12.4	238	3.1	31.4	10.7	2.2

HASH BROWNS

Regular, Burger King*	1 Regular/102g	276	19.2	270	2.4	21.7	18.8	2.4

MAYONNAISE

Heinz, Sachet, Burger King*	1 Sachet/12g	80	9.0	667	0.0	0.0	75.0	0.0

MILK

Semi Skimmed, Kids, Burger King*	1 Carton/258g	117	3.9	47	3.5	4.6	1.6	0.0

MILK SHAKE

Chocolate, Large, Burger King*	1 Serving/519g	612	10.4	118	3.0	22.0	2.0	0.0
Chocolate, Regular, Burger King*	1 Serving/401g	449	8.0	112	3.0	20.0	2.0	0.1
Chocolate, Small, Burger King*	1 Serving/276g	301	8.3	109	3.0	19.0	3.0	0.1
Strawberry, Large, Burger King*	1 Serving/519g	581	10.4	112	3.0	20.0	2.0	0.0
Strawberry, Regular, Burger King*	1 Serving/401g	433	8.0	108	3.0	19.0	2.0	0.0
Strawberry, Small, Burger King*	1 Serving/276g	293	8.3	106	3.0	18.0	3.0	0.0
Vanilla, Large, Burger King*	1 Shake/519g	460	11.5	89	2.7	14.2	2.2	0.0
Vanilla, Regular, Burger King*	1 Reg/401g	371	9.3	93	2.8	14.8	2.3	0.0

ONION RINGS

Large, Burger King*	1 Serving/180g	535	26.5	297	5.1	34.2	14.7	3.7
Regular, Burger King*	1 Serving/120g	356	17.6	297	5.1	34.2	14.7	3.7
Super, Burger King*	1 Serving/240g	713	35.3	297	5.1	34.2	14.7	3.7

SALAD

Chicken, Flame Grilled, Burger King*	1 Salad/240g	127	2.4	53	8.0	3.0	1.0	1.0
Chicken, Flame Grilled, French Dressing, Burger King*	1 Serving/280g	134	2.8	48	7.0	3.0	1.0	1.0
Garden, Burger King*	1 Serving/165g	33	1.6	20	1.0	4.0	1.0	1.0

SANDWICH

Butty, Bacon, & Egg, with Heinz Ketchup, Burger King*	1 Butty/140g	362	17.0	259	12.9	25.0	12.1	11.4
Butty, Bacon, & Egg, with HP Sauce, Burger King*	1 Butty/140g	363	17.0	259	12.9	25.0	12.1	1.4
Butty, Bacon, with Heinz Ketchup, Burger King*	1 Butty/77g	270	6.2	351	13.6	57.3	8.0	3.2
Butty, Bacon, with HP Sauce, Burger King*	1 Butty/77g	222	6.0	288	13.0	41.6	7.8	2.0
Butty, Big Breakfast, with Heinz Ketchup, Burger King*	1 Butty/297g	849	50.5	286	14.0	18.0	17.0	1.0
Butty, Egg, & Cheese, with Heinz Ketchup, Burger King*	1 Butty/126g	346	12.4	275	12.9	32.9	9.8	1.8
Butty, Sausage, & Egg, with HP Sauce, Burger King*	1 Butty/182g	454	24.0	249	13.2	19.2	13.2	1.1
Butty, Sausage, with Heinz Ketchup, Burger King*	1 Butty/119g	312	13.0	262	13.4	26.9	10.9	1.7
Butty, Sausage, with HP Sauce, Burger King*	1 Butty/119g	313	13.0	263	13.4	26.9	10.9	1.7

TEA

Regular, White, No Sugar, Burger King*	1 Reg/200ml	22	4.0	11	1.0	1.0	2.0	0.0

WRAP

Chicken, Sweet Chilli, Burger King*	1 Wrap/160g	298	6.9	186	14.4	22.1	4.3	1.3
Veggie, Burger King*	1 Wrap/231g	493	21.0	214	4.2	27.6	9.1	2.7

CAFFE NERO

BARS

Fruit & Seed, Caffe Nero*	1 Serving/65g	197	5.8	303	7.5	48.2	8.9	8.7
Granola, Organic, Caffe Nero*	1 Serving/64g	278	14.3	434	6.7	51.5	22.4	4.8

BISCOTTI

Almond, Organic, Caffe Nero*	1 Serving/37g	147	5.9	397	9.0	54.6	15.9	2.7
Chocolate, Organic, Caffe Nero*	1 Serving/37g	136	4.3	369	7.0	59.1	11.6	2.7

BISCUITS

Amaretti, Caffe Nero*	1 Biscuit/10g	40	1.2	401	3.9	70.1	11.7	10.6
Double Chocolate, Caffe Nero*	1 Biscuit/25g	126	6.8	505	5.5	57.4	27.3	3.7
Palmine, Caffe Nero*	1 Biscuit/14g	75	4.3	540	6.6	55.5	31.0	1.6

BREAD

Ciabatta, Roll, Caffe Nero*	1 Roll/70g	180	2.7	257	8.7	46.9	3.9	1.7

	Measure INFO/WEIGHT	per Measure KCAL	FAT	Nutrition Values per 100g / 100ml KCAL	PROT	CARB	FAT	FIBRE
CAFFE NERO								
BREAKFAST CEREAL								
Porridge, Semi Skim Milk, no Topping, Caffe Nero*	1 Serving/239g	234	6.7	98	4.8	13.9	2.8	1.5
Porridge, with Skimmed Milk, no Topping, Caffe Nero*	1 Serving/239g	210	3.8	88	4.8	14.0	1.6	1.5
Porridge, with Soya Milk, no Topping, Caffe Nero*	1 Serving/239g	232	7.7	97	4.9	12.1	3.2	2.0
BROWNIES								
Chocolate, Belgian, Caffe Nero*	1 Serving/75g	314	14.7	419	4.6	54.6	19.6	2.9
Chocolate, Double, GF, Organic, Caffe Nero*	1 Serving/75g	318	15.5	425	4.3	55.4	20.7	2.0
CAKE								
Cappuccino, Caffe Nero*	1 Serving/120g	486	22.7	405	3.7	56.2	18.9	0.5
Carrot, & Raisin, Organic, Wrapped, Caffe Nero*	1 Serving/70g	290	17.5	414	4.5	43.4	25.0	3.9
Carrot, & Raisin, Wheat Free, Organic, Caffe Nero*	1 Serving/70g	295	17.7	421	4.1	44.8	25.3	3.4
Chocolate Crunch, Caffe Nero*	1 Serving/65g	308	16.5	473	6.2	54.3	25.3	4.2
Chocolate Fudge, Caffe Nero*	1 Serving/124g	526	26.9	424	5.2	52.2	21.7	1.2
Lemon Drizzle, Organic, Caffe Nero*	1 Serving/73g	247	9.9	338	3.3	50.5	13.6	0.5
Lemon Drizzle, Slice, Organic, Wrapped, Caffe Nero*	1 Pack/70g	248	11.1	354	4.2	48.5	15.9	0.8
Red Velvet, Caffe Nero*	1 Slice/100g	414	19.9	414	4.2	54.7	19.9	0.9
CHEESECAKE								
Chocolate, White & Dark, Truffle, Caffe Nero*	1 Serving/131g	533	35.6	407	4.8	35.7	27.2	0.5
Sicilian Lemon, Caffe Nero*	1 Serving/107g	400	26.0	374	5.0	33.0	24.3	1.4
CHOCOLATE								
Bar, Dark, 50% Cocoa, Caffe Nero*	1 Serving/40g	213	12.4	534	6.4	53.6	31.1	7.0
Bar, Milk, Caffe Nero*	1 Serving/40g	223	13.5	561	8.0	55.0	34.0	1.5
Bar, Milk, with Hazelnuts, Caffe Nero*	1 Serving/40g	229	15.2	572	8.0	49.5	38.0	1.8
Coin, Caffe Nero*	1 Serving/25g	129	7.0	516	6.3	59.7	27.8	2.1
Penguin, Milk, Paolo Pinguino, Caffe Nero*	1 Serving/45g	246	14.8	547	6.6	55.5	32.8	1.8
COFFEE								
Cappuccino, Grande, Semi Skimmed, Caffe Nero*	1 Grande/263g	92	3.4	35	2.7	3.6	1.3	0.0
Cappuccino, Grande, Skimmed Milk, Caffe Nero*	1 Grande/262g	68	0.5	26	2.7	3.7	0.2	0.0
Cappuccino, Grande, Soya Milk, Caffe Nero*	1 Grande/258g	90	4.4	35	2.8	1.9	1.7	0.5
Cappuccino, Regular, Semi Skimmed Milk, Caffe Nero*	1 Regular/142g	37	1.4	26	2.0	2.7	1.0	0.0
Cappuccino, Regular, Skimmed Milk, Caffe Nero*	1 Regular/142g	27	0.3	19	2.0	2.7	0.2	0.0
Cappuccino, Regular, Soya Milk, Caffe Nero*	1 Regular/138g	36	1.8	26	2.1	1.4	1.3	0.3
Caramelatte, Semi Skimmed Milk, Caffe Nero*	1 Serving/422g	485	25.3	115	2.3	12.3	6.0	0.0
Latte, Grande, Semi Skimmed Milk, Caffe Nero*	1 Grande/363g	138	5.1	38	2.9	3.9	1.4	0.0
Latte, Grande, Skimmed Milk, Caffe Nero*	1 Grande/364g	102	1.1	28	2.9	4.0	0.3	0.0
Latte, Grande, Soya Milk, Caffe Nero*	1 Grande/355g	135	6.4	38	3.1	2.1	1.8	1.8
Latte, Iced, Semi Skim, Caffe Nero*	1 Latte/397g	616	15.1	155	7.9	23.4	3.8	0.0
Latte, Regular, Semi Skim, Shot of Syrup, Caffe Nero*	1 Regular/245g	191	2.4	78	2.1	15.2	1.0	0.0
Latte, Regular, Semi Skim Milk, Caffe Nero*	1 Regular/209g	69	2.5	33	2.5	3.4	1.2	0.0
Latte, Regular, Skim Milk, Caffe Nero*	1 Regular/212g	51	0.4	24	2.5	3.4	0.2	0.0
Latte, Regular, Soya Milk, Caffe Nero*	1 Regular/212g	68	3.4	32	2.6	1.8	1.6	0.4
Mocha, Regular, no Cream, Semi Skim, Caffe Nero*	1 Regular/231g	150	3.2	65	2.8	10.3	1.4	0.8
Mocha, Regular, no Cream, Skimmed Milk, Caffe Nero*	1 Serving/232g	132	1.2	57	2.8	10.3	0.5	0.8
Mocha, Regular, no Cream, Soya, Caffe Nero*	1 Regular/231g	148	3.9	64	2.9	8.8	1.7	1.1
Mocha, White Chocolate, Semi Skim Milk, Caffe Nero*	1 Serving/402g	414	25.3	103	2.4	6.1	6.3	0.0
COFFEE BEANS								
Chocolate Coated, Caffe Nero*	1 Serving/25g	117	6.6	469	8.5	50.0	26.6	11.9
COOKIES								
Chocolate, Triple, Caffe Nero*	1 Serving/72g	333	17.5	463	5.6	55.6	24.3	3.3
Chocolate Chip, Organic, Caffe Nero*	1 Serving/60g	263	12.1	438	4.5	56.6	20.1	1.5
Chocolate Chunk, Milk, Caffe Nero*	1 Serving/72g	338	17.9	470	5.8	55.8	24.9	1.7
Oat & Raisin, Organic, Caffe Nero*	1 Serving/60g	282	14.0	470	4.4	60.5	23.4	2.6

	Measure INFO/WEIGHT	per Measure KCAL	FAT	Nutrition Values per 100g / 100ml KCAL	PROT	CARB	FAT	FIBRE
CAFFE NERO								
CRISPS								
Mature Cheddar & Spring Onion, Caffe Nero*	1 Serving/40g	192	11.4	481	6.1	54.0	28.6	4.4
Sea Salt, Caffe Nero*	1 Serving/40g	197	10.8	493	7.0	54.0	27.1	4.5
Sea Salt & Balsamic Vinegar, Caffe Nero*	1 Serving/40g	192	11.0	482	7.0	54.1	27.5	4.0
CROISSANT								
Almond, Caffe Nero*	1 Serving/83g	350	19.8	422	10.0	41.7	23.9	2.6
Butter, Caffe Nero*	1 Serving/50g	204	11.6	408	8.5	40.9	23.3	1.7
Cheese Twist, Caffe Nero*	1 Serving/76g	316	18.4	416	13.4	36.1	24.2	2.6
Chocolate Twist, Caffe Nero*	1 Serving/79g	320	15.4	405	7.7	49.7	19.5	1.6
Pain au Chocolat, Caffe Nero*	1 Serving/65g	270	15.1	415	8.1	43.4	23.2	1.7
CUPCAKES								
Chocolate, Caffe Nero*	1 Serving/68g	311	19.1	457	3.1	48.7	28.1	0.5
Lemon, Caffe Nero*	1 Serving/72g	340	19.6	472	2.9	54.0	27.2	0.3
Raspberry, Caffe Nero*	1 Serving/67g	295	15.1	440	3.4	55.7	22.5	0.5
DANISH PASTRY								
Maple Pecan, Caffe Nero*	1 Pastry/82g	312	25.0	381	5.2	42.3	30.5	2.1
FRUIT SALAD								
Caffe Nero*	1 Serving/190g	103	0.2	54	0.6	12.1	0.1	1.5
HOT CHOCOLATE								
Milano, with Whipped Cream, Caffe Nero*	1 Serving/241g	424	22.6	176	3.5	19.3	9.4	2.0
Regular, No Cream, Skimmed Milk, Caffe Nero*	1 Serving/236g	217	1.9	92	3.3	17.6	0.8	1.5
Regular, No Cream, Soya Milk, Caffe Nero*	1 Serving/234g	229	4.4	98	3.4	15.9	1.9	1.9
Regular, Whipped Cream, Semi Skim Milk, Caffe Nero*	1 Serving/250g	352	18.2	141	3.1	15.3	7.3	1.3
JUICE								
Apple, Organic, Carton, Caffe Nero*	1 Carton/200g	94	0.0	47	0.5	11.2	0.0	0.0
Apple, Pressed, 100% Premium, Caffe Nero*	1 Bottle/250g	120	0.0	48	0.1	11.8	0.0	0.0
Apple & Mango Juice, Caffe Nero*	1 Serving/250g	125	0.0	50	0.2	12.3	0.0	0.1
Mango & Passion Fruit, Booster, Caffe Nero*	1 Serving/597g	191	0.6	32	0.4	7.8	0.1	0.6
Orange, 100% Squeezed, Fresh, Caffe Nero*	1 Serving/250g	95	0.0	38	0.5	8.8	0.0	0.1
Orange, Lemon & Lime, Booster, Caffe Nero*	1 Serving/591g	207	0.6	35	0.5	7.6	0.1	0.9
Strawberry & Raspberry, Booster, Caffe Nero*	1 Serving/589g	206	1.8	35	0.4	7.5	0.3	1.6
LEMONADE								
Italian, Sicilian, Still, Caffe Nero*	1 Serving/666g	320	0.7	48	0.1	11.3	0.1	0.3
MILK SHAKE								
Frappe, Banana, Semi Skimmed, Caffe Nero*	1 Frappe/420g	315	4.6	75	3.0	13.5	1.1	0.0
Frappe, Banana, Skimmed, Caffe Nero*	1 Frappe/419g	285	1.3	68	3.0	13.6	0.3	0.0
Frappe, Banana, with Cream & Sprinkles, Caffe Nero*	1 Frappe/347g	402	21.8	116	2.9	12.2	6.3	0.0
Frappe, Double Choc, Cream, & Sprinkles, Caffe Nero*	1 Frappe/345g	411	21.4	119	2.9	13.4	6.2	0.2
Frappe, Double Choc, Skimmed Milk, Caffe Nero*	1 Frappe/453g	290	1.4	64	2.9	12.3	0.3	0.5
Frappe, Double Chocolate, Caffe Nero*	1 Frappe/453g	317	4.5	70	2.9	12.3	1.0	0.5
Frappe, Latte, Cream, & Sprinkles, Caffe Nero*	1 Frappe/344g	334	21.0	97	2.7	7.9	6.1	0.1
Frappe, Latte, Semi Skimmed Milk, Caffe Nero*	1 Frappe/424g	225	3.8	53	2.8	8.5	0.9	0.1
Frappe, Latte, Skimmed Milk, Caffe Nero*	1 Frappe/430g	198	0.9	46	2.8	8.6	0.2	0.1
Frappe, Latte, Soya Milk, Caffe Nero*	1 Frappe/388g	101	5.0	26	2.2	1.5	1.3	0.4
Frappe, Mint, Cream, & Sprinkles, Caffe Nero*	1 Frappe/347g	399	21.9	115	2.9	12.0	6.3	0.0
Frappe, Mint, Semi Skimmed, Caffe Nero*	1 Frappe/419ml	310	4.6	74	3.0	13.3	1.1	0.0
Frappe, Mint, Semi Skimmed Milk, Caffe Nero*	1 Frappe/419g	310	4.6	74	3.0	13.3	1.1	0.0
Frappe, Mocha Frappe Latte, Skim Milk, Caffe Nero*	1 Frappe/453g	290	1.4	64	2.9	12.3	0.3	0.5
Frappe, Mocha Latte, Cream, & Sprinkles, Caffe Nero*	1 Frappe/345g	386	21.4	112	2.8	11.2	6.2	0.5
Frappe, Mocha Latte, Semi Skimmed Milk, Caffe Nero*	1 Frappe/459g	317	4.5	70	2.9	12.3	1.0	0.5
Frappe, Strawberry, Caffe Nero*	1 Frappe/416g	316	4.6	76	3.0	13.6	1.1	0.0
Frappe, Vanilla, Caffe Nero*	1 Frappe/420g	315	4.6	75	3.0	13.6	1.1	0.0
Frappe Cream, Banana & Caramel, Caffe Nero*	1 Frappe/446g	460	22.3	103	2.0	11.7	5.0	0.0

CAFFE NERO

MILK SHAKE

	Measure INFO/WEIGHT	KCAL	FAT	KCAL	PROT	CARB	FAT	FIBRE
Frappe Creme, Coconut & Chocolate, Caffe Nero*	1 Frappe/473g	516	25.1	109	2.2	13.2	5.3	0.4
Frappe Creme, Strawberry & Vanilla, Caffe Nero*	1 Frappe/446g	469	21.4	105	2.0	13.7	4.8	0.0
Latte, Caramel, Semi Skimmed Milk, Caffe Nero*	1 Latte/428g	274	3.9	64	2.8	11.4	0.9	0.1

MINTS

Peppermints, Sugar Free, Caffe Nero*	1 Serving/14g	35	0.1	249	0.6	97.0	0.8	0.0

MUFFIN

Apple, & Pecan, Spiced, Caffe Nero*	1 Muffin/120g	474	26.5	395	4.7	43.5	22.1	1.5
Bacon, & Tomato Sauce, English, Caffe Nero*	1 Muffin/106g	277	7.5	261	13.4	34.8	7.1	2.2
Blueberry, Caffe Nero*	1 Muffin/121g	463	24.6	382	5.0	44.1	20.3	1.3
Blueberry, Reduced Fat, Caffe Nero*	1 Muffin/115g	351	11.0	305	5.6	47.3	9.6	3.3
Chocolate, & Hazelnut, Filled, Caffe Nero*	1 Muffin/120g	528	27.8	440	5.6	51.5	23.2	1.5
Chocolate, Belgian, Triple, Caffe Nero*	1 Muffin/120g	530	28.1	441	6.2	49.5	23.4	2.2
Cranberry, & Orange, Reduced Fat, Caffe Nero*	1 Muffin/120g	322	9.8	269	4.5	44.3	8.2	3.1
Egg Mayo, Cheese, & Mustard, English, Caffe Nero*	1 Muffin/134g	314	12.2	234	11.3	25.9	9.1	1.7
Ham, & Egg Mayo, with Cheese, English, Caffe Nero*	1 Muffin/134g	314	12.2	234	11.3	25.9	9.1	1.7
Lemon, Poppy Seed, Caffe Nero*	1 Muffin/121g	478	24.1	394	6.3	46.7	19.9	1.2
Raspberry, & White Chocolate, Caffe Nero*	1 Muffin/120g	493	25.4	411	5.1	48.1	21.2	1.0

PANINI

All Day Breakfast, Caffe Nero*	1 Serving/196g	389	15.9	198	9.0	21.3	8.1	1.6
Bacon, & Tomato Sauce, Breakfast, Caffe Nero*	1 Serving/105g	263	9.7	251	11.1	30.6	9.3	1.4
Brie, Bacon, & Caramelised Onion, Caffe Nero*	1 Serving/185g	478	20.6	258	10.3	28.8	11.1	1.2
Cheddar, Mozzarella, & Tomato, Tostati, Caffe Nero*	1 Serving/88g	215	8.7	244	11.7	26.4	9.9	1.2
Chicken, Bacon, & Arrabbiata Sauce, Caffe Nero*	1 Serving/204g	363	6.5	178	12.3	24.4	3.2	1.4
Chicken Pesto, Caffe Nero*	1 Serving/210g	385	13.3	183	11.8	19.7	6.3	1.1
Ham, & Egg Mayo, Breakfast, Caffe Nero*	1 Serving/146g	326	16.4	223	10.8	19.9	11.2	1.2
Ham, Mozzarella & Emmental, Tostati, Caffe Nero*	1 Serving/93g	218	8.3	235	14.2	24.2	9.0	1.2
Meatball, & Mozzarella, Napoletana, Caffe Nero*	1 Serving/213g	511	23.8	240	11.7	22.6	11.2	1.2
Mushroom, Mozzarella & Cheddar, Caffe Nero*	1 Serving/195g	348	11.9	178	8.4	21.8	6.1	1.3
Napoli Salami, & Mozzarella, Caffe Nero*	1 Serving/193g	404	17.8	209	10.1	21.5	9.2	1.2
Pepperoni, Mozzarella, & Tomato, Caffe Nero*	1 Serving/193g	472	23.4	244	11.1	22.1	12.1	1.1
Tomato, Vine, Mozzarella, & Basil, Caffe Nero*	1 Serving/212g	398	17.4	188	8.3	20.3	8.2	1.3
Tuna Melt, Caffe Nero*	1 Serving/201g	389	13.4	194	11.6	21.2	6.7	1.1

PASTA

Red Pepper Penne, Caffe Nero*	1 Serving/303g	197	3.0	65	2.8	11.4	1.0	1.3

POPCORN

Sea Salt, Caffe Nero*	1 Serving/23g	115	6.5	501	8.2	53.6	28.2	10.9
Sweet & Salt, Caffe Nero*	1 Serving/25g	123	6.2	492	7.1	60.0	24.6	9.5

SALAD

Chicken with Caesar Dressing, Caffe Nero*	1 Serving/170g	156	9.8	92	6.2	3.2	5.8	0.9

SANDWICH

BLT, Caffe Nero*	1 Sandwich/171g	471	27.2	275	10.4	21.6	15.9	2.0
Chicken, Salad & Pesto, Roll, GF, Caffe Nero*	1 Roll/154g	357	19.2	232	9.7	18.4	12.5	3.4
Chicken Salad, Less than 300 Calories, Caffe Nero*	1 Sandwich/191g	272	4.2	142	9.8	19.9	2.2	1.6
Egg Mayonnaise, Free Range, Caffe Nero*	1 Sandwich/157g	323	13.7	205	9.4	21.2	8.7	2.5
Ham, & Cheddar, Caffe Nero*	1 Sandwich/179g	418	17.8	233	15.2	20.8	9.9	1.4
Mature Cheddar & Pickle, Caffe Nero*	1 Sandwich/191g	421	20.3	220	9.1	21.2	10.6	1.6
Tuna Mayo, Cucumber, 300 Calories, Caffe Nero*	1 Sandwich/166g	258	4.7	155	10.5	21.0	2.8	2.0
Tuna Salad, Caffe Nero*	1 Sandwich/147g	268	5.3	182	11.7	25.8	3.6	1.8

SCONES

Fruit, Traditional, Caffe Nero*	1 Serving/99g	336	9.1	339	7.2	55.5	9.2	2.8

SHORTBREAD

Buttery, Crunchy, Caffe Nero*	1 Pack/50g	245	14.4	490	5.0	52.9	28.7	1.2

	Measure INFO/WEIGHT	per Measure		Nutrition Values per 100g / 100ml				
		KCAL	FAT	KCAL	PROT	CARB	FAT	FIBRE
CAFFE NERO								
SOUP								
Potato & Leek, Low Fat, Caffe Nero*	1 Serving/300g	114	4.2	38	1.0	4.9	1.4	0.6
Tomato, Sundried, & Basil, Organic, Caffe Nero*	1 Serving/300g	129	4.8	43	1.3	5.4	1.6	1.1
SYRUP								
Vanilla, Caffe Nero*	1 Shot/36g	122	0.0	339	0.0	84.2	0.0	0.0
Vanilla, Sugar Free, Caffe Nero*	1 Shot/38g	5	0.0	13	0.0	10.2	0.0	0.0
TART								
Apple & Blackcurrant, Caffe Nero*	1 Serving/101g	279	12.9	276	2.9	37.4	12.8	2.2
Custard, Portuguese, Caffe Nero*	1 Serving/69g	184	6.5	266	3.9	41.5	9.4	2.4
TEA								
Chai Latte, Semi Skimmed Milk, Caffe Nero*	1 Serving/401g	281	10.0	70	3.8	8.6	2.5	0.1
Chai Latte, Skimmed Milk, Caffe Nero*	1 Serving/405g	239	5.3	59	3.8	8.4	1.3	0.0
TIRAMISU								
Caffe Nero*	1 Serving/95g	311	20.6	327	3.9	28.4	21.7	1.0
TOPPING								
Berry Compote, for Porridge, Caffe Nero*	1 Serving/40g	47	0.1	117	0.6	29.3	0.2	1.9
Maple Sauce, for Porridge, Caffe Nero*	1 Serving/40g	94	0.0	234	0.0	58.4	0.1	0.1
WAFFLES								
Caramel, Caffe Nero*	1 Waffle/39g	177	8.2	453	3.5	62.0	21.0	1.0
WRAP								
Chicken Caesar, Caffe Nero*	1 Serving/165g	434	22.8	263	12.8	21.9	13.8	0.8
Falafel, Caffe Nero*	1 Serving/157g	424	21.8	270	8.7	29.4	13.9	1.8
YOGHURT								
Blackcurrant, Bio, Greek Style, Caffe Nero*	1 Serving/150g	235	12.9	157	5.3	14.2	8.6	0.2
Blueberry, Greek Style, Brunch Pot, Caffe Nero*	1 Serving/130g	198	6.1	152	6.2	20.8	4.7	1.2
Honey, Greek, Bio, Caffe Nero*	1 Serving/149g	231	13.0	155	5.0	14.0	8.7	0.0
Strawberry, Greek Style, Brunch Pot, Caffe Nero*	1 Serving/130g	197	6.1	151	6.2	20.6	4.7	1.1
COSTA								
BISCOTTI								
Almond, Costa*	1 Biscotti/50g	165	6.3	330	7.6	46.0	12.6	1.0
BISCUITS								
Almond, Mini, Bag, Costa*	1 Bag/78g	383	23.8	491	14.3	40.0	30.5	0.0
Bourbon, The Ultimate, Costa*	1 Biscuit/85g	427	22.8	502	6.0	57.3	26.8	3.7
Chocolate, Costa*	1 Serving/16g	76	5.0	448	4.9	41.1	29.3	0.0
Custard Cream, The Ultimate, Costa*	1 Biscuit/85g	410	18.2	482	4.4	67.2	21.4	1.4
Fruit & Oat, Costa*	1 Biscuit/30g	140	5.5	465	4.9	69.2	18.2	2.0
Garibaldi, Costa*	1 Biscuit/34g	158	8.1	464	5.3	57.3	23.8	2.9
BREAKFAST								
Bacon Roll, Costa*	1 Pack/130g	367	11.0	282	15.6	35.8	8.5	1.7
Egg & Mushroom Roll, Costa*	1 Pack/155g	354	12.3	228	8.4	30.9	7.9	1.8
BROWNIES								
Bites, Costa*	1 Serving/72g	342	22.1	475	5.4	44.3	30.7	0.0
CAKE								
Carrot, Costa*	1 Slice/138g	514	23.4	374	5.1	48.6	17.0	0.0
Chocolate, Christmas, Costa*	1 Serving/162g	616	25.8	380	4.9	53.0	15.9	2.5
Chocolate, Costa*	1 Slice/150g	575	23.6	383	4.8	76.7	15.7	0.0
Lemon, Costa*	1 Slice/144g	576	25.4	399	3.6	56.0	17.6	0.0
Victoria Sandwich, Costa*	1 Slice/136g	546	25.6	401	3.5	54.0	18.8	0.0
COFFEE								
Americano, Full Fat Milk, Massimo, Costa*	1 Massimo/600ml	44	2.2	7	0.4	0.7	0.4	0.0
Americano, Full Fat Milk, Medio, Costa*	1 Medio/480ml	40	2.1	8	0.5	0.7	0.4	0.0
Americano, Full Fat Milk, Primo, Costa*	1 Primo/380ml	40	2.3	11	0.7	1.1	0.6	0.0
Americano, Massimo, Iced, Costa*	1 Massimo/600ml	62	0.4	10	0.1	2.4	0.1	0.0

COSTA

	Measure INFO/WEIGHT	per Measure KCAL	per Measure FAT	Nutrition Values per 100g / 100ml KCAL	PROT	CARB	FAT	FIBRE
COFFEE								
Americano, Medio, Iced, Costa*	1 Medio/480ml	480	0.3	100	0.1	2.0	0.1	0.0
Americano, no Added Milk, Massimo, Costa*	1 Massimo/600ml	12	0.4	2	0.1	0.3	0.1	0.0
Americano, no Added Milk, Medio, Costa*	1 Medio/480ml	8	0.3	2	0.1	0.2	0.1	0.0
Americano, no Added Milk, Primo, Costa*	1 Primo/360ml	6	0.2	2	0.1	0.2	0.1	0.0
Americano, Primo, Iced, Costa*	1 Primo/360ml	23	0.2	6	0.1	1.4	0.1	0.0
Americano, Skimmed Milk, Medio, Costa*	1 Medio/480ml	25	0.3	5	0.5	0.8	0.1	0.0
Americano, Skimmed Milk, Primo, Costa*	1 Primo/360ml	23	0.3	6	0.6	0.9	0.1	0.0
Americano, Soya Milk, Massimo, Costa*	1 Serving/600ml	31	1.3	5	0.4	0.5	0.2	0.0
Americano, Soya Milk, Medio, Costa*	1 Serving/480ml	27	1.2	6	0.4	0.5	0.2	0.0
Americano, Soya Milk, Primo, Costa*	1 Serving/200ml	14	0.6	7	0.5	0.6	0.3	0.0
Babyccino, Chocolate, Full Fat Milk, Costa*	1 Solo/30ml	138	5.0	460	16.0	60.7	16.7	0.0
Babyccino, Chocolate, Skimmed Milk, Solo, Costa*	1 Solo/30ml	102	0.8	340	16.7	62.0	2.7	0.0
Babyccino, Chocolate, Soya Milk, Solo, Costa*	1 Serving/30ml	107	2.8	357	15.0	51.0	9.3	0.0
Babyccino, Full Fat Milk, Solo, Costa*	1 Solo/30ml	109	4.4	363	14.3	43.3	14.7	0.0
Babyccino, Skimmed Milk, Solo, Costa*	1 Solo/30ml	73	0.2	243	14.7	44.7	0.7	0.0
Babyccino, Soya Milk, Solo, Costa*	1 Solo/30ml	78	2.3	260	13.3	34.0	7.7	0.0
Caffe Latte, Full Fat Milk, Massimo, Costa*	1 Massimo/600ml	260	14.4	43	2.2	3.2	2.4	0.0
Caffe Latte, Full Fat Milk, Medio, Costa*	1 Latte/480ml	202	11.2	42	2.2	3.2	2.3	0.0
Caffe Latte, Full Fat Milk, Primo, Costa*	1 Primo/360ml	151	8.5	42	2.2	3.1	2.4	0.0
Caffe Latte, Skimmed Milk, Massimo, Costa*	1 Massimo/600ml	149	0.7	25	2.4	3.6	0.1	0.0
Caffe Latte, Skimmed Milk, Medio, Costa*	1 Medio/480ml	114	0.5	24	2.3	3.5	0.1	0.0
Caffe Latte, Skimmed Milk, Primo, Costa*	1 Primo/360ml	86	0.3	24	2.4	3.5	0.1	0.0
Caffe Latte, Soya Milk, Massimo, Costa*	1 Massimo/600ml	165	7.7	28	2.2	1.8	1.3	0.0
Caffe Latte, Soya Milk, Medio, Costa*	1 Medio/480ml	124	5.8	26	2.0	1.7	1.2	0.0
Caffe Latte, Soya Milk, Primo, Costa*	1 Primo/360ml	93	4.4	26	2.0	1.6	1.2	0.0
Cappuccino, Full Fat Milk, Massimo, Costa*	1 Massimo/655ml	223	7.7	34	1.1	1.6	1.2	0.0
Cappuccino, Full Fat Milk, Massimo, Iced, Costa*	1 Massimo/600ml	124	3.6	21	0.6	3.3	0.6	0.0
Cappuccino, Full Fat Milk, Medio, Costa*	1 Medio/480ml	167	8.9	35	1.8	2.8	1.8	0.0
Cappuccino, Full Fat Milk, Medio, Iced, Costa*	1 Medio/360ml	70	2.2	20	0.6	3.0	0.6	0.0
Cappuccino, Full Fat Milk, Primo, Costa*	1 Primo/360ml	101	5.2	28	1.4	2.4	1.4	0.0
Cappuccino, Full Fat Milk, Primo, Iced, Costa*	1 Primo/360ml	62	2.1	17	0.6	2.5	0.6	0.0
Cappuccino, Skimmed Milk, Massimo, Costa*	1 Massimo/600ml	121	0.8	20	1.8	3.0	0.1	0.0
Cappuccino, Skimmed Milk, Massimo, Iced, Costa*	1 Massimo/600ml	99	0.6	16	0.6	3.4	0.1	0.0
Cappuccino, Skimmed Milk, Medio, Costa*	1 Medio/480ml	99	0.6	21	1.8	3.1	0.1	0.0
Cappuccino, Skimmed Milk, Medio, Iced, Costa*	1 Medio/360ml	55	0.4	15	0.6	3.0	0.1	0.0
Cappuccino, Skimmed Milk, Primo, Costa*	1 Primo/360ml	64	0.5	18	1.5	2.7	0.1	0.0
Cappuccino, Skimmed Milk, Primo, Iced, Costa*	1 Primo/360ml	47	0.4	13	0.6	2.5	0.1	0.0
Cappuccino, Soya Milk, Massimo, Costa*	1 Massimo/600ml	134	5.9	22	1.6	1.7	1.0	0.0
Cappuccino, Soya Milk, Massimo, Iced, Costa*	1 Massimo/600ml	102	2.0	17	0.6	3.0	0.3	0.0
Cappuccino, Soya Milk, Medio, Costa*	1 Medio/480ml	108	4.7	22	1.6	1.7	1.0	0.0
Cappuccino, Soya Milk, Medio, Iced, Costa*	1 Medio/480ml	76	1.6	16	0.6	2.6	0.3	0.0
Cappuccino, Soya Milk, Primo, Costa*	1 Primo/360ml	69	3.0	19	1.4	1.6	0.8	0.0
Cappuccino, Soya Milk, Primo, Iced, Costa*	1 Primo/360ml	49	1.2	14	0.6	2.1	0.3	0.0
Cooler, Chocolate, Full Fat Milk, Medio, Creamy, Costa*	1 Medio/480ml	514	17.4	107	1.6	17.0	3.6	0.0
Cooler, Chocolate, Full Fat Milk, Primo, Creamy, Costa*	1 Primo/360ml	366	13.0	102	1.6	15.6	3.6	0.0
Cooler, Chocolate, Skim Milk, Medio, Creamy, Costa*	1 Medio/480ml	465	11.6	97	1.6	17.1	2.4	0.0
Cooler, Chocolate, Skim Milk, Primo, Creamy, Costa*	1 Primo/360ml	328	8.6	91	1.6	15.7	2.4	0.0
Cooler, Chocolate, Soya Milk, Medio, Creamy, Costa*	1 Medio/480ml	472	14.4	98	1.5	16.2	3.0	0.0
Cooler, Chocolate, Soya Milk, Primo, Creamy, Costa*	1 Primo/360ml	333	10.8	92	1.4	14.8	3.0	0.0
Cooler, Full Fat Milk, Massimo, Costa*	1 Massimo/568ml	297	4.4	52	0.8	10.5	0.8	0.0
Cooler, Full Fat Milk, Medio, Costa*	1 Medio/455ml	232	3.9	51	0.8	10.0	0.8	0.0
Cooler, Full Fat Milk, Primo, Costa*	1 Primo/341ml	170	2.2	50	1.0	9.2	0.6	0.0

	Measure INFO/WEIGHT	per Measure KCAL	FAT	Nutrition Values per 100g / 100ml KCAL	PROT	CARB	FAT	FIBRE

COSTA

COFFEE

	Measure INFO/WEIGHT	KCAL	FAT	KCAL	PROT	CARB	FAT	FIBRE
Cooler, Mocha, Full Fat Milk, Massimo, Costa*	1 Massimo/600ml	481	6.7	80	1.1	16.4	1.1	0.0
Cooler, Mocha, Full Fat Milk, Medio, Costa*	1 Medio/480ml	370	5.5	77	1.1	15.5	1.2	0.0
Cooler, Mocha, Skimmed Milk, Massimo, Costa*	1 Massimo/600ml	445	2.5	74	1.1	16.4	0.4	0.0
Cooler, Mocha, Skimmed Milk, Medio, Costa*	1 Medio/480ml	339	1.9	71	1.1	15.6	0.4	0.0
Cooler, Mocha, Skimmed Milk, Primo, Costa*	1 Primo/360ml	233	1.2	65	1.2	14.2	0.3	0.0
Cooler, Mocha, Soya Milk, Massimo, Costa*	1 Massimo/600ml	450	4.5	75	1.0	15.9	0.8	0.0
Cooler, Mocha, Soya Milk, Medio, Costa*	1 Medio/480ml	343	3.7	71	1.0	15.0	0.8	0.0
Cooler, Mocha, Soya Milk, Primo, Costa*	1 Primo/360ml	237	2.9	66	1.1	13.4	0.8	0.0
Cooler, Skimmed Milk, Massimo, Costa*	1 Massimo/568ml	261	0.4	46	0.8	10.6	0.1	0.0
Cooler, Skimmed Milk, Medio, Costa*	1 Medio/455ml	201	0.3	44	0.9	10.1	0.1	0.0
Cooler, Skimmed Milk, Primo, Costa*	1 Primo/360ml	141	0.2	39	1.0	8.8	0.1	0.0
Cooler, Soya Milk, Massimo, Costa*	1 Massimo/568ml	266	2.4	47	0.7	10.0	0.4	0.0
Cooler, Soya Milk, Medio, Costa*	1 Medio/455ml	205	2.1	45	0.8	9.4	0.5	0.0
Cooler, Soya Milk, Primo, Costa*	1 Primo/341ml	145	1.9	43	0.9	8.5	0.6	0.0
Cooler, Strawberry, Full Fat Milk, Medio, Creamy, Costa*	1 Medio/480ml	489	15.8	102	1.3	16.8	3.3	0.0
Cooler, Strawberry, Full Fat Milk, Primo, Creamy, Costa*	1 Prino/360ml	348	11.9	97	1.3	15.5	3.3	0.0
Cooler, Strawberry, Skim Milk, Medio, Creamy, Costa*	1 Medio/480ml	439	10.0	91	1.3	16.9	2.1	0.0
Cooler, Strawberry, Skim Milk, Primo, Creamy, Costa*	1 Primo/360ml	310	7.5	86	1.3	15.6	2.1	0.0
Cooler, Strawberry, Soya Milk, Medio, Creamy, Costa*	1 Medio/480ml	446	12.8	93	1.2	16.0	2.7	0.0
Cooler, Strawberry, Soya Milk, Primo, Creamy, Costa*	1 Primo/360ml	315	9.6	88	1.2	14.7	2.7	0.0
Cooler, Toffee, Full Fat, Primo, Creamy, Costa*	1 Primo/360ml	420	16.6	117	1.4	17.4	4.6	0.0
Cooler, Toffee, Full Fat Milk, Medio, Creamy, Costa*	1 Medio/480ml	572	21.9	119	1.4	18.1	4.6	0.0
Cooler, Toffee, Skimmed Milk, Medio, Creamy, Costa*	1 Medio/480ml	522	16.2	109	1.4	18.2	3.4	0.0
Cooler, Toffee, Skimmed Milk, Primo, Creamy, Costa*	1 Primo/360ml	383	12.2	106	1.5	17.5	3.4	0.0
Cooler, Toffee, Soya Milk, Medio, Creamy, Costa*	1 Medio/480ml	529	19.0	110	1.3	17.3	4.0	0.0
Cooler, Toffee, Soya Milk, Primo, Creamy, Costa*	1 Primo/360ml	388	14.4	108	1.3	16.6	4.0	0.0
Cooler, Vanilla, Full Fat Milk, Medio, Creamy, Costa*	1 Medio/480ml	316	6.0	66	1.2	12.5	1.2	0.0
Cooler, Vanilla, Full Fat Milk, Primo, Creamy, Costa*	1 Primo/360ml	220	4.5	61	1.2	11.3	1.2	0.0
Cooler, Vanilla, Skimmed Milk, Medio, Creamy, Costa*	1 Medio/480ml	266	0.2	55	1.2	12.6	0.0	0.0
Cooler, Vanilla, Skimmed Milk, Primo, Creamy, Costa*	1 Primo/360ml	183	0.2	51	1.2	11.4	0.1	0.0
Cooler, Vanilla, Soya Milk, Medio, Creamy, Costa*	1 Medio/480ml	256	3.0	53	1.0	10.8	0.6	0.0
Cooler, Vanilla, Soya Milk, Primo, Creamy, Costa*	1 Primo/360ml	188	2.3	52	1.1	10.5	0.6	0.0
Cortado, Full Fat Milk, Solo, Costa*	1 Solo/30ml	74	4.1	247	13.0	18.7	13.7	0.0
Cortado, Skimmed Milk, Solo, Costa*	1 Serving/30ml	42	0.2	140	13.7	20.7	0.7	0.0
Cortado, Soya Milk, Solo, Costa*	1 Solo/30ml	46	2.2	153	12.0	10.0	7.3	0.0
Espresso, Ristretto, Doppio, Costa*	1 Doppio/60ml	6	0.2	10	0.7	1.3	0.3	0.0
Espresso, Ristretto, Solo, Costa*	1 Solo/30ml	3	0.1	10	0.7	1.3	0.3	0.0
Flat White, Full Fat Milk, Primo, Costa*	1 Primo/360ml	135	7.6	38	1.9	2.8	2.1	0.0
Flat White, Skimmed Milk, Primo, Costa*	1 Primo/360ml	77	0.3	21	2.1	3.1	0.1	0.0
Flat White, Soya Milk, Primo, Costa*	1 Primo/360ml	85	4.0	24	1.9	1.5	1.1	0.0
Latte, Caramel, Ful Fat, Medio, Costa*	1 Medio/480ml	251	11.2	52	2.2	5.7	2.3	0.0
Latte, Caramel, Full Fat Milk, Massimo, Costa*	1 Massimo/600ml	325	14.4	54	2.2	5.9	2.4	0.0
Latte, Caramel, Full Fat Milk, Primo, Costa*	1 Primo/360ml	184	8.5	51	2.2	5.4	2.4	0.0
Latte, Caramel, no Sugar, Soya Milk, Massimo, Costa*	1 Massimo/600ml	169	7.7	28	2.2	2.1	1.3	0.0
Latte, Caramel, Skimmed Milk, Massimo, Costa*	1 Massimo/600ml	215	0.7	36	2.4	6.3	0.1	0.0
Latte, Caramel, Skimmed Milk, Medio, Costa*	1 Medio/480ml	164	0.5	34	2.3	6.0	0.1	0.0
Latte, Caramel, Skimmed Milk, Primo, Costa*	1 Primo/360ml	118	0.3	33	2.4	5.7	0.1	0.0
Latte, Caramel, Soya Milk, Massimo, Costa*	1 Massimo/600ml	231	7.7	38	2.2	4.4	1.3	0.0
Latte, Caramel, Soya Milk, Medio, Costa*	1 Medio/480ml	173	5.8	36	2.0	4.2	1.2	0.0
Latte, Caramel, Soya Milk, Primo, Costa*	1 Primo/360ml	126	4.4	35	2.0	3.9	1.2	0.0
Latte, Caramel, Sugar Free, Full Fat, Massimo, Costa*	1 Massimo/600ml	263	14.4	44	2.2	3.6	2.4	0.0
Latte, Caramel, Sugar Free, Full Fat Milk, Medio, Costa*	1 Serving/480ml	205	11.2	43	2.2	3.5	2.3	0.0

COSTA
COFFEE

	Measure INFO/WEIGHT	per Measure KCAL	FAT	Nutrition Values per 100g / 100ml KCAL	PROT	CARB	FAT	FIBRE
Latte, Caramel, Sugar Free, Skim Milk, Massimo, Costa*	1 Massimo/600ml	153	0.7	26	2.4	4.0	0.1	0.0
Latte, Caramel, Sugar Free, Skim Milk, Primo, Costa*	1 Primo/360ml	88	0.3	24	2.4	3.8	0.1	0.0
Latte, Caramel, Sugar Free, Skim Milk, Primo, Costa*	1 Medio/480ml	117	0.5	24	2.3	3.8	0.1	0.0
Latte, Caramel, Sugar Free, Soya Milk, Primo, Costa*	1 Primo/360ml	95	4.4	26	2.0	1.9	1.2	0.0
Latte, Caramel. Sugar Free, Soya Milk, Medio, Costa*	1 Medio/480ml	127	5.8	26	2.0	2.0	1.2	0.0
Latte, Cinnamon, Full Fat Milk, Massimo, Costa*	1 Massimo/600ml	325	14.4	54	2.2	5.9	2.4	0.0
Latte, Cinnamon, Full Fat Milk, Medio, Costa*	1 Medio/480ml	173	9.7	36	2.0	4.2	2.0	0.0
Latte, Cinnamon, Full Fat Milk, Medio, Costa*	1 Medio/480ml	251	11.2	52	2.2	5.7	2.3	0.0
Latte, Cinnamon, Full Fat Milk, Primo, Costa*	1 Primo/360ml	184	8.5	51	2.2	5.4	2.4	0.0
Latte, Cinnamon, Skimmed Milk, Massimo, Costa*	1 Massimo/600ml	215	0.7	36	2.4	6.3	0.1	0.0
Latte, Cinnamon, Skimmed Milk, Medio, Costa*	1 Medio/480ml	164	0.5	34	2.3	6.0	0.1	0.0
Latte, Cinnamon, Skimmed Milk, Primo, Costa*	1 Primo/360ml	121	0.3	34	2.4	5.7	0.1	0.0
Latte, Cinnamon, Soya Milk, Massimo, Costa*	1 Massimo/600ml	231	7.7	38	2.2	4.4	1.3	0.0
Latte, Cinnamon, Soya Milk, Primo, Costa*	1 Primo/360ml	126	4.4	35	2.0	3.9	1.2	0.0
Latte, Full Fat Milk, Massimo, Costa*	1 Massimo/600ml	240	10.5	40	1.6	4.5	1.8	0.0
Latte, Full Fat Milk, Medio, Iced, Costa*	1 Medio/480ml	184	8.3	38	1.6	4.2	1.7	0.0
Latte, Full Fat Milk, Primo, Iced, Costa*	1 Primo/360ml	132	6.3	37	1.7	3.6	1.8	0.0
Latte, Gingerbread, Full Fat Milk, Massimo, Costa*	1 Massimo/600ml	328	14.4	55	2.2	6.0	2.4	0.0
Latte, Gingerbread, Full Fat Milk, Medio, Costa*	1 Medio/480ml	253	11.2	53	2.2	5.8	2.3	0.0
Latte, Gingerbread, Full Fat Milk, Primo, Costa*	1 Primo/360ml	185	8.5	51	2.2	5.5	2.4	0.0
Latte, Gingerbread, Skimmed Milk, Massimo, Costa*	1 Massimo/600ml	218	0.7	36	2.4	6.4	0.1	0.0
Latte, Gingerbread, Skimmed Milk, Medio, Costa*	1 Medio/480ml	166	0.5	35	2.3	6.1	0.1	0.0
Latte, Gingerbread, Skimmed Milk, Primo, Costa*	1 Primo/360ml	120	0.3	33	2.4	5.8	0.1	0.0
Latte, Gingerbread, Soya Milk, Medio, Costa*	1 Medio/480ml	175	5.8	36	2.0	4.3	1.2	0.0
Latte, Roasted Hazelnut, Full Fat Milk, Massimo, Costa*	1 Massimo/600ml	323	14.4	54	2.2	5.9	2.4	0.0
Latte, Roasted Hazelnut, Full Fat Milk, Medio, Costa*	1 Medio/480ml	249	11.2	52	2.2	5.6	2.3	0.0
Latte, Roasted Hazelnut, Full Fat Milk, Primo, Costa*	1 Primo/360ml	183	8.5	51	2.2	5.3	2.4	0.0
Latte, Roasted Hazelnut, Skim Milk, Massimo, Costa*	1 Massimo/600ml	213	0.7	36	2.4	4.6	0.1	0.0
Latte, Roasted Hazelnut, Skimmed Milk, Medio, Costa*	1 Medio/480ml	162	0.5	34	2.3	5.9	0.1	0.0
Latte, Roasted Hazelnut, Skimmed Milk, Primo, Costa*	1 Primo/360ml	117	0.3	32	2.4	5.7	0.1	0.0
Latte, Roasted Hazelnut, Soya Milk, Medio, Costa*	1 Medio/480ml	172	5.8	36	2.0	4.1	1.2	0.0
Latte, Roasted Hazelnut, Soya Milk, Primo, Costa*	1 Primo/360ml	125	4.4	35	2.0	3.8	1.2	0.0
Latte, Skimmed Milk, Massimo, Iced, Costa*	1 Massimo/600ml	155	0.6	26	1.7	4.7	0.1	0.0
Latte, Skimmed Milk, Medio, Iced, Costa*	1 Medio/480ml	116	0.4	24	1.7	4.2	0.1	0.0
Latte, Skimmed Milk, Primo, Iced, Costa*	1 Primo/360ml	81	0.4	22	1.7	3.8	0.1	0.0
Latte, Soya Milk, Massimo, Iced, Costa*	1 Massimo/600ml	166	5.4	28	1.5	3.4	0.9	0.0
Latte, Soya Milk, Medio, Iced, Costa*	1 Medio/480ml	125	4.3	26	1.5	3.0	0.9	0.0
Latte, Soya Milk, Primo, Iced, Costa*	1 Primo/360ml	87	3.3	24	1.5	2.5	0.9	0.0
Latte, Vanilla, Full Fat Milk, Medio, Costa*	1 Medio/480ml	253	11.2	53	2.2	5.8	2.3	0.0
Latte, Vanilla, Skimmed Milk, Massimo, Costa*	1 Massimo/600ml	217	0.7	36	2.4	6.4	0.1	0.0
Latte, Vanilla, Skimmed Milk, Medio, Costa*	1 Medio/480ml	165	0.5	34	2.3	6.1	0.1	0.0
Latte, Vanilla, Skimmed Milk, Primo, Costa*	1 Primo/360ml	120	0.3	33	2.4	5.8	0.1	0.0
Latte, Vanilla, Soya Milk, Massimo, Costa*	1 Massimo/600ml	233	7.7	39	2.2	4.6	1.3	0.0
Latte, Vanilla, Soya Milk, Medio, Costa*	1 Medio/480ml	175	5.8	36	2.0	4.3	1.2	0.0
Latte, Vanilla, Soya Milk, Primo, Costa*	1 Primo/360ml	127	4.4	35	2.0	4.0	1.2	0.0
Light, Massimo, Costa*	1 Massimo/600ml	98	0.5	16	1.6	2.4	0.1	0.0
Light, Medio, Costa*	1 Medio/480ml	88	0.4	18	1.8	2.7	0.1	0.0
Light, Primo, Costa*	1 Primo/360ml	65	0.3	18	1.8	2.7	0.1	0.0
Mocha, Full Fat Milk, Massimo, Costa*	1 Massimo/600ml	381	15.8	64	2.5	7.3	2.6	0.0
Mocha, Full Fat Milk, Massimo, Iced, Costa*	1 Massimo/600ml	332	9.8	55	1.6	8.5	1.6	0.0
Mocha, Full Fat Milk, Medio, Costa*	1 Medio/480ml	324	12.7	68	2.5	8.2	2.6	0.0
Mocha, Full Fat Milk, Medio, Iced, Costa*	1 Medio/480ml	259	7.9	54	1.6	8.2	1.6	0.0

INFO/WEIGHT	Measure	per Measure		Nutrition Values per 100g / 100ml				
		KCAL	FAT	KCAL	PROT	CARB	FAT	FIBRE

COSTA

COFFEE

	Measure INFO/WEIGHT	KCAL	FAT	KCAL	PROT	CARB	FAT	FIBRE
Mocha, Full Fat Milk, Primo, Costa*	1 Primo/360ml	213	8.5	59	2.2	7.0	2.4	0.0
Mocha, Full Fat Milk, Primo, Iced, Costa*	1 Primo/360ml	186	5.8	52	1.6	7.6	1.6	0.0
Mocha, Skimmed Milk, Massimo, Costa*	1 Massimo/600ml	272	3.4	45	2.5	7.4	0.6	0.0
Mocha, Skimmed Milk, Massimo, iced, Costa*	1 Massimo/600ml	272	2.8	45	1.6	8.6	0.5	0.0
Mocha, Skimmed Milk, Medio, Costa*	1 Medio/480ml	250	3.2	52	2.7	8.6	0.7	0.0
Mocha, Skimmed Milk, Medio, Iced, Costa*	1 Massimo/480ml	210	2.1	44	1.6	8.3	0.4	0.0
Mocha, Skimmed Milk, Primo, Costa*	1 Primo/360ml	161	2.0	45	2.4	6.9	0.6	0.0
Mocha, Skimmed Milk, Primo, Iced, Costa*	1 Primo/360ml	148	1.5	41	1.6	7.8	0.4	0.0
Mocha, Soya Milk, Massimo, Costa*	1 Massimo/600g	293	9.7	49	2.4	5.9	1.6	0.0
Mocha, Soya Milk, Massimo, Iced, Costa*	1 Massimo/600ml	280	6.2	47	1.5	7.7	1.0	0.0
Mocha, Soya Milk, Medio, Costa*	1 Medio/480ml	265	8.4	55	2.5	6.9	1.8	0.0
Mocha, Soya Milk, Medio, Iced, Costa*	1 Medio/480ml	288	6.5	60	1.9	9.8	1.4	0.0
Mocha, Soya Milk, Primo, Costa*	1 Primo/360ml	172	5.5	48	2.2	5.9	1.5	0.0
Mocha, Soya Milk, Primo, Iced, Costa*	1 Primo/360ml	153	3.6	42	1.4	6.8	1.0	0.0
Mocha Cordato, Skimmed Milk, Solo, Costa*	1 Solo/30ml	78	0.8	260	16.0	42.3	2.7	0.0
Mocha Cortado, Full Fat Milk, Solo, Costa*	1 Solo/30ml	111	4.8	370	15.0	40.7	16.0	0.0
Mocha Cortado, Skimmed Milk, Solo, Costa*	1 Solo/30ml	78	0.8	260	16.0	42.3	2.7	0.0
Mocha Cortado, Soya Milk, Solo, Costa*	1 Solo/30g	82	2.8	273	14.3	31.7	9.3	0.0
Mocha Flake, Full Fat Milk, Massimo, Costa*	1 Massimo/600ml	552	29.8	92	2.8	8.8	5.0	0.0
Mocha Flake, Full Fat Milk, Medio, Costa*	1 Medio/480ml	495	26.8	103	2.8	10.2	5.6	0.0
Mocha Flake, Full Fat Milk, Primo, Costa*	1 Primo/360ml	360	20.1	100	2.7	9.6	5.6	0.0
Mocha Flake, Skimmed Milk, Massimo, Costa*	1 Massimo/600ml	443	17.4	74	2.8	9.0	2.9	0.0
Mocha Flake, Skimmed Milk, Medio, Costa*	1 Medio/480ml	421	17.3	88	3.0	10.5	3.6	0.0
Mocha Flake, Skimmed Milk, Primo, Costa*	1 Primo/360ml	308	13.6	85	2.8	9.9	3.8	0.0
Mocha Flake, Soya Milk, Massimo, Costa*	1 Massimo/600ml	464	23.7	77	2.6	7.5	4.0	0.0
Mocha Flake, Soya Milk, Medio, Costa*	1 Medio/480ml	436	22.4	91	2.8	8.9	4.7	0.0
Mocha Flake, Soya Milk, Primo, Costa*	1 Primo/360ml	319	17.1	89	2.6	8.4	4.8	0.0
Mocha Latte, Full Fat, Massimo, Costa*	1 Massimo/600ml	393	16.9	66	2.6	7.2	2.8	0.0
Mocha Latte, Full Fat Milk, Medio, Costa*	1 Medio/480ml	304	13.1	63	2.6	7.0	2.7	0.0
Mocha Latte, Full Fat Milk, Primo, Costa*	1 Primo/380ml	231	10.2	61	2.5	6.5	2.7	0.0
Mocha Latte, Skimmed Milk, Massimo, Costa*	1 Massimo/600ml	284	3.2	47	2.8	7.6	0.5	0.0
Mocha Latte, Skimmed Milk, Medio, Costa*	1 Medio/480ml	222	2.5	46	2.7	7.5	0.5	0.0
Mocha Latte, Skimmed Milk, Primo, Costa*	1 Primo/360ml	155	1.6	43	2.7	6.9	0.4	0.0
Mocha Latte, Soya Milk, Massimo, Costa*	1 Massimo/600ml	303	10.3	50	2.6	5.9	1.7	0.0
Mocha Latte, Soya Milk, Medio, Costa*	1 Medio/480ml	235	7.9	49	2.4	5.8	1.6	0.0
Mocha Latte, Soya Milk, Primo, Costa*	1 Primo/380ml	175	6.0	46	2.4	5.2	1.6	0.0
Strawberry, Skimmed Milk, Primo, Costa*	1 Primo/360ml	310	7.5	86	1.3	15.6	2.1	0.0

COOKIES

	Measure	KCAL	FAT	KCAL	PROT	CARB	FAT	FIBRE
Choc Chunk, Double, Costa*	1 Pack/60g	296	15.2	493	5.2	61.1	25.3	3.7
Fruit & Oat, Costa*	1 Pack/60g	283	12.7	472	5.1	65.2	21.2	2.0

CROISSANT

	Measure	KCAL	FAT	KCAL	PROT	CARB	FAT	FIBRE
Almond, Costa*	1 Croissant/88g	336	16.9	382	9.3	43.0	19.2	0.0
Butter, Costa*	1 Croissant/64g	276	16.7	431	8.3	40.6	26.1	0.0
Tomato & Emmental, Costa*	1 Croissant/98g	342	21.0	349	9.0	30.0	21.4	0.0

CUPCAKES

	Measure	KCAL	FAT	KCAL	PROT	CARB	FAT	FIBRE
Banoffee, Costa*	1 Cupcake/112g	431	17.7	385	3.7	56.7	15.8	0.0
Lemon, Costa*	1 Cupcake/97g	512	32.5	528	2.8	53.2	33.5	0.0
Rocky Road, Costa*	1 Cupcake/101g	427	17.7	421	5.1	58.9	17.5	0.0

FLAPJACK

	Measure	KCAL	FAT	KCAL	PROT	CARB	FAT	FIBRE
Fruity, Costa*	1 Serving/85g	353	12.1	415	4.9	67.0	14.2	12.5
Nutty, Costa*	1 Serving/85g	391	20.0	460	7.4	54.8	23.5	5.0

COSTA

	Measure INFO/WEIGHT	per Measure KCAL	FAT	Nutrition Values per 100g / 100ml KCAL	PROT	CARB	FAT	FIBRE
FLATBREAD								
Cajun Chicken, Costa*	1 Pack/168g	310	5.1	184	12.7	26.6	3.0	0.0
Cheddar & Caramelised Onion Chutney, Costa*	1 Pack/118g	340	13.3	288	11.9	34.8	11.3	0.0
Chicken, Green Thai, Costa*	1 Pack/173g	325	6.4	188	12.2	26.6	3.7	0.0
Emmenthal & Mushroom, Costa*	1 Pack/158g	391	16.1	248	13.1	25.9	10.2	0.0
FLAVOURING FOR COFFEE								
Caramel, Massimo, Costa*	1 Massimo/600ml	66	0.0	11	0.0	2.7	0.0	0.0
Caramel, Medio, Costa*	1 Medio/480ml	49	0.0	10	0.0	2.5	0.0	0.0
Caramel, Primo, Costa*	1 Primo/360ml	33	0.0	9	0.0	2.2	0.0	0.0
Cinnamon, Massimo, Costa*	1 Massimo/600ml	66	0.0	11	0.0	2.7	0.0	0.0
Cinnamon, Medio, Costa*	1 Medio/480ml	49	0.0	10	0.0	2.5	0.0	0.0
Cinnamon, Primo, Costa*	1 Primo/360ml	33	0.0	9	0.0	2.2	0.0	0.0
Gingerbread, Massimo, Costa*	1 Massimo/600ml	68	0.0	11	0.0	2.8	0.0	0.0
Gingerbread, Medio, Costa*	1 Medio/480ml	51	0.0	11	0.0	2.6	0.0	0.0
Gingerbread, Primo, Costa*	1 Primo/360ml	34	0.0	9	0.0	2.3	0.0	0.0
Roasted Hazelnut, Massimo, Costa*	1 Massimo/600ml	63	0.0	10	0.0	2.6	0.0	0.0
Roasted Hazelnut, Medio, Costa*	1 Medio/480ml	48	0.0	10	0.0	2.4	0.0	0.0
Roasted Hazelnut, Primo, Costa*	1 Primo/360ml	32	0.0	9	0.0	2.2	0.0	0.0
Vanilla, Massimo, Costa*	1 Massimo/600ml	68	0.0	11	0.0	2.8	0.0	0.0
Vanilla, Medio, Costa*	1 Medio/480ml	51	0.0	11	0.0	2.6	0.0	0.0
Vanilla, Primo, Costa*	1 Primo/360ml	34	0.0	9	0.0	2.3	0.0	0.0
FRESCATO								
Coffee, Full Fat Milk, Medio (Coffee Only), Costa*	1 Medio454ml	423	7.9	93	1.5	17.9	1.7	0.0
Coffee, Full Fat Milk, Primo, (Coffee Only), Costa*	1 Primo/340ml	302	5.6	89	1.4	17.1	1.6	0.0
Coffee, Skimmed Milk, Medio (Coffee Only), Costa*	1 Medio/454ml	359	0.5	79	1.6	18.0	0.1	0.0
Coffee, Skimmed Milk, Primo (Coffee Only), Costa*	1 Primo/340ml	256	0.5	75	1.5	17.2	0.2	0.0
Coffee, Soya Milk, Medio (Coffee Only), Costa*	1 Medio/454ml	375	3.9	83	1.5	17.1	0.9	0.0
Coffee, Soya Milk, Primo, (Coffee Only), Costa*	1 Primo/340ml	267	2.8	79	1.4	16.3	0.8	0.0
Coffee Caramel, Full Fat Milk, Medio, Costa*	1 Medio/454ml	488	7.9	107	1.5	21.5	1.7	0.0
Coffee Caramel, Skimmed Milk, Primo, Costa*	1 Primo/340ml	289	0.5	85	1.5	19.6	0.2	0.0
Coffee Caramel, Soya Milk, Primo, Costa*	1 Primo/340ml	300	2.8	88	1.4	18.6	0.8	0.0
Coffee Mocha, Full Fat Milk, Medio, Costa*	1 Medio/454ml	540	8.3	119	1.6	24.0	1.8	0.0
Coffee Mocha, Skimmed Milk, Medio, Costa*	1 Medio/454ml	477	1.2	105	1.7	24.1	0.3	0.0
Coffee Mocha, Skimmed Milk, Primo, Costa*	1 Primo/340ml	335	0.8	99	1.6	22.6	0.2	0.0
Coffee Vanilla, Full Fat Milk, Medio, Costa*	1 Medio/454ml	491	7.9	108	1.5	21.6	1.7	0.0
Coffee Vanilla, Full Fat Milk, Primo, Costa*	1 Primo/340ml	336	5.6	99	1.4	19.6	1.6	0.0
Coffee Vanilla, Skimmed Milk, Medio, Costa*	1 Medio/454ml	427	0.7	94	1.6	21.7	0.2	0.0
Coffee Vanilla, Skimmed Milk, Primo, Costa*	1 Primo/340ml	290	0.5	85	1.5	19.7	0.2	0.0
FRUIT COOLERS								
Mango & Passionfruit, Massimo, Costa*	1 Massimo/600ml	290	0.6	48	0.2	11.6	0.1	0.0
Mango & Passionfruit, Medio, Costa*	1 Medio/480ml	232	0.5	48	0.2	11.6	0.1	0.0
Mango & Passionfruit, Primo, Costa*	1 Primo/360ml	173	0.3	48	0.1	11.6	0.1	0.0
Peach, Massimo, Costa*	1 Massimo/600ml	406	0.3	68	0.2	16.3	0.0	0.0
Peach, Medio, Costa*	1 Medio/480ml	325	0.2	68	0.2	16.3	0.0	0.0
Peach, Primo, Costa*	1 Primo/360ml	243	0.2	68	0.2	16.3	0.1	0.0
Red Berry, Massimo, Costa*	1 Massimo/600ml	409	0.6	68	0.2	16.3	0.1	0.0
Red Berry, Medio, Costa*	1 Medio/480ml	327	0.5	68	0.2	16.3	0.1	0.0
Red Berry, Primo, Costa*	1 Primo/360ml	245	0.3	68	0.2	16.3	0.1	0.0
HOT CHOCOLATE								
Full Fat, Massimo, Costa*	1 Massimo/600ml	432	19.3	72	3.0	7.6	3.2	0.0
Full Fat, Medio, Costa*	1 Medio/480ml	327	14.6	68	2.8	7.2	3.0	0.0
Full Fat, Primo, Costa*	1 Primo/360ml	225	10.1	62	2.6	6.6	2.8	0.0
Marshmallows & Cream, Skim, Massimo, Costa*	1 Massimo/600ml	441	12.7	74	3.2	10.2	2.1	0.0

	Measure INFO/WEIGHT	per Measure KCAL	FAT	Nutrition Values per 100g / 100ml KCAL	PROT	CARB	FAT	FIBRE

COSTA

HOT CHOCOLATE

	Measure INFO/WEIGHT	KCAL	FAT	KCAL	PROT	CARB	FAT	FIBRE
Marshmallows & Cream, Skim, Medio, Costa*	1 Medio/480ml	380	12.1	79	3.2	10.7	2.5	0.0
Marshmallows & Cream, Skim, Primo, Costa*	1 Primo/360ml	277	8.8	77	3.0	10.6	2.4	0.0
Marshmallows & Cream, Soya Milk, Massimo, Costa*	1 Massimo/600ml	468	21.0	78	3.0	8.2	3.5	0.0
Marshmallows & Cream, Soya Milk, Medio, Costa*	1 Medio/480ml	401	18.7	84	3.0	8.8	3.9	0.0
Marshmallows & Cream, Soya Milk, Primo, Costa*	1 Primo/360ml	294	13.4	82	2.8	8.9	3.7	0.0
Skimmed, Massimo, Costa*	1 Massimo/600ml	296	3.0	49	3.1	7.9	0.5	0.0
Skimmed, Medio, Costa*	1 Medio/480ml	235	2.4	49	3.0	7.9	0.5	0.0
Skimmed, Primo, Costa*	1 Primo/360ml	156	1.5	43	2.8	7.0	0.4	0.0
Soya Milk, Massimo, Costa*	1 Massimo/600ml	323	11.3	54	2.8	6.0	1.9	0.0
Soya Milk, Medio, Costa*	1 Medio/480ml	256	9.0	53	2.8	6.0	1.9	0.0
Soya Milk, Primo, Costa*	1 Primo/360ml	172	6.1	48	1.5	5.3	1.7	0.0

ICE DESSERTS

	Measure INFO/WEIGHT	KCAL	FAT	KCAL	PROT	CARB	FAT	FIBRE
Double Choc Flake, Full Fat Milk, Medio, Costa*	1 Medio/454ml	786	29.9	173	2.1	26.4	6.6	0.0
Simply Vanilla, Full Fat Milk, Medio, Costa*	1 Medio/454ml	421	7.8	93	1.4	17.9	1.7	0.0
Simply Vanilla, Full Fat Milk, Primo, Costa*	1 Primo/340ml	301	5.6	89	1.4	17.1	1.6	0.0
Simply Vanilla, Skimmed Milk, Primo, Costa*	1 Primo/340ml	255	0.5	75	1.5	17.2	0.2	0.0
Simply Vanilla, Soya Milk, Medio, Costa*	1 Medio/454ml	373	3.8	82	1.4	17.0	0.8	0.0
Simply Vanilla, Soya Milk, Primo, Costa*	1 Primo/340ml	267	2.7	79	1.4	16.2	0.8	0.0
Strawberry Shortcake, Full Fat Milk, Primo, Costa*	1 Primo/340ml	569	23.9	167	1.8	24.3	7.0	0.0
Strawberry Shortcake, Skimmed Milk, Medio, Costa*	1 Medio/454ml	694	19.0	153	1.9	27.2	4.2	0.0

JUICE DRINK

	Measure INFO/WEIGHT	KCAL	FAT	KCAL	PROT	CARB	FAT	FIBRE
Orange & Raspberry, Fruit Cooler, Medio, Costa*	1 Medio/480ml	320	0.2	67	0.2	15.9	0.0	0.0
Orange & Raspberry, Fruit Cooler, Primo, Costa*	1 Primo/360ml	241	0.2	67	0.2	16.1	0.1	0.0
Orange & Raspberry, Juice Drink, Massimo, Costa*	1 Massimo/600ml	403	0.3	67	0.2	16.1	0.0	0.0
Tropical Fruit, Fruit Cooler, Massimo, Costa*	1 Massimo/600ml	400	2.6	67	0.2	15.3	0.4	0.0
Tropical Fruit, Fruit Cooler, Medio, Costa*	1 Medio/480ml	317	2.0	66	0.2	15.2	0.4	0.0
Tropical Fruit, Fruit Cooler, Primo, Costa*	1 Primo/360ml	240	1.5	67	0.1	15.2	0.4	0.0

LEMONADE

	Measure INFO/WEIGHT	KCAL	FAT	KCAL	PROT	CARB	FAT	FIBRE
Iced, Massimo, Costa*	1 Massimo/600ml	196	0.0	33	0.0	7.9	0.0	0.0
Iced, Medio, Costa*	1 Medio/480ml	147	0.0	31	0.0	7.4	0.0	0.0
Iced, Primo, Costa*	1 Serving/360ml	98	0.0	27	0.0	6.6	0.0	0.0
Peach, Iced, Massimo, Costa*	1 Massimo/600ml	172	0.0	29	0.0	7.0	0.0	0.0
Peach, Iced, Medio, Costa*	1 Medio/480ml	129	0.0	27	0.0	6.6	0.0	0.0
Peach, Iced, Primo, Costa*	1 Primo/360ml	86	0.0	24	0.0	5.8	0.0	0.0
Raspberry & Cranberry, Iced, Massimo, Costa*	1 Massimo/600ml	179	0.0	30	0.0	7.3	0.0	0.0
Raspberry & Cranberry, Iced, Medio, Costa*	1 Medio/480ml	134	0.0	28	0.0	6.8	0.0	0.0
Raspberry & Cranberry, Iced, Primo, Costa*	1 Primo/360ml	89	0.0	25	0.0	6.1	0.0	0.0
Strawberry, Iced, Massimo, Costa*	1 Massimo/600ml	175	0.0	29	0.0	7.1	0.0	0.0
Strawberry, Iced, Medio, Costa*	1 Medio/480ml	131	0.0	27	0.0	6.7	0.0	0.0
Strawberry, Iced, Primo, Costa*	1 Primo/360ml	87	0.0	24	0.0	5.9	0.0	0.0

MUFFIN

	Measure INFO/WEIGHT	KCAL	FAT	KCAL	PROT	CARB	FAT	FIBRE
Banana & Pecan Breakfast Loaf, Costa*	1 Muffin/113g	442	23.4	391	5.1	44.0	20.7	0.0
Blueberry, Costa*	1 Muffin/132g	475	20.9	360	4.0	50.4	15.8	0.0
Chocolate, Mini, Costa*	1 Muffin/19g	73	3.9	383	4.3	44.5	20.5	0.0
Chocolate, Triple, Costa*	1 Muffin/130g	530	27.8	408	5.3	48.6	21.4	0.0
Lemon & Orange, Low Fat, Costa*	1 Muffin/135g	319	3.1	236	4.6	49.4	2.3	1.1
Lemon & Poppyseed, Costa*	1 Muffin/131g	532	28.0	406	4.3	49.0	21.4	0.0
Lemon & White Chocolate, Costa*	1 Muffin/129g	472	20.4	366	5.4	52.3	15.8	0.0
Original, Breakfast Loaf, Costa*	1 Serving/128g	443	18.6	346	5.0	48.9	14.5	0.0
Raspberry, & White Chocolate, Costa*	1 Muffin/135g	511	26.0	376	4.8	46.4	19.1	0.0
Raspberry, & White Chocolate, Mini, Costa*	1 Muffin/19g	72	3.7	379	4.1	45.9	19.4	0.0

	Measure INFO/WEIGHT	per Measure KCAL	FAT	Nutrition Values per 100g / 100ml KCAL	PROT	CARB	FAT	FIBRE
PAIN AU RAISIN								
Costa*	1 Pastry/119g	356	13.7	299	5.1	43.7	11.5	0.0
PANINI								
Brie & Tomato Chutney, Costa*	1 Panini/177g	453	16.5	256	9.8	33.3	9.3	2.8
Chicken & Pesto, Costa*	1 Serving/209g	419	21.4	200	22.5	57.9	10.2	0.0
Chicken Roasted Pepper & Rocket, Costa*	1 Pack/185g	338	7.6	183	10.4	26.0	4.1	3.2
Goats Cheese & Caramelised Onion Chutney, Costa*	1 Panini/172g	431	5.3	251	4.9	19.5	3.1	0.0
Goats Cheese & Pepper, Costa*	1 Serving/197g	424	11.0	215	9.9	30.3	5.6	0.0
Ham & Cheese, Costa*	1 Panini/175g	461	21.2	263	12.5	26.2	12.1	0.0
Mozzarella, Tomato & Basil, Costa*	1 Panini/190g	400	11.0	211	8.3	29.8	5.8	0.0
Ragu Meatball, Costa*	1 Serving/190g	477	15.8	251	11.7	31.2	8.3	0.0
Steak & Cheese, Costa*	1 Serving/228g	492	16.4	216	11.3	25.7	7.2	0.0
Tuna Melt, Costa*	1 Panini/190g	462	14.3	243	14.4	29.5	7.5	0.0
ROLL								
All Day Breakfast, Costa*	1 Roll/230g	663	33.6	288	11.7	27.5	14.6	0.0
SALAD								
Chargrilled Vegetable & Cous Cous, Costa*	1 Serving/291g	352	7.6	121	3.0	21.5	2.6	0.0
Chicken & Pasta, Costa*	1 Serving/270g	427	11.1	158	8.4	21.9	4.1	0.0
Chicken & Pesto Pasta, Costa*	1 Pack/271g	420	11.4	155	7.8	21.3	4.2	1.7
Cous Cous, Moroccan Styles, Costa*	1 Pack/290g	392	7.3	135	3.6	24.6	2.5	2.2
Sunblush Tomato & Feta Pasta, Costa*	1 Pack/267g	360	13.6	135	4.4	17.1	5.1	2.2
Tuna, Costa*	1 Pack/181g	274	4.0	151	10.3	22.6	2.2	0.0
SANDWICH								
Bacon & Tomato Sauce, Tostato, Costa*	1 Tostato/132g	316	6.6	239	8.5	40.2	5.0	0.0
BLT, Costa*	1 Pack/169g	397	15.7	235	11.0	26.8	9.3	0.0
Brie, Apple & Grape, Costa*	1 Serving/225g	536	24.5	238	8.3	28.7	10.9	0.0
Chicken, Coronation, Costa*	1 Pack/258g	600	26.1	232	12.5	23.0	10.1	2.5
Chicken, Roast, Costa*	1 Pack/177g	325	7.1	184	13.0	23.8	4.0	0.0
Club, All Day Breakfast, Costa*	1 Pack/243g	592	20.9	244	11.0	30.6	8.6	0.0
Club, Chicken & Bacon, Costa*	1 Pack/213g	484	13.2	227	13.6	29.3	6.2	0.0
Egg, Free Range, Costa*	1 Pack/172g	377	14.6	219	9.7	25.9	8.5	0.0
Egg Mayonnaise & Tomato, Free Range, Costa*	1 Pack/174g	389	24.1	223	8.6	18.3	13.8	0.0
Ham Hock & Mustard Pickle, Roll, Costa*	1 Pack/163g	286	5.2	176	10.6	26.1	3.2	0.0
Houmous, Costa*	1 Pack/165g	263	4.7	160	6.4	25.9	2.8	0.0
Ploughmans, Cheese, Roll, Costa*	1 Pack/175g	431	21.3	247	9.4	25.0	12.2	0.0
Prawn, Tiger, with Lime & Chilli Dressing, Costa*	1 Pack/185g	367	19.0	198	8.2	21.2	10.2	0.0
Prawn Mayonnaise, on Wholemeal, Costa*	1 Pack/163g	291	7.7	178	9.0	23.6	4.7	0.0
Salmon, & Salad, Poached, Oatmeal, Costa*	1 Pack/151g	224	4.2	148	7.7	22.9	2.8	0.0
Sausage, Chorizo, & Vine Ripened Tomato, Costa*	1 Pack/181g	315	3.8	174	15.5	26.1	2.1	0.0
Tuna, & Salad, Costa*	1 Pack/177g	289	4.1	163	11.9	25.7	2.3	0.0
SCONE								
Fruit, Costa*	1 Serving/110g	370	11.8	336	5.6	55.1	10.7	0.0
SHORTBREAD								
Mini, Bag, Costa*	1 Bag/65g	316	15.7	486	4.1	63.0	24.1	0.0
SHORTCAKE								
Raspberry, Costa*	1 Shortcake/45g	215	10.7	477	2.4	63.5	23.7	0.0
SLICES								
Cheese, Twist, Pastry, Costa*	1 Pastry/103g	346	20.4	336	11.1	29.5	19.8	0.0
Cinnamon Swirl, Pastry, Costa*	1 Pastry/92g	341	22.8	369	4.0	31.9	24.7	0.0
Pecan, Pastry, Costa*	1 Pastry/105g	465	29.9	443	5.6	42.1	28.5	3.0
SOUP								
Fish, Bouillabaisse, Costa*	1 Serving/400g	180	5.6	45	5.8	2.2	1.4	0.0

	Measure INFO/WEIGHT	per Measure KCAL	FAT	Nutrition Values per 100g / 100ml KCAL	PROT	CARB	FAT	FIBRE
COSTA								
TART								
Chocolate & Orange, Costa*	1 Serving/78g	357	18.5	458	5.8	56.3	23.8	2.3
TEA								
Iced, Lemon, Costa*	1 Bottle/275ml	91	0.0	33	0.0	8.0	0.0	0.0
Iced, Original, Massimo, Costa*	1 Massimo/600ml	179	0.0	30	0.0	9.1	0.0	0.0
Iced, Original, Medio, Costa*	1 Medio/480ml	135	0.0	28	0.0	6.9	0.0	0.0
Iced, Original, Primo, Costa*	1 Primo/360ml	88	0.0	24	0.0	6.0	0.0	0.0
Iced, Peach, Massimo, Costa*	1 Massimo/600ml	121	0.0	20	0.0	4.8	0.0	0.0
Iced, Peach, Medio, Costa*	1 Medio/480ml	91	0.0	19	0.0	4.5	0.0	0.0
Iced, Peach, Primo, Costa*	1 Primo/360ml	60	0.0	17	0.0	4.0	0.0	0.0
Iced, Raspberry, Massimo, Costa*	1 Massimo/600ml	133	0.0	22	0.0	5.4	0.0	0.0
Iced, Raspberry, Medio, Costa*	1 Medio/480ml	100	0.0	21	0.0	5.1	0.0	0.0
Iced, Raspberry, Primo, Costa*	1 Primo/360ml	67	0.0	19	0.0	4.5	0.0	0.0
Latte, Chai, Full Fat, Massimo, Costa*	1 Massimo/600ml	429	16.9	72	2.6	9.0	2.8	0.0
Latte, Chai, Full Fat, Medio, Costa*	1 Medio/480ml	325	12.7	68	2.5	8.6	2.6	0.0
Latte, Chai, Full Fat, Medio, Costa*	1 Medio/480ml	325	12.7	68	2.5	8.6	2.6	0.0
Latte, Chai, Full Fat, Primo, Costa*	1 Primo/360ml	223	8.9	62	2.3	7.8	2.5	0.0
Latte, Chai, Skimmed, Massimo, Costa*	1 Massimo/600ml	293	0.6	49	2.8	9.4	0.1	0.0
Latte, Chai, Skimmed, Medio, Costa*	1 Medio/480ml	232	0.5	48	2.7	9.3	0.1	0.0
Latte, Chai, Skimmed, Primo, Costa*	1 Primo/360ml	154	0.3	43	2.5	8.2	0.1	0.0
Latte, Chai, Soya Milk, Massimo, Costa*	1 Massimo/600ml	320	8.9	53	2.5	7.5	1.5	0.0
Latte, Chai, Soya Milk, Medio, Costa*	1 Medio/480ml	254	7.0	53	2.5	7.4	1.5	0.0
Latte, Chai, Soya Milk, Primo, Costa*	1 Primo/360ml	170	4.8	47	2.3	6.6	1.3	0.0
TRAYBAKE								
Chocolate Tiffin Triangle, Costa*	1 Serving/85g	433	25.7	509	4.9	54.6	30.2	0.0
Fruit, Seed, Nut & Honey Bar, Costa*	1 Serving/75g	317	15.2	423	7.5	52.5	20.3	0.0
Granola Bar, Costa*	1 Bar/75g	317	15.2	423	7.5	52.5	20.3	0.0
Shortbread, Caramel, Costa*	1 Serving/77g	426	26.5	553	4.7	55.9	34.4	0.0
WRAP								
Chicken Caesar, Costa*	1 Pack/194g	420	15.6	216	11.8	24.1	8.0	1.4
Chicken Fajita, Costa*	1 Wrap/186g	416	12.9	223	12.1	28.0	6.9	0.0
Spicy Three Bean, Costa*	1 Pack/235g	456	14.3	194	7.1	27.7	6.1	0.0
YOGHURT								
Honey & Granola, Costa*	1 Pot/190g	303	6.1	159	5.3	27.3	3.2	0.0
Strawberry & Granola, Costa*	1 Pot/190g	253	7.4	133	5.4	19.0	3.9	0.0
DOMINO'S PIZZA								
DIP								
Garlic & Herb, Domino's Pizza*	1 Pot/28g	194	21.1	693	1.1	1.9	75.4	0.1
PIZZA								
American Hot, Classic, Delight, Large, Domino's Pizza*	1 Slice/75g	189	6.9	252	15.1	26.2	9.2	2.0
American Hot, Classic, Delight, Med, Domino's Pizza*	1 Slice/68g	175	6.5	255	15.2	26.1	9.5	2.0
American Hot, Classic, Delight, Small, Domino's Pizza*	1 Slice/61g	157	6.3	259	11.7	28.9	10.4	1.9
American Hot, Classic, Large, Domino's Pizza*	1 Slice/315g	823	35.0	261	10.9	28.7	11.1	1.9
American Hot, Classic, Medium, Domino's Pizza*	1 Slice/288g	761	32.9	264	11.0	28.5	11.4	1.9
American Hot, Classic, Personal, Domino's Pizza*	1 Slice/204g	536	19.8	262	11.2	31.4	9.7	2.2
American Hot, Classic, Small, Domino's Pizza*	1 Slice/253g	669	28.1	264	12.2	27.7	11.1	1.9
American Hot, GF, Delight, Small, Domino's Pizza*	1 Slice/53g	138	5.8	258	12.2	26.8	10.9	2.1
American Hot, GF, Smal, Domino's Pizza*	1 Slice/53g	134	6.5	251	8.7	25.5	12.1	2.4
American Hot, Italian, Delight, Large, Domino's Pizza*	1 Slice/66g	173	6.6	263	11.9	30.2	10.1	2.1
American Hot, Italian, Delight, Medium, Domino's Pizza*	1 Slice/58g	155	6.2	266	12.0	29.7	10.6	2.1
American Hot, Italian, Delight, Small, Domino's Pizza*	1 Slice/51g	137	5.8	269	12.1	28.9	11.3	2.0
American Hot, Italian, Large, Domino's Pizza*	1 Slice/274g	643	28.0	234	10.6	24.1	10.2	1.8
American Hot, Italian, Medium, Domino's Pizza*	1 Slice/58g	138	6.2	237	10.8	23.7	10.7	1.8

DOMINO'S PIZZA

PIZZA

	Measure INFO/WEIGHT	per Measure KCAL	FAT	Nutrition Values per 100g / 100ml KCAL	PROT	CARB	FAT	FIBRE
American Hot, Italian, Small, Domino's Pizza*	1 Slice/51g	123	5.8	241	10.9	23.1	11.4	1.8
American Hot, Personal Pizza, Domino's Pizza*	1 Slice/61g	161	5.1	264	14.7	32.6	8.3	2.2
Americano, Classic, Delight, Large, Domino's Pizza*	1 Slice/73g	213	6.7	290	15.1	36.0	9.1	2.1
Americano, Classic, Delight, Medium, Domino's Pizza*	1 Slice/67g	197	6.3	292	15.1	35.8	9.4	2.1
Americano, Classic, Delight, Personal, Domino's Pizza*	1 Slice/203g	590	17.2	291	13.7	38.9	8.5	2.3
Americano, Classic, Delight, Small, Domino's Pizza*	1 Slice/60g	184	5.9	304	14.9	37.8	9.8	2.5
Americano, Classic, Large, Domino's Pizza*	1 Slice/73g	221	8.1	301	14.3	35.3	11.0	2.4
Americano, Classic, Medium, Domino's Pizza*	1 Slice/68g	205	7.6	303	14.3	35.1	11.3	2.4
Americano, Classic, Personal, Domino's Pizza*	1 Slice/202g	609	20.8	301	15.1	36.0	10.3	2.4
Americano, Classic, Small, Domino's Pizza*	1 Slice/60g	183	7.3	305	15.5	32.4	12.1	2.5
Americano, GF, Delight, Small, Domino's Pizza*	1 Slice/53g	159	5.9	302	13.7	35.5	11.2	2.5
Americano, GF, Small, Domino's Pizza*	1 Slice/52g	166	6.9	315	12.4	35.9	13.1	2.4
Americano, Italian, Delight, Large, Domino's Pizza*	1 Slice/64g	192	6.7	300	18.4	31.8	10.4	2.8
Americano, Italian, Delight, Medium, Domino's Pizza*	1 Slice/57g	172	6.2	303	18.5	31.3	10.9	2.8
Americano, Italian, Delight, Small, Domino's Pizza*	1 Slice/50g	153	5.8	306	18.7	30.6	11.6	2.7
Americano, Italian, Large, Domino's Pizza*	1 Slice/64g	197	7.8	307	15.5	33.0	12.1	2.4
Americano, Italian, Small, Domino's Pizza*	1 Slice/50g	157	6.6	313	15.9	31.7	13.2	2.4
Americano, Personal Pizza, Domino's Pizza*	1 Slice/64g	184	4.9	287	19.4	35.0	7.7	2.5
Carolina, Classic, Delight, Large, Domino's Pizza*	1 Slice/79g	212	6.7	268	13.3	33.8	8.5	1.9
Carolina, Classic, Delight, Medium, Domino's Pizza*	1 Slice/72g	194	6.2	269	13.4	33.7	8.6	1.9
Carolina, Classic, Delight, Personal, Domino's Pizza*	1 Slice/220g	605	19.9	274	11.9	35.5	9.0	2.0
Carolina, Classic, Delight, Small, Domino's Pizza*	1 Slice/64g	176	5.5	277	12.9	35.7	8.7	2.3
Carolina, Classic, Large, Domino's Pizza*	1 Slice/79g	220	8.2	278	12.6	33.0	10.3	2.1
Carolina, Classic, Medium, Domino's Pizza*	1 Slice/72g	201	7.5	280	12.6	33.0	10.4	2.1
Carolina, Classic, Personal, Domino's Pizza*	1 Slice/220g	624	23.4	283	13.3	32.9	10.6	2.0
Carolina, Classic, Small, Domino's Pizza*	1 Slice/63g	177	6.9	279	13.5	30.7	10.9	2.3
Carolina, GF, Small, Domino's Pizza*	1 Slice/56g	160	6.6	284	10.3	33.7	11.7	2.1
Carolina, Italian, Delight, Large, Domino's Pizza*	1 Slice/69g	190	6.7	274	16.1	29.5	9.7	2.5
Carolina, Italian, Delight, Medium, Domino's Pizza*	1 Slice/61g	169	6.1	275	16.2	29.2	9.9	2.5
Carolina, Italian, Delight, Small, Domino's Pizza*	1 Slice/54g	147	5.5	274	16.1	28.6	10.2	2.4
Carolina, Italian, Large, Domino's Pizza*	1 Slice/69g	195	7.8	281	13.4	30.7	11.3	2.1
Carolina, Italian, Medium, Domino's Pizza*	1 Slice/61g	173	7.1	282	13.5	30.3	11.5	2.1
Carolina, Italian, Small, Domino's Pizza*	1 Slice/53g	150	6.2	281	13.5	29.6	11.7	2.1
Cheese & Tom, Classic, Delight, Med, Domino's Pizza*	1 Slice/53g	138	3.3	262	17.0	33.0	6.3	2.4
Cheese & Tomato, Classic, Large, Domino's Pizza*	1 Slice/57g	158	5.1	274	11.5	36.2	8.8	2.2
Cheese & Tomato, Classic, Medium, Domino's Pizza*	1 Slice/53g	144	4.6	274	11.5	36.2	8.8	2.2
Cheese & Tomato, Classic, Personal, Domino's Pizza*	1 Slice/161g	435	11.3	270	11.6	38.9	7.0	2.5
Cheese & Tomato, Classic, Small, Domino's Pizza*	1 Slice/45g	122	3.5	269	12.9	35.8	7.7	2.3
Cheese & Tomato, GF, Small, Domino's Pizza*	1 Slice/73g	185	6.2	252	8.2	34.2	8.4	3.0
Cheese & Tomato, Italian, Large, Domino's Pizza*	1 Slice/48g	115	3.4	239	11.3	31.5	7.1	2.2
Cheese & Tomato, Italian, Medium, Domino's Pizza*	1 Slice/42g	100	3.0	239	11.3	31.5	7.1	2.2
Cheese & Tomato, Italian, Small, Domino's Pizza*	1 Slice/35g	85	2.5	239	11.3	31.5	7.1	2.2
Chicken Feast, Classic, Delight, Small, Domino's Pizza*	1 Slice/72g	165	3.7	228	16.5	29.0	5.1	2.3
Chicken Feast, Classic, Large, Domino's Pizza*	1 Slice/89g	201	5.6	226	14.6	27.8	6.3	2.1
Chicken Feast, Classic, Medium, Domino's Pizza*	1 Slice/81g	183	5.1	226	14.6	27.8	6.3	2.1
Chicken Feast, Classic, Personal, Domino's Pizza*	1 Slice/62g	153	3.8	247	15.7	32.3	6.1	2.1
Chicken Feast, Classic, Small, Domino's Pizza*	1 Slice/72g	163	4.5	226	14.6	27.8	6.3	2.1
Chicken Feast, Italian, Large, Domino's Pizza*	1 Slice/69g	195	8.0	283	16.5	28.1	11.6	2.4
Chicken Feast, Italian, Medium, Domino's Pizza*	1 Slice/64g	181	7.4	283	16.5	28.1	11.6	2.4
Meateor, Classic, Large, Domino's Pizza*	1 Slice/87g	278	11.1	319	14.5	36.7	12.7	1.8
Meateor, Classic, Medium, Domino's Pizza*	1 Slice/80g	255	10.2	319	14.5	36.7	12.7	1.8
Meateor, Classic, Personal, Domino's Pizza*	1 Slice/66g	204	7.8	310	18.4	32.5	11.8	2.3

DOMINO'S PIZZA

PIZZA

	Measure INFO/WEIGHT	per Measure KCAL	FAT	KCAL	PROT	CARB	FAT	FIBRE
Meateor, Classic, Small, Domino's Pizza*	1 Slice/73g	233	9.3	319	14.5	36.7	12.7	1.8
Meateor, Italian, Large, Domino's Pizza*	1 Slice/67g	236	11.9	352	15.3	32.8	17.7	1.7
Meateor, Italian, Medium, Domino's Pizza*	1 Slice/63g	247	12.2	392	16.0	38.6	19.3	2.0
Mighty Meaty, Classic, Delight, Small, Domino's Pizza*	1 Slice/80g	202	7.3	253	16.5	26.1	9.1	2.2
Mighty Meaty, Classic, Large, Domino's Pizza*	1 Slice/95g	243	9.7	256	15.0	26.1	10.2	2.0
Mighty Meaty, Classic, Medium, Domino's Pizza*	1 Slice/87g	218	8.9	251	14.7	25.0	10.3	1.9
Mighty Meaty, Classic, Personal, Domino's Pizza*	1 Slice/66g	179	6.6	270	15.5	29.7	9.9	2.0
Mighty Meaty, Classic, Small, Domino's Pizza*	1 Slice/80g	206	8.5	257	15.3	25.2	10.6	2.0
Mighty Meaty, Italian, Large, Domino's Pizza*	1 Slice/75g	222	11.8	296	16.2	22.6	15.7	2.3
Mighty Meaty, Italian, Medium, Domino's Pizza*	1 Slice/70g	216	11.2	309	16.5	24.6	16.0	2.1
New Yorker, Classic, Delight, Large, Domino's Pizza*	1 Slice/87g	225	7.1	258	17.5	27.9	8.1	2.2
New Yorker, Classic, Delight, Medium, Domino's Pizza*	1 Slice/80g	207	6.5	258	17.5	27.9	8.1	2.2
New Yorker, Classic, Delight, Personal, Domino's Pizza*	1 Slice/60g	151	4.5	252	13.7	31.4	7.5	2.2
New Yorker, Classic, Delight, Small, Domino's Pizza*	1 Slice/73g	188	5.9	258	17.5	27.9	8.1	2.2
New Yorker, Classic, Large, Domino's Pizza*	1 Slice/88g	225	8.2	257	15.5	26.7	9.4	2.0
New Yorker, Classic, Medium, Domino's Pizza*	1 Slice/80g	206	7.5	257	15.5	26.7	9.4	2.0
New Yorker, Classic, Personal, Domino's Pizza*	1 Slice/60g	165	5.1	275	16.3	32.1	8.5	2.0
New Yorker, Classic, Small, Domino's Pizza*	1 Slice/73g	188	6.9	257	15.5	26.7	9.4	2.0
New Yorker, Italian, Large, Domino's Pizza*	1 Slice/67g	217	10.4	322	17.6	26.7	15.5	2.2
New Yorker, Italian, Medium, Domino's Pizza*	1 Slice/63g	203	9.8	322	17.6	26.7	15.5	2.2
Pepperoni Passion, Classic, Large, Domino's Pizza*	1 Slice/78g	228	9.1	292	16.7	28.7	11.6	2.0
Pepperoni Passion, Classic, Medium, Domino's Pizza*	1 Slice/72g	210	8.3	292	16.7	28.7	11.6	2.0
Pepperoni Passion, Classic, Personal, Domino's Pizza*	1 Slice/59g	182	7.0	307	17.9	30.8	11.8	1.9
Pepperoni Passion, Classic, Small, Domino's Pizza*	1 Slice/65g	190	7.5	292	16.7	28.7	11.6	2.0
Pepperoni Passion, Italian, Large, Domino's Pizza*	1 Slice/58g	210	10.9	362	19.0	27.5	18.8	2.2
Pepperoni Passion, Italian, Medium, Domino's Pizza*	1 Slice/55g	199	10.3	362	19.0	27.5	18.8	2.2
Tandoori Hot, Classic, Delight, Small, Domino's Pizza*	1 Slice/73g	159	3.6	218	15.0	28.4	4.9	2.4
Tandoori Hot, Classic, Large, Domino's Pizza*	1 Slice/89g	198	5.6	223	13.4	28.1	6.3	2.2
Tandoori Hot, Classic, Medium, Domino's Pizza*	1 Slice/81g	176	5.0	217	13.0	27.2	6.2	2.2
Tandoori Hot, Classic, Personal, Domino's Pizza*	1 Slice/62g	149	3.7	240	14.5	31.9	6.0	2.2
Tandoori Hot, Classic, Small, Domino's Pizza*	1 Slice/73g	162	4.6	222	13.5	27.9	6.3	2.3
Tandoori Hot, Italian, Large, Domino's Pizza*	1 Slice/69g	177	7.6	257	14.3	24.9	11.1	2.6
Tandoori Hot, Italian, Medium, Domino's Pizza*	1 Slice/64g	173	7.3	270	14.5	27.4	11.4	2.5
Texas BBQ, Classic, Delight, Personal, Domino's Pizza*	1 Slice/61g	156	3.4	256	14.2	36.4	5.5	1.9
Texas BBQ, Classic, Delight, Small, Domino's Pizza*	1 Slice/71g	170	3.9	240	13.0	33.4	5.5	2.2
Texas BBQ, Classic, Large, Domino's Pizza*	1 Slice/87g	240	7.0	276	14.4	36.6	8.0	1.8
Texas BBQ, Classic, Medium, Domino's Pizza*	1 Slice/79g	218	6.3	276	14.4	36.6	8.0	1.8
Texas BBQ, Classic, Personal, Domino's Pizza*	1 Slice/61g	171	4.0	280	18.4	35.6	6.6	2.5
Texas BBQ, Classic, Small, Domino's Pizza*	1 Slice/71g	196	5.7	276	14.4	36.6	8.0	1.8
Texas BBQ, Italian, Large, Domino's Pizza*	1 Slice/63g	183	7.3	289	15.3	30.8	11.6	1.7
Texas BBQ, Italian, Medium, Domino's Pizza*	1 Slice/59g	206	8.0	351	15.6	40.3	13.7	2.1
The Sizzler, Classic, Large, Domino's Pizza*	1 Slice/95g	271	10.6	285	14.7	31.5	11.2	2.2
The Sizzler, Classic, Medium, Domino's Pizza*	1 Slice/87g	248	9.7	285	14.7	31.5	11.2	2.2
The Sizzler, Classic, Personal, Domino's Pizza*	1 Slice/65g	177	5.7	271	15.6	32.6	8.7	2.4
The Sizzler, Classic, Small, Domino's Pizza*	1 Slice/78g	222	8.7	285	14.7	31.5	11.2	2.2
The Sizzler, Italian, Large, Domino's Pizza*	1 Slice/75g	227	10.9	303	14.7	28.4	14.5	2.2
The Sizzler, Italian, Medium, Domino's Pizza*	1 Slice/70g	243	12.0	347	16.1	32.1	17.1	2.4
Veg Supreme, Classic, Delight, Large, Domino's Pizza*	1 Slice/88g	188	4.3	214	13.1	29.5	4.9	2.5
Veg Supreme, Classic, Delight, Med, Domino's Pizza*	1 Slice/80g	171	3.9	214	13.1	29.5	4.9	2.5
Veg Supreme, Classic, Delight, Small, Domino's Pizza*	1 Slice/72g	154	3.5	214	13.1	29.5	4.9	2.5
Veg Supreme, Classic, Large, Domino's Pizza*	1 Slice/88g	192	5.5	218	11.5	29.1	6.3	2.3
Veg Supreme, Classic, Medium, Domino's Pizza*	1 Slice/80g	170	4.9	213	11.0	28.3	6.1	2.3

	Measure INFO/WEIGHT	per Measure KCAL	per Measure FAT	Nutrition Values per 100g / 100ml KCAL	PROT	CARB	FAT	FIBRE

DOMINO'S PIZZA

PIZZA

	Measure INFO/WEIGHT	KCAL	FAT	KCAL	PROT	CARB	FAT	FIBRE
Veg Supreme, Classic, Personal, Domino's Pizza*	1 Slice/61g	144	3.7	236	12.7	32.8	6.0	2.2
Veg Supreme, Classic, Small, Domino's Pizza*	1 Slice/72g	156	4.5	217	11.5	28.9	6.2	2.3
Veg Supreme, Italian, Large, Domino's Pizza*	1 Slice/68g	171	7.5	252	11.8	26.1	11.1	2.7
Veg Supreme, Italian, Medium, Domino's Pizza*	1 Slice/63g	168	7.3	266	12.0	28.7	11.5	2.6

WRAP

	Measure INFO/WEIGHT	KCAL	FAT	KCAL	PROT	CARB	FAT	FIBRE
Meatball Mayhem, Wrapzz, Domino's Pizza*	1 Wrap/137g	384	17.4	280	9.6	30.7	12.7	1.8
Pepperoni Passion, Wrapzz, Domino's Pizza*	1 Wrap/95g	293	14.8	308	12.6	28.3	15.6	1.9
Tandoori Hot, Wrapzz, Domino's Pizza*	1 Wrap/115g	267	9.7	232	12.5	25.7	8.4	2.1
Vegetarian Supreme, Wrapzz, Domino's Pizza*	1 Wrap/110g	234	8.0	211	8.3	27.0	7.2	2.6

EAT

BAGEL

	Measure INFO/WEIGHT	KCAL	FAT	KCAL	PROT	CARB	FAT	FIBRE
BLT, EAT*	1 Bagel/222g	567	20.5	255	14.7	28.8	9.2	1.8
Cheese & Chilli Jam, EAT*	1 Bagel/224g	583	21.1	260	11.1	33.5	9.4	1.8
Egg, Free Range & Chorizo, EAT*	1 Bagel/240g	561	24.0	234	10.7	25.9	10.0	1.6
Pastrami, New York, EAT*	1 Bagel/217g	468	11.7	216	13.6	29.1	5.4	1.5
Salmon, Smoked, Scottish & Soft Cheese, EAT*	1 Bagel/199g	444	10.8	223	13.0	31.2	5.4	1.7

BAGUETTE

	Measure INFO/WEIGHT	KCAL	FAT	KCAL	PROT	CARB	FAT	FIBRE
Beef & Rocket, EAT*	1 Baguette/228g	556	18.2	244	13.2	29.2	8.0	1.8
Brie, Tomato & Basil, EAT*	1 Baguette/191g	455	17.2	238	9.2	29.1	9.0	1.9
Chicken, Bacon & Avocado, EAT*	1 Baguette/252g	552	19.9	219	13.2	23.8	7.9	1.9
Chicken, Thai, EAT*	1 Baguette/201g	432	12.3	215	11.9	28.4	6.1	1.8
Chicken Banh Mi, EAT*	1 Pack/261g	465	10.7	178	8.6	25.6	4.1	1.7
Egg & Bacon, Half, EAT*	1 Serving/112g	311	12.2	278	13.5	30.5	10.9	1.8
Ham & Jarlsberg, EAT*	1 Serving/218g	566	23.3	260	15.4	24.9	10.7	1.4
Ham & Tomato, EAT*	1 Baguette/245g	422	10.3	172	9.6	23.2	4.2	1.6
Ham Brie & Cranberry, EAT*	1 Baguette/245g	583	25.1	239	11.0	25.8	10.3	1.4

EAT

BAGUETTE

	Measure INFO/WEIGHT	KCAL	FAT	KCAL	PROT	CARB	FAT	FIBRE
Mature Cheddar & Sweet Chilli Jam, Eat*	1 Baguette/201g	577	25.1	287	10.4	33.1	12.5	1.7

EAT

BAGUETTE

	Measure INFO/WEIGHT	KCAL	FAT	KCAL	PROT	CARB	FAT	FIBRE
Sticky BBQ Banh Mi, EAT*	1 Roll/269g	473	2.4	176	7.9	33.1	0.9	1.8
The Big Salami, EAT*	1 Baguette/254g	569	26.9	224	9.2	22.5	10.6	1.5
Tuna & Cucumber, EAT*	1 Baguette/208g	511	22.7	245	10.9	25.0	10.9	1.5

BAGUETTE

	Measure INFO/WEIGHT	KCAL	FAT	KCAL	PROT	CARB	FAT	FIBRE
Egg & Tomato, EAT*	1 Serving/140g	304	12.2	217	9.0	24.8	8.7	1.7

BREAD

	Measure INFO/WEIGHT	KCAL	FAT	KCAL	PROT	CARB	FAT	FIBRE
Brown Roll, for Soup, EAT*	1 Roll/69g	187	3.5	271	8.5	47.4	5.1	2.0
Chunk of Freshly Baked Brown Bread, EAT*	1 Serving/67g	141	1.3	211	7.4	44.0	1.9	2.7
Chunk of Freshly Baked White Bread, EAT*	1 Serving/67g	162	2.9	242	7.3	46.4	4.3	1.9
Wheat Free Seeded Rye Bread, EAT*	1 Serving/144g	331	6.0	230	6.7	48.0	4.2	6.7
White Roll, for Soup, EAT*	1 Roll/69g	185	3.3	268	8.3	47.1	4.8	1.7

BREAKFAST CEREAL

	Measure INFO/WEIGHT	KCAL	FAT	KCAL	PROT	CARB	FAT	FIBRE
Bircher, Mango & Passionfruit, EAT*	1 Pot/225g	336	9.2	149	3.1	25.2	4.1	2.2
Granola, & Full Fat Milk, EAT*	1 Serving/230g	476	17.7	207	5.7	29.9	7.7	4.1
Granola, & Full Fat Milk, with Chocolate Syrup, EAT*	1 Serving/239g	509	18.4	213	5.7	31.2	7.7	4.4
Granola, & Skimmed Milk, EAT*	1 Serving/230g	435	13.3	189	5.7	30.0	5.8	4.1
Granola, & Skimmed Milk, with Chocolate Syrup, EAT*	1 Serving/239g	466	13.9	195	5.7	31.4	5.8	4.4
Granola, & Soya Milk, EAT*	1 Serving/230g	435	15.9	189	5.8	27.3	6.9	4.5
Granola, & Soya Milk, with Chocolate Syrup, EAT*	1 Serving/239g	468	16.7	196	5.9	28.7	7.0	4.7
Grapenuts, Banana & Honey, EAT*	1 Serving/228g	349	6.4	153	6.3	25.4	2.8	1.5
Muesli, Apple, Almond & Cinnamon, Bircher, EAT*	1 Serving/210g	361	12.2	172	6.1	23.3	5.8	2.3

	Measure INFO/WEIGHT	per Measure KCAL	FAT	Nutrition Values per 100g / 100ml KCAL	PROT	CARB	FAT	FIBRE
EAT								
BREAKFAST CEREAL								
Muesli, Swiss, Bircher, EAT*	1 Serving/205g	246	3.1	120	4.7	21.7	1.5	2.0
Porridge, Apple & Blackberry, Compote, Small, EAT*	1 Serving/231g	210	2.3	91	3.6	17.2	1.0	1.7
Porridge, Banana & Maple Syrup, Super, Small, EAT*	1 Serving/254g	196	3.6	77	5.6	13.4	1.4	1.7
Porridge, Plain, Big, EAT*	1 Serving/280g	213	3.1	76	4.4	11.9	1.1	1.1
Porridge, Plain, Small, EAT*	1 Serving/180g	137	2.0	76	4.4	11.9	1.1	1.2
Porridge, Plain, Super, Small, EAT*	1 Serving/219g	136	3.5	62	2.4	9.0	1.6	1.8
Porridge, Super with Banana, Big, EAT*	1 Serving/350g	224	5.2	64	2.3	9.8	1.5	1.8
Porridge, Super with Banana, Small, EAT*	1 Serving/240g	156	3.6	65	2.3	10.1	1.5	1.9
Porridge, Super with Banana & Maple Syrup, Big, EAT*	1 Serving/364g	266	5.5	73	2.2	12.0	1.5	1.8
Porridge, with Apple & Blackberry, Compote, Big, EAT*	1 Serving/331g	291	3.6	88	3.9	16.0	1.1	1.5
Porridge, with Banana, Big, EAT*	1 Serving/300g	234	0.9	78	4.1	12.8	0.3	1.2
Porridge, with Banana, Small, EAT*	1 Serving/200g	162	2.2	81	4.0	13.5	1.1	1.3
Porridge, with Banana & Maple Syrup, Big, EAT*	1 Serving/315g	308	6.9	98	4.0	15.1	2.2	1.2
Porridge, with Banana & Maple Syrup, Small, EAT*	1 Serving194g	177	1.9	91	4.1	16.0	1.0	1.0
Porridge, with Berry Compote, Super, Small, EAT*	1 Serving/30g	205	2.3	89	3.6	16.4	1.0	1.2
Porridge, with Berry Compote, Super, Big, EAT*	1 Serving/330g	284	3.3	86	3.8	15.5	1.0	1.2
Porridge, with Maple Syrup, Big, EAT*	1 Serving/294g	253	3.2	86	4.2	14.6	1.1	1.0
Porridge, with Maple Syrup, Small, EAT*	1 Serving/195g	185	2.1	95	4.1	17.3	1.1	1.1
Porridge, with Maple Syrup, Super, EAT*	1 Serving/344g	244	5.5	71	2.3	11.4	1.6	1.7
Porridge, with Maple Syrup, Super, Small, EAT*	1 Serving/235g	176	3.5	75	2.3	12.6	1.5	1.7
Porridge with Berry Compote, Small, EAT*	1 Serving/230g	196	2.1	85	3.6	15.3	0.9	1.1
BRIOCHE								
Fruited without Butter, Toasted, EAT*	1 Serving/120g	414	13.4	345	7.3	50.2	11.2	2.2
BROWNIES								
Chocolate, Belgian, EAT*	1 Serving/73g	330	20.0	452	5.1	46.2	27.4	1.0
CAKE								
Banana, Toffee, & Pecan, EAT*	1 Serving/79g	247	10.8	313	3.3	45.1	13.7	0.9
Carrot, EAT*	1 Serving/100g	319	20.0	319	2.8	33.1	20.0	1.6
Chocolate, EAT*	1 Serving/63g	236	13.0	374	4.1	43.8	20.6	1.5
Chocolate Caramel Crispie, Slice, EAT*	1 Slice/61g	279	17.4	458	3.9	53.6	28.5	0.9
Lemon Curd, Slice, EAT*	1 Slice/75g	300	12.9	400	3.2	59.0	17.2	1.6
Lemon Drizzle, EAT*	1 Serving/70g	232	10.8	332	3.5	44.8	15.5	0.8
Red Velvet, EAT*	1 Pack/128g	500	24.3	391	4.7	50.0	19.0	0.9
Tiffin, Caramel, EAT*	1 Serving/73g	351	18.9	481	3.6	60.0	25.9	0.7
Victoria Sponge EAT*	1 Serving/72g	166	7.9	230	2.5	30.5	10.9	0.6
CHEESECAKE								
Lemon, EAT*	1 Serving/114g	446	34.7	391	2.9	25.7	30.4	0.4
CHERRIES								
Bag of, EAT*	1 Serving/125g	55	0.1	44	0.8	9.0	0.1	1.8
COFFEE								
Cappuccino, Skimmed Milk, EAT*	1 Tall/12oz	118	4.0	33	2.4	3.4	1.1	0.0
Cappuccino, Soya Milk, EAT*	1 Tall/12oz	131	4.9	37	3.2	3.5	1.4	0.9
Cappuccino, Whole Milk, Big, EAT*	1 Big/474ml	159	8.4	34	2.3	2.3	1.8	0.0
Cappuccino, Whole Milk, Small, EAT*	1 Tall/12oz	130	6.5	37	2.6	2.4	1.8	0.0
Espresso, Macchiato, Skimmed Milk, EAT*	1 Espresso/4oz	8	0.3	7	0.5	0.6	0.3	0.0
Espresso, Macchiato, Soya Milk, EAT*	1 Espresso/4oz	9	0.4	8	0.6	0.7	0.3	0.2
Espresso, Macchiato, Whole Milk, Double, EAT*	1 Double/8oz	20	0.4	8	1.4	0.4	0.2	0.0
Espresso, Macchiato, Whole Milk, Single, EAT*	1 Single/4oz	13	0.3	11	1.5	0.6	0.2	0.0
Latte, Chai, Skimmed Milk, EAT*	1 Tall/12oz	305	1.0	86	3.2	17.7	0.3	0.0
Latte, Chai, Soya Milk, EAT*	1 Tall/12oz	279	5.3	79	2.4	13.9	1.5	0.5
Latte, Chai, Whole Milk, Big, EAT*	1 Big/16oz	332	12.8	70	2.7	9.0	2.7	0.0
Latte, Chai, Whole Milk, Small, EAT*	1 Small/12oz	262	10.2	74	2.9	9.3	2.9	0.0

EAT

	Measure INFO/WEIGHT	per Measure KCAL	FAT	Nutrition Values per 100g / 100ml KCAL	PROT	CARB	FAT	FIBRE
COFFEE								
Latte, Chiller, Skimmed Milk, EAT*	1 Tall/12oz	241	3.3	68	3.1	11.9	0.9	0.0
Latte, Chiller, Whole Milk, EAT*	1 Tall/12oz	412	14.8	116	1.8	17.8	4.2	0.2
Latte, Iced, Skimmed Milk, EAT*	1 Tall/12oz	95	3.2	27	1.9	2.7	0.9	0.0
Latte, Iced, Soya Milk, EAT*	1 Tall/12oz	105	3.9	30	2.5	2.8	1.1	0.7
Latte, Matcha, Skimmed Milk, EAT*	1 Tall/12oz	204	1.0	57	3.0	10.6	0.3	0.3
Latte, Matcha, Soya Milk, EAT*	1 Tall/12oz	201	5.8	57	3.0	7.4	1.6	0.3
Latte, Matcha, Whole Milk, EAT*	1 Tall/12oz	297	11.8	84	3.0	10.4	3.3	0.3
Latte, Skimmed Milk, EAT*	1 Small/12oz	99	3.4	42	3.0	4.2	1.4	0.0
Latte, Soya Milk, EAT*	1 Tall/12oz	157	5.9	46	4.0	4.3	1.7	1.1
Latte, Whole Milk, Big, EAT*	1 Big/16oz	224	11.6	47	3.1	3.2	2.4	0.0
Latte, Whole Milk, Small, EAT*	1 Small/12oz	173	9.0	49	3.3	3.2	2.5	0.0
Matcha, Chiller, Whole Milk, EAT*	1 Tall/12oz	418	14.9	118	1.9	18.2	4.2	0.3
Mocha, Chiller, Skimmed Milk, EAT*	1 Tall/12oz	243	3.4	68	2.5	12.6	1.0	0.0
Mocha, Chiller, Whole Milk, EAT*	1 Tall/12oz	283	7.5	80	2.5	12.6	2.1	0.0
Mocha, Skimmed Milk, EAT*	1 Tall/12oz	157	5.0	44	3.0	4.8	1.4	0.0
Mocha, Soya Milk, EAT*	1 Tall/12oz	173	6.1	49	4.0	5.0	1.7	1.2
Mocha, Whole Milk, EAT*	1 Tall/12oz	219	11.4	62	3.0	4.8	3.2	0.0
White, Flat, Skimmed Milk, EAT*	1 Tall/341ml	87	0.3	26	2.6	3.7	0.1	0.0
White, Flat, Soya Milk, EAT*	1 Tall/341ml	147	4.8	43	5.1	2.3	1.4	0.4
COOKIES								
Chocolate, EAT*	1 Serving/90g	401	16.8	446	6.6	61.4	18.7	2.7
Muesli, EAT*	1 Serving/90g	376	13.4	418	5.7	63.5	14.9	3.6
CROISSANT								
Almond, EAT*	1 Serving/83g	350	19.8	422	10.0	41.7	23.9	2.9
Chocolate, EAT*	1 Serving/81g	361	21.3	445	6.9	45.4	26.2	3.0
EAT*	1 Serving/71g	305	17.1	427	9.4	43.4	23.9	2.7
Egg, Cheese & Tomato, EAT*	1 Pack/149g	434	25.1	291	9.0	20.8	16.8	1.6
Egg & Bacon, EAT*	1 Pack/138g	497	31.8	361	13.2	24.8	23.1	1.7
Ham & Jarlsberg Croissant, EAT*	1 Serving/128g	339	21.1	265	15.6	20.8	16.5	0.0
Tomato & Jarlsberg, EAT*	1 Serving/123g	291	19.1	236	9.0	22.6	15.5	0.4
DANISH PASTRY								
Maple Pecan, Plait, EAT*	1 Serving/83g	377	26.0	454	4.7	38.4	31.3	5.2
FROZEN YOGHURT								
Brownie Sundae, EAT*	1 Serving/176g	308	6.0	175	3.6	34.1	3.4	2.0
Plain, EAT*	1 Serving/140g	169	0.3	121	3.5	29.0	0.2	2.0
with Fresh Berries, EAT*	1 Serving/200g	190	0.4	95	2.7	22.0	0.2	2.5
FRUIT SALAD								
Big, EAT*	1 Serving/279g	120	0.3	43	0.6	10.9	0.1	1.8
Fresh, EAT*	1 Serving/160g	77	0.2	48	0.6	11.3	0.1	0.5
Rainbow, EAT*	1 Serving/141g	86	0.6	61	0.8	12.5	0.4	2.6
Summer Berries, EAT*	1 Serving/130g	48	0.3	37	0.8	6.8	0.2	3.1
GRAPES								
Bag, EAT*	1 Serving/133g	80	0.1	60	0.4	15.4	0.1	1.0
HOT CHOCOLATE								
Whole Milk, Big, EAT*	1Big/16oz	380	15.6	80	3.1	9.7	3.3	1.2
HOT POT								
BBQ Pulled Pork, EAT*	1 Pack/340g	510	15.0	150	9.7	17.3	4.4	0.8
Burmese Chicken Curry, EAT*	1 Bowl/385g	462	18.5	120	5.4	12.3	4.8	1.2
Cumberland Sausage, Mash & Onion Gravy, EAT*	1 Pack/470g	658	40.4	140	4.8	10.1	8.6	1.2
Mexican Chicken, EAT*	1 Pot/315g	476	24.6	151	11.8	11.0	7.8	0.6
Sweet Potato & Spinach Dal, EAT*	1 Pot/380g	380	6.1	100	3.6	17.0	1.6	1.8
Texan Chilli, EAT*	1 Pack/378g	386	9.5	102	5.8	13.6	2.5	1.9

	Measure INFO/WEIGHT	per Measure KCAL	FAT	Nutrition Values per 100g / 100ml KCAL	PROT	CARB	FAT	FIBRE
EAT								
HOT POT								
Thai Green Chicken Curry, EAT*	1 Pack/386g	491	22.0	127	5.9	11.3	5.7	0.9
ICE CREAM								
Chocolate, Belgian, Haagen Das, EAT*	1 Serving/100g	227	18.4	227	3.9	23.8	18.4	1.7
Cookies & Cream, Haagen Das, EAT*	1 Serving/100g	225	14.4	225	3.7	20.0	14.4	0.7
Strawberries & Cream, Haagen Das, EAT*	1 Serving/100g	221	14.1	221	3.5	20.0	14.1	0.3
Vanilla, Haagen Das, EAT*	1 Serving/100g	225	15.2	225	3.8	18.1	15.2	0.0
JELLY								
Elderflower & Berry, EAT*	1 Pack/150g	110	0.2	73	1.1	16.3	0.1	0.9
Plum & Apple Jelly, EAT*	1 Pot/130g	143	0.1	110	1.8	25.7	0.1	0.5
JUICE DRINK								
Mango & Lime, Blast, EAT*	1 Tall/12oz	253	0.3	71	0.3	17.7	0.1	0.1
Peach & Mint, Blast, EAT*	1 Tall/12oz	216	0.2	61	0.2	15.1	0.1	0.0
Wild Berry, Blast, EAT*	1 Tall/12oz	330	0.2	93	0.2	23.5	0.1	0.5
MUFFIN								
Bacon Butty, Hot Toasted, EAT*	1 Serving/90g	291	10.9	324	17.1	36.1	12.1	0.8
Bacon Butty, Toasted, Hot, Large, EAT*	1 Serving/190g	589	18.4	310	15.4	39.7	9.7	0.9
Blueberry, Low Fat, EAT*	1 Muffin/119g	383	13.4	322	5.8	47.9	11.3	2.5
Chocolate, Belgian, EAT*	1 Serving/124g	511	26.4	412	5.0	48.9	21.3	2.1
Egg, Mushroom & Cheddar, Hot Toasted, EAT*	1 Serving/125g	240	6.9	192	9.1	26.2	5.5	1.0
Eggs Benedict, Hot Toasted, EAT*	1 Serving/120g	265	8.9	220	10.2	27.6	7.4	0.8
Fruit & Bran, EAT*	1 Muffin/124g	498	25.1	402	5.7	47.2	20.3	3.8
Full English Breakfast, EAT*	1 Serving/295g	687	24.5	233	10.7	28.4	8.3	0.7
Smoked Salmon & Egg, Hot Toasted, EAT*	1 Serving/126g	325	10.0	258	11.8	37.1	7.9	1.5
Sunshine, EAT*	1 Serving/124g	498	25.1	402	5.7	47.2	20.3	3.8
NOUGAT								
EAT*	1 Serving/30g	126	2.7	420	3.7	80.5	9.1	0.5
NUTS								
Honey & Chilli, EAT*	1 Serving/100g	496	31.7	496	15.9	44.4	31.7	5.6
OLIVES								
Chilli & Herb, EAT*	1 Serving/75g	99	10.1	132	0.8	1.8	13.5	3.5
PAIN AU CHOCOLATE								
EAT*	1 Serving/78g	329	18.4	422	9.8	42.6	23.6	3.6
PANCAKES								
American Buttermilk, Maple & Berry Compote, EAT*	1 Serving/171g	328	3.2	192	3.4	40.0	1.9	0.9
American Buttermilk, with Maple, EAT*	1 Serving/100g	239	2.2	238	3.6	55.5	2.2	1.0
American Buttermilk, with Maple & Bacon, EAT*	1 Serving/106g	292	4.9	275	8.5	50.0	4.6	0.8
American Buttermilk, with Maple & Banana, EAT*	1 Serving/113g	260	2.1	231	3.2	50.0	1.9	1.2
PASTRY								
Cheese Twist, EAT*	1 Serving/74g	313	19.0	421	14.0	33.7	25.6	2.2
Cinnamon Swirl, EAT*	1 Serving/77g	360	24.5	470	5.1	40.4	32.0	4.4
PEAS								
Wasabi, EAT*	1 Serving/38g	158	4.6	416	20.0	57.0	12.0	7.0
PIE								
Banoffee, EAT*	1 Serving/112g	395	24.1	353	3.7	36.0	21.5	1.4
PIES								
Beef & Stilton, Pie Only, EAT*	1 Pie/270g	629	31.6	233	10.2	21.1	11.7	1.6
Beef & Stilton with Mash & Gravy, EAT*	1 Pie/560g	885	40.3	158	5.9	15.9	7.2	1.9
Cheese & Onion, Pie Only, EAT*	1 Pie/270g	856	58.9	317	8.5	21.5	21.8	1.8
Cheese & Onion with Mash & Gravy, EAT*	1 Pie/560g	1098	67.8	196	4.9	16.2	12.1	1.9
Chicken & Mushroom Pie Only, EAT*	1 Pie/250g	685	37.8	274	11.3	22.6	15.1	1.4
Chicken & Mushroom with Mash & Gravy, EAT*	1 Pie/540g	929	47.0	172	6.1	16.5	8.7	1.7
Goats Cheese & Sweet Potato, Mash & Gravy, EAT*	1 Pie/560g	946	45.9	169	4.1	18.4	8.2	2.0

EAT

	INFO/WEIGHT	KCAL	FAT	KCAL	PROT	CARB	FAT	FIBRE
PIES								
Goats Cheese & Sweet Potato, Pie Only, EAT*	1 Pie/270g	694	36.7	257	6.6	26.2	13.6	1.9
Steak & Ale, Pie Only, EAT*	1 Pie/250g	670	37.8	268	10.4	22.1	15.1	1.5
Steak & Ale with Mash & Gravy, EAT*	1 Pie/540g	913	47.0	169	5.7	16.3	8.7	1.7
SALAD								
Chicken, Simple, without Dressing, EAT*	1 Pack/345g	376	19.0	109	6.4	7.8	5.5	1.2
Chicken, Tandoori, Mango, & Rice, with Dressing, EAT*	1 Serving/206g	251	5.6	122	8.3	15.6	2.7	1.6
Chicken, with Dressing, Simple, EAT*	1 Pack/366g	501	32.2	137	6.0	7.9	8.8	1.1
Chicken Tandoori, Mango, & Rice, no Dressing, EAT*	1 Serving/186g	227	3.9	122	8.7	16.5	2.1	1.7
Chipotle, Chicken Tortilla,with Dressing, Bold EAT*	1 Pack/370g	541	19.3	146	8.5	17.0	5.2	2.6
Chipotle, Chicken Tortilla,without Dressing, Bold EAT*	1 Pack/345g	515	19.4	149	9.0	16.2	5.6	2.7
Coleslaw, Vietnamese, with Dressing, Side, EAT*	1 Pack/156g	150	9.1	96	3.0	7.2	5.8	2.2
Coleslaw, Vietnamese, without Dressing, Side, EAT*	1 Pack/137g	81	2.9	59	2.4	7.4	2.1	2.3
Ham, & Potato, with Dressing, Summer, EAT*	1 Serving/331g	480	36.7	145	6.0	4.9	11.1	0.8
Ham, Mediterranean Serrano, no Dressing, EAT*	1 Pack/304g	368	14.9	121	9.3	9.1	4.9	2.1
Ham, Mediterranean Serrano, with Dressing, Bold EAT*	1 Pack/331g	501	28.2	151	8.6	9.1	8.5	2.0
Ham, Summer, & Potato, without Dressing, EAT*	1 Serving/303g	370	26.4	122	6.4	4.3	8.7	0.9
Houmous, & Falafel, Mezze, without Dressing, EAT*	1 Box/353g	395	16.9	112	3.2	12.8	4.8	4.6
Houmous Detox Box, with Dressing, EAT*	1 Pack/254g	478	40.9	188	3.1	7.4	16.1	3.3
Houmous Detox Box, without Dressing, EAT*	1 Pack/262g	414	33.3	158	3.3	7.5	12.7	3.6
Mexican Bean Pot, Less Than 5% Fat, Vegetarian, EAT*	1 Salad/172g	192	4.0	111	5.2	17.1	2.3	4.1
Mezze, with Dressing, EAT*	1 Serving/306g	425	26.6	139	3.6	12.0	8.7	2.7
Mezze, without Dressing, EAT*	1 Serving/286g	349	20.3	122	3.8	11.0	7.1	2.9
Noodles, Chicken, Spicy, less than 5% Fat, EAT*	1 Serving/325g	419	9.1	129	8.9	16.8	2.8	1.6
Noodles, Crayfish, Spicy, Less Than 5% Fat, EAT*	1 Serving/285g	348	8.0	122	6.6	18.2	2.8	1.6
Pea & Mint, Pot, No Dressing, EAT*	1 Salad/106g	98	2.6	92	6.8	7.4	2.4	3.0
Pea & Mint, Pot with Dressing, EAT*	1 Salad/125g	171	9.8	136	5.9	7.5	7.8	2.7
Prawn Cocktail, Pot, EAT*	1 Salad/129g	218	17.2	169	9.9	2.1	13.3	0.6
Prawn Cocktail, Side, EAT*	1 Serving/166g	345	29.4	208	9.4	2.4	17.7	0.7
Rainbow, Superfood, with Dressing, EAT*	1 Serving/340g	520	24.8	153	5.4	15.2	7.3	2.6
Rainbow, Superfood, without Dressing, EAT*	1 Serving/340g	439	16.0	129	5.9	14.2	4.7	2.8
Salmon, Omega Booster, Box, with Dressing, EAT*	1 Pack/194g	392	34.9	202	6.6	2.3	18.0	1.9
Salmon, Omega Booster, Box, without Dressing, EAT*	1 Pack/173g	281	23.6	162	7.4	1.3	13.6	2.1
Salmon, Sushi, with Dressing, Bold, EAT*	1 Pack/340g	493	11.9	145	5.5	24.1	3.5	1.0
Salmon Sushi, without Dressing, Bold, EAT*	1 Pack/308g	434	9.8	141	6.0	23.2	3.2	1.1
Tuna, with Dressing, Simple, EAT*	1 Pack/322g	316	17.7	98	6.9	4.6	5.5	0.8
Tuna, without Dressing, Simple, EAT*	1 Pack/292g	193	5.8	66	7.4	4.3	2.0	0.9
SANDWICH								
Bacon, Butty, EAT*	1 Butty/170g	600	15.5	353	17.8	53.3	9.1	2.2
Bacon, Butty, Small, EAT*	1 Butty/93g	330	9.2	355	18.6	51.0	9.9	2.2
Bacon, Lettuce & Tomato, EAT*	1 Pack/204g	479	25.1	235	11.1	19.9	12.3	1.7
Cheddar Salad, Simple, EAT*	1 Pack/188g	405	18.8	215	9.4	21.7	10.0	1.8
Chicken, & Chipotle Salsa, Toastie, EAT*	1 Sandwich/284g	486	11.4	171	10.6	23.3	4.0	1.7
Chicken, & Chorizo, EAT*	1 Sandwich/209g	416	17.4	199	12.3	19.7	8.3	1.7
Chicken, Avocado & Basil, EAT*	1 Pack/233g	452	24.0	194	10.3	17.9	10.3	2.7
Chicken, Pork, Sage & Onion, Roast, Bloomer, EAT*	1 Sandwich/238g	569	25.9	239	11.8	24.7	10.9	1.8
Chicken, Tomato & Pesto, Smoked, Bloomer, EAT*	1 Pack/244g	454	15.4	186	12.4	20.4	6.3	2.2
Chicken & Bacon, EAT*	1 Pack/229g	472	21.5	206	12.3	18.0	9.4	1.6
Chicken & Bacon, Very Small, EAT*	1 Pack/114g	241	11.5	211	12.2	17.7	10.1	1.6
Chicken & Basil, Smoked, Toastie, EAT*	1 Pack/240g	550	24.7	229	12.1	22.3	10.3	1.2
Chicken Salad, less than 5% Fat, Simple EAT*	1 Pack/203g	327	9.7	161	10.1	19.3	4.8	1.9
Club, EAT*	1 Pack/296g	624	28.7	211	12.9	17.7	9.7	1.3
Crayfish, Lemon & Rocket, EAT*	1 Pack/188g	333	13.9	177	9.5	20.9	7.4	1.6

	Measure INFO/WEIGHT	per Measure KCAL	FAT	Nutrition Values per 100g / 100ml KCAL	PROT	CARB	FAT	FIBRE
EAT								
SANDWICH								
Crayfish, Lemon & Rocket, Very Small, EAT*	1 Pack/99g	174	6.8	176	9.4	19.9	6.9	1.4
Egg, Free Range, & Roast Tomato, Bloomer, EAT*	1 Pack/215g	525	25.6	244	11.1	23.4	11.9	2.8
Egg Mayo, Free Range, & Tomato Bloomer, EAT*	1 Pack/262g	627	38.8	239	7.3	19.1	14.8	1.5
Egg Mayonnaise, Chunky, & Watercress, EAT*	1 Pack/204g	462	25.2	227	8.8	20.0	12.4	1.7
Egg Mayonnaise, Free Range, & Cress, Simple, EAT*	1 Pack/183g	410	20.9	224	8.7	21.6	11.4	1.8
Ham, & Cheese, Simply, Toastie, EAT*	1 Serving/240g	588	31.2	245	11.8	21.4	13.0	1.0
Ham, & Free Range Egg, Bloomer, EAT*	1 Pack/246g	573	28.5	233	13.0	19.4	11.6	2.0
Ham, Cheddar & Piccalilli, EAT*	1 Pack/246g	448	17.7	182	11.2	19.1	7.2	1.4
Ham, Simple, Kids, EAT*	1 Sandwich/121g	318	13.4	263	10.8	30.4	11.1	2.2
Ham, Tomato & Mustard, EAT*	1 Pack/203g	394	17.5	194	9.8	19.3	8.6	1.6
Houmous, Avocado & Harissa, EAT*	1 Pack/213g	396	15.1	186	6.1	25.2	7.1	3.8
Mozzarella, Tomato & Pesto, Toastie, EAT*	1 Toastie/249g	545	26.9	219	9.6	20.8	10.8	1.2
Pastrami, New York, Bloomer, EAT*	1 Pack/240g	513	20.7	213	11.3	22.3	8.6	0.3
Pastrami, New York, EAT*	1 Pack/224g	358	11.4	160	9.9	18.6	5.1	1.3
Pork, Pulled, Brioche Bun, EAT*	1 Pack/235g	456	12.5	194	12.7	24.6	5.3	0.8
Salmon, Egg & Watercress, Smoked, EAT*	1 Pack/211g	477	25.3	226	10.8	18.7	12.0	1.6
Salmon & Soft Cheese, Smoked Scottish, EAT*	1 Pack/165g	380	16.5	230	12.1	22.9	10.0	1.6
Steak & Cheese Melt, Toastie, EAT*	1 Pack/265g	552	24.9	208	10.8	21.2	9.4	1.3
The Hot Cubano, Toastie, EAT*	1 Pack/270g	521	22.4	193	10.8	20.0	8.3	0.9
Tuna & Cheddar Melt, Toastie, EAT*	1 Pack/255g	594	28.6	233	13.9	20.7	11.2	1.0
Tuna & Cucumber, less than 5% Fat, EAT*	1 Pack/187g	305	7.1	163	10.8	21.3	3.8	1.7
Tuna & Mayo, Simple, Kids, EAT*	1 Sandwich/138g	371	17.0	269	12.4	27.4	12.3	1.9
Tuna Mayonnaise, & Cucumber, Simple, EAT*	1 Sandwich/199g	338	11.1	170	9.6	20.1	5.6	1.6
Turkey, & Cranberry, less than 5% Fat, Very Small, EAT*	1 Pack/109g	184	4.4	169	11.1	22.4	4.0	1.5
Turkey & Cranberry, less than 5% Fat, EAT*	1 Pack/223g	381	10.0	171	11.8	22.2	4.5	1.5
SHORTBREAD								
Millionares, EAT*	1 Cake/85g	396	21.2	466	3.5	57.6	25.0	0.8
SLICES								
Coconut & Raspberry, EAT*	1 Slice/75g	306	17.6	408	5.9	44.1	23.4	4.5
Coconut & Raspberry, EAT*	1 Serving/75g	306	17.6	408	5.9	44.1	23.4	4.5
Oat & Fruit, EAT*	1 Serving/73g	292	11.7	400	4.1	61.2	16.0	3.3
SOUP								
Chicken, Creamy, Small, Simple, EAT*	1 Small/300ml	237	14.4	79	4.2	4.5	4.8	0.6
Bacon, & Lentil, Smokey, Small, Simple, EAT*	1 Small/300ml	249	3.9	83	5.9	11.4	1.3	1.2
Bacon, & Sweetcorn Chowder with Garnish, Small, EAT*	1 Small/314g	371	25.5	118	3.0	8.7	8.1	1.1
Beef, & Barley, with Garnish, Big, Bold, EAT*	1 Pack/400g	249	6.4	62	4.2	6.6	1.6	2.1
Beef, & Barley, with Garnish, Small, Bold, EAT*	1 Pack/300g	187	4.8	62	4.2	6.6	1.6	2.1
Beef, & Barley, with Garnish, Very Big, Bold, EAT*	1 Pack/600g	373	9.6	62	4.2	6.6	1.6	2.1
Beef, & Barley, without Garnish, Big, Bold, EAT*	1 Pack/400g	248	6.4	62	4.2	6.6	1.6	2.1
Beef, & Barley, without Garnish, Very Big, Bold, EAT*	1 Pack/600g	372	9.6	62	4.2	6.6	1.6	2.1
Beef, & Potato Massaman, no Garnish, Small, EAT*	1 Small/300g	255	11.1	85	3.8	8.7	3.7	0.9
Beef, & Potato Massaman, with Garnish, Small, EAT*	1 Pack/312g	259	11.2	83	3.7	8.4	3.6	0.9
Beef Rendang, Malaysian, with Garnish, Small, EAT*	1 Small/302g	263	12.7	87	4.2	7.5	4.2	1.1
Beef Rendang, Malaysian, without Garnish, Small, EAT*	1 Small/300g	261	12.6	87	4.2	7.5	4.2	1.1
Butternut Squash, Thai, Simple, EAT*	1 Small/300ml	168	6.6	56	1.0	6.9	2.2	1.5
Carrot, Cumin & Coriander, Small, Simple, EAT*	1 Pack/300g	135	3.0	45	1.1	7.2	1.0	1.9
Carrot, Cumin & Coriander, Very Big, Simple, EAT*	1 Pack/625g	281	6.2	45	1.1	7.2	1.0	1.9
Carrot, Parsnip & Ginger, Small, Simple, EAT*	1 Small/300g	150	4.2	50	1.0	7.8	1.4	1.8
Cauliflower Cheese, Small, Simple, EAT*	1 Small/300ml	216	13.8	72	2.5	5.1	4.6	1.0
Chana Dal, Super, Small, EAT*	1 Small/300g	198	3.6	66	3.9	10.0	1.2	3.0
Chicken, & Garden Vegetable with Garnish, Small, EAT*	1 Small/320g	131	1.6	41	4.5	4.5	0.5	0.7
Chicken, & Rice Noodles, Pho, Pot, EAT*	1 Pot/875g	315	1.8	36	3.0	5.2	0.2	0.4

EAT

SOUP

	Measure INFO/WEIGHT	per Measure KCAL	FAT	Nutrition Values per 100g / 100ml KCAL	PROT	CARB	FAT	FIBRE
Chicken, Jerk, with Garnish, Big, Bold, EAT*	1 Pack/440g	436	18.1	99	4.9	11.1	4.1	1.1
Chicken, Jerk, with Garnish, Small, Bold, EAT*	1 Pack/340g	340	13.9	100	4.8	11.6	4.1	1.1
Chicken, Jerk, with Garnish, Very Big, Bold, EAT*	1 Pack/680g	680	27.9	100	4.8	11.6	4.1	1.1
Chicken, Jerk, without Garnish, Small, Bold, EAT*	1 Pack/300g	282	12.9	94	5.1	9.2	4.3	1.1
Chicken, Jerk, without Garnish, Very Big, Bold, EAT*	1 Pack/600g	564	25.8	94	5.1	9.2	4.3	1.1
Chicken, Leek & Bacon Risotto with Garnish, EAT*	1 Serving/370ml	359	18.9	97	4.7	8.1	5.1	0.5
Chicken, Leek & Bacon Risotto without Garnish, EAT*	1 Serving/400ml	344	23.2	86	5.2	3.0	5.8	0.4
Chicken, Pot Pie with Garnish, Small, Bold, EAT*	1 Small/330ml	343	17.8	104	4.8	9.0	5.4	1.0
Chicken, Pot Pie without Garnish, Small, Bold, EAT*	1 Small/300g	216	9.0	72	4.6	6.8	3.0	1.0
Chicken & Barley, Hearty, Bold, no Garnish, Small, EAT*	1 Small/300g	159	2.1	53	4.3	6.4	0.7	1.5
Chicken & Barley, Hearty, with Garnish, Small, EAT*	1 Small/306g	187	3.1	61	4.4	7.7	1.0	1.5
Chicken Chilli, Mexican, with Garnish, EAT*	1 Serving/300ml	264	7.5	88	6.1	10.2	2.5	1.4
Chicken Chilli, Mexican, without Garnish, EAT*	1 Serving/300ml	282	8.1	94	6.5	10.8	2.7	1.4
Chicken Curry, Thai Green, with Garnish, Small, EAT*	1 Small/340ml	309	14.3	91	4.4	8.1	4.2	0.6
Chicken Curry, Thai Green, without Garnish, Small, EAT*	1 Small/300ml	252	13.2	84	4.6	5.2	4.4	0.5
Chicken Harira, with Garnish, Bold, Small, EAT*	1 Small/310g	254	3.4	82	6.6	11.1	1.1	1.9
Chicken Harira, without Garnish, Bold, Small, EAT*	1 Small/300g	219	1.5	73	6.6	10.1	0.5	1.7
Chicken Laksa, without Garnish, Small, Bold, EAT*	1 Small/300g	273	15.0	91	5.0	5.1	5.0	0.1
Chicken Laksa with Garnish, Small, Bold, EAT*	1 Small/310ml	276	15.2	89	4.9	5.0	4.9	0.2
Chicken Laksa without Garnish, Big, EAT*	1 Serving/625ml	569	31.3	91	5.0	5.1	5.0	0.1
Chicken Pho, EAT*	1 Serving/786ml	291	4.7	37	3.7	3.6	0.6	0.3
Chicken Tortilla, Mexican, no Garnish, Bold, Small, EAT*	1 Small/300g	120	0.9	40	4.6	4.4	0.3	1.0
Chicken Tortilla, Mexican, with Garnish, Simple, EAT*	1 Small/320g	176	6.1	55	4.2	4.7	1.9	1.2
Chicken Tortilla, Mexican, with Garnish, Small, EAT*	1 Small/320g	189	5.4	59	5.1	5.5	1.7	1.0
Chicken Tortilla, Mexican, without Garnish, Simple, EAT*	1 Small/336g	138	2.7	41	4.2	3.6	0.8	1.0
Chorizo, & Chickpea, EAT*	1 Serving/402ml	358	16.5	89	5.0	8.1	4.1	1.6
Chunky Minestrone with Pesto with Garnish, EAT*	1 Small/319ml	188	7.6	59	2.1	7.0	2.4	1.4
Duck Gyoza, Dumpling, Hoisin, EAT*	1 Serving/847ml	432	7.6	51	2.3	8.4	0.9	0.5
Duck Gyoza, Dumpling & Egg Noodles Pho, Pot, EAT*	1 Pot/849g	382	5.1	45	2.1	7.8	0.6	0.6
French Onion with Garnish, EAT*	1 Serving/316ml	136	3.8	43	1.6	6.2	1.2	0.5
French Onion without Garnish, EAT*	1 Serving/400ml	112	1.2	28	0.7	5.4	0.3	0.5
Gazpacho, EAT*	1 Serving/279ml	78	1.4	28	1.0	4.5	0.5	1.0
Goan, Potato, Small, Simple, EAT*	1 Small/300g	246	13.2	82	2.0	6.9	4.4	1.2
Haddock Chowder, Smoked, no Garnish, Small, EAT*	1 Small/300g	234	10.8	78	3.8	7.1	3.6	0.8
Haddock Chowder, Smoked, with Garnish, Small, EAT*	1 Small/302g	236	10.9	78	3.8	7.1	3.6	0.8
Ham, Pea, & Mint with Garnish, EAT*	1 Serving/321ml	202	4.5	63	4.8	7.5	1.4	1.1
Ham, Pea, & Mint without Garnish, EAT*	1 Serving/626ml	388	8.8	62	4.7	7.4	1.4	0.6
Hungarian Goulash with Garnish, Big, EAT*	1 Serving/403ml	314	8.5	78	7.7	7.2	2.1	0.8
Hungarian Goulash with Garnish, Small, EAT*	1 Small/302g	995	6.4	329	7.7	7.2	2.1	0.8
Hungarian Goulash without Garnish, Big, EAT*	1 Serving/400ml	312	8.4	78	7.7	7.2	2.1	0.8
Hungarian Goulash without Garnish, Small, EAT*	1 Small/300g	234	6.3	78	7.7	7.2	2.1	0.8
Lobster Bisque, Simple, EAT*	1 Small/300g	267	21.6	89	1.5	4.1	7.2	1.1
Meatball, Italian, with Garnish, Small, EAT*	1 Small/310g	254	8.1	82	4.8	9.2	2.6	2.1
Meatball, Italian, without Garnish, Small, EAT*	1 Small/300g	225	6.0	75	4.1	9.5	2.0	2.2
Minestrone, with Pesto, without Garnish, Chunky, EAT*	1 Small/300ml	123	1.2	41	1.8	7.3	0.4	1.5
Mushroom, & Chestnut, Wild, Simple, EAT*	1 Small/300g	240	14.1	80	1.4	8.1	4.7	1.1
Mushroom, Wild, Forest, EAT*	1 Serving/300ml	150	8.7	50	2.0	3.7	2.9	0.8
Prawn Tom Yum, EAT*	1 Serving/814ml	285	9.0	35	1.8	4.1	1.1	0.5
Prawn Tom Yum Pho, Pot, EAT*	1 Pack/839g	369	10.1	44	3.0	5.3	1.2	0.7
Red Pepper, Fire Roasted, & Goats Cheese, EAT*	1 Small/300ml	141	6.9	47	1.9	4.6	2.3	0.9
Squash, & Maple, EAT*	1 Small/300g	198	9.0	66	0.9	8.4	3.0	1.1
Steak, & Ale, Pot Pie with Garnish, EAT*	1 Serving/415ml	415	13.3	100	8.3	9.2	3.2	1.2

	Measure INFO/WEIGHT	per Measure		Nutrition Values per 100g / 100ml				
		KCAL	FAT	KCAL	PROT	CARB	FAT	FIBRE

EAT
SOUP
Steak, & Ale, Pot Pie without Garnish, EAT*	1 Serving/625ml	550	13.8	88	8.4	8.3	2.2	1.2
Sweet Potato, & Chilli, Simple, EAT*	1 Small/300ml	261	13.2	87	1.3	9.6	4.4	1.7
Sweetcorn, Creamy, Simple, EAT*	1 Small/300g	315	15.3	105	2.5	12.1	5.1	1.3
Tomato, Slow Roasted, Small, Simple, EAT*	1 Small/300ml	240	18.3	80	1.2	4.7	6.1	1.1
Tomato & Basil, Spicy, Simple, EAT*	1 Small/300ml	78	0.9	26	0.9	4.6	0.3	0.9
Veg, Gyoza Dumpling & Egg Noodles Pho, Pot, EAT*	1 Pot/855g	402	9.4	47	2.1	6.9	1.1	0.6
Vegetable, Garden, EAT*	1 Small/300ml	165	8.7	55	0.9	6.1	2.9	1.2
Vegetable, Spicy Moroccan, Simple, EAT*	1 Small/300ml	138	2.1	46	1.7	7.8	0.7	1.9
Vegetarian, Gyoza Dumpling, EAT*	1 Serving/798ml	431	11.2	54	2.3	7.6	1.4	0.6

SUSHI
Fish, without Soy Sauce, EAT*	1 Serving/289g	474	9.8	164	6.4	26.0	3.4	2.2
Vegetarian, without Soy Sauce, EAT*	1 Serving/165g	253	2.3	153	2.5	31.7	1.4	1.6

TEA
Chai Latte, Soya, EAT*	1 Cup/355ml	208	6.4	59	4.2	7.1	1.8	0.0

TOAST
Cheese, & Marmite, EAT*	1 Pack/120g	344	13.4	287	13.1	33.5	11.2	2.2
Cheese, & Tomato, EAT*	1 Toast/148g	305	10.4	206	10.0	25.6	7.0	2.1
Nutella, & Banana, EAT*	1 Serving/153g	393	10.9	257	6.0	41.8	7.1	2.4

WAFFLES
Toffee, EAT*	1 Serving/65g	301	11.7	463	3.5	71.7	18.0	2.2

WRAP
Chicken, Mexican, EAT*	1 Pack/215g	396	13.6	184	9.9	22.1	6.3	2.0
Chicken, Roast, Simple, EAT*	1 Wrap/185g	409	20.5	221	10.0	19.9	11.1	1.2
Houmous, & Falafel, EAT*	1 Wrap/244g	471	21.2	193	5.9	22.9	8.7	3.7
Houmous, & Salad, Simple, EAT*	1 Wrap/202g	362	17.0	179	4.9	21.1	8.4	2.6
Peking Duck, EAT*	1 Wrap/208g	433	16.2	208	11.3	22.9	7.8	1.3
Tuna Nicoise, Naked,EAT*	1 Wrap/238g	457	19.0	192	10.6	19.2	8.0	1.8

YOGHURT
& Granola, EAT*	1 Bowl/197g	313	11.4	159	7.7	19.6	5.8	1.9
Granola, & Mixed Red Berries, EAT*	1 Serving/180g	306	8.8	170	5.8	26.1	4.9	2.4
Mango, & Passionfruit, EAT*	1 Serving/124g	145	3.6	117	5.6	17.1	2.9	0.2
Red Berries, Mixed, EAT*	1 Serving/124g	131	3.6	106	5.6	14.1	2.9	0.3

GREGGS
BAGUETTE
Chicken, & Sweetcorn, Greggs*	1 Baguette/235g	480	11.0	204	10.2	29.8	4.7	0.0
Chicken, Club, Chargrilled, Hot, Greggs*	1 Roll/167g	510	23.5	305	15.9	27.0	14.1	0.0
Chicken, Club, Greggs*	1 Baguette/265g	600	18.5	226	10.6	29.1	7.0	0.0
Chicken, Fajita, Hot, Greggs*	1 Roll/165g	410	11.0	248	12.7	33.3	6.7	0.0
Chicken, Pesto, Greggs*	1 Baguette/214g	520	16.0	243	11.7	32.5	7.5	0.0
Chicken, Sweet Chilli, Greggs*	1 Baguette/237g	520	3.0	219	10.3	39.7	1.3	0.0
Chicken, Tandoori, Greggs*	1 Baguette/200g	490	16.0	245	10.5	36.0	8.0	0.0
Chicken, Tikka, Greggs*	1 Baguette/250g	490	10.5	196	10.2	29.0	4.2	0.0
Chicken Mayonnaise, Greggs*	1 Baguette/200g	510	16.0	255	10.5	33.8	8.0	0.0
Egg Mayonnaise, & Tomato, Free Range, Greggs*	1 Baguette/237g	480	13.0	203	8.2	29.3	5.5	0.0
Ham, & Cheese, Greggs*	1 Baguette/216g	580	19.0	269	14.4	32.2	8.8	0.0
Ham, & Cheese, Hot, Greggs*	1 Roll/156g	430	17.5	276	16.4	26.9	11.2	0.0
Ham, & Coleslaw, Greggs*	1 Baguette/193g	450	10.5	233	9.3	35.8	5.4	0.0
Meatball, Melt, Hot, Greggs*	1 Roll/175g	390	12.5	223	9.4	29.1	7.1	0.0
Mexican Bandit, Greggs*	1 Baguette/265g	640	22.0	242	10.9	30.0	8.3	0.0
Mozzarella, & Tomato, Hot, Greggs*	1 Roll/149g	460	20.5	309	12.8	31.2	13.8	0.0
Prawn Mayonnaise, Greggs*	1 Baguette/235g	500	15.0	213	8.7	4.5	6.4	0.0
Tuna, Crunch, Greggs*	1 Baguette/235g	530	12.5	226	10.6	32.6	5.3	0.0

GREGGS

INFO/WEIGHT	Measure	per Measure		Nutrition Values per 100g / 100ml				
		KCAL	FAT	KCAL	PROT	CARB	FAT	FIBRE
BAGUETTE								
Tuna, Crunch, Melt, Hot, Greggs*	1 Roll/187g	440	13.0	235	13.4	30.0	7.0	0.0
BAKE								
Chicken, Greggs*	1 Bake/138g	450	32.0	326	8.7	20.6	23.2	0.0
Chicken Curry, Greggs*	1 Bake/131g	400	25.5	305	7.6	21.4	19.5	0.0
Sausage, Bean & Cheese, Melt, Greggs*	1 Bake/140g	430	27.5	307	7.1	25.4	19.6	0.0
Steak, Greggs*	1 Bake/139g	430	27.5	309	12.2	20.5	19.8	0.0
The Spicy One, Fajita Flavour Chicken, Greggs*	1 Bake/143g	430	27.5	301	8.0	24.5	19.2	0.0
BROWNIES								
Chocolate, Mini, Greggs*	1 Brownie/18g	90	5.0	500	8.3	58.3	27.8	0.0
BUNS								
Belgian, Greggs*	1 Bun/135g	420	5.0	311	4.8	64.1	3.7	0.0
Iced, Christmas Ring, Greggs*	1 Bun/60g	210	5.0	350	4.2	62.5	8.3	0.0
Iced, Finger, Greggs*	1 Bun/35g	111	3.0	316	7.0	52.4	8.7	1.6
CAKE								
Christmas Slice, Greggs*	1 Slice/86g	360	11.5	419	5.8	67.4	13.4	0.0
Gingerbread, Cupcake, Greggs*	1 Cake/97g	426	19.2	440	3.3	60.4	19.8	0.6
Sweet Lemon Cupcake, Greggs*	1 Cake/81g	380	16.0	469	0.0	71.6	19.8	0.0
COFFEE								
Black, Regular, Greggs*	1 Cup/455ml	20	0.6	4	0.3	0.3	0.1	0.0
CROISSANT								
All Butter, Greggs*	1 Croissant/55g	250	14.5	455	9.1	45.4	26.4	0.0
DOUGHNUT								
Blueberry Burst, Greggs*	1 Doughnut/96g	340	10.5	355	6.3	57.0	11.0	0.0
Cinnamon, Greggs*	1 Doughnut/96g	380	16.5	396	6.2	54.7	17.2	0.0
Finger, Creamed Filled, Topped with Jam, Greggs*	1 Finger/109g	390	26.5	358	5.5	27.5	24.3	0.0
Jaffa Cake, Greggs*	1 Doughnut/95g	320	8.5	337	5.3	58.4	9.0	0.0
Jam Filled, Greggs*	1 Doughnut/74g	250	7.5	338	7.4	53.4	10.1	0.0
Lemon Drizzle, Greggs*	1 Doughnut/105g	360	11.5	343	5.2	55.7	11.0	0.0
Strawberry Milkshake Filled, Greggs*	1 Doughnut/91g	360	15.0	396	6.3	53.8	16.5	0.0
Sugar, Mini, Greggs*	1 Doughnut/25g	59	3.2	236	0.0	28.0	12.8	0.0
Triple Chocolate, Vanilla Filled, Greggs*	1 Doughnut/91g	337	11.6	370	6.3	57.0	12.7	0.0
Yum Yum, Greggs*	1 Yum Yum/79g	340	20.5	430	5.1	42.4	26.0	0.0
Yum Yum, Toffee Topping, Greggs*	1 Yum Yum/73g	290	16.5	397	5.5	43.2	22.6	0.0
ECLAIR								
Chocolate, with Cream, Greggs*	1 Eclair/93g	350	24.5	376	4.8	29.6	26.3	0.0
FLAPJACK								
Fruity, Mini, Greggs*	1 Flapjack/22g	110	5.0	500	6.8	59.1	22.7	0.0
FRUIT								
Tropical, Greggs*	1 Serving/150g	80	0.0	53	0.7	11.3	0.0	0.0
GINGERBREAD								
Man with Chocolate Beans, Greggs*	1 Man/47g	210	5.5	452	6.4	78.5	11.8	0.0
MUFFIN								
Chocolate, Rainbow, Greggs*	1 Muffin/92g	370	16.5	402	4.4	53.8	17.9	0.0
Chocolate, Triple, Greggs*	1 Muffin/139g	570	31.0	410	5.0	46.8	22.3	0.0
Lemon, Sicilian, Greggs*	1 Muffin/126g	500	24.5	397	5.2	48.8	19.4	0.0
Sticky Toffee, Greggs*	1 Muffin/128g	530	27.0	414	5.1	49.2	21.1	0.0
PAIN AU CHOCOLAT								
with Belgian Chocolate, Greggs*	1 Pain/81g	340	18.5	420	8.6	45.1	22.8	0.0
PASTA								
Cheese & Tomato, with Mixed Herbs, Pot, Greggs*	1 Pack/300g	380	11.0	127	5.2	18.0	3.7	0.0
Fajita Chicken, in Tomato Sauce, Spicy, Pot, Greggs*	1 Pack/300g	360	8.0	120	5.7	17.8	2.7	0.0

GREGGS

INFO/WEIGHT	Measure		per Measure KCAL	FAT	Nutrition Values per 100g / 100ml KCAL	PROT	CARB	FAT	FIBRE

PASTY

Cheese & Onion, Freshly Baked, Greggs*	1 Pasty/126g		390	26.0	310	6.0	23.4	20.6	0.0
Cornish, Greggs*	1 Pasty/190g		560	32.0	295	7.4	21.0	16.8	0.0
Ham & Cheese Past, Greggs*	1 Pasty/140g		420	28.0	300	7.0	22.0	20.0	0.0

PIE

Mince, Sweet, Greggs*	1 Pie/70g		290	11.0	414	4.3	61.4	15.7	0.0
Mince, Sweet, Iced, Greggs*	1 Pie/63g		230	6.5	365	2.4	62.7	10.3	0.0

PIZZA

Cheese & Tomato, Greggs*	1 Serving/111g		290	10.5	261	9.5	32.0	9.5	0.0
Chicken, Chargrilled, Greggs*	1 Serving/111g		340	11.5	306	14.9	36.5	10.4	0.0
Chicken, Spicy, Greggs*	1 Serving/183g		450	11.5	246	12.3	36.9	6.3	0.0
Pepperoni, Greggs*	1 Serving/121g		350	14.0	289	11.6	33.1	11.6	0.0

PORRIDGE

Golden Syrup Flavour, Greggs*	1 Pot/234g		260	3.5	111	3.6	19.7	1.5	0.0
Plain Oats, Creamy, Greggs*	1 Pot/234g		260	5.0	111	3.6	20.1	2.1	0.0
Sultanna, Apple & Cinnamon Flavour, Greggs*	1 Pot/238g		270	4.5	113	4.0	21.2	1.9	0.0

ROLLS

Bacon, & Sausage, Corn Topped, Breakfast, Greggs*	1 Roll/182g		460	23.5	253	12.4	20.9	12.9	0.0
Bacon, Corn Topped Roll, Breakfast, Greggs*	1 Roll/152g		380	19.5	250	11.5	22.4	12.8	0.0
Sausage, Corn Topped Roll, Breakfast, Greggs*	1 Roll/164g		410	19.0	250	11.9	24.4	11.6	0.0

SALAD

Chicken & Bacon, Layered, Greggs*	1 Pack/211g		250	9.5	118	6.9	10.9	4.5	0.0

SANDWICH

BLT, Sweetcure Bacon, Malt Brown, Classic, Greggs*	1 Serving/100g		258	13.2	258	8.9	24.2	13.2	0.0
Cheese, & Tomato, Cheddar, on Oatmeal, Greggs*	1 Sandwich/187g		490	23.0	262	9.9	26.7	12.3	0.0
Cheese, Savoury, on Seeded White, Greggs*	1 Pack/166g		480	22.0	289	10.8	31.0	13.2	0.0
Cheese Ploughman's, Oval Bite, Greggs*	1 Pack/201g		420	20.0	209	8.7	20.9	10.0	0.0
Chicken, & Mango, on Malted Brown, Bloomer, Greggs*	1 Bloomer/217g		510	18.5	235	11.3	28.3	8.5	0.0
Chicken, & Mango, on White, Bloomer, Greggs*	1 Bloomer/217g		510	19.5	235	11.3	26.7	9.0	0.0
Chicken, & Salsa, Chargrilled, on Oatmeal, Greggs*	1 Sandwich/216g		340	3.5	157	12.0	22.2	1.6	0.0
Chicken, Bacon, & Sweetcorn, White, Bloomer, Greggs*	1 Bloomer/235g		520	18.5	221	11.1	27.0	7.9	0.0
Chicken, BBQ, Oval Bite, Greggs*	1 Roll/204g		340	6.0	167	10.8	23.0	2.9	0.0
Chicken, Chargrilled, Oval Bite, Greggs*	1 Roll/211g		440	19.0	209	11.6	19.2	9.0	0.0
Chicken, Chilli, Double, Oval Bite, Greggs*	1 Roll/219g		390	9.5	178	11.0	22.4	4.3	0.0
Chicken, Mexican, Oval Bite, Greggs*	1 Roll/179g		420	15.0	235	14.2	24.0	8.4	0.0
Chicken, Sweet Chilli, on White, Bloomer, Greggs*	1 Sandwich/255g		460	3.0	180	10.8	31.0	1.2	0.0
Chicken Salad, Classic, on Malted Brown, Greggs*	1 Sandwich/248g		520	23.0	210	9.9	20.6	9.3	0.0
Chicken Salad, Low Fat Mayo, Malted Brown, Greggs*	1 Pack/218g		380	7.0	174	10.8	25.2	3.2	0.0
Christmas Dinner, Greggs*	1 Pack/205g		570	18.5	278	12.2	35.4	9.0	0.0
Egg Mayonnaise, on Seeded White, Greggs*	1 Pack/174g		420	17.5	241	11.2	26.7	10.1	0.0
Egg Mayonnaise, with Cracked Black Pepper, Greggs*	1 Sandwich/166g		420	12.0	253	9.9	35.5	7.2	0.0
Festive, Oval Bite, Greggs*	1 Sandwich/160g		410	18.0	256	13.4	23.8	11.2	0.0
Ham, & Egg, Honey Roast, Salad, on Oatmeal, Greggs*	1 Sandwich/243g		450	15.5	185	9.9	21.0	6.4	0.0
Ham, Cheese, & Pickle, On White, Bloomer, Greggs*	1 Bloomer/228g		510	18.0	224	11.2	27.4	7.9	0.0
Ham, Cheese, Pickle, Malted Brown, Bloomer, Greggs*	1 Bloomer/228g		540	19.0	237	11.2	29.0	8.3	0.0
Ham Salad, Oval Bite, Greggs*	1 Sandwich/175g		320	10.5	183	9.1	21.7	6.0	0.0
Prawn Mayonnaise, Reduced Fat, on Oatmeal, Greggs*	1 Sandwich/166g		300	7.5	181	10.2	23.8	4.5	0.0
Sub, Chicken, & Mayonnaise, on White, Greggs*	1 Sub/186g		400	15.0	215	11.6	22.3	8.1	0.0
Sub, Egg Mayonnaise, & Bacon, Plain White, Greggs*	1 Roll/181g		430	16.5	238	12.2	26.2	9.1	0.0
Sub, Ham, & Egg, with Salad, on White, Greggs*	1 Sub/220g		390	14.5	177	9.8	19.1	6.6	0.0
Sub, Tuna Mayonnaise, on Seeded White, Greggs*	1 Sub/222g		410	12.0	185	11.7	21.0	5.4	0.0
Sub, Tuna Mayonnaise, on White, Greggs*	1 Roll/202g		350	10.0	173	11.6	19.6	5.0	0.0
Tuna, Sweet Chilli, & Red Pepper, on Oatmeal, Greggs*	1 Sandwich/206g		370	4.5	180	11.2	27.2	2.2	0.0

	Measure INFO/WEIGHT	per Measure KCAL	FAT	Nutrition Values per 100g / 100ml KCAL	PROT	CARB	FAT	FIBRE
GREGGS								
SANDWICH								
Tuna Crunch, on Brown, Bloomer, Greggs*	1 Sandwich/235g	520	15.0	221	11.1	28.9	6.4	0.0
Tuna Mayo, & Sweetcorn, Low Fat, Oatmeal, Greggs*	1 Sandwich/166g	310	5.5	187	13.0	24.7	3.3	0.0
Tuna Mayonnaise, & Cucumber, on Oatmeal, Greggs*	1 Sandwich/194g	400	11.0	206	12.1	25.5	5.7	0.0
Tuna Mayonnaise, On Malted Brown, Greggs*	1 Sandwich/203g	440	13.5	217	12.3	26.6	6.6	0.0
SAUSAGE ROLL								
Freshly Baked, Greggs*	1 Serving/103g	360	25.5	350	8.2	22.8	24.8	0.0
Mini, Greggs*	1 Roll/26g	81	6.5	310	8.5	21.5	25.0	0.0
SLICES								
Toffee Apple, Lattice, Greggs*	1 Slice/77g	277	15.0	360	4.0	41.0	19.5	0.0
SOUP								
Lentil & Bacon, Greggs*	1 Serving/300g	180	5.5	60	3.5	7.7	1.8	0.0
Tomato, Heinz, Greggs*	1 Pot/296g`	200	7.4	68	0.9	10.5	2.5	0.0
TART								
Egg Custard, Greggs*	1 Tart/90g	257	13.0	286	5.5	33.2	14.5	0.0
Strawberry, Greggs*	1 Tart/65g	180	7.5	277	2.3	41.5	11.5	0.0
Strawberry, with Fresh Cream, Greggs*	1 Tart/94g	300	16.5	319	3.2	35.1	17.6	0.0
TEACAKES								
Bakery, Greggs*	1 Teacake/74g	210	3.5	284	7.4	52.0	4.7	0.0
TURNOVER								
Apple, Fresh Cream, Greggs*	1 Turnover/176g	540	32.5	307	2.8	34.1	18.5	0.0
WRAP								
Bacon & Cheese, Greggs*	1 Wrap/98g	410	31.0	421	14.4	19.0	31.8	0.0
Chicken, & Bacon, Caesar, Greggs*	1 Wrap/189g	450	23.5	238	10.8	20.4	12.4	0.0
Chicken, Chargrilled, Greggs*	1 Wrap/192g	410	18.5	214	10.2	20.8	9.6	0.0
YOGHURT								
Raspberry, & Granola, Natural, Greggs*	1 Pot/190g	228	4.8	120	5.0	18.5	2.5	0.0
J D WETHERSPOON								
BAGUETTE								
BLT, Malted Grain, J D Wetherspoon*	1 Baguette/399g	823	45.5	206	8.3	17.8	11.4	1.3
Club, Malted Grain, J D Wetherspoon*	1 Baguette/388g	768	36.8	198	9.8	18.5	9.5	1.4
Crayfish, Malted Grain, J D Wetherspoon*	1 Baguette/314g	594	25.5	189	6.1	23.2	8.1	1.7
Hot Sausage & Tomato Chutney, J D Wetherspoon*	1 Meal/250g	839	33.4	336	14.1	40.7	13.4	3.8
Ploughmans, Lloyds, J D Wetherspoon*	1 Baguette/346g	778	34.3	225	8.6	25.5	9.9	2.2
Tuna Mayonnaise, Malted Grain, J D Wetherspoon*	1 Baguette/401g	710	31.3	177	8.9	18.1	7.8	1.3
Wiltshire Ham, J D Wetherspoon*	1 Baguette/346g	536	13.1	155	9.9	20.4	3.8	1.5
BHAJI								
Onion, J D Wetherspoon*	1 Bhaji/30g	43	2.2	143	5.3	18.7	7.3	5.7
BIRYANI								
Chicken, without Naan, J D Wetherspoon*	1 Meal/614g	700	24.6	114	4.7	14.8	4.0	1.3
BREAD								
Garlic, Ciabatta, J D Wetherspoon*	1 Serving/142g	406	17.9	286	8.0	1.0	12.6	1.5
Naan, J D Wetherspoon*	1 Naan/90g	197	2.5	219	7.6	41.0	2.8	1.4
BREAKFAST								
Baguette, Quorn Sausage, J D Wetherspoon*	1 Baguette/285g	622	18.3	218	10.5	29.4	6.4	3.4
Blueberry Muffin, J D Wetherspoon*	1 Muffin/124g	467	25.8	374	4.7	43.2	20.7	0.4
Bran, Fruit & Nut Muffin, J D Wetherspoon*	1 Serving/145g	571	31.7	394	7.2	43.0	21.9	1.1
Children's, J D Wetherspoon*	1 Serving/341g	613	37.1	180	10.4	10.8	10.9	2.3
Chocolate Muffin, J D Wetherspoon*	1 Muffin/125g	490	28.4	392	5.0	43.6	22.7	4.8
Eggs Benedict, J D Wetherspoon*	1 Serving/100g	573	30.9	573	38.7	33.6	30.9	2.4
Farmhouse, with Toast, J D Wetherspoon*	1 Serving/796g	1647	101.8	207	9.4	14.0	12.8	1.9
Morning Roll, with Bacon, J D Wetherspoon*	1 Roll/183g	546	34.6	298	11.1	21.7	18.9	1.1
Morning Roll, with Fried Egg, J D Wetherspoon*	1 Roll/143g	400	21.3	280	9.7	27.8	14.9	1.4

	Measure INFO/WEIGHT	per Measure KCAL	per Measure FAT	Nutrition Values per 100g / 100ml KCAL	PROT	CARB	FAT	FIBRE
J D WETHERSPOON								
BREAKFAST								
Morning Roll, with Quorn Sausage, J D Wetherspoon*	1 Roll/143g	367	16.1	257	10.1	29.5	11.3	2.6
Morning Roll, with Sausage, J D Wetherspoon*	1 Roll/158g	517	28.0	327	13.8	30.1	17.7	2.3
Scrambled Egg, on Toast, J D Wetherspoon*	1 Serving/265g	503	24.9	190	8.4	17.4	9.4	1.1
Toast & Preserves, J D Wetherspoon*	1 Serving/148g	420	15.2	284	5.7	41.8	10.3	3.2
Traditional, J D Wetherspoon*	1 Breakfast/523g	904	60.1	173	8.4	9.4	11.5	1.8
Vegetarian, J D Wetherspoon*	1 Breakfast/562g	804	47.2	143	6.7	10.2	8.4	2.1
BURGERS								
Beef, Double, & Chips, J D Wetherspoon*	1 Serving/598g	1382	81.6	231	16.8	11.4	13.6	0.5
Beef, Double, Cheese, & Chips, J D Wetherspoon*	1 Serving/654g	1565	91.4	239	17.2	10.7	14.0	0.5
Beef, with Bacon, Cheese & Chips, J D Wetherspoon*	1 Serving/531g	1295	78.9	244	15.2	12.6	14.8	0.5
Beef, with Cheese, & Chips, J D Wetherspoon*	1 Serving/456g	966	53.8	212	13.7	13.8	11.8	0.5
Beef, with Chips, J D Wetherspoon*	1 Serving/428g	881	46.4	206	12.8	15.7	10.8	0.6
Chicken, Fillet, with Chips, J D Wetherspoon*	1 Serving/465g	727	17.1	156	10.9	16.7	3.7	0.8
Lamb, Double, Minted, with Chips, J D Wetherspoon*	1 Serving/598g	1077	47.2	180	14.6	14.1	7.9	0.9
Lamb, Minted, with Chips, J D Wetherspoon*	1 Serving/428g	712	27.8	166	11.3	17.2	6.5	0.9
Vegetable, with Chips, J D Wetherspoon*	1 Meal/488g	839	25.9	172	4.7	27.2	5.3	2.0
BUTTY								
Bacon, Brown Bloomer, J D Wetherspoon*	1 Serving/309g	869	39.6	281	23.3	18.3	12.8	1.2
Bacon & Egg, Brown Bloomer, J D Wetherspoon*	1 Serving/269g	702	31.1	261	18.2	21.0	11.6	1.4
Bacon & Egg, White Bloomer, J D Wetherspoon*	1 Serving/269g	689	32.7	256	16.7	20.9	12.2	1.2
Chip, Brown Bloomer, J D Wetherspoon*	1 Serving/204g	478	14.7	234	7.6	35.7	7.2	1.9
Chip, White Bloomer, J D Wetherspoon*	1 Serving/204g	465	16.3	228	5.6	35.6	8.0	1.6
Chip & Cheese, Brown Bloomer, J D Wetherspoon*	1 Serving/232g	593	24.4	256	9.7	31.4	10.5	1.6
Chip & Cheese, White Bloomer, J D Wetherspoon*	1 Serving/232g	580	26.0	250	7.9	31.3	11.2	1.4
Sausage & Egg, Brown Bloomer, J D Wetherspoon*	1 Serving/331g	885	49.0	268	16.8	20.8	14.8	1.3
Sausage & Egg, White Bloomer, J D Wetherspoon*	1 Serving/331g	872	50.6	264	11.4	20.7	15.3	1.1
CAKE								
Chocolate Fudge, & Ice Cream, J D Wetherspoon*	1 Serving/239g	822	47.3	344	4.0	37.6	19.8	0.4
CAULIFLOWER CHEESE								
J D Wetherspoon*	1 Portion/220g	275	15.2	125	4.1	3.6	6.9	0.8
CHEESECAKE								
Chocolate Chip, J D Wetherspoon*	1 Serving/100g	270	11.5	270	4.9	36.8	11.5	0.5
White Chocolate & Raspberry, J D Wetherspoon*	1 Serving/175g	656	36.9	375	5.6	40.8	21.1	0.9
CHICKEN								
Wings, Buffalo, J D Wetherspoon*	1 Portion/328g	636	42.9	194	15.2	4.0	13.1	0.5
CHICKEN ALFREDO								
Pasta, with Dressed Side Salad, J D Wetherspoon*	1 Meal/576g	950	52.4	165	8.7	12.0	9.1	0.3
Pasta, with Garlic Bread, J D Wetherspoon*	1 Meal/501g	1007	47.6	201	10.8	13.0	9.5	0.3
Pasta, without Garlic Bread, J D Wetherspoon*	1 Meal/430g	804	38.7	187	11.3	15.0	9.0	0.1
CHICKEN FORESTIERRE								
J D Wetherspoon*	1 Serving/684g	626	26.0	92	7.7	8.7	3.8	1.0
CHICKEN ROAST								
& Chips, Peas, Toms, Mushrooms, J D Wetherspoon*	1 Meal/742g	904	38.6	122	13.0	5.6	5.2	1.2
with BBQ Sauce, J D Wetherspoon*	1 Meal/742g	948	37.5	128	11.3	9.2	5.0	0.6
with Chips & BBQ Sauce, J D Wetherspoon*	1 Meal/768g	1183	53.0	154	11.5	12.2	6.9	0.9
with Chips & Salad, J D Wetherspoon*	1 Meal/695g	983	52.1	141	13.1	5.9	7.5	0.6
with Jacket Potato, Salad, & Salsa, J D Wetherspoon*	1 Meal/785g	1193	57.3	152	12.2	10.2	7.3	1.3
with Piri Piri Sauce, J D Wetherspoon*	1 Serving/994g	994	47.1	100	8.4	5.8	4.7	0.8
with Side Salad & BBQ Sauce, J D Wetherspoon*	1 Meal/666g	913	46.0	137	12.2	6.0	6.9	0.9
CHICKEN VINDALOO								
J D Wetherspoon*	1 Meal/500g	704	19.0	141	6.4	21.0	3.8	1.3

J D WETHERSPOON

	Measure INFO/WEIGHT	per Measure KCAL	per Measure FAT	Nutrition Values per 100g / 100ml KCAL	PROT	CARB	FAT	FIBRE
CHILLI								
Con Carne, with Rice, & Tortilla, J D Wetherspoon*	1 Serving/585g	744	20.0	127	6.5	17.8	3.4	1.6
CHIPS								
Bowl, J D Wetherspoon*	1 Serving/300g	750	30.4	250	3.5	36.5	10.1	2.9
with Cheese, J D Wetherspoon*	1 Serving/501g	1002	51.6	200	5.2	21.9	10.3	1.8
with Roast Gravy, J D Wetherspoon*	1 Serving/400g	392	12.4	98	2.5	17.6	3.1	0.0
CHUTNEY								
Mango, J D Wetherspoon*	1 Serving/25g	47	0.2	188	0.4	44.8	0.8	0.4
CIABATTA								
BBQ Chicken & Bacon Melt, J D Wetherspoon*	1 Ciabatta/333g	716	33.6	215	11.3	20.4	10.1	1.8
BLT, J D Wetherspoon*	1 Ciabatta/390g	789	47.3	202	8.2	15.4	12.1	1.5
Club, J D Wetherspoon*	1 Ciabatta/378g	734	38.6	194	9.7	16.1	10.2	1.6
Crayfish, J D Wetherspoon*	1 Ciabatta/305g	561	27.4	184	5.8	20.3	9.0	1.9
Mature Cheddar Cheese & Pickle, J D Wetherspoon*	1 Ciabatta/350g	662	31.5	189	7.8	19.4	9.0	1.7
Tuna Mayonnaise, J D Wetherspoon*	1 Ciabatta/391g	676	32.8	173	8.8	15.8	8.4	1.5
Wiltshire Ham, J D Wetherspoon*	1 Ciabatta/335g	503	14.8	150	9.8	17.7	4.4	1.7
CURRY								
Beef, Malaysian, Rendang, Naan, J D Wetherspoon*	1 Meal/706g	1144	41.0	162	6.8	20.1	5.8	1.1
Goan, Vegetable, without Naan, J D Wetherspoon*	1 Meal/748g	1017	41.9	136	3.1	18.3	5.6	1.3
Kashmiri, Lamb, with Naan, J D Wetherspoon*	1 Meal/704g	1021	33.1	145	7.2	19.5	4.7	1.2
Kashmiri, Lamb, without Naan, J D Wetherspoon*	1 Meal/615g	824	30.7	134	7.1	16.3	5.0	1.1
Kerala, Fish, with Naan, J D Wetherspoon*	1 Meal/706g	1066	36.0	151	7.0	20.0	5.1	1.0
Kerala, Fish, without Naan, J D Wetherspoon*	1 Meal/616g	869	33.3	141	6.9	16.9	5.4	0.9
Mushroom Dopiaza, with Naan, J D Wetherspoon*	1 Serving/719g	899	24.5	125	3.5	21.5	3.4	1.5
Royal Thali, with Naan, J D Wetherspoon*	1 Meal/948g	1336	48.3	141	7.1	16.8	5.1	1.3
Thai, Green Chicken, without Naan, J D Wetherspoon*	1 Meal/617g	1037	46.9	168	7.5	17.6	7.6	0.5
Vegetable, Goan, with Naan Bread, J D Wetherspoon*	1 Meal/707g	1032	36.8	146	3.6	21.2	5.2	1.3
Vegetarian, Thali, with Naan, J D Wetherspoon*	1 Meal/950g	1320	42.7	139	5.3	20.3	4.5	2.4
DHANSAK								
Lamb, Meal, J D Wetherspoon*	1 Serving/720g	983	26.1	137	7.2	19.6	3.6	0.8
FISH & CHIPS								
Haddock, J D Wetherspoon*	1 Meal/496g	806	40.7	162	7.2	14.4	8.2	2.4
Plaice, Breaded, & Peas, J D Wetherspoon*	1 Serving/460g	550	15.6	120	6.8	15.0	3.4	1.7
Traditional, J D Wetherspoon*	1 Serving/495g	804	40.6	162	7.2	14.4	8.2	2.4
FISH CAKES								
Salmon & Lime, with Tartare Sauce, J D Wetherspoon*	1 Serving/355g	569	31.3	160	5.8	14.5	8.8	1.0
GAMMON								
Steak, 8oz, Eggs, Chips & Pineapple, J D Wetherspoon*	1 Meal/609g	1036	51.8	170	13.4	10.2	8.5	0.8
Steak, Egg, Chips & Side Salad, J D Wetherspoon*	1 Meal/593g	801	41.5	135	10.2	9.0	7.0	0.3
GAMMON &								
Chips, Peas, Tomato, & Egg, J D Wetherspoon*	1 Meal/564g	844	41.2	150	15.0	6.7	7.3	1.3
Chips, Peas, Tomato, & Pineapple, J D Wetherspoon*	1 Meal/575g	799	36.2	139	13.6	7.8	6.3	1.4
HAGGIS								
with Neeps & Tatties, J D Wetherspoon*	1 Meal/682g	982	52.5	144	4.6	15.0	7.7	1.9
HAM								
& Eggs, J D Wetherspoon*	1 Serving/396g	253	12.7	64	4.9	3.5	3.2	0.0
ICE CREAM								
Bombe, Mint Chocolate, J D Wetherspoon*	1 Portion/135g	300	13.4	222	2.6	30.6	9.9	0.8
Chocolate, Bomb, J D Wetherspoon*	1 Portion/100g	259	13.4	259	5.9	34.3	13.4	5.4
Neopolitan, Movenpick, J D Wetherspoon*	1 Bowl/100g	181	9.6	181	3.0	20.0	9.6	0.0
JALFREZI								
Chicken, Meal, with Naan Bread, J D Wetherspoon*	1 Meal/705g	916	19.7	130	6.8	19.9	2.8	1.3
Chicken, without Naan Bread, J D Wetherspoon*	1 Meal/615g	719	17.2	117	6.7	16.9	2.8	1.3

	Measure INFO/WEIGHT	per Measure KCAL	FAT	Nutrition Values per 100g / 100ml KCAL	PROT	CARB	FAT	FIBRE
J D WETHERSPOON								
KORMA								
Chicken, Meal, without Naan, J D Wetherspoon*	1 Meal/617g	944	38.2	153	6.4	17.0	6.2	0.8
Chicken, with Naan, J D Wetherspoon*	1 Meal/704g	1141	40.8	162	6.6	20.1	5.8	0.9
LASAGNE								
Al Forno with Dressed Side Salad, J D Wetherspoon*	1 Meal/658g	823	40.8	125	5.5	11.4	6.2	0.8
MASALA								
Chicken, Hot, with Naan, J D Wetherspoon*	1 Meal/707g	1033	31.1	146	6.9	20.1	4.4	1.2
Chicken, Hot, without Naan, J D Wetherspoon*	1 Meal/614g	835	28.2	136	6.8	17.1	4.6	1.1
Vegetable, Tandoori, Meal, J D Wetherspoon*	1 Serving/720g	1020	36.0	142	3.4	20.7	5.0	2.3
MEATBALLS								
with Linguine Pasta, J D Wetherspoon*	1 Serving/512g	614	24.0	120	6.3	13.1	4.7	1.9
MELT								
BBQ Chicken, & Chips, & Salad, J D Wetherspoon*	1 Serving/643g	849	42.4	132	10.4	8.2	6.6	0.4
MIXED GRILL								
with Chips, & Dressed Side Salad, J D Wetherspoon*	1 Serving/784g	1324	87.0	169	12.0	5.6	11.1	0.3
MOUSSAKA								
Vegetarian, J D Wetherspoon*	1 Serving/555g	582	38.8	105	2.7	7.6	7.0	2.7
NACHOS								
J D Wetherspoon*	1 Serving/366g	1139	67.3	311	7.0	29.2	18.4	3.2
with Chilli Con Carne, J D Wetherspoon*	1 Meal/570g	1505	88.9	264	8.6	22.2	15.6	1.8
with Fajita Chicken, J D Wetherspoon*	1 Serving/486g	1225	70.5	252	5.7	24.7	14.5	2.9
with Five Bean Chilli, J D Wetherspoon*	1 Serving/571g	1399	81.1	245	7.3	21.8	14.2	2.7
PANINI								
BBQ Chicken & Bacon, Melt, J D Wetherspoon*	1 Panini/337g	650	27.6	193	9.9	19.9	8.2	1.7
Cheese, Tomato, & Bacon, J D Wetherspoon*	1 Panini/261g	630	29.0	241	14.3	21.6	11.1	0.8
Cheese & Tuna, J D Wetherspoon*	1 Panini/221g	551	22.3	249	15.5	24.9	10.1	0.7
Club, J D Wetherspoon*	1 Panini/378g	734	38.6	194	9.7	16.1	10.2	1.6
Fajita Chicken, J D Wetherspoon*	1 Panini/235g	359	6.1	153	4.4	28.8	2.6	1.7
Mature, Cheddar Cheese & Tomato, J D Wetherspoon*	1 Panini/330g	750	27.1	227	10.4	18.0	8.2	1.7
Pepperoni & Mozzarella, J D Wetherspoon*	1 Panini/205g	617	33.4	301	11.6	27.5	16.3	1.0
Tomato, Mozzarella & Green Pesto, J D Wetherspoon*	1 Panini/245g	502	22.9	205	7.3	23.0	9.4	1.4
PASTA BAKE								
Mediterranean, J D Wetherspoon*	1 Serving/450g	577	22.1	128	4.3	16.4	4.9	0.9
PEAS								
& Ham, White Poppy Seed Bloomer, J D Wetherspoon*	1 Portion/456g	474	17.8	104	4.4	12.5	3.9	2.0
PIE								
Aberdeen Angus, Chips, & Veg, J D Wetherspoon*	1 Serving/780g	1356	86.6	174	5.5	15.7	11.1	0.9
Cottage, with Chips & Peas, J D Wetherspoon*	1 Meal/682g	846	33.4	124	3.7	15.6	4.9	1.9
Fish, Carrot & Broccoli, Herb Butter, J D Wetherspoon*	1 Serving/550g	612	38.0	111	4.6	9.7	6.9	2.4
Scotch, J D Wetherspoon*	1 Serving/145g	302	15.4	208	13.1	7.8	10.6	0.9
Scotch, with Chips & Beans, J D Wetherspoon*	1 Serving/435g	603	22.2	139	6.8	14.9	5.1	1.5
PLATTER								
Italian Style, J D Wetherspoon*	1 Platter/1020g	1985	75.5	195	10.4	22.9	7.4	0.6
Mexican, Chilli, Sour Cream, J D Wetherspoon*	1 Platter/1062g	2560	141.2	241	7.5	22.6	13.3	2.8
Mexican, with Five Bean Chilli, J D Wetherspoon*	1 Platter/1002g	2358	123.2	235	6.2	25.6	12.3	3.6
Western, J D Wetherspoon*	1 Platter/1454g	2973	168.7	204	16.9	9.1	11.6	0.4
POPPADOMS								
& Dips, J D Wetherspoon*	1 Serving/134g	425	10.9	317	4.6	28.4	8.1	2.5
POTATO BOMBAY								
J D Wetherspoon*	1 Serving/300g	285	14.7	95	1.8	10.8	4.9	2.5
POTATO SKINS								
Cheese & Bacon, Loaded, J D Wetherspoon*	1 Serving/439g	949	58.4	216	8.9	15.2	13.3	1.5
Cheese & Red Onion, Loaded, J D Wetherspoon*	1 Serving/414g	835	51.3	202	6.0	16.5	12.4	1.6

J D WETHERSPOON

	Measure INFO/WEIGHT	per Measure KCAL	FAT	Nutrition Values per 100g / 100ml KCAL	PROT	CARB	FAT	FIBRE
POTATO SKINS								
Chilli Con Carne, Loaded, J D Wetherspoon*	1 Serving/503g	735	35.7	146	5.0	15.7	7.1	1.9
POTATO WEDGES								
Spicy, J D Wetherspoon*	1 Serving/270g	434	15.7	161	2.2	27.7	5.8	1.8
Spicy, with Sour Cream, J D Wetherspoon*	1 Serving/330g	558	27.4	169	2.3	23.4	8.3	1.5
POTATOES								
Baked, Jacket, Coleslaw, J D Wetherspoon*	1 Meal/596g	918	48.9	154	2.3	17.1	8.2	1.8
Mashed, Creamy, J D Wetherspoon*	1 Portion/279g	349	21.2	125	1.5	15.0	7.6	1.1
Roast, J D Wetherspoon*	1 Portion/200g	290	9.4	145	2.5	23.0	4.7	2.3
RIBS								
Double, J D Wetherspoon*	1 Serving/350g	767	40.9	219	16.7	11.9	11.7	0.4
Double, with Chips, J D Wetherspoon*	1 Serving/500g	949	46.5	190	12.5	14.9	9.3	0.3
Double, with Jacket Potato, J D Wetherspoon*	1 Serving/590g	1159	50.7	196	11.4	19.2	8.6	1.3
RICE								
Basmati, Yellow, J D Wetherspoon*	1 Portion/200g	286	1.2	143	3.4	31.1	0.6	0.2
J D Wetherspoon*	1 Serving/200g	274	0.4	137	2.9	30.9	0.2	0.2
ROGAN JOSH								
Lamb, Meal, without Naan, J D Wetherspoon*	1 Meal/617g	820	27.7	133	7.1	17.0	4.5	1.0
Lamb, with Naan, J D Wetherspoon*	1 Meal/706g	1017	30.4	144	7.2	20.1	4.3	1.1
SALAD								
Caesar, Chicken, J D Wetherspoon*	1 Meal/230g	507	36.4	220	14.3	5.1	15.8	0.8
Caesar, J D Wetherspoon*	1 Meal/211g	448	38.0	212	6.8	5.8	18.0	1.1
Chicken, BBQ, Croutons & Dressing, J D Wetherspoon*	1 Portion/350g	315	8.4	90	9.4	7.5	2.4	0.8
Chicken & Bacon, Warm, J D Wetherspoon*	1 Meal/426g	600	41.3	141	9.8	3.8	9.7	0.6
Crayfish, J D Wetherspoon*	1 Meal/317g	247	18.0	78	4.4	2.7	5.7	0.6
Side, No Dressing, J D Wetherspoon*	1 Salad/195g	125	4.5	64	2.0	8.9	2.3	1.1
Side, with Dressing, J D Wetherspoon*	1 Salad/215g	263	19.6	122	2.2	8.1	9.1	1.0
Side, with Dressing & Croutons, J D Wetherspoon*	1 Portion/140g	221	18.3	158	2.1	8.6	13.1	1.1
Side, with Dressing & No Croutons, J D Wetherspoon*	1 Portion/129g	145	14.0	112	1.0	3.2	10.8	0.9
Side, without Croutons, J D Wetherspoon*	1 Portion/111g	157	10.8	141	9.8	3.8	9.7	0.6
Thai Noodle, J D Wetherspoon*	1 Portion/393g	433	21.3	110	2.7	12.7	5.4	1.4
Thai Noodle, with Chicken, J D Wetherspoon*	1 Meal/554g	637	27.7	115	9.2	9.6	5.0	1.4
Tiger Prawn, Dressing, & Chilli Jam, J D Wetherspoon*	1 Portion/340g	500	33.0	147	4.7	10.1	9.7	0.9
Tuna, with Eggs, Olives, & Croutons, J D Wetherspoon*	1 Portion/395g	679	51.7	172	10.3	3.2	13.1	0.7
SAMOSAS								
Lamb, J D Wetherspoon*	1 Samosa/90g	160	3.8	178	7.9	29.9	4.2	3.9
Vegetable, J D Wetherspoon*	1 Samosa/50g	92	3.1	184	5.4	28.4	6.2	2.2
SANDWICH								
Beef, Hot, Brown Bloomer, J D Wetherspoon*	1 Sandwich/299g	618	27.2	207	11.4	19.9	9.1	1.3
BLT, Brown Bloomer, J D Wetherspoon*	1 Sandwich/404g	885	39.6	219	18.0	14.6	9.8	1.2
BLT, White Bloomer, J D Wetherspoon*	1 Sandwich/404g	872	32.7	216	17.0	14.6	8.1	1.0
Cheddar, & Pickle, Brown Bloomer, J D Wetherspoon*	1 Sandwich/260g	665	31.9	256	11.0	25.4	12.3	1.9
Cheddar, & Pickle, White Bloomer, J D Wetherspoon*	1 Sandwich/260g	638	32.8	245	9.2	0.0	12.6	1.5
Chicken, Half Fat Mayo, Brown, Hot, J D Wetherspoon*	1 Sandwich/289g	628	28.3	217	11.8	20.7	9.8	1.7
Chicken, Half Fat Mayo, White, Hot, J D Wetherspoon*	1 Sandwich/289g	615	29.8	213	11.3	20.6	10.3	1.5
Egg Mayonnaise, Brown Bloomer, J D Wetherspoon*	1 Sandwich/295g	704	39.5	239	10.1	19.7	13.4	1.3
Egg Mayonnaise, White Bloomer, J D Wetherspoon*	1 Sandwich/295g	692	41.0	235	8.7	19.6	13.9	1.1
Ham, & Tomato, Brown Bloomer, J D Wetherspoon*	1 Sandwich/239g	514	17.2	215	11.4	24.4	7.2	1.8
Ham, & Tomato, White Bloomer, J D Wetherspoon*	1 Sandwich/239g	501	18.6	210	9.7	24.4	7.8	1.5
Prawn Mayonnaise, Brown Bloomer, J D Wetherspoon*	1 Sandwich/244g	579	26.6	237	11.0	23.8	10.9	1.6
Prawn Mayonnaise, White Bloomer, J D Wetherspoon*	1 Sandwich/244g	567	28.3	232	9.3	23.7	11.6	1.4
Salmon, Lemon Mayo, Brown, J D Wetherspoon*	1 Sandwich/229g	637	33.7	278	11.4	25.4	14.7	1.7
Tuna Mayo, Half Fat Mayo, White, J D Wetherspoon*	1 Sandwich/389g	828	47.1	213	11.2	15.6	12.1	1.0

J D WETHERSPOON

Measure		per Measure		Nutrition Values per 100g / 100ml				
INFO/WEIGHT		KCAL	FAT	KCAL	PROT	CARB	FAT	FIBRE
SAUSAGE & MASH								
with Red Wine Gravy, J D Wetherspoon*	1 Portion/677g	887	50.8	131	6.0	10.2	7.5	1.8
SAUSAGES WITH								
Bacon & Egg, J D Wetherspoon*	1 Serving/582g	1040	57.6	179	11.7	11.3	9.9	1.0
Chips & Beans, J D Wetherspoon*	1 Meal/554g	897	42.6	162	7.3	16.4	7.7	2.3
SCAMPI								
Breaded, Chips, Peas, Tartare, J D Wetherspoon*	1 Serving/561g	987	43.7	176	5.2	19.9	7.8	2.3
SORBET								
Mango & Passionfruit, J D Wetherspoon*	1 Serving/135g	115	0.1	85	0.2	20.0	0.1	0.2
SOUP								
Leek & Potato, no Bread & Butter, J D Wetherspoon*	1 Bowl/420	105	0.8	25	0.9	5.1	0.2	1.0
Mushroom, No Bread, J D Wetherspoon*	1 Serving/305g	252	16.5	83	2.8	5.5	5.4	0.4
Mushroom, with Brown Bloomer, J D Wetherspoon*	1 Serving/429g	561	23.7	131	3.4	16.0	5.5	1.2
Mushroom, with White Bloomer, J D Wetherspoon*	1 Serving/429g	549	25.2	128	3.4	15.9	5.9	1.1
Tomato, No Bread, J D Wetherspoon*	1 Serving/305g	198	14.0	65	0.9	3.9	4.6	0.6
Tomato, with Brown Bloomer, J D Wetherspoon*	1 Serving/429g	576	25.8	134	3.7	15.7	6.0	1.3
Tomato, with White Bloomer, J D Wetherspoon*	1 Serving/429g	563	27.3	131	2.8	15.6	6.4	1.2
Tomato & Basil, Organic, J D Wetherspoon*	1 Serving/491g	584	23.1	119	2.9	15.8	4.7	1.2
Tomato & Basil, Organic, no Bread, J D Wetherspoon*	1 Bowl/350g	200	15.0	57	0.7	3.0	4.3	0.6
SPONGE PUDDING								
Treacle, with Hot Custard, J D Wetherspoon*	1 Serving/515g	1267	71.1	246	2.3	41.8	13.8	0.2
SQUASH								
Butternut, Roast Dinner, J D Wetherspoon*	1 Meal/847g	1211	55.9	143	4.9	17.5	6.6	2.9
STEAK								
Ribeye, 8oz, Chips & Side Salad, J D Wetherspoon*	1 Meal/562g	1006	71.9	179	8.0	8.9	12.8	0.3
STEAK &								
Breaded Scampi, Chips, & Peas, J D Wetherspoon*	1 Serving/816g	1369	72.6	168	10.1	11.3	8.9	1.2
STEAK WITH								
Chips, & Dressed Side Salad, Rump, J D Wetherspoon*	1 Meal/634g	922	60.2	145	9.5	6.3	9.5	0.3
Chips, & Dressed Side Salad, Sirloin, J D Wetherspoon*	1 Meal/577g	979	73.3	170	7.6	6.9	12.7	0.3
Jacket Pot, Salad, & Salsa, Rump, J D Wetherspoon*	1 Meal/724g	1132	64.4	156	9.0	10.9	8.9	1.1
Jacket Pot, Salad, & Salsa, Sirloin, J D Wetherspoon*	1 Meal/667g	1189	77.4	178	7.3	11.8	11.6	1.2
STEW								
Irish, J D Wetherspoon*	1 Serving/600g	516	23.4	86	7.3	5.6	3.9	0.9
STUFFING BALLS								
Sage & Onion, J D Wetherspoon*	1 Portion/70g	137	1.1	196	6.6	32.3	1.6	3.6
TART								
Apple, with Ice Cream, J D Wetherspoon*	1 Serving/235g	464	20.0	197	1.6	29.8	8.5	0.4
TIKKA								
Mixed Grill, Starter, J D Wetherspoon*	1 Portion/374g	460	23.9	123	13.4	3.2	6.4	0.9
TIKKA MASALA								
Chicken with Rice & No Naan Bread, J D Wetherspoon*	1 Meal/614g	872	33.2	142	6.9	16.9	5.4	1.2
WAFFLES								
Belgian, Ice Cream & Maple Syrup, J D Wetherspoon*	1 Serving/395g	934	33.6	236	13.8	28.4	8.5	0.8
WRAP								
Caesar Wetherwrap, J D Wetherspoon*	1 Wrap/159g	478	32.6	301	7.0	23.1	20.5	1.5
Caesar Wetherwrap, Tortillas & Salsa, J D Wetherspoon*	1 Serving/244g	624	38.8	256	5.7	23.4	15.9	1.6
Caesar Wetherwrap & Wedges, J D Wetherspoon*	1 Serving/289g	687	40.2	238	5.0	25.2	13.9	1.6
Chicken, Cheese, & Potato Wedges, J D Wetherspoon*	1 Serving/401g	762	34.1	190	8.0	22.2	8.5	1.5
Chicken, Guacamole, Tortillas, Salsa, J D Wetherspoon*	1 Serving/273g	474	16.9	174	8.2	21.9	6.2	2.0
Chicken, Guacamole, Wedges, J D Wetherspoon*	1 Serving/318g	537	18.4	169	7.2	23.7	5.8	2.0
Chicken, with Chicken Breast, J D Wetherspoon*	1 Wrap/292g	450	21.6	154	9.4	14.5	7.4	1.5
Chicken, with Potato Wedges, J D Wetherspoon*	1 Serving/373g	647	24.2	174	6.7	23.9	6.5	1.7

	Measure INFO/WEIGHT	per Measure KCAL	FAT	Nutrition Values per 100g / 100ml KCAL	PROT	CARB	FAT	FIBRE

J D WETHERSPOON

WRAP

	Measure INFO/WEIGHT	KCAL	FAT	KCAL	PROT	CARB	FAT	FIBRE
Chicken, with Tortilla Chips & Salsa, J D Wetherspoon*	1 Serving/328g	584	23.0	178	7.5	22.3	7.0	1.6
Chicken & Cheese, J D Wetherspoon*	1 Wrap/271g	553	26.3	204	10.7	19.6	9.7	1.4
Club Wetherwrap, with Wedges, J D Wetherspoon*	1 Serving/381g	822	43.1	216	10.9	19.2	11.3	1.2
Fajita Chicken, J D Wetherspoon*	1 Wrap/228g	345	14.1	151	3.8	21.2	6.2	1.9
Fajita Chicken, Tortilla Chips, Salsa, J D Wetherspoon*	1 Serving/313g	491	20.3	157	3.5	21.9	6.5	1.9
Fajita Chicken, with Potato Wedges, J D Wetherspoon*	1 Serving/358g	554	21.8	155	3.2	23.5	6.1	1.9
Poached Salmon, with Wedges, J D Wetherspoon*	1 Serving/298g	656	34.3	220	7.1	24.2	11.5	1.5
Poached Salmon & Prawn Salad, J D Wetherspoon*	1 Wrap/355g	512	34.1	144	9.8	4.5	9.6	0.5
Reggae Reggae Chicken, Breast, J D Wetherspoon*	1 Meal/100g	364	9.6	364	24.4	42.0	9.6	2.7

YORKSHIRE PUDDING

J D Wetherspoon*	2 Puddings/56g	132	4.6	236	8.2	32.9	8.2	1.1

KFC

BEANS

BBQ, Large, KFC*	1 Serving/188g	158	1.4	84	5.3	15.1	0.7	0.0
BBQ, Regular, KFC*	1 Serving/130g	200	1.5	154	6.2	30.0	1.2	6.9

BURGERS

Fillet, KFC*	1 Burger/245g	479	19.8	196	11.1	19.6	8.1	0.0
Fillet, Mini, KFC*	1 Burger/114g	275	11.2	241	14.8	24.0	9.8	0.0
Fillet Tower Burger, KFC*	1 Burger/163g	617	21.0	378	24.3	41.4	12.9	0.0
Mini Fillet, Kids, KFC*	1 Burger/114g	253	6.4	222	15.8	27.0	5.6	0.0
Tower, KFC*	1 Burger/210g	628	20.8	299	15.9	30.0	9.9	0.0
Tower, Zinger, KFC*	1 Burger/264g	655	32.7	248	11.2	24.4	12.4	0.0
Zinger, Fillet, KFC*	1 Burger/185g	445	19.6	241	13.9	22.4	10.6	1.4
Zinger, KFC*	1 Burger/219g	481	20.8	220	12.2	22.0	9.5	0.0

CHEESECAKE

Boysenberry, Chateau, KFC*	1 Serving/85g	196	9.4	230	4.0	30.0	11.0	0.0
Cookies & Cream, KFC*	1 Serving/80g	261	17.1	326	4.3	29.1	21.4	0.0

CHICKEN

Breast, Original Recipe, KFC*	1 Breast/137g	285	13.3	207	24.9	5.6	9.7	0.0
Drumsticks, Original Recipe, KFC*	1 Drumstick/95g	162	9.5	170	11.9	9.1	10.0	0.0
Fillet, Mini, Not In a Bun, KFC*	1 Fillet/50g	116	4.0	232	26.6	14.0	8.0	0.0
Popcorn, Kids, KFC*	1 Portion/66g	144	8.4	219	14.1	13.2	12.7	0.0
Popcorn, Large, KFC*	1 Serving/189g	494	29.8	262	17.5	13.5	15.8	0.0
Ribs, Original Recipe, KFC*	1 Rib/126g	238	13.4	188	19.8	4.2	10.6	0.0
Strips, Crispy, KFC*	1 Strip/46g	112	5.4	243	15.4	20.4	11.7	0.0
Thighs, Original Recipe, KFC*	1 Thigh/134g	218	14.2	162	12.6	4.4	10.6	0.0
Wings, Hot, KFC*	1 Wing/58g	102	7.0	175	9.4	7.6	12.1	0.0
Wings, Original Recipe, KFC*	1 Wing/48g	126	3.8	262	25.0	8.3	8.0	0.0

COLESLAW

Large, KFC*	1 Serving/200g	268	22.4	134	0.8	9.5	11.2	0.0
Regular, KFC*	1 Serving/100g	134	11.2	134	0.8	9.5	11.2	0.0

CORN

Cobs, Cobette, KFC*	1 Serving/70g	141	8.5	201	4.3	20.1	12.1	0.0

DRESSING

Caesar, KFC*	1 Sachet/35g	103	10.9	295	19.2	2.7	31.1	0.0
French, KFC*	1 Sachet/45g	30	1.3	66	0.2	2.9	2.9	0.0
Vinaigrette, Low Fat, KFC*	1 Sachet/35g	21	0.8	59	0.5	8.9	2.2	0.0
Yoghurt, Coriander & Chilli, KFC*	1 Sachet/45g	166	16.2	369	2.2	9.3	36.0	0.0

FRIES

Large, KFC*	1 Serving/162g	375	19.3	232	3.1	32.4	11.9	0.0
Regular, KFC*	1 Serving/111g	257	13.2	232	3.1	32.4	11.9	0.0

	Measure INFO/WEIGHT	per Measure KCAL	FAT	Nutrition Values per 100g / 100ml KCAL	PROT	CARB	FAT	FIBRE
KFC								
GRAVY								
Large, KFC*	1 Serving/204g	144	8.0	71	2.4	7.4	3.9	0.0
Regular, KFC*	1 Serving/102g	72	4.0	71	2.4	7.4	3.9	0.0
ICE CREAM								
Avalanche, KFC*	1 Pot/28g	114	5.1	407	10.4	51.4	18.2	0.0
Soft, KFC*	1 Serving/110g	171	7.0	155	3.7	20.6	6.4	0.0
PIE								
Apple Slice, Colonel's Pies, KFC*	1 Slice/113g	310	13.9	274	1.7	38.9	12.3	0.0
Strawberry Creme, Slice, KFC*	1 Slice/78g	279	15.0	358	5.4	41.0	19.2	2.5
SALAD								
Chicken, Original Recipe, No Dressing, KFC*	1 Salad/292g	270	9.5	92	9.0	7.0	3.3	0.0
Chicken, Zinger, No Dressing, KFC*	1 Salad/285g	307	14.8	108	7.8	8.0	5.2	0.0
Potato, KFC*	1 Portion/160g	229	13.9	143	2.5	14.3	8.7	1.8
WRAP								
Twister, Salsa, Toasted, KFC*	1 Wrap/222g	516	24.9	232	8.7	24.6	11.2	0.0
Twister, Toasted, KFC*	1 Wrap/217g	509	24.8	235	8.9	24.6	11.5	0.0
Wrapstar, KFC*	1 Wrapstar/239g	642	36.6	269	11.4	25.9	15.3	0.0
KRISPY KREME								
DOUGHNUTS								
Apple Pie, Krispy Kreme*	1 Doughnut/80g	311	17.6	389	6.0	41.0	22.0	1.9
Blueberry, Powdered, Filled, Krispy Kreme*	1 Doughnut/86g	307	17.2	357	7.0	36.0	20.0	5.0
Butterscotch Fudge, Krispy Kreme*	1 Doughnut/93g	372	16.7	400	6.0	53.0	18.0	0.0
Chocolate, Glazed, Krispy Kreme*	1 Doughnut/80g	309	13.6	387	4.0	55.0	17.0	3.0
Chocolate Dreamcake, Krispy Kreme*	1 Doughnut/95g	390	19.0	411	6.0	51.0	20.0	3.0
Chocolate Iced, Creme Filled, Krispy Kreme*	1 Doughnut/87g	372	20.0	428	6.0	46.0	23.0	2.0
Chocolate Iced, Custard Filled, Krispy Kreme*	1 Doughnut/87g	318	16.5	366	5.0	41.0	19.0	1.8
Chocolate Iced, Ring, Glazed, Krispy Kreme*	1 Doughnut/66g	278	13.2	422	5.0	54.0	20.0	1.5
Chocolate Iced, with Creme Filling, Krispy Kreme*	1 Doughnut/87g	350	20.9	402	3.0	42.0	24.0	1.0
Chocolate Iced, with Sprinkles, Krispy Kreme*	1 Doughnut/71g	298	12.7	421	6.0	55.0	18.0	1.6
Chocolate Praline Fudge Cake, Krispy Kreme*	1 Doughnut/73g	346	21.2	474	6.0	43.0	29.0	5.6
Cinnamon Apple, Filled, Krispy Kreme*	1 Doughnut/81g	269	14.6	332	7.0	37.0	18.0	5.0
Cookie Crunch, Krispy Kreme*	1 Doughnut/73g	316	14.6	433	4.0	56.0	20.0	5.0
Cookies & Kreme, Krispy Kreme*	1 Doughnut/93g	379	16.7	408	4.0	57.0	18.0	0.0
Cruller, Glazed, Krispy Kreme*	1 Doughnut/54g	254	15.6	471	4.0	49.0	29.0	3.0
Glazed, with a Creme Filling, Krispy Kreme*	1 Doughnut/86g	309	15.5	359	5.0	44.0	18.0	4.0
Lemon Filled, Glazed, Krispy Kreme*	1 Doughnut/66g	218	10.5	331	5.0	41.0	16.0	4.0
Lemon Meringue Pie, Krispy Kreme*	1 Doughnut/83g	339	19.7	412	6.0	40.0	24.0	1.8
Maple Iced, Krispy Kreme*	1 Doughnut/66g	279	15.2	422	5.0	49.0	23.0	3.0
Orange Sundae Gloss, Krispy Kreme*	1 Doughnut/81g	338	17.0	418	5.0	50.0	21.0	3.0
Original, Glazed, Krispy Kreme*	1 Doughnut/52g	222	11.9	428	6.0	48.0	23.0	1.1
Raspberry, Glazed, Krispy Kreme*	1 Doughnut/86g	350	17.2	407	6.0	48.0	20.0	1.8
Sour Cream, Krispy Kreme*	1 Doughnut/80g	340	18.4	425	4.0	53.0	23.0	1.0
Strawberries & Kreme, Krispy Kreme*	1 Doughnut/91g	381	20.9	419	5.0	47.0	23.0	1.8
Strawberry Filled, Powdered, Krispy Kreme*	1 Doughnut/74g	248	13.3	335	7.0	36.0	18.0	5.0
Strawberry Gloss, Krispy Kreme*	1 Doughnut/62g	253	12.4	409	5.0	50.0	20.0	1.6
Vanilla, Krispy Kreme*	1 Doughnut/80g	315	13.7	391	4.0	57.0	17.0	2.0
White Chocolate & Almond, Krispy Kreme*	1 Doughnut/93g	421	24.2	453	8.0	45.0	26.0	1.9
MCDONALD'S								
BAGEL								
Toasted, with Strawberry Jam, McDonald's*	1 Bagel/105g	260	1.0	248	8.0	52.0	1.0	3.0
with Bacon, Egg & Cheese, McDonald's*	1 Bagel/173g	455	22.5	263	13.0	26.0	13.0	2.0
with Butter & Jam, McDonald's*	1 Bagel/122g	399	10.2	326	5.9	58.8	8.3	2.2
with Flora & Jam, McDonald's*	1 Bagel/120g	369	6.9	305	6.0	59.4	5.7	2.2

	Measure INFO/WEIGHT	per Measure KCAL	FAT	Nutrition Values per 100g / 100ml KCAL	PROT	CARB	FAT	FIBRE
MCDONALD'S								
BAGEL								
with Philadelphia, McDonald's*	1 Bagel/125g	318	5.9	254	7.7	47.5	4.7	2.1
with Sausage, Egg & Cheese, McDonald's*	1 Bagel/203g	540	28.4	266	14.0	22.0	14.0	2.0
with Sausage & Egg, McDonald's*	1 Bagel/207g	551	26.5	266	13.3	23.3	12.8	1.6
BREAD								
Bagel, Plain, Toasted, McDonald's*	1 Bagel/85g	210	0.8	248	9.0	50.0	1.0	3.0
BREAKFAST								
Big Breakfast, McDonald's*	1 Breakfast/264g	595	37.0	225	11.0	15.0	14.0	1.0
Big Breakfast Bun, McDonald's*	1 Bun/242g	571	32.2	236	13.0	15.1	13.3	0.9
BREAKFAST CEREAL								
Porridge, Oatso Simple, & Jam, McDonald's*	1 Serving/232g	246	5.3	106	4.0	17.0	2.3	0.9
Porridge, Oatso Simple, & Sugar, McDonald's*	1 Serving/215g	205	5.4	95	4.3	13.7	2.5	0.9
Porridge, Oatso Simple, Plain, McDonald's*	1 Serving/212g	195	4.2	92	5.0	13.0	2.0	1.0
BROWNIE								
Belgian Bliss, McDonald's*	1 Serving/85g	390	22.1	459	6.0	51.0	26.0	2.0
BURGERS								
1955 Burger, McDonald's*	1 Burger/281g	655	33.7	233	14.0	18.0	12.0	2.0
Bacon, Chicken & Onion, McDonald's*	1 Burger/255g	660	33.1	259	14.0	22.0	13.0	2.0
Big Mac, Bigger, McDonald's*	1 Burger/324g	714	34.0	220	12.9	18.5	10.5	1.6
Big Mac, McDonald's*	1 Burger/214g	491	25.7	229	13.0	19.0	12.0	2.0
Big Mac, No Sauce, No Cheese, McDonald's*	1 Burger/181g	400	16.0	221	12.2	23.8	8.8	1.1
Big Tasty, McDonald's*	1 Burger/346g	835	52.0	241	13.0	14.0	15.0	1.0
Big Tasty, with Bacon, McDonald's*	1 Burger/359g	890	57.4	248	14.0	14.0	16.0	1.0
Cheeseburger, Bacon, McDonald's*	1 Burger/127g	336	15.3	264	16.0	24.0	12.0	2.0
Cheeseburger, Double, McDonald's*	1 Burger/169g	440	23.7	260	17.0	19.0	14.0	1.0
Cheeseburger, McDonald's*	1 Burger/119g	300	12.0	253	14.4	26.2	10.1	2.5
Chicken Fiesta, McDonald's*	1 Burger/240g	610	26.4	254	14.0	24.0	11.0	2.0
Chicken Legend, with Bacon, Cool Mayo, McDonald's*	1 Burger/227g	590	22.7	260	15.0	27.0	10.0	2.0
Festive, Deluxe, McDonald's*	1 Burger/284g	770	45.5	271	16.0	17.0	16.0	1.0
Filet-O-Fish, McDonald's*	1 Burger/150g	350	18.1	232	10.0	24.0	12.0	1.0
Filet-O-Fish, No Tartar Sauce, McDonald's*	1 Burger/124g	290	9.0	234	12.1	30.6	7.3	0.8
Hamburger, McDonald's*	1 Burger/104g	250	8.3	240	13.0	29.0	8.0	2.0
Mayo Chicken, McDonald's*	1 Burger/122g	310	13.4	254	10.0	30.0	11.0	2.0
McChicken Sandwich, McDonald's*	1 Sandwich/171g	385	17.2	224	9.0	26.0	10.0	2.0
Quarter Pounder, Bacon with Cheese, McDonald's*	1 Burger/230g	592	33.2	259	16.5	15.4	14.5	1.3
Quarter Pounder, Deluxe, McDonald's*	1 Burger/253g	521	26.8	206	11.4	16.1	10.6	1.7
Quarter Pounder, Double, with Cheese, McDonald's*	1 Burger/275g	710	40.3	259	19.5	12.2	14.7	1.1
Quarter Pounder, McDonald's*	1 Burger/178g	424	19.0	238	14.5	20.9	10.7	2.1
Quarter Pounder, with Cheese, McDonald's*	1 Burger/194g	490	25.3	252	16.0	19.0	13.0	2.0
Summer Chorizo, McDonald's*	1 Burger/238g	650	35.7	273	17.0	17.0	15.0	1.0
The M, McDonald's*	1 Serving/240g	580	28.8	242	16.0	18.0	12.0	1.0
The M with Bacon, McDonald's*	1 Serving/249g	620	32.4	249	17.0	18.0	13.0	1.0
BURGERS VEGETARIAN								
Vegetable, Deluxe, McDonald's*	1 Burger/181g	411	16.3	227	6.0	30.0	9.0	6.0
BUTTER								
Country Life, McDonald's*	1 Pack/11g	85	9.0	752	0.0	0.0	80.0	0.0
CAKE								
Birthday, McDonald's*	1 Portion/158g	640	22.6	405	2.7	65.4	14.3	1.0
CARROTS								
Sticks, McDonald's*	1 Bag/80g	30	0.0	38	0.0	8.0	0.0	2.0
CHEESE								
Soft, Philadelphia, Light, McDonald's*	1 Serving/35g	55	3.9	157	9.0	3.0	11.0	0.0

MCDONALD'S

	Measure INFO/WEIGHT	per Measure KCAL	FAT	Nutrition Values per 100g / 100ml KCAL	PROT	CARB	FAT	FIBRE
CHICKEN								
McNuggets, 4 Pieces, McDonald's*	4 Pieces/70g	170	9.3	238	13.0	19.0	13.0	1.0
McNuggets, 6 Pieces, McDonald's*	6 Pieces/105g	250	13.7	238	13.0	19.0	13.0	1.0
McNuggets, 9 Pieces, McDonald's*	9 Pieces/157g	375	20.5	238	13.0	19.0	13.0	1.0
Selects, 3 Pieces, McDonald's*	3 Pieces/130g	365	19.6	280	16.0	20.0	15.0	1.0
Selects, 5 Pieces, McDonald's*	5 Pieces/219g	612	32.8	280	16.0	20.0	15.0	1.0
COFFEE								
Black, Large, McDonald's*	1 Serving/428ml	0	0.0	0	0.0	0.0	0.0	0.0
Black, Regular, McDonald's*	1 Serving/312ml	0	0.0	0	0.0	0.0	0.0	0.0
Cappuccino, Large, McDonald's*	1 Serving/307ml	120	3.1	39	3.0	4.0	1.0	0.0
Cappuccino, Regular, McDonald's*	1 Serving/231ml	90	2.3	39	3.0	4.0	1.0	0.0
Caramel Frappe, Regular, McDonald's*	1 Serving/312ml	450	19.0	144	2.2	20.5	6.1	0.0
Espresso, Single Shot, McDonald's*	1 Serving/30ml	0	0.0	0	0.0	0.0	0.0	0.0
Latte, Large, McDonald's*	1 Serving/451ml	185	4.5	41	3.0	4.0	1.0	0.0
Latte, Regular, McDonald's*	1 Serving/337ml	135	3.4	40	3.0	4.0	1.0	0.0
White, Large, McDonald's*	1 Serving/428ml	30	0.0	7	0.0	1.0	0.0	0.0
White, Regular, McDonald's*	1 Serving/313ml	25	0.0	8	1.0	1.0	0.0	0.0
COLA								
Coca-Cola, Diet, McDonald's*	1 Med/405ml	4	0.0	1	0.0	0.0	0.0	0.0
Coca-Cola, McDonald's*	1 Med/405ml	170	0.0	42	0.0	10.0	0.0	0.0
Coke, Zero, McDonald's*	1 Serving/200ml	2	0.0	1	0.0	0.0	0.0	0.0
CREAMER								
Uht, McDonald's*	1 Cup/14ml	17	1.4	123	4.2	4.2	10.0	0.0
CROUTONS								
McDonald's*	1 Sachet/14g	60	2.0	426	11.8	63.4	14.0	2.7
DIP								
BBQ, McDonald's*	1 Pot/50g	83	0.0	166	0.0	37.0	0.0	0.0
Caramelised Onion, McDonald's*	1 Dip/31g	45	1.9	144	3.0	19.0	6.0	3.0
Sour Cream & Chive, McDonald's*	1 Pot/50g	150	16.0	300	2.0	2.0	32.0	4.0
Sweet Chilli, McDonald's*	1 Pot/31g	80	0.9	256	0.0	58.0	3.0	0.0
DOUGHNUTS								
Chocolate Donut, McDonald's*	1 Donut/79g	345	16.2	437	5.7	43.8	20.5	1.0
Chocolate Donut, McMini, McDonald's*	1 Donut/17g	64	3.0	375	6.8	46.9	17.8	1.6
Cinnamon Donut, McDonald's*	1 Donut/72g	302	18.1	419	5.1	43.1	25.1	3.8
Sugared Donut, McDonald's*	1 Donut/49g	205	14.7	418	6.0	35.0	30.0	4.0
DRESSING								
Balsamic, Low Fat, McDonald's*	1 Sachet/33g	20	1.0	60	0.0	9.0	3.0	0.0
Caesar, Low Fat, McDonald's*	1 Sachet/80g	55	1.6	68	2.0	10.0	2.0	0.0
French, Low Fat, McDonald's*	1 Serving/22g	13	0.6	58	0.5	7.1	2.6	1.0
FANTA								
Orange, McDonald's*	1 Super/750ml	315	0.0	42	0.0	10.0	0.0	0.0
FISH FINGERS								
McDonald's*	3 Fingers/84g	195	9.2	232	15.0	19.0	11.0	1.0
FRIES								
French, Large, McDonald's*	1 Serving/160g	460	22.4	288	3.0	38.0	14.0	4.0
French, Medium, McDonald's*	1 Serving/114g	330	16.0	289	3.0	37.0	14.0	4.0
French, Small, McDonald's*	1 Serving/80g	230	11.2	288	2.0	38.0	14.0	4.0
FRUIT								
Bag, McDonald's*	1 Pack/80g	40	0.8	50	0.0	12.0	1.0	2.0
FRUIT DRINK								
Fruitizz, Sparkling, McDonald's*	1 Drink/250ml	160	0.0	64	0.4	15.6	0.0	0.0
FRUIT SHOOT								
Robinsons, McDonald's*	1 Bottle/200ml	10	0.0	5	0.0	1.0	0.0	0.0

MCDONALD'S

	Measure INFO/WEIGHT	per Measure KCAL	FAT	Nutrition Values per 100g / 100ml KCAL	PROT	CARB	FAT	FIBRE
HASH BROWNS								
McDonald's*	1 Hash Brown/53g	140	9.0	264	2.0	26.0	17.0	2.0
HOT CHOCOLATE								
McDonald's*	1 Serving/330ml	164	3.6	50	0.7	8.8	1.1	0.0
HOT DOG								
& Ketchup, McDonald's*	1 Serving/116g	296	14.6	255	9.6	25.8	12.6	1.3
ICE CREAM								
Smartie, McDonald's*	1 Pot/120g	260	9.5	216	3.4	33.3	7.9	1.0
ICE CREAM CONE								
McDonald's*	1 Cone/90g	141	4.5	156	4.5	24.4	5.0	0.0
with Flake, McDonald's*	1 Cone/107g	204	7.7	191	4.8	27.0	7.2	0.0
JAM								
Strawberry, McDonald's*	1 Pack/20g	50	0.0	250	0.0	60.0	0.0	0.0
JUICE								
Tropicana, McDonald's*	1 Bottle/250ml	108	0.0	43	1.0	9.0	0.0	0.4
KETCHUP								
Tomato, McDonald's*	1 Portion/23g	25	0.0	109	0.0	26.0	0.0	0.0
LEMONADE								
Sprite, Z, McDonald's*	1 Lge/500ml	5	0.0	1	0.0	0.0	0.0	0.0
MARGARINE								
Flora, Original, McDonald's*	1 Portion/10g	55	6.0	550	0.0	0.0	60.0	0.0
MCFLURRY								
After Eight, McDonald's*	1 McFlurry/206g	400	16.5	194	3.0	27.0	8.0	1.0
Cadbury, Shortcake, Limited Edition, McDonald's*	1 McFlurry/205g	385	14.4	187	3.0	28.0	7.0	1.0
Chocolate, Cornetto, McDonald's*	1 Serving/207g	400	16.6	193	3.0	29.0	8.0	1.0
Cornetto, Mint Choc, McDonald's*	1 Serving/207g	400	16.6	193	3.0	29.0	8.0	1.0
Creme Egg, Cadbury's, McDonald's*	1 McFlurry/203g	381	12.9	188	2.9	29.8	6.3	0.5
Crunchie, McDonald's*	1 McFlurry/185g	330	11.1	178	3.0	28.0	6.0	1.0
Dairy Milk, McDonald's*	1 McFlurry/184g	340	12.9	184	3.0	28.0	7.0	1.0
Dairy Milk, with Caramel, McDonald's*	1 McFlurry/206g	385	13.0	187	2.9	29.1	6.3	0.0
Flake, Chocolate, McDonald's*	1 Mcflurry/206ml	400	14.4	194	3.0	29.0	7.0	0.0
Flake, Raspberry, McDonald's*	1 McFlurry/205ml	370	12.3	180	3.0	27.0	6.0	0.0
Jammie Dodger, McDonald's*	1 McFlurry/128g	256	8.2	200	3.9	33.6	6.4	0.3
Raspberry, McDonald's*	1 McFlurry/206ml	370	12.3	180	3.0	27.0	6.0	0.0
Rolo, McDonald's*	1 McFlurry/205g	390	13.3	190	4.0	29.2	6.5	0.1
Smarties, McDonald's*	1 McFlurry/185g	330	11.1	178	3.0	28.0	6.0	1.0
Strawberry, Cornetto, McDonald's*	1 McFlurry/207g	375	12.4	181	3.0	29.0	6.0	0.0
Terry's Chocolate Orange, McDonald's*	1 McFlurry/203g	405	16.3	199	3.0	28.0	8.0	0.0
Toffee Swirl, Oreo Cookie, McDonald's*	1 McFlurry/206ml	400	12.4	194	3.0	31.0	6.0	1.0
Wispa Gold, McDonald's*	1 McFlurry/206g	395	14.0	192	2.9	29.1	6.8	0.5
Yorkie, McDonald's*	1 McFlurry/204g	379	14.9	186	3.4	27.0	7.3	0.8
MCMUFFIN								
Bacon & Egg, Double, McDonald's*	1 McMuffin/161g	395	21.0	244	15.0	16.0	13.0	1.0
Bacon & Egg, McDonald's*	1 McMuffin/146g	345	17.5	237	14.0	18.0	12.0	1.0
Sausage & Egg, Double, McDonald's*	1 McMuffin/222g	560	35.6	252	16.0	12.0	16.0	1.0
Sausage & Egg, McDonald's*	1 McMuffin/174g	420	24.3	242	14.0	16.0	14.0	1.0
Scrambled Egg, McDonald's*	1 McMuffin/147g	294	14.1	200	10.9	17.5	9.6	1.3
MELT								
Toasted Ham & Cheese, McDonald's*	1 Serving/100g	239	8.0	239	11.2	30.6	8.0	1.8
MILK								
Fresh, Portion, McDonald's*	1 Portion/14ml	10	0.0	69	0.0	7.0	0.0	0.0
Organic, McDonald's*	1 Bottle/250ml	118	5.0	47	4.0	5.0	2.0	0.0

MCDONALD'S

INFO/WEIGHT	Measure	per Measure KCAL	FAT	Nutrition Values per 100g / 100ml KCAL	PROT	CARB	FAT	FIBRE
MILKSHAKE								
Banana, Large, McDonald's*	1 Serving/432ml	545	13.0	126	3.0	21.0	3.0	0.0
Banana, Medium, McDonald's*	1 Serving/338ml	425	10.1	126	3.0	21.0	3.0	0.0
Banana, Small, McDonald's*	1 Serving/178ml	226	5.3	127	3.0	21.0	3.0	0.0
Cadburys Dairy Milk, Caramel, Large, McDonald's*	1 Serving/417ml	505	16.7	121	3.0	19.0	4.0	1.0
Cadburys Dairy Milk, Caramel, Medium, McDonald's*	1 Serving/394ml	480	15.8	122	3.0	19.0	4.0	1.0
Chocolate, Large, McDonald's*	1 Serving/431ml	530	12.9	123	3.0	20.0	3.0	0.0
Chocolate, Medium, McDonald's*	1 Serving/337ml	425	10.1	126	3.0	21.0	3.0	0.0
Chocolate, Small, McDonald's*	1 Serving/177ml	225	5.3	127	3.0	21.0	3.0	0.0
Starburst Mixed Berry Flavour, McDonald's*	1 Small/177ml	200	4.0	113	2.8	20.3	2.3	0.0
Strawberry, Large, McDonald's*	1 Serving/432ml	540	13.0	125	3.0	21.0	3.0	0.0
Strawberry, Medium, McDonald's*	1 Serving/336ml	420	10.1	125	3.0	21.0	3.0	0.0
Strawberry, Small, McDonald's*	1 Serving/177ml	220	5.3	124	3.0	21.0	3.0	0.0
Vanilla, Large, McDonald's*	1 Serving/431ml	535	12.9	124	3.0	21.0	3.0	0.0
Vanilla, Medium, McDonald's*	1 Serving/336ml	420	10.1	125	3.0	21.0	3.0	0.0
Vanilla, Small, McDonald's*	1 Serving/177ml	220	5.3	124	3.0	21.0	3.0	0.0
MOZZARELLA								
Dippers, McDonald's*	3 Dippers/85g	265	13.6	312	13.0	27.0	16.0	1.0
MUFFIN								
Blueberry, Low Fat, McDonald's*	1 Muffin/126g	300	3.8	238	5.0	50.0	3.0	2.0
Double Chocolate, McDonald's*	1 Muffin/123g	515	28.3	419	6.0	46.0	23.0	2.0
ONION RINGS								
McDonald's*	1 Serving/99g	245	11.9	247	4.0	31.0	12.0	3.0
PANCAKE								
& Sausage, with Syrup, McDonald's*	1 Portion/223g	615	20.1	275	8.0	42.0	9.0	2.0
& Syrup, McDonald's*	1 Pack/175g	515	14.0	294	4.0	52.0	8.0	2.0
PIE								
Apple, McDonald's*	1 Pie/80g	231	12.8	289	2.0	35.0	16.0	0.0
POTATO WEDGES								
McDonald's*	1 Portion/177g	349	17.7	197	3.3	23.3	10.0	2.8
QUORN*								
Burger, Premiere, McDonald's*	1 Burger/210g	311	6.1	148	9.1	24.2	2.9	2.7
ROLL								
Bacon, McBacon, McDonald's*	1 Roll/122g	349	14.0	286	13.5	30.5	11.5	1.7
Bacon, with Brown Sauce, McDonald's*	1 Roll/126g	350	8.8	278	15.0	37.0	7.0	2.0
Bacon, with Tomato Ketchup, McDonald's*	1 Roll/126g	345	8.8	273	15.0	36.0	7.0	2.0
SALAD								
Chicken, No Bacon, Grilled, McDonald's*	1 Salad/255g	115	2.6	45	7.0	2.0	1.0	1.0
Chicken, with Bacon, Grilled, McDonald's*	1 Salad/266g	164	5.3	62	9.0	2.0	2.0	1.0
Crispy Chicken, No Bacon, McDonald's*	1 Salad/281g	270	11.2	96	8.0	6.0	4.0	1.0
Crispy Chicken, with Bacon, McDonald's*	1 Serving/292g	326	14.6	111	10.0	7.0	5.0	1.0
Garden, Side, No Dressing, McDonald's*	1 Salad/91g	10	0.0	11	1.0	2.0	0.0	1.0
Garden, Side, with Balsamic Dressing, McDonald's*	1 Salad/128g	91	3.8	71	1.0	11.0	3.0	1.0
SANDWICH								
Deli, Chicken, Salad, McDonald's*	1 Sandwich/216g	350	8.6	162	7.0	24.0	4.0	2.0
Deli, Chicken, Sweet Chilli, McDonald's*	1 Sandwich/250g	570	22.5	228	12.0	28.0	9.0	2.0
Deli, Chicken & Bacon, McDonald's*	1 Sandwich/192g	405	13.4	211	10.0	27.0	7.0	2.0
Deli, Spicy Veggie, McDonald's*	1 Sandwich/216g	555	21.6	257	6.0	36.0	10.0	4.0
SAUCE								
Barbeque, McDonald's*	1 Portion/50g	85	1.0	170	0.0	38.0	2.0	0.0
Curry, Sweet, McDonald's*	1 Portion/29g	50	0.9	171	0.0	38.0	3.0	3.0
Mustard, Mild, McDonald's*	1 Portion/30g	64	3.6	212	1.0	24.8	12.1	0.0
Sweet & Sour, McDonald's*	1 Portion/29g	50	0.0	172	0.0	38.0	0.0	0.0

	Measure INFO/WEIGHT	per Measure KCAL	FAT	Nutrition Values per 100g / 100ml KCAL	PROT	CARB	FAT	FIBRE
MCDONALD'S								
SUNDAE								
Hot Caramel, McDonald's*	1 Sundae/189g	357	8.3	189	3.8	33.9	4.4	0.0
Hot Fudge, McDonald's*	1 Sundae/187g	352	10.7	188	4.5	30.0	5.7	0.0
No Topping, McDonald's*	1 Sundae/149g	219	7.6	147	4.2	21.6	5.1	0.0
Strawberry, McDonald's*	1 Sundae/214g	360	8.6	168	2.0	33.0	4.0	0.0
Toffee, McDonald's*	1 Sundae/182g	350	9.1	192	3.0	34.0	5.0	1.0
SYRUP								
Pancake, McDonald's*	1 Pot/55g	190	0.0	345	0.0	84.0	0.0	0.0
TEA								
with Milk, McDonald's*	1 Serving/333ml	10	3.3	3	0.0	1.0	1.0	0.0
WRAP								
Breakfast, with Brown Sauce, McDonald's*	1 Wrap/229g	595	30.0	260	10.9	2358.0	13.1	1.7
Breakfast, with Tomato Ketchup, McDonald's*	1 Wrap/229g	595	30.0	260	10.9	23.6	13.1	1.7
Chicken, BBQ, Snack, McDonald's*	1 Wrap/115g	300	12.0	261	10.4	30.4	10.4	1.7
Chicken, Cajun, McDonald's*	1 Wrap/22g	585	33.4	263	9.0	22.0	15.0	2.0
Chicken, Cheese & Bacon Snack, McDonald's*	1 Wrap/100g	360	18.0	360	14.0	33.0	18.0	2.0
Chicken, Fajita, McDonald's*	1 Wrap/259g	647	31.1	250	8.9	26.7	12.0	1.2
Chicken, Grilled, Salad, McDonald's*	1 Wrap/221g	335	11.0	152	7.2	19.9	5.0	1.8
Chicken, Snack, McDonald's*	1 Wrap/112g	266	11.2	237	10.0	29.0	10.0	2.0
Garlic & Herb, Snack, McDonald's*	1 Serving/121g	335	18.2	276	12.0	25.0	15.0	2.0
Oriental, Snack, McDonald's*	1 Wrap/127g	265	10.1	209	10.0	25.0	8.0	2.0
Vegetable, Spicy, McDonald's*	1 Wrap/203g	445	16.3	219	5.0	29.0	8.0	5.0
NANDO'S								
BREAD								
Garlic, Nando's*	1 Regular/90g	321	15.7	357	7.1	43.4	17.5	2.0
BURGERS								
Bean, Nando's*	1 Burger/235g	470	13.9	200	8.7	27.4	5.9	2.2
Chicken Breast Fillet, Nando's*	1 Burger/195g	333	5.3	171	15.9	21.0	2.7	1.9
Double Chicken Breast, Nando's*	1 Burger/275g	446	6.9	162	20.2	15.0	2.5	0.8
Veggie, Nando's*	1 Burger/235g	433	9.9	184	8.4	28.4	4.2	2.8
CHICKEN								
¼ Breast, Peri Peri, Nando's*	¼ Breast/90g	135	2.4	150	28.1	3.4	2.7	0.0
¼ Leg, Peri Peri, Nando's*	1 Portion/95g	218	13.2	229	25.9	0.1	13.9	0.0
½ Peri Peri, Nando's*	½ Chicken/185g	353	15.6	191	27.0	1.7	8.4	0.0
Breast, Fillet Strips, Nando's*	1 Serving/108g	153	2.2	141	30.6	0.2	2.0	0.0
Butterfly, Peri Peri, Flame Grilled, Nando's*	1 Portion/190g	310	8.9	163	30.1	0.1	4.7	0.5
Whole, Nando's*	1 Chicken/370g	705	31.3	191	27.0	1.7	8.5	0.0
Wings, 10, Nando's*	10 Wings/236g	630	37.6	267	30.8	0.1	15.9	0.5
Wings, 3, Nando's*	3 Wings/71g	190	11.3	268	30.8	0.1	15.9	0.6
Wings, 5, Nando's*	5 Wings/123g	296	17.3	241	28.4	0.1	14.1	0.0
CHIPS								
Large, Nando's*	1 Serving/480g	1241	49.7	259	2.8	36.8	10.4	3.8
Per Peri, Regular, Nando's*	1 Portion/161g	359	14.6	223	2.9	33.5	9.1	2.6
Peri Peri, Large, Nando's*	1 Serving/482g	1074	43.7	223	2.9	33.6	9.1	2.5
Regular, Nando's*	1 Serving/160g	414	16.6	259	2.8	36.8	10.4	3.8
COLESLAW								
Large, Nando's*	1 Serving/300g	498	45.9	166	0.8	6.3	15.3	1.1
Regular, Nando's*	1 Serving/150g	249	23.0	166	0.8	6.3	15.3	1.1
CORN								
On The Cob, Large, Nando's*	1 Serving/138g	138	3.7	100	5.7	22.0	2.7	4.6
CRISPS								
Hot Peri Peri, Nando's*	1 Bag/40g	206	10.8	514	5.1	57.4	27.0	3.4
Smoky Barbeque Peri Peri, Nando's*	½ Pack/75g	375	20.2	500	5.1	57.4	27.0	3.4

NANDO'S

INFO/WEIGHT	Measure	per Measure		Nutrition Values per 100g / 100ml				
		KCAL	FAT	KCAL	PROT	CARB	FAT	FIBRE
DESSERT								
Carrot Cake, Nando's*	1 Serving/215g	839	62.0	390	3.7	26.7	28.8	0.9
Choc-a-Lot Cake, Nando's*	1 Serving/182g	650	44.0	357	4.5	33.0	24.2	1.7
Chocolate Cheesecake, Nando's*	1 Serving/159g	612	47.5	385	5.3	24.7	29.8	0.8
Gooey Caramel Cheesecake, Nando's*	1 Serving/158g	582	41.9	368	5.3	28.9	26.5	0.8
Nata, Custard Tart, Nando's*	1 Serving/60g	168	6.5	280	5.5	40.3	10.8	2.0
FROZEN YOGHURT								
Banana, Nando's*	1 Serving/100g	87	0.1	87	3.3	18.2	0.1	0.1
Chocolate, Nando's*	1 Serving/100g	78	0.2	78	2.5	16.3	0.2	0.6
Strawberry, Nando's*	1 Serving/100g	71	0.2	71	2.5	15.2	0.2	0.1
Vanilla, Nando's*	1 Serving/100ml	70	0.1	70	2.5	15.0	0.1	0.1
HOUMOUS								
with Peri Peri Drizzle & Pitta, Nando's*	1 Serving/295g	776	29.2	263	7.4	35.1	9.9	3.3
ICE CREAM								
Chocolate, Nando's*	1 Serving/90g	191	10.0	212	2.2	24.0	11.1	1.0
Passion Fruit, Nando's*	1 Serving/90g	122	0.0	136	0.3	32.9	0.0	2.5
Strawberry, Nando's*	1 Serving/90g	164	6.3	182	2.4	24.8	7.0	0.5
Toffee, Nando's*	1 Serving/90g	178	7.3	198	3.9	20.8	8.1	1.0
Vanilla, Nando's*	1 Serving/90g	199	10.4	221	3.8	20.7	11.6	0.0
ICED LOLLY								
Chilly Billy, Nando's*	1 Lolly/70g	30	0.1	43	0.1	10.1	0.1	0.0
MASH								
Creamy, Large, Nando's*	1 Large/400g	540	31.6	135	1.7	13.0	7.9	2.5
Creamy, Regular, Nando's*	1 Regular/200g	270	15.8	135	1.7	13.0	7.9	2.5
Sweet Potato, Fino Side, Nando's*	1 Serving/200g	248	4.2	124	2.2	22.7	2.1	2.7
NUTS								
Peri-Peri, Nando's*	1 Serving/100g	627	53.6	627	23.6	7.9	53.6	9.2
OLIVES								
Spicy, Mixed, Nando's*	1 Bowl/125g	133	13.0	106	0.9	0.6	10.4	3.0
PEAS								
Macho, Large, Nando's*	1 Serving/280g	336	20.7	120	4.7	7.0	7.4	4.2
Macho, Regular, Nando's*	1 Serving/140g	168	10.4	120	4.7	7.0	7.4	4.2
PITTA								
Bean, Nando's*	1 Pitta/235g	484	13.1	206	8.5	29.4	5.6	2.2
Chicken Breast, Nando's*	1 Pitta/195g	347	4.5	178	15.7	23.3	2.3	1.0
Double Chicken with Mayonnaise, Nando's*	1 Serving/275g	460	6.1	167	20.0	16.6	2.2	0.7
Veggie, Nando's*	1 Pitta/235g	447	9.1	190	8.2	30.3	3.9	2.8
RATATOUILLE								
Fino Side, Nando's*	1 Serving/180g	108	6.5	60	1.3	3.8	3.6	3.4
RICE								
Spicy, Large, Nando's*	1 Serving/300g	546	10.8	182	3.0	32.8	3.6	3.4
Spicy, Regular, Nando's*	1 Serving/150g	273	5.4	182	3.0	32.8	3.6	3.4
ROLL								
Portuguese with Chicken Livers, Nando's*	1 Serving/220g	485	14.8	220	17.5	23.2	6.8	2.0
Prego Steak, Nando's*	1 Roll/220g	573	24.1	260	19.4	22.2	11.0	2.6
SALAD								
Avocado & Green Bean, Nando's*	1 Serving/245g	305	25.8	124	2.4	3.4	10.5	3.3
Ceaser, No Chicken, Nando's*	1 Salad/226g	287	22.0	127	3.4	6.5	9.8	1.1
Mediterranean, Nando's*	1 Salad/290g	294	18.5	101	3.3	3.9	6.4	1.6
Mixed Leaf, Nando's*	1 Portion/115g	22	0.4	19	1.4	2.0	0.3	1.3
Side, Regular, Nando's*	1 Salad/53g	10	0.2	19	1.8	1.5	0.3	1.1
VEGETABLES								
Roasted, Saucy, Nando's*	1 Serving/103g	62	3.7	60	1.3	3.8	3.6	3.4

	Measure INFO/WEIGHT	per Measure KCAL	FAT	Nutrition Values per 100g / 100ml KCAL	PROT	CARB	FAT	FIBRE
NANDO'S								
WRAP								
Beanie, Nando's*	1 Wrap/320g	716	30.1	224	7.2	26.2	9.4	2.1
Chicken, Breast, Fillet, Double, Nando's*	1 Wrap/360g	670	23.0	186	16.2	16.8	6.4	1.0
Chicken, Breast, Fillet, Nando's*	1 Wrap/280g	577	21.5	206	12.1	21.5	7.7	1.2
Portabello Mushroom & Halloumi Cheese, Nando's*	1 Wrap/339g	780	47.3	230	6.8	18.5	14.0	1.3
Veggie, Nando's*	1 Wrap/320g	677	26.1	212	7.0	26.9	8.2	2.5
PIZZA EXPRESS								
ANTIPASTO								
Italian, Classic, Sharing Starter, Pizza Express*	½ Serving/252g	562	29.7	223	11.1	19.1	11.8	2.1
BREAD								
Garlic, Starter, Pizza Express*	1 Serving/105g	239	4.9	228	7.8	39.8	4.7	2.5
Garlic, With Mozzarella, Starter, Pizza Express*	1 Serving/131g	304	9.3	232	11.2	32.1	7.1	2.0
BROWNIES								
Gluten Free, Dolcetti, Pizza Express*	1 Serving/55g	216	11.9	392	4.6	43.6	21.6	0.1
Piccolo, Pizza Express*	1 Serving/55g	216	11.9	392	4.6	43.6	21.6	0.1
BRUSCHETTA								
Con Funghi, Starter, Pizza Express*	1 Serving/272g	367	13.3	135	4.0	19.2	4.9	1.3
Starter, Pizza Express*	1 Serving/218g	392	19.6	180	4.5	21.2	9.0	1.6
CAKE								
Chocolate Fudge, & Ice Cream, Pizza Express*	1 Serving/161g	423	18.5	263	4.7	34.9	11.5	1.2
Chocolate Fudge, Mini, Dolcetti, Pizza Express*	1 Serving/85g	251	11.2	295	4.5	39.1	13.2	1.6
CALZONE								
Salami E Salsiccia, Main, Pizza Express*	1 Calzone/518g	984	50.8	190	8.7	17.5	9.8	1.4
Verdure, Main, Pizza Express*	1 Calzone/564g	1280	80.7	227	6.4	19.0	14.3	1.4
CAVATAPPI								
Formaggi, Main, Pizza Express*	1 Serving/544g	1093	56.0	201	9.0	17.9	10.3	0.9
CHEESECAKE								
& Ice Cream, Pizza Express*	1 Serving/164g	464	28.9	283	4.8	26.6	17.6	0.5
CHIPS								
Polenta, Side, Pizza Express*	1 Serving/183g	441	23.4	241	3.7	27.4	12.8	1.2
DESEERT								
Chocolate Glory, Pizza Express*	1 Serving/309g	686	23.5	222	4.2	34.1	7.6	1.1
DESSERT								
Caffe Reale, Dolcetti, Pizza Express*	1 Serving/65g	190	11.7	293	3.1	29.9	18.0	1.9
Semi Freddo Reale, Dolcetti, Pizza Express*	1 Serving/40g	134	8.8	336	2.6	29.0	22.1	0.3
Toffee Fudge Glory, Pizza Express*	1 Serving/295g	631	20.1	214	3.7	34.6	6.8	0.4
DOUGH BALLS								
& Garlic Butter, With Side Salad, Piccolo, Pizza Express*	1 Serving/158g	186	8.2	118	3.1	15.1	5.2	1.4
Doppio, Sharing Starter, Pizza Express*	½ Serving/130g	376	19.0	289	7.5	32.8	14.6	2.1
Starter, Pizza Express*	1 Serving/120g	347	16.8	289	7.0	35.0	14.0	2.2
GELATO								
Chocolate, Coppa, Pizza Express*	1 Serving/125g	252	10.5	202	4.5	27.6	8.4	1.8
Strawberry, Coppa, Pizza Express*	1 Serving/125g	215	3.4	172	0.7	35.8	2.7	0.3
Vanilla, Choc Sauce & Cone, Piccolo, Pizza Express*	1 Serving/72g	153	4.8	213	4.2	34.3	6.6	0.9
Vanilla, Coppa, Pizza Express*	1 Serving/125g	245	9.1	196	4.7	28.1	7.3	0.5
Vanilla, Fruit Coulis, & Cone, Piccolo, Pizza Express*	1 Serving/72g	132	4.7	183	4.0	27.4	6.5	0.7
Vanilla, Piccolo, Pizza Express*	1 Serving/60g	113	4.5	188	4.5	25.7	7.5	0.5
Vanilla, Toffee Sauce & Cone, Piccolo, Pizza Express*	1 Serving/72g	150	4.6	208	3.9	35.7	6.4	0.5
Vanilla, with Chocolate Sauce, Piccolo, Pizza Express*	1 Serving/70g	146	4.6	209	4.1	33.3	6.6	0.9
Vanilla, with Cone, Piccolo, Pizza Express*	1 Serving/62g	120	4.6	194	4.6	27.0	7.5	0.6
Vanilla, with Fresh Strawberry, Piccolo, Pizza Express*	1 Serving/62g	120	4.6	194	4.6	27.0	7.5	0.6
Vanilla, with Fruit Coulis, Piccolo, Pizza Express*	1 Serving/70g	125	4.6	178	3.9	26.3	6.5	0.7
Vanilla, with Fudge Cubes, Piccolo, Pizza Express*	1 Serving/70g	153	5.8	219	4.1	32.0	8.3	0.4

	Measure INFO/WEIGHT	per Measure KCAL	per Measure FAT	Nutrition Values per 100g / 100ml KCAL	PROT	CARB	FAT	FIBRE

PIZZA EXPRESS

GELATO

	Measure INFO/WEIGHT	KCAL	FAT	KCAL	PROT	CARB	FAT	FIBRE
Vanilla, with Toffee Sauce, Piccolo, Pizza Express*	1 Serving/70g	143	4.5	204	3.9	32.7	6.4	0.4

LASAGNE

Classica, Main, Pizza Express*	1 Serving/427g	623	32.9	146	9.0	10.4	7.7	0.1
Verde, Main, Pizza Express*	1 Serving/468g	744	52.4	159	4.4	9.7	11.2	0.2

PARMIGIANA

Melanzane, Main, Pizza Express*	1 Serving/428g	728	56.1	170	4.9	7.9	13.1	0.8

PASTA

Bianca, Piccolo, Main, Pizza Express*	1 Serving/219g	385	15.8	176	4.4	23.0	7.2	1.2
Bolognese, Piccolo, Main, Pizza Express*	1 Serving/256g	333	7.4	130	5.8	20.0	2.9	1.0
Burro, Piccolo, Main, Pizza Express*	1 Serving/115g	310	12.1	270	6.3	37.7	10.5	2.2
Napoletana, Piccolo, Main, Pizza Express*	1 Serving/219g	311	7.2	142	4.1	24.1	3.3	1.5
Pollo, Main, Pizza Express*	1 Serving/573g	923	47.0	161	7.9	14.0	8.2	0.8

PIE

Banoffee, & Ice Cream, Pizza Express*	1 Serving/142g	524	38.9	369	2.1	28.4	27.4	2.6

PIZZA

American, Classic, GF, Pizza Express*	1 Pizza/381g	1020	45.5	268	6.6	33.4	12.0	0.8
American, Classic, Main, Pizza Express*	1 Pizza/376g	805	33.5	214	10.3	24.2	8.9	1.6
American, Hot, Classic, GF, Pizza Express*	1 Pizza/401g	1023	45.6	255	6.3	31.7	11.4	0.8
American, Hot, Leggera, Main, Pizza Express*	1 Pizza/269g	395	15.6	147	8.1	16.5	5.8	1.3
American, Light Mozzarella, Piccolo, GF, Pizza Express*	1 Pizza/180g	408	14.8	227	7.0	31.2	8.2	0.8
American, Light Mozzarella, Piccolo, Pizza Express*	1 Pizza/190g	338	9.7	178	10.4	24.0	5.1	1.6
American, Piccolo, GF, Pizza Express*	1 Pizza/171g	424	23.0	248	6.3	32.8	13.5	0.8
American, Piccolo, Pizza Express*	1 Pizza/181g	355	11.9	196	9.9	25.3	6.6	1.7
American Hot, Classic, Main, Pizza Express*	1 Pizza/396g	808	33.3	204	9.8	23.2	8.4	1.6
American Hot, Romana, Main, Pizza Express*	1 Pizza/417g	863	37.5	207	10.4	22.1	9.0	1.5
Caprina Rossa, Romana, Main, Pizza Express*	1 Pizza/524g	901	39.3	172	7.7	19.4	7.5	1.5
Da Morire, Romana, Main, Pizza Express*	1 Pizza/537g	940	44.0	175	7.7	17.9	8.2	2.1
Diavolo, Romana, Main, Pizza Express*	1 Pizza/477g	978	42.9	205	11.0	20.2	9.0	1.6
Etna, Romana, Main, Pizza Express*	1 Pizza/502g	1039	46.7	207	11.3	20.1	9.3	1.4
Fiorentina, Classic, GF, Pizza Express*	1 Pizza/493g	1045	45.1	212	6.2	26.2	9.1	0.7
Fiorentina, Classic, Main, Pizza Express*	1 Pizza/488g	830	32.7	170	9.0	19.1	6.7	1.4
Four Seasons, Classic, GF, Pizza Express*	1 Pizza/380g	894	35.0	235	4.3	33.4	9.2	1.0
Four Seasons, Classic, Main, Pizza Express*	1 Pizza/375g	679	22.9	181	8.0	24.4	6.1	1.9
Giardiniera, Classic, GF, Pizza Express*	1 Pizza/525g	1115	55.8	212	4.1	25.0	10.6	1.3
Giardiniera, Classic, Main, Pizza Express*	1 Pizza/520g	900	43.7	173	6.7	18.4	8.4	1.9
Il Padrino, Romana, Main, Pizza Express*	1 Pizza/532g	1123	59.1	211	9.7	18.6	11.1	1.4
La Reine, Classic, GF, Pizza Express*	1 Pizza/418g	954	38.2	228	6.0	30.4	9.1	0.9
La Reine, Classic, Main, Pizza Express*	1 Pizza/413g	739	26.0	179	9.4	22.1	6.3	1.7
La Reine, Light Mozzarella, Piccolo, GF, Pizza Express*	1 Pizza/203g	396	12.9	195	6.7	27.8	6.4	0.8
La Reine, Light Mozzarella, Piccolo, Pizza Express*	1 Pizza/213g	326	7.7	153	9.7	21.6	3.6	1.6
La Reine, Piccolo, GF, Pizza Express*	1 Pizza/193g	411	15.2	213	6.1	29.2	7.9	0.9
La Reine, Piccolo, Pizza Express*	1 Pizza/203g	341	9.9	168	9.3	22.6	4.9	1.7
Margherita, Classic, GF, Pizza Express*	1 Pizza/359g	899	45.5	250	5.5	35.1	12.7	0.8
Margherita, Classic, Main, Pizza Express*	1 Pizza/354g	683	22.7	193	9.4	25.7	6.4	1.7
Margherita, Lite Mozzarella, Piccolo, GF, Pizza Express*	1 Pizza/170g	359	10.6	211	6.1	32.9	6.2	0.8
Margherita, Lite Mozzarella, Piccolo, Pizza Express*	1 Pizza/180g	290	5.4	161	9.6	25.3	3.0	1.6
Margherita, Piccolo, GF, Pizza Express*	1 Pizza/165g	388	14.0	235	5.9	33.8	8.5	0.8
Margherita, Piccolo, Pizza Express*	1 Pizza/175g	318	8.8	182	9.5	25.9	5.0	1.7
Margherita, Romana, Piccolo, GF, Pizza Express*	1 Pizza/220g	495	21.4	225	8.2	26.3	9.7	0.6
Margherita, Romana, Piccolo, Pizza Express*	1 Pizza/230g	426	16.1	185	10.9	20.6	7.0	1.4
Mushroom, Light Mozzarella, Piccolo, Pizza Express*	1 Pizza/201g	293	5.6	146	8.9	22.8	2.8	1.6
Mushroom, Lite Mozzarella, Piccolo, GF, Pizza Express*	1 Pizza/191g	363	10.7	190	5.6	29.4	5.6	0.8

	Measure INFO/WEIGHT	per Measure KCAL	FAT	Nutrition Values per 100g / 100ml KCAL	PROT	CARB	FAT	FIBRE
PIZZA EXPRESS								
PIZZA								
Mushroom, Piccolo, GF, Pizza Express*	1 Pizza/180g	377	13.0	210	4.9	31.0	7.2	0.8
Mushroom, Piccolo, Pizza Express*	1 Pizza/190g	308	7.8	162	8.4	23.2	4.1	1.7
Padana, Leggera, Main, Pizza Express*	1 Pizza/322g	415	10.0	129	4.1	21.6	3.1	1.4
Padana Romana, Main, Pizza Express*	1 Pizza/459g	831	27.1	181	7.4	25.4	5.9	1.5
Pollo, Light Mozzarella, Piccolo, GF, Pizza Express*	1 Pizza/190g	382	10.8	201	8.1	29.4	5.7	0.7
Pollo, Light Mozzarella, Piccolo, Pizza Express*	1 Pizza/200g	312	5.6	156	11.2	22.8	2.8	1.5
Pollo, Piccolo, GF, Pizza Express*	1 Pizza/180g	396	13.1	220	7.5	31.0	7.3	0.7
Pollo, Piccolo, Pizza Express*	1 Pizza/190g	327	7.8	172	10.8	23.9	4.1	1.6
Pollo Ad Astra, Leggera, Main, Pizza Express*	1 Pizza/367g	418	8.8	114	9.6	14.1	2.4	1.1
Pollo Ad Astra, Romana, Main, Pizza Express*	1 Pizza/491g	800	22.1	163	11.2	20.1	4.5	1.4
Polpette Bolognese, Romana, Main, Pizza Express*	1 Pizza/580g	1160	58.6	200	10.1	17.6	10.1	1.0
Pomodoro, Pesto, Leggera, Main, Pizza Express*	1 Pizza/316g	401	17.4	127	5.7	14.7	5.5	1.3
Pomodoro, Pesto, Romana, Main, Pizza Express*	1 Pizza/543g	1151	60.3	212	11.5	17.1	11.1	1.1
Quattro Formaggi, Romana, Main, Pizza Express*	1 Pizza/424g	886	39.0	209	10.9	21.6	9.2	1.4
Rustichella, Romana, Main, Pizza Express*	1 Pizza/511g	1022	46.5	200	9.8	20.5	9.1	1.8
Sloppy Giuseppe, Classic, Main, Pizza Express*	1 Pizza/469g	952	39.4	203	11.3	20.9	8.4	1.1
Sloppy Guiseppe, Classic, GF, Pizza Express*	1 Pizza/474g	1167	51.3	246	8.3	28.1	10.8	1.1
Toscana Romana, Main, Pizza Express*	1 Pizza/524g	1169	62.4	223	11.9	17.8	11.9	1.2
Veneziana, Romana, Main, Pizza Express*	1 Pizza/423g	795	30.0	188	9.1	23.0	7.1	1.7
RISOTTO								
Pollo Funghi, Starter, Pizza Express*	1 Serving/237g	367	21.8	155	6.4	11.3	9.2	0.4
SALAD								
Bosco, Main, Pizza Express*	1 Serving/362g	652	38.7	180	6.5	14.7	10.7	2.1
Caesar, Side, Pizza Express*	1 Serving/129g	313	25.4	243	8.1	8.1	19.7	0.9
Chicken Caesar, Grande, Main, Pizza Express*	1 Serving/350g	630	25.9	180	12.1	16.5	7.4	1.4
Leggara, Chicken, Superfood, Main, Pizza Express*	1 Serving/407g	338	19.9	83	6.1	3.8	4.9	1.2
Mixed Leaf, Side, Pizza Express*	1 Serving/411g	185	14.4	45	0.8	2.9	3.5	0.8
Mozzarella & Tomato, Starter, Pizza Express*	1 Serving/240g	458	38.9	191	9.5	2.0	16.2	0.4
Pollo Pancetta, Main, Pizza Express*	1 Serving/467g	425	8.4	91	6.2	12.2	1.8	1.0
Vegetable, & Goats Cheese, Warm, Pizza Express*	1 Serving/406g	690	43.4	170	4.3	14.1	10.7	1.8
SORBET								
Raspberry, Dolcetti, Pizza Express*	1 Serving/65g	86	1.9	132	1.0	25.4	2.9	1.6
Raspberry, Piccolo, Pizza Express*	1 Serving/60g	61	0.2	101	0.6	23.7	0.4	1.1
Raspberry, Pizza Express*	1 Serving/130g	172	3.8	132	1.0	25.4	2.9	1.6
TALEGGIO								
Oven Baked, Sharing Starter, Pizza Express*	½ Serving/164g	377	16.6	230	11.3	24.0	10.1	1.6
TIRAMISU								
Dessert, Pizza Express*	1 Serving/199g	553	32.0	278	3.5	26.6	16.1	0.2
TORTA								
Double Chocolate Espresso, Dolcetti, Pizza Express*	1 Serving/81g	363	26.8	448	3.9	33.1	33.1	3.3
Lemon, & Mascarpone, Pizza Express*	1 Serving/167g	529	32.7	317	5.1	32.1	19.6	0.3
Lemon Meringue, Dolcetti, Pizza Express*	1 Serving/51g	185	10.0	362	5.9	40.6	19.6	0.9
PIZZA HUT								
BACON BITS								
Pizza Hut*	1 Serving/12g	60	3.6	496	8.3	48.7	29.8	0.0
BEANS								
Chocolate Coated, Ice Cream Factory, Pizza Hut*	1 Serving/30g	142	5.4	475	5.5	72.2	18.1	0.0
BEETROOT								
Pizza Hut*	1 Portion/25g	14	0.0	55	0.9	12.0	0.1	0.0
BREAD								
Garlic, Ciabatta, Pizza Hut*	2 Pieces/253g	820	32.1	324	9.1	43.4	12.7	0.0
Garlic, Dipsters, Pizza Hut*	1 Piece/90g	308	14.2	342	6.8	43.1	15.8	0.0

	Measure INFO/WEIGHT	per Measure KCAL	per Measure FAT	Nutrition Values per 100g / 100ml KCAL	PROT	CARB	FAT	FIBRE
PIZZA HUT								
BREAD								
Garlic, Pizza Hut*	1 Slice/30g	95	4.6	318	6.8	38.1	15.4	0.0
Garlic, with Cheese, Pizza Hut*	4 Pieces/187g	568	34.0	304	15.9	19.0	18.2	0.0
BREADSTICKS								
Garlic, Pizza Hut*	1 Stick/50g	174	6.7	347	9.8	46.9	13.4	1.0
BRUSCHETTA								
Light Lunch, Pizza Hut*	3 Pieces/211g	369	16.0	175	4.1	22.4	7.6	0.0
CAKE								
Chocolate Fudge, Dessert, Pizza Hut*	1 Piece/178g	684	31.9	384	4.2	51.4	17.9	0.0
CARBONARA								
Ham, Buffet, Pizza Hut*	1 Portion/200g	180	4.6	90	3.4	14.4	2.3	0.0
CHEESE								
4 & Vegetable, Buffet, Pizza Hut*	1 Portion/200g	210	8.6	105	4.0	12.6	4.3	0.0
Hard, Grated, Pizza Hut*	1 Serving/30g	121	9.0	404	33.0	0.1	30.0	0.0
Parmesan Reggiano, Grated at Table, Pizza Hut*	1 Serving/5g	20	1.4	400	34.0	0.0	28.0	0.0
Three Cheese Melt, Starter, Pizza Hut*	3 Pieces/209g	546	38.1	261	11.2	12.3	18.2	0.0
CHEESECAKE								
Chocolate, Pizza Hut*	1 Serving/63g	228	11.1	360	5.6	44.9	17.5	0.0
Clotted Cream, Pizza Hut*	1 Serving/64g	205	10.4	323	4.6	39.3	16.4	0.0
Lemon & Ginger, Pizza Hut*	1 Serving/64g	205	9.7	323	4.2	42.4	15.2	0.0
New York Style, Baked, Pizza Hut*	1 Slice/113g	442	16.2	391	6.6	62.3	14.3	0.0
Vanilla, Madagascan, Dessert, Pizza Hut*	1 Serving/133g	397	18.1	298	4.8	39.2	13.6	0.0
CHICKEN								
Cheesy Jalapeno Poppers, Pizza Hut*	6 Pieces/150g	408	20.0	272	5.2	32.8	13.3	0.0
Dippin, Pizza Hut*	1 Serving/155g	332	14.4	214	15.7	17.1	9.3	0.0
Goujons, Pizza Hut*	5 Pieces/169g	311	13.5	184	17.0	11.0	8.0	1.5
Strips, Breaded, (Five Strips), Pizza Hut*	5 Pieces/175g	283	13.2	162	16.0	8.9	7.5	0.0
Strips, Breaded, with Wedges, 2, Kids, Pizza Hut*	1 Serving/231g	386	11.6	167	6.7	23.9	5.0	0.0
Strips, Breaded, with Wedges, 3, Kids, Pizza Hut*	1 Serving/265g	451	14.3	170	8.1	22.2	5.4	0.0
Strips, Breaded, Wrap Factory, 2, Kids, Pizza Hut*	1 Serving/246g	434	12.1	176	8.3	24.8	4.9	0.0
Strips, Breaded, Wrap Factory, 3, Kids, Pizza Hut*	1 Serving/324g	617	17.9	190	9.2	25.9	5.5	0.0
Strips, Hot n Kicking, Pizza Hut*	7 Pieces/140g	276	12.6	197	17.0	12.0	9.0	0.0
Wings, BBQ, (Delivery Only), Pizza Hut*	6 Pieces/156g	303	14.4	194	23.2	4.6	9.2	0.0
Wings, BBQ, Pizza Hut*	6 Pieces/171g	306	14.5	179	21.4	4.4	8.5	0.0
Wings, BBQ, Saucy, Pizza Hut*	6 Wings/159g	355	21.8	223	21.4	3.6	13.7	0.0
Wings, Buffalo, Saucy, Pizza Hut*	6 Wings/181g	380	22.2	209	21.0	3.7	12.2	0.0
Wings, Spicy, Crunch, (Delivery Only), Pizza Hut*	1 Portion/218g	510	30.5	234	17.0	10.0	14.0	0.0
Wings, Texan BBQ Chicken, Pizza Hut*	6 Pieces/159g	355	21.8	223	21.4	3.6	13.7	0.0
Wings, with Sour Cream & Chive Dip, Pizza Hut*	1 Pack/178g	680	56.1	382	22.8	1.9	31.5	1.3
COLESLAW								
Pizza Hut*	1 Pot/38g	54	4.6	143	0.9	7.1	12.3	0.0
Pots, (Delivery Only), Pizza Hut*	1oz/28g	38	3.1	134	0.8	7.4	11.2	0.0
COUS COUS								
Pizza Hut*	1 Serving/100g	219	9.0	219	5.0	30.0	9.0	0.0
CREAM								
Single, Dessert, Pizza Hut*	1 Serving/40g	75	7.2	188	2.6	3.9	18.0	0.0
UHT, Portion, Pizza Hut*	1 Portion/12g	23	2.2	188	2.7	3.9	18.0	0.0
CROUTONS								
Pizza Flavoured, Pizza Hut*	1 Serving/12g	23	3.1	196	10.1	55.2	26.1	0.0
Salad, Large, Pizza Hut*	1 Portion/20g	94	4.2	470	11.0	59.1	21.1	0.0
DESSERT								
Cherries in Sauce, Pizza Hut*	1 Serving/19g	28	0.0	142	0.5	34.9	0.1	0.0
Chocolate Obsession, Pizza Hut*	1 Serving/100g	157	6.8	157	2.0	22.1	6.8	0.0

PIZZA HUT

INFO/WEIGHT	Measure	per Measure KCAL	FAT	Nutrition Values per 100g / 100ml KCAL	PROT	CARB	FAT	FIBRE
DESSERT								
Toffee Apple Meltdown, Pizza Hut*	1 Serving/120g	325	11.0	271	3.3	43.7	9.2	0.0
DIP								
BBQ Sauce Portion, in Restaurant, Pizza Hut*	1 Pot/28g	34	0.0	121	1.4	29.3	0.1	0.0
BBQ Tabasco, Pizza Hut*	1 Serving/25g	36	0.1	142	1.2	33.6	0.2	0.0
Garlic & Herb, Pizza Hut*	1 Serving/28g	93	9.2	331	1.4	7.6	32.6	0.0
Mayonnaise, Light, Restaurant Only, Pizza Hut*	1 Dippot/50g	163	16.5	326	0.6	6.0	33.0	0.0
Sour Cream & Chive, Restaurant Only, Pizza Hut*	1 Serving/28g	83	8.7	296	0.7	3.6	31.1	0.0
Sweet Chilli Sauce, Restaurant Only, Pizza Hut*	1 Pot/28g	48	0.2	171	0.4	32.9	0.7	0.0
Tomato Ketchup, Restaurant Only, Pizza Hut*	1 Pot/28g	39	0.0	139	1.4	34.3	0.0	0.0
DOUGH BALLS								
Cheese & Jalapeno, (Delivery Only), Pizza Hut*	1 Portion/198g	495	16.2	250	9.7	33.8	8.2	0.0
DRESSING								
1000 Island, Pizza Hut*	1 Serving/38g	107	9.7	280	0.7	11.5	25.5	0.0
Blue Cheese, Pizza Hut*	1 Serving/35g	91	8.0	258	1.7	11.5	22.7	0.0
Caesar, Pizza Hut*	1 Serving/40g	27	1.1	68	1.5	8.9	2.8	0.0
Ranch, Pizza Hut*	1 Serving/32g	163	18.0	510	1.2	1.5	56.4	0.0
Vinaigrette, Low Fat, Pizza Hut*	1 Serving/30ml	23	0.2	77	0.3	17.2	0.5	0.0
FISH								
Goujons (5 Strips), Pizza Hut*	5 Strips/210g	416	20.9	198	10.0	17.1	10.0	0.0
FRIES								
Seasoned, Savoury, (Express Only), Pizza Hut*	1 Portion/145g	247	11.1	171	2.3	23.0	7.7	0.0
Seasoned, Savoury, Pizza Hut*	1 Serving/144g	238	11.5	165	2.4	20.8	8.0	0.0
FRUIT SALAD								
Apple & Grape, Fresh, Mix, Pizza Hut*	1 Portion/80g	39	0.8	49	0.4	12.0	1.0	0.0
FUDGE BROWNIE								
Pizza Hut*	1 Serving/105g	418	16.4	398	4.3	60.1	15.6	0.0
ICE CREAM								
Coco Mango, Pizza Hut*	1 Serving/100g	88	1.8	88	0.6	17.3	1.8	0.0
Cookie Craving, Pizza Hut*	1 Serving/100g	149	6.9	149	1.6	20.1	6.9	0.0
Dairy, Dessert, Pizza Hut*	1 Portion/142g	272	12.6	192	4.6	23.3	8.9	0.2
Mix, Pizza Hut*	1 Serving/100g	147	6.2	147	4.0	18.8	6.2	0.0
Traditional, Dessert, Pizza Hut*	1 Serving/130g	251	13.5	193	2.6	22.4	10.4	0.0
Traditional, Kids, Pizza Hut*	1 Serving/89g	171	9.2	193	2.6	22.4	10.4	0.0
Traditional, Pizza Hut*	1 Serving/132g	254	13.7	193	2.6	22.4	10.4	0.0
KETCHUP								
Heinz, Pizza Hut*	1 Serving/12g	14	0.0	119	0.5	28.4	0.1	0.0
LETTUCE								
Cos, Fresh, Pizza Hut*	1 Serving/80g	10	0.2	13	0.7	1.9	0.3	0.0
MACARONI CHEESE								
Pizza Hut*	1 Serving/41g	57	2.4	140	4.9	16.6	6.0	0.0
MARSHMALLOWS								
Mini, Ice Cream Factory, Pizza Hut*	1 Serving/30g	96	0.0	320	5.4	74.3	0.0	0.0
MAYONNAISE								
Sachet, Pizza Hut*	1 Sachet/12g	88	9.8	731	1.3	1.8	81.2	0.0
MEATBALLS								
in Pomodoro Sauce, Light Lunch, Pizza Hut*	1 Portion/253g	342	18.2	135	6.6	11.0	7.2	0.0
MELON								
Pieces, Fresh, Pizza Hut*	1 Serving/80g	27	0.0	34	0.8	8.2	0.0	0.0
MILK								
Half Fat, Portions, Millac Maid, Pizza Hut*	1 Portion/14g	6	0.2	45	6.0	5.1	1.6	0.0
MILKSHAKE								
Strawberry Cheesecake, Pizza Hut*	1 Serving/236g	371	14.1	157	3.4	22.3	6.0	0.0

	Measure INFO/WEIGHT	per Measure KCAL	FAT	Nutrition Values per 100g / 100ml KCAL	PROT	CARB	FAT	FIBRE
PIZZA HUT								
MILKSHAKE								
The Chocoholic, Pizza Hut*	1 Serving/248g	442	20.4	178	3.6	22.8	8.2	0.0
Toffee Banoffee Shake, Pizza Hut*	1 Serving/404g	763	22.6	189	2.4	32.3	5.6	0.0
MUFFIN								
Cheesecake, Sicilian Lemon, Pizza Hut*	1 Portion/130g	508	24.2	391	5.1	50.9	18.6	0.0
Fruity, Pizza Hut*	1 Serving/115g	366	13.7	318	4.1	48.4	11.9	0.0
Mixed Berry, Pizza Hut*	1 Muffin/108g	402	22.6	372	4.4	41.6	20.9	0.0
Sicilian Lemon Cheesecake, Pizza Hut*	1 Serving/130g	508	24.2	391	5.1	50.9	18.6	0.0
Strawberry & White Chocolate, Pizza Hut*	1 Muffin/108g	402	22.6	372	4.4	41.6	20.9	0.0
MUSHROOMS								
Blue Cheese, Pizza Hut*	1 Serving/256g	514	40.7	201	7.2	7.5	15.9	0.0
Breaded, Pizza Hut*	6 Pieces/180g	410	14.4	228	4.5	26.1	8.0	0.0
Garlic, 2, Pizza Hut*	1 Serving/230g	570	43.4	248	7.9	7.0	18.9	0.0
Garlic, Crispy Coated, Pizza Hut*	1 Portion/135g	240	10.1	178	4.1	23.4	7.5	0.0
Garlic, with BBQ Dip, Pizza Hut*	1 Portion/112g	263	11.2	234	6.2	30.5	10.0	3.4
Garlic, with Sour Cream & Chive Dip, Pizza Hut*	1 Portion/112g	426	34.6	380	6.4	20.0	30.8	3.4
NACHOS								
Chilli, Pizza Hut*	1 Serving/190g	550	33.1	289	8.8	27.2	17.4	0.0
Sharing Starters, Pizza Hut*	1 Serving/356g	1087	76.3	305	7.9	24.6	21.4	0.0
Side, Delivery Only, Pizza Hut*	1 Serving/222g	669	40.3	301	7.7	30.2	18.1	0.0
OLIVES								
Mixed, Pizza Hut*	1 Serving/70g	140	9.0	200	1.5	19.6	12.8	0.0
ONION RINGS								
Chilli, (Delivery Only), Pizza Hut*	1 Ring/13g	26	1.2	212	3.2	28.2	9.6	0.0
Chilli, Pizza Hut*	8 Rings/100g	212	9.6	212	3.2	28.2	9.6	0.0
ONIONS								
White, Pizza Hut*	1 Serving/24g	10	0.0	42	1.0	10.0	0.0	0.0
PANCAKE								
Fruity, Kids, Pizza Hut*	1 Serving/156g	227	3.3	146	1.9	30.6	2.1	0.0
PASTA								
3 Cheese & Vegetable, Pizza Hut*	1 Serving/300g	315	12.9	105	4.0	12.6	4.3	0.0
4 Cheese, Sharing, Pizza Hut*	1 Serving/1200g	1860	102.0	155	6.1	13.5	8.5	0.0
Adults, Pizza Hut*	1 Serving/100g	250	10.9	250	5.7	16.8	10.9	0.0
Alfredo, Chicken, Sharing, (Delivery Only), Pizza Hut*	1 Pack/1200g	1680	40.8	140	8.1	19.1	3.4	0.0
Alfredo, Light Lunch, Pizza Hut*	1 Portion/226g	294	5.0	130	4.1	23.3	2.2	0.0
Alfredo, Pizza Hut*	1 Portion/400g	520	8.8	130	4.1	23.3	2.2	0.0
Arrabiata, Pizza Hut*	1 Portion/450g	441	13.0	98	2.9	15.0	2.9	0.0
Bolognese, Sharing, (Delivery Only), Pizza Hut*	1 Pack/1200g	1500	64.8	125	7.2	11.9	5.4	0.0
Bolognese, Sharing, Pizza Hut*	1 Serving/1200g	1500	64.8	125	7.2	11.9	5.4	0.0
Cannelloni, Spinach & Ricotta, Pizza Hut*	1 Portion/404g	566	27.5	140	6.2	13.1	6.8	0.0
Chicken Alfredo, Sharing, Pizza Hut*	1 Serving/1200g	1680	40.8	140	8.1	19.1	3.4	0.0
Gemelli, Pizza Hut*	1 Serving/100g	155	4.4	155	4.3	26.0	4.4	0.0
Ham & Mushroom, Pizza Hut*	1 Serving/450g	473	10.4	105	4.2	17.0	2.3	0.0
Kids, Pizza Hut*	1 Serving/100g	180	9.4	180	6.9	16.5	9.4	0.0
Lasagne, Traditional, Pizza Hut*	1 Portion/460g	589	26.7	128	5.9	13.0	5.8	0.0
Macaroni Cheese, Kids, Pizza Hut*	1 Portion/250g	332	16.2	133	4.0	14.8	6.5	0.0
Mezzaluna, Tomato & Mozzarella, Pizza Hut*	1 Serving/351g	340	10.2	97	3.1	14.7	2.9	0.0
Mezzaluna, Tomato & Mozzarella, Pizza Hut*	1 Portion/350g	340	10.2	97	3.1	14.7	2.9	0.0
Salmone Penne Al Forno, Pizza Hut*	1 Serving/496g	832	49.1	168	7.5	10.6	9.9	0.0
Spaghetti Bolognese, Kids, New, Pizza Hut*	1 Serving/234g	211	3.5	90	7.6	14.6	1.5	0.0
Tagliatelle, Alla Carbonara, Pizza Hut*	1 Serving/400g	548	32.4	137	5.6	10.4	8.1	0.0
Tagliatelle, Meatball, Italian Recipe, Pizza Hut*	1 Portion/240g	324	10.6	135	6.9	16.6	4.4	0.0
Tomato, Pizza Hut*	1 Serving/80g	149	7.4	186	3.7	21.8	9.3	0.0

PIZZA HUT

	Measure INFO/WEIGHT	per Measure KCAL	FAT	Nutrition Values per 100g / 100ml KCAL	PROT	CARB	FAT	FIBRE
PASTA								
Tomato & Pepperoni, Pizza Hut*	1 Serving/300g	312	8.1	104	3.6	16.3	2.7	0.0
PASTA BAKE								
Salmon, Pizza Hut*	1 Portion/400g	692	42.8	173	7.9	11.3	10.7	0.0
PASTA SALAD								
Sweetcorn & Pepper, Pizza Hut*	1 Serving/47g	75	2.5	159	4.6	23.1	5.3	0.0
Tomato, Dressed, Med, Pizza Hut*	1 Serving/100g	112	1.5	112	3.5	21.2	1.5	0.0
Tomato & Basil, Pizza Hut*	1 Serving/50g	50	0.8	100	3.7	17.8	1.5	0.0
PENNE								
Mediterranean Vegetable, Pizza Hut*	1 Portion/448g	592	19.7	132	3.7	18.3	4.4	0.0
PEPPERS								
Mixed, Fresh, Pizza Hut*	1 Serving/80g	12	0.2	15	0.8	2.6	0.3	0.0
Red & Green Wedges, Pizza Hut*	1 Serving/40g	6	0.1	15	0.8	2.6	0.3	0.0
Romano, Stuffed, Pizza Hut*	1 Serving/208g	250	13.3	120	2.7	13.3	6.4	0.0
PIE								
Banoffee, Dessert, Pizza Hut*	1 Serving/125g	428	25.3	340	2.5	37.3	20.1	0.0
Banoffee, Pizza Hut*	1 Serving/100g	350	21.5	350	4.2	34.9	21.5	0.0
PIZZA								
BBQ Deluxe, Cheesy Bites, Pizza Hut*	1 Slice/143g	358	11.6	251	11.7	34.4	8.1	0.0
BBQ Deluxe, Italian, Individual, Pizza Hut*	1 Slice/78g	185	6.1	238	10.9	34.3	7.9	0.0
BBQ Deluxe, Italian, Large, Pizza Hut*	1 Slice/95g	239	8.0	252	14.3	29.7	8.4	0.0
BBQ Deluxe, Italian, Medium, Pizza Hut*	1 Slice/105g	253	8.0	241	12.0	31.1	7.6	0.0
BBQ Deluxe, Pan, Individual, Pizza Hut*	1 Slice/79g	200	7.9	253	12.7	28.0	10.0	0.0
BBQ Deluxe, Pan, Large, Pizza Hut*	1 Slice/122g	306	12.1	251	11.8	28.6	9.9	0.0
BBQ Deluxe, Pan, Medium, Pizza Hut*	1 Slice/107g	276	11.3	257	11.7	28.8	10.5	0.0
BBQ Deluxe, Stuffed Crust, Pizza Hut*	1 Serving/155g	337	10.4	217	11.6	31.9	6.7	0.0
Cajun Chicken, Hot One, Italian, Medium, Pizza Hut*	1 Slice/100g	250	9.3	250	12.5	29.1	9.3	0.0
Cajun Chicken, Hot One, Pan, Large, Pizza Hut*	1 Slice/125g	321	14.7	257	12.9	24.7	11.8	0.0
Cajun Chicken, Hot One, Pan, Medium, Pizza Hut*	1 Slice/105g	273	12.3	259	12.7	25.6	11.7	0.0
Cajun Chicken, Hot One, Stuffed Crust, Pizza Hut*	1 Slice/135g	331	10.8	245	13.3	30.0	8.0	0.0
Cheese Feast, Italian, Medium, Pizza Hut*	1 Slice/96g	260	11.3	272	12.3	29.1	11.8	0.0
Cheese Feast, Pan, Medium, Pizza Hut*	1 Slice/106g	299	15.0	283	14.6	24.2	14.2	0.0
Cheese Feast, Stuffed Crust, Pizza Hut*	1 Slice/132g	361	13.8	273	14.3	30.5	10.4	0.0
Chicken, Hi Light, Medium, Pizza Hut*	1 Slice/83g	189	5.5	230	13.2	29.2	6.7	0.0
Chicken Feast, Italian, Medium, Pizza Hut*	1 Slice/100g	249	8.6	248	14.1	28.6	8.6	0.0
Chicken Feast, Pan, Medium, Pizza Hut*	1 Slice/109g	283	12.0	259	15.5	24.6	11.0	0.0
Chicken Feast, Stuffed Crust, Pizza Hut*	1 Slice/133g	337	12.6	254	14.8	27.3	9.5	0.0
Chicken Supreme, Cheesy Bites, Pizza Hut*	1 Slice/148g	322	10.0	218	11.8	29.5	6.8	0.0
Chicken Supreme, Express, Pizza Hut*	1 Serving/65g	143	5.8	221	10.1	28.1	9.0	0.0
Chicken Supreme, Italian, Individual, Pizza Hut*	1 Slice/74g	169	4.4	229	10.7	35.4	5.9	0.0
Chicken Supreme, Italian, Large, Pizza Hut*	1 Slice/111g	217	6.4	196	9.8	29.3	5.8	0.0
Chicken Supreme, Italian, Medium, Pizza Hut*	1 Slice/102g	220	6.3	215	10.3	31.9	6.2	0.0
Chicken Supreme, Pan, Individual, Pizza Hut*	1 Slice/81g	186	8.0	231	11.6	26.9	9.9	0.0
Chicken Supreme, Pan, Large, Pizza Hut*	1 Slice/124g	271	11.6	219	10.9	26.1	9.4	0.0
Chicken Supreme, Pan, Medium, Pizza Hut*	1 Slice/115g	251	9.9	219	11.2	26.6	8.6	0.0
Chicken Supreme, Stuffed Crust, Pizza Hut*	1 Slice/153g	367	11.0	240	11.6	34.8	7.2	0.0
Country Feast, Italian, Medium, Pizza Hut*	1 Slice/109g	252	9.6	232	9.7	28.6	8.8	0.0
Country Feast, Pan, Medium, Pizza Hut*	1 Slice/115g	279	12.1	243	11.4	25.8	10.5	0.0
Country Feast, Stuffed Crust, Pizza Hut*	1 Slice/144g	326	10.8	227	11.5	28.4	7.5	0.0
Express, Supreme, Pizza Hut*	1 Serving/68g	165	7.6	242	10.7	27.8	11.2	0.0
Farmhouse, Cheesy Bites, Pizza Hut*	1 Slice/133g	332	12.6	250	13.2	30.7	9.5	0.0
Farmhouse, Italian, Individual, Pizza Hut*	1 Slice/74g	188	6.0	253	11.8	33.1	8.1	0.0
Farmhouse, Italian, Large, Pizza Hut*	1 Slice/92g	206	6.7	224	10.2	34.0	7.3	0.0

PIZZA HUT

PIZZA

INFO/WEIGHT		KCAL	FAT	KCAL	PROT	CARB	FAT	FIBRE
Farmhouse, Italian, Medium, Pizza Hut*	1 Slice/84g	192	5.4	229	10.2	35.7	6.4	0.0
Farmhouse, Pan, Individual, Pizza Hut*	1 Slice/70g	179	7.4	256	11.3	31.6	10.6	0.0
Farmhouse, Pan, Large, Pizza Hut*	1 Slice/106g	257	11.0	242	11.4	29.7	10.4	0.0
Farmhouse, Pan, Medium, Delivery, Pizza Hut*	1 Slice/75g	182	7.8	242	11.3	28.6	10.4	0.0
Farmhouse, Pan, Medium, Pizza Hut*	1 Slice/100g	242	10.4	242	11.3	28.6	10.4	0.0
Farmhouse, Stuffed Crust, Pizza Hut*	1 Slice/132g	387	10.0	293	11.8	30.0	7.6	0.0
Ham, Hi Light, Medium, Pizza Hut*	1 Slice/82g	184	5.5	225	12.1	29.1	6.7	0.0
Happy Hour, Chicken & Mushroom, Pizza Hut*	1 Serving/80g	165	5.4	207	9.6	27.6	6.8	0.0
Happy Hour, Ham & Sweetcorn, Pizza Hut*	1 Serving/86g	174	5.6	202	9.4	27.0	6.5	0.0
Happy Hour, Pepper & Tomato, Pizza Hut*	1 Serving/86g	163	5.4	189	8.0	26.1	6.3	0.0
Happy Hour, Pepperoni & Onion, Pizza Hut*	1 Serving/80g	179	6.9	224	9.4	28.2	8.6	0.0
Hawaiian, Cheesy Bites, Pizza Hut*	1 Slice/136g	316	10.6	232	11.6	31.2	7.8	0.0
Hawaiian, Express, Pizza Hut*	1 Serving/60g	147	6.4	245	10.5	29.9	10.6	0.0
Hawaiian, Italian, Individual, Pizza Hut*	1 Serving/71g	164	4.2	229	9.8	37.9	5.8	0.0
Hawaiian, Italian, Large, Pizza Hut*	1 Slice/99g	221	7.0	223	10.0	33.2	7.1	0.0
Hawaiian, Italian, Medium, Pizza Hut*	1 Slice/92g	201	5.6	219	9.8	33.3	6.1	0.0
Hawaiian, Pan, Individual, Pizza Hut*	1 Serving/73g	175	6.5	240	10.9	32.2	8.9	0.0
Hawaiian, Pan, Large, Delivery, Pizza Hut*	1 Serving/89g	234	10.2	262	10.6	32.6	11.4	0.0
Hawaiian, Pan, Large, Pizza Hut*	1 Slice/112g	293	12.7	262	10.6	32.6	11.4	0.0
Hawaiian, Pan, Medium, Pizza Hut*	1 Slice/109g	245	9.7	224	10.1	28.5	8.9	0.0
Hawaiian, Stuffed Crust, Pizza Hut*	1 Slice/141g	306	10.3	217	11.0	30.7	7.3	0.0
Hot 'n' Spicy, Cheesy Bites, Pizza Hut*	1 Slice/127g	331	12.6	261	12.6	33.7	9.9	0.0
Hot 'n' Spicy, Italian, Individual, Pizza Hut*	1 Slice/66g	180	6.9	272	11.0	36.5	10.4	0.0
Hot 'n' Spicy, Italian, Large, Pizza Hut*	1 Slice/93g	236	9.4	254	11.2	32.7	10.1	0.0
Hot 'n' Spicy, Italian, Medium, Pizza Hut*	1 Slice/86g	222	8.4	259	11.0	34.5	9.8	0.0
Hot 'n' Spicy, Pan, Individual, Pizza Hut*	1 Slice/71g	183	7.9	259	10.9	30.4	11.2	0.0
Hot 'n' Spicy, Pan, Large, Pizza Hut*	1 Slice/105g	266	11.4	254	12.0	30.2	10.9	0.0
Hot 'n' Spicy, Pan, Medium, Pizza Hut*	1 Slice/93g	237	10.6	254	11.5	29.2	11.4	0.0
Hot 'n' Spicy, Stuffed Crust, Pizza Hut*	1 Slice/139g	329	11.0	236	11.8	33.1	7.9	0.0
Margherita, Cheesy Bites, Pizza Hut*	1 Serving/128g	337	12.9	263	12.8	33.1	10.1	0.0
Margherita, Fingers, Kids, Pizza Hut*	1 Serving/95g	258	12.1	273	11.0	28.4	12.8	0.0
Margherita, Italian, Individual, Pizza Hut*	1 Slice/67g	177	5.4	264	11.9	39.2	8.0	0.0
Margherita, Italian, Large, Pizza Hut*	1 Slice/91g	229	8.6	252	10.4	34.2	9.5	0.0
Margherita, Italian, Medium, Pizza Hut*	1 Slice/80g	205	7.0	256	11.0	35.7	8.8	0.0
Margherita, Pan, Individual, Pizza Hut*	1 Slice/71g	189	8.1	268	11.6	32.4	11.5	0.0
Margherita, Pan, Large, Pizza Hut*	1 Slice/105g	273	12.4	261	11.6	29.8	11.9	0.0
Margherita, Pan, Medium, Pizza Hut*	1 Serving/97g	256	11.4	265	11.6	30.6	11.8	0.0
Margherita, Stuffed Crust, Pizza Hut*	1 Slice/140g	349	12.4	248	14.0	31.6	8.8	0.0
Margherita, Thick, Kids, Pizza Hut*	1 Serving/202g	506	17.9	251	9.0	33.0	8.9	0.0
Meat Feast, Cheesy Bites, Pizza Hut*	1 Slice/142g	387	16.2	272	13.9	30.3	11.4	0.0
Meat Feast, Italian, Individual, Pizza Hut*	1 Slice/81g	220	8.8	270	13.9	32.3	10.8	0.0
Meat Feast, Italian, Large, Pizza Hut*	1 Slice/111g	279	12.7	251	12.9	27.3	11.4	0.0
Meat Feast, Italian, Medium, Pizza Hut*	1 Slice/100g	257	11.0	258	13.0	30.0	11.0	0.0
Meat Feast, Pan, Individual, Pizza Hut*	1 Slice/84g	220	9.9	262	13.3	27.6	11.8	0.0
Meat Feast, Pan, Large, Pizza Hut*	1 Slice/124g	344	16.4	277	12.6	29.1	13.2	0.0
Meat Feast, Pan, Medium, Pizza Hut*	1 Slice/112g	294	13.9	262	12.2	28.0	12.4	0.0
Meat Feast, Stuffed Crust, Pizza Hut*	1 Slice/152g	376	15.8	247	13.5	28.0	10.4	0.0
Meaty, The Edge, Medium, Pizza Hut*	1 Slice/36g	110	5.7	308	17.0	20.4	16.1	0.0
Meaty BBQ, Cheesy Bites, Delivery, Pizza Hut*	1 Serving/115g	282	10.8	245	11.3	31.1	9.4	0.0
Meaty BBQ, Italian, Medium, Delivery, Pizza Hut*	1 Serving/70g	154	5.0	220	10.9	30.0	7.2	0.0
Meaty BBQ, Pan, Medium, Delivery, Pizza Hut*	1 Serving/92g	215	8.7	234	11.1	25.9	9.5	0.0
Mediterranean Meat Deluxe, Italian, Medium, Pizza Hut*	1 Slice/91g	245	9.4	270	12.8	33.5	10.4	0.0

PIZZA HUT

PIZZA

	Measure INFO/WEIGHT	per Measure KCAL	FAT	Nutrition Values per 100g / 100ml KCAL	PROT	CARB	FAT	FIBRE
Mediterranean Meat Deluxe, Pan, Individual, Pizza Hut*	1 Slice/75g	212	10.4	284	13.5	29.5	13.9	0.0
Mediterranean Meat Deluxe, Pan, Medium, Pizza Hut*	1 Slice/98g	245	11.2	249	11.7	28.1	11.4	0.0
Mountain Fantastico, Italian, Individual, Pizza Hut*	1 Slice/75g	183	6.3	245	9.3	36.4	8.5	0.0
Pepperoni Feast, Cheesy Bites, Pizza Hut*	1 Slice/135g	382	16.7	284	15.8	29.6	12.4	0.0
Pepperoni Feast, Italian, Individual, Pizza Hut*	1 Slice/73g	205	8.4	282	11.4	36.3	11.6	0.0
Pepperoni Feast, Italian, Large, Delivery, Pizza Hut*	1 Serving/68g	195	9.5	286	12.0	30.8	14.0	0.0
Pepperoni Feast, Italian, Large, Pizza Hut*	1 Slice/103g	286	13.3	278	12.2	30.9	12.9	0.0
Pepperoni Feast, Italian, Medium, Pizza Hut*	1 Slice/93g	254	9.8	273	12.3	35.0	10.5	0.0
Pepperoni Feast, Pan, Individual, Pizza Hut*	1 Slice/79g	227	10.8	286	12.3	30.3	13.6	0.0
Pepperoni Feast, Pan, Large, Pizza Hut*	1 Slice/115g	347	20.2	302	12.0	26.4	17.6	0.0
Pepperoni Feast, Pan, Medium, Pizza Hut*	1 Slice/106g	297	15.9	279	12.6	26.2	14.9	0.0
Pepperoni Feast, Stuffed Crust, Pizza Hut*	1 Slice/143g	375	16.2	261	13.1	30.4	11.3	0.0
Seafood Fantastico, Italian, Individual, Pizza Hut*	1 Slice/81g	173	4.6	213	15.3	25.1	5.7	0.0
Seafood Fantastico, Italian, Large, Pizza Hut*	1 Slice/106g	228	6.6	215	15.1	24.6	6.2	0.0
Seafood Lovers, Italian, Individual, Pizza Hut*	1 Slice/66g	170	5.4	258	9.8	38.4	8.2	0.0
Seafood Lovers, Italian, Large, Pizza Hut*	1 Slice/90g	215	6.8	239	10.2	35.3	7.6	0.0
Seafood Lovers, Italian, Medium, Pizza Hut*	1 Slice/82g	202	6.6	245	10.1	35.3	8.0	0.0
Seafood Lovers, Pan, Individual, Pizza Hut*	1 Slice/69g	160	6.0	232	10.7	31.3	8.7	0.0
Seafood Lovers, Pan, Medium, Pizza Hut*	1 Slice/98g	233	10.4	237	9.7	28.3	10.6	0.0
Seafood Lovers, Stuffed Crust, Pizza Hut*	1 Slice/131g	314	10.9	239	12.3	31.8	8.3	0.0
Spicy, Hot One, Pan, Medium, Pizza Hut*	1 Slice/115g	274	13.0	239	11.2	23.1	11.3	0.0
Super Supreme, Cheesy Bites, Pizza Hut*	1 Slice/162g	393	16.2	242	12.4	26.9	10.0	0.0
Super Supreme, Italian, Individual, Pizza Hut*	1 Slice/97g	260	11.0	267	13.9	27.3	11.3	0.0
Super Supreme, Italian, Large, Pizza Hut*	1 Slice/128g	281	13.2	219	10.6	24.4	10.3	0.0
Super Supreme, Italian, Medium, Pizza Hut*	1 Slice/119g	267	11.5	225	11.1	26.3	9.7	0.0
Super Supreme, Pan, Individual, Pizza Hut*	1 Slice/96g	228	10.9	237	11.9	24.8	11.3	0.0
Super Supreme, Pan, Large, Pizza Hut*	1 Slice/148g	346	17.7	234	11.4	22.5	12.0	0.0
Super Supreme, Pan, Medium, Pizza Hut*	1 Slice/127g	323	18.5	255	11.4	22.8	14.6	0.0
Super Supreme, Stuffed Crust, Pizza Hut*	1 Slice/165g	397	14.3	241	11.7	29.0	8.7	0.0
Super Supreme, Stuffed Crust, Pizza Hut*	1 Serving/165g	366	16.5	222	11.9	25.2	10.0	0.0
Supreme, Italian, Individual, Pizza Hut*	1 Slice/81g	204	7.5	251	10.9	33.5	9.2	0.0
Supreme, Italian, Large, Pizza Hut*	1 Slice/113g	264	11.0	233	9.7	29.6	9.7	0.0
Supreme, Pan, Individual, Pizza Hut*	1 Slice/84g	209	9.6	248	11.0	28.0	11.4	0.0
Supreme, Stuffed Crust, Pizza Hut*	1 Slice/160g	371	13.8	232	11.9	29.7	8.6	0.0
The Sizzler, Cajun Chicken, Italian, Large, Pizza Hut*	1 Serving/83g	177	6.1	213	11.2	28.1	7.4	0.0
The Sizzler, Cajun Chicken, Italian, Medium, Pizza Hut*	1 Serving/67g	147	4.8	220	11.8	30.2	7.2	0.0
The Sizzler, Cajun Chicken, Pan, Large, Pizza Hut*	1 Serving/90g	215	7.9	238	10.8	27.2	8.8	0.0
The Sizzler, Cajun Chicken, Pan, Medium, Pizza Hut*	1 Serving/75g	166	7.0	221	10.3	27.3	9.3	0.0
The Sizzler, Cajun Chicken, Stuffed Crust, Pizza Hut*	1 Serving/114g	270	9.8	236	11.7	31.7	8.6	0.0
The Sizzler, Spicy Beef, Italian, Large, Pizza Hut*	1 Serving/80g	179	5.9	223	9.6	33.1	7.4	0.0
The Sizzler, Spicy Beef, Italian, Medium, Pizza Hut*	1 Serving/68g	163	6.1	240	10.9	31.6	9.0	0.0
The Sizzler, Spicy Beef, Pan, Large, Pizza Hut*	1 Serving/96g	240	11.0	250	10.5	29.1	11.5	0.0
The Sizzler, Spicy Beef, Pan, Medium, Pizza Hut*	1 Serving/76g	173	7.7	228	10.3	32.0	10.1	0.0
The Sizzler, Spicy Mushroom, Italian, Large, Pizza Hut*	1 Serving/79g	165	5.5	209	9.3	31.2	7.0	0.0
The Sizzler, Spicy Mushroom, Stuffed Crust, Pizza Hut*	1 Serving/116g	244	7.9	210	9.7	31.7	6.8	0.0
The Works, The Edge, Medium, Pizza Hut*	1 Slice/64g	150	6.7	235	12.7	19.5	10.4	0.0
Tortilla, Thin, Kids, Pizza Hut*	1 Serving/108g	264	14.4	245	9.1	20.9	13.4	0.0
Tuscani, Chicken & Mushroom, Pizza Hut*	1 Serving/491g	1032	55.0	210	10.5	16.9	11.2	0.0
Tuscani, Mediterranean Meat, Pizza Hut*	1 Pizza/379g	1065	56.8	281	13.6	21.8	15.0	0.0
Tuscani, Verde, Pizza Hut*	1 Serving/460g	878	42.3	191	8.0	18.6	9.2	0.0
Tuscani Caprina, Pizza Hut*	1 Pizza/474g	990	45.5	209	9.0	20.6	9.6	0.0
Vegetable Supreme, Cheesy Bites, Pizza Hut*	1 Slice/145g	312	10.0	215	10.0	30.7	6.9	0.0

	Measure INFO/WEIGHT	per Measure KCAL	FAT	Nutrition Values per 100g / 100ml KCAL	PROT	CARB	FAT	FIBRE
PIZZA HUT								
PIZZA								
Vegetable Supreme, Italian, Individual, Pizza Hut*	1 Slice/77g	160	4.7	207	8.7	32.4	6.1	0.0
Vegetable Supreme, Italian, Large, Pizza Hut*	1 Slice/111g	222	6.3	200	7.4	32.5	5.7	0.0
Vegetable Supreme, Italian, Medium, Pizza Hut*	1 Slice/99g	196	6.0	198	8.3	30.7	6.1	0.0
Vegetable Supreme, Pan, Individual, Pizza Hut*	1 Slice/84g	180	7.6	214	8.6	27.7	9.0	0.0
Vegetable Supreme, Pan, Large, Pizza Hut*	1 Slice/126g	258	11.6	204	8.1	25.7	9.2	0.0
Vegetable Supreme, Pan, Medium, Pizza Hut*	1 Slice/109g	263	11.2	241	9.9	30.0	10.3	0.0
Vegetable Supreme, Stuffed Crust, Pizza Hut*	1 Slice/156g	307	10.8	197	9.3	27.8	6.9	0.0
Vegetarian, Hi Light, Medium, Pizza Hut*	1 Slice/77g	170	5.1	221	10.3	30.0	6.6	0.0
Vegetarian Hot One, Cheesy Bites, Pizza Hut*	1 Slice/142g	302	10.1	212	9.8	30.3	7.1	0.0
Vegetarian Hot One, Italian, Individual, Pizza Hut*	1 Slice/78g	164	4.5	211	8.1	34.6	5.8	0.0
Vegetarian Hot One, Italian, Large, Pizza Hut*	1 Slice/114g	165	6.7	145	7.5	19.1	5.9	0.0
Vegetarian Hot One, Italian, Medium, Pizza Hut*	1 Slice/98g	188	5.4	192	9.3	29.5	5.5	0.0
Vegetarian Hot One, Pan, Individual, Pizza Hut*	1 Slice/82g	174	6.0	211	8.8	29.6	7.3	0.0
Vegetarian Hot One, Pan, Large, Pizza Hut*	1 Slice/126g	290	12.1	231	9.4	29.7	9.6	0.0
Vegetarian Hot One, Pan, Medium, Pizza Hut*	1 Slice/115g	234	9.9	204	8.4	26.6	8.6	0.0
Vegetarian Hot One, Stuffed Crust, Pizza Hut*	1 Slice/161g	334	11.1	208	10.1	30.2	6.9	0.0
Veggie, The Edge, Medium, Pizza Hut*	1 Slice/60g	136	5.4	227	11.2	22.2	9.0	0.0
PLATTER								
Favourites, Pizza Hut*	1 Platter/732g	1385	82.4	189	8.7	13.5	11.3	0.0
POTATO SKINS								
Cheese & Bacon (6 Skins), Pizza Hut*	6 Skins/246g	408	17.8	166	6.4	20.1	7.2	0.0
Jacket, Loaded, with Cheese, Pizza Hut*	1 Portion/267g	571	34.2	214	13.6	11.2	12.8	0.0
Jacket, Pizza Hut*	1 Portion/224g	571	37.2	255	3.4	23.0	16.6	2.1
Jacket, with Sour Cream & Chive Dip, Pizza Hut*	1 Portion/224g	311	24.1	139	1.4	9.3	10.8	0.8
POTATO WEDGES								
without Dip, Pizza Hut*	1 Serving/390g	569	23.8	146	2.5	20.3	6.1	0.0
POTATOES								
Baby, Pizza Hut*	1 Serving/80g	63	1.4	79	1.2	14.6	1.8	0.0
PROFITEROLES								
Dessert, Pizza Hut*	1 Serving/100g	381	31.3	381	4.6	20.1	31.3	0.0
Pizza Hut*	1 Serving/100g	381	31.3	381	4.6	20.1	31.3	0.0
PUDDING								
Sticky Toffee, Pizza Hut*	1 Serving/105g	400	18.2	380	5.5	50.6	17.3	0.0
RAISINS								
Chocolate, Ice Cream Factory, Pizza Hut*	1 Serving/30g	122	4.3	405	5.4	63.3	14.2	0.0
SALAD								
4 Leaf Mix, Pizza Hut*	1 Serving/100g	14	0.5	14	0.8	1.7	0.5	0.0
Beetroot & Carrot, with Balsamic Vinaigrette, Pizza Hut*	1 Serving/80g	24	0.2	30	1.1	5.7	0.3	0.0
Caesar, Chicken, Pizza Hut*	1 Sm/172g	263	12.7	153	14.1	7.4	7.4	0.0
Caesar, Classic, Pizza Hut*	1 Portion/194g	367	23.1	189	7.2	13.0	11.9	0.0
Caesar, Classic, Small, Pizza Hut*	1 Serving/97g	183	11.5	189	7.2	13.0	11.9	0.0
Caesar, Pizza Hut*	1 Salad/195g	344	20.2	177	6.0	14.8	10.4	0.0
Caesar, Prawn, Pizza Hut*	1 Portion/345g	459	24.2	133	9.6	7.6	7.0	0.0
Caesar, with Chicken & Bacon, Pizza Hut*	1 Serving/375g	588	29.6	157	14.4	6.8	7.9	0.0
Carrot Batons, Fresh, Pizza Hut*	1 Serving/80g	28	0.2	35	0.6	7.9	0.3	0.0
Cheese, Goats, Pizza Hut*	1 Serving/341g	525	40.2	154	7.5	4.4	11.8	0.0
Cheese, Hard, Grated, Pizza Hut*	1 Serving/50g	202	15.0	404	33.0	0.0	30.0	0.0
Chicken, Warm, Pizza Hut*	1 Salad/342g	403	17.4	118	11.0	6.8	5.1	0.0
Chicken & Bacon, Pizza Hut*	1 Serving/323g	514	32.0	159	10.3	6.9	9.9	0.0
Coleslaw, Pizza Hut*	1 Serving/80g	149	14.6	186	1.1	4.5	18.2	0.0
Dressed, Tabbouleh, Pizza Hut*	1 Serving/100g	189	8.1	189	4.2	24.9	8.1	0.0
Fresh, Carrot, Grated, Pizza Hut*	1 Serving/17g	5	0.1	30	0.7	6.0	0.5	0.0

	Measure INFO/WEIGHT	per Measure KCAL	FAT	Nutrition Values per 100g / 100ml KCAL	PROT	CARB	FAT	FIBRE
PIZZA HUT								
SALAD								
Fresh, Cucumber, Slices, Pizza Hut*	1 Serving/80g	8	0.1	10	0.7	1.5	0.1	0.0
Fresh, Onion, Red, Slices, Pizza Hut*	1 Portion/80g	29	0.2	36	1.2	7.9	0.2	0.0
Fresh, Seasonal, Pizza Hut*	1 Serving/80g	12	0.5	15	0.7	1.8	0.6	0.0
Fresh, Tomatoes, Cherry, Pizza Hut*	1 Serving/80g	15	0.3	19	0.8	3.0	0.4	0.0
Leaf Mix, Pizza Hut*	1 Serving/41g	7	0.5	17	2.9	6.3	1.1	0.0
Mozzarella & Tomato, Light Lunch, Pizza Hut*	1 Serving/188g	387	30.6	206	12.3	2.4	16.3	0.0
Mozzarella & Tomato, Pizza Hut*	1 Salad/160g	234	19.0	146	7.8	2.1	11.9	0.0
Olive & Feta, Pizza Hut*	1 Portion/406g	345	26.0	85	3.8	3.6	6.4	0.0
Potato, Whole, Pizza Hut*	1 Serving/100g	154	10.1	154	1.6	13.5	10.1	0.0
Tuna, Pizza Hut*	1 Portion/461g	378	8.8	82	10.4	5.9	1.9	2.0
SAUCE								
Caramel, Ice Cream Factory, Pizza Hut*	1 Serving/25g	77	1.0	307	0.7	67.2	3.9	0.0
Chocolate, Ice Cream Factory, Pizza Hut*	1 Serving/25g	74	0.6	298	2.0	66.8	2.5	0.0
Strawberry, Ice Cream Factory, Pizza Hut*	1 Serving/25g	70	0.0	280	0.0	69.5	0.0	0.0
SMOOTHIE								
BananaBerry Split, Pizza Hut*	1 Serving/171g	258	0.4	151	1.5	33.6	0.2	0.0
Truly Tropical, Pizza Hut*	1 Serving/239g	234	0.3	98	0.6	24.0	0.1	0.0
Very Berry, Pizza Hut*	1 Serving/220g	189	0.3	86	0.6	20.4	0.1	0.0
SPAGHETTI BOLOGNESE								
Pizza Hut*	1 Portion/475g	745	31.3	157	6.2	17.8	6.6	0.0
SUNDAE								
Double Chocolate, Pizza Hut*	1 Sundae/145g	307	16.2	212	3.1	27.0	11.2	0.0
SWEETCORN								
Pizza Hut*	1 Serving/30g	24	0.2	79	1.8	16.8	0.8	0.0
TIRAMISU								
Delivery, Pizza Hut*	1 Serving/75g	223	10.3	297	3.9	39.5	13.7	0.0
Pizza Hut*	1 Serving/84g	248	11.4	297	3.9	39.5	13.7	0.0
TOMATO								
Spicy & Red Pepper, Buffet, Pizza Hut*	1 Portion/200g	170	1.8	85	3.1	16.7	0.9	0.0
TOMATOES								
Slices, Fresh, Pizza Hut*	1 Serving/80g	14	0.2	17	0.7	3.1	0.3	0.0
TOPPINGS								
Caramel Sauce, Pizza Hut*	1 Serving/100g	307	3.9	307	0.7	67.2	3.9	0.0
Chocolate Raisins, Pizza Hut*	1 Serving/100g	405	14.2	405	5.4	63.3	14.2	0.0
Chocolate Sauce, Pizza Hut*	1 Serving/100g	298	2.5	298	2.0	66.8	2.5	0.0
Coated Chocolate Beans, Pizza Hut*	1 Serving/100g	475	18.1	475	5.5	72.2	18.1	0.0
Lemon Sauce, Pizza Hut*	1 Serving/100g	280	0.0	280	0.1	69.0	0.0	0.0
Mini Marshmallows, Pizza Hut*	1 Serving/100g	320	0.0	320	5.4	74.3	0.0	0.0
Strawberry Sauce, Pizza Hut*	1 Serving/100g	280	0.0	280	0.0	69.5	0.0	0.0
TUSCANI PLATTER								
Pizza Hut*	1 Serving/462g	1223	89.5	265	8.8	13.2	19.4	0.0
POD FOODS								
SALAD								
Crunchy Indian Slaw, Side, Pod Foods*	1 Portion/199g	355	21.5	178	5.3	15.9	10.8	2.8
PRET & MANGER								
SALAD								
Salmon, & Quinoa, Protien Pot, Pret & Manger*	1 Pack/140g	145	4.0	104	7.8	11.9	2.9	2.0
PRET A MANGER								
BAGUETTE								
Avocado, & Basil, Pret a Manger*	1 Pack/254g	163	7.2	163	4.6	19.8	7.2	2.8
Brie, Tomato & Basil, Pret a Manger*	1 Pack/209g	418	17.3	200	8.2	23.2	8.3	1.6
Cheddar, & Pickle, Posh, Artisan, Pret a Manger*	1 Baguette/243g	590	27.1	243	9.1	29.2	11.2	2.6

PRET A MANGER

	Measure INFO/WEIGHT	per Measure KCAL	FAT	Nutrition Values per 100g / 100ml KCAL	PROT	CARB	FAT	FIBRE
BAGUETTE								
Chicken, Sweet Chilli, & Coriander, Pret a Manger*	1 Pack/210g	390	11.4	186	10.2	23.8	5.4	1.5
Chicken Caesar, & Bacon on Artisan, Pret a Manger*	1 Pack/230g	584	25.8	254	13.5	24.3	11.2	1.8
Prawn,Thai, Pret a Manger*	1 Baguette/237g	374	9.6	158	7.8	22.5	4.0	1.6
Prosciutto, Italian, Artisan, Pret a Manger*	1 Pack/246g	545	24.7	222	9.8	25.8	10.0	2.0
Salmon, & Watercress, on Artisan, Pret a Manger*	1 Baguette/234g	472	12.9	202	12.1	27.4	5.5	2.3
Salmon, Smoked, & Egg, Breakfast, Pret a Manger*	1 Pack/153g	350	17.8	229	10.6	20.5	11.6	1.2
BISCUITS								
Fruit & Oat, Pret a Manger*	1 Pack/40g	187	9.8	468	8.2	50.0	24.5	6.2
BREAD								
Artisan Soup, Pret a Manger*	1 Serving/80g	168	0.6	210	7.0	43.8	0.8	2.0
Baguette, White, for Soup, Pret a Manger*	1 Baguette/142g	336	1.7	237	8.3	48.3	1.2	2.7
BREAKFAST CEREAL								
Bircher Muesli Bowl, Pret a Manger*	1 Bowl/206g	304	9.7	148	6.3	20.2	4.7	1.4
Granola, & Honey, Pret Pot, Pret a Manger*	1 Pot/133g	263	7.8	198	7.3	28.8	5.9	1.3
Granola, Hot & Cold, Pret a Manger*	1 Serving/226g	579	19.9	256	6.4	38.4	8.8	3.5
Porridge, no Topping, Pret a Manger*	1 Serving/300g	243	8.4	81	3.0	9.6	2.8	1.7
Porridge, with Compote, Pret a Manger*	1 Serving/332g	276	8.4	83	2.8	11.1	2.5	1.6
Porridge, with Honey, Pret a Manger*	1 Serving/335g	350	8.4	104	2.7	16.6	2.5	1.5
CAKE								
Apple, Slice, Pret a Manger*	1 Slice/100g	303	14.7	303	3.8	38.8	14.7	1.9
Banana, Slice, Pret a Manger*	1 Slice/82g	275	11.9	335	3.5	47.3	14.5	1.5
Carrot, Slice, Pret a Manger*	1 Slice/112g	400	22.2	357	3.9	40.6	19.8	2.4
Chocolate, Slice, Pret a Manger*	1 Slice/88g	354	20.9	402	5.3	41.7	23.8	1.4
Lemon Slice, Pret a Manger*	1 Slice/70g	257	10.6	367	4.1	52.4	15.1	2.1
CHEESECAKE								
Lemon, Pot, Pret a Manger*	1 Pot/120g	390	25.9	325	2.7	29.3	21.6	1.4
CHOCOLATE								
Dark with Sea Salt, Pret a Manger*	1 Bar/25g	136	9.0	544	4.0	44.0	36.0	8.0
COFFEE								
Americano, Pret a Manger*	1 Serving/360ml	35	1.3	10	0.7	0.9	0.4	0.0
Americano White, Semi Skimmed, Pret a Manger*	1 Cup/350g	14	0.5	4	0.3	0.4	0.1	0.0
Cappuccino, Pret a Manger*	1 Serving/231ml	88	3.1	38	2.7	3.8	1.3	0.0
Espresso, Pret a Manger*	1 Serving/137ml	0	0.0	0	0.0	0.0	0.0	0.0
Filter Coffee, Semi Skimmed Milk, Pret a Manger*	1 Serving/350ml	14	0.5	4	0.3	0.4	0.1	0.0
Flat White, Pret a Manger*	1 Serving/210ml	75	2.7	36	2.6	3.4	1.3	0.0
Latte, Merry, Very Berry, Pret a Manger*	1 Regular/295g	145	0.6	49	2.4	9.1	0.2	0.0
Latte, Skimmed Milk, Pret a Manger*	1 Serving/285ml	110	4.0	39	2.8	3.7	1.4	0.0
Macchiato, Pret a Manger*	1 Serving/60ml	5	0.2	8	0.5	0.8	0.3	0.0
Mocha, Semi Skimmed Milk, Pret a Manger*	1 Serving/293ml	175	5.0	60	3.0	8.0	1.7	0.0
COOKIES								
Chocolate, Chunk, Pret a Manger*	1 Cookie/90g	381	13.9	423	5.3	64.6	15.4	2.6
Oat, Apple & Raisin, Pret a Manger*	1 Cookie/90g	353	10.3	392	6.3	62.2	11.4	3.1
White Chocolate & Orange, Pret a Manger*	1 Cookie/90g	365	11.6	406	5.4	65.7	12.9	2.4
CRISPS								
Cheddar & Onion, Double, Topcorn, Pret a Manger*	1 Pack/25g	123	6.5	492	8.0	55.6	26.0	9.6
Cheese & Red Onion, Croxton Manor, Pret a Manger*	1 Pack/40g	210	12.8	525	6.2	49.8	32.0	5.2
Sea Salt, Maldon, Pret a Manger*	1 Pack/40g	218	14.3	545	5.2	48.0	35.8	5.5
Sea Salt & Cider Vinegar, Pret a Manger*	1 Pack/40g	204	12.2	510	5.2	51.8	30.5	5.5
CROISSANT								
Almond, Pret a Manger*	1 Croissant/95g	387	20.1	407	8.7	47.0	21.2	3.5
Chocolate, Pret a Manger*	1 Croissant/95g	420	23.2	442	7.7	46.5	24.4	2.9
French, Butter, Pret a Manger*	1 Croissant/80g	324	18.9	405	8.2	39.5	23.6	2.4

PRET A MANGER

	Measure INFO/WEIGHT	per Measure KCAL	FAT	Nutrition Values per 100g / 100ml KCAL	PROT	CARB	FAT	FIBRE
CROISSANT								
Ham, Bacon & Cheese, Pret a Manger*	1 Croissant/110g	351	22.7	319	12.2	19.8	20.6	1.2
Mozzarella, & Tomato, Pret a Manger*	1 Croissant/110g	373	24.6	339	13.4	20.2	22.4	1.3
DRESSING								
for Crayfish & Avocado, Pret a Manger*	1 Serving/28g	144	14.8	514	0.7	8.2	52.9	0.0
for Greens & Grains, No Bread, Pret a Manger*	1 Pot/45g	41	3.0	91	4.0	3.8	6.7	0.2
for Pole & Line Caught Tuna Nicoise, Pret a Manger*	1 Pot/45g	231	23.8	513	0.7	8.0	52.9	0.0
for Roasted Vegetable & Feta, Pret a Manger*	1 Dressing/45g	231	23.8	513	0.7	8.0	52.9	0.0
for Sesame Chicken & Noodle Salad, Pret a Manger*	1 Pot/45g	140	9.8	311	12.0	16.0	21.8	0.0
for Superfood Salad, Pret a Manger*	1 Pot/45g	231	23.8	513	0.7	8.0	52.9	0.0
GINGER BEER								
Pure Pret, Pret a Manger*	1 Serving/330ml	152	0.0	46	0.0	11.4	0.0	0.0
GINGERBREAD								
Godfrey, Pret's Gingerbread Man, Pret a Manger*	1 Serving/54g	195	7.3	361	4.6	55.4	13.5	1.7
HOT CHOCOLATE								
Pret a Manger*	1 Serving/285ml	237	5.9	83	3.4	12.7	2.1	0.0
JUICE								
Carrot, Pret a Manger*	1 Serving/250ml	60	0.3	24	0.5	5.7	0.1	0.0
Orange, Pret a Manger*	1 Serving/260ml	114	0.0	44	0.6	11.0	0.0	0.1
JUICE DRINK								
Apple, Pure, Pret a Manger*	1 Serving/330ml	159	0.0	48	0.1	11.6	0.0	0.0
Orange, Pure, Pret a Manger*	1 Serving/330ml	200	0.0	61	0.1	3.1	0.0	0.0
LEMONADE								
Still, Pure, Pret a Manger*	1 Bottle/500ml	171	0.0	34	0.0	8.3	0.0	0.0
MANGO								
Dried, Pret a Manger*	1 Serving/35g	116	0.1	331	1.4	84.6	0.3	3.7
MOUSSE								
Chocolate, Pret a Manger*	1 Serving/100g	375	29.2	375	3.4	24.6	29.2	1.2
MUFFIN								
Double Berry, Pret a Manger*	1 Muffin/145g	498	23.8	343	5.2	44.5	16.4	2.3
High Fibre, Pret a Manger*	1 Muffin/130g	442	24.4	340	8.0	28.6	18.8	9.0
NECTARINE								
Pret a Manger*	1 Fruit/1133g	53	0.1	40	1.4	9.0	0.1	1.1
POPCORN								
Rock Salt, Light, Pret a Manger*	1 Pack/29g	138	7.1	476	6.6	63.8	24.5	15.2
Sweet & Salt, Light, Pret a Manger*	1 Pack/30g	138	5.8	460	7.1	64.3	19.3	6.7
PRETZELS								
Pret a Manger*	1 Serving/105g	333	7.6	317	8.7	52.8	7.2	3.0
SALAD								
Beef, & Noodle, Asian, no Dressing, Pret a Manger*	1 Pack/266g	309	6.3	116	7.3	16.4	2.4	1.4
Ceasar, Chicken, Pret a Manger*	1 Pack/252g	370	16.0	147	11.9	9.1	6.4	0.8
Chicken, Chef's Italian, no Dressing, Pret a Manger*	1 Serving/282g	306	21.2	109	7.6	2.6	7.5	2.0
Edamame, Bowl, Pret a Manger*	1 Serving/125g	94	4.2	76	6.3	4.9	3.4	0.0
Hoisin Duck, no Bread, Pret a Manger*	1 Pack/202g	138	10.6	68	7.5	7.5	5.2	1.7
Salmon, & Sweet Pickle, Smoked, Pret a Manger*	1 Serving/271g	481	22.5	177	8.2	16.8	8.3	2.0
Superfood, no Dressing, Pret a Manger*	1 Serving/337g	375	17.8	111	4.3	11.9	5.3	4.2
Tuna Nicoise, no Dressing, Pret a Manger*	1 Serving/275g	168	5.8	61	9.2	1.4	2.1	0.9
Vegetable, & Feta, Roasted, no Dressing, Pret a Manger*	1Pack/285g	187	7.6	66	3.1	6.7	2.7	1.3
SANDWICH								
BLT, Beech Smoked, Pret a Manger*	1 Pack/229g	431	21.0	188	8.0	17.8	9.2	1.8
Cheddar, & Pret Pickle, Mature, Pret a Manger*	1 Pack/246g	479	24.3	195	7.6	18.4	9.9	1.7
Cheese, Edam, Salad, Pret a Manger*	1 Pack/212g	473	26.6	223	8.8	18.7	12.6	1.8
Cheese, Emmental, Salad, Pret a Manger*	1 Pack/239g	494	28.2	207	8.3	16.9	11.8	1.8

PRET A MANGER

	Measure INFO/WEIGHT	per Measure KCAL	FAT	Nutrition Values per 100g / 100ml KCAL	PROT	CARB	FAT	FIBRE
SANDWICH								
Cheese, Kid's, Pret a Manger*	1 Pack/127g	399	20.2	314	13.9	28.9	15.9	2.2
Chicken, & Pesto, Bloomer, Pret a Manger*	1 Pack/273g	477	17.1	175	10.2	18.0	6.3	1.9
Chicken, Avocado, Pret a Manger*	1 Pack/246g	469	23.4	191	9.7	16.1	9.5	2.7
Club, Classic, Super, Pret a Manger*	1 Pack/255g	505	24.8	198	11.1	15.7	9.7	1.5
Corned Beef, Bloomer, Pret a Manger*	1 Pack/289g	536	21.4	185	10.7	18.5	7.4	1.9
Crayfish, & Mango, Sweet Chilli, Bloomer, Pret a Manger*	1 Pack/215g	401	12.2	187	9.3	24.6	5.7	2.3
Crayfish, & Rocket, Wild, Pret a Manger*	1 Pack/194g	374	15.0	193	10.6	19.4	7.7	1.5
Egg Mayo, Free-Range, Pret a Manger*	1 Pack/189g	426	23.5	225	8.9	19.6	12.4	1.6
Egg Salad, Cracking, Pret a Manger*	1 Pack/241g	430	23.1	178	7.0	16.2	9.6	1.5
Eggs Florentine, Bloomer, Pret a Manger*	1 Pack/254g	545	26.8	215	9.8	19.4	10.6	2.1
Falafel & Humous, Moroccan, Pret a Manger*	1 Pack/285g	525	17.6	184	5.8	23.0	6.2	3.3
Falafel Salad, Moroccan, Pret a Manger*	1 Sandwich/278g	417	8.8	150	5.5	21.2	3.2	1.4
Ham, & Pickle, Wiltshire, on Granary, Pret a Manger*	1 Pack/240g	367	12.2	153	7.4	18.8	5.1	1.7
Ham, Kid's, Pret a Manger*	1 Pack/127g	289	8.2	228	13.4	28.9	6.5	2.2
Ham & Egg, Classic, Bloomer, Pret a Manger*	1 Pack/225g	547	25.2	243	14.7	20.9	11.2	1.9
Humous, Crunchy, Bloomer, Pret a Manger*	1 Pack/224g	511	17.5	228	10.1	30.1	7.8	7.0
Jambon Beurre, Pret a Manger*	1 Pack/144g	359	13.1	249	11.3	29.6	9.1	1.9
Salmon, Smoked, Scottish, Pret a Manger*	1 Pack/156g	366	14.2	235	14.5	23.6	9.1	1.8
The New York Bloomer, Pret a Manger*	1 Pack/227g	507	22.0	223	13.0	22.0	9.7	2.2
Tuna Mayo, Kid's, Pret a Manger*	1 Pack/150g	372	17.3	248	10.9	24.9	11.5	1.9
SMOOTHIE								
Mango, Pret a Manger*	1 Serving/250ml	143	0.5	57	0.6	13.7	0.2	3.0
Strawberry, Pret a Manger*	1 Serving/250ml	128	0.8	51	0.9	11.2	0.3	0.0
Vitamin Volcano, Pret a Manger*	1 Serving/250ml	138	0.8	55	0.6	12.4	0.3	1.3
SOUP								
Broccoli, & Italian Cheese, Pret a Manger*	1 Pack/370g	226	14.1	61	2.2	3.8	3.8	1.3
Butternut Squash, & Sage, Pret a Manger*	1 Pot/370g	104	3.0	28	0.9	3.9	0.8	0.0
Cashew, Butternut & Spice, Pret a Manger*	1 Pack/370g	266	14.4	72	1.9	7.0	3.9	1.4
Chicken, & Roasted Corn, Chowder, Pret a Manger*	1 Soup/370g	259	8.9	70	3.5	7.6	2.4	1.0
Chicken, Broccoli, & Brown Rice, Pret a Manger*	1 Serving/370g	134	2.2	36	2.7	4.6	0.6	0.0
Chicken, Moroccan, Pret a Manger*	1 Serving/370g	304	9.9	82	4.5	8.8	2.7	2.4
Chicken Curry, Malaysian, Pret a Manger*	1 Serving/370g	270	14.8	73	2.7	5.5	4.0	2.0
Chilli, with a Hint of Chocolate, Mexican, Pret a Manger*	1 Pack/370g	344	8.9	93	3.8	12.4	2.4	3.2
Ham, Hock, Pret a Manger*	1 Serving/370g	410	18.9	111	6.0	8.9	5.1	2.6
Lentil, & Coconut Curry, Pret a Manger*	1 Pack/370g	403	15.9	109	5.4	11.5	4.3	1.5
Meatball, Italian, Pret a Manger*	1 Serving/370g	263	15.5	71	2.4	5.8	4.2	1.0
Minestrone, Pret a Manger*	1 Pack/370g	218	10.7	59	2.0	5.3	2.9	1.5
Miso, Pret a Manger*	1 Serving/20g	32	1.0	160	10.0	0.0	5.0	0.0
Mushroom, Cream of, Pret a Manger*	1 Pack/370g	159	8.9	43	1.3	3.2	2.4	0.6
Mushroom, Risotto, Pret a Manger*	1 Serving/370g	259	13.7	70	2.4	6.4	3.7	0.0
Pea & Ham, Pret a Manger*	1 Pack/370g	233	10.7	63	4.5	3.8	2.9	2.0
Pork, BBQ, Pulled, & Bean, Pret a Manger*	1 Pack/370g	341	7.4	92	6.4	10.8	2.0	2.4
Red Pepper, & Creme Fraiche, Pret a Manger*	1 Pack/370g	215	15.2	58	1.1	3.7	4.1	0.9
Sausage Hot Pot, Pret a Manger*	1 Serving/370g	230	13.0	62	4.0	2.6	3.5	2.0
Tomato, & Saffron, Sweet, Pret a Manger*	1 Pack/370g	255	14.8	69	1.7	5.9	4.0	0.7
Tomato, Classic, Pret a Manger*	1 Serving/370g	218	10.7	59	1.8	6.0	2.9	0.8
Veg, & Bean, Smoky Root, Pret a Manger*	1 Serving/370g	192	3.0	52	2.3	7.4	0.8	3.2
SUSHI								
California Rolls, Pret a Manger*	1 Pack/206g	354	9.3	172	5.1	27.5	4.5	1.4
Deluxe, Pret a Manger*	1 Pack/232g	382	9.3	165	6.2	25.8	4.0	1.3
Deluxe Bento Box, Pret a Manger*	1 Serving/256g	353	10.0	138	6.4	19.5	3.9	1.7
Maki & Nigiri, Pret a Manger*	1 Serving/200g	314	8.4	157	5.4	23.4	4.2	1.0

	Measure INFO/WEIGHT	KCAL	FAT	KCAL	PROT	CARB	FAT	FIBRE
PRET A MANGER								
SUSHI								
Salmon & Prawn Sushi, Pret a Manger*	1 Serving/232g	382	9.3	165	6.2	25.8	4.0	1.3
Veggie, Pret a Manger*	1 Pack/226g	333	5.8	147	3.6	27.7	2.6	2.0
TART								
Bakewell, Pret a Manger*	1 Serving/68g	318	18.1	468	7.6	49.7	26.6	2.5
TEA								
Breakfast, Ceylon, Pret a Manger*	1 Serving/360ml	14	0.5	4	0.3	0.4	0.1	0.0
Green, Tropical, Pret a Manger*	1 Serving/60ml	0	0.0	0	0.0	0.0	0.0	0.0
Peach, Iced, Still Pret a Manger*	1 Serving/500ml	78	0.0	16	0.0	3.8	0.0	0.0
Red Berries, Pret a Manger*	1 Serving/60ml	0	0.0	0	0.0	0.0	0.0	0.0
Vanilla Chai, Pret a Manger*	1 Cup/360g	14	0.5	4	0.3	0.4	0.1	0.0
TOASTIE								
Chicken, & Bacon, Pret a Manger*	1 Pack/254g	533	21.2	210	14.2	19.1	8.4	2.0
Halloumi, & Red Pepper, Pret a Manger*	1 Pack/233g	543	25.5	233	11.7	21.6	10.9	2.9
Ham, Cheese, & Mustard, Pret a Manger*	1 Serving/215g	588	27.6	273	17.8	21.8	12.8	2.0
Mozzarella & Pesto, Italian, Pret a Manger*	1 Serving/234g	511	24.3	218	10.3	20.8	10.4	2.2
Tuna Melt, Pret a Manger*	1 Serving/219g	555	24.0	253	16.8	21.5	11.0	2.4
WRAP								
Avocado, & Herb Salad, Pret a Manger*	1 Wrap/246g	460	30.5	187	4.8	13.6	12.4	2.6
Beef Samosa, Hot, Pret a Manger*	1 Wrap/235g	531	29.1	226	8.3	20.2	12.4	2.3
Chicken, Jalapeno, Hot, Pret a Manger*	1 Wrap/262g	430	14.5	164	12.7	15.1	5.5	1.9
Chicken, Sesame, Sushi, Pret a Manger*	1 Pack/227g	400	16.2	176	10.8	16.9	7.1	2.4
Chicken Raita, with Salad, Pret a Manger*	1 Wrap/233g	314	7.1	135	9.7	16.3	3.0	2.2
Falafel & Halloumi, Hot, Pret a Manger*	1 Wrap/244g	578	22.8	237	7.4	24.8	9.3	1.7
Hoisin Duck, Pret a Manger*	1 Wrap/212g	341	19.5	161	8.4	19.8	9.2	1.5
Humous, Salad, Chunky, Pret a Manger*	1 Pack/209g	446	20.9	213	7.2	24.0	10.0	5.8
Italian Pizza Hot, Pret a Manger*	1 Wrap/200g	391	17.2	196	8.7	20.8	8.6	2.4
Nori, Super Veg, Pret a Manger*	1 Pack/180g	292	11.4	162	5.6	20.6	6.3	3.2
O'mega Salmon Salad, Pret a Manger*	1 Pack/200g	319	13.2	160	9.2	15.8	6.6	1.6
Swedish Meatball, Hot, Pret a Manger*	1 Wrap/233g	674	41.3	289	14.1	17.9	17.7	1.8
YOGHURT								
Yoghurt Nuts, Pret a Manger*	1 Pack/75g	430	33.2	573	6.9	29.7	44.3	6.9
YOGHURT DRINK								
Blueberry, Probiotic, Pret a Manger*	1 Serving/250ml	185	4.3	74	2.3	12.4	1.7	0.0
Vanilla, Probiotic, Pret a Manger*	1 Serving/250ml	203	6.3	81	2.9	9.7	2.5	0.0
STARBUCKS								
BAGEL								
Salmon, with Cream Cheese, Smoked, Starbucks*	1 Bagel/165g	370	11.1	224	12.7	27.2	6.7	1.7
BARS								
Chocolate, Dark, Fairtrade, Starbucks*	1 Bar/45g	259	20.8	575	6.7	27.6	46.3	10.7
Chocolate, Milk, Fairtrade, Starbucks*	1 Bar/45g	242	17.4	537	6.4	49.0	38.6	2.2
Granola, Starbucks*	1 Bar/85g	398	22.0	468	7.2	48.9	25.9	5.1
BISCUITS								
Ginger Snaps, Starbucks*	1 Biscuit/30g	134	4.6	445	4.8	71.9	15.4	1.5
BREAKFAST CEREAL								
Maple & Honey Granola, Topping, Starbucks*	1 Serving/25g	112	4.0	448	9.0	64.5	15.9	5.6
Maple & Honey Sauce, Topping, Starbucks*	1 Serving/40g	120	0.0	300	0.1	74.8	0.1	0.2
Porridge Dairy, Starbucks*	1 Serving/230g	244	6.2	106	4.1	17.4	2.7	1.8
Porridge Soy, Starbucks*	1 Serving/230g	205	4.8	89	4.6	13.9	2.1	2.2
Very Berry Compote, Topping, Starbucks*	1 Serving/50g	59	0.1	119	0.6	29.7	0.2	2.1
BROWNIES								
Belgian Chocolate, GF, Fairtrade, Starbucks*	1 Cake/72g	370	22.8	514	4.1	51.9	31.7	2.6

	Measure INFO/WEIGHT	per Measure		Nutrition Values per 100g / 100ml				
		KCAL	FAT	KCAL	PROT	CARB	FAT	FIBRE

STARBUCKS

BUTTIE

Bacon, Starbucks*	1 Buttie/118g	414	18.2	351	19.1	33.3	15.4	1.4

CAKE

Chocolate Chilli, Petite, Starbucks*	1 Piece/38g	170	8.7	448	5.3	57.6	22.8	4.4
Chocolate Chilli, Starbucks*	1 Cake/38g	170	8.7	448	5.3	57.6	22.8	4.4
Loaf, Banana Nut, Starbucks*	1 Cake/103g	431	25.8	418	6.5	40.5	25.0	2.8
Loaf, Lemon, Starbucks*	1 Cake/86g	365	20.2	424	5.0	47.3	23.5	1.6
Loaf, Raspberry & Coconut, Starbucks*	1 Cake/89g	402	22.8	452	4.5	49.9	25.6	2.1
Loaf Cake Chocolate Hazelnut, Starbucks*	1 Cake/85g	331	20.8	389	4.0	38.4	24.5	3.2
Marshmallow Twizzle, Chocolate, Starbucks*	1 Cake/40g	193	8.6	483	4.4	66.9	21.6	1.8
Marshmallow Twizzle, Red White & Blue, Starbucks*	1 Cake/35g	147	4.9	421	4.4	68.8	13.9	1.6
Rocky Road, Starbucks*	1 Cake/78g	423	27.1	542	4.3	51.5	34.8	2.7

CHEWING GUM

Sugar Free, Starbucks*	1 Chew/3g	5	0.0	166	0.0	80.0	0.0	0.0

COFFEE

Caffe Americano, Grande, Starbucks*	1 Grande/473ml	17	0.0	4	0.2	0.6	0.0	0.0
Caffe Americano, Short, Starbucks*	1 Short/236ml	6	0.0	2	0.2	0.4	0.0	0.0
Caffe Americano, Tall, Starbucks*	1 Tall/355ml	11	0.0	3	0.2	0.6	0.0	0.0
Caffe Americano, Venti, Starbucks*	1 Venti/591ml	23	0.0	4	0.2	0.7	0.0	0.0
Caffe Latte, Grande, Semi Skimmed Milk, Starbucks*	1 Grande/473ml	188	7.0	40	2.6	3.9	1.5	0.0
Caffe Latte, Grande, Skimmed Milk, Starbucks*	1 Grande/473ml	131	0.3	28	2.7	4.1	0.1	0.0
Caffe Latte, Grande, Soy, Starbucks*	1 Grande/473ml	148	5.3	31	2.2	2.7	1.1	0.3
Caffe Latte, Grande, Whole Milk, Starbucks*	1 Grande/473ml	223	11.5	47	2.6	3.8	2.4	0.0
Caffe Latte, Short, Semi Skimmed Milk, Starbucks*	1 Short/236ml	95	3.5	40	2.7	4.0	1.5	0.0
Caffe Latte, Short, Skimmed Milk, Starbucks*	1 Short/236ml	67	0.1	28	2.7	4.2	0.0	0.0
Caffe Latte, Short, Soy, Starbucks*	1 Short/236ml	75	2.7	32	2.2	2.8	1.1	0.3
Caffe Latte, Short, Whole Milk, Starbucks*	1 Short/236ml	113	5.8	48	2.6	3.9	2.5	0.0
Caffe Latte, Tall, Semi Skimmed Milk, Starbucks*	1 Tall/355ml	143	5.1	40	2.7	4.2	1.4	0.0
Caffe Latte, Tall, Skimmed Milk, Starbucks*	1 Tall/355ml	102	0.2	29	2.7	4.3	0.1	0.0
Caffe Latte, Tall, Soy, Starbucks*	1 Tall/355ml	110	4.0	31	2.2	2.8	1.1	0.3
Caffe Latte, Tall, Whole Milk, Starbucks*	1 Tall/355ml	172	8.4	48	2.6	4.2	2.4	0.0
Caffe Latte, Venti, Semi Skimmed Milk, Starbucks*	1 Venti/591ml	248	9.2	42	2.8	4.2	1.6	0.0
Caffe Latte, Venti, Skimmed Milk, Starbucks*	1 Venti/591ml	174	0.4	29	2.8	4.4	0.1	0.0
Caffe Latte, Venti, Soy, Starbucks*	1 Venti/591ml	184	6.7	31	2.2	2.8	1.1	0.3
Caffe Latte, Venti, Whole Milk, Starbucks*	1 Venti/591ml	299	15.0	51	2.6	4.2	2.5	0.0
Caffe Misto, Grande, Semi Skimmed Milk, Starbucks*	1 Grande/473ml	106	4.1	22	1.5	2.1	0.9	0.0
Caffe Misto, Grande, Skimmed Milk, Starbucks*	1 Grande/473ml	73	0.2	15	1.5	2.2	0.0	0.0
Caffe Misto, Grande, Soy, Starbucks*	1 Grande/473ml	82	3.2	17	1.2	1.4	0.7	0.2
Caffe Misto, Grande, Whole Milk, Starbucks*	1 Grande/473ml	126	6.8	27	1.5	2.0	1.4	0.0
Caffe Misto, Short, Semi Skimmed Milk, Starbucks*	1 Short/236ml	54	2.1	23	1.5	2.1	0.9	0.0
Caffe Misto, Short, Skimmed Milk, Starbucks*	1 Short/236ml	37	0.1	16	1.6	2.2	0.0	0.0
Caffe Misto, Short, Soy, Starbucks*	1 Short/236ml	42	1.6	18	1.3	1.4	0.7	0.2
Caffe Misto, Short, Whole Milk, Starbucks*	1 Short/236ml	65	3.5	28	1.5	2.0	1.5	0.0
Caffe Misto, Tall, Semi Skimmed Milk, Starbucks*	1 Tall/355ml	81	3.2	23	1.5	2.1	0.9	0.0
Caffe Misto, Tall, Skimmed Milk, Starbucks*	1 Tall/355ml	56	0.2	16	1.6	2.2	0.1	0.0
Caffe Misto, Tall, Soy, Starbucks*	1 Tall/355ml	63	2.4	18	1.3	1.4	0.7	0.2
Caffe Misto, Tall, Whole Milk, Starbucks*	1 Tall/355ml	97	5.2	27	1.5	2.0	1.5	0.0
Caffe Misto, Venti, Semi Skimmed Milk, Starbucks*	1 Venti/591ml	134	5.2	23	1.5	2.1	0.9	0.0
Caffe Misto, Venti, Skimmed Milk, Starbucks*	1 Venti/591ml	92	0.3	16	1.6	2.2	0.1	0.0
Caffe Misto, Venti, Soy, Starbucks*	1 Venti/591ml	104	4.0	18	1.3	1.4	0.7	0.2
Caffe Misto, Venti, Whole Milk, Starbucks*	1 Venti/591ml	160	8.6	27	1.5	2.0	1.5	0.0
Caffe Mocha, Cream, Grande, Semi Skim, Starbucks*	1 Grande/473ml	335	15.0	71	2.8	9.1	3.2	0.4
Cappuccino, Grande, Semi Skimmed Milk, Starbucks*	1 Grande/473ml	115	4.1	24	1.6	2.5	0.9	0.0

STARBUCKS

	Measure INFO/WEIGHT	per Measure KCAL	FAT	Nutrition Values per 100g / 100ml KCAL	PROT	CARB	FAT	FIBRE
COFFEE								
Cappuccino, Grande, Skimmed Milk, Starbucks*	1 Grande/473ml	82	0.2	17	1.6	2.6	0.0	0.0
Cappuccino, Grande, Soy, Starbucks*	1 Grande/473ml	92	3.2	19	1.4	1.8	0.7	0.2
Cappuccino, Grande, Whole Milk, Starbucks*	1 Grande/473ml	136	6.8	29	1.6	2.4	1.4	0.0
Cappuccino, Short, Semi Skimmed Milk, Starbucks*	1 Short/236ml	78	2.8	33	2.2	3.3	1.2	0.0
Cappuccino, Short, Skimmed Milk, Starbucks*	1 Short/236ml	55	0.1	23	2.2	3.4	0.0	0.0
Cappuccino, Short, Soy, Starbucks*	1 Short/236ml	62	2.2	26	1.8	2.3	0.9	0.3
Cappuccino, Short, Whole Milk, Starbucks*	1 Short/236ml	92	4.7	39	2.1	3.2	2.0	0.0
Cappuccino, Tall, Semi Skimmed Milk, Starbucks*	1 Tall/355ml	97	3.4	27	1.8	2.9	1.0	0.0
Cappuccino, Tall, Skimmed Milk, Starbucks*	1 Tall/355ml	69	0.1	20	1.8	3.0	0.0	0.0
Cappuccino, Tall, Soy, Starbucks*	1 Tall/355ml	74	2.5	21	1.4	2.0	0.7	0.2
Cappuccino, Tall, Whole Milk, Starbucks*	1 Tall/355ml	116	5.6	33	1.7	2.9	1.6	0.0
Cappuccino, Venti, Semi Skimmed Milk, Starbucks*	1 Venti/591ml	161	5.7	27	1.8	2.8	1.0	0.0
Cappuccino, Venti, Skimmed Milk, Starbucks*	1 Venti/591ml	115	0.2	19	1.8	2.9	0.0	0.0
Cappuccino, Venti, Soy, Starbucks*	1 Venti/591ml	123	4.2	21	1.4	1.9	0.7	0.2
Cappuccino, Venti, Whole Milk, Starbucks*	1 Venti/591ml	192	9.3	33	1.7	2.8	1.6	0.0
Espresso, Con Panna, Doppio, Starbucks*	1 Doppio/60ml	36	2.5	61	1.5	4.5	4.2	0.0
Espresso, Con Panna, Solo, Starbucks*	1 Solo/30ml	31	2.5	103	1.7	5.7	8.3	0.0
Espresso, Doppio, Starbucks*	1 Doppio/60ml	11	0.0	19	1.2	3.3	0.0	0.0
Espresso, Solo, Starbucks*	1 Solo/30ml	6	0.0	19	1.3	3.3	0.0	0.0
Espresso Macchhiato, Doppio, Semi Skim, Starbucks*	1 Doppio/60ml	14	0.1	24	1.5	3.8	0.2	0.0
Espresso Macchhiato, Doppio, Skimmed, Starbucks*	1 Doppio/60ml	13	0.0	22	1.7	4.0	0.0	0.0
Espresso Macchhiato, Doppio, Soy, Starbucks*	1 Doppio/60ml	14	0.1	22	1.5	3.3	0.2	0.0
Espresso Macchhiato, Doppio, Whole Milk, Starbucks*	1 Doppio/60ml	15	0.2	24	1.5	3.8	0.3	0.0
Espresso Macchhiato, Solo, Semi Skim Milk, Starbucks*	1 Solo/30ml	8	0.1	27	1.7	4.0	0.3	0.0
Espresso Macchhiato, Solo, Skimmed Milk, Starbucks*	1 Solo/30ml	7	0.0	24	1.7	4.0	0.0	0.0
Espresso Macchhiato, Solo, Soy, Starbucks*	1 Solo/30ml	7	0.1	25	1.7	3.7	0.3	0.0
Espresso Macchhiato, Solo, Whole Milk, Starbucks*	1 Solo/30ml	8	0.2	28	1.7	4.0	0.7	0.0
Filter, Grande, Starbucks*	1 Grande/473ml	5	0.1	1	0.1	0.0	0.0	0.0
Filter, Short, Starbucks*	1 Short/236ml	3	0.1	1	0.1	0.0	0.0	0.0
Filter, Tall, Starbucks*	1 Tall/355ml	4	0.1	1	0.1	0.0	0.0	0.0
Filter, Venti, Starbucks*	1 Venti/591ml	6	0.1	1	0.1	0.0	0.0	0.0
Flat White, Short Size as Standard, Whole, Starbucks*	1 Short/236ml	119	5.8	50	2.8	4.3	2.5	0.0
Iced, Caffe Americano, Grande, Starbucks*	1 Grande/473ml	17	0.0	4	0.2	0.6	0.0	0.0
Iced, Caffe Americano, Tall, Starbucks*	1 Tall/335ml	11	0.0	3	0.2	0.6	0.0	0.0
Iced, Caffe Americano, Venti, Starbucks*	1 Venti/591ml	23	0.0	4	0.2	0.7	0.0	0.0
Iced, Caffe Mocha, & Whip, Grande, Skim, Starbucks*	1 Grande/473ml	289	13.6	61	2.0	8.2	2.9	0.4
Iced, Caffe Mocha, & Whip, Grande, Soy, Starbucks*	1 Grande/473ml	300	16.1	63	1.8	7.6	3.4	0.6
Iced, Caffe Mocha, & Whip, Grande, Whole, Starbucks*	1 Grande/473ml	333	18.9	70	2.0	8.1	4.0	0.4
Iced, Caffe Mocha, & Whip, Tall, Semi Skim, Starbucks*	1 Tall/335ml	225	11.8	67	1.9	8.4	3.5	0.4
Iced, Caffe Mocha, & Whip, Tall, Skim Milk, Starbucks*	1 Tall/335ml	208	9.8	62	2.0	8.5	2.9	0.4
Iced, Caffe Mocha, & Whip, Tall, Soy, Starbucks*	1 Tall/335ml	214	11.3	64	1.8	7.9	3.4	0.5
Iced, Caffe Mocha, & Whip, Tall, Whole Milk, Starbucks*	1 Tall/335ml	236	13.1	71	1.9	8.4	3.9	0.4
Iced, Caffe Mocha, & Whip, Venti, Skim Milk, Starbucks*	1 Venti/591ml	315	14.1	53	1.7	7.7	2.4	0.4
Iced, Caffe Mocha, & Whip, Venti, Soy, Starbucks*	1 Venti/591ml	325	16.4	55	1.5	7.2	2.8	0.5
Iced, Caffe Mocha, & Whip, Venti, Whole, Starbucks*	1 Venti/591ml	357	19.0	60	1.6	7.6	3.2	0.4
Iced, Caramel Macchiato, Grande, Soy, Starbucks*	1 Grande/473ml	206	5.3	43	1.8	6.3	1.1	0.2
Iced, Caramel Macchiato, Tall, Soy, Starbucks*	1 Tall/335ml	134	3.3	40	1.4	6.1	1.0	0.2
Iced, Caramel Macchiato, Tall, Whole Milk, Starbucks*	1 Tall/335ml	161	5.5	48	1.5	6.8	1.6	0.0
Iced, Caramel Macchiato, Venti, Semi Skim, Starbucks*	1 Venti/591ml	221	5.0	37	1.3	6.1	0.8	0.0
Iced, Caramel Macchiato, Venti, Skimmed, Starbucks*	1 Venti/591ml	189	1.2	32	1.3	6.2	0.2	0.0
Iced, Caramel Macchiato, Venti, Soy, Starbucks*	1 Venti/591ml	201	4.2	34	1.1	5.6	0.7	0.1
Iced, Caramel Macchiato, Venti, Whole Milk, Starbucks*	1 Venti/591ml	243	7.5	41	1.3	6.1	1.3	0.0

STARBUCKS

	Measure INFO/WEIGHT	per Measure KCAL	FAT	Nutrition Values per 100g / 100ml KCAL	PROT	CARB	FAT	FIBRE
COFFEE								
Iced, Grande, Starbucks*	1 Grande/473ml	4	0.1	1	0.1	0.0	0.0	0.0
Iced, Tall, Starbucks*	1 Tall/335ml	3	0.1	1	0.1	0.0	0.0	0.0
Iced, Venti, Starbucks*	1 Venti/591ml	5	0.1	1	0.1	0.0	0.0	0.0
Iced Caffe Latte, Grande, Semi Skimmed, Starbucks*	1 Grande/473ml	126	4.5	27	1.8	2.7	1.0	0.0
Iced Caffe Latte, Grande, Skimmed Milk, Starbucks*	1 Grande/473ml	90	0.2	19	1.8	2.8	0.0	0.0
Iced Caffe Latte, Grande, Soy, Starbucks*	1 Grande/473ml	104	3.6	22	1.5	2.0	0.8	0.2
Iced Caffe Latte, Grande, Whole Milk, Starbucks*	1 Grande/473ml	149	7.5	32	1.7	2.6	1.6	0.0
Iced Caffe Latte, Tall, Semi Skimmed Milk, Starbucks*	1 Tall/335ml	87	3.0	26	1.7	2.8	0.9	0.0
Iced Caffe Latte, Tall, Skimmed Milk, Starbucks*	1 Tall/335ml	63	0.1	19	1.7	2.8	0.0	0.0
Iced Caffe Latte, Tall, Soy, Starbucks*	1 Tall/335ml	71	2.4	21	1.5	2.0	0.7	0.2
Iced Caffe Latte, Tall, Whole Milk, Starbucks*	1 Tall/335ml	104	4.9	31	1.6	2.8	1.5	0.0
Iced Caffe Latte, Venti, Semi Skimmed Milk, Starbucks*	1 Venti/591ml	132	4.6	22	1.5	2.4	0.8	0.0
Iced Caffe Latte, Venti, Skimmed Milk, Starbucks*	1 Venti/591ml	95	0.2	16	1.5	2.4	0.0	0.0
Iced Caffe Latte, Venti, Soy, Starbucks*	1 Venti/591ml	109	3.7	18	1.3	1.7	0.6	0.2
Iced Caffe Latte, Venti, Whole Milk, Starbucks*	1 Venti/591ml	158	7.5	27	1.4	2.4	1.3	0.0
Iced Cappuccino, Grande, Semi Skimmed, Starbucks*	1 Grande/473ml	135	4.9	29	1.9	2.9	1.0	0.0
Iced Cappuccino, Grande, Skimmed Milk, Starbucks*	1 Grande/473ml	96	0.2	20	1.9	3.0	0.0	0.0
Iced Cappuccino, Grande, Soy, Starbucks*	1 Grande/473ml	111	4.0	23	1.6	2.1	0.8	0.2
Iced Cappuccino, Grande, Whole Milk, Starbucks*	1 Grande/473ml	163	8.1	34	1.8	2.9	1.7	0.0
Iced Cappuccino, Tall, Semi Skimmed Milk, Starbucks*	1 Tall/335ml	94	3.3	28	1.9	3.0	1.0	0.0
Iced Cappuccino, Tall, Skimmed Milk, Starbucks*	1 Tall/335ml	68	0.1	20	1.9	3.0	0.0	0.0
Iced Cappuccino, Tall, Soy, Starbucks*	1 Tall/335ml	78	2.7	23	1.6	2.2	0.8	0.2
Iced Cappuccino, Tall, Whole Milk, Starbucks*	1 Tall/335ml	113	5.4	34	1.8	3.0	1.6	0.0
Iced Cappuccino, Venti, Semi Skimmed, Starbucks*	1 Venti/591ml	141	4.9	24	1.6	2.5	0.8	0.0
Iced Cappuccino, Venti, Skimmed Milk, Starbucks*	1 Venti/591ml	101	0.2	17	1.6	2.6	0.0	0.0
Iced Cappuccino, Venti, Soy, Starbucks*	1 Venti/591ml	116	3.9	20	1.4	1.8	0.7	0.2
Iced Cappuccino, Venti, Whole Milk, Starbucks*	1 Venti/591ml	168	8.1	28	1.5	2.5	1.4	0.0
Macchiato, Caramel, Grande, Semi Skim, Starbucks*	1 Grande/473ml	240	6.7	51	2.2	7.2	1.4	0.0
Macchiato, Caramel, Grande, Skimmed, Starbucks*	1 Grande/473ml	193	1.1	41	2.3	7.4	0.2	0.0
Macchiato, Caramel, Grande, Soy, Starbucks*	1 Grande/473ml	207	5.3	44	1.9	6.2	1.1	0.2
Macchiato, Caramel, Grande, Whole Milk, Starbucks*	1 Grande/473ml	269	10.5	57	2.2	7.1	2.2	0.0
Macchiato, Caramel, Short, Semi Skimmed, Starbucks*	1 Short/236ml	122	3.8	52	2.3	6.9	1.6	0.0
Macchiato, Caramel, Short, Skimmed Milk, Starbucks*	1 Short/236ml	97	0.9	41	2.4	7.1	0.4	0.0
Macchiato, Caramel, Short, Soy, Starbucks*	1 Short/236ml	104	3.0	44	1.9	5.9	1.3	0.3
Macchiato, Caramel, Short, Whole Milk, Starbucks*	1 Short/236ml	137	5.7	58	2.2	6.8	2.4	0.0
Macchiato, Caramel, Tall, Semi Skimmed, Starbucks*	1 Tall/355ml	209	6.3	59	2.8	7.9	1.8	0.0
Macchiato, Caramel, Tall, Skimmed Milk, Starbucks*	1 Tall/355ml	165	1.0	46	2.9	8.1	0.3	0.0
Macchiato, Caramel, Tall, Soy, Starbucks*	1 Tall/355ml	167	4.6	47	2.1	6.5	1.3	0.3
Macchiato, Caramel, Tall, Whole Milk, Starbucks*	1 Tall/355ml	240	9.8	68	2.7	7.9	2.8	0.0
Macchiato, Caramel, Venti, Semi Skimmed, Starbucks*	1 Venti/591ml	329	9.3	56	2.6	7.8	1.6	0.0
Macchiato, Caramel, Venti, Skimmed Milk, Starbucks*	1 Venti/591ml	261	1.2	44	2.6	8.0	0.2	0.0
Macchiato, Caramel, Venti, Soy, Starbucks*	1 Venti/591ml	280	7.4	47	2.1	6.6	1.3	0.3
Macchiato, Caramel, Venti, Whole Milk, Starbucks*	1 Venti/591ml	376	14.6	64	2.5	7.8	2.5	0.0
Mocha, & Cream, Short, Skim Milk, Starbucks*	1 Short/236ml	161	6.4	68	2.9	9.5	2.7	0.4
Mocha, & Cream, Short, Whole Milk, Starbucks*	1 Short/236ml	198	11.0	84	2.8	9.2	4.7	0.4
Mocha, & Cream, Tall, Semi Skim Milk, Starbucks*	1 Tall/355ml	273	12.7	77	2.8	9.4	3.6	0.4
Mocha, & Whip Cream, Grande, Skim Milk, Starbucks*	1 Grande/473ml	288	9.5	61	2.8	9.3	2.0	0.4
Mocha, & Whip Cream, Grande, Soy, Starbucks*	1 Grande/473ml	302	13.7	64	2.4	8.1	2.9	0.6
Mocha, & Whip Cream, Grande, Whole Milk, Starbucks*	1 Grande/473ml	364	18.7	77	2.8	9.0	4.0	0.4
Mocha, & Whip Cream, Short, Soy, Starbucks*	1 Short/236ml	167	8.5	71	2.5	8.4	3.6	0.6
Mocha, & Whip Cream, Tall, Skim Milk, Starbucks*	1 Tall/355ml	238	8.5	67	2.8	9.5	2.4	0.4
Mocha, & Whip Cream, Tall, Soy, Starbucks*	1 Tall/355ml	247	11.8	70	2.5	8.4	3.3	0.7

STARBUCKS

	Measure INFO/WEIGHT	per Measure KCAL	FAT	Nutrition Values per 100g / 100ml KCAL	PROT	CARB	FAT	FIBRE
COFFEE								
Mocha, & Whip Cream, Tall, Whole Milk, Starbucks*	1 Tall/355ml	297	15.5	84	2.7	9.4	4.4	0.4
Mocha, & Whip Cream, Venti, Semi Skim, Starbucks*	1 Venti/591ml	417	17.7	70	2.7	9.2	3.0	0.4
Mocha, & Whip Cream, Venti, Skim Milk, Starbucks*	1 Venti/591ml	359	10.9	61	2.8	9.3	1.8	0.4
Mocha, & Whip Cream, Venti, Soy, Starbucks*	1 Venti/591ml	373	15.8	63	2.5	8.4	2.7	0.7
Mocha, & Whip Cream, Venti, Whole Milk, Starbucks*	1 Venti/591ml	456	22.3	77	2.7	9.2	3.8	0.4
Mocha, White Choc, Whip, Grande, Skim, Starbucks*	1 Grande/473ml	425	12.9	90	3.2	13.4	2.7	0.0
Mocha, White Choc, Whip, Grande, Soy, Starbucks*	1 Grande/473ml	439	17.0	93	2.8	12.3	3.6	0.2
Mocha, White Choc, Whip, Grande, Whole, Starbucks*	1 Grande/473ml	500	22.1	106	3.1	13.2	4.7	0.0
Mocha, White Choc, Whip, Short, Skimmed, Starbucks*	1 Short/236ml	229	8.0	97	3.3	13.7	3.4	0.0
Mocha, White Choc, Whip, Short, Soy, Starbucks*	1 Short/355ml	236	10.1	66	1.9	8.3	2.8	0.2
Mocha, White Choc, Whip, Short, Whole, Starbucks*	1 Short/236ml	267	12.7	113	3.2	13.4	5.4	0.0
Mocha, White Choc, Whip, Tall, Semi Skim, Starbucks*	1 Tall/355ml	323	14.5	91	3.2	13.4	4.1	0.0
Mocha, White Choc, Whip, Tall, Skimmed, Starbucks*	1 Tall/355ml	327	10.4	92	3.2	13.6	2.9	0.0
Mocha, White Choc, Whip, Tall, Soy, Starbucks*	1 Tall/355ml	465	20.4	131	4.7	15.3	5.8	0.2
Mocha, White Choc, Whip, Tall, Whole Milk, Starbucks*	1 Tall/355ml	385	17.1	108	3.1	13.4	4.8	0.0
Mocha, White Choc, Whip, Venti, Skimmed, Starbucks*	1 Venti/591ml	515	14.3	87	3.2	13.4	2.4	0.0
Mocha, White Choc, Whip, Venti, Soy, Starbucks*	1 Venti/591ml	530	19.5	90	2.8	12.2	3.3	0.2
Mocha, White Choc, Whip, Venti, Whole, Starbucks*	1 Venti/591ml	613	25.8	104	3.1	13.3	4.4	0.2
Refresha, Cool Lime, Grande, Starbucks*	1 Grande/475ml	50	0.0	11	0.0	13.0	0.0	0.0
Refresha, Cool Lime, Tall, Starbucks*	1 Tall/355ml	40	0.0	11	0.0	2.9	0.0	0.0
Refresha, Cool Lime, Trenta, Starbucks*	1 Trenta/918ml	100	0.0	11	0.0	2.7	0.0	0.0
Refresha, Cool Lime, Venti, Starbucks*	1 Venti/710ml	80	0.0	11	0.0	2.8	0.0	0.0
Refresha, Valencia Orange, Grande, Starbucks*	1 Grance/473ml	71	0.0	15	0.0	3.8	0.0	0.0
Refresha, Valencia Orange, Short, Starbucks*	1 Short/236ml	63	0.0	27	0.0	5.9	0.0	0.0
Refresha, Valencia Orange, Tall, Starbucks*	1 Tall/254ml	93	0.0	37	0.0	7.9	0.0	0.0
Refresha, Valencia Orange, Venti, Starbucks*	1 Venti/200ml	51	0.0	26	0.0	5.6	0.0	0.0
COOKIES								
Chocolate Chunk, Starbucks*	1 Cookie/107g	499	20.5	466	7.4	65.0	19.2	1.7
Fruit & Oat, Starbucks*	1 Cookie/50g	216	8.8	433	4.4	64.3	17.6	3.1
CRISPS								
Pepperoni, Potato Chips, Starbucks*	1 Pack/50g	239	14.1	478	6.0	53.6	28.2	4.9
Sea Salt, Potato Chips, Starbucks*	1 Pack/50g	244	15.0	488	5.6	53.3	30.0	4.5
Sea Salt & Cider Vinegar, Potato Chips, Starbucks*	1 Pack/50g	248	14.2	496	6.2	54.2	28.3	4.3
CROISSANT								
Almond, Starbucks*	1 Croissant/104g	433	21.8	416	6.4	50.1	21.0	2.0
Butter Croissant, Starbucks*	1 Croissant/70g	267	15.8	381	5.8	38.2	22.5	1.3
Cinnamon Swirl, Starbucks*	1 Croissant/115g	371	11.7	323	7.4	49.1	10.2	2.6
Ham & Emmental Croissant, Starbucks*	1 Croissant/120g	378	21.0	315	13.8	25.2	17.5	0.9
DOUGHNUT								
Apple Fritter, Starbucks*	1 Doughnut/115g	473	24.3	411	6.0	47.5	21.1	3.1
DRIED FRUIT								
, Starbucks*	1 Serving/30g	90	0.1	299	1.9	73.0	0.4	2.0
FRAPPUCCINO								
Caramel, No Whip, Grande, Skimmed Milk, Starbucks*	1 Grande/473ml	134	0.1	28	0.7	6.3	0.0	0.0
Caramel, No Whip, Tall, Skimmed Milk, Starbucks*	1 Tall/335ml	96	0.1	29	0.7	6.3	0.0	0.1
Caramel, No Whip, Venti, Skimmed Milk, Starbucks*	1 Venti/591ml	165	0.1	28	0.7	6.2	0.0	0.1
Caramel with Whip, Grande, Semi Skim Milk, Starbucks*	1 Grande/473ml	390	13.7	82	0.9	13.3	2.9	0.0
Caramel with Whip, Grande, Semi Skim Milk, Starbucks*	1 Grande/473ml	338	14.4	72	1.1	10.1	3.0	0.0
Caramel with Whip, Grande, Skimmed Milk, Starbucks*	1 Grande/473ml	375	11.9	79	0.9	13.4	2.5	0.0
Caramel with Whip, Grande, Skimmed Milk, Starbucks*	1 Grande/473ml	317	11.9	67	1.1	10.2	2.5	0.0
Caramel with Whip, Grande, Soy, Starbucks*	1 Grande/473ml	380	13.4	80	0.8	13.0	2.8	0.1
Caramel with Whip, Grande, Soy, Starbucks*	1 Grande/473ml	325	13.9	69	0.9	9.7	2.9	0.1

STARBUCKS

FRAPPUCCINO

	Measure INFO/WEIGHT	per Measure KCAL	FAT	Nutrition Values per 100g / 100ml KCAL	PROT	CARB	FAT	FIBRE
Caramel with Whip, Grande, Whole Milk, Starbucks*	1 Grande/473ml	400	15.0	85	0.8	13.3	3.2	0.0
Caramel with Whip, Grande, Whole Milk, Starbucks*	1 Grande/473ml	351	16.0	74	1.0	10.1	3.4	0.0
Caramel with Whip, Tall, Semi Skimmed, Starbucks*	1 Tall/335ml	286	10.2	85	1.0	13.6	3.0	0.0
Caramel with Whip, Tall, Semi Skimmed, Starbucks*	1 Tall/335ml	255	10.7	76	1.2	10.7	3.2	0.0
Caramel with Whip, Tall, Skimmed Milk, Starbucks*	1 Tall/335ml	273	8.7	82	1.0	13.7	2.6	0.0
Caramel with Whip, Tall, Skimmed Milk, Starbucks*	1 Tall/335ml	238	8.7	71	1.2	10.8	2.6	0.0
Caramel with Whip, Tall, Soy, Starbucks*	1 Tall/335ml	278	9.9	83	0.9	13.3	3.0	0.1
Caramel with Whip, Tall, Soy, Starbucks*	1 Tall/335ml	244	10.3	73	1.0	10.3	3.1	0.1
Caramel with Whip, Tall, Whole Milk, Starbucks*	1 Tall/335ml	294	11.2	88	1.0	13.6	3.3	0.0
Caramel with Whip, Tall, Whole Milk, Starbucks*	1 Tall/335ml	265	12.1	79	1.2	10.7	3.6	0.0
Caramel with Whip, Venti, Semi Skimmed, Starbucks*	1 Venti/591ml	444	13.0	75	0.8	13.2	2.2	0.0
Caramel with Whip, Venti, Semi Skimmed, Starbucks*	1 Venti/591ml	393	14.0	67	1.0	10.4	2.4	0.0
Caramel with Whip, Venti, Skimmed, Starbucks*	1 Venti/591ml	427	10.9	72	0.8	13.2	1.8	0.0
Caramel with Whip, Venti, Skimmed, Starbucks*	1 Venti/591ml	368	11.0	62	1.0	10.5	1.9	0.0
Caramel with Whip, Venti, Soy, Starbucks*	1 Venti/591ml	433	12.6	73	0.7	12.9	2.1	0.1
Caramel with Whip, Venti, Soy, Starbucks*	1 Venti/591ml	377	13.4	64	0.9	10.0	2.3	0.1
Caramel with Whip, Venti, Whole, Starbucks*	1 Venti/591ml	455	14.3	77	0.7	13.1	2.4	0.0
Caramel with Whip, Venti, Whole, Starbucks*	1 Venti/591ml	409	16.0	69	1.0	10.4	2.7	0.0
Choc Cream, & Whip, Grande, Semi Skim, Starbucks*	1 Grande/473ml	335	14.7	71	1.2	10.2	3.1	0.2
Choc Cream, & Whip, Grande, Skimmed, Starbucks*	1 Grande/473ml	314	12.2	66	1.3	10.3	2.6	0.2
Choc Cream, & Whip, Grande, Soy, Starbucks*	1 Grande/473ml	322	14.2	68	1.1	9.8	3.0	0.3
Choc Cream, & Whip, Grande, Whole, Starbucks*	1 Grande/473ml	349	16.3	74	1.2	10.2	3.4	0.2
Choc Cream, & Whip, Tall, Semi Skim, Starbucks*	1 Tall/335ml	243	10.7	72	1.3	10.3	3.2	0.2
Choc Cream, & Whip, Tall, Skimmed, Starbucks*	1 Tall/335ml	226	8.7	67	1.4	10.4	2.6	0.2
Choc Cream, & Whip, Tall, Soy, Starbucks*	1 Tall/335ml	232	10.3	69	1.2	9.9	3.1	0.3
Choc Cream, & Whip, Tall, Whole, Starbucks*	1 Tall/335ml	253	12.0	75	1.3	10.3	3.6	0.2
Choc Cream, & Whip, Venti, Semi Skim, Starbucks*	1 Venti/591ml	386	14.4	65	1.2	10.3	2.4	0.2
Choc Cream, & Whip, Venti, Skim, Starbucks*	1 Venti/591ml	361	11.5	61	1.2	10.4	2.0	0.2
Choc Cream, & Whip, Venti, Soy, Starbucks*	1 Venti/591ml	370	13.8	63	1.0	9.9	2.3	0.3
Choc Cream, & Whip, Venti, Whole, Starbucks*	1 Venti/591ml	401	16.4	68	1.2	10.3	2.8	0.2
Coffee, No Whip, Grande, Semi Skimmed, Starbucks*	1 Grande/473ml	232	1.9	49	0.7	10.6	0.4	0.0
Coffee, No Whip, Grande, Skimmed Milk, Starbucks*	1 Grande/473ml	216	0.1	46	0.7	10.6	0.0	0.0
Coffee, No Whip, Grande, Soy, Starbucks*	1 Grande/473ml	222	1.6	47	0.6	10.3	0.3	0.1
Coffee, No Whip, Grande, Whole Milk, Starbucks*	1 Grande/473ml	241	3.2	51	0.7	10.5	0.7	0.0
Coffee, No Whip, Tall, Semi Skimmed Milk, Starbucks*	1 Tall/335ml	169	1.6	51	0.8	10.7	0.5	0.0
Coffee, No Whip, Tall, Skimmed Milk, Starbucks*	1 Tall/335ml	157	0.1	47	0.9	10.8	0.0	0.0
Coffee, No Whip, Tall, Soy, Starbucks*	1 Tall/335ml	162	1.3	48	0.7	10.4	0.4	0.1
Coffee, No Whip, Tall, Whole Milk, Starbucks*	1 Tall/335ml	177	2.6	53	0.8	10.7	0.8	0.0
Coffee, No Whip, Venti, Semi Skimmed Milk, Starbucks*	1 Venti/591ml	286	2.1	48	0.6	10.6	0.4	0.0
Coffee, No Whip, Venti, Skimmed Milk, Starbucks*	1 Venti/591ml	268	0.1	45	0.7	10.7	0.0	0.0
Coffee, No Whip, Venti, Soy, Starbucks*	1 Venti/591ml	275	1.7	46	0.6	10.3	0.3	0.1
Coffee, No Whip, Venti, Whole Milk, Starbucks*	1 Venti/591ml	296	3.5	50	0.6	10.6	0.6	0.0
Espresso, No Whip, Grande, Semi Skim Milk, Starbucks*	1 Grande/473ml	210	1.3	44	0.6	9.9	0.3	0.0
Espresso, No Whip, Grande, Skimmed Milk, Starbucks*	1 Grande/473ml	200	0.1	42	0.6	9.9	0.0	0.0
Espresso, No Whip, Grande, Soy, Starbucks*	1 Grande/473ml	204	1.1	43	0.5	9.7	0.2	0.1
Espresso, No Whip, Grande, Whole Milk, Starbucks*	1 Grande/473ml	217	2.1	46	0.6	9.9	0.4	0.0
Espresso, No Whip, Tall, Semi Skimmed, Starbucks*	1 Tall/335ml	143	0.9	43	0.6	9.5	0.3	0.0
Espresso, No Whip, Tall, Skimmed Milk, Starbucks*	1 Tall/335ml	136	0.0	41	0.6	9.5	0.0	0.0
Espresso, No Whip, Tall, Soy, Starbucks*	1 Tall/335ml	139	0.7	41	0.5	9.3	0.2	0.1
Espresso, No Whip, Tall, Whole Milk, Starbucks*	1 Tall/335ml	148	1.5	44	0.6	9.4	0.4	0.0
Espresso, No Whip, Venti, Semi Skimmed, Starbucks*	1 Venti/591ml	262	1.5	44	0.5	9.9	0.3	0.0
Espresso, No Whip, Venti, Skimmed Milk, Starbucks*	1 Venti/591ml	250	0.1	42	0.5	10.0	0.0	0.0

STARBUCKS

INFO/WEIGHT	Measure	per Measure		Nutrition Values per 100g / 100ml				
		KCAL	FAT	KCAL	PROT	CARB	FAT	FIBRE
FRAPPUCCINO								
Espresso, No Whip, Venti, Soy, Starbucks*	1 Venti/591ml	254	1.2	43	0.5	9.8	0.2	0.1
Espresso, No Whip, Venti, Whole Milk, Starbucks*	1 Venti/591ml	270	2.5	46	0.5	9.9	0.4	0.0
Light, No Whip, Grande, Skimmed Milk, Starbucks*	1 Grande/473ml	118	0.1	25	0.7	5.4	0.0	0.1
Light, No Whip, Tall, Skimmed Milk, Starbucks*	1 Tall/335ml	83	0.1	25	0.8	5.3	0.0	0.1
Light, No Whip, Venti, Skimmed Milk, Starbucks*	1 Venti/591ml	139	0.1	24	0.7	5.0	0.0	0.1
Mango Passion, Tea, Grande, Starbucks*	1 Grande/473ml	191	0.3	40	0.2	9.8	0.1	0.3
Mango Passion, Tea, Tall, Starbucks*	1 Tall/335ml	157	0.2	47	0.2	11.4	0.1	0.3
Mango Passion, Tea, Venti, Starbucks*	1 Venti/591ml	228	0.3	39	0.2	9.4	0.1	0.3
Mocha, No Whip, Grande, Skimmed Milk, Starbucks*	1 Grande/473ml	143	0.8	30	0.8	6.7	0.2	0.2
Mocha, No Whip, Tall, Skimmed Milk, Starbucks*	1 Tall/335ml	96	0.5	29	0.9	6.3	0.1	0.1
Mocha, No Whip, Venti, Skimmed Milk, Starbucks*	1 Venti/591ml	179	0.9	30	0.9	6.7	0.2	0.2
Mocha with Whip, Grande, Semi Skimmed, Starbucks*	1 Grande/473ml	361	13.7	76	1.0	12.2	2.9	0.1
Mocha with Whip, Grande, Skimmed Milk, Starbucks*	1 Grande/473ml	346	12.0	73	1.0	12.2	2.5	0.1
Mocha with Whip, Grande, Soy, Starbucks*	1 Grande/473ml	352	13.3	74	0.9	11.9	2.8	0.2
Mocha with Whip, Grande, Whole Milk, Starbucks*	1 Grande/473ml	370	14.8	78	1.0	12.1	3.1	0.1
Mocha with Whip, Tall, Semi Skimmed Milk, Starbucks*	1 Tall/335ml	266	10.0	79	1.1	12.6	3.0	0.1
Mocha with Whip, Tall, Skimmed Milk, Starbucks*	1 Tall/335ml	254	8.6	76	1.1	12.7	2.6	0.1
Mocha with Whip, Tall, Soy, Starbucks*	1 Tall/335ml	258	9.7	77	1.0	12.3	2.9	0.2
Mocha with Whip, Tall, Whole Milk, Starbucks*	1 Tall/335ml	274	11.0	82	1.1	12.6	3.3	0.1
Mocha with Whip, Venti, Semi Skimmed, Starbucks*	1 Venti/591ml	427	13.2	72	0.9	12.7	2.2	0.1
Mocha with Whip, Venti, Skimmed Milk, Starbucks*	1 Venti/591ml	410	11.3	69	0.9	12.7	1.9	0.2
Mocha with Whip, Venti, Soy, Starbucks*	1 Venti/591ml	416	12.8	70	0.8	12.4	2.2	0.2
Mocha with Whip, Venti, Whole Milk, Starbucks*	1 Venti/591ml	437	14.6	74	0.9	12.7	2.5	0.2
Raspberry, Tea, Grande, Starbucks*	1 Grande/473ml	192	0.1	41	0.1	10.0	0.0	0.1
Raspberry, Tea, Venti, Starbucks*	1 Venti/591ml	229	0.1	39	0.1	9.5	0.0	0.1
Raspberry, Tea, Tall, Starbucks*	1 Tall/335ml	158	0.1	47	0.1	11.6	0.0	0.2
Strawb & Cream, Whip, Grande, Semi Skim, Starbucks*	1 Grande/473ml	404	13.6	85	1.0	14.1	2.9	0.1
Strawb & Cream, Whip, Grande, Skim Milk, Starbucks*	1 Grande/473ml	384	11.3	81	1.0	14.2	2.4	0.1
Strawb & Cream, Whip, Grande, Soy, Starbucks*	1 Grande/473ml	391	13.1	83	0.9	13.7	2.8	0.2
Strawb & Cream, Whip, Grande, Whole Milk, Starbucks*	1 Grande/473ml	415	15.1	88	1.0	14.1	3.2	0.1
Strawb & Cream, Whip, Tall, Semi Skim Milk, Starbucks*	1 Tall/335ml	316	9.9	94	1.2	16.0	3.0	0.1
Strawb & Cream, Whip, Tall, Skim Milk, Starbucks*	1 Tall/335ml	300	8.1	90	1.2	16.1	2.4	0.1
Strawb & Cream, Whip, Tall, Soy, Starbucks*	1 Tall/335ml	306	9.6	91	1.0	15.6	2.9	0.2
Strawb & Cream, Whip, Tall, Whole Milk, Starbucks*	1 Tall/335ml	326	11.2	97	1.1	16.0	3.3	0.1
Strawb & Cream, Whip, Venti, Semi Skim, Starbucks*	1 Venti/591ml	445	13.0	75	0.9	13.1	2.2	0.1
Strawb & Cream, Whip, Venti, Skim Milk, Starbucks*	1 Venti/591ml	422	10.3	71	1.0	13.2	1.7	0.1
Strawb & Cream, Whip, Venti, Whole Milk, Starbucks*	1 Venti/591ml	459	14.9	78	0.9	13.1	2.5	0.1
Strawberries & Cream, & Whip, Venti, Soy, Starbucks*	1 Venti/591ml	431	12.5	73	0.8	12.8	2.1	0.2
Vanilla with Whip, Grande, Semi Skimmed, Starbucks*	1 Grande/473ml	327	13.9	69	1.1	9.7	2.9	0.0
Vanilla with Whip, Grande, Skimmed Milk, Starbucks*	1 Grande/473ml	305	11.3	65	1.1	9.8	2.4	0.0
Vanilla with Whip, Grande, Soy, Starbucks*	1 Grande/473ml	313	13.4	66	0.9	9.3	2.8	0.1
Vanilla with Whip, Grande, Whole Milk, Starbucks*	1 Grande/473ml	341	15.6	72	1.1	9.7	3.3	0.0
Vanilla with Whip, Tall, Semi Skimmed Milk, Starbucks*	1 Tall/335ml	233	10.0	69	1.2	9.6	3.0	0.0
Vanilla with Whip, Tall, Skimmed Milk, Starbucks*	1 Tall/335ml	216	8.1	64	1.2	9.6	2.4	0.0
Vanilla with Whip, Tall, Soy, Starbucks*	1 Tall/335ml	222	9.7	66	1.0	9.1	2.9	0.1
Vanilla with Whip, Tall, Whole Milk, Starbucks*	1 Tall/335ml	243	11.4	73	1.1	9.5	3.4	0.0
Vanilla with Whip, Venti, Semi Skimmed Milk, Starbucks*	1 Venti/591ml	372	13.4	63	1.0	9.7	2.3	0.0
Vanilla with Whip, Venti, Skimmed Milk, Starbucks*	1 Venti/591ml	347	10.4	59	1.0	9.8	1.8	0.0
Vanilla with Whip, Venti, Soy, Starbucks*	1 Venti/591ml	346	12.4	59	0.7	9.2	2.1	0.1
Vanilla with Whip, Venti, Whole Milk, Starbucks*	1 Venti/591ml	388	15.4	66	1.0	9.7	2.6	0.0
FRUIT								
Fairtrade Banana, Starbucks*	1 Banana/120g	108	0.5	90	0.8	22.6	0.4	2.7

	INFO/WEIGHT	KCAL	FAT	KCAL	PROT	CARB	FAT	FIBRE
STARBUCKS								
FRUIT SALAD								
Starbucks*	1 Pot/183g	95	0.4	52	0.6	11.1	0.2	1.6
HOT CHOCOLATE								
Classic with Whip, Grande, Semi Skimmed, Starbucks*	1 Grande/473ml	323	15.0	68	2.6	8.7	3.2	0.4
Classic with Whip, Grande, Skimmed Milk, Starbucks*	1 Grande/473ml	277	9.5	58	2.7	8.8	2.0	0.4
Classic with Whip, Grande, Soy, Starbucks*	1 Grande/473ml	291	13.7	62	2.3	7.7	2.9	0.6
Classic with Whip, Grande, Whole Milk, Starbucks*	1 Grande/473ml	352	18.7	74	2.6	8.6	4.0	0.4
Classic with Whip, Short, Semi Skimmed, Starbucks*	1 Short/236ml	178	9.1	75	2.7	8.9	3.9	0.4
Classic with Whip, Short, Skimmed Milk, Starbucks*	1 Short/236ml	155	6.4	66	2.8	9.1	2.7	0.4
Classic with Whip, Short, Soy, Starbucks*	1 Short/236ml	162	8.5	69	2.3	7.9	3.6	0.6
Classic with Whip, Short, Whole Milk, Starbucks*	1 Short/236ml	193	11.0	82	2.6	8.8	4.7	0.4
Classic with Whip, Tall, Semi Skimmed Milk, Starbucks*	1 Tall/335ml	260	12.5	78	3.0	9.5	3.7	0.4
Classic with Whip, Tall, Skimmed Milk, Starbucks*	1 Tall/335ml	222	8.0	66	3.0	9.7	2.4	0.4
Classic with Whip, Tall, Soy, Starbucks*	1 Tall/335ml	234	11.4	70	2.6	8.4	3.4	0.7
Classic with Whip, Tall, Whole Milk, Starbucks*	1 Tall/335ml	284	15.5	85	3.0	9.4	4.6	0.4
Classic with Whip, Venti, Semi Skimmed, Starbucks*	1 Venti/591ml	398	17.5	67	2.8	8.7	3.0	0.4
Classic with Whip, Venti, Skimmed Milk, Starbucks*	1 Venti/591ml	336	10.2	57	2.8	8.9	1.7	0.4
Classic with Whip, Venti, Soy, Starbucks*	1 Venti/591ml	355	15.7	60	2.4	7.7	2.7	0.6
Classic with Whip, Venti, Whole Milk, Starbucks*	1 Venti/591ml	437	22.5	74	2.7	8.6	3.8	0.4
Signature with Whip, Grande, Semi Skim, Starbucks*	1 Grande/473ml	537	30.7	113	3.2	12.4	6.5	1.4
Signature with Whip, Grande, Skimmed Milk, Starbucks*	1 Grande/473ml	505	27.0	107	3.3	12.6	5.7	1.4
Signature with Whip, Grande, Soy, Starbucks*	1 Grande/473ml	515	29.8	109	3.0	11.8	6.3	1.6
Signature with Whip, Grande, Whole Milk, Starbucks*	1 Grande/473ml	556	33.5	118	3.2	12.5	7.1	1.4
Signature with Whip, Short, Semi Skimmed, Starbucks*	1 Short/236ml	283	16.9	120	3.3	12.6	7.2	1.4
Signature with Whip, Short, Skimmed Milk, Starbucks*	1 Short/236ml	267	15.0	113	3.3	12.7	6.4	1.4
Signature with Whip, Short, Soy, Starbucks*	1 Short/236ml	272	16.4	115	3.1	11.9	6.9	1.6
Signature with Whip, Short, Whole Milk, Starbucks*	1 Short/236ml	293	18.1	124	3.2	12.5	7.7	1.4
Signature with Whip, Tall, Semi Skimmed, Starbucks*	1 Tall/335ml	418	24.2	125	3.5	13.5	7.2	1.5
Signature with Whip, Tall, Skimmed Milk, Starbucks*	1 Tall/335ml	393	21.3	117	3.6	13.6	6.4	1.5
Signature with Whip, Tall, Soy, Starbucks*	1 Tall/335ml	401	23.5	120	3.3	12.8	7.0	1.7
Signature with Whip, Tall, Whole Milk, Starbucks*	1 Tall/335ml	433	26.1	129	3.5	13.4	7.8	1.5
Signature with Whip, Venti, Semi Skimmed, Starbucks*	1 Venti/591ml	665	37.2	113	3.3	12.7	6.3	1.4
Signature with Whip, Venti, Skimmed Milk, Starbucks*	1 Venti/591ml	624	32.4	106	3.3	12.7	5.5	1.4
Signature with Whip, Venti, Soy, Starbucks*	1 Venti/591ml	637	36.0	108	3.0	12.0	6.1	1.6
Signature with Whip, Venti, Whole Milk, Starbucks*	1 Venti/591ml	690	40.4	117	3.2	12.5	6.8	1.4
LOLLIPOPS								
Starbucks*	1 Lolly/13g	50	0.0	388	0.0	97.0	0.0	0.0
MILK								
Steamed, Grande, Semi Skimmed Milk, Starbucks*	1 Grande/473ml	203	8.0	43	2.8	4.0	1.7	0.0
Steamed, Grande, Skimmed Milk, Starbucks*	1 Grande/473ml	138	0.3	29	2.9	4.2	0.1	0.0
Steamed, Grande, Soy, Starbucks*	1 Grande/473ml	157	6.1	33	2.3	2.7	1.3	0.3
Steamed, Grande, Whole Milk, Starbucks*	1 Grande/473ml	244	13.2	52	2.8	3.9	2.8	0.0
Steamed, Short, Semi Skimmed Milk, Starbucks*	1 Short/236ml	102	4.0	43	2.9	4.1	1.7	0.0
Steamed, Short, Skimmed Milk, Starbucks*	1 Short/236ml	70	0.2	30	2.9	4.3	0.1	0.0
Steamed, Short, Soy, Starbucks*	1 Short/236ml	79	3.1	34	2.4	2.7	1.3	0.3
Steamed, Short, Whole Milk, Starbucks*	1 Short/236ml	123	6.7	52	2.8	3.9	2.8	0.0
Steamed, Tall, Semi Skimmed Milk, Starbucks*	1 Tall/335ml	155	6.1	46	3.1	4.4	1.8	0.0
Steamed, Tall, Skimmed Milk, Starbucks*	1 Tall/335ml	106	0.3	32	3.1	4.6	0.1	0.0
Steamed, Tall, Soy, Starbucks*	1 Tall/335ml	120	4.7	36	2.5	2.9	1.4	0.4
Steamed, Tall, Whole Milk, Starbucks*	1 Tall/335ml	187	10.1	56	3.0	4.2	3.0	0.0
Steamed, Venti, Semi Skimmed Milk, Starbucks*	1 Venti/591ml	258	10.2	44	2.9	4.1	1.7	0.0
Steamed, Venti, Skimmed Milk, Starbucks*	1 Venti/591ml	175	0.4	30	2.9	4.3	0.1	0.0
Steamed, Venti, Soy, Starbucks*	1 Venti/591ml	199	7.8	34	2.4	2.7	1.3	0.3

STARBUCKS

	Measure INFO/WEIGHT	per Measure KCAL	per Measure FAT	KCAL	PROT	CARB	FAT	FIBRE
MILK								
Steamed, Venti, Whole Milk, Starbucks*	1 Venti/591ml	309	16.7	52	2.8	3.9	2.8	0.0
MINTS								
After Coffee, Starbucks*	1 Mint/2g	5	0.0	250	0.0	100.0	0.0	0.0
MUFFIN								
Chocolate & Belgian Choc Sauce, Starbucks*	1 Muffin/119g	430	17.8	361	6.6	48.7	15.0	2.6
Classic Blueberry, Starbucks*	1 Muffin/110g	481	18.6	437	5.6	47.4	16.9	1.6
Rise & Shine, Starbucks*	1 Muffin/124g	448	18.8	361	7.1	47.8	15.2	2.3
Skinny Blueberry Muffin, Starbucks*	1 Muffin/141g	372	5.5	264	4.1	51.9	3.9	2.3
Skinny Lemon & Poppyseed Iced, Starbucks*	1 Muffin/139g	399	6.1	287	3.9	56.6	4.4	2.6
Skinny Peach & Raspberry, Starbucks*	1 Muffin/136g	369	3.9	271	6.2	53.9	2.9	2.3
NUTS								
Mixed, Starbucks*	1 Pack/75g	401	25.2	535	17.7	41.1	33.6	6.7
Roasted Almonds, Starbucks*	1 Pack/75g	484	41.4	646	21.2	17.7	55.2	10.5
PAIN AU CHOCOLAT								
Starbucks*	1 Pastry/65g	269	15.9	414	5.7	42.2	24.4	2.6
PAIN AU RAISINS								
Starbucks*	1 Pastry/110g	373	19.2	339	4.7	40.3	17.5	1.4
PANCAKES								
Buttermilk, Starbucks*	1 Pack/90g	227	2.4	252	4.6	51.9	2.7	1.2
PANINI								
All Day Breakfast, Starbucks*	1 Panini/158g	338	15.2	214	11.5	19.7	9.6	1.4
Cheese & Marmite, Starbucks*	1 Panini/130g	373	17.8	287	14.3	26.0	13.7	1.1
Croque Monisieur, Starbucks*	1 Panini/190g	456	17.7	240	12.8	25.9	9.3	0.9
Italian Mozzarella & Slow Roast Tomato, Starbucks*	1 Panini/178g	470	20.5	264	11.2	28.0	11.5	1.5
Meatball, Starbucks*	1 Panini/216g	521	22.5	241	11.2	25.0	10.4	1.4
Roast Chicken & Tomato, Starbucks*	1 Panini/223g	375	8.0	168	10.2	23.1	3.6	1.4
Roast Chicken & Tomato, Starbucks*	1 Panini/207g	321	7.5	155	9.4	21.4	3.6	1.2
Steak, Cheese & Caramelised Onion, Starbucks*	1 Panini/210g	525	20.4	250	14.9	25.3	9.7	1.0
Tuna Melt & Mature Cheddar, Starbucks*	1 Panini/200g	492	21.0	246	13.3	24.2	10.5	0.9
SALAD								
Chicken & Red Pesto, Bistro Box, Starbucks*	1 Salad/296g	275	13.9	93	5.1	7.1	4.7	1.1
Cured Ham Hock, Bistro Box, Starbucks*	1 Salad/302g	387	20.5	128	7.9	8.2	6.8	1.3
Falafel Mezze, Bistro Box, Starbucks*	1 Salad/329g	494	14.5	150	5.0	20.9	4.4	3.6
Tuna, Potato & Pea, Bistro Box, Starbucks*	1 Salad/286g	320	14.6	112	6.3	9.5	5.1	1.7
SANDWICH								
Cheese & Pickle, GF, Starbucks*	1 Sandwich/197g	552	32.5	280	7.5	23.9	16.5	2.9
Free Range Egg Mayonnaise, Starbucks*	1 Sandwich/191g	365	15.3	191	10.3	18.6	8.0	1.9
Roasted Chicken with Herb Mayonnaise, Starbucks*	1 Sandwich/201g	314	7.2	156	10.6	19.2	3.6	2.1
SHORTBREAD								
Chocolate Chunk, Fairtrade, Starbucks*	1 Shortbread/96g	497	29.0	518	6.2	53.5	30.2	3.1
SYRUP								
1 Pump - 1/4 fl oz 10g, Starbucks*	1 Pump/10g	20	0.0	202	0.0	50.0	0.0	0.0
2 Pumps - 1/2 fl oz - 20g, Starbucks*	2 Pumps/20g	40	0.0	202	0.0	50.5	0.0	0.0
3 Pumps - 3/4 fl oz - 30g, Starbucks*	3 Pumps/30g	61	0.0	202	0.0	50.3	0.0	0.0
4 Pumps - 1 fl oz - 40g, Starbucks*	4 Pumps/40g	81	0.0	202	0.0	50.2	0.0	0.0
5 Pumps - 1 1/4 fl oz - 50g, Starbucks*	5 Pumps/50g	101	0.0	202	0.0	50.2	0.0	0.0
Bar Mocha, 1 Pump - 1/2 fl oz - 17g, Starbucks*	1 Pump/17g	26	0.6	156	3.5	37.6	3.5	5.9
Bar Mocha, 2 Pumps - 1 fl oz - 34g, Starbucks*	2 Pumps/34g	53	1.1	156	3.8	37.6	3.2	5.9
Bar Mocha, 3 Pumps - 1 1/2 fl oz - 51g, Starbucks*	3 Pumps/51g	79	1.7	156	3.7	37.5	3.3	5.9
Bar Mocha, 4 Pumps - 2 fl oz - 68g, Starbucks*	4 Pumps/68g	106	2.3	156	3.7	37.5	3.4	5.7
Bar Mocha, 5 Pumps - 2 1/2 fl oz - 85g, Starbucks*	5 Pumps/85g	132	2.8	156	3.6	37.5	3.3	5.8

	Measure INFO/WEIGHT	per Measure KCAL	FAT	Nutrition Values per 100g / 100ml KCAL	PROT	CARB	FAT	FIBRE
STARBUCKS								
TEA								
Brewed, Grande, Starbucks*	1 Grande/473ml	0	0.0	0	0.0	0.0	0.0	0.0
Brewed, Short, Starbucks*	1 Short/236ml	0	0.0	0	0.0	0.0	0.0	0.0
Brewed, Tall, Starbucks*	1 Tall/335ml	0	0.0	0	0.0	0.0	0.0	0.0
Brewed, Venti, Starbucks*	1 Venti/591ml	0	0.0	0	0.0	0.0	0.0	0.0
Chai, Latte, Grande, Semi Skimmed Milk, Starbucks*	1 Grande/473ml	236	4.0	50	1.6	9.3	0.8	0.0
Chai, Latte, Grande, Skimmed Milk, Starbucks*	1 Grande/473ml	204	0.2	43	1.6	9.4	0.0	0.0
Chai, Latte, Grande, Soy, Starbucks*	1 Grande/473ml	213	3.2	45	1.3	8.6	0.7	0.2
Chai, Latte, Grande, Whole Milk, Starbucks*	1 Grande/473ml	255	6.5	54	1.5	9.2	1.4	0.0
Chai, Latte, Short, Semi Skimmed Milk, Starbucks*	1 Short/236ml	119	2.0	50	1.6	9.3	0.8	0.0
Chai, Latte, Short, Skimmed Milk, Starbucks*	1 Short/236ml	103	0.1	44	1.7	9.4	0.0	0.0
Chai, Latte, Short, Soy, Starbucks*	1 Short/236ml	108	1.6	46	1.4	8.6	0.7	0.2
Chai, Latte, Short, Whole Milk, Starbucks*	1 Short/236ml	129	3.3	55	1.6	9.3	1.4	0.0
Chai, Latte, Tall, Semi Skimmed Milk, Starbucks*	1 Tall/335ml	179	3.0	53	1.7	9.9	0.9	0.0
Chai, Latte, Tall, Skimmed Milk, Starbucks*	1 Tall/335ml	154	0.2	46	1.7	10.0	0.1	0.0
Chai, Latte, Tall, Soy, Starbucks*	1 Tall/335ml	162	2.4	48	1.4	9.1	0.7	0.2
Chai, Latte, Tall, Whole Milk, Starbucks*	1 Tall/335ml	194	5.0	58	1.6	9.8	1.5	0.0
Chai, Latte, Venti, Semi Skimmed Milk, Starbucks*	1 Venti/591ml	296	5.0	50	1.6	9.3	0.8	0.0
Chai, Latte, Venti, Skimmed Milk, Starbucks*	1 Venti/591ml	256	0.3	43	1.6	9.4	0.1	0.0
Chai, Latte, Venti, Soy, Starbucks*	1 Venti/591ml	268	4.0	45	1.3	8.6	0.7	0.2
Chai, Latte, Venti, Whole Milk, Starbucks*	1 Venti/591ml	322	8.3	54	1.5	9.2	1.4	0.0
Iced, Chai, Latte, Grande, Semi Skimmed, Starbucks*	1 Grande/473ml	238	4.2	50	1.6	9.3	0.9	0.0
Iced, Chai, Latte, Grande, Skimmed Milk, Starbucks*	1 Grande/473ml	205	0.2	43	1.6	9.4	0.0	0.0
Iced, Chai, Latte, Grande, Soy, Starbucks*	1 Grande/473ml	219	3.4	46	1.4	8.6	0.7	0.2
Iced, Chai, Latte, Grande, Whole Milk, Starbucks*	1 Grande/473ml	259	6.9	55	1.5	9.2	1.5	0.0
Iced, Chai, Latte, Tall, Semi Skimmed Milk, Starbucks*	1 Tall/335ml	176	3.0	52	1.6	9.7	0.9	0.0
Iced, Chai, Latte, Tall, Skimmed Milk, Starbucks*	1 Tall/335ml	152	0.2	45	1.6	9.9	0.1	0.0
Iced, Chai, Latte, Tall, Soy, Starbucks*	1 Tall/335ml	162	2.4	48	1.4	9.1	0.7	0.2
Iced, Chai, Latte, Tall, Whole Milk, Starbucks*	1 Tall/335ml	191	5.0	57	1.6	9.7	1.5	0.0
Iced, Chai, Latte, Venti, Semi Skimmed Milk, Starbucks*	1 Venti/591ml	277	4.4	47	1.3	9.0	0.7	0.0
Iced, Chai, Latte, Venti, Skimmed Milk, Starbucks*	1 Venti/591ml	242	0.3	41	1.4	9.0	0.1	0.0
Iced, Chai, Latte, Venti, Soy, Starbucks*	1 Venti/591ml	256	3.5	43	1.2	8.5	0.6	0.2
Iced, Chai, Latte, Venti, Whole Milk, Starbucks*	1 Venti/591ml	299	7.2	51	1.3	9.0	1.2	0.0
TOPPING								
Caramel - 4g, Starbucks*	1 Serving/4ml	15	0.6	372	0.0	62.5	15.0	0.0
Chocolate - 4g, Starbucks*	1 Serving/4ml	6	0.1	152	2.5	37.5	2.5	2.5
Sprinkles - 1g, Starbucks*	1 Serving/1g	4	0.0	380	0.0	100.0	0.0	0.0
Whipped Cream, Cold, Grande, Starbucks*	1 Grande/32g	114	11.2	356	1.9	9.4	35.0	0.0
Whipped Cream, Cold, Tall, Starbucks*	1 Tall/25g	81	8.0	324	1.6	8.0	32.0	0.0
Whipped Cream, Cold, Venti, Starbucks*	1 Venti/35g	104	10.2	297	1.7	8.6	29.1	0.0
Whipped Cream, Hot, Grande/Venti, Starbucks*	1 Serving/21g	72	7.0	343	1.9	9.5	33.3	0.0
Whipped Cream, Hot, Short, Starbucks*	1 Short/16g	52	5.1	325	1.9	6.2	31.9	0.0
Whipped Cream, Hot, Tall Beverage - 19g, Starbucks*	1 Tall/19g	62	6.1	326	1.6	10.5	32.1	0.0
WAFFLES								
Caramel, Large, Starbucks*	1 Waffle/80g	354	16.2	443	3.2	62.2	20.3	1.1
YOGHURT								
Apple, Oats & Berries, Breakfast Pot, Starbucks*	1 Pot/180g	319	11.9	177	4.1	24.3	6.6	2.1
Natural, Creamy, Starbucks*	1 Serving/140g	132	6.4	94	5.5	7.5	4.6	0.0
SUBWAY								
BACON								
2 Strips, Subway*	2 Strips/9g	40	2.9	444	33.3	0.0	32.2	0.0
BREAD								
Flatbread, Subway*	1 Flatbread/85g	203	2.5	239	9.4	42.4	2.9	3.1

SUBWAY

	Measure INFO/WEIGHT	per Measure KCAL	FAT	Nutrition Values per 100g / 100ml KCAL	PROT	CARB	FAT	FIBRE
BREAD								
Rolls, Sub, Honey Oat, 9 Grain, 6 Inch, Subway*	1 Sub/78g	198	1.5	254	11.5	44.9	1.9	6.7
Rolls, Sub, Italian, Hearty, 6 Inch, Subway*	1 Bread/75g	201	1.5	268	10.7	50.7	2.0	2.8
Rolls, Sub, Italian, Herbs & Cheese, 6 Inch, Subway*	1 Sub/82g	234	4.3	285	12.2	46.3	5.2	2.3
Rolls, Sub, Wheat, 9 Grain, 6 Inch, Subway*	1 Bread/78g	198	1.5	254	11.5	44.9	1.9	6.7
Rolls, Sub, White, Italian, 6 Inch, Subway*	1 Sub/71g	190	1.3	268	9.9	50.7	1.8	2.2
CANDY								
Chocolate Chip, Subway*	1 Serving/45g	211	9.7	469	4.4	66.7	21.6	2.0
CHEESE								
American, Subway*	1 Serving/11g	40	3.4	364	18.2	9.1	30.9	0.0
Cheddar, Monterey, Subway*	1 Serving/14g	57	4.4	407	25.0	0.0	31.4	0.0
Peppered, Subway*	1 Serving/11g	39	3.1	355	18.2	0.0	28.2	0.0
COOKIES								
Chocolate Chip, Subway*	1 Cookie/45g	218	10.3	484	4.4	64.4	22.9	2.4
Chocolate Chunk, Subway*	1 Cookie/45g	214	10.2	476	4.4	66.7	22.7	2.0
Double Choc Chip, Subway*	1 Cookie/45g	221	11.7	491	4.4	60.0	26.0	2.7
Oatmeal Raisin, Subway*	1 Cookie/45g	196	8.1	436	6.7	66.7	18.0	1.1
Rainbow, Subway*	1 Cookie/45g	211	9.7	469	4.4	66.7	21.6	2.0
White Chip, Mac Nut, Subway*	1 Cookie/45g	218	11.0	484	4.4	62.2	24.4	1.1
DOUGHNUTS								
Chocolate, Subway*	1 Doughnut/55g	243	15.5	442	7.3	38.2	28.2	2.2
Sugared, Subway*	1 Doughnut/49g	207	11.6	422	6.1	42.9	23.7	1.0
DRESSING								
Ranch, Subway*	1 Serving/21g	44	4.5	210	0.0	4.8	21.4	0.0
FLATBREAD								
Bacon, Breakfast, Subway*	1 Flatbread/113g	276	7.3	244	13.7	31.9	6.5	2.3
Bacon, Egg, & Cheese, Breakfast, Subway*	1 Flatbread/145g	335	12.4	231	11.7	25.9	8.6	1.9
Beef, Melt, Big, Subway*	1 Flatbread/247g	418	17.9	169	8.5	16.4	7.2	2.0
Beef, Subway*	1 Flatbread/226g	287	4.0	127	9.9	17.2	1.8	1.6
Chicken, & Bacon, Ranch, Melt, Subway*	1 Flatbread/299g	508	20.2	170	12.4	13.8	6.8	1.2
Chicken, Breast, Subway*	1 Flatbread/240g	309	4.0	129	11.0	16.7	1.7	1.5
Chicken, Tandoori, Subway*	1 Flatbread/261g	320	4.7	123	10.3	14.9	1.8	1.4
Chicken, Temptation, Subway*	1 Flatbread/269g	411	9.7	153	9.8	19.8	3.6	1.3
Chicken, Teriyaki, & Sweet Onion, Subway*	1 Flatbread/283g	359	4.2	127	9.6	18.2	1.5	1.4
Chicken, Tikka, Subway*	1 Flatbread/240g	128	1.7	128	11.0	16.4	1.7	1.5
Club, Subway*	1 Flatbread/259g	315	4.4	122	10.9	15.2	1.7	1.4
Egg, & Cheese, Breakfast, Subway*	1 Flatbread/131g	299	10.0	228	10.0	28.6	7.6	2.1
Ham, Subway*	1 Sandwich/226g	274	4.5	121	8.3	17.6	2.0	1.6
Italian, BMT, Subway*	1 Flatbread/233g	401	17.7	172	8.8	16.9	7.6	1.6
Italian, Spicy, Subway*	1 Flatbread/229g	476	26.3	208	8.9	17.0	11.5	1.6
Meatball, Marinara, Subway*	1 Flatbread/307g	440	16.5	143	7.5	16.4	5.4	2.2
Mega Melt, Breakfast, Subway*	1 Flatbread/221g	512	23.5	232	12.8	20.4	10.6	1.6
Sausage, Breakfast, Subway*	1 Flatbread/161g	379	13.6	235	12.1	27.1	8.4	2.1
Sausage, Egg, & Cheese, Breakfast, Subway*	1 Flatbread/207g	475	21.1	229	11.9	21.8	10.2	1.7
Steak, & Cheese, Subway*	1 Flatbread/252g	348	9.5	138	9.9	16.4	3.8	1.6
Subway Melt, with Cheese, Subway*	1 Flatbread/256g	364	10.2	142	10.6	15.6	4.0	1.4
Tuna, Subway*	1 Flatbread/240g	364	13.6	152	8.4	16.9	5.7	1.5
Turkey, & Ham, Subway*	1 Flatbread/235g	283	4.0	120	9.2	16.7	1.7	1.5
Turkey, Breast, Subway*	1 Flatbread/226g	274	3.2	121	9.2	17.2	1.4	1.6
Veggie Delite, Subway*	1 Flatbread/169g	218	2.6	129	5.2	22.7	1.5	2.1
Veggie Patty, Subway*	1 Flatbread/254g	385	9.7	152	8.2	18.6	3.8	1.4
MAYONNAISE								
Light, Subway*	1 Serving/15g	56	6.0	373	0.0	6.7	40.0	0.0

SUBWAY

INFO/WEIGHT	Measure	per Measure KCAL	FAT	Nutrition Values per 100g / 100ml KCAL	PROT	CARB	FAT	FIBRE
MEATBALLS								
Bowl, Subway*	1 Bowl/206g	317	19.1	154	9.2	9.2	9.3	2.0
MUFFIN								
Blueberry, Subway*	1 Muffin/111g	352	20.6	317	4.5	36.0	18.6	2.7
Chocolate Chunk, Subway*	1 Muffin/111g	394	22.9	355	5.4	39.6	20.6	2.6
Double Chocolate Chunk, Subway*	1 Muffin/111g	389	22.0	350	5.4	40.5	19.8	2.8
NACHOS								
Cheese, Melted, Subway*	1 Serving/126g	415	24.3	329	8.7	28.6	19.3	2.1
SALAD								
Beef, Subway*	1 Salad/328g	118	2.4	36	4.9	1.8	0.7	1.1
Chicken, Breast, Subway*	1 Salad/342g	139	2.4	41	5.8	2.0	0.7	1.0
Chicken, Teriyaki, & Sweet Onion, Subway*	1 Salad/385g	189	2.6	49	5.4	4.9	0.7	1.0
Chicken, Tikka, Subway*	1 Salad/342g	137	2.4	40	5.8	1.8	0.7	1.0
Club, Subway*	1 Salad/361g	145	2.8	40	6.1	1.9	0.8	1.0
Garden, Side, Subway*	1 Salad/135g	21	0.2	16	0.7	2.2	0.2	1.3
Ham, Subway*	1 Salad/328g	104	2.9	32	3.7	2.1	0.9	1.1
Turkey, & Ham, Subway*	1 Salad/338g	113	2.3	33	4.7	1.8	0.7	1.1
Turkey, Breast, Subway*	1 Salad/328g	104	1.6	32	4.6	1.8	0.5	1.1
Veggie Delite, Subway*	1 Salad/271g	49	1.0	18	1.1	1.8	0.4	1.3
SAUCE								
BBQ, Low Fat, Subway*	1 Serving/21g	37	0.1	176	0.0	42.9	0.5	1.0
Chipotle Southwest, Subway*	1 Serving/21g	90	9.2	429	0.0	9.5	43.8	0.5
Honey Mustard, Low Fat, Subway*	1 Serving/21g	32	0.2	152	0.0	33.3	1.0	0.5
Sweet Onion, Low Fat, Subway*	1 Serving/21g	34	0.1	162	0.0	38.1	0.5	0.5
SOUP								
Beef Goulash, Subway*	1 Serving/250g	199	11.8	80	3.3	6.0	4.7	0.9
Carrot and Coriander, Subway*	1 Serving/250g	81	1.8	32	0.9	5.6	0.7	1.1
Country Chicken & Vegetable, Subway*	1 Serving/250g	168	11.0	67	2.7	4.2	4.4	0.2
Cream of Chicken, Subway*	1 Serving/250g	160	11.3	64	2.7	3.1	4.5	0.0
Cream of Mushroom, Subway*	1 Serving/250g	150	10.8	60	1.0	4.4	4.3	0.3
Highland Vegetable, Subway*	1 Serving/250g	73	0.3	29	1.5	5.5	0.1	0.9
Leek & Potato, Subway*	1 Serving/250g	124	3.0	50	1.7	8.0	1.2	1.1
Lentil, & Potato, Subway*	1 Pot/250g	182	5.0	73	4.4	9.3	2.0	1.1
Lentil & Bacon, Subway*	1 Serving/250g	182	5.0	73	4.4	9.3	2.0	1.1
Minestrone, Subway*	1 Pot/250g	125	3.0	50	1.7	7.8	1.2	1.0
Red Pepper, & Tomato, Subway*	1 Pot/250g	100	4.0	40	1.4	6.0	1.6	0.9
Thai Style Vegetable, Subway*	1 Serving/250g	87	1.0	35	1.1	6.7	0.4	0.8
Tomato, Subway*	1 Serving/250g	103	3.8	41	0.8	6.1	1.5	0.3
Wild Mushroom, Subway*	1 Serving/250g	101	5.5	40	1.0	4.1	2.2	0.3
SUBS								
Bacon, Breakfast, Subway*	1 Sub/106g	271	6.3	256	15.1	33.0	5.9	4.9
Bacon, Egg, & Cheese, Breakfast, Subway*	1 Sub/138g	330	11.4	239	13.0	26.1	8.3	3.9
Beef, Kids Pak, Subway*	1 Sub/156g	210	2.2	135	10.3	18.6	1.4	3.1
Beef, Low Fat, Subway*	1 Sub/219g	282	3.0	129	10.5	17.4	1.4	2.9
Chicken, & Bacon, Ranch Melt, Subway*	1 Sub/292g	503	19.2	172	13.0	13.7	6.6	2.2
Chicken, & Jalapeño, Melt, Subway*	1 Sub/249g	345	6.4	139	11.7	15.7	2.6	2.6
Chicken, Breast, Low Fat, Subway*	1 Sub/233g	304	3.0	130	11.6	16.7	1.3	2.7
Chicken, Tandoori, Low Fat, Subway*	1 Sub/254g	315	3.7	124	11.0	15.0	1.5	2.5
Chicken, Temptation, Subway*	1 Sub/262g	406	8.7	155	10.3	19.8	3.3	2.4
Chicken, Teriyaki, Sweet Onion, Low Fat, Subway*	1 Sub/276g	354	3.3	128	10.1	18.1	1.2	2.4
Chicken, Tikka, Low Fat, Subway*	1 Sub/233g	302	3.0	130	11.6	16.3	1.3	2.7
Club, Low Fat, Subway*	1 Sub/252g	310	3.4	123	11.5	15.1	1.4	2.5
Egg, & Cheese, Breakfast, Subway*	1 Sub/124g	294	9.0	237	11.3	29.0	7.3	4.4

	Measure INFO/WEIGHT	per Measure		Nutrition Values per 100g / 100ml				
		KCAL	FAT	KCAL	PROT	CARB	FAT	FIBRE
SUBWAY								
SUBS								
Ham, Kids Pak, Subway*	1 Sub/147g	192	2.2	131	8.2	19.7	1.5	3.3
Ham, Low Fat, Subway*	1 Sub/219g	269	3.5	123	8.7	17.4	1.6	2.9
Italian BMT, Subway*	1 Sub/226g	396	16.8	175	9.3	16.8	7.4	2.8
Meatball Marinara, Subway*	1 Sub/300g	435	15.5	145	8.0	16.3	5.2	3.1
Mega Melt, Breakfast, Subway*	1 Sub/214g	507	22.5	237	13.6	20.6	10.5	2.9
Sausage, Breakfast, Subway*	1 Sub/154g	374	12.6	243	13.0	27.3	8.2	4.0
Sausage, Egg, & Cheese, Breakfast, Subway*	1 Sub/200g	470	20.1	235	12.5	22.0	10.0	3.1
Spicy Italian, Subway*	1 Sub/222g	471	25.3	212	9.5	17.1	11.4	2.8
Steak & Cheese, Subway*	1 Sub/245g	343	8.5	140	10.6	16.3	3.5	2.7
Subway Melt, Includes Cheese, Subway*	1 Sub/249g	359	9.3	144	11.2	15.7	3.7	2.5
Tuna, Subway*	1 Sub/233g	359	12.6	154	9.0	16.7	5.4	2.7
Turkey, & Ham, Low Fat, Subway*	1 Sub/228g	278	3.0	122	9.6	16.7	1.3	2.8
Turkey, Breast, Kids Pak, Subway*	1 Sub/156g	201	1.6	129	9.6	18.6	1.0	3.1
Turkey, Breast, Low Fat, Subway*	1 Sub/219g	269	2.2	123	10.0	17.4	1.0	2.9
Veggie Delite, Kids Pak, Subway*	1 Sub/118g	164	1.2	139	5.9	24.6	1.0	4.1
Veggie Delite, Low Fat, Subway*	1 Sub/162g	213	1.6	131	5.6	22.8	1.0	3.9
Veggie Patty, Subway*	1 Sub/247g	380	8.7	154	8.9	18.6	3.5	2.6
TOASTIE								
Cheese, Subway*	1 Toastie/64g	210	9.5	328	17.2	29.7	14.8	1.2
Pepperoni Pizza, Subway*	1 Toastie/93g	247	12.4	266	11.8	23.7	13.3	1.4
WRAPS								
Beef, Subway*	1 Wrap/242g	412	8.1	170	9.1	25.6	3.3	1.3
Chicken & Bacon Ranch Melt, Subway*	1 Wrap/315g	633	24.3	201	11.7	20.6	7.7	1.0
Chicken Breast, Subway*	1 Wrap/256g	434	8.1	170	10.2	24.6	3.2	1.2
Chicken Temptation, Subway*	1 Wrap/285g	536	13.8	188	9.1	27.0	4.8	1.1
Chicken Tikka, Subway*	1 Wrap/256g	432	8.1	169	10.2	24.6	3.2	1.2
Ham, Subway*	1 Wrap/242g	399	8.6	165	7.9	26.0	3.6	1.3
Italian B.M.T., Subway*	1 Wrap/249g	526	21.8	211	8.4	25.3	8.8	1.2
Meatball Marinara, Subway*	1 Wrap/323g	561	20.2	174	7.1	22.9	6.3	1.9
Spicy Italian, Subway*	1 Wrap/245g	602	30.4	246	8.2	25.3	12.4	1.3
Steak & Cheese, with Peppers & Onions, Subway*	1 Wrap/268g	473	13.6	176	9.3	24.3	5.1	1.3
Subway Club, Subway*	1 Wrap/275g	440	8.5	160	10.2	22.9	3.1	1.1
Subway Melt with Cheese, Subway*	1 Wrap/272g	489	14.3	180	9.9	23.2	5.3	1.1
Sweet Onion Chicken Teriyaki, Subway*	1 Wrap/299g	484	8.3	162	9.0	25.1	2.8	1.2
Tuna, Subway*	1 Wrap/256g	489	17.7	191	7.8	25.0	6.9	1.2
Turkey Breast, Subway*	1 Wrap/242g	399	7.3	165	8.7	25.6	3.0	1.3
Turkey Breast & Ham, Subway*	1 Wrap/251g	408	8.1	163	8.8	25.1	3.2	1.2
Veggie Delite, Subway*	1 Wrap/185g	343	6.7	185	4.9	33.5	3.6	1.7
Veggie Patty, Subway*	1 Wrap/270g	510	13.8	189	7.8	26.3	5.1	1.1
WAGAMAMA								
BEANS								
Edamame with Salt, Wagamama*	1 Serving/202g	179	6.3	89	6.6	3.7	3.1	9.9
BEEF								
Teriyaki Soba, Wagamama*	1 Serving/607g	829	38.5	137	8.1	11.2	6.3	1.0
CAKE								
Chocolate Fudge with Vanilla Ice Cream, Wagamama*	1 Serving/203g	671	36.9	331	4.0	37.6	18.2	0.4
CHA HAN								
Chicken & Prawn, Rice, Wagamama*	1 Dinner/778g	972	24.9	125	5.1	18.6	3.2	0.8
Mini Chicken, Fried Rice & Vegetables, Wagamama*	1 Serving/245g	429	11.5	175	8.2	24.9	4.7	0.4
CHEESECAKE								
White Chocolate Ginger, Wagamama*	1 Serving/142g	460	22.2	324	5.2	40.3	15.6	0.6

	Measure INFO/WEIGHT	per Measure KCAL	FAT	Nutrition Values per 100g / 100ml KCAL	PROT	CARB	FAT	FIBRE
WAGAMAMA								
CHICKEN								
Firecracker, Stir Fried with Vegetables, Wagamama*	1 Portion/720g	1056	27.4	147	7.7	20.1	3.8	0.6
Grilled, Katsu Curry, Wagamama*	1 Serving/569g	871	30.2	153	6.0	20.1	5.3	0.5
Mini with Sauce & Rice, Wagamama*	1 Serving/295g	484	13.9	164	8.0	22.2	4.7	0.5
Raisukaree in Coconut Curry Sauce, Wagamama*	1 Serving/774g	1276	58.0	165	5.7	18.4	7.5	0.5
Tama Rice, Wagamama*	1 Meal/810g	917	25.9	113	4.5	16.4	3.2	0.5
Tebasaki, Wagamama*	1 Serving/105g	274	15.5	261	21.7	9.8	14.8	1.3
Teriyaki Donburi, Wagamama*	1 Serving/580g	934	17.0	161	9.1	24.2	2.9	0.6
Tori Kara Age, Wagamama*	1 Serving/171g	494	30.4	289	25.9	6.3	17.8	0.1
CHICKEN								
Itame, & Noodles in Green Coconut Soup, Wagamama*	1 Portion/829g	850	51.4	103	4.5	6.6	6.2	1.1
COD								
Cubes, Deep Fried, with Rice & Veg, Wagamama*	1 Serving/344g	582	19.3	169	6.4	22.9	5.6	0.7
CURRY								
Chicken, Chu Chee, Wagamama*	1 Serving/824g	1350	61.7	164	4.9	18.8	7.5	0.7
Chicken, Kastu, Wagamama*	1 Serving/619g	1103	45.2	178	7.5	20.5	7.3	0.5
EBI KATSU								
Prawns, Deep Fried in Panko Crumbs, Wagamama*	1 Serving/129g	289	18.2	224	9.4	14.5	14.1	0.9
FROZEN YOGHURT								
Chocolate, Chilli & Ginger, Wagamama*	1 Serving/195g	300	3.7	154	5.0	28.7	1.9	1.4
Citrus Yuzu, Wagamama*	1 Serving/133g	196	2.8	147	4.7	27.3	2.1	0.2
Strawberry & Five Spices, Wagamama*	1 Serving/133g	224	2.5	168	4.5	33.2	1.9	0.2
GYOZA								
Chicken & Vegetable, Dumplings, Wagamama*	1 Serving/149g	236	10.6	158	7.6	15.0	7.1	2.0
Duck Dumplings with Hoi Sin Sauce, Wagamama*	1 Serving/115g	299	12.3	260	10.4	29.2	10.7	2.8
Ebi, Prawn & Vegetable Dumplings, Wagamama*	1 Serving/112g	219	8.4	196	8.3	22.0	7.5	3.2
Sweet Ginger & Apple, Dumplings, Wagamama*	5 Dumplings/135g	358	9.6	265	3.3	46.4	7.1	1.2
Yasai, Vegetable Dumplings, Wagamama*	1 Serving/150g	301	19.0	201	3.1	17.5	12.7	2.3
ICE CREAM								
Coconut Reika, Wagamama*	1 Serving/195g	417	21.4	214	3.5	25.0	11.0	0.7
ITAME								
Prawn, Wagamama*	1 Bowl/769g	746	49.2	94	2.0	6.9	6.2	1.1
JUICE								
Apple, Mint, Celery & Lime, Wagamama*	1 Serving/273g	153	0.3	56	0.2	13.8	0.1	0.3
Apple & Orange, Wagamama*	1 Serving/271g	129	0.3	48	0.4	11.2	0.1	0.6
Blueberry, Apple & Ginger, Wagamama*	1 Serving/359g	183	0.4	51	0.4	11.2	0.1	2.0
Carrot with a Hint of Ginger, Wagamama*	1 Serving/312g	72	0.0	23	0.2	5.0	0.0	1.1
Fruit, Refreshing Cleansing Blend, Wagamama*	1 Serving/311g	128	0.0	41	0.4	9.9	0.0	0.3
KUSHIYAKI								
Lollipop Prawn, Wagamama*	1 Serving/122g	228	16.6	187	10.4	5.6	13.6	0.4
NOODLES								
Amai Udon, Teppan Fried, Wagamama*	1 Serving/676g	865	35.1	128	5.5	13.9	5.2	1.7
Chicken, Spicy, & Soba Noodles, Wagamama*	1 Serving/703g	944	40.8	134	6.0	14.2	5.8	0.8
Chicken Ramen with Vegetables in Soup, Wagamama*	1 Serving/810g	519	13.0	64	5.1	7.0	1.6	0.4
Ginger Chicken Udon, Wagamama*	1 Serving/605g	752	28.4	124	7.0	12.6	4.7	1.6
Grilled Mini Chicken Breast with Veg, Wagamama*	1 Serving/273g	373	7.4	137	12.1	15.9	2.7	0.4
Grilled Mini Fish & Vegetables, Wagamama*	1 Serving/248g	309	6.7	125	7.5	17.4	2.7	0.5
Pad Thai, Chicken & Prawn, Wagamama*	1 Serving/648g	794	31.0	123	5.4	13.8	4.8	1.4
Yaki Udon, Wagamama*	1 Serviing/619g	716	26.0	116	5.8	12.8	4.2	1.8
Yasai Chilli Men, Wagamama*	1 Bowl/673g	923	44.2	137	3.6	15.4	6.6	1.1
Yasai Pad Thai, Wagamama*	1 Portion/632g	820	36.7	130	4.4	14.3	5.8	1.4
PRAWNS								
Firecracker, Stir fried with Vegetables, Wagamama*	1 Serving/659g	906	24.4	138	3.8	21.9	3.7	0.7

	Measure	per Measure		Nutrition Values per 100g / 100ml				
	INFO/WEIGHT	KCAL	FAT	KCAL	PROT	CARB	FAT	FIBRE
WAGAMAMA								
RAMEN								
Chilli Beef, Wagamama*	1 Serving/989g	680	22.7	69	5.1	6.7	2.3	0.6
Chilli Chicken, Wagamama*	1 Serving/949g	597	16.1	63	4.6	6.9	1.7	0.6
Grilled Fish, Seafood & Noodles, Wagamama*	1 Bowl/685g	463	4.8	68	5.6	9.5	0.7	0.4
SALAD								
Chicken Mandarin & Sesame, Wagamama*	1 Serving/393g	790	54.2	201	11.0	7.7	13.8	1.1
Ginger Beef & Coriander, Wagamama*	1 Serving/433g	686	54.6	158	8.4	2.5	12.6	1.0
SOUP								
Teriyaki Salmon Ramen, Wagamama*	1 Serving/913g	711	22.9	78	5.6	7.8	2.5	0.8
Yasai Itame, Wagamama*	1 Serving/799g	845	58.8	106	2.3	7.0	7.4	1.2
SQUID								
Deep Fried with Shichimi & Chilli Sauce, Wagamama*	1 Serving/208g	493	33.3	237	8.7	14.3	16.0	0.4
SUSHI								
California Roll, Inside Out with Surimi, Wagamama*	1 Serving/93g	132	3.3	142	2.0	25.1	3.5	0.8
Cucumber Hosomaki, Wagamama*	1 Serving/108g	138	0.6	129	1.5	29.2	0.6	0.5
Hosomaki, Avocado, Wagamama*	1 Serving/113g	176	4.5	157	1.7	28.0	4.0	1.0
Tuna Hosomaki, Wagamama*	1 Serving/118g	171	0.9	145	8.0	26.5	0.8	0.0
Tuna Nigiri, Wagamama*	1 Serving/72g	102	0.7	142	10.1	23.1	1.0	0.0
Uramaki, Mango, Avocado & Cucumber, Wagamama*	1 Serving/84g	114	2.4	136	1.7	25.2	2.9	0.9
Uramaki, Salmon Skin with Avocado, Wagamama*	1 Serving/95g	169	6.3	178	6.0	23.3	6.7	0.7
Yasai Selection, Wagamama*	1 Serving/249g	345	6.3	139	1.7	26.8	2.5	0.9
TUNA								
Sashimi, Raw, Wagamama*	1 Serving/91g	109	1.9	120	21.6	3.7	2.1	0.0
Tataki, Wagamama*	1Serving/98g	95	1.1	96	17.4	3.6	1.1	1.4
WASABI CO LTD								
BEEF								
Sukiyaki Don, Wasabi Co Ltd*	1 Portion/592g	758	16.0	128	7.4	18.4	2.7	0.0
CHICKEN								
Gyoza, Steamed, Side Dish, Wasabi Co Ltd*	1 Portion/20g	43	2.6	215	8.3	16.3	13.0	0.0
Karaage, Wasabi Co Ltd*	1 Portion/210g	468	18.5	223	24.5	11.4	8.8	0.0
Katsu, Wasabi Co Ltd*	1 Portion/160g	421	9.0	263	26.9	26.3	5.6	0.0
Spicy, Don, Wasabi Co Ltd*	1 Portion/671g	825	18.8	123	7.8	16.5	2.8	0.0
Sweet Chilli, Wasabi Co Ltd*	1 Portion/350g	844	18.6	241	24.7	23.7	5.3	0.0
Sweet Chilli Don, Wasabi Co Ltd*	1 Portion/652g	991	28.0	152	7.6	20.7	4.3	0.0
Teriyaki, Wasabi Co Ltd*	1 Portion/350g	388	7.7	111	14.7	8.2	2.2	0.0
Teriyaki Don, Wasabi Co Ltd*	1 Portion/684g	732	9.6	107	6.9	16.6	1.4	0.0
with Spicy Sauce, Wasabi Co Ltd*	1 Portion/350g	402	8.4	115	14.0	9.3	2.4	0.0
CHICKEN								
Karaage, Side Dish, Wasabi Co Ltd*	1 Portion/70g	156	6.2	223	24.5	11.4	8.8	0.0
Yakitori, Side Dish, Wasabi Co Ltd*	1 Portion/40g	65	5.2	163	0.0	11.8	12.9	0.0
CURRY								
Chicken, Katsu Don, Wasabi Co Ltd*	1 Portion/668g	1136	34.7	170	8.3	22.5	5.2	0.0
Chicken, Wasabi Co Ltd*	1 Portion/350g	536	30.4	153	11.0	7.7	8.7	0.0
Chicken Katsu, Wasabi Co Ltd*	1 Portion/360g	774	33.5	215	13.4	19.5	9.3	0.0
Tofu, Wasabi Co Ltd*	1 Portion/350g	536	37.4	153	3.6	10.5	10.7	0.0
Tofu Don, Wasabi Co Ltd*	1 Portion/552g	707	25.4	128	2.9	18.9	4.6	0.0
NOODLES								
Roasted Veg Yakisoba, Wasabi Co Ltd*	1 Portion/630g	554	19.5	88	3.6	11.5	3.1	0.0
Stir Fry, Chicken Katsu Yakisoba, Wasabi Co Ltd*	1 Portion/568g	710	8.0	125	13.7	14.2	1.4	0.0
Stir Fry, Chicken Yakisoba, Wasabi Co Ltd*	1 Portion/450g	459	3.6	102	12.4	11.3	0.8	0.0
Stir Fry, Tofu Yakisoba, Wasabi Co Ltd*	1 Portion/450g	554	24.3	123	7.1	11.4	5.4	0.0
PRAWN								
Fried Don, Wasabi Co Ltd*	1 Portion/555g	666	15.0	120	2.2	21.8	2.7	0.0

	Measure INFO/WEIGHT	per Measure KCAL	FAT	Nutrition Values per 100g / 100ml KCAL	PROT	CARB	FAT	FIBRE

WASABI CO LTD

RICE

	Measure INFO/WEIGHT	KCAL	FAT	KCAL	PROT	CARB	FAT	FIBRE
Steamed, Wasabi Co Ltd*	1 Portion/250g	298	0.8	119	2.3	26.6	0.3	0.0

SALMON

Teriyaki, Wasabi Co Ltd*	1 Portion/150g	339	19.2	226	20.5	7.0	12.8	0.0

SOUP

Miso, Side Dish, Wasabi Co Ltd*	1 Portion/170ml	17	0.5	10	0.6	1.3	0.3	0.0

SUSHI

	Measure INFO/WEIGHT	KCAL	FAT	KCAL	PROT	CARB	FAT	FIBRE
Avocado Hosomaki, Wasabi Co Ltd*	1 Portion/40g	2	0.0	6	0.1	1.5	0.1	0.0
California Hand Roll, Wasabi Co Ltd*	1 Portion/119g	23	0.2	19	0.3	2.8	0.2	0.0
California Roll, Wasabi Co Ltd*	1 Portion/59g	4	0.1	7	0.1	2.9	0.2	0.0
Chicken Karaage Set, Wasabi Co Ltd*	1 Portion/818g	520	28.6	64	17.7	36.4	3.5	0.0
Chicken Katsu Salad, Wasabi Co Ltd*	1 Portion/858g	770	29.2	90	15.3	29.1	3.4	0.0
Chicken Teriyaki Hand Roll, Wasabi Co Ltd*	1 Portion/107g	21	0.2	20	2.1	2.3	0.2	0.0
Chicken Teriyaki Onigiri, Wasabi Co Ltd*	1 Portion/147g	47	0.6	32	6.8	1.1	0.4	0.0
Chicken Teriyaki Roll, Wasabi Co Ltd*	1 Portion/54g	4	0.1	7	1.0	2.5	0.2	0.0
Chirashi Sushi with Japanese Dressing, Wasabi Co Ltd*	1 Portion/660g	484	8.6	73	12.2	26.4	1.3	0.0
Crabmeat & Cucumber Roll, Wasabi Co Ltd*	1 Portion/60g	5	0.2	8	0.2	2.5	0.4	0.0
Cucumber Hosomaki, Wasabi Co Ltd*	1 Portion/29g	2	0.0	6	0.1	0.2	0.1	0.0
Edamame, Wasabi Co Ltd*	1 Portion/208g	25	6.0	12	1.1	9.2	2.9	0.0
Fried Prawn Hand Roll, Wasabi Co Ltd*	1 Portion/115g	26	0.6	22	0.3	1.9	0.5	0.0
Fried Prawn Roll, Wasabi Co Ltd*	1 Portion/46g	3	0.1	7	0.4	1.6	0.3	0.0
Hana Set, Wasabi Co Ltd*	1 Portion/538g	411	6.5	76	1.9	16.1	1.2	0.0
Harmony Set, Wasabi Co Ltd*	1 Portion/534g	403	7.5	75	3.1	17.1	1.4	0.0
Japanese Omelette Nigiri, Wasabi Co Ltd*	1 Portion/38g	3	0.1	7	0.8	0.7	0.2	0.0
Mini Chirashi Set, Wasabi Co Ltd*	1 Portion/487g	248	9.3	51	13.6	22.0	1.9	0.0
Mixed California Roll Set, Wasabi Co Ltd*	1 Portion/470g	248	15.5	53	7.5	20.5	3.3	0.0
Mixed Maki Set, Wasabi Co Ltd*	1 Portion/393g	205	4.3	52	2.9	14.4	1.1	0.0
Mixed Veg Set, Wasabi Co Ltd*	1 Portion/312g	149	3.1	48	10.1	9.8	1.0	0.0
Prawn Mayo Gunkan, Wasabi Co Ltd*	1 Portion/48g	3	0.2	5	0.1	1.7	0.5	0.0
Pumpkin Korokke Set, Wasabi Co Ltd*	1 Portion/517g	299	15.0	58	22.6	26.6	2.9	0.0
Rainbow Set, Wasabi Co Ltd*	1 Portion/618g	436	7.4	70	1.8	24.7	1.2	0.0
Salmon & Masago Roll, Wasabi Co Ltd*	1 Portion/59g	4	0.2	7	0.1	2.8	0.3	0.0
Salmon Hosomaki, Wasabi Co Ltd*	1 Portion/35g	2	0.0	6	0.1	0.6	0.1	0.0
Salmon Nigiri, Wasabi Co Ltd*	1 Portion/42g	2	0.0	6	0.1	1.1	0.1	0.0
Salmon Nigiri Set, Wasabi Co Ltd*	1 Portion/255g	96	1.8	38	2.4	6.7	0.7	0.0
Salmon Onigiri, Wasabi Co Ltd*	1 Portion/168g	44	0.7	26	0.5	3.7	0.4	0.0
Salmon Sesame Gunkan, Wasabi Co Ltd*	1 Portion/58g	3	0.1	5	0.1	3.5	0.1	0.0
Sashimi Set, Wasabi Co Ltd*	1 Portion/251g	230	10.8	92	9.8	3.4	4.3	0.0
Seaweed Onigiri, Wasabi Co Ltd*	1 Portion/172g	46	1.2	27	1.1	3.6	0.7	0.0
Seaweed Salad Gunkan, Wasabi Co Ltd*	1 Portion/39g	3	0.2	8	2.7	0.5	0.5	0.0
Shrimp Nigiri, Wasabi Co Ltd*	1 Portion/28g	2	0.1	6	0.1	0.1	0.2	0.0
Snomono Salad, Wasabi Co Ltd*	1 Portion/279g	83	14.2	30	14.6	9.6	5.1	0.0
Spicy Chirashi Sushi, Wasabi Co Ltd*	1 Portion/660g	519	9.2	79	12.6	23.5	1.4	0.0
Spicy Mini Chirashi Set, Wasabi Co Ltd*	1 Portion/487g	291	9.7	60	14.2	17.3	2.0	0.0
Spicy Salmon Gunkan, Wasabi Co Ltd*	1 Portion/54g	4	0.2	7	1.7	1.7	0.4	0.0
Spicy Salmon Roll, Wasabi Co Ltd*	1 Portion/60g	4	0.1	6	0.4	2.7	0.1	0.0
Sweet & Spicy Chicken Bento, Wasabi Co Ltd*	1 Portion/917g	923	22.9	101	15.1	21.4	2.5	0.0
Tobiko Cucumber Gunkan, Wasabi Co Ltd*	1 Portion/26g	2	0.1	6	0.7	0.1	0.2	0.0
Tofu Nigiri, Wasabi Co Ltd*	1 Portion/49g	3	0.0	6	0.2	1.7	0.1	0.0
Tofu Roll, Wasabi Co Ltd*	1 Portion/46g	3	0.0	6	0.5	1.6	0.1	0.0
Tuna & Mustard Onigiri, Wasabi Co Ltd*	1 Portion/171g	48	0.7	28	2.2	2.5	0.4	0.0
Tuna & Sweetcorn Roll, Wasabi Co Ltd*	1 Portion/51g	3	0.2	7	0.5	0.7	0.3	0.0
Tuna Hosomaki, Wasabi Co Ltd*	1 Portion/33g	2	0.0	6	0.1	0.3	0.1	0.0

	Measure INFO/WEIGHT	per Measure KCAL	FAT	Nutrition Values per 100g / 100ml KCAL	PROT	CARB	FAT	FIBRE
WASABI CO LTD								
SUSHI								
Tuna Nigiri, Wasabi Co Ltd*	1 Portion/38g	2	0.0	6	0.1	0.5	0.1	0.0
Wakame Seaweed Salad, Wasabi Co Ltd*	1 Portion/150g	339	8.7	226	15.2	28.2	5.8	0.0
Wasabi Special Bento, Wasabi Co Ltd*	1 Portion/614g	423	18.4	69	7.4	22.9	3.0	0.0
TANMEN								
Chicken, Wasabi Co Ltd*	1 Portion/833g	425	11.7	51	3.4	6.1	1.4	0.0
Chicken Dumpling, Wasabi Co Ltd*	1 Portion/833g	458	14.2	55	1.9	7.9	1.7	0.0
Prawn Tempura, Wasabi Co Ltd*	1 Portion/813g	382	9.8	47	1.1	8.0	1.2	0.0
Spicy Chicken, Wasabi Co Ltd*	1 Portion/864g	475	13.0	55	3.4	7.0	1.5	0.0
Veg, Wasabi Co Ltd*	1 Portion/819g	385	9.8	47	1.9	7.1	1.2	0.0
TEMPURA								
Prawn, Side Dish, Wasabi Co Ltd*	1 Portion/20g	38	2.1	189	0.0	23.0	10.7	0.0
WIMPY								
BREAKFAST								
Bacon & Egg Breakfast Roll, Wimpy*	1 Roll/194g	368	12.1	190	13.4	18.3	6.2	0.0
Bacon Breakfast Roll, Wimpy*	1 Roll/144g	278	5.1	193	13.3	24.7	3.5	0.0
Hashbrown, Wimpy*	1 Serving/424g	545	41.1	129	4.1	8.7	9.7	1.9
Sausage & Egg Breakfast Roll, Wimpy*	1 Roll/211g	527	28.4	250	11.8	20.3	13.5	0.0
Sausage Breakfast Roll, Wimpy*	1 Roll/161g	437	21.5	271	11.3	26.6	13.4	0.0
The Country Breakfast, Wimpy*	1 Serving/271g	392	23.1	145	9.4	6.9	8.5	1.7
The Great Wimpy Breakfast, Wimpy*	1 Serving/459g	910	53.6	198	10.7	12.7	11.7	1.2
Toast with Jam, Extra, Wimpy*	1 Serving/89g	276	8.3	310	7.3	52.6	9.3	1.7
Wimpy Club, Wimpy*	1 Serving/330g	767	38.6	232	14.7	18.2	11.7	0.8
BURGERS								
BBQ Burger, Wimpy*	1 Burger/236g	644	30.5	273	14.2	24.6	12.9	1.6
Bender in a Bun with Cheese, Wimpy*	1 Burger/170g	424	23.4	249	10.2	20.8	13.8	1.2
Chicken & Bacon Melt, Wimpy*	1 Burger/172g	443	20.2	258	12.6	25.4	11.7	0.0
Chicken Fillet, in a Bun, Savoury, Wimpy*	1 Burger/218g	356	13.8	163	10.4	16.1	6.3	1.1
Chicken Fillet, Wimpy*	1 Burger/327g	380	16.8	116	6.7	11.1	5.1	0.0
Chicken Fillet in a Bun, Hot & Spicy, Wimpy*	1 Burger/193g	398	18.5	206	10.6	19.1	9.6	1.8
Chicken in a Bun, Wimpy*	1 Burger/191g	449	21.4	235	10.4	22.7	11.2	1.3
Classic, Wimpy*	1 Burger/159g	337	15.1	212	12.4	19.9	9.5	0.0
Classic Bacon Cheeseburger, Wimpy*	1 Burger/192g	405	19.0	211	13.6	16.8	9.9	0.0
Classic Kingsize, Wimpy*	1 Burger/227g	551	31.1	243	16.2	14.2	13.7	0.0
Classic with Cheese, Wimpy*	1 Burger/175g	379	18.5	217	12.7	17.3	10.6	1.1
Halfpounder with Bacon & Cheese, Wimpy*	1 Burger/312g	892	50.5	286	19.2	15.5	16.2	0.8
Mega Burger, Wimpy*	1 Burger/206g	594	36.0	288	15.3	18.0	17.5	0.0
Quarterpounder, Wimpy*	1 Burger/200g	538	31.3	269	15.0	18.0	15.6	0.0
Quarterpounder with Bacon & Cheese, Wimpy*	1 Burger/237g	658	33.4	278	16.8	20.5	14.1	1.1
Quarterpounder with Cheese, Wimpy*	1 Burger/213g	578	34.6	271	15.1	17.2	16.2	0.0
Spicy Bean, Wimpy*	1 Burger/233g	611	29.4	262	5.9	30.5	12.6	2.7
Spicy Bean with Cheese, Wimpy*	1 Burger/245g	1459	98.3	596	24.2	35.5	40.1	2.7
CHICKEN								
Chicken Chunks with Chips, Wimpy*	1 Serving/333g	779	46.8	234	8.3	19.0	14.0	1.5
CHOCOLATE								
Crushed Flake (for Desserts), Wimpy*	1 Serving/20g	104	6.1	520	7.5	57.0	30.5	1.0
DESSERT								
Brown Derby with Dairy Ice Cream, Wimpy*	1 Serving/180g	431	20.6	239	4.5	31.3	11.4	1.4
Brownie Sundae, Wimpy*	1 Sundae/252g	574	21.8	228	3.8	34.7	8.6	0.6
Cheese Cake, Wimpy*	1 Serving/144g	412	18.3	286	4.5	38.5	12.7	0.0
Chocolate Fudge Cake, Wimpy*	1 Serving/100g	371	12.4	371	4.7	60.2	12.4	0.0
Chocolate Waffle with Dairy Ice Cream, Wimpy*	1 Serving/178g	691	37.0	388	5.1	45.3	20.8	0.0
Chocolate Waffle with Squirty Cream, Wimpy*	1 Serving/158g	667	36.9	422	5.1	47.7	23.4	0.0

WIMPY

INFO/WEIGHT	Measure	per Measure KCAL	per Measure FAT	Nutrition Values per 100g / 100ml KCAL	PROT	CARB	FAT	FIBRE

DESSERT

	Measure INFO/WEIGHT	KCAL	FAT	KCAL	PROT	CARB	FAT	FIBRE
Dairy Ice Cream with Chocolate Sauce, Wimpy*	1 Serving/88g	200	8.1	227	3.4	32.5	9.2	0.0
Dairy Ice Cream with Strawberry Sauce, Wimpy*	1 Serving/88g	199	7.9	226	3.0	34.3	9.0	0.0
Deep Filled Apple Tart, Wimpy*	1 Serving/164g	339	10.2	207	1.7	36.2	6.2	0.0
Eskimo Waffle, Wimpy*	1 Serving/228g	694	30.2	304	4.6	42.7	13.2	1.3
Half Chocolate Waffle with Dairy Ice Cream, Wimpy*	1 Serving/116g	395	18.8	341	4.0	44.7	16.2	0.0
Ice Cream Sundae, Plain, Wimpy*	1 Sundae/170g	190	8.8	112	3.1	15.0	5.2	0.0
Mini Knickerbocker Glory with Dairy Ice Cream, Wimpy*	1 Serving/194g	190	8.5	98	1.6	13.2	4.4	0.0
Spotted Dick Pudding, Wimpy*	1 Serving/130g	400	16.5	308	4.1	44.2	12.7	0.0
Toffee Sundae, Wimpy*	1 Sundae/239g	537	23.6	225	3.8	30.8	9.9	0.8
Treacle Sponge Pudding, Wimpy*	1 Serving/130g	504	21.3	388	3.9	56.1	16.4	0.0

EXTRAS

Bacon, Wimpy*	1 Serving/91g	267	22.0	294	24.2	0.0	24.2	0.0
Cheese, Slice, Wimpy*	1 Slice/12g	40	3.3	333	18.3	5.0	27.5	0.0
Chips Large Portion, Wimpy*	1 Portion/143g	333	17.1	233	3.0	30.4	12.0	3.0
Chips Standard Portion, Wimpy*	1 Portion/114g	267	13.7	234	3.0	30.5	12.0	3.0
Coleslaw, Wimpy*	1 Serving/50g	49	3.8	98	1.4	6.2	7.6	0.8
Egg, Wimpy*	1 Egg/50g	90	7.0	180	13.6	0.0	14.0	0.0
Hash Browns, Wimpy*	1 Serving/55g	93	7.8	169	2.2	19.6	14.2	1.8
Heinz Baked Beans, Wimpy*	1 Portion/110g	85	0.2	77	4.4	12.6	0.2	3.6
Mozarella Meltz 3, Wimpy*	3 Meltz/79g	253	15.4	320	15.4	25.7	19.5	2.5
Mozarella Meltz 6, Wimpy*	6 Meltz/157g	506	30.8	322	15.6	25.9	19.6	2.5
Onion Rings Large (12), Wimpy*	1 Portion/180g	401	23.2	223	3.2	23.6	12.9	3.0
Onion Rings Standard (6), Wimpy*	1 Portion/90g	201	11.6	223	3.2	23.6	12.9	3.0
Side Salad, Wimpy*	1 Portion/145g	44	0.3	30	1.4	6.1	0.2	0.8

FISH

Haddock, Peas & Chips, Wimpy*	1 Serving/314g	674	37.9	215	6.6	21.2	12.1	2.4
Scampi & Chips with Peas, Wimpy*	1 Serving/303g	577	29.8	190	5.2	22.7	9.8	2.3

GRILL

BBQ Rib Rack Platter, Wimpy*	1 Serving/439g	713	35.2	162	5.6	17.5	8.0	1.4
Classic Bacon Grill, Wimpy*	1 Serving/321g	722	45.3	225	11.5	14.0	14.1	0.0
Gourmet Chicken Platter, Wimpy*	1 Serving/392g	525	21.4	134	11.4	10.0	5.5	1.4
Sausage, Egg & Chips, Wimpy*	1 Serving/244g	597	38.8	245	9.0	17.4	15.9	1.7
Steak Platter, Wimpy*	1 Serving/424g	719	38.0	170	9.9	12.9	9.0	0.0
The International Grill, Wimpy*	1 Serving/416g	1010	71.3	243	13.9	10.0	17.1	0.9
Wimpy All-Day Breakfast, Wimpy*	1 Serving/410g	731	39.7	178	8.3	14.5	9.7	0.0

ICE CREAMS

Banana Longboat with Soft Ice Cream, Wimpy*	1 Serving/209g	260	6.0	124	2.3	23.9	2.9	0.0
Brown Derby with Dairy Ice Cream, Wimpy*	1 Serving/125g	397	19.7	318	5.6	38.9	15.8	0.0
Choc Nut Sundae, Wimpy*	1 Serving/83g	196	6.2	236	4.6	38.4	7.5	0.0
Fruit & Nut Sundae, Wimpy*	1 Serving/83g	138	5.8	166	4.2	23.3	7.0	0.0
Ice Cream Portion, Soft with Chocolate Sauce, Wimpy*	1 Serving/71g	137	3.2	193	2.8	36.1	4.5	0.0
Ice Cream Portion, Soft with Strawberry Sauce, Wimpy*	1 Serving/71g	137	3.0	193	2.4	38.3	4.2	0.0
Knickerbockerglory with Soft Ice Cream, Wimpy*	1 Serving/138g	196	6.0	142	2.7	24.7	4.4	0.0
Triple Strawberry Sundae with Soft Ice Cream, Wimpy*	1 Serving/170g	123	3.3	72	1.4	13.1	1.9	0.0

KIDS

Cheese Toastie with Salad, Wimpy*	1 Serving/250g	367	8.8	147	5.9	24.2	3.5	1.2
Chicken Chunks Meal with Chips, Wimpy*	1 Serving/172g	440	26.1	256	8.4	22.2	15.2	1.8
Chicken Chunks Meal with Salad, Wimpy*	1 Serving/187g	265	16.8	142	6.8	8.4	9.0	0.8
Fish Bites Meal with Chips, Wimpy*	1 Serving/160g	380	20.9	238	6.7	24.7	13.1	2.1
Fish Bites Meal with Salad, Wimpy*	1 Serving/175g	205	11.6	117	5.2	9.8	6.6	0.9
Hamburger Meal with Chips, Wimpy*	1 Serving/184g	457	20.0	248	9.0	29.9	10.9	0.0
Hamburger Meal with Salad, Wimpy*	1 Serving/199g	283	10.7	142	7.5	16.4	5.4	0.0

WIMPY

	Measure INFO/WEIGHT	per Measure		Nutrition Values per 100g / 100ml				
		KCAL	FAT	KCAL	PROT	CARB	FAT	FIBRE
KIDS								
Junior Cheeseburger Meal with Chips, Wimpy*	1 Serving/191g	497	23.5	260	10.0	27.8	12.3	2.1
Sausage Meal with Chips, Wimpy*	1 Serving/160g	428	27.7	268	8.9	19.9	17.3	1.9
Wimpy Hot Dog with Salad, Wimpy*	1 Serving/241g	425	21.1	176	7.0	17.3	8.8	0.0
MUFFIN								
Giant Blueberry, Wimpy*	1 Muffin/108g	470	25.6	435	5.9	48.9	23.7	0.0
NUTS								
Nibbed (for Desserts), Wimpy*	1 Serving/5g	32	2.8	640	26.0	6.0	56.0	12.0
PANINI								
Cheese & Tomato, Wimpy*	1 Panini/225g	694	25.1	309	14.6	37.4	11.1	2.2
Cheese with Red Onion, Wimpy*	1 Panini/205g	673	22.8	329	14.6	42.7	11.1	1.9
Ham, Tomato & Cheese, Wimpy*	1 Panini/275g	1145	39.0	417	33.0	38.4	14.2	2.2
Ham & Cheese, Wimpy*	1 Panini/235g	944	33.3	402	32.0	35.7	14.2	1.4
Steak, Cheese & Onion, Wimpy*	1 Panini/305g	688	28.6	226	13.8	21.4	9.4	1.0
POTATO JACKET								
Plain with Butter, Wimpy*	1 Serving/327g	453	7.6	139	3.5	27.7	2.3	2.4
with Baked Beans, Wimpy*	1 Serving/452g	549	7.9	121	3.4	23.5	1.8	2.7
with Beans & Cheese, Wimpy*	1 Serving/577g	1069	51.5	185	8.4	18.4	8.9	2.1
with Coleslaw, Wimpy*	1 Serving/452g	576	17.1	127	2.9	21.7	3.8	2.0
with Grated Cheese, Wimpy*	1 Serving/452g	973	51.2	215	9.6	20.0	11.3	1.8
with Tuna Mayo, Wimpy*	1 Serving/452g	764	34.2	169	5.9	20.6	7.6	1.8
RIBS								
Pork Rib, Wimpy*	1 Rib/189g	463	22.4	245	13.0	21.6	11.9	0.0
ROLL								
Bacon & Egg, in a Bun, Wimpy*	1 Roll/155g	702	41.7	453	29.6	22.6	26.9	1.4
Bacon in a Bun, Wimpy*	1 Roll/125g	341	16.1	273	16.0	22.6	12.9	1.4
SALAD								
Fish, Wimpy*	1 Serving/356g	389	21.3	109	4.6	9.9	6.0	0.0
Gourmet Chicken, Wimpy*	1 Serving/358g	251	4.3	70	11.9	2.7	1.2	0.4
Hot & Spicy Chicken, Wimpy*	1 Serving/290g	283	15.2	98	6.1	6.7	5.2	0.9
Scampi, Wimpy*	1 Serving/356g	376	19.1	106	4.2	10.7	5.4	0.0
Steak, Wimpy*	1 Serving/355g	329	16.9	93	10.0	2.7	4.8	0.4
SAUCE								
Chocolate (for Sundae), Wimpy*	1 Serving/28g	80	0.4	286	1.4	66.1	1.4	1.1
Maple Flavoured Syrup (for Dessert), Wimpy*	1 Serving/28g	74	0.1	264	0.0	67.9	0.4	0.0
Strawberry (for Dessert), Wimpy*	1 Serving/28g	78	0.0	279	0.0	69.6	0.0	0.4
SWEETS								
Mini Marshmallows (for Desserts), Wimpy*	1 Serving/10g	33	0.0	330	4.0	83.0	0.0	0.0
TEACAKE								
Toasted with Butter, Wimpy*	1 Teacake/66g	227	2.3	344	1.7	10.4	3.4	0.4
VEGETARIAN								
Lemon Pepper Quorn, Wimpy*	1 Serving/239g	586	26.5	245	8.0	29.2	11.1	0.0
Spicy Beanburger, Wimpy*	1 Serving/233g	593	29.2	255	5.4	30.8	12.5	0.0
WRAPID								
WRAP								
All Day Breakfast (W22), Wrapid*	1 Wrap/223g	569	27.9	255	14.0	23.1	12.5	1.5
Breakfast Panini (W35), Wrapid*	1 Wrap/181g	466	20.2	257	12.9	27.6	11.2	1.8
Chicken Fajita (W18), Wrapid*	1 Wrap/226g	485	19.2	215	13.3	22.0	8.5	1.3
Chicken Tikka Balti (W15), Wrapid*	1 Wrap/266g	476	13.7	179	8.5	24.4	5.2	1.5
Chicken Tikka Massala Pot (WPOT004), Wrapid*	1 Pot/310g	487	14.7	157	5.4	20.8	4.7	1.2
Chilli Cheese Bean (T8 & W46), Wrapid*	1 Wrap/189g	411	13.9	217	7.8	29.9	7.3	2.8
Chilli Con Carne & Rice (W19), Wrapid*	1 Wrap/286g	505	13.9	176	3.9	28.8	4.8	1.2
Chilli Con Carne Pot (WPOT001), Wrapid*	1 Wrap/310g	412	12.9	133	2.2	20.9	4.2	0.4

WRAPID

WRAP

	Measure INFO/WEIGHT	per Measure KCAL	FAT	Nutrition Values per 100g / 100ml KCAL	PROT	CARB	FAT	FIBRE
Croques Monsier, Ham & Cheese (W30), Wrapid*	1 Wrap/231g	648	30.5	281	15.4	27.1	13.2	0.8
Fajita Chicken Panini (W39), Wrapid*	1 Wrap/181g	336	8.4	186	10.0	25.5	4.6	1.6
Ham & Cheddar Panini (W34), Wrapid*	1 Wrap/176g	501	21.4	284	13.1	30.9	12.2	1.5
Ham & Pineapple Pizza (W28), Wrapid*	1 Wrap/270g	510	17.6	189	12.5	21.3	6.5	2.1
Meat Balls Pasta Pot (WPOT002), Wrapid*	1 Pot/291g	349	9.1	120	4.8	19.0	3.1	1.4
Mushroom, Cheese & Egg (W20), Wrapid*	1 Wrap/210g	531	29.6	253	9.6	22.0	14.1	1.4
Pepperoni Pizza (W26), Wrapid*	1 Wrap/249g	688	36.8	276	16.5	21.2	14.8	2.3
Pepperoni Pizza Panini (W37), Wrapid*	1 Wrap/194g	570	30.7	294	13.9	25.0	15.8	1.8
Roast Vegetable Pasta Pot (WPOT003), Wrapid*	1 Pot/311g	294	3.5	94	3.4	18.1	1.1	1.7
Roasted Peppers Pizza (W27), Wrapid*	1 Wrap/261g	502	18.7	192	11.9	21.3	7.2	2.5
Steak & Mash, Wrapid*	1 Wrap/246g	424	9.7	172	6.6	26.2	4.0	1.0
Stir Fry Chicken with Noodles (W23), Wrapid*	1 Wrap/251g	411	8.6	164	8.0	24.8	3.4	1.5
Tuna Melt (W29), Wrapid*	1 Wrap/237g	538	21.3	227	16.3	21.2	9.0	1.3
Tuna Melt Panini (W33), Wrapid*	1 Wrap/178g	430	15.1	241	14.2	27.7	8.5	1.3
Vegetable, Breakfast Panini (W43), Wrapid*	1 Wrap/204g	366	11.0	180	7.0	25.8	5.4	1.8
Vegetable, Red Thai Panini (W45), Wrapid*	1 Wrap/185g	360	12.8	194	6.8	30.1	6.9	2.1

Useful Resources

Weight Loss
Weight Loss Resources is home to the UK's largest calorie and nutrition database along with diaries, tools and expert advice for weight loss and health.
Tel: 01733 345592 Email: helpteam@weightlossresources.co.uk
Website: www.weightlossresources.co.uk

Exercise Equipment for Home
Diet and Fitness Resources has a range of equipment for exercise at home, from pedometers to treadmills and fitballs to weights. As well as diet tools such as food diaries, a weight loss kit and diet plates.
Tel: 01733 345592 Email: helpteam@dietandfitnessresources.co.uk
Website: www.dietandfitnessresources.co.uk

Dietary Advice
The British Dietetic Association has helpful food fact leaflets and information on how to contact a registered dietitian.
Tel: 0121 200 8080 Email: webmaster@bda.uk.com
Website: www.bda.uk.com

Healthy Eating
The British Nutrition Foundation has lots of in depth scientifically based nutritional information, knowledge and advice on healthy eating for all ages.
Tel: 0207 404 6504 Email: postbox@nutrition.org.uk
Website: www.nutrition.org.uk

Healthy Heart
The British Heart Foundation provides advice and information for all on all heart aspects from being healthy, to living with heart conditions, research and fundraising.
Tel: 0207 554 000   Email: via their website
Website: www.bhf.org.uk

Cancer Research
Cancer Research UK is the leading UK charity dedicated to research, education and fundraising for all forms of cancer.
Tel: 0207 242 0200 Email: via their website
Website: www.cancerresearchuk.org

Diabetes Advice
Diabetes UK is the leading charity working for people with diabetes. Their mission is to improve the lives of people with diabetes and to work towards a future without diabetes
Tel : 0845 120 2960 Email: info@diabetes.org.uk
Website: www.diabetes.org.uk

Beating Bowel Cancer
Beating Bowel Cancer is a leading UK charity for bowel cancer patients, working to raise awareness of symptoms, promote early diagnosis and encourage open access to treatment choice for those affected by bowel cancer.Tel: 08450 719301   Email: nurse@beatingbowelcancer.org
Website: http://www.beatingbowelcancer.org

Safety and Standards
The Food Standards Agency is an independent watchdog, set up to protect the public's health and consumer interests in relation to food.
Tel: 0207 276 8829 Email: helpline@foodstandards.gsi.gov.uk
Website: www.food.gov.uk

Feedback

If you have any comments or suggestions about The Calorie, Carb & Fat Bible, or would like further information on Weight Loss Resources, please call, email, or write to us:

Tel: 01733 345592
Email: helpteam@weightlossresources.co.uk
Address: Laurence Beeken,
            Weight Loss Resources Ltd,
            2C Flag Business Exchange,
            Vicarage Farm Road,
            Peterborough,
            PE1 5TX.

Reviews for The Calorie Carb & Fat Bible

'What a brilliant book. I know I'll be sinking my teeth into it.'
GMTV Nutritionist Amanda Ursell, BSc RD

'To help you make low-cal choices everyday, invest in a copy.'
ZEST magazine

'There is no doubt that the food listings are extremely helpful
for anyone wishing to control their calorie intake in order to lose
pounds or maintain a healthy weight.'
Women's Fitness magazine

'Useful if you don't want to exclude any overall food groups.'
Easy Living magazine

'Quite simply an astonishing achievement by the authors.'
Evening Post, Nottingham

'The book gives you all the basic information so you can work out
your daily calorie needs.'
Woman magazine

'This is a welcome resource in view of the 'national epidemic of obesity.'

Bryony Philip, Bowel Cancer UK

'The authors seem to understand the problems of slimming.'

Dr John Campion

'Jam-packed with info on dieting, and full to bursting point with the calorie, carbohydrate and fat values of thousands of different foods, it's the perfect weight loss tool.'

Evening Express, Aberdeen

'Excellent resource tool - used by myself in my role as a Practice Nurse.'

Pam Boal, Sunderland

'I recently bought your book called the Calorie, Carb & Fat Bible and would love to tell you what a brilliant book it is. I have recently started a weight management programme and I honestly don't know where I'd be without your book. It has helped me a lot and given me some really good advice.'

Rachel Mitchell

About Weight Loss Resources

weightlossresources.co.uk

"What this does is put you in control with no guilt, no awful groups and no negativity! Fill in your food diary, get support on the boards and watch it fall off!"

LINDAB, Weight Loss Resources Member

How Does It Work?

Weight Loss Resources is home to the UK's biggest online calorie and nutrition database. You simply tap in your height, weight, age and basic activity level - set a weight loss goal, and the programme does all the necessary calculations.

What Does It Do?

The site enables you to keep a food diary which keeps running totals of calories, fat, fibre, carbs, proteins and portions of fruit and veg. You can also keep an exercise diary which adds the calories you use during exercise. At the end of a week, you update your weight and get reports and graphs on your progress.

How Will It Help?

You'll learn a great deal about how your eating and drinking habits affect your weight and how healthy they are. Using the diaries and other tools you'll be able to make changes that suit your tastes and your lifestyle. The result is weight loss totally tailored to your needs and preferences. A method you can stick with that will help you learn how to eat well for life!

Try It Free!

Go to **www.weightlossresources.co.uk** and take a completely free, no obligation, 24 hour trial. If you like what you see you can sign up for membership from £6.95 per month.